CLINICAL BEHAVIORAL
MEDICINE FOR SMALL ANIMALS

Dr. Karen Overall received her B.A. and M.A. degrees concomitantly from the University of Pennsylvania in 1978. After a year spent at the Smithsonian Tropical Research Institute in Panama, she was awarded her V.M.D. from the University of Pennsylvania, School of Veterinary Medicine, in 1983. She completed a residency in Behavioral Medicine at Penn in 1989 after returning to graduate school at the University of Wisconsin–Madison to continue her Ph.D. work in behavioral ecology. Her Ph.D. research dealt with mating systems and egg physiology of a protected species of lizard. Dr. Overall is the author of numerous articles on behavioral medicine and lizard behavioral ecology and is a regular columnist for the journals *Canine Practice, Feline Practice,* and *DVM Magazine*. She is a Diplomate of the American College of Veterinary Behavior (ACVB) and is certified by the Animal Behavior Society (ABS) as an Applied Animal Behaviorist. Dr. Overall is currently on the staff of the University of Pennsylvania School of Veterinary Medicine, where she runs the Behavior Clinic. She lectures frequently on behavioral medicine both nationally and internationally. Her research interests focus on the development of animal models for human psychiatric illness. Dr. Overall was awarded the 1993 Randy Award for excellence and creativity in research. Other interests include integration of conservation biology into veterinary medicine and international outreach.

CLINICAL BEHAVIORAL MEDICINE FOR SMALL ANIMALS

KAREN L. OVERALL, M.A., V.M.D., Ph.D.
Diplomate, American College of Veterinary Behavior
Department of Clinical Studies
School of Veterinary Medicine
University of Pennsylvania
Philadelphia, Pennsylvania

with 135 illustrations

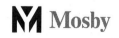
Mosby

St. Louis Baltimore Boston Carlsbad Chicago Naples New York Philadelphia Portland
London Madrid Mexico City Singapore Sydney Tokyo Toronto Wiesbaden

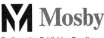

Dedicated to Publishing Excellence

A Times Mirror
Company

Vice President and Publisher: Don Ladig
Editor: Linda L. Duncan
Developmental Editor: Jo Salway
Project Manager: Patricia Tannian
Project Specialist: Ann E. Rogers
Manuscript Editor: Judy Ahlers
Book Design Manager: Gail Morey Hudson
Manufacturing Manager: Dave Graybill
Cover Design: Donna Wilkerson

Printed in the United States of America
Composition and lithography by Progressive Information Technologies
Printing/binding by Maple-Vail Book Mfg Group

Mosby–Year Book, Inc.
11830 Westline Industrial Drive
St. Louis, Missouri 63146

Library of Congress Cataloging in Publication Data

Overall, Karen L.
    Clinical behavioral medicine for small animals /Karen L. Overall.
       p.   cm.
    Includes bibliographical references and index.
    ISBN 0-8016-6820-4
     1. Dogs—Behavior.   2. Cats—Behavior.   3. Dogs—Psychology.
4. Cats—Psychology.   5. Animal behavior therapy.   I. Title.
SF433.094   1997
636.7'089689—dc20   96-18753
                                      CIP

96 97 98 99 00 / 9 8 7 6 5 4 3 2 1

This book is dedicated to the memory of
my much loved *Australian Shepherd,*

"Maggie"

who died suddenly, at the age of almost 11 years, in July of 1995
when I was completing the final revision of the manuscript.
The quintessential dog, Maggie was completely honest
and possessed of great dignity, grace, and humor.
She was my soulmate, and I fear the
allotment for those is one
per lifetime.
Maggie taught me how to
love completely and brought great joy to
everyone who knew her. Were all pets like Maggie,
this book would be unnecessary.

····· Preface

···

OVERVIEW

This book is intended to be a practical text on Behavioral Medicine; its purpose is to acquaint the practitioner with the principles of clinical behavioral medicine. The book is *not* intended to be a comprehensive overview of either the fields of Ethology or Animal Behavior, or of the complete research that has been done in Behavioral Medicine. The focus of this book is *clinical* behavioral medicine. For those interested, there are excellent extant treatises on comparative behavior, behavioral ecology, evolution of behavior, and wild versus domestic behaviors (Clutton-Brock, 1989; Sibly and Smith, 1985; Fisher, 1993; Turner and Bateson, 1988; Sheldon, 1992; Bradshaw, 1992; Krebs and Davies, 1991; Slobodchikoff, 1988).

This book focuses on diagnostic and treatment approaches for the major classes of problems that are seen in cats and dogs. Emphasis is placed on the more common and more serious problems, rather than on what might be more intellectually stimulating but less common problems. For example, a large amount of attention is paid to canine aggression and feline elimination disorders since these are the two most prominent problems in dogs and cats. Other disorders that are less well understood but that are intellectually challenging, such as stereotypies, are also addressed, but not in the same detail. There are also large sections on normal dog and cat behavior; these sections are intended to allow the practitioner to understand the etiology of problematical behavior. Again, the sections on normal behavior are not comprehensive dissertations on the subjects, but rather they focus on issues that will allow practitioners to address the prevention of behavioral disorders and to understand their development and treatment.

This text is designed with two goals in mind: (1) to provide practical clinical information for practitioners and veterinary students, and (2) to set the intellectual framework for understanding future growth, development, and changes in the field. While designed primarily to help practitioners become familiar with behavioral medicine, the text is also intended to act as a survey compendium for specialists. Specialists in behavioral medicine vary in their approaches, and I have tried to include the most recent, up to date, and occasionally, unpublished research in the field with the intent of providing a nidus for further discussion. I have tried to place all of this information in a logical structure so that the theory involved in behavioral medicine is apparent.

REFERENCES AND APPENDICES

A word on the references and appendixes is warranted.

First, the references are not cited by number in the text. They are cited by the author's name and the date when the paper was published because this method is user friendly. Second, all of the references are at the back of the book rather than following each chapter. This allows the reader to go to an alphabetized list of all the references contained in the book and find them in one place in case there is a need to return to them; it also saves paper. I made a concession to this being a practical text by limiting the number of references cited. I tried to cite the sentinel reference for the topic because practitioners told me that, while they were interested in the references, their needs were practical rather than academic. Accordingly, the reference list is not exhaustive.

The appendixes are intended to provide accompanying information for the chapters, but may be ancillary. For instance, for the chapter on Treatment, the sources for all of the gizmos discussed are listed in Appendix C. The protocols that are discussed within the chapters are in Appendix B in a form that can be photocopied. I hope that further editions will contain any modifications that practitioners suggest to make these more usable.

This book is meant to be a vital, *practical* volume that will allow the practitioner to better prevent, diagnose, and treat behavioral cases in general practice, and to competently refer them, if need be. In fact, if, after the practitioner reviews the text, he or she decides to consult or refer to a specialist, I will have done a service. Behavioral medicine is difficult and time consuming. Some aspects of it are, like other specialties, best practiced by specialists.

Chapters are accompanied by specific case histories germane to their topics. None of these case histories is fictitious; all have been taken from the files of the Behavior Clinic at VHUP, although some identifying features have been changed.

This is a vital, developing, ongoing project. Suggestions from practitioners are not only welcomed; they are solicited. A great many practitioners made suggestions that were directly incorporated into this volume, and they are listed in the Acknowledgments. If there are aspects that practitioners would like to see developed more fully or in a manner that is more usable for them in practice, those changes will be made in future editions, and practitioners who contribute to those will, of course, also be acknowledged.

Finally, this is a young field, and more is unknown than is known. I have tried to indicate when issues are not clear, what is not known, and what steps are required to know what is necessary. While I have reported previously unpublished data from the Behavior Clinic at VHUP, I have also attempted to indicate whenever something is my opinion and whether data are available that may substantiate or refute that opinion. I know I have made mistakes and that in places time will prove me wrong; science advances by pursuing and correcting those wrongs. While writing this I made the conscious attempt to develop the intellectual framework for how to think about complex behavioral problems, so that the groundwork is laid for correcting errors in interpretation and for the future development of the field by specialists. I hope that this endeavor becomes a dynamic part of my academic career and that in future editions I will be able to report on the corrections and advances.

Karen L. Overall

····· Acknowledgments

···

My first thanks are due to the practitioners, clinicians, and veterinary students who have waited so long for this book. Novice book authors have no idea of the time commitment that is involved in writing a book, and I appreciate everyone's anticipatory patience. The book has undergone two complete and many partial revisions based on the input from practitioners, my colleagues in the American College of Veterinary Behavior, and veterinary students: they all had topics they wanted covered in more depth. Hence the altered, larger than planned (and delayed) manuscript. I thank my editor, Linda Duncan, at Mosby for her faith, encouragement, and understanding; and Ann Rogers for the care she took with the preparation of this text.

I am indebted to the veterinary students at the University of Pennsylvania School of Veterinary Medicine, particularly those in the graduating classes of 1990 through 1997. Their questions, interest, and enthusiasm were essential for the development of parts of this text and are responsible for my continuing presence at Penn Vet. Certain students who have worked in the Behavior Clinic are notable for their help in preparation of some of the client handouts, critiques of chapters, and commentary on cases. Special thanks go to Tracy Barlup (Penn Vet 1996), Emily Elliot (Penn Vet 1997), Christina Fantoni, Reina Fuji (Penn Vet 1996), Caroline Garzotti (Penn Vet 1996), Hue Karreman (Penn Vet 1995), Serena Liu (Penn Vet 1993), Nirit Rosenberg (Penn Vet 1997), Rhonda Schulman (Davis Vet 1994), Laurie Sponza (Penn Vet 1996), Michelle Trammell (Penn Vet 1993), and Mel Wilkins (Penn Vet 1995). Lois Vogelpohl-Hall and Emily Elliot (Penn Vet 1997) were essential in initiating and running the puppy clinics. Laurie Sponza (Penn Vet 1996) patiently read, edited, and suggested corrections for many parts of various drafts of the manuscript. During my time at Penn Vet there has never been the much-needed complete funding for Behavioral Medicine that some other veterinary schools enjoy. All of these students have run the Clinic and have risen to the huge challenge involved in that. I am enormously grateful to them, for without their efforts I would have had no time at all to think.

This book was written primarily with practitioners in mind, and I have benefitted emotionally from the support that they have shown the field, and intellectually from the questions they ask. They have forced me to say things more clearly, more logically, and in a more applicable manner. The participants in the Behavioral Seminars at Eastern States/North American Veterinary Conference during 1991, 1992, 1994, and 1995 set the tone for this book. Some practitioners commented on some of the client handouts and are frequent users of the VHUP Behavior Clinic's telephone consultation service for veterinarians. I am sure that I am omitting some practitioners who spurred clear writing, but the following practitioners have earned my gratitude for their enthusiasm, belief, faith, and help: Drs. Patty Boge (California), Gail Bowman (North Carolina), Danny Brass (Arizona), Glen Deckert (Virginia), Diane Eigner (Pennsylvania), Patty Gaylord (Maine), Larry Gerson (Pennsylvania), Debbie Horwitz (Missouri), Wayne Hunthausen (Kansas), Gary Landsberg (Ontario), Lisa Levy (Illinois), Jo Moorer (Maryland), Ralph Pope (Tennessee), Pam Reppert (New York), Richard Rogers (Maryland), Gary Selmonsky (New York), Margo Schwag (Pennsylvania), Rae Ann Van Pelt (Illinois), Karen Wolfscheimer (Louisiana).

New fields, like Behavioral Medicine, gain wider focus and recognition when they are featured at major conferences. Dr. Colin Burrows and his colleagues at Eastern States/North American Veterinary Conference have made it a point to provide practitioners with state-of-the-art continuing education and have fully integrated Behavioral Medicine into that. Dr. Burrows has also encouraged his compatriots at the BSAVA and the WVA/WSAVA to do the same. This has given the field a broad visibility it otherwise would not have. I am grateful to him for this professional and personal support.

Some of my colleagues in academia have been particularly helpful and supportive. They have both recognized the importance of the field (for which they deserve kudos) and have asked probing questions. While the list is not exhaustive, special thanks are due to Drs. Greg Acland, John August, Ken Bovée, Tony Buffington, Colin Harvey, Peter Ihrke, Peter Jezyk, Alan Klide, Meryl Littman, Vicki Meyers-Wallen, Don Patterson, Alan Paul, Rob Schwartzman, Kevin Shanley, Shel Steinberg, Steve Thompson, Charles Vite, and Alice Wolf. European, Australian, and Canadian colleagues have also been helpful and enthusiastic, and those deserving particular thanks include Dr. Diane Frank, Dr. Bruce Fogle, Mrs. Sarah

Heath, Dr. Robert Holmes, Mr. Danny Mills, Dr. Roger Mugford, Dr. Peter Neville, Dr. Maria Cristina Osella, and Dr. Kersti Seksel.

Without the people who created and fought for the discipline of the specialty of Behavioral Medicine in Veterinary Medicine, attention to the field would still lag. Accordingly, Drs. R.K. Anderson, Bonnie Beaver, Leslie Cooper, Sharon Crowell-Davis, Ben Hart, Kathe Houpt, Andrew Luescher, Ilana Reisner, Elizabeth Shull, Barbara Simpson, Victoria Voith, and Tom Wolfle deserve special thanks. I was fortunate to be Dr. Voith's last resident when she was at Penn Vet and I benefitted immeasurably from the experience. Dr. R.K. Anderson has been particularly encouraging of young members of the field, and has served as a model for how this should be done.

Penn Vet is a unique intellectual environment. While the powers that be at Penn Vet have not yet made the necessary commitment to Behavioral Medicine, they have provided me with the chance to develop my own resources. Only when veterinary schools make the needed financial and logistic commitment to Behavioral Medicine will the discipline have fully arrived and earned its protection from pseudo-science. This type of decision requires the leadership and courage to allocate the appropriate resources.

During the course of writing this book I was diagnosed with two exhausting, painful, and potentially debilitating immune-mediated conditions. They have sapped my strength and energy, and have forced me to begin to restructure my life; hence, they are part of the reason this book was so delayed. Regardless, under any circumstances it is extremely difficult for a junior faculty member to find and take the time necessary to write a book. Universities do not facilitate such endeavours at that academic level. It is even harder for someone like myself, who is in a "soft money" position that is predicated on the expectation that the clinician will do no research or writing, to make the time to accomplish such a task. I delayed the writing and publication of my Ph.D. thesis, and some of my

own work in behavioral medicine to complete this work because I thought it might be more important. Accordingly, I would have been able to complete none of this without the help and support of two people: my resident and great friend, Dr. Ann Beebe, and my husband, Dr. Art Dunham.

It is an honor and a responsibility to train a resident. It has been a pleasure to see Ann blossom intellectually, and I realize that this surely must be one of the rewards of academic medicine. At times, Ann has single-handedly run the Clinic, and she has been there at every step to help because she believes the field is important. I am indebted to her.

My husband, Arthur, is one of a kind, and a rare gem. He has restructured some of his academic life to take care of me and has been there whenever I have needed him. Art has been unwavering in his belief in me, my skills, and my pursuits. He has given me courage that I may not have otherwise had, and he did so simply by being one of the best in his field, and being one of the most inherently ethical and generous scientists I have ever known. His contribution to this text is invisible and immeasurable.

Finally, many people have helped in some unpredictable ways. Our clients are truly the best of the best, and their pets provide the source material for many of my ideas. Ken Mullin, head of VHUP's Medical Information Section, is incredibly smart, organized, and resourceful. Few retrospective or prospective studies can be done at Penn without his help. VHUP's pharmacists, Sue Celani, Pat Reichle, and Alice Verity, have learned more than they wanted to know about psychotropic medication and have gone out of their way to help me, Ann, and our clients. They also make our lives unceasingly amusing. The person who typed the manuscript, Jim Hostetter, is notable for his terrific typing and pithy verbal badinage. He named the manuscript "the behemoth" and commented that if reading the advice contained in it did not help, it was sufficiently heavy that throwing it at the dog might. I hope it doesn't come to that.

..... Contributors

Deidre E. Gannon, Esq., is a practicing attorney in Cherry Hill, New Jersey. She has successfully combined her J.D. from Rutgers University with more than 20 years of experience in the sport of purebred dogs. She is the author of *The Complete Guide to Dog Law* (Howell Book House, 1994). Her two editions of *The Rare Breed Handbook* (Golden Boy Press, 1991, 1987) have become the foundation works for breeds yet to be recognized by the American Kennel Club. She is also a contributing editor to Lawyers Cooperative Publishing, as well as a number of national canine magazines.

Robin Lee Schurr Stawasz, M.S.W., received her Bachelor of Animal Science degree from Cornell University and her Master of Social Work degree from the University of Pennsylvania. While at Penn, she acted as a social worker at the Veterinary Hospital of the University of Pennsylvania, 2 years of which were spent at the Behavior Clinic with Dr. Overall. She also has extensive experience in the field of pet-facilitated psychotherapy and the grief reaction to pet loss. She now has a private behavior consulting practice in the Elmira, New York, area and serves on the Board of Directors of the Chemung County Humane Society and S.P.C.A. She would like to dedicate this work to her loving family who mean so much to her.

Contents

1 ····· The Veterinary Importance of Clinical Behavioral Medicine

HISTORICAL PERSPECTIVE OF BEHAVIORAL MEDICINE

As was true with human psychiatry and medicine, clinical behavioral medicine has been resisted as a mainstream specialty until recently. This is understandable—it is a relatively young field (Beaver, 1992; Voith, 1991). Furthermore, the discipline was likened to dog training and handling, or to obedience work. This perception was partly because of ignorance, but also because dog trainers and handlers were the people who earnestly tried, with varying degrees of training and success, to solve animal behavioral problems. Until recently, anyone with any degree of training (or lack thereof) could designate himself or herself as qualified to treat pet behavior problems. This is part of the reason that it has taken so long for the field to gain legitimacy and one of the reasons the field has been viewed as "flaky" and "soft."

Primarily because of the efforts of Bonnie Beaver, DVM, at Texas A&M University School of Veterinary Medicine, behavioral medicine is now (since 1995) a board-certified discipline. This designation should be a welcome development for all practitioners, because it will facilitate the addition of behavioral medicine to the veterinary curriculum and provide a rigorous, consistent standard by which specialists will be trained. Board certification should greatly facilitate the growth of the field in the next decade.

In another attempt to legitimize the field before the approval of board certification, the Animal Behavior Society (ABS) attempted to standardize requirements for those calling themselves pet behaviorists. Recognizing that nonveterinarians could make valuable contributions to the field, the ABS created two categories of standardization and certification to acknowledge this: Applied Animal Behaviorist (includes veterinarians) and Associate Applied Animal Behaviorist (those with master's degrees) (contact information is found in Appendix C). Although this certification will never provide veterinarians with the same level of rigor and status as will board certification, it provides an opportunity to recognize individuals who wish to pursue advanced behavioral training. My personal preference, both because of the degree of rigor involved, and because of the frequent need for pharmacological therapy in behavioral medicine, is that difficult cases be referred to board-certified or board-eligible specialists in veterinary behavior, or specialists at university veterinary teaching and research hospitals, particularly if these are readily available.

Currently six to nine veterinary schools in the United States and Canada provide some type of program in behavioral medicine (the count discrepancy results from whether the program is both a clinical and a vital, required part of the veterinary curriculum). Four veterinary schools have, or have recently had, residencies or fellowships in behavioral medicine. The Morris Animal Foundation has been essential in funding residencies in behavioral medicine, providing funds for the first resident in the 1992-1993 academic year.

OVERCOMING MYTHS

The inclusion of behavioral medicine in veterinary medicine is important for the following reasons. First, general practitioner veterinarians are committed to providing total patient care. They should be in the position to evaluate deviations from normal behavior and to suggest solutions before the problem worsens. Obedience trainers, dog handlers, and private handlers have their roles; these are discussed in Chapter 14. However, the activities of each of these groups are predicated on normal behavior and on the assumption that all problems are management related. Although management may play a role in both the expression of behavioral problems and their resolutions, it is inexcusable and irresponsible to advance poor management as the primary cause of behavioral disorders. The majority of animals with behavioral problems are not poorly behaved or misbehaved; they are abnormal or are responding to an abnormal social system. Ian Dunbar (1991) has attempted to discuss this division. He divided problems into three classifications: temperament problems, behavior problems, and obedience problems. "Obedience problems" involve poorly behaved or misbehaved dogs. The other two categories encompass pets that are abnormal, or pets that experience either abnormal social systems or problematic responses to normal social systems.

Veterinarians must be taught to understand normal behavior and to anticipate or recognize when deviations from it have occurred. Using a cooperative effort with a good obedience club or school, the veterinarian can accomplish this effectively and provide individual help and advice that is not available in other settings (Myles, 1991). This cooperative effort implies education on both sides and acknowledges that obedience is not a substitute for behavioral therapy. Veterinarians should not relinquish their responsibility because of ignorance.

Second, veterinarians are expected by their clients to provide care for their pets. In a survey of all the faculty, residents, and interns at the Veterinary Hospital of the University of Pennsylvania (VHUP), I found that *every* individual admitted that he or she had denied the preferred standard of care to an animal, at some time, because the animal's behavior rendered it intractable or dangerous. Animals who are ill or in pain are more difficult to handle, behaviorally, than those who are well; therefore the pet's problem and the veterinarian's helplessness spiral. The acceptance of clinical behavioral medicine as a legitimate specialty in veterinary medicine should obviate these difficulties and allow veterinarians to exercise their skill to the utmost. There is also a beneficial financial component. It has been estimated that up to 15% of patients are lost to practices annually because of behavioral problems (Sigler, 1991); financial losses concurrent with this have been estimated to be at least $17,000 per annum. Cuts, bites, and scratches are responsible for a $25 million per year human health industry, and the insurance costs from dog bites may exceed $1 billion annually (Daristotle, 1994).

Third, veterinarians, not trainers (and not most individuals with only master's or doctoral degrees) are trained in diagnosis and treatment. Implicit in this training is some degree of freedom from prejudice, favoritism, and mythology. The nature of breed clubs and the work of handlers and trainers may preclude such freedom. The majority of canine patients visiting the Behavior Clinic at VHUP (more than 90% in 1993) have had some type of obedience training. Some patients have obedience or conformation titles or both. For the individual who is interested in becoming an applied animal behaviorist without the veterinary degree, there are few, if any, rigorous, university-affiliated applied animal behavior programs. This lack of educational opportunity exists for both trainers and owners.

At the Behavior Clinic at VHUP, more than 50% of the cases have underlying medical complications that need to be treated, behavioral problems that require medication, or both conditions. Furthermore, rather than being pets that are misbehaving and thus are management problems, many pets with behavioral problems are truly abnormal or have an organic cause for the problem. The definition of an *organic cause* is changing; even disorders of serotonin metabolism could become accepted organic disorders within the next decade.

These abnormal pets *are* treatable; however, their problems will not be resolved with handlers, obedience instructors, or trainers. For a veterinarian to rely solely on such aids in a behavioral problem is akin to using alchemy to treat hepatopathy: it is no longer necessary. Most future advances in behavioral medicine will probably be pharmacological. Currently pharmacological adjuvants for treating behavioral problems are becoming well accepted and successfully used. They are not quick fixes, and, given that the medications used are the same psychotropic medications used in human medicine, such treatment must be used responsibly. Some of these medications are useful to break the cycle of inappropriate response so that behavior modification can be better instituted, whereas others are maintenance drugs with a role analogous to that of insulin for treatment of diabetics. Medicine advances—and this is a nascent area of veterinary medicine—will allow veterinarians to hone their skills and further their intellectual endeavors.

Fourth, a knowledge of behavioral medicine is essential for knowing when to refer difficult cases to teaching and research institutions. Such referrals are the basis of much medical progress. The issue of liability is more complex, but as the field advances it is reasonable to begin to hold veterinarians to higher standards of competence in behavioral cases than was true in the past. This issue is fully explored in Chapter 15.

Finally, behavioral medicine provides the clinician and practitioner with the opportunity to be more than an executioner. For no other broad class of veterinary problems has death been a primary option. Between 15 and 20 million animals are euthanized in humane shelters each year (Anderson & Foster, 1995; Sigler, 1991). Estimates indicate that the majority of these animals were brought to shelters because of behavioral problems (Anderson & Foster, 1995; Sigler, 1991). There is no accurate estimate of the number of pets euthanized at veterinary practices each year for behavioral problems, but the number is not insubstantial. Were there an infectious disease epidemic of this magnitude, there would be no doubt as to its import. Behavioral problems are complex and multifactorial, and often not easily solvable. These factors have led to the slow spread and acclamation of the field of behavioral medicine. Because euthanasia is accepted as a normal part of veterinary medicine, we have not been without a "solution" for a problem pet; on the other hand, since euthanasia is frowned on in human medicine, it is not surprising that psychiatry was accepted considerably earlier than was veterinary behavioral medicine.

Thirty percent of dog owners and 18% of cat owners who bring their pets to the Behavior Clinic at VHUP have considered euthanasia because of the problem that prompted their clinic visit. For 100% of all canine patients seen within the past 2 years, someone had recommended euthanasia before their visit.

After evaluation and treatment, fewer than 10% of canine patients were euthanized within a year of their visit, and fewer than 1% of feline patient were euthanized within 1 year of the visit. *Treatment makes a difference.* For clients who ultimately do choose euthanasia, access to the full range of options and attendant ramifications has been provided. These issues are discussed in Chapters 12 and 16.

TERMINOLOGY

The terminology used in this book, particularly that for aggression, follows that of Moyer (1968). Moyer used a functional classification of aggression; with modification, that classification is used in this text. The utility of a functional classification of aggression has been debated. Unfortunately, functional classifications may be the most amenable for use in practical texts. They are not useful for understanding underlying mechanisms. The issues of diagnosis in both human and veterinary medicine is problematic. A diagnosis does not necessarily imply an underlying mechanistic phenomenon. An ideal diagnosis *does* imply underlying causality or mechanism; for most conditions it is not necessary to understand all mechanistic levels (Box 1-1).

The more common diseases for which this is true are infectious diseases, such as malaria, and endocrine diseases, such as diabetes mellitus. However, as more is learned about diabetes, it appears that a singular genetic or functional mechanism does not exist. Clearly, diagnosis or treatment can be misled because the correct *level* of mechanism is not considered. Once the

genetic and the cellular levels are studied more closely, deeper insight into disease processes not provided by an overview of the organismal or organ level can be gained. When an aggressive dog is the problem, the level of the complete organism is considered; this is the manifestation of all integrated systems. It is impossible to pinpoint with any certainty the underlying neurotransmitter defects that may be interacting to produce the behaviors of that animal, hence the development of a *functional* classification of aggression.

Psychiatric and behavioral conditions are more problematic to diagnose than are infectious and metabolic ones. As more is learned about neurochemical perturbations associated with problem behaviors, the distinction between "organic" and "behavioral" etiologies has blurred. Defects in serotonin metabolism may be recognized as a level of organic disease in the future; however, such recognition may not put us any closer to a mechanistic basis for the "disease" process. Serotonin is variously active in a wide variety of neuroanatomical regions and affects a wide variety of behaviors. The same is true for other neurotransmitters. Many of these neurotransmitters exert their effect, not just by their presence, but because of the amount of the transmitter that is available. A paradoxical effect can be generated by an amount of neurotransmitter in excess of that necessary for normal functioning. We are beginning to learn about such patterns for serotonin. Some of the newer developments in neurotransmitter research are highlighted in Chapter 13.

The American Psychiatric Association (1994) uses functional classifications for human psychiatry. The Association publishes *The Diagnostic and Statistical Manual of Mental Disorders (DSM-IV)*, updated and revised periodically, a manifesto of functional classifications of all recognized syndromes, diseases, and psychiatric complexes. A functional classification is not a rambling collection of associated traits. Unfortunately, this is how such a classification is often viewed. A functional classification, as presented in this text (see Appendix F) and in the *DSM-IV*, enables the clinician to study constellations of signs that are highly correlated with specific behavioral traits, allowing the clinician to formulate diagnoses (hypotheses) that can be tested in a rigorous and paradigmatic manner through treatment. Correlation is not analogous to underlying causality, but it does allow grouping of behaviors that are associated with specific behavioral traits.

For example, in the case of the dominantly aggressive dog, it is known that many such dogs dislike being stared at, dislike being physically reprimanded, and become more aggressive if they are reprimanded or physically forced to do something (such as lie down or move from a piece of furniture). This does not mean that all dominantly aggressive dogs demonstrate all of the associated behaviors, nor does it mean that all dogs exhibiting any of these behaviors (e.g., staring) either are or will become dominantly aggressive. Most

---

BOX 1-1

LEVELS OF "CAUSALITY" TO CONSIDER IN ANY BEHAVIORAL DIAGNOSIS

1. Phenotype
   a. Role of underlying broad genotype × environment interactions
   b. Role of phenomenological diagnoses
2. Neuroanatomy
   a. Role of localization of activity
   b. Role of neuroanatomical diagnoses
3. Neurophysiology/Neurochemistry
   a. Role of chemical/substrate interaction
   b. Role of most mechanistic pathophysiological diagnoses
4. Molecular
   a. Role of gene regulation and interaction with substrate
   b. Role of most etiological diagnostic refinements
5. Genotype
   a. Role of heritability

dominantly aggressive dogs exhibit some manifestation of that constellation of signs. They may also exhibit other signs, but a functional classification permits unambiguous grouping of the *symptoms* into a diagnostic framework. A diagnosis is actually a hypothesis to be tested; when we suggest a diagnosis, we are also suggesting or assuming some level of mechanism for it. In the context of a dominantly aggressive dog, the mechanism can operate at the level of the social system (in which case we know that the dog is going to react inappropriately in certain social contexts, confirming the diagnosis of dominance aggression), or it could operate at the cellular or organ level. The technology for imaging brain levels of norepinephrine and serotonin is currently developing at a rapid rate, but a practical diagnostic technique does not now exist in veterinary medicine. Hence, we are deprived of exploring one level of the mechanism of the problem. Regardless, we know that if we give some of these dominantly aggressive dogs antianxiety drugs that boost serotonin levels, the dogs are better able to integrate their behavior at the social level just described. Accordingly, we have confirmed the diagnosis of dominance aggression both at the mechanistic level of cellular and organ mechanism and at the mechanistic level of the social system. By looking at a diagnosis as a hypothesis to be tested, we also can then test this hypothesis at some level by implementing treatments. If the treatment is not successful, the condition has been misdiagnosed or an inappropriate level of diagnosis has been addressed. As an alternative, we may have diagnosed the condition correctly but assumed an underlying mechanism that was refuted by the lack of response to treatment. Caution is urged unless treatments are specific at some predetermined mecha-

nistic level. The "higher" the level of diagnosis, the less likely this is to be true (see Box 1-1).

The response to treatment provides information not understood about the diagnosis in the beginning, *if* we carefully structure our thought processes. Hence, a functional classification allows progression in a specific manner every time new information is added. Parsimony should argue that functional classifications have unappreciated benefits.

A final advantage of a functional classification is perhaps its largest selling point: a functional classification of behavioral problems also provides the practitioner with the first "clue" about intervention. As detailed in Chapter 12, the first step in treatment is an attempt to avoid any circumstances in which the particular behavioral problem becomes pronounced or apparent. If you are using a classification that allows you to call the diagnosis, for example, dominance aggression, and you know that the specific things that instigate it are the constellation of behaviors affiliated with this, you can avoid them. If one calls aggressions "affective disorders," it is unclear what specific circumstances should be avoided. As one moves further down the level of diagnosis (see Box 1-1), it is harder to use the mechanistic information to employ behavior modification. Practitioners of behavioral medicine must work toward the creation of a veterinary version of the *DSM-IV*. Much of the debate in the field has centered on the rationale for nomenclature. Progress can be achieved by finalizing the definitive classifications. We can hope that Max Planck was wrong when he stated that new scientific truths do not triumph by convincing their opponents but because the opponents eventually die and the new generation is familiar with the idea from the beginning.

2 ····· Epidemiology

···

CLIENT ATTITUDES TOWARD PETS

In 1985 there were approximately 55 million dogs and 52 million cats in the United States; approximately 13 million of these were unwanted animals in shelters. The majority of these unwanted animals are euthanized. It has been estimated that as much as 20% of a U.S. city's pet population passes through an animal shelter.

It is estimated that by 1998, 34.3 million households will own a dog (Wise & Yang, 1994); this figure represents a slight decrease from the 1991 estimate that 34.6 million households were projected to own at least one dog (Wise & Yang, 1992). By 1998, 32 million households are projected to own a cat (Wise & Yang, 1994), and the biggest contribution to an increase in pet ownership is in the feline sector. A study published in 1992 (Anon, 1992a) indicated that 10% of the population in the United States had naturalistic views toward animals, 7% had ecologistic views, 35% had humanistic views, 20% viewed animals in a moralistic manner, 1% viewed animals in a scientistic manner, 15% viewed animals in an aesthetic manner, 20% viewed animals within a utilitarian context, 3% viewed them in a dominionistic context, whereas only 2% viewed them in a negativistic context. The negativistic statistics are encouraging until the last category—neutralistic—is considered; 35% of all people interviewed viewed animals in a neutralistic manner. When questioned about this, they confirmed that they were afraid of pet animals for one reason or another. Considering that only 1% viewed animals scientistically, these are frightening statistics for behavioral medicine clinicians. The smallest category, the scientistic category, encompassed knowledge about the biology of animals, normal versus abnormal behaviors, uses of animals for research purposes, and studies of the behavior of the animal and animal models for human disease. The proportion of people with the neutralistic view (people who are fearful) is equal to that portion of the population that has the humanistic view (interest in animals for pets). It behooves practitioners to understand people's views of pets and the differences between normal and abnormal behavior in pet animals given these statistics if the field is to flourish.

Seven percent of cats in the United States are purebred, and more than 50% of dogs are purebred (Beaver, 1980, 1992). Eight percent of British cats are of a recognized breed (Neville, 1992), but, unlike the situation in the U.S., these cats are overrepresented in the behavior clinic patient population. In Great Britain, the most common pedigreed strains are similar to those in the United States: Siamese represent 24% of pedigrees seen at a behavioral practice, with Burmese, Abyssinians, and Persians the next most frequent.

In the United States in 1976, 31% of female pet cats were spayed and 40% of male pet cats were castrated (Wilbur, 1976). These percentages increased greatly by 1992 (Manning & Rowan, 1992) as indoor pet cats became more popular (Wise & Yang, 1994). Many of the cats in Great Britain are indoor-outdoor cats, and many of the cats about whom public health concerns in the United States have been raised are outdoor, feral cats. Feral cats may not be truly feral, but may be free-ranging domesticated cats. Distinguishing between the two groups is rare because they present the same problems to a community. Free-ranging cats in the United States have an average lifespan in the general population of only 3 to 5 years; indoor cats have an average lifespan of 12 years and frequently live longer than 20 years (Childs & Ross, 1986; Comfort, 1956; Kolata et al., 1974). Car accidents are the biggest killers of free-ranging cats, but feline behavioral quirks earn the enmity of their human neighbors, often resulting in placement in another home or a rescue organization or euthanasia.

Complaints of free-ranging or feral cats include fouling of common areas, nocturnal fighting and caterwauling, leaving of corpses, attacks on pets and people, entering homes uninvited, flea infestations within the neighborhood, health risks from the cats in general (toxoplasmosis), killing of pet and ornamental birds and fish, and digging of gardens, possibly for elimination purposes (Ablett, 1981). In 1994, five U.S. children aged 3 to 11 years had encephalitis attributed to cat scratch disease, which has an incidence of 22,000 reported cases in the United States annually (Centers for Disease Control, *MMWR*, 1994).

Regardless, the single biggest complaint about cats, even nonpet cats, is behavior. Many of these feral and free-ranging cats are captured and taken to shelters where they comprise an unknown proportion of the 6 to 7 million cats that are brought to shelters annually. Between 1972 and 1983, euthanasia in U.S. shelters actually declined from more than 20% of cats taken into shelters to 10%. Behavior, *not* infectious disease, is the leading killer of pets.

COMMON BEHAVIORAL PROBLEMS IN CATS

Studies designed to describe the feline patient population (Morgan & Houpt, 1990; Olm & Houpt, 1988) found that the average age of pet cats was not different from that of dogs (3.7 years). Seventy-eight (64%) of the 120 cats studied were domestic short-haired cats, whereas 13 (11%) were purebred cats, the numerically dominant breed also being the most popular or common one — Siamese. The vast majority of the cats were not declawed. Forty-eight of the 58 male cats were castrated (above the national average); 58 of the 64 female cats were spayed (above the national average). Morgan and Houpt (1990) used a survey format to elucidate the types of behaviors exhibited by these cats that are often considered problem behaviors. It should be emphasized that all of the cats in this study were considered by their people to be normal, and the clients were not directly complaining about their behaviors, nor were they seeking redress for them. Seventy-two (60%) of the cats were reported by clients to scratch furniture, 51 (42%) of them ate houseplants, 44 (36%) of them were "aggressive" to other cats, 31 (25%) stole food on a regular basis, 20 (16%) "housesoiled" with no details given as to the nature of this, 20 of them (16%) vocalized at "undesirable" times, and 15 (12%) were "aggressive" to people (the specific details of the aggression were not detailed). Nine (7%) chewed fabric, 6 (5%) hissed at people (no data were provided to distinguish this from aggression to people), 5 (4%) were shy (undefined and the cats may just have been not as friendly as desired), 2 (2%) were territorially aggressive (although it was not clear whether this was to people, animals, or both), 2 (2%) were skittish or "neurotic" (and it is not clear how this was distinguished from being shy), 2 (2%) were overly affectionate, and 3 (2%) played roughly with their people and their belongings at night. It is important to remember that this population breakdown occurred in a population of cats about whom the clients had no complaints. These were clients who were seeking help for other reasons and participated in a behavior survey.

Certainly, house-soiling by cats is the most common complaint of clients who perceived they had behavior problems with their cats; aggression is the second most common complaint. That 20 of the 122 cats experienced house-soiling for which clients were not specifically seeking help is remarkable. Unlike data cited by Hart and Cooper (1984), males were no more likely to house-soil than females in this random population of cats. This leaves open the question of whether males do more frequently house-soil and, if not, if people who have male cats might be more inclined to complain about it. Declawed cats tended to jump onto counters more frequently than clawed cats but did not appear to become more aggressive by using

their teeth after they had been declawed if they had been unaggressive before declawing (Morgan & Houpt, 1990).

In a study conducted of 30 animal behaviorists by *Animal Behavior Consultant Newsletter* (1987), 29 of the behaviorists treated cats; again, elimination was the most common diagnosis (36.8% of the total). This complaint was followed by feline aggression (35.1%), spraying (12.3%), destruction (7%), separation-related problems (undefined) (3.5%), and other miscellaneous problems (3.5%). A survey of cat owners indicated that 47% of them think that their cats engage in a problem behavior (Voith, 1985), with the most common diagnosis being elimination, followed, at a distant second, by aggression to other cats (Voith, 1981d).

COMMON BEHAVIORAL PROBLEMS IN DOGS

According to Arkow and Dow (1983), the three most common reasons for placing a dog in a new home or with a rescue association include changes in the client's lifestyle, behavioral problems of the pet, and the fact that caring for the pet was too time consuming. All three of these are behavioral-associated problems, but it is interesting that behavioral problems are specifically identified. The same study noted that pet retention was not unrelated to purchase price. If the pet dog was free, it was kept an average of 17 months, whereas if the client had paid $100 or more for the pet, it was kept an average of 36 months. The average lifespan of a pet dog is considerably more than 36 months if it is provided with appropriate veterinary care and shelter. These animals are not being placed because of physical health problems—they are being placed because people either had unrealistic expectations about pets or because the pets had behavioral problems. Given that so many behavioral problems are not treated early because clients do not realize that help is available and that some behavioral problems are management related, it behooves clinicians to focus on behavioral problems in terms of preventive care in pets.

In reviewing these epidemiological data, it is important to remember that only 84% of dog owners have a veterinarian, and 78% of them have taken the dog to the vet within the year (Troutman, 1988). Hence, the incidence of problems reported through veterinary practices may be an underestimate of problems in the entire population.

The number of clients who report some behavioral problem in their pet dogs ranges between 42% (Houpt, 1985) and 90% (Sigler, 1991). Of animals that are taken to shelters, 50% to 70% are euthanized because of behavioral problems. This does not include the animals that are actually seen for behavioral problems, but for which a different reason is given by the clients for relinquishment. A minimum of 7 to 8 million animals a year are euthanized for behavioral problems in

Humane Shelters alone, and recent data indicate that that percentage is equaled or exceeded in private practice. This suggests that Sigler's (1991) estimate of an annual private practice income loss average of $17,000 to $20,000, resulting from an annual loss of 15% of patients because of behavioral problems, may be a lower boundary.

The situation does not appear to differ greatly in Great Britain. One fifth of all dogs studied by Valery O'Farrell at Edinburgh University (Royal Dick) School of Veterinary Medicine had a behavioral problem (cited in Appleby, 1993). Furthermore, 39% of non-clinical cases were euthanized for behavior problems in Scotland (Stead, 1982). This latter figure represents animals that did not have medical problems, but were euthanized regardless. This suggests that the statistics cited for the United States are not atypical for other countries. Although Great Britain and the United States share a cultural heritage, there are some differences in lifestyle between inhabitants of the countries. It is safe to conclude that behavioral problems may be ubiquitous but are not a result of our perceptions of them.

In a comprehensive survey in which clients were presented with a multiple-choice questionnaire, Campbell (1986) found that 87% of the 1422 people with dogs listed one or more behavioral problems with their pets, with a mean of 4.7 problems per dog. Jumping on people was indicated by 37% of the clients, and barking or begging was a complaint of 33% of the clients. Both of these behaviors are management related, and it would be foolish to deny that management-related (i.e., purely preventable behavioral) complaints contribute to death in pets. In a different questionnaire designed to solicit from clients pet behaviors they perceived as problems, many fewer people listed specific behavioral problems. In part, this might be because the respondents did not realize that not all dogs jump on people or that it was acceptable to complain about such things. It is interesting to note that the number one complaint was house-soiling by dogs, with 20% of the respondents indicating that this was a problem (Campbell, 1986). House-soiling is *not* one of the most common complaints about dogs seen in behavioral clinics. Canine aggression of all types is by far the most common behavioral complaint of clients, although referral and survey data *do* differ in some ranks (Box 2-1).

The most common diagnosis for the canine patients in Voith's 1981 study was aggressive behavior toward people. The second most common diagnosis for dogs was separation anxiety. Dog bites to human beings make up at least 1% of all emergency department visits and cost $30 million per year in the United States in health care costs alone (August, 1988; Fleisher & Boenning, 1981; Greene et al., 1990). Most dog bites involve younger children, and 65% of all facial bites are in children under 10 years of age (Beck &

BOX 2-1
COMMON PROBLEMS REPORTED IN DOGS

Owner Survey	**Referral Diagnosis**
Aggression	Aggression
Excessive barking/ vocalization*	House-soiling*
Destructive chewing*	Destructive chewing*
Begging*	Fears/phobias
House-soiling*	Hyperactive/excitable*
Jumping on furniture*	Separation anxiety
Jumping on people*	Submissive behavior*
Running away*	Excessive vocaliza- tion*
Fear of loud noises	Abnormal eating*
Disobedience*	Medically based prob- lems
Excited/unruly/hyperac- tive*	Others
Stealing food items*	
Destructive behavior*	
Unacceptable eating be- havior*	
Eating feces*	

(From Beaver, 1993b)
Items are listed in rank order.
*Potential for management to be at least partially causal.

Jones, 1984; Feder et al., 1987; Harris et al., 1974). More than 2 million dog bites are reported annually in the United States, encouraging the postal service to devise guidelines for letter carriers to avoid bites (the guidelines include don't run; don't scream; avoid eye contact; back away; don't approach strange or confined dogs; let animal see and sniff you before petting).

Wright and Nesselrote (1987) found that 90% of 105 dogs referred for behavioral problems had three classes of problems: aggression, a behavior they termed stimulus reactivity, and separation problems. The mean age of their patients was 3.4 years; there were more males in the aggressive categories. As is true for cats, the proportion of neutered dogs has increased during the past 20 years in the United States, but it is still more common for a female dog to be spayed than for a male to be castrated (Manning & Rowan, 1992; Wilbur, 1976).

In three practices—one in Canada and two in the United States—Landsberg (1991a) found that of 743 dogs seen for behavioral problems, 59% were aggressive. The primary diagnosis for these aggressive animals was dominance aggression, and dominantly aggressive dogs made up 62% of the aggressive dogs. The second and third most common forms of aggression were fear aggression and territorial aggression. Of the cases studied by Landsberg, 18% involved canine elimination, 14% involved destruction, 6% involved phobias and fears, 6% involved excitability (this is a poorly defined term in this study and may be a correlate of other behavioral diagnoses), and 5% involved barking. The data on the frequency of aggressive dogs in the Landsberg study concur with those collected by Borchelt (1983a), who studied 372 dogs at the Animal Medical Center in New York City. Of those dogs brought to the center for behavioral problems, 66% were aggressive.

In a survey of 30 individuals who worked as animal behaviorists that was published in the *Animal Behavior Consultant Newsletter* in 1987, aggression in dogs involved only 32% of the cases, whereas elimination was involved in 19%. Separation problems were associated with approximately 15%, destruction with approximately 11% (although it is not clear from this survey if the destruction was involved in separation anxiety–affiliated problems), phobias (undefined in this survey) with 7.6% of the cases, and barking in 5.1% of the cases; a miscellaneous category made up 10% of the cases. One of the reasons that aggression was less common in this study of 30 animal behaviorists might be that the majority of these individuals were not specialists in veterinary medicine. It could be argued that the most severe cases, among which aggression would be included, would find their way to teaching and research hospitals and veterinary specialists, so that the two pools of patients may not come from the same population distribution.

In the Landsberg study (1991a), cocker spaniels, German shepherds, golden retrievers, and Lhaso apsos appeared most commonly on all three practice lists, regardless of geographic location. These are also the dogs that appeared on the most common purebred dog lists for those years. Because the practices did not provide any data on the distributions of breeds within their patient populations, it would be inappropriate to draw any breed-specific conclusions. Few breeds are represented out of proportion to the general hospital population at VHUP. This problem with apparency is discussed in depth in both Chapters 3 and 6.

THE VETERINARIAN'S ROLE IN CLIENT EDUCATION AND PREVENTION, DIAGNOSIS, AND TREATMENT OF BEHAVIOR PROBLEMS

In a study of Canadian veterinary practices, McKeown and Luescher (1988) found that 3% to 4% of all cases in the practices focused on behavioral concerns. However, this small proportion of cases took up 20% of the veterinarian's time. This means that 96% of the cases get only 80% of the veterinarian's time, whereas 4% get 20%. This emphasizes the need for basic knowledge on the part of the practitioner, so that the practitioner can intervene to prevent problems. Interestingly, most clients *expect* that the veterinarians should be able to advise them about prevention and treatment of behavioral problems, but they do not perceive that veterinarians meet those expectations (Case, 1988).

Not only are behavioral problems a major factor in life-and-death decisions for pet animals, but they are a major factor for people who do not complain about their pets' behavior. In data I collected at VHUP and area veterinary hospitals in 1989, 68% of all clients coming to a veterinarian's office for *any* reason had a question about their pet's behavior. Questions ranged from whether the behavior was normal, whether it was abnormal, whether something could be done to improve the behavior, or whether the clients were somehow damaging the pet's "psyche." Interestingly, when these clients were asked whether they would seek help, the majority explicitly said they would *not* go to their veterinarian because their veterinarian did not know anything about animal behavior.

It is time to rectify this situation. The single biggest killer of pets is not infectious disease; it is *behavioral problems*, and the single biggest facilitator of this phenomenon is our ignorance.

3 ····· Normal Canine Behavior

···

EVOLUTIONARY OVERVIEW

In 1865 Sir Francis Galton elucidated the conditions under which animals could become domesticated: (1) they should be hearty, (2) they should have an inborn liking for man, (3) they should be comfort loving, (4) they should be useful to the savages (remember, this was 1865), (5) they should breed freely, and (6) they should be easy to tend. These reasons indicate why sheep and goats were among the first domesticated animals (by hunter-gatherers approximately 9000 years ago) and may explain why cattle and pigs were domesticated later. Galton's conditions predispose the domesticator to choose neotenic (infantile) characters; this is what we have done with our domesticated dogs and cats (Coppinger et al., 1987).

Tamed animals that are subjected to artificial, rather than natural, selection are usually favored for economic, cultural, and aesthetic reasons (Zeuner, 1963). The original domesticated dogs may have worked with people first and become companions second. Some authors have postulated that companions were developed from runts. The effects of taming and domestication produced the same physical changes in widely different groups of animals. Many of the characteristics that are so similar originate from the aforementioned retention of juvenile or neotenic characteristics, and therefore the same form may appear in a dog and a pig. Examples of neotenic traits include the deposition of fat under the skin, the shortening of jaws, and the curling of the tail (Clutton-Brock, 1987; Coppinger et al., 1987). With the exception of the cat, all domesticated animals were derived from wild species that are extremely social and easily recognized as such (Kleiman & Eisenberg, 1973). This does not imply that cats are asocial; however, their social system differs from that of the dog. Domestic cats are derived from the most social and friendliest of the wild cats, *Felis silvestris libyca*, the cat that was apparently easiest to "tame." Because domestic animals were derived from social species, general social behavior patterns probably have changed relatively little with domestication. Specific behaviors have been modified by enhancement or reduction through specific breeding and artificial selection. The extent to which such modifications were possible depends on the variation and expression of the original social pattern. All social animals (including ants) have social patterns that are based on rules and their structure.

Even signaling is a form of rule structure. Such rules and social patterns facilitate efficient allocation of effort and energy, decrease danger, encourage cohesiveness, and provide a communication system that permits animals to communicate the extent to which they are confident or confused about the aforementioned. It would behoove animal behavior clinicians to understand these patterns if they are to grasp why dogs behave as they do and understand the cause of many of their behavior problems.

The early stages of domestication have been accompanied by a decrease in body size (Bekoff et al., 1984; Gittleman et al., 1989). In fact, this change in size has been used to distinguish skeletal remains at archeological sites. In most domesticated mammals, the size of the brain becomes smaller relative to the size of the body, and the sense organs become reduced. Within a few generations of breeding, the facial region of the skull and jaw become shortened. The skull and jaw changes are the most apparent signs of domestication seen in the remains of early dogs. The compaction of the molars and the premolars in early domesticated dogs is used to distinguish their remains from those of wolves (Clutton-Brock, 1987). The same pattern is also found in teeth of modern dogs. For example, the Great Dane dog is larger than the wolf progenitor but has smaller teeth with a less complicated cusp pattern than is found in the wolf. One could question whether this was deliberate selection for a safer companion animal, because the teeth of wolves are classic predator's teeth, or whether this resulted from a change in dietary habits. In addition to the differences in the teeth, the tympanic bulla of the Great Dane is also smaller than that of the wolf. Domestication may also have altered long-distance auditory needs.

Development of Breeds

The domestic dog was first derived from a wolf, possibly the Asiatic wolf *(Canis lupus paillipes)* (Messent & Serpell, 1981; Scott, 1967a). Since the hypothesized initial domestication event, 4000 generations of breeding have produced a diversity of modern breeds. Most of the modern breeds have been developed within the last 150 years (Scott & Fuller, 1965), and this development of breeds is apparent in the paintings of the times. Remains of wolves have been found with those of humans since the middle Pleistocene and Early Paleolithic era (Olsen, 1985). Some of the first remains of domesticated dogs have been found in a cave in Iraq that dates to 12,000 years before present (Davis & Valla, 1978; Turnbull & Reed, 1974), and domestic dog remains dating from 10,000 to 15,000 years ago have been found elsewhere (Olsen, 1985). Since 6500 years before the present, dogs have been found everywhere that humans have been found (Reed, 1964).

The dog family (Canidae) has 34 species ranging in size from bush dogs, which are dachshund size, to the Arctic wolf. Canids, both wild and domesticated, inhabit a variety of environments including temperate and tropical forest, savannah, tundra, and desert. They are far more omnivorous than is usually believed (Wayne, 1993), which probably helped them in their rapid expansion in domestication worldwide. Omnivory also probably accounts for the widespread distribution of canids in a diversity of habitats.

The order Carnivora, which includes dogs and cats, originated 40 to 60 million years ago. The Canidae diverged from other carnivore families 50 to 60 million years ago; this is early in carnivore evolution and may be one of the reasons why most canids share so many attributes of their social systems (Wayne, 1993).

Much has been made of the similarities between wolves and dogs. This may become an even more forceful component of behavioral arguments now that all previous claims that dogs were derived from jackals (Lorenz, 1954) have been rejected. Wolves, wolflike canids, and dogs have the same number of diploid (2n) chromosomes—78 (Davis & Valla, 1978), as do the golden jackal (Canis aureus), the side-striped jackal (Canis adustus), and the black-backed jackal (Canis mesomelas), yet these are all small, 5 to 10 kg canids. The larger, 12 to 30 kg, wolflike canids (the Simian jackal [Canis simensis], the gray wolf [Canis lupus], the coyote [Canis latrans], the red wolf [Canis rufus], the dhole [Cuon alpinis], and the African wild dog [Lycaon pictus]) also have the same number of diploid chromosomes. Again, these species share attributes of social structure.

Allozyme and chromosomal analysis suggests several phylogenetic divergences in the Canidae. The first divergence includes the wolflike canids (dogs, gray wolves, coyotes, and jackals). The second divergence includes the South American canids; these canids have an extremely diverse morphology but are of common ancestry. The third divergence appears to have resulted in the red fox–like canids of the old and new world (red and kit foxes), whereas the fourth divergence appears to be monotypic, including only the bat-eared fox and the raccoon dog (Wayne, 1993). Phylogenetic analysis of mitochondrial cytochrome *b* gene (736 base pairs) indicates a close relationship between gray wolves, dogs, coyotes, and Simian jackals (Wayne, 1993; Wayne, 1989). The gray wolf and coyote shared a common ancestry 2 million years ago and have diverged by 4% of the mitochondrial DNA sequences (Wayne, 1993). The dog and the gray wolf diverge by, at most, 0.2% of mitochondrial DNA sequences (Wayne, 1993). It is interesting to note that when gene frequencies of red blood cell antigens are compared for dingoes and domestic dogs, the overall population frequencies are indistinguishable (Symons & Bell, 1992).

Social Patterns

All of the canid groups share certain social patterns. Differences in dog behavior when compared with wolf behavior have been attributed to domestication (Bekoff et al, 1984; Kretchmer & Fox, 1975; Scott, 1967a, 1968). Some changes attributed to domestication include changes in responses to certain thresholds. An example is the exaggerated barking observed in domestic dogs. It is unusual for either coyotes or wolves to bark or howl unless they are doing so in a group or as youngsters (Harrington & Mech, 1979, 1982). Barking is a behavior that domestication has elaborated in dogs.

Domestic dogs also appear to exhibit an increase in docility and adaptability. This docility may have been developed from a suite of behaviors that was chosen to make a potentially dangerous animal more tractable. Among such changes that occurred in domesticated dogs is the change in predatory behavior. In all domestic dogs, the sequence of behaviors demonstrated during hunting and predation has been truncated, under normal, nondeprived circumstances. Without exception, the killing bite has been inhibited. Various parts of the predation sequence have been shaped to meet the intent of the specific domesticated breed. The following breeds exhibit the noted partial hunting sequences (Bradshaw & Brown, 1990):

- Bloodhound: tracking, trailing
- Sheepdog: eyeing, stalking, chasing
- Setter, pointer: stalking, pointing
- Boarhound: attacking, killing
- Retriever: retrieving (cubs, mates)
- Protecting dogs: inhibited biting and holding

Domestic dogs also demonstrate a perpetuation of infantile (neotenic) behavior patterns as adults. Behavior patterns of persistent play and begging are concomitant with the neotenic physical patterns selected for in many breeds of dogs (Coppinger et al., 1987). Other neotenic behaviors that have been described by Schenkel (1967) include elaborations of play, passive submission, and whining behavior. The wolf has more infantile behavior as an adult than do many other canid species. That fact alone may have facilitated domestication (Bradshaw & Brown, 1990). The coupling of neotenic behaviors to human desires may have made it possible to domesticate wolves. Finally, domestic dogs have different breeding patterns from other canids. They are more promiscuous than any other canid group; the rule in most canid groups is to form pair-bonds (Kretchmer & Fox, 1975). Domestic dogs can breed every 6 months, with the exception of basenjis, who have retained the ancestral reproductive pattern of fall breeding (Fuller, 1956).

Canids exhibit the tendency to follow a leader when in a group, as well as exhibiting other group-associated deferential behaviors. It is possible that humans did not fully domesticate dogs but underwent a codomestication process with dogs. It has been postulated that wolves and the early domesticated dogs were probably attracted to early campfires because of the smell of meat (Clutton-Brock, 1987). It is not unreasonable to assume that humans were able to recognize another social system that was similar to ours. Although wolves would not have barked to the extent that domestic dogs do, the howling and group responses may have worked equally well for humans and wolves as early predator warning systems.

Humans share many aspects of their social systems with those of canids. These social systems are not derived from a shared, common ancestor, and thus are not homologous by descent, but they do appear to be analogous. The evidence for this congruence is vast and strong. Both humans and canids live in extended family groups, provide extensive parental care, share care of young with both related and nonrelated group members, give birth to altricial young that require large amounts of early care and sustained amounts of later social interaction, nurse for an extended period before weaning to semisolid food (dogs do this by regurgitation; humans use baby food, but the concept is the same), have extensive vocal and nonvocal communication (it has been estimated that up to 80% of all human communication is nonverbal; Smith, 1977), and have a sexual maturity that precedes social maturity. Dogs are sexually mature by 6 to 9 months of age and are not socially mature until beginning at 18 to 36 months of age. People are sexually mature some time between 8 and 13 years of age, and are not socially mature until well into their 20s or 30s (if such a phenomenon ever actually happens in people). In addition, the human social system is a *fluid* hierarchical one that is based on ability, age, or both, but that is grounded in the context of *deference*. Human families do not battle to determine who sits at the head of the table at holidays—in many cultures this place is usually reserved for the older member of the family or for an honored guest. Dogs are very much like this. The contests that occur are used to elucidate and test hierarchical relationships, but day-to-day interactions are largely based on deferential behaviors. Furthermore, combat in both canids and humans is not the first choice for resolution of conflict. When combat is the first choice for conflict resolution, it is an abnormal, out-of-context behavior. Instead, agonistic behavior is generally accompanied by an elaborate display structure designed to minimize damage to the individual. Communication of offensive tactics avoids the costs of outright battle and the damages that may be incurred. Both canid and human social systems use signals and displays that minimize the probability of outright battle. Deferential relationships in both dogs and humans are *not* structured as linear hierarchies. This is a point most often missed by writers of popular books about dog behavior, and by breeders. Most evidence supporting linear hierarchies is artifactual and the result of poor experimental design. In fact, the study of relationships between fewer than six animals will automatically produce a numerical rank order hierarchy that is linear (Bernstein, 1981; Boyd & Silk, 1983; Rowell, 1974; Syme, 1974); however, such ranks are unable to account for the social complexities that are noted. Instead, deferential behaviors are context dependent and are based on knowledge, age, size, and the situation in which individuals are interacting. Given this background, it is not surprising that humans were able to incorporate dogs into our social groups, as we were incorporated into theirs.

Unfortunately, because dogs and people do have such similar social systems and use so many of the same signals, it has been very easy for people to assume that when a dog gives a signal that resembles a human signal, the message is exactly the same and that it means exactly the same thing (*sensu* Smith, 1965). Nothing could be further from the truth. One of the goals of this chapter is to elucidate the extent to which canine communication is *canine* communication that *people* have adapted to human circumstances. In such cases, dogs may be communicating purely canine behaviors. The communication section discusses this concept in depth and is very useful for clients who have difficulty with the idea that the behavior they perceive as friendly is in fact, from the dog's perspective, a challenging behavior.

Reviewing the similarities between canid and human social systems also explains why cats were not selected to perform the same types of jobs for which we selected dogs, and why the domestication history of cats differs from that of dogs. Not only do cats have social systems that are much more complex in many ways and more varied than are canid social systems, but most cats were physically larger at the period when dogs were being domesticated. The inability to accurately interpret the signals of an animal that is the archetypal predator and larger than the domesticator, coupled with the inability to understand subtle, nonverbal signals in a context that would facilitate working together, would have created a far more dangerous situation than that with canids. Furthermore, it is worth remembering that all wild cats are obligate carnivores; therefore the potential for domestication was historically different. It is interesting to note that although dogs were domesticated from a large, wild canid, the wolf, and that the first domesticated dogs were slightly smaller than wolves, extant domesticated dogs range in size from 1 to 2 kg to almost 100 kg. This range far exceeds that in wild dogs. In contrast, domesticated cats are all quite small and have a far smaller size range than do extant wild felids. This size factor, in addition to the feline origins as obligate carnivores, suggests why humans' relationship with them has been rooted in a less interactive mutualism than has been our relationship with dogs.

The Development of Early Canine Behavior

Far more information is available on the development of normal behavior in dogs than on such behavior in cats. This may reflect the possibly erroneous perception that dogs are more social than cats. Regardless, most of the information is derived from laboratory situations in which dogs are kept, and from organizations interested in developing service dogs.

In the late 1940s and early 1950s, attention was paid to the development of service dogs for search and rescue, for working with handicapped individuals (primarily visually impaired), and with regard to breed predispositions for specific behaviors as dog show hobbyists increased in number. At that time, J.P. Scott and colleagues developed a laboratory colony of dogs that were rigorously examined with regard to the developmental stages of specific behaviors. Concomitantly, work was being done on German shepherd dogs in Europe, primarily those intended for use as search and rescue dogs. In addition to variation in the development of individual, within litter, and between litter behaviors, Scott and co-workers realized that there might also be some breed differences in the intensity of some of these behaviors because different breeds had been selected to do different jobs. Hence they included mixed breed dogs in their colony, with beagles, basenjis, cocker spaniels, fox terriers, shelties, and Scottish terriers. These are all breeds that differ in the tasks for which they were selected, yet are small enough to be manageable in a laboratory colony situation. The following section reviews these early findings. Specific implications of their findings for the potential development of behavior problems are then discussed.

Early General Findings from the Bar Harbor Colony

From birth to 2 weeks of age, puppies' olfactory, thermal, and tactile sensory capabilities develop; they have no auditory or visual capabilities. At approximately 2 to 3 weeks of age, eyes open, concomitant with an increase in mobility. At this stage dogs begin to exhibit social behaviors.

Before the work of Scott and colleagues, it was generally believed that in the 3- to 12-week age range dogs experienced what was called "maximum social ability." If they were isolated from other dogs during those times, they seemed to have more problems interacting with dogs. The focus of the Bar Harbor group was to test the hypothesis that a "critical" period existed, and to examine the extent to which the puppies developed responses to different types of stimuli within that period. Using standard observational techniques and trained observers, dogs were examined beginning at birth. Behavioral observations started at 3

weeks of age. In this colony, weaning occurred at about 7 weeks. Puppies were kept with their mothers until 10 weeks of age so that the separation did not coincide with changes in feeding schedules in the dogs. By 12 weeks of age, the dogs voluntarily chose to wander more widely. This is one reason that 12 weeks of age was considered to be the end of the socialization period. These pups were handled daily for weighing. Mild stress and early handling were actually beneficial for the puppies and allowed them to better cope with stresses that came later. Hans Selye (1952) noted the beneficial effects of early, mild stress in his Nobel prize–winning work on cortical steroids and stress levels. This finding might be beneficial to breeders, because early stress (daily handling) is often avoided for reasons of disease transmission. Rigorous cleaning and conscientious vaccination schedules should alleviate the latter.

Experiments confirmed that 3 weeks of age was approximately the earliest time that "socialization" began (Scott, 1970, 1962, 1958). From days 13 to 20, the "transition period," dogs become more coordinated, open their eyes, and begin to startle to sound. The change in motor abilities coincides with eruption of teeth at approximately day 20. Tail-wagging behavior follows. These behaviors were characterized by considerable between-breed variation (Table 3-1). It is interesting that there is less variation in a behavior that facilitates interaction (tail wagging) than in characteristics associated with specific breed structure. General results indicated that pups should be exposed to people at an early age to decrease development of avoidance behaviors. When placed in rooms with passive observers for 10-minute intervals at 3 weeks of age, pups approached and explored the observer. At first, such explorations were uncoordinated. If the puppies were not exposed to observers until 7 weeks of age, it took 2 days for the puppies to habituate sufficiently to the observer to approach and explore. If the puppies were kept from people until 14 weeks of age, and then placed in a room with a passive observer, they would not approach the observer. These data were confirmed in subsequent works (Bacon & Stanley, 1963, 1970a; Freedman et al., 1961; Lore & Eisenberg, 1986). Desensitization by hand feeding was necessary for dogs that

TABLE 3-1 Breed-Associated Physical and Behavioral Development

Breed	Complete Eye Opening at 2 Weeks (%)	Upper Canine Eruption at 3 Weeks (%)	Tail Wagging at 4 Weeks (%)
Basenji	65	79	27
Beagle	94	74	49
Cocker spaniel	94	22	83
Fox terrier	11	14	42
Sheltie	31	31	56

(Data from Scott and Fuller, 1965.)

were not exposed to people until 14 weeks of age (Bacon & Stanley, 1970b). Pups that were kept in kennels beyond 14 weeks were very timid and had a lack of confidence in any circumstances other than that kennel (Pfaffenberger & Scott, 1959). Once this trend was noted, the laboratory dogs were all moved outdoors at 12 to 14 weeks to aid exploration.

Although these general results are broadly applicable, breed-specific differences in response were reported (Freedman, 1958; Melzack & Scott, 1957). Beagles that were isolated from weeks 3 to 20 became fearful of unfamiliar humans. Those who were only partially isolated during this period demonstrated decreased activity. In contrast, Scottish terriers that were isolated from weeks 3 to 20 became hyperactive and insensitive to pain.

When beagles, fox terriers, shelties, and basenjis were exposed to two treatment situations—indulged (never punished, encouraged to be active and interactive) and disciplined (restrained, made to always comply with commands to obtain food)—the behavioral responses to subsequent physical corrections while offered food treats differed by breed. Basenjis ate the treat, regardless of whether they had been previously "indulged" or "disciplined." Shelties avoided the treats, regardless of previous treatment (Scott et al., 1968; Scott, 1968). Fox terriers in the "disciplined" group took the treat, but those in the "indulged" group avoided it.

Not all breeds respond the same to all circumstances, even if they are reared identically (Elliot & Scott, 1965; Fuller & Clark 1968). This strongly suggests, not that all individuals in a breed will be of a specific behavioral type, but that the gene × environment interaction will be complex. Oddly, these gene × environment interactions have been poorly studied.

Specialization and Sensitive Periods

The broad findings of Scott and colleagues led to the definition of developmental periods for dogs: at 3 to 8 weeks of age dogs do well learning about how to interact with other dogs; between week 5 and weeks 7 to 12, dogs do best learning how to interact with people; and between weeks 10 to 12 and weeks 16 to 20, dogs do extremely well in exploring novel environments. These periods were later, perhaps inappropriately, called *socialization periods*. They have achieved undeserved deity status.

The concept of developmental periods was similar to the idea of sensitive periods later articulated by Bateson (1979) and Cairns et al. (1985). The concept of a sensitive period implies some risk assessment. Part of one's response varies with genetic makeup and part of it varies with gene × environment interaction, but exposure is critical. If one is *not* exposed to the stimuli to which one can respond during the relevant periods, one may be at risk of developing problems attendant with those periods. For instance, if a dog is never

exposed to people, that dog may then be fearful of people and may not approach them later in life. If that dog had been exposed to people early, there is no guarantee that he would have been problem-free, but he would have had the opportunity to learn to react appropriately.

These periods should not be used as guides for delaying exposure. Clients should *not* wait to expose dogs to people until 5 to 7 to 12 weeks of age, for example. The specified time frame only implies that dogs are not sufficiently neurologically and behaviorally focused on people to initiate interaction with people before 5 to 7 weeks; however, there is no reason that they should not be exposed to people in novel circumstances starting as early as possible. The first focus in the dog's life is other dogs; this is logical. Dogs then expand their horizon to include first, people, and then, novel situations and objects. If the dogs are deprived of these periods, they are at risk of developing inappropriate or abnormal behaviors associated with them. The earlier dogs can learn about the environment in which they are to live (without inducing fear), the better; if they are protected from environmental stimuli, they may react inappropriately when later exposed (Scott, 1963; Stanley et al., 1970). Unfortunately, this does not mean that if everything is done "correctly" that a perfect dog will result. Some dogs, like some people, have fewer inherent coping skills than others. The extent to which this phenomenon is genetic is unknown.

Some moderate stress introduced during the first few days of life is beneficial, but excessive stress leads to an increase in adrenocorticotropic hormone (ACTH) secretion. Excessive secretion of ACTH has been correlated with a decreased ability to learn. Other studies have indicated that pups that are isolated from 3 days to 20 weeks of age, regardless of having their physiologic needs met, are disturbed for life (Agrawal et al., 1967) and have impaired learning ability (Melzack, 1968; Melzack & Scott, 1957; Thompson & Heron, 1954). In a further elaboration of earlier developmental experiments, Freedman and colleagues (1961) handled different groups of puppies at 2, 3, 5, 7, and 9 weeks of age; the control group was not handled until 14 weeks of age. The dogs handled between weeks 5 and 7 were the most responsive to humans; the control animals were fearful and never formed close attachments (Fuller & Clark, 1966; Scott, 1970). Similar situations have been reported for primate species, again underscoring the similarities in the social systems (Harlow & Harlow, 1965, Suomi et al., 1981). The extent to which this response is modulated by ACTH is unknown.

Puppies raised only with kittens during 2.5 to 13 weeks of age do not recognize dogs as conspecifics; they preferentially choose to consort with cats (Fox, 1969b, 1971c). This is not the result of nursing and feeding behaviors; machine-fed puppies become normally attached to people if given appropriate contact

(Brodbeck, 1954). Both slightly overfed and slightly underfed puppies have enhanced attachment responses (Stanley and Elliot, 1962). This may be because overfeeding or underfeeding reinforces hierarchical social structures and neotenic begging behavior. Whether these early feeding behaviors play a role in the later development of problem behaviors like separation anxiety is unknown. A mixture of punishment and reward structures induced the most rapid "socialization" to handlers when puppies were separated from other puppies (Scott & Fuller, 1965). It has been postulated that this represents a range of behaviors actually encountered in litters, where spontaneous playful aggression is finally lost by 16 weeks of age.

The role of early experience for the development of normal social behavior is supported by data using other species. For instance, laughing gull chicks (*Larus atricilla*) experience adult crooning before hatching, and they respond with an increased activity pattern and increased vocalizations when they experience crooning after hatching. Chicks who are deprived of this prehatching experience have decreased activity patterns and decreased vocalizations when presented with crooning (Impekoven, 1976). Russock and Hale (1979) examined *Gallus* chicks' responsiveness to maternal food calls. Responsiveness to food calls decreased with age if the chicks never experienced calls early in life, but a *single*, early, brief exposure to a call maintains responsiveness later. This is a very small amount of stimulation indeed. Adult mice that have had experience with mouse pups approach the sound of playbacks of pup distress calls, but those that do not have any prior experience with mouse pups do not approach the distress call playback source (Ehret & Koch, 1989).

These experiments indicate that early stimulation and early experience can influence behaviors in the distant future, including some maternal behaviors. Although there is no definitive evidence to substantiate the exact course in dogs, many authors have postulated that dogs that have problems caring for puppies were denied early maternal contact themselves. Breeders should err on the side of safety and stimulate the puppies as much as possible. It must be emphasized that the dogs should not show signs of extreme or prolonged distress when stimulated.

"Socialization" of young puppies is important for a normal range of canid behaviors to be exhibited (Markwell & Thorne, 1987); however, exposure should be nondamaging. Fox and Bekoff (1975) found that what they called the social "sense" was developed most intensely between weeks 4 and 10. Puppies at those ages approached any stimulus, but started to become fearful of some new animals at about 6 weeks of age and began to be more discriminating in their approaches. Stimuli affecting a social "sense" may involve food (Ross, 1951; Ross & Ross, 1949a, b). Aggressive behavior (defined here as barking, growling, and biting) in young puppies is limited to the context of possession of food or an object (toys or bones) in the context of a hierarchical relationship in the litter (James, 1949; Scott & Fuller, 1965). These behaviors were apparent by 5 weeks of age or earlier.

The Case Against Very Early and Very Late Puppyhood Adoption

If breeders are interested in working with their pups, they need to watch the pups' response and know the range of "normal" behaviors. Seven-week-old pups left with their mother will work in groups to attack intruders (Scott & Fuller, 1965). It is not unusual that, if left continuously with their mother by 7 weeks of age, pups functionally form a pack. At 3 to 4 weeks of age, pups start to follow each other. By 5 weeks of age, they rush at an opening as a group. The more activity there is at the opening, the more frenzied the puppies will become. If the puppies are raised in a field instead of a kennel situation, they are fully exploratory by 12 weeks of age. In both kennel and field situations, the strongest attachment to location and to their companions occurs at about 6 to 7 weeks. This period is when the most severe upset occurs and when the most destabilizing effects appear, if pups are separated from home or companion (Elliot & Scott, 1961). This response is mitigated if all littermates are exposed to a variety of fairly benign circumstances, both as an intact litter and in smaller groups early in life. Separation from each other or a place at 6 weeks of age causes recidivistic changes in the puppies' behavioral development. These findings comprise one of the strongest arguments in favor of the abolition of puppy mills. They also provide insight into why so many puppies that are placed at a very young age have behavioral problems. Some breeders believe that the optimal age to place animals is 6 to 7 weeks, and some books recommend 7 weeks of age as the optimal age to place a puppy (Campbell, 1992). Based on the research, this is too early to place a puppy. Not only will the behavioral response to separation be profound, but interstate commerce laws do not allow puppies to be shipped before 7 weeks of age. Maternal antibodies begin to wane by 6 to 8 weeks of age; vaccination schedules may not yet be established. In addition, shipping stress can make the pups more susceptible to disease.

Further evidence that social exposure should be rigorous and early is derived from work on guide dogs. Breeders are concerned that early exposure might subject their dogs to biologic risk. Guide dog puppies are vaccinated at 6 weeks of age and every third week until they are 12 to 16 weeks of age. Of the 24,000 puppies examined, fewer than half a dozen that were healthy during the vaccination series became unwell. This work (cited in Appleby, 1993) is substantiated by research by the Pediatrics and Genetics Group at the University of Pennsylvania School of Veterinary Medicine. Provided the puppies are engaged in an active immunization program, it has been suggested that some exposure to "street" virus, provided it does not occur because the dogs were exposed to critically ill animals, may be beneficial in boosting the puppies' immunity (P. Jezyk, VHUP; personal communication).

Stress at 6 to 7 weeks also affects the pups' ability to learn. This is an important consideration for housebreaking. Puppies begin to form a firm substrate and location preference for elimination by 8½ weeks. Their mothers have stimulated them to urinate and defecate up until about 3 weeks of age; from 3 to 7 to 8 weeks puppies eliminate whenever necessary, with little regard to location. Accordingly, this is an approximation of the best time to place a puppy. If breeders are willing to housebreak the puppy and encourage its independence (see discussion that follows), there may be no cost to keeping the puppy longer than 8½ weeks. Breeders may believe that this is too time consuming, yet Fuller (1967) noted that semiisolated puppies could be "socialized" with as little as two 20-minute periods a week.

Puppies respond best to objects, such as leashes, between 5 and 9 weeks of age (Scott & Fuller, 1965). Breeders can help puppies by starting to fit them with head halters, harnesses, and leashes.

Puppies separated from the dam and litter at the time of weaning display vocalizations at a rate of up to 100 per minute (Elliott & Scott, 1961). This argues that one should not concomitantly wean and place dogs. Pettijohn and co-workers (1977) provide data that indicate that toys have no effect on relieving separation distress, but that social stimuli do. Humans may be preferred to dogs for relief of the social exposure stress that occurs at 7 to 8 weeks of age, the time when dogs are apt to explore people.

Puppies have firmly developed hierarchical relationships among themselves by 11 weeks of age; these are well stabilized by 15 weeks of age. Unless the breeder is going to keep the puppies, the puppies should be placed in homes when they can most easily develop stable relationships. Most of the firm hierarchical relationships within a household do not occur until the puppy has begun to reach social maturity, at 18 to 36 months of age. The disruptive effect of breaking apart a hierarchy on which an animal has been relying has not been examined.

The extent to which breed affects behavior is little known but often queried. General patterns are recognized; for example, beagle pups seem far more motivated by food than basenjis (Scott & Fuller, 1965). This may not be surprising for a breed that has been selected to work with its nose. Furthermore, beagles have been selected to work in groups; when reared alone until 16 weeks of age, beagles lose the capacity for spontaneous play. Play can be elicited, but these dogs play differently than ones that associate with other beagles (Adler & Adler, 1977).

Postmodern Findings

Many of the studies on service dogs conducted in the United States and Europe confirm these broad findings (Fuller, 1955; Pfaffenberg & Scott, 1959; Scott & Beilfelt, 1976; Stur et al., 1989). Of the puppies that left kennels at or before 12 weeks of age, 90% graduated as successful guide dogs; if they are left only an additional 3 weeks (15 weeks of age) in the kennel, only 30% of those dogs successfully graduate as guide dogs (Appleby, 1993). The same pattern has been noted in dogs reared for Canine Companions for Independence (P. Mundell, Canine Companions for Independence; personal communication, 1994). This may relate less to exposure and socialization periods than to times when animals learn best. Language acquisition may be an analogous situation with humans. If humans are exposed to the sounds of a foreign language early, we learn it more easily than if we are not exposed until later in life. Some of the effects of socialization may be mitigated by learning, physical environments, and by the genetic environment.

In 5 of 13 tests to evaluate maternal and paternal genetic effects on puppies' ability to learn and perform tasks, there was a significant effect of sire on specific behaviors; the largest of these was on the behavior to fetch an object. The between-dam variance was very high for all of the 13 behavioral measures that were examined, and, on average, was 3 times higher than the heritability scores of the sires (cited in Fält, 1984). Similar data have been cited for the Swedish dog training center (Fält, 1984). This has some far-ranging implications for people who are training dogs for specific tasks.

Comparisons of German shepherd and beagle behavior indicate that locomotor activity is independent of other behaviors involved in the investigation of novel objects (Wright, 1983). There are no sex differences at either 5 or 8 weeks of age in locomotion or in distress calls; maximum distress, as indicated only by vocalization, occurs at the fifth week of development (Gurski et al., 1980).

Hand-reared puppies explore novel stimuli more than kennel-reared puppies when evaluated at 8½ weeks of age. This does *not* mean that pups should be separated from their mothers early and hand-reared. It *does* mean that stimulation is important for the development of exploratory behaviors. Early separation of mother and pups has been shown to be detrimental to the behavioral and physical development of pups. Slabbert and Rasa (1993) definitely demonstrated that separation of pups from their mothers at 6 weeks of age had a negative effect on the physical condition and weight of pups. Closer bonds with humans were not promoted by early separation in this study; in fact, early separation interfered with puppies' physical health.

In a study of the ontogeny of human-dog interactions from birth to 9 months of age in 47 different breeds, Feddersen-Petersen (1994) cited the effects of inadequate rearing conditions—"socially deprived" dogs were antagonistic when greeted by humans and exhibited agonistic behavior in response to human approach, whereas dogs that had adequate socialization exhibited normal, friendly greetings and were well adapted in other social circumstances.

Possession of a bone and the ability to control it changes greatly for lower ranking puppies between 5½ and 11½ weeks of age, but very assertive and controlling puppies can retain the rank and their bone (Wright, 1980). This suggests that the fluidity observed in adult social hierarchies is actually developed at quite a young age, and that breeders should be encouraged to consider that adaptability to changes in social hierarchy may be a far more valuable social skill than being "top dog."

Although the data collected by Scott and colleagues are classic in nature, it is important to remember the following: (1) sample sizes were small, (2) the number of breeds examined were few, (3) all examinations took place in a laboratory using laboratory animals—this does not reflect the possible range of normal behaviors, and (4) these studies have never been replicated or expanded. We have "progressed" to discussing and treating the "abnormal" without fully investigating the "normal." Furthermore, the data from these studies have been misused and misapplied by the lay public. Texts expound on "drives," "aptitude," and "temperament," yet no data have been rigorously collected, or statistical tests performed, to substantiate any assertions about drive, temperament, and aptitude. Thus all discussions of these attributes must be cautiously interpreted in this light.

Summary Recommendations

In summary, clients should be encouraged to handle their dogs from birth and to expose their puppies to a variety of circumstances in as positive and benign a manner as possible. It is critical that breeders start exposing their puppies to dogs by about 3 weeks of age and to people by about 5 weeks of age; puppies should be exposed to novel circumstances throughout. Clients and breeders should be reminded that these recommended times are not "etched in stone" and should be viewed in a risk assessment context: if the dogs are not allowed to experience the appropriate stimuli during the times when they are receptive to them, they *may* develop problems attendant with those periods. We must emphasize to clients that they do not need to delay exposing the animals to circumstances provided the animals are not showing any prolonged or profound signs of fear or distress. Some distress and fear can be adaptive, and learning how to handle conflict or resolve a less than advantageous interaction is an important task in social development. This is seldom examined in dogs. There is much variation in puppy behavior, and earlier exposure might be beneficial for some animals. We also need to emphasize to clients the extent to which early learning is important and that early "bad" learning (the learning of undesirable behaviors) can also be important. Clients should be aware of the fact that puppies de-

velop very strong substrate preferences for elimination by 8½ weeks of age and that they are very handleable and tractable for leash-walking from 5 to 8½ weeks of age. Finally, we should emphasize to clients that puppies are individuals and vary both within and between litters. Clients need to be aware of any signs of behavioral or physiologic stress and distress and to intervene if their "socialization program" is unduly distressing their puppy.

Classification of Specific Behaviors

Early canine behaviors can be divided into et-epimeletic (care-seeking), epimeletic (caregiving), and allelomimetic (group-activity) behaviors. Until about 4 weeks of age (at the end of the transitional period and the beginning of the time period when dogs are most amenable to social interaction) the relationship between the mother and puppies is primarily epimeletic. Epimeletic behaviors include:

1. Licking the pup's anal and genital regions and eating urine and feces
2. Grooming and licking faces
3. Pushing pups with the nose to encourage them toward warmth and feeding opportunities and to stimulate postures associated with respiration and other physical and physiologic functions
4. Carrying straying puppies
5. Guarding pups
6. Suckling
7. Regurgitation
8. Carrying food for puppies.

As they age, puppies perform rutting and whining, et-epimeletic behaviors. These include:

1. Tail-wagging, with their tail low in a deferential solicitation gesture
2. Yelping
3. Licking the mother's face, nose, and lips
4. Jumping up and pawing at the mother
5. Following the mother closely.

Group or allelomimetic behaviors that the puppies exhibit as they move into their more social periods include:

1. Sleeping together
2. Feeding
3. Walking, running, and sitting or lying together
4. Investigating things as a group
5. Barking or howling as a group
6. Grooming other group members
7. Sniffing and nosing other members of the group

VISUAL, OLFACTORY, AND AUDITORY SYSTEMS IN DOGS
Vision

Dogs, with a 97-degree binocular field, have relatively poor binocular vision. In humans, half of the fibers in the optic nerve are not decussated, or uncrossed. In the cat, this is true for a third of the fibers. In the dog, this is true for only one fourth of the fibers. Accordingly, dogs have better lateral vision than do humans.

Sheep dogs can see hand signals at a distance of 1 km, in part because of this distribution of decussated and nondecussated fibers (cited in Fogle, 1990). The tapetum reflects light to the rods and cones so that dogs actually do see better at night than people do, and dogs register low light quite well. Dogs see in rudimentary color vision and they are sensitive to short-wave light. Dog color vision is sufficiently discriminating so that they can pick out an object based on color (Neitz et al., 1989). Partly because of their ability to track moving objects and partly because of shading differences, dogs are postulated to be able to track European television, which has 625 dots per second, but not television in the United States, which has only 525 dots per second (cited in Fogle, 1990). Personal observation disputes this; clients frequently report that their dogs monitor activity on television, but no quantitative measures of tracking ability exist.

Much of canine communication is based on visual signaling, so one might expect dogs who are required to do much signaling (young puppies interacting in groups) to be modestly handicapped by a lack of vision. This appears to be true. Other inappropriate or undesirable behaviors that may be concomitant with visual problems include fearful behaviors and problems navigating a changed environment. The latter is probably more of a problem for older dogs who gradually lose their vision; young dogs who have never been visual may develop their own systems for communicating. My dog, who has congenital cataracts, gave inappropriate visual signals as a puppy. As she began to develop some vision, her signaling abilities improved, although the signals were never recognized by other dogs as apparently being wholly in context based on recipient responses.

Hearing

Dogs can hear up to 15,000 to 60,000 cycles per second (cps); cats can hear slightly better (20,000 to 100,000 cps), whereas humans can hear only up to 20,000 cycles per second (Beaver, 1992a). Both cats and dogs can discriminate one-eighth to one-tenth tones (Ewer, 1973; Neff & Diamond, 1958) and have an upper threshold of 60 to 65 kHz. Cat hearing is still slightly more acute than that in dogs; cats can hear 10 full octaves (some humans can hear 8½ octaves).

Smell

Dogs have the greatest olfactory acuity of any domestic species. They can detect concentrations of a substance at $\frac{1}{100}$th of the strength that humans can detect (Moulton et al., 1960)—at diluents of $\frac{1}{100}$ to $\frac{1}{10,000,000}$ (Becker et al., 1962). Dogs have 2.8×10^8 olfactory cells and 7000 mm² of surface area (humans have 2×10^7 olfactory cells and 500 mm² surface area). Dogs can detect fingerprints 6 weeks after they were placed on a pane of glass (King et al., 1964) and can individually identify twins based purely on odor (Kalmus, 1955; cited in Houpt, 1991b).

In a test to determine whether an individual can reliably discriminate between humans and identify an individual regardless of the origin of the body odor, gauze pads soaked with secretions from exocrine, eccrine, and sebaceous glands were tested in a rigorous experimental design (Toner & Miller, 1993). The dogs investigated were experienced police dogs; they had a 93.3% success rate in correctly discriminating not only the scent of the individual, but the body part from which the scent came. If clothing was used, the accuracy increased to 100%, suggesting that a large scent pool helps. These results are in direct contrast with those from a less complete study (Brisbin & Austad, 1991) in which no reliable association between a dog's ability to match scent left on evidence with the corresponding people was found. The mechanism of discrimination of scent is still unknown.

There is some evidence that male dogs may be better scent trackers than female dogs are, but early studies did not discriminate between dogs tested on known and possibly protected territories, and dogs tested on random territories. It has been hypothesized that male dogs must learn about estrous female dogs through their urine and about territorial occupancy through scent. There are no data to support this theory. Forty percent of field trial dogs have some impaired sense of smell (cited in Fogle, 1990); most of this has been attributed to early viral infection. Dogs apparently recover their sense of smell 6 weeks after infection with nasal respiratory viruses; however, this still may be a concern for the use of nasal vaccine in some tracking dogs. As with some other performance capabilities, the scenting ability appears heritable.

Dogs use many clues of communication to identify other dogs; only one of these is pheromonal.

Scent Marking

Very little work has been done on normal social aspects of marking in domestic dogs, including scent marking with feces and anal sac secretions. Scent marking has been more fully investigated for nondomestic species and is thought to play a profound role in intraspecific hierarchical organization (Gosling, 1982; Kleiman, 1966; Peters & Mech, 1975; Ralls, 1971; Rieger, 1979). Comparable data for domestic dogs is limited, but scent is likely to be important in subtle interactions.

Anal sac secretions are normally eliminated with the feces and leave a unique odor (Bradshaw et al., 1990; Natynczuk et al., 1989). Anal sacs can be forcefully expressed by scooting. The extent to which this would leave a physical and olfactory cue has been underinvestigated in the literature. Anal sac secretions can provide an individual identification for greetings between dogs that know each other (Fox & Bekoff, 1975). This may be the basis of part of the social role that ear sniffing can play in hierarchical interactions (Overall, 1995b). Anal sacs are often emptied when the dog is excited. This behavior has been the basis for labeling anal sac secretions as "fear pheromone," but to attribute the sole communicatory function of anal sacs to "fear" is simplistic.

Scratching may disperse scent, but dogs seldom scratch the exact area where they urinated or defecated. It is impossible to rule out the role of the interdigital glands, merocrine sweat glands (pads), or sebaceous glands (found on hairy, interdigital skins) (Bradshaw & Brown, 1990) in the role of marking by scratching. Scratching, whether accompanied by urine or feces, provides a two-pronged visual display. First, the animal exhibits a species-specific posture during the scratching. Second, the animal leaves olfactory and visual marks (Bekoff, 1979a,b). Although vaginal deposits of terahydroxybenzoate stimulate mating behavior in dogs, urine deposits of male dogs do not appear to repel conspecifics (Bekoff, 1979b; Scott & Fuller, 1965). This does not mean that urine deposits of dogs are without information. Other information may be provided by urine, including data about the specific individual involved, specific identification of the social group involved (implied by Scott & Fuller, 1965), sex, and status information (see information on behavioral correlates of metabolic screen data in aggressive dogs contained in Chapter 6), recency of visit, and duration of visit. All of these cues could allow dogs to make decisions about how to allocate their time and energy in that physical area. Furthermore, olfactory communication can act as passive social behavior and may act to decrease active agonistic interactions.

The extent to which olfaction plays a role in modulating social interactions is likely to be affected by sexual dimorphism. Males are more likely to mark with feces than are females (Sprague & Anisko, 1973). Male dogs are more strongly attracted to the urine of an estrous bitch than they are to the vaginal or anal sac secretions of the bitch (Doty & Dunbar, 1974), but males need mating experience to respond to estrous versus anestrous females (Beach & Gilmore, 1949). Males without mating experience also appear to respond to these substances, but the other attendant changes in their behavior have not been well investigated.

Nervous System Development and Body Rhythms

Myelin is completely absent from the brains of newborn puppies but appears during the first 4 weeks. This is the same time period during which ribonucleic acid synthesis is increasing at a rapid rate (Fox, 1971a). It has been postulated that deoxycholic acid, which is present in feces, may promote myelinization and intestinal immunocompetence (see Beaver, 1995). The components of the brain grow differentially for the first 4 weeks of life and reach the adult proportions by 5 to 6 weeks (Fox, 1971a), the time at which EEG activity represents that of the adult. There is a concurrent development in the complexity of canine behavior. At birth a dog's brain is only 10% dry matter; this increases to 19% in an adult dog (Fox, 1964b, 1966a, 1970d).

Approximately 85% of a pet dog's sleep is rapid eye movement (REM) sleep at 7 days of age. By 35 days, only 7% of sleep is REM sleep and 30% is slow-wave sleep (SWS). Dogs attain an adult electroencephalographic pattern by 6 months of age (Fox, 1967a, 1971).

Dogs, like most other animals, experience annual rhythms. Domestic dogs breed an average of every 6 months now, although basenjis have a seasonal breeding that occurs annually, as occurs in the wild canid situation (Fuller, 1956). One could argue that this behavior is an adaptation to seasonal food availability. Dogs have a diurnal cortisol pattern that is different from that in cats but more similar to that in people. Fluctuations in diurnal cortisol do not occur in puppies or in some older dogs; this has been associated with their restlessness (Palazzolo & Quadri, 1987). Restlessness is one of the changes that is reported for dogs that may be experiencing senescence or cognitive dysfunction (Ruehl et al., 1994). Cognitive dysfunction is poorly understood. Dogs also have body temperature circadian rhythms of approximately 23.7 hours (Kanno, 1977).

Wolves reach sexual maturity at 2 years of age. Other wild canids sexually mature in 1 year. This may be an adaptation to a social system that involves helpers at the den: the delay in maturity of some individuals within the group may be enforced socially and pheromonally (Bradshaw & Brown, 1990). In wild canids other than wolves, social and sexual maturity occur concomitantly. It has been suggested that domestication accelerated the development of the endocrine glands associated with reproduction. Whether this is an indirect effect of the artificial social situation and available food supply or a direct effect of selection for rapid breeding is unclear (Fox, 1978).

Male domestic dogs can have continual spermatogenesis; in wild dogs spermatogenesis is seasonal. Female domestic dogs usually have two seasons a year except for basenjis and dingos, which have one season a year (Scott & Fuller, 1965). The range of sexual maturity in domestic dogs is 6 to 15 months with a mean at 7 to 10 months of age (Houpt, 1991b), but may be later for some large or giant breeds. For female domestic dogs the first estrous and proestrous cycles are shorter than subsequent ones, and levels of luteinizing hormone and estradiol are lower during the first cycle than in subsequent ones (Chakraborty et al., 1980). Females are less attracted to males and less solicitous of males in their first cycle (Beach, 1970; Ghosh et al., 1984) and mating is driven by female preference (Beach, 1970). Ovarian hormones function to attract the female to the male and to make her receptive to mounting. Cats require estrogen alone to complete the sequence of estrous behavior (Houpt, 1991); however, dogs need progesterone also (Signoret, 1975). A normal bout of dog copulation lasts from 10 to 30 minutes (mean, 14 minutes) for the lock phase of copulation (Hart, 1968). Dogs may copulate up to five times per day (Fox & Bekoff, 1975).

Domestic dogs that are living within a family or in a group and are relatively high-ranking dogs usually become sexually mature at about 6 to 9 months of age; social maturity does not begin until about 18 months of age.

Only one half of all stray dogs are able to copulate; none of those younger than 1 year of age was successful in a study that examined age- and rank-specific copulatory abilities (Ghosh et al., 1984). Social hierarchical relationships may inhibit mother-son matings and sib-sib matings. Females may have personal mating preferences that are not related to hierarchy or to social relationships that occur at times other than their estrous cycle (Beach & Le Boeuf, 1967; Le Boeuf, 1967). It is not clear if this is a result of artificial constructs. Relationships may have developed during the mating season that would not have developed at other times, allowing us to think that females are making "choices" that have nothing to do with their ordinary social structure. Beach (1968) found that pups raised in isolation had trouble achieving intromission. He postulated that these pups may have had decreased mounting behavior experience that occurs in normal puppy play. Problems associated with breeding include the following:

1. Dominant males may not be able to breed an overly submissive female
2. A dominant male's presence may pose a problem for the breeding of a subordinate male
3. A male may refuse to breed in a strange environment
4. A stud dog may show a preference for some specific female through learning and social interaction
5. Frightening circumstances inhibit sexual behavior in general
6. Females may only breed with certain males

Breeders should not overlook the role of the social system in modulating domestic canid breeding.

Maternal and Caretaking Behaviors

Maternal behavior in most domestic dogs is relatively problem free. When problems develop they are usually related to human intervention or, theoretically, to a lack of early social experience in the bitch. Maternal behavior in dogs usually is flawlessly executed. Prolactin induces maternal behavior in bitches. In rats, regardless of whether they are female or virgin, the mere presence of pups induces maternal behavior. In domestic dogs, as in wolves, males and other females help the bitch, particularly if they are part of the same social group and have good social relationships. The males may even regurgitate food to the puppies or to the bitch.

Nest building begins 24 to 48 hours before parturition. The bitch becomes restless approximately 24 hours before parturition and experiences a pronounced decrease in appetite. Parturition is followed by licking of the puppies; the bitch may ignore all of the puppies until she has completed delivery. Cannibalism and infanticide *do* occur and *can* be a component of normal behavior. However, these behaviors are rare. It has been postulated that population and social factors may affect infanticide; there is some evidence to indicate that cannibalism of one's own young may be heritable. If the bitch has experienced cannibalistic episodes in the absence of upsetting external stimuli, she should *not* be bred again. By licking the puppies, bitches lead them to the saliva trail to the nipples. Teat order is not fixed in puppies, but access to specific teats can be controlled by dominant puppies. Cortisol levels in beagles are lower for puppies 8 weeks and younger than they are for mature animals (Randolph et al., 1995). Normal endogenous adrenocorticotropic hormone concentration and adequate cortisol response to exogenous adrenocorticotropic hormone indicates functional and mature pituitary and adrenal glands.

Hence, puppies experience and can handle large amounts of stress quite early. Larger amounts of stress result in engorged adrenal glands without documented pathologic effects (Fox, 1964a; Fox & Stelzner, 1966c). Dogs are more proficient in competitive situations throughout life if they are stressed and can respond with an *appropriate* adrenal enlargement. In the puppies studied by Fox, these dogs had increased growth, decreased "emotionality," and increased resistance to disease (Fox 1970b,c).

Mounting and Marking

Virtually all elimination postures can be "normal" for dogs (Sprague & Anisko, 1973) (Fig. 3-1). Mounting and marking are normal behaviors. Most mounting is *not* sexual; if one watches puppies play one realizes that mounting behavior is a normal part of puppy play and can be a manipulative behavior. It later becomes a part of normal social communicatory behavior. Mounting can be a direct challenge to another dog or can be a communicatory gesture. Because of the sexually dimorphic elaboration of communicatory behaviors, mounting and marking are dimorphic behaviors. These behaviors tend to increase in frequency as a dog approaches sexual maturity, indicating that both of these behaviors have a far stronger social than sexual component. In a study by Borchelt (1984a,b), 50% of male dogs mounted by 5½ months of age (n = 38), 50% leg-lifted by 8 months of age (n = 51), and 50% urine-marked by 13 months of age (n = 11). Clearly, urine marking is not just a sexual behavior. Ninety percent of dogs urine-marked by 24 months of age, 95% leglifted by 24 months of age, and 98% mounted by 24 months of age (Borchelt, 1984b). In this study it is not clear what percentage of dogs were intact versus castrated. Scott and Fuller (1965) reported that incomplete pelvic thrusting occurs as early as 3 to 4 weeks

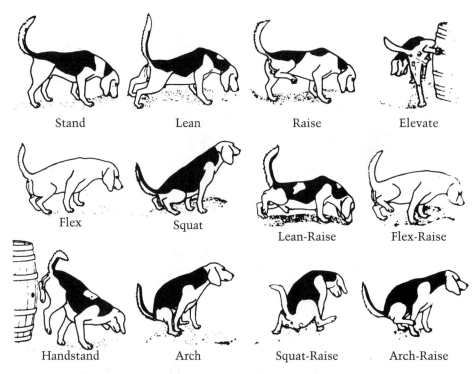

Fig. 3-1 All postures represent a range of "normal" canine elimination postures. The squat is the most common female posture, whereas the elevated posture is the most common for males. The occurrence of timing of elevation is primarily affected by the individual's role in the social hierarchy and the social context in which it occurs, not by reproductive status. Note that the female analog of this posture is the handstand. (From Sprague and Anisko, 1973.)

of age. Behaviors that are associated with sexual behavior are practiced early and are a component of social behavior. Males in artificially segregated groups show a high incidence of squatting urination (Scott & Fuller, 1965) and the most powerful stimulus for raised-leg urination is the odor of a dog from a different social group. Hence, concern for the development of leg lifting should not be an impediment to early neutering.

There may also be a size component to some behaviors that have sexually dimorphic and social components. Small to medium kenneled fox terriers leg-lift by approximately 20 to 32 weeks of age (Martins & Valle, 1948). However, in a mixed-sized dog colony, leg lifting occurs earlier, by 19 to 43 weeks of age (Berg, 1944).

Urine marking is more frequent and occurs at a greater rate in free-ranging males than in females. It is important to remember that not all marking occurs for the same reason. This difference may be partly sexual advertisement, but may also be social. Males and females can form pair-bonds in such situations and can communicate information on their location and activity to the other individual. Roaming, interdog aggression, mounting, and urine marking are all hormonally modulated. If dogs exhibiting these behaviors are castrated, roaming decreases by about 90%, inter-

dog aggression decreases by approximately 60%, mounting decreases by approximately 60%, and urine marking behavior decreases by about 50% (Hopkins et al., 1976). All of these behaviors also have a learned component; the longer castration is delayed after an animal has begun to exhibit these behaviors, the greater the extent of the learned component over the hormonal component. Castrating an animal that has been urine marking for 10 years will not have a great effect on decreasing urine marking behavior. Hormonal factors facilitate the experiences that enhance learning in these areas, but at some point the hormonal factors become far less important than the learned ones.

Females are under fewer hormonal influences until their first heat cycle; therefore early spaying would be expected to have no effect on any change in their behavior. There are two exceptions to this. Spayed dogs can experience weight gain, because estrogen is a strong appetite stimulant (Houpt et al., 1979). However, if females never experience estrogenic stimuli, as would be true for those who are spayed very early (6 to 8 weeks), they may not have the attendant problems with ovariohysterectomy (OHE) associated changes in estrogen that could promote weight gain. The second case in which early spaying can have an effect on female behavior involves bitches younger than 6 months of age that have already shown aggression to people. In a small but statistically significant study of these dogs, O'Farrell and Peachey (1990) demonstrated that aggression worsened after ovariohysterectomy. It has been hypothesized that these dogs may experience some in utero androgenization (Overall, 1995c); if so, permitting them to have one or two heat cycles may decrease their aggression.

There is no evidence that neutering affects any dog's working ability. When groups of puppies that have been spayed or castrated in an early neuter program (8 to 10 weeks of age) at Canine Companions for Independence were compared with those in the same program that were neutered at 6 to 10 months of age, no differences were noted in the dogs' abilities to work, to be trained in the program, or in failure rates for the program (P. Mundell, Canine Companions for Independence; personal communication).

Both male and female puppies develop substrate preferences for elimination at about 8½ weeks of age. Scratching is virtually always discussed in the literature in the context of accompanying urination or defecation. This is probably simplistic. The act of scratching does *not* have to be accompanied by urination or defecation, or deliberate urine or fecal marking. There are two components of the act of scratching that have received insufficient attention. Bekoff (1979a) alluded to the fact that the behavior of scratching is a species-specific identification behavior. Scratching has two components, noise and motion, which may make it more noticeable and recognizable as a long-distance signal, particularly to conspecifics. I have spent hours observing coyotes, foxes, and domestic dogs scratching. During an interaction between a coyote in Big Bend National Park in Texas and my two spayed, female pet dogs, the coyote started to scratch with its front feet while barking and moving back and forth near my dogs. At no time did the coyote urinate or defecate during this process. When one of my dogs barked at the coyote after the coyote (a female) approached within 3 feet, the coyote responded with vigorous scratching using the front feet and by frenzied patrolling back and forth while baying and yipping. My younger dog will scratch with her back feet after only smelling coyote feces, without herself urinating or defecating. One has to question whether the scratching in the absence of the other dog could contribute a disruptive or a masking scent. Scratching has been reported to be more common when other dogs can see the behavior (Bekoff, 1979a).

The same issues can be raised for rolling. Rolling is a very visual behavior and it leaves a visual disturbance. Rolling could leave scent and a visual impression of the dog doing the rolling. One of my dogs has dispersed a pile of coyote feces by rolling on it; after there were no feces left, she stayed in the area and continued to roll. The extent to which dogs that behave in this way may be dispersing their own scent is unclear. People always accuse dogs of enjoying rolling

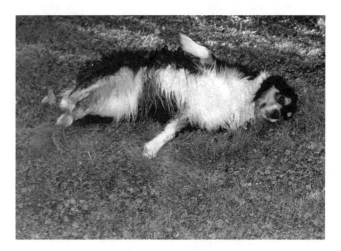

This dog is rolling after swimming. Notice the arc in the grass caused by the dependent foreleg and the depressions caused by the rubbing of the head and neck. Since 5 weeks of age this dog has had almost no vision, yet she still makes these visual displays. Rolling may be a scent marking or scent acquisition behavior, but it also helps to loosen the undercoat and aids in grooming after a bath or swim. (Photo by K.L. Overall.)

in smelly substances. Because we do not know what social stimuli they are receiving and what social cues they might be leaving, it would be inappropriate to suggest that they are simply enjoying this. It would not be surprising if rolling occurred more frequently after baths that strip dogs of their own scents and leave them with perfume scents. Rolling would make them less apparent in the olfactory background to competitors or predators and help them recover some of the scent milieu in which they function.

Dietary Concerns and Feeding Behavior

Taste and olfaction are probably closely linked in the dog, as they are for humans. Dogs are reported to be indifferent to sweets unless they are trained to like them; however, a fondness for sweets appears to be acquired with one trial learning. Sweet, sour, bitter, and salty receptors all exist on the dog's tongue. In laboratory situations, dogs prefer canned meat to fresh, cooked meat to raw meat, and meat to anything that is cereal. In pet dogs, taste, texture, and smell of food and the owner's perception all appear to be important when gauging palatability (Houpt et al., 1978, 1979). Smell appears to be more important, either alone or in interaction with taste, in ranking preferences, and if the dog is allowed to smell a preferred substance, it could be tricked into eating another substance.

Dietary problems are not common in dogs, but many of the behaviors associated with eating and hunting could lead to problematic behaviors later. Innate canine eating and hunting behaviors include:

1. Stocking and pointing
2. Herding

3. Digging
4. Scent following
5. Shaking, throwing, catching, killing
6. Returning food to a denning site
7. Regurgitation
8. Gnawing and chewing
9. Vegetable and plant eating
10. Prey carrying
11. Prey guarding
12. Prey catching behaviors (Fox, 1971a, 1972c).

Inappropriate behaviors attendant with these normal behaviors are discussed in Chapter 11.

Obesity is the most common problem associated with diet in dogs. It has been estimated that, at any point in time, 30% of dogs in Great Britain are overweight (cited in Fogle, 1990). Testosterone, as already discussed, facilitates behaviors associated with covering a wider range of territory and increased motor activity. The removal of testosterone might then facilitate more sedentary behaviors, and in the absence of reduced caloric intake, more of those calories are allocated to fat.

The second problem that occurs with diet in dogs is anorexia. This is not common, but is more frequently reported in some breeds (Yorkies) than others. The extent to which this might be associated with other nervous and anxiety-related behaviors has not been investigated.

The third problem that clients report involves ingestion of grass and vegetation. These are normal behaviors in dogs that may have some anthelmintic function. Some plants, particularly houseplants, are poisonous to dogs and cats. Pet animals are not better botanists than are their people, so indiscriminate ingestion of plants should be discouraged.

The fourth diet-related problem that clients report is pica or the ingestion of inappropriate, nonnutritive objects. Coprophagia is sometimes included in a diagnosis of pica. Some picalike behaviors may be related to learning. These problems are discussed in the miscellaneous section. Some of these behaviors may be manifestations of obsessive-compulsive disorder and are discussed in Chapter 10.

Food intake in dogs, like other species, is hormonally controlled. A gastric load just before a meal does not influence food intake for dogs, but one 20 minutes before eating does influence intake (Janowitz & Grossman, 1949). Clients could use this to limit their dog's intake. Cholecystokinin, glucagon, and naloxone decrease food intake (Levine et al., 1984). Naloxone may also stimulate food intake depending on the condition for which it is prescribed. Because naloxone is used as a behavioral drug, it may have other ramifications. Ventromedial hypothalamic lesions tend to lead to hyperphagia in dogs (Rozkowska & Fondberg, 1973), indicating that part of the regulation of food intake occurs in this region. Dogs fed *ad libitum*, under normal conditions, tend to eat small meals frequently throughout the day, primarily concentrating these

during daylight hours (Mugford, 1977). Again, clients may be able to regulate their dog's intake by following these normal patterns.

Communicatory Behaviors, the Role of Play, and the Development of Social Communication and Interaction

In a scheme developed by Scott and Fuller (1965) and outlined by Borchelt (1984a,b), a functional classification of behavior involving seven systems has been described. The first system is the **system of ingestion,** involving feeding and drinking. The second system, resting and sleeping, involves **shelter-related activities.** The third system focuses on **care of the body surface,** including autogrooming and allogrooming. The fourth system, the **reproductive system,** encompasses nesting behaviors, mating behaviors (including courtship and copulation), care of the young, and nursing and providing care for others' young. The **elimination system** involves behaviors associated with urination and defecation. Behaviors involved with the **social contact system** include investigative behavior, play behavior, and attachment behaviors (care-seeking and separation-resisting behaviors). The last system, the **agonistic system,** involves fighting, aggression, behaviors associated with the development of dominant and subordinate structures, and the defense system (fear and escape). The **communicatory and play systems** involve integration of signals inherent in all systems.

The role of play has been thoroughly discussed by Fagen (1981). Play functions to:

1. Stimulate communal behavior
2. Facilitate social interaction
3. Mold adult behavior, particularly through the role of the learning curve
4. Establish early, strong social relationships, although the role of social hierarchy and its development in play is less clear
5. Enhance physical and mental dexterity
6. Improve coordination
7. Provide a venue for safe experimentation and the first demonstration of ritual and ritualized behaviors
8. Provide puppies with an outlet to learn about social rules and predictability through sequences of events
9. Provide puppies with an outlet for exploration
10. Provide them with a safe outlet for increasingly complex problem solving

Most of the normal canid behaviors associated with pet dogs are learned during the play period. Because reflexes are functional by 6 to 9 weeks and neurologic development is completed during the next few months (Czarkowska, 1983), the role of play in communication cannot be underestimated. Puppies from litters subjected to many uninhibited bites from other dogs are less socially gregarious with other dogs and people, and play less with toys later in life. This emphasizes the role of play in encouraging dogs to learn social skills (Wilsson, Swedish Dog Training Center, cited in Fogle, 1990, from a study of 600 puppies). Play has not been investigated in dogs that are less social than others. Such a study would be useful because it allows us to evaluate the extent to which play might function in the development of normal social behavior.

There is evidence that the hunting dog *(Lycaon pictus)*, a highly social carnivore that lives and hunts in packs, has a poorly developed hierarchical social system. In this canid, social behavior is more dependent on mutual regurgitation of food and less on communication by facial expression and posturing than it is in the wolf (Clutton-Brock, 1987). The extent to which play may be involved in this early development has not been identified. Feral domestic dogs are thought to be solitary (Berman & Dunbar, 1983; Daniels, 1983a,b; Rubin & Beck, 1982). This may be related to food—garbage distribution may not be sufficient for more than one dog at a time. Structured social groups have been noted in some studies of feral dogs (Carr, 1985; Daniels & Bekoff, 1989), but there are no data available on the early development of play and its role in facilitating structured social groups in feral dogs. Social behaviors of feral dogs have been characterized by small recognizable components (social ethograms), which show that most social behaviors occur in predatory sequences for dogs (Bradshaw & Brown, 1990). The role of play in the development of these predatory sequences has not been well studied in dogs, as it has for cats.

Canine Communication

Before discussing the details of normal domestic dog communicatory structures, it is useful to define the terms used in this field.

A **context** is a set of events, conditions, and changeable recipient characteristics that modify the effect of a signal on a recipient's behavior. Context includes both immediate and historical factors. Sources of contextual information include the characteristics of the recipient and the sources external to the recipient (i.e., the signaler and the setting). If the signal itself does not provide enough information, the role of context is absolutely critical. This is an important concept for both practitioners and clients to grasp because *context* is the best determinant of whether a behavior is abnormal or normal. One of the criteria by which abnormal behaviors are gauged is whether they are contextually appropriate. Some behaviors about which clients complain could be normal, appropriate, in-context behaviors, but undesirable. These comprise a different class of behavioral problems.

The second definition that requires some thought is that of an **informed decision.** An informed decision is a response that is characteristic of the recipient of communicatory signals. We usually assume that any decision that is made is "informed" (Green & Marler,

1979; Hailman, 1977; Markl, 1985; Smith, 1977, 1985). This may not always be the case, particularly in an abnormal, out-of-context situation (the sphere of most behavioral problems) (Moynihan, 1970, 1982). The recipient is important (McGregor, 1991). This leads to the question, "What do received signals mean for abnormal animals?" This is important particularly in the discussion of treatment of these animals, and is an area on which future research should focus.

The **distance** at which the signal is delivered interacts with the quality of the signal. This interaction is underexplored in domestic animals, but it has been investigated in nondomestic species. For gulls *(Larus glaucescens)*, attack is more likely for a remote-control gull (the signaler) that is sitting in a horizontal position than for an upright remote-control gull. If the remote-control gull (the signaler) is moved toward the recipient of the signal, rather than away, a more vigorous reaction is elicited (Amlaner & Stout, 1978). Paton (1986) looked at the role of distance and skuas. Certain agonistic movements of the signaler lead to escape of the recipient only if the signaler faced the recipient; otherwise escape was only probable if the signaler was nearby. Such behaviors have been underinvestigated in applied behavioral medicine. They probably warrant investigation more for abnormal animals than they do for normal animals.

The role of groups has been investigated in both domestic and nondomestic animals. Packs of wolves with pups are more likely to howl in response to howls than are packs of wolves without pups (Harrington & Mech, 1979). There have been no studies that have examined whether social facilitation in barking in household pets is common, but in my personal household, my older dog, who seldom barks, barks more since we obtained the younger dog, who is visually impaired and who barks quite frequently. Barking is a domestic dog characteristic. Basenji dogs are among the only breeds of domestic dogs who do not innately bark, but they can learn to do so. Most dogs have a low threshold of arousal to bark; this may be one of the traits that we selected to develop in domestic dogs. Barking has at least two main functions: guarding (alerting behaviors) and attention-seeking behaviors. The attention-seeking behaviors can include play solicitation, hunting solicitation (particularly if hunting in groups is beneficial), and may have aggressive connotations. Further evidence that wolves, rather than jackals, are the ancestors of the domestic dogs is found in their voice analysis. Wolves fulfill the aforementioned characteristics, whereas jackals do not (Clutton-Brock, 1987).

The importance of location of vocal signals has been investigated for other nondomesticated species, such as birds, but this factor has not been well investigated for domestic dogs. Territorial birds may react only when their neighbors' song is played within the territory holder's realm of habitation (Falls & Brooks, 1975); otherwise, the territory holder responds weakly to playback calls of neighbors. Gibbons *(Hylobates lar)* are more likely to approach neighbors who are giving loud calls when those calls are played from territorial boundaries (Raemaekers & Raemaekers, 1985). Wolves with rendezvous sites are most likely to respond to howls (Harrington & Mech, 1979), and wolves attending a kill, especially a recent one with lots of food, are more responsive to howls than are packs without a kill (Harrington & Mech, 1979). These are clues about the role of the interactions between the social environment and the physical environment. In experimental situations, wolf pups have different reactions to a howl depending on whether a human, a dog, or a container of live mice is present in a room with a pup when the howl is played (Shalter et al., 1977).

Characteristics of vocal display may depend on the extent to which ambiguity could be damaging. Marler and Hamilton (1966) noted that the more solitary primates had more highly stereotyped calls. More social primates had calls that were more variable *unless* the cost of minimizing any errors in communication became important, as would be the case in a mating season. Domestic dogs may be governed by the same rules affecting potential problems and ambiguity.

The final issue that has been underinvestigated in behavioral medicine focuses on the addition of various components that may result in differences in response when combined, rather than when viewed separately. For example, in common grackles *(Quiscalus quiscula)*, the message and the response become graded in intensity when signals are combined. In cichlid fish *(Haplochromis burtoni)* individuals are more readily attacked if a blue eye bar appears; the attack increases further if the fish simultaneously assumes a head-down posture. In contrast, orange pectoral spots decrease the probability of an attack, partly because these colors indicate sexual identity. It is important to notice that a combination of signaling components can be achieved by changing intensity of frequency or of the signals, and by combining two communicatory systems, as in the cichlids. These types of combination behaviors in dogs and in cats warrant study.

Canine vocal communication has been categorized into five basic sound groups (Fox, 1972c):

1. Infantile sounds, including crying, whimpering, and whining
2. Warning sounds, including barking and growling
3. Eliciting sounds, including howling
4. Withdrawal sounds including yelping
5. Pleasure sounds including moans

Wolves bark when strangers approach a pack and growl when challenged or when eating, but they whine when greeting each other. Howling acts as a social coordinator in wolves. The preservation of neotenic behaviors that has occurred in domestic dogs has exaggerated this role. Barking in domestic dogs tends to be an announcement of a presence, of a territorial clue, or of an identification of an individual. My visually impaired dog barks when she arrives anywhere. It is interesting that stray dogs seldom bark (Beck, 1973). Barking is an example of a signal that has a warning value but is variable in character.

Whining and howling behaviors are et-epimeletic behaviors. Whining is among the first sounds a puppy makes. Howls carry a long distance; it is possible that the reason dogs howl for fire engines is that the sounds generated by the engines are similar to group sounds—they are mimicking them. According to Harrington and Mech (1982), wolves can distinguish strange adult howls from strange pup howls and answer only the former. In domestic dogs howling is seen in anxiety or attention-seeking behaviors; this could be a holdover from soliciting group interactions. Growling is seen in domestic dogs primarily in agonistic situations.

Some of the best work on canine vocalization has been done by Patricia McConnell. McConnell (1990a, b) looked at two specific signals that are frequently used by trainers and that are asserted to cause dogs to commit specific classes of behaviors: short, rapidly repeated, rising notes that are postulated to elicit a "come" response, and one long note that has been asserted to elicit a "stay" response. Short, rapidly repeated notes *did* elicit a "come" response, but, in contrast to what most handlers believe, one long note *did not* elicit a "stay" response, although it did decrease motor activity. Signals that inhibit behavior probably should be divided into two categories (McConnell, 1990b). Handlers use signals that are designed to slow or soothe, like the long continuous notes that have little frequency modulation, and signals that are designed to stop, which consist of one, short, rapidly descending note (McConnell & Baylis, 1985).

Canids use short, rapidly repeated whines to elicit an approach by conspecifics (Cohen & Fox, 1976). Equid and ovid species also use low repetitious notes ("nickers" and "gurgles") to elicit approach from their young (Houpt & Wolski, 1982; Waring, 1983). The long squeal of a mare who is unreceptive to a stallion or the long squeal that takes place between two stallions who are interacting inhibits approach and decreases motor activity (Waring, 1983).

Krebs and Dawkins (1984) maintain that the primary function of animal communication is manipulation of the behavior of the receiver by the signaler. It is clear from McConnell's work that this is exactly what is achieved by handlers of herding dogs.

In addition to vocal communication, which tends to reach long distances, short-distance postural and visual communication is critically important to the dog (Figs. 3-2 and 3-3). Postural and visual communication tends to reach a shorter distance and tends to be more immediate than is olfactory signaling, which can last a long time, or vocal signaling, which occurs over a long distance. The latter type of signaling does not generally allow for a quick response time. Postural and visual communication in domestic dogs includes

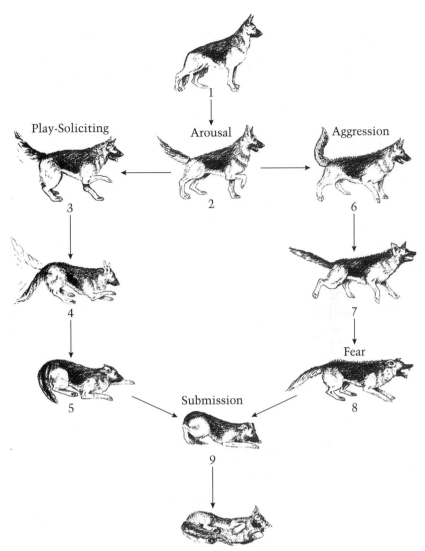

Fig. 3-2 Facets to note about body posture include relative placement of head and neck, posture of dorsum *(top line)*, placement of feet, posture and activity of tail, and pelage activity (piloerection). Breed differences in "normal" relaxed postures are important. A German shepherd is pictured, with a gentle slope to the hip and a relaxed tail. In a sight hound, a "normal" relaxation posture would include a squared hip and tucked tail. (From the Monks of New Skete, 1991; adapted from Fox, 1972c).

As the dog becomes more aroused and more agonistically reactive (2), the intention movement of the paw becomes more definitive and angular and less solicitous. The hind feet are more broadly spread and the tail is less arched and more rigid. The neck is stiffer and the head is raised.

The approach into a play bow is shown in 3. Note the elevated right forepaw in a solicitation gesture, the forward and gently arched neck, and the broadly flagging tail.

As the dog becomes more volitionally and assertively antagonistic (6), the hind feet are more broadly spread, providing a better base for pivoting; the tail is flagged, plumed, arched, and vibrating or stiffly wagging at the

tip; the hair is piloerected along the entire dorsum, connoting reactivity; the neck and shoulders are set and squared; the head is high and forward; and the dog is leaning forward or into its forequarters (a position selected for in the conformation ring, along with the correlated assertive and often aggressive behaviors).

As the dog becomes more fearful (8), the piloerection—a sign of reactivity—persists, but is now predominantly bimodal and most pronounced over the shoulders and hips, the tail is lowered as confidence or willingness to define the volitional parts of the contest change, the head and neck are no longer arched over the back, but are in line with the plane of the dorsum, the feet are closer together, and the legs are lower to the ground.

5 and 9 represent the non-antagonistic version of the continuum that is represented in an antagonistic form in 8. The head and neck are tucked into the plane of the dorsum; the ventrum is flush with the ground; the tail is tucked; the coat is flattened; and as the dog withdraws more from active involvement in the interaction, it rolls on its back (10) with feet and limbs flexed, tail tucked, neck hunched, and belly exposed. Urination and salivation may accompany this posture. Facial signals are portrayed and discussed in Fig. 3-3.

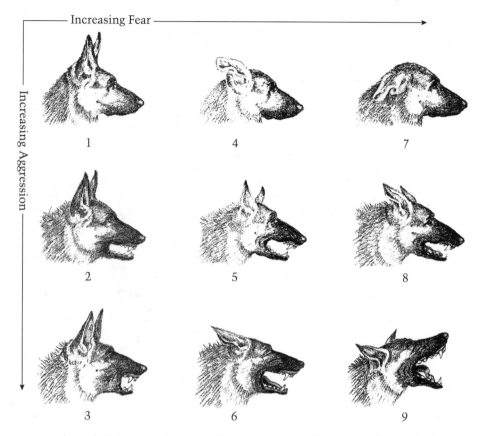

Fig. 3-3 Facets to note about facial expression include the position and orientation of the ears, the set of the head and neck, the pelage on the neck and around the head, the set of the jaw and relative apparency of the teeth, the posture of the corner of the mouth, the position of the ventral neck and the oral cavity, the set of the eyes and position of the skin around the eyes ("eyebrows"), the size of the pupils, and the position and shape of the nares. Breed differences in these features can be important: cocked ears in a dachshund will not look like those of the German shepherd portrayed. Changes in relative degree are important.

As one moves from 1 to 7 the dog is becoming more fearful, distressed, concerned, or anxious, and less actively assertive. The head lowers relative to the ventral neck; the ears are pulled back, droop, and become more flaccid; the line of the mouth or lips becomes less firm and more loose (drooling may accompany this) the eyebrows are arched; the brow furrowed; and the facial skin around the eyes becomes less taut. None of the teeth are exposed at all. Posture 7 represents a dog that is subdued, deferential, passive, and volitionally solicitous.

Moving from 1 to 3, the head and neck become more set and more angular, the hair is piloerected on the dorsum of the neck; the ears are cocked forward; the brow is rigid, hooded, and set; the jaw is square, with minimal exposure of the ventral neck and oral cavity; the nostrils and pupils are dilated; and the teeth are set in line and exposed rostrally. Posture 3 represents a dog that is confident and assertive in its active aggression and that would not hesitate to attack should the other individual in the interaction fail to back down.

Posture 9 represents an animal that is actively attempting to deflect an antagonistic situation. The hair on the neck is piloerected, and the ventral neck is fully exposed, as is the oral cavity. The ears are neither cocked nor flaccid; the skin on the face is loose; the nares are dilated but flared and may be dripping; the skin around the eyes is pulled ventrally; and while the pupils are dilated, the field of vision is not unobstructed as in 3. The teeth, including all of the molars, are displayed. This is the classic posture representing a conflict between aggression and fear. The dog may not have the confidence to engage in an aggression interaction or may not have the physical ability. The dog is not simply deferring to the approacher (more clearly conveyed in 7) but is communicating capitulation. The extent to which the signaler is not a threat is conveyed by complete disclosure about equipment (i.e., the teeth and neck that are completely bared). One can believe that this dog, based on the tongue posture, is also vocalizing using relatively sharp, high-pitched, repetitive sounds. (From the Monks of New Skete, 1991; adapted from Fox, 1972c.)

posturing of the ears, the mouth, facial expressions, hair on the shoulders and rump, and the overall body position and stance. Alert dogs tend to stand with their tail and ears up and a foot out, indicating an intention movement and possibly a willingness, intent, or ability to approach others. We should be aware of the role of artificial selection and manipulation in affecting the ability to visually communicate intention. We have artificially influenced all parts of the body involved in signaling: coat shape and thickness, tail length, and ear structure. Domestic dog body posture has been compared with wolf body posture (Lorenz, 1954). Other models include a two-dimensional model of confident (assertive) versus aggressive behaviors in domestic dogs based on body postures (Goddard & Beilharz, 1985a) and a wolf model of relative roles in interactions using two-dimensional dominant versus subordinate behaviors derived from body postures (Abrantes, 1967).

Friendly postures of domestic dogs decrease their size relative to that of other dogs and decrease their potential threat through physical posturing to others (Beaver, 1981). Dogs exhibiting passive submission behaviors tend to have an averted gaze, lower their neck and ears, lick, groom, and paw. These are included among the most friendly behaviors of dogs noted by Fox and Bekoff (1975). An averted glance is an important gesture for an animal that can communicate threats by staring. It signals that the signaler is putting itself at risk by not visually following a circumstance that could change rapidly. Only a very confident, or a very submissive or deferential animal, would avert their gaze. Dogs are considered most sub-

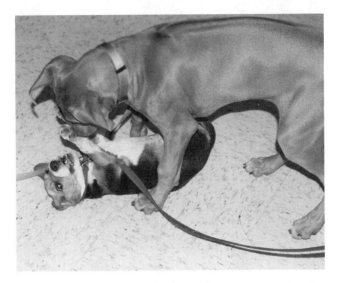

Less passive inguinal and ventral exposure, as play intensifies. Note the set jaw of the beagle puppy and compare with posture 3 in Fig. 3-3. Also note that the beagle is covering his inguinal area with his hind legs and pushing with his forepaws. The Rhodesian ridgeback puppy is in a clear solicitous posture. This is a game. (Photo by K.L. Overall.)

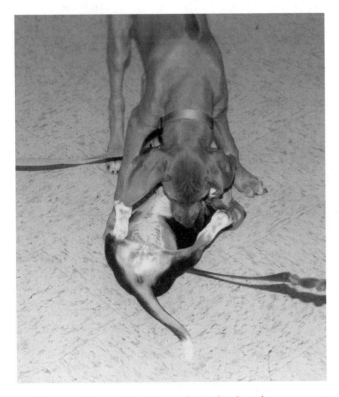

Two puppies, on-lead in a class, display the exposure of the ventrum and inguinal region in a play bout. (Photo by K.L. Overall.)

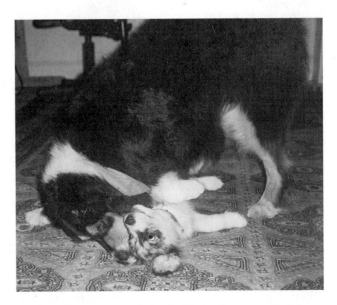

Flaccid exposure of the belly is demonstrated by a young puppy in response to pinning by the neck—a gesture that signals a request for deference—by an adult dog. (Photo by K.L. Overall.)

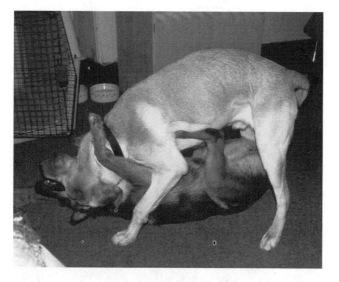

The same posture reflected in the previous photo is demonstrated between two adult dogs in play. Again, the response of the dog on the bottom is not passive (see the photo on p. 27, top right), but the postures are stereotyped ones for canids involved in play or challenge. (Photo by Liz Krug.)

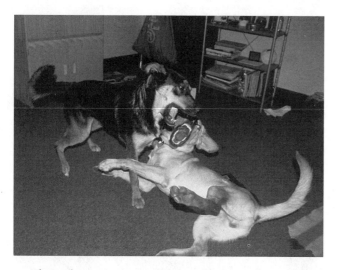

The roles are reversed from those in the previous photo, and both dogs have widely opened jaws (indicating the playful, nonagonistic nature of the encounter). Dogs in play grab at necks, cheeks, jowls, and teeth, and flag and wag their tails, as demonstrated here. (Photo by Liz Krug.)

missive when they roll on their back and present their inguinal region, with or without urination. Again, this is a neotenic behavior that is a holdover from behaviors that pups exhibit to adults in the group. In a passive situation, the tail is held lower than the horizon in dogs. In extremely submissive situations, the tail is not only held lower than the horizon, but it is held between the legs (Blackshaw, 1985b).

Many training books report that dogs will "grin" or "smile" in submissive or in happy situations. The "happy" situations are more likely to be those associated with interactive, deferential behavior. The "grin" observed in dogs is a grimace that shows their teeth; it is usually accompanied by other signals of submission (Bradshaw & Brown, 1990). This grin is almost uniformly only directed toward people; humans labeled it a "smile" because it resembles a human signal. Dogs do not have the muscles necessary to contort their faces in a true smile as do humans, and not all human cultures view the smile as a friendly gesture. This is another case in which we have uncritically transferred a human term to a similar canine behavior. Unfortunately, we have transferred with it the underlying motivational states that we attribute to humans. It would be inappropriate to think that when dogs "smile" they are happy or are being compliant; there is far more evidence to indicate that they are simply mimicking the humans who are doing those behaviors back to them. Puppies and some very deferential or anxious dogs "grin" with their lips retracted, showing a lot of gum. Puppies lick their lips, possibly sneeze, and show their incisors. These are all canine deferential behaviors, but they are not "smiles."

The importance of deference in puppy behavior is supported by the wealth of these behaviors in the puppy communicatory repertoire. Puppies roll on their back in a more exaggerated, deferential behavior. When puppies lie on their side and lift their hindleg and show their genitals, they are also exhibiting a deferential behavior. Even urination and defecation in response to the nudge of an older dog can be considered a deferential or submissive behavior. Puppies remain stationary when an aggressor mounts or paws them.

Normal Canine Communication

Puppy development involves the development of agonistic behavior. Agonistic behavior is a normal social behavior—when it is in context. Agonistic behavior encompasses outright aggression, but also includes many displays and signals that act to avoid outright aggression. It would be inappropriate to assume that agonistic behavior alone defines a dominant-subordinate relationship or a pack relationship. Terminology affiliated with packs, pack behavior, and rules about social organization within packs is unduly simplistic and should not be used uncritically. Behaviors associated with the development of agonistic behavior in young puppies are those also associated with play and include the following:

1. Stalking other pups with the head and tail down and the hindquarters up with ears erect
2. Chasing, ambushing, and pouncing on littermates
3. Standing over a littermate with the head and tail erect and the neck arched (this is a perpendicular posture with the head over the neck and shoulders and is discussed for adult dogs later)

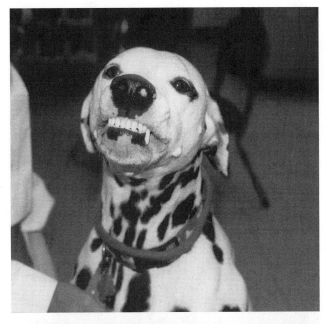

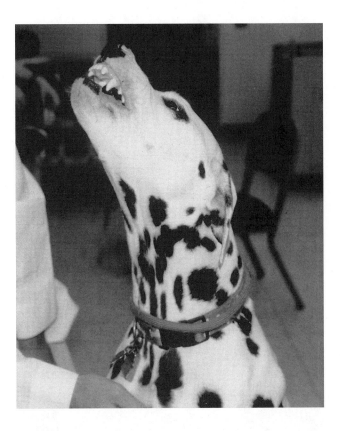

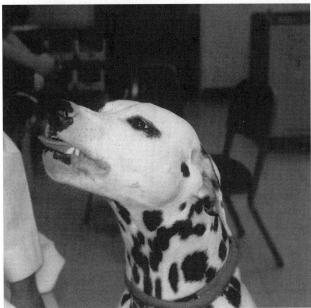

Dalmatian exhibiting "grinning" behavior in response to a request for passive interaction (the request for sit) from a human. The dog did sit and then proceeded to grin, which is how the clients say he first responds to any interaction. The dog was being seen for problem behaviors associated with anxiety. Whether there is a connection between these and contextually "excessive" grinning or solicitous behavior is unknown, but likely. This dog not only grinned, but gently licked the air in a manner consistent with begging licking seen in puppies (second photo) and proceeded to elevate his neck more extensively and to show his palate with the continued request that he stay (last photo). (Photos by Liz Krug and K.L. Overall.)

4. Circling a littermate while wagging the tail with an erect, assertive walk
5. Attacking and biting, primarily around the littermate's neck and face
6. Piloerection, primarily on the back of the neck (please note that the total amount of piloerection or puffiness, especially around the rump area, is important, and that it can be associated with fear)
7. Snarling and showing teeth, primarily the canines
8. A direct stare at littermates without dilation of the pupil; this is often referred to as "showing eye"

9. Shoulder and hip slams
10. Forepaws on a littermate's back
11. Boxing
12. Mounting with or without pelvic thrusts
13. Wagging only the tip of an erect tail
14. Ears completely erect or completely flattened
15. Excessive play fighting

It is important to note that many of these behaviors are behaviors we also associate with play.

Data from Bekoff (1972, 1974, 1977) indicate that the play bow appears to be an innate behavior and is not learned, because it appears in hand-raised puppies. Fagen (1981) indicates that many play behaviors are innate across species—this emphasizes the role of

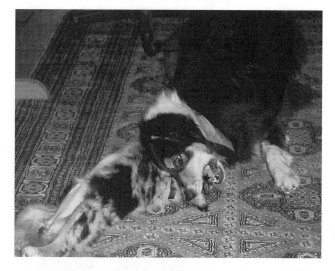

Puppy and older dog playing. Adult biting puppy's head and neck. Note puppy's totally exposed belly and flaccid hindlegs. Were this interaction to become agonistic, the puppy would tense and roll over, closing the open inguinal area. (Photo by K.L. Overall.)

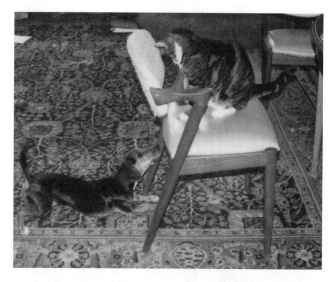

Play bows can be given to other species. Here the dog is attempting to solicit play from the cat, who actually *is* playing with the dog, although in a different style than the rough-and-tumble one the dog is seeking. (Photo by Emily Elliot and Nirit Rosenberg.)

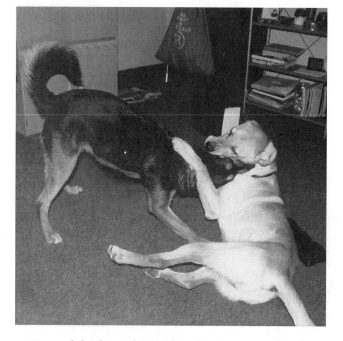

Two adult dogs playing by chewing at each other's necks. Concomitant mutual neck chewing is more common when two adults play than when two puppies play. (Photo by Liz Krug.)

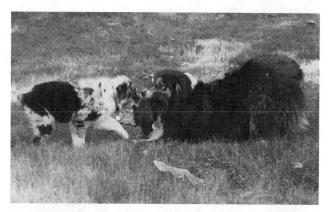

Play bow given by adult to puppy as adult offers puppy a toy and waits while she takes it. (Photo by K.L. Overall.)

play in social communication. Note that mounting behavior and pelvic thrusting relate more to ordering a social system and learning how to communicate with others in the group than to sexual behavior. Bekoff (1974, 1977) emphasized that play behaviors may have other roles that function immediately, in addition to later, in the social system to avoid conflict. In his discussion of the "play-invitation bow," he ascertains that subsequent behaviors are modified by play bows in a situation that might otherwise invoke an intensification of agonistic reaction.

Other behaviors are also associated with reduction of potential aggression. Most of the work in this area has focused on the importance of intention movements. Haölldobler (1977) found that ants (*Camponotus socius*) will not follow a trail of hind-gut material unless the recruiter in the ant nest first performs a stereotypic waggle display. Similar information exists for pigeons *(Columba livia)* performing intention

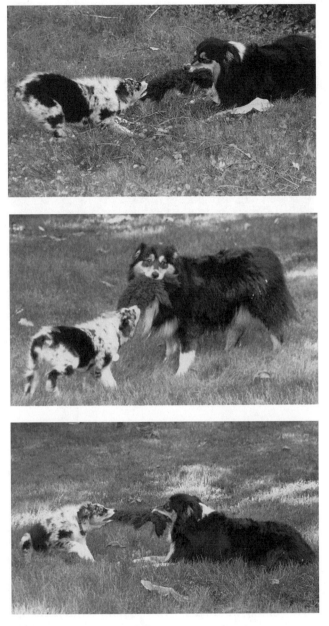

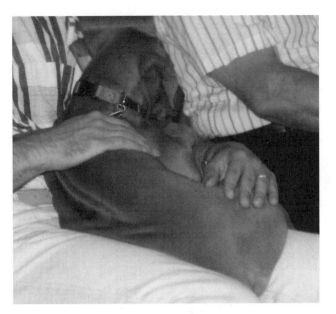

The role of pelage characteristic is underinvestigated. Dogs raised only with their own breed may require an "adjustment" period to understand the signaling of another breed in extreme circumstances. This Rhodesian ridgeback puppy could seem chronically aroused to the uninitiated. (Photo by K.L. Overall.)

Sequence of normal play that followed play-bow solicitation. Notice that the adult dog lets the puppy set the rate and intensity of play (second photo). The adult dog could take the toy any time she wanted. That she is letting the puppy tug on the toy and control the game (third photo) is indicative of a contextually appropriate response given the age and size mismatch. (Photos by K.L. Overall.)

movements. In the presence of these movements, the flock does not fly; without these movements, the flock leaves as a group (Davis, 1975). This approach to the understanding of canine and feline behavior has been largely underexplored. Interactions between dogs and those involving dogs and people are very complex, but a good analysis of intention movements would help clients with problem animals. This is one of the techniques that we use in the Behavior Clinic at the University of Pennsylvania.

Morton (1977) argues that agonistic signals often convey the deceptive notion that the signaler is larger and more dangerous than he actually is. This is certainly one of the possible interpretations for piloerection in domestic dogs. Clients should be forewarned, however, that breed variation can be very important. Some breeds that have been selected to have shorter coats may communicate a signal somewhat differently than do breeds with longer coats. No comparative work has been done on this issue. Dogs that are behaving antagonistically may do so to "probe" the social environment to acquire contextual information (Burk, 1988; Smith, 1981). Piloerection and mounting displays that are learned early in puppyhood may function in this manner as behavioral probes. One of the problems in complex social hierarchies like those of canids and felids is that as the repertoire of displays increases, recipients begin to have some difficulty decoding the displays and discriminating among them (Moynihan, 1970). This complexity is an important factor when explaining to clients how to work with a problem dog. One of the problems that clients encounter is that they often overwhelm dogs with signals that the dogs are incapable of processing at the rate presented. This problem worsens if a dog is stressed because of problems.

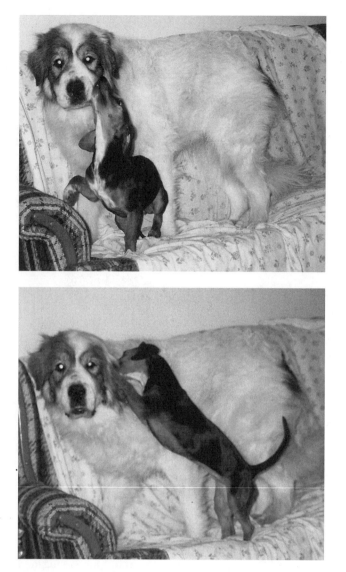

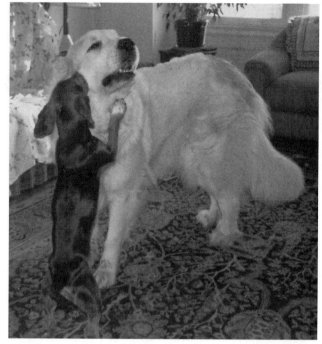

Licking can be an et-epimeletic, solicitous, or deferential behavior. The smaller dog is an adult but is soliciting the two larger great Pyrenees dogs. The ear licking in the second photo is also a deferential behavior. Note that the large dogs are soliciting this deferential licking just by standing there. That offers a clue about status in the household. (Photos by Emily Elliot and Nirit Rosenberg.)

Given the above general discussion of aspects of communication, it would be worthwhile to look at the specific classifications of signals that have been published in the literature. One of the earliest of these was compiled by Scott and Fuller (1965) and has been summarized and expanded by Fox (1969a, 1972c). Three categories of nonvocal communication are generally identified: distance-decreasing signals, distance-increasing signals, and ambivalent or mixed system signals.

Distance-decreasing signals include the avoidance of eye contact, a submissive "grin" or "grimace" with the lips pulled back horizontally, flattening of the ears, lowering of the body, wagging of the tail, flicking or licking of the tongue, raising a forepaw in a solicitation gesture (but not to the extent that the stance sets the individual off balance), and rolling (Beaver, 1982b). All of these behaviors are shown to people, but not all of them are shown to dogs. As mentioned,

the vertical retraction "grin" is restricted to canine interactions with humans and has not been reported on a regular basis in dog-dog interactions. This may be a mimicry behavior by the dog because we humans are constantly approaching them face to face and grinning.

Licking at the mouth of humans is an associated sequence and may be derived from early canine etepimetetic behaviors. These behaviors continue into adulthood and are displayed in deferential contexts. They should not be considered the homolog of human kissing, and may represent a challenge in certain contexts (see Chapter 6).

Distance-increasing signals are those designed to minimize contact and interactions. These signals include staring; snarling (distinguished by lips that are held horizontally forward and vertical, so as to expose the canine teeth); ears that are erect and forward or absolutely flat against the head; an increased perception

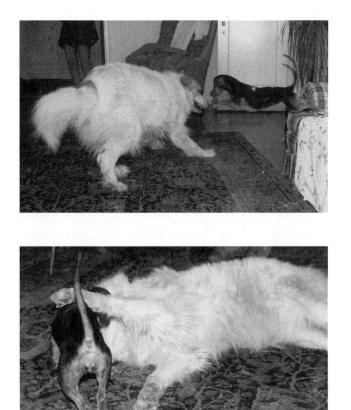

Note the relative tail postures of the dogs in the first photo. The small dog is very confident and the assertive individual in this interaction; his tail is arched over his back. The large dog in the first photo is willing to interact and has a flagged tail with a modified play posture. The small dog is in control of the pursuit of the interaction as indicated by the elevated and flagging tail (second photo), although a modulating paw, which could be a challenge, is being levied by the larger dog. (Photos by Emily Elliot and Nirit Rosenberg.)

of body size that is portrayed by changes in stance, including changes of head posture, piloerection, and a stiffening and contraction of the muscles; urination and ground scratching; a tail that is held straight and vertically or arched over the back; and flagging or wagging of just the tip of the tail held as described.

Ambivalent signals of mixed systems usually include a mixture of the signals described above, but the positions of the head and body are not concordant. The safest recommendation is to tell clients that if they perceive they are getting conflicting facial and body signals, they should believe the worst. If they are not satisfied with that explanation, it is always a good idea to believe the teeth-end of the dog.

The specific behaviors tabulated by Scott and Fuller (1965) identify functional categories of behavior and specify the behaviors within those. These include epimeletic behavior, et-epimeletic behavior, and agonistic behavior. Agonistic behavior is generally associated with intraspecific conflict, but it is usually an adaptive behavior. Agonistic behaviors can include aggression and status-related behaviors, defense and subordination-associated behaviors, active defense, and passive defense. Many epimeletic and et-epimeletic behaviors have relevance for behavioral problems. There may be an association between problematic behaviors that have been derived from care-seeking origins, and selection for more neotenic traits in pet animals.

The aggressive component of agonistic behavior includes stalking, with the head and tail down but with the ears pricked, the back arched, or the hindquarters raised; chasing, pouncing, and spraying; the perpendicular or T posture already described where one dog stands with his or her head or neck over another dog (Fig. 3-4); walking around an adversary in a stiff-legged gait with neck arched and neck and tail raised with or without a stiffly wagging tail (this appears to be a very common vertebrate agonistic display and is even found in lizards); overt attacking and biting; specific attacking of the face and shoulder with seizure and shaking; piloerection; baring of teeth with the vertical retraction already described; and turning the head away from an adversary. The latter has been characterized as an appeasement gesture; this is probably inaccurate. Fox (1972c) has described it as a "dare" to other animals to attack. Only a very confident animal can afford to back down at the apex of a disagreement, so this signal is better understood as one that communicates to the receiver that if he or she will do the dominant animal's (or aggressor's) bidding, the aggressor is willing to not let the aggressive act escalate further. Vocal agonistic displays include growling, barking, snapping of the teeth, gaping (which is a sort of a noisy, yawning display), and pawing with or without growling. These behaviors are most commonly seen in animals that perceive that they are high-status animals, or in animals that are actively engaging in aggression. The wrestling or boxing with forepaws and adversary's backs; mounting, usually without pelvic thrusts; wagging of the tip of the tail with the tail erect; ears flattened against the side of the head or alternately acutely erect; a direct gaze with pupillary dilation; and other components of the play fighting already described for early puppyhood also are components of aggressive or status-related agonistic behavior. Defense and deference behaviors usually involve submissive approaches in greetings: the forequarters of the body are lower than the hindquarters and the head and neck are usually extended and swung from side to side, baring the side or the dorsum of the neck. When used by a subordinate animal, this display is designed to truncate the interaction before any aggression intensifies. If such defensive or deferential behaviors are successful, the behavioral sequence proceeds through flexing of the back, going down on one hip,

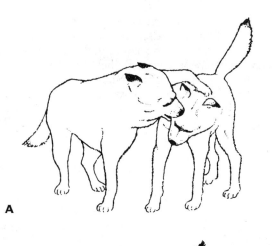

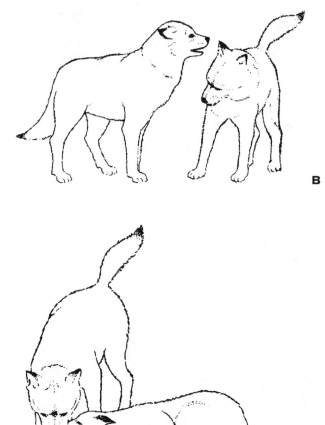

Fig. 3-4   The series of four drawings demonstrates the stereotyped approach, assertion, and deference postures associated with canine interaction. (From Clutton-Brock, 1987; adapted from Schenkel, 1967.)

A, The dog on the left is grabbing the other by the jowls while placing a paw over the shoulder. This is an extremely active challenge. Note that the challenger's tail is down, and there is no piloerection. The recipient has a flagged tail, which in this context indicates that he still perceives that he has an assertive, nonsolicitous, nondeferential role.

B, The dog on the left is using the perpendicular T-approach—nose and head to shoulders—that characterizes the first response phase of an interaction involving challenge. The dog on the left is now soliciting information from the dog on the right. Note that the challenger still has a lowered tail, that his ears are down, and that his

mouth is slightly gaped. He is not actively aggressive. The receiver turns his neck—a deferential gesture—but still does not back down.

C, The challenger has increased the intensity of the challenge by aligning in a parallel manner with the recipient of the challenge. At this point the challenger cocks his ears, stiffens his neck and back, and raises his tail. The recipient's response is finally to defer actively by spreading his hind legs, lowering his haunches, dropping his tail, putting his ears back, and exposing his neck and teeth in a deferential grimace.

D, The challenger presents his face for deferential licking, which is directed at the commissures of the mouth. The dog deferring is now flush with the ground and has tucked his tail. Notice that throughout the encounter no frank aggression occurred.

and, ultimately, rolling over and presenting the neck and the inguinal region for sniffing or licking by the other animal.

Signaling behavior involved in active defense indicates that the recipient of the initial aggressive display meets the challenge, should it continue. Behaviors such as piloerection and snarling with visible teeth

are common under these circumstances. Piloerection and snarling are exaggerated behaviors; exaggeration may indicate that the signaler is not willing to actively aggress, but *will* actively defend itself. These animals will also turn their heads away and, while baring their teeth and showing eyes, bare their neck. This is not a contradictory signal. The signaler is con-

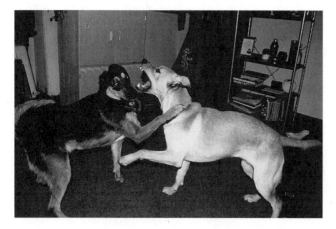

Play boxing using the classic canine challenge of a paw on the shoulder. (Photo by Liz Krug.)

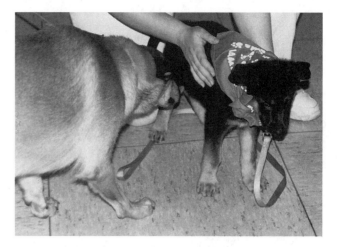

Immobile posture and averted gaze displayed by puppy in response to approach to inguinal region by older dog. (Photo by K.L. Overall.)

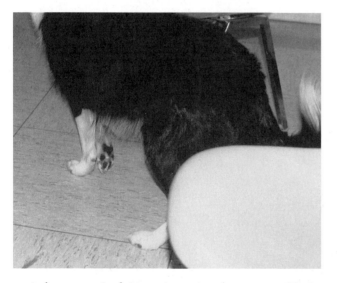

A forepaw raised in an intention movement. Notice the anticipatory curl of the border collie's tail. A toy is being held just off camera. (Photo by K.L. Overall.)

veying a message to the aggressor that the signaler is willing to allow the aggressor to have the higher rank, but if the aggressor pursues the attack, the signaler will retaliate rather than acquiesce.

Passive defensive behavior can involve sitting, crouching, and running away; licking of the lips and showing of teeth (this is also a behavior that appears in anxiety-provoking situations; it may be that many of the passive behaviors have been mischaracterized and they are less passive than they are anxious); the submissive "grin" with the lips retracted horizontally, the tail between the legs, the ears depressed and an indirect gaze; forepaw raising; rolling onto the back with the legs extended; lateral recumbency with an elevation of the topmost hindleg to give access to the inguinal region; recumbency and complete inhibition of

movement in a tonic immobility; urination and defecation; and a silent, quiet stance while the aggressor places its feet on the animal's back. The latter signal is a signal by default—what the animal is really doing is not meeting a challenge. It is important to remember that when animals *do not* do something, they are still conveying information. Absence of a signal can function as a signal itself.

All of these behaviors are elaborations of early behaviors seen in puppies. Accordingly, how these behaviors are shaped in puppies may be very important.

To briefly review, the following categories are critical in canine communication: body posture in threats and challenges, tail position, and eye and facial gestures. These signaling categories are outlined in Table 3-2 and shown in Figs. 3-2 and 3-3.

Body postures are probably among the most visible long-distance communicatory displays in threat and challenge situations (see Fig. 3-4 for a sequence displaying these. Notice the use of the classic approach interaction postures: challenger approaches perpendicular to shoulder; intensification is indicated by change to perpendicular position. See Table 3-2 for specific signal interpretation). The subordinate respondent, recipient of the aggressive or agonistic display, or the victim usually shifts the body weight backward and lowers the body in response to a threat. Following this response, the aggressor usually moves forward and higher. These are large, visible displays that can be seen at almost any distance. The vocalizations that accompany these behaviors often increase in pitch, frequency, and volume and may involve both barking and growling. This is a dual signaling system that can indicate that the recipient of the aggression is no threat to the other individual. The point of most agonistic behavior is not to have outright battle, but to ensure that battle is used as a last resort. In a hierar-

TABLE 3-2 SIGNALING CATEGORIES

Signal	Circumstance Information	Signal	Circumstance Information
Barking	Alerting/warning	Tail wag	Willingness to interact
	Attention-seeking	Tail tip wag; stiff	Confident
Growling	Warning		Assertive
	Distance-increasing		Offensively interactive
Crying	Et-epimeletic	Neck erect or arched	Confident
Whimpering			Challenging
Whining		Ears erect	Alert
Howling	Elicit social contact		Confident
	Anxiety situations (social contact = reassurance)	Ears back	Fear
		Ears vertically dropped	Deference
Moans	Pleasure, contentment		Submission
Tail and ears up; forefoot in front of other	Alert, ready to participate		Low rank
			Anxiety
Direct gaze	Challenge	Snarl/growl with only incisors and canines apparent	Confidence
	Confidence		Offensively aggressive
	Absence of threat		Distance-increasing
	Distance-increasing	Snarl/growl with all teeth and back of throat apparent	Defensively aggressive
Averted gaze	Fear		Fearful
	Cowardice		Distance-increasing
	Deference	Body lowered	Defensive
	Absence of challenge (not the same as deference for confident, high-ranking dogs)		Distance-decreasing
			Fear
			Deference
	Distance-decreasing signal		Relaxed
Belly presented	Deference	Licking lips, flicking tongue	Appeasement
	Relaxation		Et-epimeletic
Tail tucked when belly presented	Fear/submission		Distance-decreasing
			Anxious (and solicitation of reassurance; derived from et-epimeletic)
Tail tucked when belly presented with urination	Profound fear/submission	Raising forepaw	Distance-decreasing
Grin	Deference		Solicitation of attention
	Distance-decreasing signal		Deference (off balance)
Piloerection	Arousal associated with anxiety, fear, aggression	Paws out, front end down, rump up, tail wagging	Body bow, invitation to play
	Distance-increasing	Perpendicular posture	Challenge
Piloerection restricted to neck or tail region	Confident dog		Confidence
		Mounting or pressing on back or shoulders of another dog	Challenge
Rigid stance, stiff torso musculature	Confidence and intent to interact (may not be aggressive)		
		Licking at corner of another dog's (or person's) mouth	Et-epimeletic
	Distance-increasing		Deference
Tail above horizon	Confident		Solicitation
	High status	Blowing out lips/cheeks	Anticipation (positive or negative)
Tail below horizon	Less confident		Anxiety (if very fast)
	Lower status	Popping or snapping of upper and lower jaws ("bill" pops)	Capitulation, intention to comply as a last resort
	Deference		
	Fear		
	Caution for sighthounds for whom a lowered tail is normal carriage		

chical situation most individuals would avoid outright battles because profound costs (not the least of which is loss of life) are associated with them.

When one individual challenges another, the challenger's first behaviors involve body posture signals. Dogs that are challenging another dog lean forward and piloerect, following this with growling and baring of teeth. The extent to which the latter behaviors are exhibited depends on the response that they receive. If the challenger is unsuccessful in controlling the behavior of the other dog, the challenge behaviors may intensify by addition of more signals or by intensifying the gestures themselves. Intensification may include flattening the ears and lowering the head and neck. These types of behaviors are also correlated with protective behaviors. They may function secondarily to indicate that the animal is intensifying aggression. Flattening the ears and lowering the neck expose the aggressor to far less physical damage than behaviors that leave the neck up. A lowered neck is associated with the ability to deliver a blow with more force. Erect ears are at risk for more damage in a fight (Fox, 1970a).

Aggressors who have already made the decision to attack usually do so with a stealthy approach. This approach may include crouching body posture and a lowered head, and changes in ear postures. As aggression intensifies, ear postures change from erect to flattened. The first clue that an individual might become aggressive to another animal is the intense nature of the physical orientation demonstrated toward the potential victim. In contrast, friendly approaches include bounding, a head position that is level with or above the body, decreased body tension (again, this is probably a correlate of not tensing muscles for attack), loose ears that possibly may be folded back and down, and a very loosely carried body (Fox & Bekoff, 1975).

Tail position is important in dogs. For dogs that have docked, bobbed, or short tails, no good comparative studies have been done to ascertain whether their rump assumes signaling potential. There are also no studies that indicate whether these dogs are at a disadvantage in group communication with other dogs, or whether their owners are disadvantaged at understanding their signaling. The latter may be important if the dog begins to have behavioral problems. Tails held below the horizon are highly correlated with submissive postures or passive behaviors (Bradshaw & Brown, 1990). Tails held between the legs are correlated with extreme submission (Blackshaw, 1985b). An individual dog can signal its intent to threaten another dog by holding the tail above the level of the horizon; in an extreme circumstance the tail is arched either over the back or held straightly vertical (Bradshaw & Brown, 1990). The degree of arch or of vertical hold can be a measure of relative rank among dogs. It is important to realize that a wagging tail is only an indication of a willingness to interact. In Bradshaw and Brown's (1990) study, most of the interactions as-

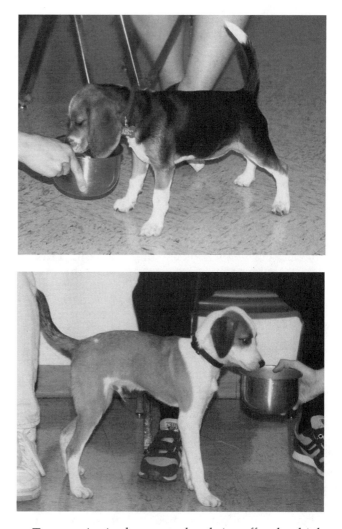

Two puppies in the puppy class being offered a drink after a play session. In the first photo, the beagle is showing all the signs of a confident, assertive dog: tail arched over back, legs spread, ears forward, and neck set. In the second photo, the beagle mix is showing signals consistent with a less confident dog: tail slightly lowered, back arched, feet closely spaced, ears back and down, and neck slightly retracted. It is interesting that these relative postures were so clearly displayed in passive circumstances, since the beagle mix puppy was the most timid in all interactions with people and the other dogs. (Photos by K.L. Overall.)

sociated with wagging tails were aggressive interactions, but the extent of the sweep of the tail is also important. A tail that is wagging very loosely below the horizon usually correlates with a dog that is friendly in approach. Brown and Bradshaw (1990) postulated that the greater the frequency of wagging, the more agitated the individual was becoming. This is probably true both for dogs that are aggressive and dogs that are giving submissive, subordinate, or et-epimeletic signals. Frenzied tail wagging of very submissive dogs is frequently reported. Tail wagging is not well understood (Bradshaw & Brown, 1990; Fox & Bekoff, 1975) because it is a complex behavior that may involve both visual and olfactory cues. For very large dogs that displace a lot of air, it could also involve auditory cues. The tail at least acts as a visual flag and is a behavior that can be seen from a great distance with larger dogs.

Eye contact is critical for most social species. Eye contact can be an indication of a warm, friendly interaction, or of a profound threat. One of the most intense, initial aggressive displays by cats involves direct eye contact. The first response in canine interaction is usually some degree of establishment of eye contact. The dog who is of a higher rank (this can be determined by age, by social status, or by the unsureness of one of the participants in the interaction) usually maintains eye contact longer. Younger or lower ranking dogs look away or make no direct eye contact. It has been postulated that the extent to which a dog can maintain eye contact with another dog functions to set social priorities (Beaver, 1981a, 1982b; Blackshaw, 1985a,b). Chance (1967) noted that high-ranking animals both elicit *and* receive attention. This is consistent with the finding that low-ranking baboons often initiate displays, but that displays of dominance are elicited rather than emitted (Rowell, 1966, 1974). The same pattern of control has been noted for wolves, coyotes, and hyenas (Bekoff, 1972; Bekoff et al., 1981; Fox, 1968b, 1969a, 1971c, 1973a; Lockwood, 1979; Owens & Owens, 1996).

Training books tend to focus on eye contact. Clients are frequently advised to maintain eye contact with their dogs until the dog looks away. This can be a terrible suggestion if the dog is aggressive, because staring is perceived by the dog as a challenge. Maintaining eye contact puts the client in the role of challenger. When eye contact fails to establish an instantaneous social relationship, the situation becomes one of challenge. Not all stares must result in full-fledged challenge. Eye contact is reinforced by another communicatory system—the vocal or auditory one. A growl or a snarl usually accompanies eye contact when it is used as a challenge. Visual displays are enhanced by the baring of teeth, piloerection, stiffening of the legs, and holding the head and the ears erect. This integration of signaling systems is important. It would be unfortunate to rely on only one system to obtain relevant information.

Canine social hierarchies are actually multitiered or multilayered (Abrantes, 1967). They are not rigid dominant-subordinate systems as asserted in many training manuals. Not only does subdominance occur, but the social hierarchy is a fluid one that is responsive to the contextual situation. The literature has been saturated with assertions about absolute dominant and submissive behaviors and ranks, in the absence of data to support such a rigid approach (Alt-

mann, 1962; Syme, 1974). Before accepting conclusions about relative social ranks, one must consider the role of experimental artifact. Single causality experiments can be inherently flawed and may result in the observation of linear ranks where none exist (Appleby, 1983; Boyd & Silk, 1983; Richards, 1974). The more likely scenario is one in which relative "rank" is determined by the ongoing behavioral and social context, within the milieu created by the interactions of the demographic, genetic, resource, and physiological environments (Beaudet et al., 1994; Bekoff & Mech, 1984; Chase, 1974; Dewsbury, 1990; Dunham et al., 1989; Fox et al., 1970; James, 1949; Landau, 1951; Netto et al., 1992; Scott, 1956; Stur, 1987). Dog social systems resemble human ones: the individual that is in charge in one circumstance may not be in charge in another (Fox & Stelzner, 1967). This does not occur because one individual competed with the former leader for control and won. The choice *not* to control an event can be a sign of high status or of confidence. Selection has acted to enhance a variety of contextual responses.

Submission involves effort on the part of an inferior or lower-ranking animal toward creating friendly and harmonic social integration (Clutton-Brock, 1987; Schenkel, 1967). Ritualized behaviors involved in submission are characterized by combinations of signals conveying inferiority (i.e., lack of threat) and positive social tendencies. Most submissive behaviors contain no elements of hostility, but the onus of modulating the social interaction is on the deferential or submissive individual. The form that this modulation takes depends on the attitude and behavior of the superior or aggressive individual (Clutton-Brock, 1987). If that individual is intolerant, the more subordinate animal usually does not persist. If the superior animal is friendly toward the more subordinate animal after receiving these signals, harmonic social integration usually ensues. This describes the puppylike behavior that develops into the adult behavior. The more inquisitive or severe the superior is, the more the inferior, subordinate animal acts passively. This response may occur because the subordinate animal is unsure of the intent of the superior animal and is giving the other animal a chance to convey additional information. By a process of repeated testing of each other, the exact hierarchical relationship *in that context* can be defined. As with most social interactions, the context itself is defined by a ritualization of the displays; this ritualization is actually a rule structure for communication. Social systems follow rules. Problems develop with social animals when the rule structure is either not understood, not communicated, or the responses to it are abnormal.

It is critical that clients realize that although wolves are "wild" ancestors of dogs, aggression is the exception in wolves. In 43.5% of 120 relationships involving 16 wolves, the subordinate attacked the dominant animal (Van Hooff & Wensing, 1987). Thirty-three percent of more than 7000 aggressive acts were directed toward a higher ranking individual. Very few actions resulted in outright fights. Dogs differ from wolves in the extent to which their fear response is part of the repertoire of a social contest. Wolves develop a very early fear response; this is probably what inhibits their socialization to humans (Fox, 1972b). Accordingly, when wolves must be accustomed to humans, they must be exposed to them within the first days of life (Fox & Andrews, 1973b; Klinghammer & Goodman, 1987). Domestic dogs have a delayed fear period (Fox & Spencer, 1969; Fox & Stelzner, 1966a,b). The extent to which this is involved in modulation of the signaling associated with the interactions discussed above has not been fully studied.

Domestic dogs have altered prey-catching behavior when compared with that of wolves. The temporal sequence of prey-catching, killing, dissection, and ingestion is present in coyotes by about 8 weeks of age. This sequence is truncated in the domestic dog. In dog-coyote hybrids the behavioral sequence is very disorganized, although all the individual behaviors are present (Fox, 1969c). In most breeds of domestic dogs the actual killing bite has been selected to be inhibited. Loss of this inhibition is a very good indication of when a behavior has become abnormal in a domestic animal. Even dog breeds that were selected for their ability to help humans hunt have been selected to inhibit biting. This is true for breeds that nip or bite as part of their herding, guarding, or hunting sequence. Very few dogs that are truly abnormal and exhibit predatory aggression toward humans ingest their "prey," so the predation sequence is also truncated in these abnormal animals.

Border collies represent an excellent example of the extent to which domestication has modified the predation sequence. The first predatory sequence is retained in the eye-stalk-chase sequence of behavior. Instead of progressing to the next stage in the predatory sequence, border collies repeat these types of behaviors (Coppinger et al., 1987). These patterns appear to be strongly heritable, and the extent to which they can be influenced by training also appears to be strongly heritable (McConnell & Baylis, 1985). Another example is found in Mediterranean breeds that were designed to guard, not herd, stock (the Anatolian dog). These individuals exhibit very few predatory patterns, but in a study by Green and Woodruff (1988), many guarding dogs were responsible for predation on lambs in sheep flocks. Factors associated with this were not investigated in this study, but in most cases the guarding dogs were responsible for more lamb deaths than were coyotes. Coppinger et al. (1987) concluded that there is selection for inhibition very early in development, as evidenced by puppy play. Some of this inhibition is present in wolves.

The Role of Breeds in Domestic Dog Behavior

A *breed* is best defined as a group of animals selected by man to possess uniform appearance that is heritable and that distinguishes that breed from other groups of animals within the same species. Canine breeds were probably first developed by the Romans. The first breeds may have been large, heavy mastifflike hunting dogs that date from approximately 2000 BC in Western Asia and Egypt (Clutton-Brock, 1987). The ancient Egyptian hunting dogs looked like modern greyhounds; these ancient dogs were postulated to also have been developed at approximately 2000 BC (Clutton-Brock, 1987). Russian breeders discovered in the early 1900s that it was possible to tame silver foxes in 12 generations of controlled breeding that relied solely on selecting for subtle temperament and for tractability (cited in Fogle, 1990).

Roman dogs were identified by their actual tasks. House-guarding dogs were called *Villa tici*, shepherd dogs were *Pastorales pecuaru*, sporting dogs were *Venatici*, pugnacious or war dogs were *Pugnaces* or *Bellicosi*, scent dogs were *Nares sagaces*, and sight hounds or swift dogs were *Pedibus celeres* (Turner, 1962). Domestic dogs have existed for at least 1000 generations, and modern breeds represent the same work distribution as did Roman breeds. Retrievers have been selected to demonstrate an elaboration of the retrieving behaviors associated with a hunting sequence and with behaviors affiliated with caring for a mate and young. Protecting dogs or guarding dogs have been selected to demonstrate behaviors associated with inhibition of killing and mutilation associated with the final predation sequence. The basis for successful selection for bite inhibition is found in the variable behavior of wild canids. Most wild canids hunt large game as a group or pack. To make this successful, inhibition of biting by some members of the group (and it may not always be the same member) is necessary. Group behaviors associated with inhibited bites are common in dogs selected for protection, guarding of people and flocks, and in herding coupled with guarding of flocks.

Some of the mythology surrounding breeds probably arises from the Pavlovian classification of nervous system types (Pavlov, 1927). In this classification, there were five nervous system types that were associated with classic behaviors. The excitable (extreme) type of nervous system was associated with wildly active and choleric dogs. Mildly excitable dogs were happy-go-lucky, active, sanguine dogs. These were considered fairly normal, but slightly rambunctious dogs. The balanced type of nervous system was associated with a poised and assured dog. The inhibited type of nervous system was associated with a reserved, stoic, phlegmatic type of dog, whereas the extremely inhibited nervous system type was associated with stiff, withdrawn and lethargic behavior. However, this type of classification is not this simple. Behavioral and physical patterns can vary.

Although the Pavlovian classification of dog personality types is slightly simplistic and a bit anthropomorphic, it *is* a classification that allows identification of a personality type of a dog that would be compatible with a particular lifestyle. This type of matching paradigm is further discussed in the section on aptitude testing and temperament testing in Chapter 14. In Pavlov's scheme, the middle three groups are all types of dogs that exhibit relatively normal behaviors and desirable traits, whereas the two on the end represent extremes of undesirable and possibly abnormal behavior. The personality types discussed by Pavlov are apparent to some extent in all breeds. The characteristics that define some breed behaviors are

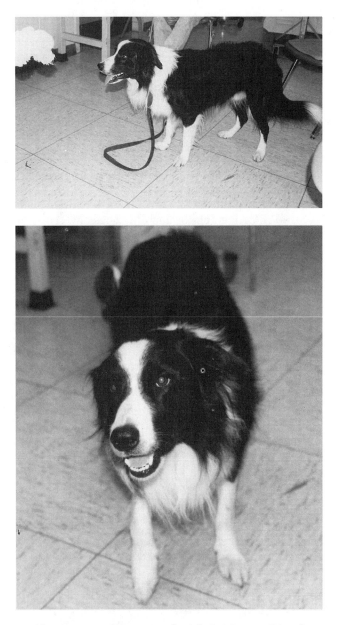

Classic postures associated with "giving eye" in a border collie. Notice the focus on the toy, the slightly lowered and pulled back ears, and the open mouth and raised forepaw associated with anticipation (bottom photo). These are part of a behavioral sequence that has been highly selected within the breed. (Photos by K.L. Overall.)

elaborations or diminutions of some of those types of patterns. For instance, Bradshaw and Brown (1990, after Fox, 1978) describe how many of the breeds of dogs have been developed from personality traits involved in hunting sequences. Many of the breed "personalities" and breed-associated suites of behaviors are elaborations of specific parts of the hunting sequence. For instance, bloodhounds and sighthounds are dogs that have been developed through selection for elaboration of the tracking and trailing sequences of prey-catching. Sheepdogs have been selected for the eye, stalk, and chase sequences, whereas setters and pointers have been selected for the stalking without the eye and the chasing—the latter has been replaced by the characteristic pointing behavior. Boarhounds are among the few breeds that have actually been selected for the attacking and killing sequences of predatory behavior. The extent to which this feature may be implicated in abnormal behavior to people is unknown.

When selecting for specific suites of behavior within a breed, physical traits may be selected for either directly, or indirectly, as correlates of the behavior. Physical patterns and traits have an influence on behavior. For example, patterns of movement are not the same in bulldogs as they are in borzois. The physical trait of stockiness and the disproportionate distribution of mass in the forequarters correlate with a less fluid walk, less speed, and a lower center of gravity. These are the opposite behavioral traits associated with the slight, the very tall, and high-necked sighthounds. Sighthounds also have eyes that may be more widely spaced than those of bulldogs when scaled for shape of head. Prospective owners of specific breeds should realize that physical traits and behavioral traits covary in ways that are not well understood or well researched. Physical features, such as long hair on the face, docked tails, pendant ears, or black color can influence the transfer of intraspecific and interspecific information. Long-haired faces can obscure signaling that uses eyes, whereas a coat that is heavy and has a lot of mass might affect an individual's ability to piloerect (Bradshaw & Brown, 1990; Fox, 1970a). Dark irises hide the pupil, prohibiting the recipient of the signal from gauging the extent to which the animal is dilating the pupil. Coat and eye color or pattern may play an underappreciated role in behavioral problems or in suites of patterned behavioral responses. Agitation under stress has been reported to be more common among cattle with specific whorl patterns (Grandin et al., 1995). Scalp whorls in humans have been associated with handedness and schizophrenia (Ortize de Zarate & Ortize de Zarate, 1991; Alexander et al., 1992). The phenotypic genetic patterns of Wardburg's syndrome in humans is not unlike that of the merling trait in dogs (Willis, 1989). A double dose of the recessive allele is correlated with deafness. The neuroectoderm gives rise to both dermatological and neurological features in ontogeny (Smith & Gong, 1974), so it is likely that coat color patterns may have some relevance for the understanding of behavior that has been widely appreciated.

Some of the earliest experiments of breed-specific behaviors were conducted by James (1951, 1952). In a colony of dogs comprised of cocker spaniels, beagles, and fox terriers, the author noted breed differences in "assertiveness" of breed. Fox terriers sired virtually all of the pups from various litters regardless of the dam's breed. This variation in reproductive success is a correlate of the suites of behaviors for which we have selected in terriers: tenacity, scrappiness, and the ability to push themselves forward among other dogs. This does not mean that the fox terrier's sperm is any more viable than that of any other breed, that they are the better dog, or that all fox terriers will be equal in siring capabilities. It *does* suggest that when in selection for suites of behaviors, correlates of those behaviors that were not anticipated are also selected.

Recent studies have examined the association of specific suites of behaviors with breed (Hart & Hart, 1984, 1985b; Hart and Miller, 1985). In these studies, 56 breeds and 13 behavioral traits were examined. Interviews were conducted with owners, breeders, veterinarians, and obedience show judges. Such studies are not objective or controlled, which is problematic in generalizing the results. The specific dogs were not asked to demonstrate specific behaviors. No baseline was set for abilities as puppies, which would help to ascertain the extent to which various environments might have influenced the expression of behaviors. The 13 categories of behavioral traits were as follow:

1. Affection demand
2. Excitability
3. Excessive barking
4. Snapping at children
5. General activity
6. Territorial defense
7. Watchdog barking
8. Aggression to dogs
9. Dominance over owner
10. Obedience training
11. Housebreaking ease
12. Destructiveness
13. Playfulness

Before discussing the results of this study, some caveats are needed.

It is important to realize that owners, breeders, and obedience show judges may favor some breeds. Veterinarians are not immune to this. In the list of 13 behavioral traits above, many of the traits are associated with each other and may not be independent. No tests for independence were conducted, and specific behaviors themselves were not assessed. For example, "affection demand" can involve a series of behaviors that are undefined; furthermore, the term can have different meanings for different observers. This is a problem inherent in subjective survey studies. Conclusions of such studies must be viewed with a considerable amount of caution. The classification of behaviors in a way that they can be recognized by unbiased observers and coded in a manner that is meaningful without bias is very difficult. Anyone who has conducted any studies of normal behavior and influences of extraneous sources, such as anesthesia, drug therapy, the stress of caging, or the stress of people has experienced these problems.

The authors of both of the above studies realized that many of these traits were associated; therefore they classified factors 1 through 5 in a group that they determined was reflective of the general "reactivity" of the animal.

Traits 6 through 10 were classified in a factor that reflected what was globally called "aggressiveness." It is important to remember that aggression is both a description and a diagnosis; "aggressiveness," as used in these studies, is liberally categorized. The conclusions of the studies do *not* imply that dogs who exhibit the behaviors represented by traits 6 through 10 will be aggressive. The third factor that was examined involved traits 10 and 11; these were said to reflect the individual's trainability.

The last two traits, "destructiveness" and "playfulness," were grouped together as a fourth factor. When a cluster analysis was performed on these data, seven clusters were identified. They are listed below:

Cluster 1. High reactivity, low trainability, and medium aggressiveness

Cluster 2. Very low reactivity, low trainability, very low aggressiveness

Cluster 3. Low reactivity, low trainability, high aggressiveness

Cluster 4. High reactivity, very high trainability, and medium aggressiveness

Cluster 5. Low reactivity, high trainability, low aggressiveness

Cluster 6. Very low reactivity, very high trainability, very high aggressiveness

Cluster 7. High reactivity, medium trainability, and very high aggressiveness

Dog breeds that clustered within these groups are:

Cluster 1. Lhasa apso, Pomeranian, Maltese, cocker spaniel, Boston terrier, Pekinese, beagle, Yorkshire terrier, weimaraner, pug, and Irish setter

Cluster 2. English bulldog, Old English sheepdog, Norwegian elkhound, bloodhound, and basset hound

Cluster 3. Samoyed, Alaskan malamute, Siberian husky, St. Bernard, Afghan hound, boxer, dalmatian, great Dane, and chow chow

Cluster 4. Shetland sheepdog, shih tzu, miniature poodle, toy poodle, bichon frise, standard poodle, English springer spaniel, and Welsh corgi

Cluster 5. Labrador retriever, vizsla, Brittany spaniel, German short-haired pointer, Newfoundland, Chesapeake Bay retriever, keeshond, collie, golden retriever, and Australian shepherd

Cluster 6. German shepherd dog, Akita, Doberman pinscher, and rottweiler

Cluster 7. Cairn terrier, West Highland white terrier, chihuahua, fox terrier, Scottish terrier, dachshund, miniature schnauzer, silky terrier, and Airedale terrier

In a similar study, Stur et al. (1989) divided dogs into four groups based on temperament as judged by owners:

1. Low aggression, high irritability
2. Low aggression, low irritability
3. High aggression, high irritability
4. High aggression, low irritability

In this study, *irritability* was defined to be a measurement of reaction to noises like explosives. This is not the standard definition of irritability (Beaver, 1995); however, Stur et al. were interested in finding lines of dogs that did not react adversely to gunshot noises.

A brief discussion of the limitations of the studies is warranted. First, people who are familiar with the breeds and who may have breed preferences may base their opinions about breed-specific behaviors on myth rather than unbiased rankings of actual behaviors that contribute to the suites of behaviors. Second, the terms (e.g., reactivity, aggressiveness) are undefined. Third, many of the behavioral traits listed include undesirable behaviors without reference to context. The assumption would be that the behaviors that have negative connotations would always be inappropriate behaviors. There is no way to tell from the data if this is true, or if the data influenced the way people ranked the individual breeds. Finally, whenever breeds are involved, vogue and fashion change. There is no way to ascertain the effect of fashion on such studies.

In a survey study that I conducted at Penn and at practices in the greater Philadelphia area, respondents (interns, residents, faculty, and practitioners) were asked to list breeds that they perceived were more or less aggressive, and to list their top three "most aggressive" and "least aggressive" breeds. Results varied according to the proportion of breeds to which that individual practitioner was exposed. Popular, up-and-coming breeds that were then receiving much media coverage found their way onto both lists (rottweilers). When the same group of respondents was asked to identify behaviors that were associated with diagnoses of aggression, most respondents did not accurately identify behaviors that were affiliated with, or were precursors to, behaviors indicative of diagnoses of aggression. Caution is urged for any interpretation of assertions about breed-specific aggression.

In the studies cited (Hart & Hart, 1985b; Hart & Miller, 1983), females ranked higher than males, regardless of breed, in obedience training, housebreaking ease, and affection demand. Males ranked higher than females, regardless of breed, for dominance over owners, aggression to other dogs, general activity, territorial defense, destructiveness, and playfulness. These conclusions require qualification. Associations between sex and activity levels, territorial defense, destructiveness, and playfulness do not appear to be true for the population studied at Penn. Part of the reason for this could be that this population examined at Penn involved dogs brought to the Behavior Clinic because of behavioral problems. The percentile ranking of dogs by sex for behavioral traits is shown in Table 3-3 (Hart & Hart, 1984, 1985b; Hart & Miller, 1985).

Individuals who evaluate dogs may have different expectations for males and females and may treat them differently. Although it is true that dominance aggression is far more common in male dogs than in female dogs, one of the reasons this trait may worsen in male dogs is that owners delay seeking treatment because they believe the myth that a male dog should be more aggressive. Inherent in the myth is the implication that no distinction is made between behaviors that are appropriate and in context and those that are inappropriate and out of context. Practitioners must discuss normal behavior with their clients and encourage *early* intervention when clients begin to believe that a specific behavior has deviated from normal.

Other authors have studied behaviors associated with patterns that have breed-affiliated connotations (Green & Woodruff, 1988; Willis, 1987, 1989). Collies tend to nip and not bite, so that there is little damage to the sheep. German shepherd × puli crosses slashed and tore at sheep when they were dispersed from the flock, causing serious wounds. Turkish dogs grabbed and actually held sheep without any tearing or injury.

Patterns of fearful and shy behavior have frequently been examined in the framework of genetics. In 1944 Thorne identified individual dogs that were "shy" when approached by strangers. Of 178 dogs that were related, 82 were extremely shy. Forty-three (52%) of the 82 were *direct* descendants of an exceedingly shy basset hound bitch. Other descendants of that bitch

TABLE 3-3 RANKING OF DOGS FOR BEHAVIORAL TRAITS

Sex	Trait	Percentile Rank
Female	Obedience training	55
Female	Housebreaking ease	45
Female	Affection demand	25
Female	Watchdog barking	0
Male	Excessive barking	0
Male	Excitability	0
Male	Playfulness	15
Male	Destructiveness	20
Male	Snapping at children	20
Male	Territorial defense	35
Male	General activity	40
Male	Aggression with dogs	65
Male	Dominance over owners	70

(Data from Hart & Hart, 1984, 1985b; Hart & Mueller, 1985.)

yielded approximately 73% shy or unfriendly dogs. It appeared that the "trait" for "shyness" was inherited in a simple dominant manner.

Other studies of "shyness" or "nervousness" have suggested more complex modes of heritability (Murphree, 193; Murphree et al., 1967, 1969, 1974, 1977; Murphree & Dykman, 1965; Murphree & Newton, 1971a,b; Walls et al., 1976) and some complex associations with other traits, such as deafness (Klein et al., 1988). The extent to which dogs become shy or fearful is important for guide dogs (Goddard & Beilharz, 1986). These dogs and other service dogs have a high rate of failure to complete their training programs (Goddard and Beilharz, 1985b). Much of the failure is associated with fear that may not become apparent until the dog's second year of life (i.e., social maturity) (Goddard & Beilharz, 1974, 1982, 1983).

Service and field trial dogs have been the foci of studies that examine the effects of breed on specific behaviors. Pointing appears to be inherited independently of head structure, and air-scenting with the head held up was dominant to air-scenting behavior with the head held low (Marchlewski, 1930, cited in MacKenzie et al., 1986). The tendency toward gunshyness (fear of the sound or sight of guns, or both) was controlled by a single locus; the tendency to not be shy around guns is actually an "under"-sensitivity to the auditory stimulus (Humphrey & Warner, 1934). Dogs that are undersensitive are homozygous for the non-gunshy locus (NN); dogs that are of medium sensitivity are heterozygous (Nn), and dogs that are gunshy or oversensitive are homozygous for the sensitivity locus (nn). This work was done early in the history of behavioral genetics; the extent to which epistatic or polygenic effects may modify such behaviors has not been explored. It is startling that in light of the frequency of noise phobias, including thunderstorm phobia, that such studies have not been done on pet dogs. It is possible that there is a genetic basis to many of these problems, and that the tendency to develop them may be heritable. This is another area that demands examination of the genetic basis to understand the factors that modulate inappropriate behaviors and help such animals.

Animals that are stick-shy (animals who are uneasy about having a stick held in front of them when movements are made) have a similar heritability pattern (Humphrey & Warner, 1934). Accordingly, the authors defined temperament as a reflection of shyness. High scores in their study reflected dogs that were not shy. Willingness to interact was defined in terms of the reaction to humans. The energy of the animal in the experimental situation was defined as the speed and the extent of movements in response to a stimulus. Aggression was defined as a behavior that was high in dogs that would attack easily. Distrust was defined as an aloofness that was not associated with fear.

In a long-term study conducted by the National Institutes of Health (Brown et al., 1978; Murphree et al.,

1967, 1969, 1977; Newton et al., 1978), the use of both behavioral and autonomic measurements could separate two strains of pointers (normal and "nervous" pointers) with absolute certainty. Either measurement (behavioral or autonomic) alone was 95% accurate. More studies that identify such traits are needed.

A colony of dogs kept at the Veterinary Hospital of the University of Pennsylvania for the purposes of studying retinal disease produces animals with intractable, unresponsive fear to unfamiliar humans. Breeding experiments confirm that the tendency to exhibit this profound behavior is inherited in a simple dominant manner (Acland, Aguirre, Overall; unpublished data, 1996). None of these animals responds to treatment with antianxiety agents, suggesting that profoundly abnormal behavioral physiologic conditions can be heritable.

The "collie-eye" herding behavior score progeny is near the parent's score (Burns & Frazier, 1966). Many additive genetic effects probably also influence this similarity in a polygenic manner.

In studies of affiliation preference, James (1951) found that beagles preferred beagles, but terriers also preferred beagles. This could be because terriers are more assertive. If an individual wants an arena in which to be assertive, it is not one in which there is competition for that behavior. Beagles might prefer beagles because they are hounds and have been selected to live harmoniously in groups, and terriers could prefer them because they could push them around, partly because of their grouping tendencies.

Burns and Frazier (1966) note that of 2000 dogs that were biters, dogs that guarded sheep were the most aggressive. They were followed by gun dogs, and then by hunting dogs. Terriers were irritable, but were only of medium aggressiveness, whereas mastiffs and bulldogs looked aggressive but did not behave that way. The authors of these early studies were well aware of the problems that have been pointed out for other studies (Hart and Hart, 1985b; Hart and Miller, 1985).

Dogs have been postulated to be more aggressive to dogs of the same sex and the same breed. This finding pertains to sexual competition, but it could be related to the ability to read the signals of the same breed with fewer errors than those of a different breed. No data on gauging these types of problems have ever been collected.

In a small study, Ginsberg (1958) found that working strains of border collies that were subjected to rigorous selection for behavior were more highly uniform with regard to their behavior than they were with regard to body characteristics. The reverse was true for dogs selected for conformation. Although border collies may appear to be more uniform with regard to performance variables, the predictability for behavioral traits based on specific breeding may be no higher than it is for race horses (Huey & Dunham, 1987). Race horses tend to have high repeatability in racing times, but low predictability of heritability of those performance times. In other words, the individual horse is quite predictable on the track, but you cannot predict how well the offspring will perform. The best example of this is Secretariat, who, to date, has not sired an animal nearly as athletic as he was. Secretariat's sons are also being born into a different performance environment.

Fear

Heritability estimates of behavioral traits with dachshunds were higher for dams than they were for sires. This pattern is not consistently true for suites of behavioral traits in Australian guide dogs. Goddard and Beilharz (1974, 1982) found that fearfulness was the most important behavioral trait for predicting which dogs would not make good guide dogs. *Absence* of fearfulness was the most highly heritable component of success. Their data are reflected in Table 3-4.

The heritability of Labrador retrievers in Australia for nervousness was 0.58 (Goddard & Bielharz 1983). In American guide dogs, the heritability for hip conformation appears to be 0.72 for males, 0.46 for females, and 0.54 for the combination (Bartlett, 1976). In such indices of heritability, it is important to remember that heritability (h2) is the result of the additive genetic variance divided by the total phenotypic variance or V_A/V_P. The additive genetic variance is the amount of genetic variance that is available for selective breeding and, hence for the traits that are shaped by selective breeding.

Smiley et al. (1977) examined components of communication systems and the heritability of the individual components with a domestic breed (beagles) and a nondomestic canid (coyotes). The intent was to look at specific signals; therefore beagles were chosen because they are fairly uniform in appearance. The results indicated that the F_1 offspring are mosaics of parental combinations. In crossbreeding experiments, the classic gape-hiss behavior of the coyote was recessive to the beagle's snarl. Although these data have few direct applications for normal behavior or for problem dogs, it is interesting to note that specific components of behavior were identifiable as attributable to coyotes or to beagles. More studies such as this are needed, both between and within breeds, to identify the underlying genetic basis of the traits of behaviors for which we have selected, and of the correlates of those behaviors that appear to produce problems.

Fält (1984) reported a high heritability for a separation response that is apparent by 8 weeks of age in German shepherd dogs raised for service programs. The separation response is both vocal and physical. Heritability estimates are highest for the mother (dam) of the puppies. In other words, there appears to be a very strong maternal effect for the extent to which puppies become distressed when separated for service at 8 weeks of age. This is a sufficiently young

TABLE 3-4 HERITABILITY ESTIMATES

	Sire	Dam	Combination
Success	0.46	0.42	0.44
Fear	0.67	0.25	0.46
Dog distribution	−0.04	0.23	0.09

(Data from Goddard & Bellharz, 1974, 1982.)

age that there do not appear to be any long-standing effects on trainability for service, but the important message from this study is that behavioral effects of heritability are identifiable as early as months of age.

Given the above, what can be stated about the heritability of specific behaviors, or of suites of behaviors, that may be appropriate or inappropriate, and what is known about the behaviors of specific breeds? *All* behavior has environmental and genetic components. The variation in the genetic component is sufficient to produce a wide array of behavioral phenotypes in the absence of any specific breed. Hence, not all mixed-breed dogs look alike or demonstrate identical behaviors in response to identical situations. This variation applies within and between litters, as noted above. Evolutionary biologists since and including Darwin have recognized these differences. The extent to which behavioral plasticity is a function of genetics is still hotly debated and, as indicated above, very few competent genetic studies have been conducted. This is particularly true for behaviors that are relevant to problems experienced by dogs, or for traits that clients would like to have in their pets. Some recent experimental evidence on desert toads living in highly variable environments indicates that natural selection may be operating to maintain developmental and concomitant behavioral plasticity, rather than selecting for one or a few modes, each of which would persevere only under limited conditions (Newman, 1989). This finding is one that is probably applicable to either mixed-breed dogs or to nondomestic canid ancestors such as wolves. One of the functions of selective breeding and the development of breeds is to select for one or a few modes, often in direct competition to selection for overall variance. These issues are important and relevant in discussing the issue of breeds.

A final comment on breed-specific behaviors is warranted. Campbell (1992) recommends that "a prospective dog owner should consult the various breed atlases to select a visually appealing breed" (p. 46) and then look at the genetic-based health and behavior problems attendant with that breed. The fact that as late as 1992 people who have been publishing in the field recommend selecting an individual or a breed on the basis of *appearance* rather than of its behavior is an appalling testimony to the lack of progress in the field in 30 years.

4 ···· Normal Feline Behavior

EVOLUTIONARY OVERVIEW

The domestic cat was probably derived from *Felis silvestris libyca,* the subspecies of the African wildcat that has been known to tame when taken into a household. This subspecies contrasts with the northern wildcat, which is fierce, regardless of handling and exposure (Serpell, 1988). It has been estimated that the first domestication of *Felis silvestris libyca* that produced *Felis catus libyca* occurred 6,000 to 10,000 years ago. One can infer that cats were more troublesome or less valued for domestication or were more useful in symbiosis without extensive domestication than were other animals, because the Egyptians, who had been quite successful in their domestication concerns, did not establish domesticated cats until 1600 BC (Zeuner, 1963). After this, exportation from Egypt was forbidden for 100 years, possibly for religious reasons (consider the goddess Bastet). It is ironic that the cat radiated worldwide with the spread of Christianity, the same religion that later vilified it as a helpmate of the devil.

It is probable that the association between people and cats that led to this domestication was serendipitous and mutualistic, with less outright selection for specific behaviors occurring than was true for dogs. Cats were probably attracted to human settlements because they attracted potential prey like rodents; humans were probably grateful to the cat for controlling rodent populations and so did not discourage their presence. This mutualism did not require that humans expand or modify innate feline behavior. Accordingly, feline predatory behavior, and most of the other attendant social behaviors that cats exhibit in human households, have been only slightly changed in their structure and behavioral elements since the cat was "domesticated." Because cats have had little direct influence on human economics, compared with that of hunting or herding dogs, for example, there has been little intervention in their behavior by humans in the past hundred years (Young, 1985). This lack of intervention is supported by coat color patterns. One of the most common feline coat colors, the tabby, has radiated worldwide, yet this color is extremely similar to that of the European wild cat and Norwegian forest cat (Clark, 1975; Searle, 1949). It is unknown the extent to which domesticated cats interbred with these wild cats but interbreeding could account for some of the variability in feline behavior.

The histories of canine and feline domestication differ. The association between dogs and people has been more symbiotic; humans and dogs may have "codomesticated" with each other. Very specific dog behaviors have been shaped to the needs of humans because humans were able to recognize "like" social systems. This shaping of and selecting for specific suites of behaviors resulted in the behavior patterns associated with specific breeds or with breeds in specific groups. For instance, hounds are expected to be good at detecting smells, and herding dogs to be less superb at being able to track a specific smell but excellent at working with an ungulate to keep it from fleeing. This type of symbiotic relationship was facilitated by the similar patterns of human and canine social systems.

In contrast, cats do not have social systems that are readily identifiable as being analogs or homologs of human social systems. Social relationships between humans and cats probably developed as mutualistic events; humans apparently did not shape or select for behaviors but expanded on the innate behaviors that were exploited. Lack of selection for specific domesticated behaviors also may be reflected in the range of body sizes for present-day cats. In the wild, the range of body sizes of wild cat species greatly exceeds the range of size of wild dog species; however, the range of body sizes of domesticated dogs is tremendous and far surpasses that reported in the wild, whereas the size range of domestic cats is relatively small and well within the range of body sizes reported for their wild counterparts. Even large domestic cats are relatively small in comparison with their wild relatives. Given the difference between human social systems and cat social systems, humans may be less able to extrapolate their signals to the cat and to directly communicate their desires to cats in a communal working relationship. Both cats and humans would be at risk for miscommunication. Cats are model carnivores. It might have been far too dangerous to attempt a symbiotic relationship with a cat species larger than *Felis silvestris libyca.*

Since at least 1600 BC, when the first evidence for tight, familiar associations between humans and domestic cats was recorded, domestic cats have been an integral part of most societies' households (Serpell, 1988; Turner & Stammach-Geering, 1990). They have recently risen in popularity in the United States. In

1983 there were 52.2 million cats in U.S. households, and 28.4% of all households had cats. By 1987, 54.6 million cats occupied 30.5% of U.S. households. Recent data estimate that the U.S. pet population included 55 million dogs and 60 million cats (Patronek & Rowan, 1995; AVMA, 1992). This pattern of increasing popularity of domestic pet felines occurred concomitant with a decrease in the numbers of domestic pet dogs (Anon 1990, 1992a; Bradshaw, 1992a; Troutman, 1988; Wise & Yang, 1992, 1994). This might reflect a change in economic conditions and a change in workplace structure, but it is also clear, based on the number of publications on cats that have appeared in recent years, that the fondness for cats is reaching a new level. More information on cats is available, and that information is superior to what has been published in the past.

Unfortunately, the prevalent image in the literature is one of the cat as an asocial, at worst, or solitary, at best, animal (Beaver, 1982, 1992; Kleiman & Eisenberg, 1973). Many authors feel that the only wild felids exhibiting any type of social behavior are African lions (Packer, 1986; Packer & Pusey, 1983; Scheel & Packer, 1991). This is inaccurate; felids that show long-term group associations complete with complex social structures include not only the lion (*Panthera leo*), but also the cheetah (*Acinonyx jubatus*), and the domestic cat (*Felis silvestris catus*).

Although it has been emphasized that domestic cats are primarily solitary (Leyhausen, 1979), being solitary neither precludes social behavior nor diminishes its potential complexity (Kling et al., 1969; Leyhausen, 1965; Robinson, 1992b; Voith & Borchelt, 1986). Most carnivores *do* live socially (Gittleman, 1989), although the degree to which they are *facultatively* [emphasis added] solitary can vary (Todd, 1978).

Social living provides any animal with the following:
1. A defense against predators
2. An ability to exploit food resources that might not be exploitable were one asocial
3. Reproductive access to conspecifics
4. Facilitation of learning about the environment
5. A collective resistance to harsh environments.

Because cats often hunt alone, unlike wild canids, it has been mistakenly believed that this is the basis for an asocial system. What is often missed is that the logic for solitary hunting relies on patterns involving body size and metabolic rate. Small cats mainly hunt small prey, primarily small rodents. A small rodent might be a sufficient meal for that one animal, whereas a large ungulate would probably be more than the animal could eat and would be unattainable by the animal hunting by itself.

Contrast the situation in small, wild or domestic cats with that of lions and the body size: metabolic rate argument becomes pellucid. Lions do not hunt large ungulates by themselves—group cooperation is imperative. The individuals in a pride take turns in

running down and cutting the ungulate from the herd (Bertram, 1975; Scheel & Packer, 1991; Schaller, 1972). Because the version of the North African wild cat that was domesticated was small, we have inadvertently selected for, with domestication, the propensity for solitary hunting. It would be wrong to mistake this as evidence for asociality.

Domestic Cat Social Grouping and Reproduction

The focus of feline social groups is invariably the female and her kittens. Most studies have concentrated on matrilineal relationships as the focus of the social grouping. Like lion prides, domestic cat groups are often composed of females, who may be related, and their juvenile offspring. It has been postulated that this social pattern is driven by the reproductive pattern of female cats.

Domestic cats reach puberty at about 10 months of age, although females born in the late spring may not cycle until the following year (Burke, 1976; Fox, 1975; Prescott, 1973). Peaks in sexual activity occur from mid-January through March and from May to June. Domestic cats are seasonally polyestrous and generally experience two cycles per year if not bred. They can cycle every 3 weeks for several months. Estrus in cats lasts 9 to 10 days in the absence of copulation, but only 4 days if copulation occurs. This difference is a function of induced ovulation. Cats can show a complete sequence of estrus behaviors if subjected to only estrogen (Houpt, 1991), unlike dogs, who also need progesterone (Signoret, 1975).

Gestation in female domestic cats is approximately 63 days. This is longer, by 3 to 7 days, than the gestation period for *Felis silvestris libyca* (Hemmer, 1979; Schmidt et al., 1983). Litter sizes vary from 1 to 10 kittens with a mean of 4.5 kittens per litter. Most domestic cats have two litters per year (Liberg, 1984a, b; Liberg & Sandell, 1988; Robinson & Cox, 1970).

Cats usually have eight nipples. Only three pairs of these nipples may produce sufficient milk to provide nourishment for a kitten, and the back nipples are preferred by kittens (Rosenblatt, 1976). Teat preference is established by 1 to 3 days, when present, and up to 80% of all kittens develop a teat preference (Rosenblatt et al., 1961).

Females form stable matriarchal groups and may join in communal nests (Macdonald & Apps, 1978; Macdonald et al., 1987). The queen moves the kittens if the nest is fouled by feces, if undigested prey remains as the kittens get older, or if the site is disturbed by a strange male cat (Leyhausen, 1979). Queens stimulate kittens to eliminate by the anogenital reflex until 23 to 39 days, and kittens can usually eliminate voluntarily by 3 weeks. This developmental change may be associated with the queen's mobile behaviors. Cats move kittens most frequently between 25 and 35 days (Schneirla et al., 1963). A familiar male may be such an integral part of the social group that he will guard against disturbances of foreign males

(Macdonald et al., 1987). Communal nests may function in part to repel intruder males; however, they may also function to ensure that all kittens receive nourishment, should the number of nipples or the production of the milk be insufficient to support large litters. In a large farm study, males would provide care and succor for the kittens, if these males were residents within the larger social group (Macdonald et al., 1987).

One of the social constructs that may facilitate communal care, particularly that involving males, is the presence of several reproductive males (Kerby & Macdonald, 1988; Turner & Mertens, 1986). In such cases, no dominant male monopolizes all the matings (Natoli & de Vito, 1988). If males can neither monopolize all matings nor guarantee paternity, it might be advantageous for them to contribute to communal care.

Females may further add to the stability of such social systems through their behavior during proestrus. During proestrus, females are attracted to males, but are not receptive to their courtship behavior and reject attempts at copulation (Whalen, 1963). It has been postulated that this is a device to enhance male-male competition (Bradshaw, 1992a). This mechanism also provides females with the opportunity to assess the staying power of males. In colonies that are sufficiently large, a proestrus that allows the females to evaluate males that are attracted to them would be one mechanism by which they could identify resident males. Furthermore, if the females are attractive to a number of males and those males are *all* part of the colony, that behavioral interaction could help facilitate communal care. In such cases there may be an element of uncertainty of paternity, but copulation could then act to solidify social relationships where individuals "within" the group are treated differently than individuals considered "outside" the group.

Unfortunately, there are no data on whether animals known to the group are less likely to practice infanticide or more likely to provide communal care; there are even fewer data on whether the extent of a genetic or social relationship makes a difference for either of these factors. It has been postulated that males within colonies could be related. If this were the case, infanticide would not be an appropriate genetic strategy to enhance any single male cat's genetic contribution, because insemination resulting from a brother would not be genetically disadvantageous to a related individual.

Relatedness has become a fascinating issue because ovulation is induced and estrus for any queen lasts only about 4 to 5 days (Natoli & de Vito, 1988, 1991; Paape et al., 1975; Schmidt et al., 1983). Liberg (1983) noted that at the peak of fertilization the queen was monopolized by the dominant male in the group. A 24-hour capacitance period is necessary for cat sperm (Hamner et al., 1970). Twenty-four hours after copulation the female ovulates (Hamner et al., 1970); there-fore one copulation might *not* be sufficient to induce females to ovulate and to ensure that sperm capacitance occurs at the time of ovulation (Aronson & Copper, 1967, 1974; Hart & Melese-d'Hospital, 1983; Sojka et al., 1970). This physiological pattern could argue strongly for either the guarding effect noted by Liberg (1983), or the effect hinted at by Bradshaw (1992a) in which multiple males might possibly contribute to insemination and, indirectly, to the stability of the social group in groups where males provide a portion of the communal care for the young. It is conceivable that both modes function depending on the demography of the group. Social structure is influenced by both the age and sex structure of the group and will interact with the resource, predation, and physical and biophysical environments to affect behaviors (Dunham et al., 1989).

The issue of infanticide has received attention because of the apparent similarity of domestic cats and African lions (Bertram, 1975). In domestic cats, weaning normally starts at approximately day 30 and continues through day 60 of the kitten's life (Scott, 1970). If kittens die, regardless of the cause of death, the queen enters estrus approximately 15 days later (Liberg, 1980; Liberg & Sandell, 1988). Under normal circumstances cats might have two litters a year; if there is a litter death, the interbirth interval can be as short as 133 days (Schmidt et al., 1983). Infanticide in domestic cats has been rarely observed directly (for exceptions see Dards [1983] and Liberg [1983]). Infanticide has been anecdotally discussed for 2000 years (Herodotus in 423 BC, cited in Macdonald et al., 1987). An evolutionary argument can be made for the occurrence of infanticide in unstable groups, or in groups that experience a cataclysmic change in the social structure; female domestic cats are induced ovulators, and the basis of social communal relationships may be influenced by the relatedness of the colony (Packer et al., 1991). There are no hard data to support this theory. It would be inappropriate to assume that all of the social relationships with feline groups are driven strictly by direct genetic relationships. However, the latter is supported to some extent by the finding that in cat colonies that contain several reproductive males, no single male monopolizes all the matings (Kerby & Macdonald, 1988; Natoli & de Vito, 1988).

It is important to consider induced ovulation from the evolutionary standpoint. We tend to think of induced ovulation as benefiting males. It might be more appropriate to study induced ovulation in a sex-blind manner and study whether becoming pregnant is a problem. Anybody who has watched young cats supports the contention that becoming pregnant is seldom a problem for cats; however, avoiding pregnancy might be a problem. There has been very little study of whether induced ovulation is a mechanism for retaining reproductive capabilities in uncertain resource environments. If cats experiencing a profound period of resource stress were able to benefit, in terms of energetic stores (fat), from a resource flush, they might be able to bring kittens into a more favorable environment. Induced ovulation could function as a mechanism to allow such exploitation. Animals that are not induced ovulators (e.g., humans, squirrel monkeys) adjust litter size in response to changing resource environments and environmental conditions, but do so through abortion or cannibalism at parturition (Day & Galef, 1977). Induced ovulation might be a mechanism that, in an uncertain mate environment, allows the queen to balance her own energetic constraints by timing the ability to reproduce with the presence of both adequate mates and resources. No research has been done on this, but it is an alternative interpretation that is supported by more recent work on allocation algorithms (Dunham et al., 1989; Dunham, 1993).

The amount of variation in data collected from different study populations suggests that the issue is far more complicated than any mode of single causality suggests. This is particularly true because no data exist that confirm or refute whether the last male to mate displaces the previous male's sperm, or if the last male's sperm has a fertilization advantage, but such effects have been reported for both Syrian golden hamsters and the laboratory rat (Dewsbury & Hartung, 1980).

In general, males do not appear to form close bonds with any single female (but there are exceptions as reported). Males seldom provide lactating females with food or bring food directly to the kittens (Liberg, 1980). Regardless, the social organization is flexible; social groups may include lone females and females in groups with other females, with or without communal nursing and midwife behavior (Baerends-van Roon & Baerends, 1979; Kerby & Macdonald, 1988). Further work is necessary to elucidate the complexity of domestic feline social systems.

It is safe to say that the variation in behavior discussed is not representative of a group of animals that could be called asocial.

Weaning is complete at approximately 60 days, and by week 12, milk quality has substantially changed. The kittens then begin to accompany their mother on hunting expeditions and do so with increasing frequency between 8 and 16 weeks of age (Wolski, 1982). Kittens in wild groupings often stay with their mother until at least 6 months or a year of age and then disperse. During this intermediate period, should they stay with the mother or with the mother's social grouping, the kittens often form independent social associations (Leyhausen, 1979; Macdonald et al., 1987; Wolski, 1982). After approximately 10 to 14 months of close association with the mother and her social coterie, the kittens experience what has been described as a "social" weaning from the group (Wolski, 1982). It has been postulated that this extended "weaning" period provides protection from harassment from the breeding tom(s) in the group. This explanation appears

somewhat simple given the complexity of the social and breeding groups already described. It is more likely that dispersal is regulated by the same factors that govern dispersal in other free-ranging populations of nondomestic animals, namely, the interaction of the demographic, predation, resource, and physical and biophysical environments (Dunham, 1993). There are no data currently available to indicate whether the demographic environment or the social environment affects dispersal.

Developmental Effects: Feeding, Prey Behavior, and Early Play

The tactile sense is present quite early in gestation. Kittens are born unable to see, but locomote freely. Eye-opening is affected both by the environment and by genetics. Kittens of young mothers appear to open their eyes earlier than those of older mothers; female kittens tend to open their eyes slightly earlier than males, but there also appears to be a strong *paternal* genetic effect on timing of eye opening (Bateson & Turner, 1988; Turner et al., 1986). This is probably not independent of the paternal effect on "boldness" (McCune, 1995).

Cats isolated from other cats from birth until 7 months of age are slow to accept introduced cats (Kolb & Nonneman, 1975; Konrad Bagshaw, 1970). Kittens that are isolated from other kittens until late in their first year of life display exaggerated autonomic responses characterized by galvanic skin responses and disruption of regular sleep rhythms (Wenzel, 1959). Neonatal isolation leads to changes in normal pain response in dogs (Melzack & Scott, 1957), but it is correlated with increased aggression in cats and rats (Guyot et al., 1983).

Singleton kittens are quicker to emerge from nest boxes between 3 and 7 weeks (Mendl, 1988) and appear to show little distress when left alone. Two kittens, when left by their mother, appear all right while together, but if separated and then left by their mother, appear more distressed than a singleton kitten that is left alone (Mendl, 1988). Most variation in individual behavior is probably not attributable to litter composition (Deag et al., 1988).

Feeding behaviors have been extensively studied with regard to developmental phase. By the time the kittens are about 4 weeks of age, the queen starts to bring them solid food, representing the beginning of the weaning phase (Ewer, 1961; Kovach & Kling, 1967; Martin & Bateson, 1988). This phase is completed by 7 weeks of age. Concomitant with this, by about 5 to 6 weeks of age, the kittens are totally independent in their ability to both eliminate and to start to find substrates resembling the ancestral substrate for elimination. For the first 3 to 5 weeks, the queen stimulates the kittens to eliminate and cleans up after them. By 3 to 5 or 6 weeks of age, kittens begin to seek out open, well-drained substrates and uses them for both urination and defecation (Fox, 1975). Covering of urine or feces may not occur—the ancestral condition is to spray urine a large percentage of the time, and feces may not be covered in many arid environments. Feces are often used as signposts for territorial delineation (Wemmer & Scow, 1977), but it may also be possible to make a case for disease control: by leaving feces exposed, disease transmission is decreased and parasites are killed in arid environments. If the cats are going to cover their urine and feces, they appear to start to do so about the same time they are able to respond fully to an olfactory challenge, at approximately 7 weeks of age. No quantitative data exist for age-specific elimination behaviors in cats.

Kittens artificially separated from their mothers at about 2 weeks of age become fearful and aggressive toward both other cats and people, demonstrate random locomotion, and learn poorly (Bacon, 1973; Seitz, 1959). Kittens who are nursed on a breeder nipple nurse normally, but will not be permitted to nurse on a lactating queen because they give inappropriate social responses to her (Rosenblatt et al., 1961). These kittens can form social attachments to other kittens, but they do so slowly. The extent to which these slow social attachments and inappropriate social responses to lactating queens may affect their own ability to raise kittens has not been investigated. Unfortunately, such scenarios might be an important factor in the abandoned, feral cat population in which a decreased plane of nutrition and early abandonment may be common.

Kittens that are weaned early also develop predatory behavior far earlier than do normally weaned kittens and are more likely to be mouse killers (Tan & Counsilman, 1985; Warren & Levy, 1979). Late weaning of kittens appears to delay predatory behavior and decreases the propensity to kill mice. This association may be indicative of nonspecific learning in response to the most common prey (mice), but the implications of this are important for people who are going to hand-rear cats. People who hand-raise early-weaned kittens might experience problems with earlier predatory behavior.

The most significant side effect of early weaning might be on play behavior. Under normal conditions, object play increases by the second month (Bateson, 1978; Dumas, 1992), but under early-weaning conditions studied by gradual separation, the administration of bromocriptine (a dopamine antagonist that stops lactation) (Bateson et al., 1981), or by a decrement in the maternal food supply, there is an early increase in certain types of play (Bateson & Young, 1981; Martin, 1984; Martin & Bateson, 1985). This may be an adaptive response to forced independence. Queens fed 50% of their *ad libitum* intake during the second half of gestation and during the first 6 weeks postpartum produce kittens with abnormal play behavior. For all of these kittens, there are more accidents in play, the males demonstrate increased aggression during social play, the females demonstrate less

climbing and more running behavior, and the cerebrum, cerebellum, and brain stem do not appear to grow at the same rate as the rest of the brain. The brain and body appear to achieve normal size once rehabilitated with food, but the extent to which there might be long-lasting effects on attachment has not been fully explored (Smith & Jansen, 1977a,b,c). Fifty percent of normal maternal food intake at gestation produces kittens with delays in postural corrections, crawling, suckling, eye-opening, running and walking, and play and climbing (Simonson, 1979). These kittens also have delayed predatory and exploratory behaviors and experience the growth stunting that becomes apparent only after weaning. The greatest behavioral delays appear in behaviors that regulate coordination, and these kittens have poor learning ability, increased reactivity, abnormal fear and aggression, and a decreased responsivity to normal environments.

Low-protein diets late in gestation and during lactation correlate delayed development with kittens that experienced these restricted diets are uncoordinated and exhibit fewer social interactions with their mothers and poorer attachment responses to their mothers (Gallo et al., 1980, 1984). Under normal conditions, feline tactile sensitivity is fully developed by the twenty-fourth day of gestation and the vestibular righting reflex is developed by the fifty-fourth day of gestation. It is not known how early in gestation the effects of dietary restriction are manifest. Cats that are abandoned and may become feral, or those born to mothers that are abandoned and possibly feral, develop abnormal social behaviors. The combination of poor learning, increased reactivity, out of context and more intense than normal reaction in any foreign circumstance, abnormal fear accompanied by aggression, and decreased ability to respond in normal situations, makes these animals poor candidates for both rehabilitation and for pets. "Good samaritans" should be aware of these associations and have realistic expectations.

Social relationships that provide the context for future communal suckling develop within the first 2 months after birth (Macdonald & Apps, 1978). These relationships are adversely affected by the nutritional situations outlined previously. Well-nourished male and female kittens are similar in mass and behavior until about 8 weeks of age. Thereafter males are larger than females (Liberg, 1983); males take 3 years to reach their adult weight whereas females only take 2 years. This occurrence is associated with the period during which cats mature socially. Sex differences appear in social play by 12 to 16 weeks of age, but are not present between weeks 4 and 12 (Barrett & Bateson, 1978). Females who play with males become more malelike in their play behavior than do females who play with females (Caro, 1981a,b). Whether this factor affects later aggressive play behavior for females raised with male siblings only has not been investigated.

The role of play has been intensively studied because of the potential association between play and predatory behavior in cats. Normal social play starts at approximately 3 to 4 weeks of age when the animal is able to get up and ambulate. It is honed when eye-paw coordination is developed at approximately 7 to 8 weeks of age after birth (Barrett & Bateson, 1978; Martin & Bateson, 1985). Complex motor activity is fully functional by 10 to 11 weeks (Villablanca & Olmstead, 1979).

Social play begins to decline at about 12 to 14 weeks of age (Caro, 1981a; West, 1974, 1979). Social play patterns become more associated with predatory behavior and social fighting by the third month, possibly concomitant with a change in motivational systems that control motor behavior (Caro, 1980b, 1981b; Pellis et al., 1988; West, 1979; Voith, 1980a). Many motor patterns in play resemble those for hunting (Caro, 1979, 1980a,c), but there is no definitive link with play as "practice" behavior for predatory skills, and the development of those skills later in life, except to the extent that we all learn from experience in any social situation in which we are placed (Martin, 1984). Cats deprived of play still develop predatory behavior (Baerends-van Roon & Baerends, 1979). Cats that did not or could not play with small objects as kittens appear in experiments to be no different than other cats when examined with regard to predatory skills at 6 months of age (Caro, 1980b), but cats are still more likely to kill the types of prey that they had known since kittenhood (Caro, 1980a). The predisposition to respond defensively toward large and difficult prey develops some time during the second month (Adamec et al., 1983). Free-ranging domestic cats start to bring their kittens live prey about 4 weeks of age, coincident with the beginning of the weaning. Kittens can actually start to kill mice on their own at approximately 5 weeks of age (Baerends-van Roon & Baerends, 1979). Weanling kittens eat food preferred by their mother even though that food may not be a common food in cat diets (Wyrwicka, 1978). Kittens appear to be able to learn to kill a rat by watching another cat do it (Kuo, 1930). They also learn a preference at this stage and restrict their preference to the *strain* of rat with which they are familiar. Competition within litters may also hone some predatory skills (Caro, 1980a,b,c), and some cats appear to be able to "catch up" to more skilled litter mates during ontogeny (Caro, 1980b).

Cats can learn about a variety of tasks through observation and may learn more quickly if it is their mother they are observing.

The tendency for cats to retrieve their young in response to high-pitched vocalization peaks at 1 week after parturition (Schneirla et al., 1963). Early in life (during the first 3 weeks) kittens use ultrasonic calls as they explore their nest (cited Deag et al., 1988); these calls may function in helping their caretakers locate them and keep them together. The patterns of communication used for eliciting social play in normal litters have been the focus of much study (West, 1979). Eight kitten play postures have been identified (West, 1974):

1. Belly-up
2. Stand-up
3. Side-step
4. Pounce
5. Vertical stance
6. Chase
7. Horizontal leap
8. Face-off

Behaviors, some of which are associated with later predatory behavior, that are most successful in eliciting play from another kitten are the pounce (39% of all play-eliciting behaviors), the belly-up display (14% of all play-eliciting behaviors), and the stand-up (16% of all play-eliciting behaviors). These behaviors are 90% effective in obtaining a response from another kitten between 6 and 12 weeks of age. As the cat matures, other behaviors become important in the play elicitation communication repertoire. The vertical stance elicits play behavior only 8% of the time at 6 weeks of age, but by 12 weeks of age it elicits play response from another littermate 24% of the time. The side-step posture, in contrast, elicits play 20% of the time at 6 weeks of age, but only 3% of the time at 12 weeks of age (West, 1979). It is important to emphasize these normal changes in communicatory and play behavior to clients because potential problems in communication could arise when people play too roughly with their kittens. Clients need to know appropriate, age-specific play behaviors.

In his study of singleton litters, Mendl (1988) found that single kittens did not engage more frequently in self- or object play than did kittens in litters of two. This suggests that social and object play must be separately motivated. Solitary kittens directed all of their play toward the mother; given that the mother is more likely to be absent from the nest than a sibling would, singleton kittens might experience less social play. Between 2 and 4 weeks of age, the particular closeness experienced by kittens to other kittens has a calming effect (Rosenblatt et al., 1962). Physical contact with the dam, particularly that involved with nuzzling of the face, has a calming effect on the kittens (Beaver, 1992). These observations have implications for early weaning. Kittens are weaned early if the queen cannot provide enough food; this results in stimulation of the early development of both object and social play (Bateson et al., 1990). In the case of early weaning, the siblings and the mother are still present; their presence could have a significant effect on the extent to which rough play might be modulated. In the usual, nonexperimental situation involving early weaning, the mother is no longer present. No studies have been done on whether these two types of early weaning have different effects on inappropriate play behavior or the early development of predatory aggression in cats. It is likely that early weaning that also precludes the social interaction of an older, experienced cat could foster more inappropriate play behavior and play aggression.

Feral cats often abandon kittens by about 4 months of age. At this time the kittens increase their environmental exploration. Barrett and Bateson (1978) noticed that males engage in twice the object play as do females by 7 weeks of age, and by 19 weeks of age these free-ranging males are demonstrating sexual behavior. Female kittens usually do not demonstrate sexual behavior until 23 weeks of age. Litters composed solely of females appear to be less aggressive in their play than are all-male litters; this difference is recognizable by weeks 12 to 16.

West (1979) postulates that the function of play, rather than teaching cats to be better predators later in life, might be to keep litters together when the litter is vulnerable. This would enhance their ability to develop good social relationships that might serve to redress vulnerability later in life. No studies have directly addressed this issue, but the work of Macdonald and co-workers (1987) suggests that this might be so.

It is not inevitable that cats will hunt, especially if they are not weaned early and if they are not taught by their mothers to be predatory. The presentation of palatable food starting at kittenhood may inhibit hunting, although the behaviors of killing and eating are separately, centrally controlled (Adamec, 1975b, 1976a, b). Although individually controlled, there is some interaction between killing and eating, which is substantiated by interactions between areas of the lateral and ventromedial hypothalamus. Regardless, the ability to inhibit hunting through the presentation of palatable foods early in life and throughout life may be important for clients who do not wish their cats to hunt. The tendency to kill when hunting, or to exhibit hunting behavior, increases with hunger (Biben, 1979) and decreases when prey is more difficult to capture. Population control at the community level is also important. Females with kittens to feed tend to be far more adept hunters than are females who do not have kittens (Turner & Meister, 1988). It has been postulated that this facilitation is a dopaminergic prolactin response.

Odor is sufficiently important for feline feeding behavior that the odor of a palatable food (cooked rabbit) can initiate feeding in the absence of any change in food offered (Robinson, 1992a). This may be partially attributable to the wide variety of substances, including those bitter and sweet, that cats seek and ingest (Robinson, 1992a).

Recent data (Robinson, 1992a) indicate that moisture determines meal size and eating speed. If a cat's diet is diluted with water, the cat compensates by eating more (Castonguay, 1981; Mugford, 1977). This effect is *not* found if inert substances such as kaolin or cellulose are added to the diet (Hirsch et al., 1978; Kanarek, 1975); hence the basis for low-calorie cat

foods. Wet food is initially consumed quickly, followed by a subsequent decrease in feeding rate. Dry, calorically dense food is consumed at a slower, more consistent rate. It is not clear whether the costs of handling affect this comparison. The preferred food temperature is 35° C—this may be the temperature that most effectively releases volatile fatty acids.

Cats gain and lose mass cyclically (Randall & Lasko, 1968). This pattern may be associated with their annual cycles of corticosteroid, thyroxine, and epinephrine, which peak in the winter (Andersen, 1973; Randall et al., 1975). Regardless, cats appear to regulate the intake of energy, not volume or mass (Robinson, 1992a). For commercial dry foods (360 kcal/100 g), an average meal contains 22.7 to 31.3 kcal. Cats eat an average meal of 35.5 kcal from fresh meat (136 kcal/100 g), 30.2 to 44.8 kcal from canned meat (80 to 90 kcal/100 g), 19.8 to 32.5 kcal from canned meat and cereal (115 kcal/100 g), and 30.1 kcal from semimoist food (320 kcal/g) (Robinson, 1992a).

One unpleasant food experience can lead to rejection of that food for months (Everett, 1944; Houpt, 1982; Macdonald et al., 1984, 1985). Cats have a requirement for thiamine (particularly with a carbohydrate-rich diet). The first symptom of thiamine deficiency could be anorexia. A single arginine-deficient meal can lead to ammonium intoxication, causing emesis and lethargy. Such factors are usually redressed by commercial cat foods, but young animals with abnormal eating patterns may not ingest sufficient food to modulate these concerns. A thorough investigation is certainly warranted in the case of any young kitten that does not eat and thrive.

Early Social Development: Age-Specific Effects on Friendliness and Exploratory Behaviors

In 1937 Lorenz defined a "critical period" with regard to imprinting. Implicit in the definition was a definitive onset and offset. During these critical periods animals were postulated to be able to learn to respond to certain stimuli; before and after these periods, Lorenz maintained, animals were unable to respond to the stimuli.

The concept of a critical period was modified by Bateson (1979). Bateson defined a "sensitive period" as an age range during which particular events are especially likely to have long-term effects on individual development. This concept is particularly relevant for developing parts of the nervous system (i.e., the visual cortex) that rely on stimuli to direct their development (Rauschecker & Marler, 1987). For example, exposure to contours of only one orientation can have long-term effects on the propensity of the visual system.

Although the concept of a sensitive period can be useful when applied to the ontogeny of neural development, it has been grossly misapplied in discussing the development of kitten and puppy behavior. This concept has been transferred, almost without critical thought, to be synonymous with a "socialization period." It is perhaps most valuable to use the concept of a sensitive period in terms of risk assessment. Animals are not behaviorally or developmentally able to respond to all stimuli when they are born. They can *begin* to respond to certain stimuli within certain broad periods. There is a considerable amount of variability in response to specific stimuli both within and between litters. Missing the appropriate stimuli (those to which the individual is now capable of responding) during these periods certainly does not guarantee a "poorly socialized" animal; however, the *risk* of inappropriate contextual responses *increases* with increased deprivation. Animals should be exposed to all relevant social stimuli early and in a nontraumatic manner. When the individual animal is developmentally ready to learn from the stimulus, it will do so. No harm results from the presence of any stimulus (i.e., other cats, humans) before the time that the animal is best able to attend to it, provided no undue trauma or fear is involved. Animals experiencing all of the appropriate "socialization" may still have behavioral problems. Although sensitive periods have been less emphasized in the importance of the development of good pet cat behavior than have sensitive periods in the importance of good pet dog behavior, feline sensitive periods may be shorter, more discreet, and more frequently legitimately implicated in the development of behavioral problems such as play aggression, inappropriate play behavior, and fear aggression.

Karsh (1983, 1984) provided baseline data about "sensitive" periods and defined the specific behavioral changes that can occur within the time frames outlined above for kittens reared in a laboratory situation. Kittens that were handled by people for only 15 minutes a day from birth through 12 to 14 weeks of age spent more time exploring the person and giving head rubs, and would leave and return several times. Kittens in home-reared litters that were held 1 to 2 hours a day, if brought to the laboratory, would go directly to people and climb onto their lap, purr, and go to sleep. These behaviors were *not* seen in the laboratory kittens, although laboratory kittens certainly were not fearful of people. The home-reared kittens were handled four to eight times longer than were the laboratory kittens, but they were also exposed to a more varied and unpredictable environment than were the laboratory kittens. It would be inappropriate to overinterpret these results, but it is probably fair to say that the earlier the kittens are handled and the more they are handled, the more friendly they are likely to be.

It is not known whether this observation hints at differences in long-term social development that are dependent on litter size. The number of handlers that each kitten experiences appears to influence the extent to which it is "friendly" (Collard, 1967). When kittens are handled regularly for the first 45 days of their life, they approach unfamiliar objects more

rapidly and spend more time with them at 4 to 7 months of age than will nonhandled kittens (Wilson et al., 1965). Handling also appears to affect developmental rate: the age at eye-opening, the age at which the nest box was left, and the rate at which Siamese kittens develop the classic Siamese coloration is earlier or faster for kittens that are handled (Meier, 1961; Meier & Stuart, 1959). This effect is enhanced with fewer kittens in the litter. Karsh and Turner (1988) postulate that these developmental effects could be due, in part, to increased maternal attention. Kittens handled by five people compared with one or none from 5.5 to 9.5 weeks of age show less fear toward people, play more with people, and are more affectionate to them. These kittens purr more, rub more, and mouth the people with whom they are playing.

Such effects also appear to be generalizable to species other than humans. Kittens are more likely to attach to conspecifics; dogs and other animals are accepted in the absence of conspecifics or if introduced early (Kuo, 1930, 1960). Fox (1969b) demonstrated that kittens exposed to Chihuahua pups from 4 weeks of age showed absolutely no fear of them at 12 weeks of age. Kittens with no exposure to the puppies avoided them and behaved defensively when they were approached by them at 12 weeks of age.

Kittens can recognize their mothers by sight, as well as smell, by the end of the third week of age (Martin & Bateson, 1988). By about 6 weeks of age kittens demonstrate an adultlike response to visual and olfactory social stimuli, including silhouettes of adult cats and the scent of adult cat urine (Kolb & Nonneman, 1975). At about this time, the gape (Flehmen) response to cat urine appears; this becomes fully expressed by 7 weeks of age. It has been postulated that the gape response, in its full adult form, is an indication of the maturation of the vomeronasal organ. The classic adult threat posture of tail down, arched back, and erect ears is often seen concomitant with this and appears at about the same time (Kolb & Nonneman, 1975).

Kittens can learn from firsthand, trial-and-error experience and by watching other cats. They are quicker at observational learning if they are watching their mother (Chesler, 1969; John et al., 1968), suggesting that there may be a role for very elegant, complex, and detailed signaling behaviors that have not been studied. The role of early social exposure in learning is also suggested by experimental results derived from maze problemsolving tests (Hebb-Williams closed field test). Alley cats achieve much higher scores than do house cats, but they also make more errors (Pollard et al., 1971).

Three rigorous experiments elucidate the time periods during the first few months of life in which kittens are most susceptible to learning specific sets of behaviors, and the effects on these of varying amounts of exposure and handling by people (Karsh & Turner, 1988) (Table 4-1).

TABLE 4-1 IMPORTANT PERIODS IN THE DEVELOPMENT OF CAT BEHAVIOR

Behavior	Period Learned
Predatory behavior taught	3 weeks
Independent predatory behavior	5 weeks
Response to social and olfactory threats	6-8 weeks
Weaning completed	7 weeks
Object play (eye-paw coordination)	7-8 weeks
Social fighting	14+ weeks
Social play	
Early	3-4 weeks
Middle	4-7 weeks
Late	6-10 or 12 weeks

Data from Karsh and Turner, 1988.

TABLE 4-2 EFFECTS OF HANDLING ON STAYING AND APPROACH LATENCY FOR CATS HANDLED 15 MINUTES PER DAY

	Group 1	Group 2	Group 3
Duration of stay	41 sec[a,b]	24 sec[a,c]	15 sec[b,c]
Approach latency	11 sec[a,b]	42 sec[a]	39 sec[b]

Data from Karsh and Turner, 1988.
Pairwise comparisons are statistically significant at the following levels: a, p ≤ 0.001; b, p ≤ 0.025; c, p ≤ 0.075.

TABLE 4-3 EFFECTS OF HANDLING ON STAYING AND APPROACH LATENCY FOR CATS HANDLED 40 MINUTES PER DAY

	Group 1	Group 2
Duration of stay	77 sec	70 sec
Approach latency	9 sec	13 sec

Data from Karsh and Turner, 1988.

In a comparison of cats kept in maternity cages and exposed to different amounts of attention, kittens were petted for 15 minutes a day from 3 to 14 weeks of age (Group 1), were petted for 15 minutes a day from 7 to 14 weeks of age (Group 2), or experienced no handling at all for the entire period, from 3 to 14 weeks of age (Group 3). Cats were evaluated first at 14 weeks of age and every 2 to 4 weeks thereafter until the cats were a year of age. An unfamiliar experimenter could hold and lightly restrain a cat and the amount of time it took the cat to approach an unfamiliar person. The results indicated that early-handled cats stayed twice as long as the nonhandled cats (41 seconds versus 15 seconds; $p ≤ 0.001$) and longer than the late-handled cats (24 seconds; $p ≤ 0.025$). The results for the latency of approach indicated that early-handled cats would approach within 11 seconds, whereas nonhandled cats approached within 39 seconds ($p ≤ 0.025$). There was no statistically significant difference between the late-handled and the nonhandled cats in terms of latency of approach (42 seconds versus 39 seconds). A larger study would be required to determine whether the direction (late-handled have a longer latency than nonhandled) is significant and indicative of age-dependent learning about avoidance. The results suggest that, regardless, if the effect *is* reflective of reality, it is *not* insurmountable (Table 4-2).

When exposure time per day was increased to 40 minutes from 15 minutes for cats handled between weeks 3 and 14, they permitted holding for 77 seconds compared with 41 seconds when they were only handled for 15 minutes a day. Cats handled from 7 to 14 weeks of age (Group 2) allowed themselves to be handled for 70 seconds compared with 15 seconds when they were handled only 15 minutes a day (Table 4-3). It appears that the greatest effect of increased handling time occurs between 7 and 14 weeks of age.

The same pattern is apparent for approach latency (11 seconds versus 9 seconds) for cats handled between 3 and 14 weeks of age, but the difference is not statistically significant (Table 4-3). For cats handled from 7 to 14 weeks of age, increased exposure decreases approach latency from 42 to 13 seconds. This is statistically indistinguishable from the change found in cats handled very early. In addition, both of the age-groups (those handled from 3 to 14 weeks of age and those handled from 7 to 14 weeks of age) spent approximately the same amount of time (1.5 minutes) with an unknown individual. These results emphasize that early handling is important, and indicate that increasing the amount of time has the greatest effect for the slightly older and more coordinated kitten. Kittens 2 to 4 weeks exhibit plasticity physiologically and behaviorally: exposure to low temperature can influence the rate of temperature regulation development at 2 weeks of age, but this effect is lost by 4 weeks (Jensen et al., 1980). This observation reinforces the extent to which early ontogeny is important in cats.

Kittens handled only during the discrete periods of weeks 1 to 5, 2 to 6, 3 to 7, and 4 to 8 most definitely demonstrate the age-specific effects of handling. The mean holding scores of cats handled from 2 to 6 weeks of age and 3 to 7 weeks of age are significantly greater than those for cats handled at 1 to 5 weeks of age and 4 to 8 weeks of age (Table 4-4). There are no statistically significant differences between the handling scores for weeks 2 to 6 and 3 to 7, or for handling scores for weeks 1 to 5 and 4 to 8, but the handling scores for the former versus the latter groups *are* statistically significantly different from each other (see Table 4-4).

These differences are exaggerated for cats classified as non-timid cats, with the same statistical patterns apparent. The data are particularly interesting for cats

TABLE 4-4 MEAN HOLDING SCORES (DURATION OF STAY) IN SECONDS OF KITTENS IN CERTAIN AGE-GROUPS

	Time Handled (in seconds)			
	Weeks 1-5	Weeks 2-6	Weeks 3-7	Weeks 4-8
All cats	87	109	108	87
n	18	21	19	17
Non-timid cats	110*,†	126*,†	120*,†	104*,†
n	13	17	16	13
Timid cats	27	36	42	35
n	5	4	3	4

Seconds rounded to nearest integer.
*NS
†Weeks 1-5 + 4-8 v 2-6 + 3-7 $p < 0.05$

classified as genetically timid or unfriendly. Although the general pattern of the changes is similar to that for both the nontimid cats and the group composed of all cats, there are *no* statistically significant differences for the handling scores between *any* of the four periods. In part, this is because the sample sizes are quite small. Regardless, this indicates that even were the curve not relatively flat, the magnitude of the differences in handling scores for any of the periods, in comparisons of the timid cats with either of the other cats for those periods, is large, and timidity is a significant factor ($p < 0.001$, F < 1) that does not interact with handling periods (Karsh & Turner, 1988). This suggests a gene × environment effect. These data strongly suggest that not only should cats be handled early and often, but that if the cat is genetically predisposed to being timid or less friendly, handling may modulate the behavior to some extent, but that such cats will never respond to the same extent as will nontimid cats. This finding has profound implications for people wishing to choose cats as excellent pets. These results have been confirmed by McCune (1995).

The gene × environment interaction is further emphasized in comparisons of "shy" versus "nonshy" animals (Martin & Bateson, 1985). Cats that used the top of a complex climbing apparatus had *mothers* that spent the most time on the frame in the first sessions (John et al., 1968). There is much variation both within and among litters, but this result suggests that further work is needed on both maternal genetic effects and on the effects of the mothers' skills on observational learning in kittens. If litters stay with the queen for a protracted time in a social setting, the queen continues to show maternal behavior, even when her offspring are adults (Deag et al., 1988). This pattern is more apparent if offspring are *daughters*. Again, this may be indicative of a gene × environment interaction that can serve as a mechanism for facilitating the structure of female social groups. No studies exist that examine this possibility.

There is some evidence that if kittens are totally hand-reared from birth, they may have problems with successful reproduction when they are adults (Mellen, 1988). Baerends-van Roon and Baerends (1979) report that hand-rearing may contribute to later social problems even if such rearing occurs in the presence of the queen, but no specific behaviors have been identified that might be affected by hand-rearing. Clients should recognize age-specific, appropriate behaviors so they can encourage these and discourage inappropriate age-specific behaviors. It is unclear if the problems reported (Baerends-van Roon & Baerends, 1979) are amenable to behavioral modification or to early intervention and subsequent reshaping.

Karsh's studies suggest that adverse effects of early weaning could be modulated by the human environment. She postulates that one-person cats (a common correlation of early weaning) might be held longer and get more quality of attention (Karsh, 1984). Early weaning in a cattery situation can be part of a well-designed program to prevent the transmission of corona virus. In combination with Karsh's work, this suggests that breeders in cattery situations can produce not only healthy cats, but behaviorally well-adjusted cats if they are able to combine early weaning with intensive handling of the young kittens, starting at 2 weeks of age. Clients should be encouraged to learn to understand the types of behaviors associated with play as previously described and as described in the "Communication" section in this chapter, so that they can recognize when the cats are deviating from normal, age-specific play behavior. This helps them to shape any tendencies (related to early weaning) for earlier predatory and rough play behavior into more suitable behavior for pets.

The topic of timid versus nontimid cats warrants discussion. Personality types have been identified for domestic felines. Feaver and colleagues (1986) described some cats as "sociable, confident, and easy-going." This designation is equivalent to Karsh's (1983a,b) "confident" cat and to Meier and Turner's (1985) "trusting" cat. Feaver et al. (1986) also characterized some cats as "timid, nervous," which is equivalent to Karsh's (1983, 1984) "timid" cat and Turner's "shy, unfriendly" cat (1985). Feaver et al.'s (1986) classification of "active, aggressive" is analogous to Karsh's (1983, 1984) "active" and Pavlov's (1927) "excitatory temperament." Turner (1991) reported two types of "friendly" personalities in house cats. He characterized these as the "play" type versus the "petting" type. McCune (1995) has recharacterized friendliness as boldness. No association between age, sex, client, or household type was noted, but these "types" may be relevant in discussions of cats with status-related aggression and play-related aggression.

Although cat *breeds* comprise only a minority of pet cats (6%-7%; Bradshaw, 1992a), breed-specific generalizations have been made. Siamese have been considered "friendlier" than other cats, but some of this "friendliness" may be because they seek heat because of a thin coat (Bradshaw, 1992a). Such reasoning may not be sufficient to account for why Siamese males are considered more paternal than other breeds (Beaver, 1992). Hart and Hart (1984) polled cat show judges and found that judges considered Siamese cats the most outgoing, whereas Russian blues were viewed as the most shy and withdrawn. Kuiat females have been described as more aggressive than males (Beaver, 1992). It is important to realize that such generalizations are not based on any quantification or qualification of actual behaviors but on subjective opinions. Even if such opinions were based on quantification of actual behaviors, such quantification would still be subject to an evaluation of the variability both within and among litters, and within and among breeds. These data are not available. Still, genetic effects have been postulated in some lines of blue-eyed, white cats. Many of these cats, particularly females, have been reported to be timid (Beaver, 1990, 1992). It has been suggested that this timidity is associated with deafness and an inability to perceive sudden changes in the auditory environment (Robinson, 1977). Coat-color effects have been noted for both mink and foxes with regard to heritable tendencies toward fear and aggression (Bradshaw, 1992a), and coat pelage characteristics have been associated with tractability and startle responses in cattle (Grandin et al., 1995). The full extent of the interaction between coat characteristics and behavior is not understood but may be important given the fate of neuroectoderm in ontogeny (Smith & Gong, 1974). Observations of patterns of behaviors within and between litters have suggested that temperament of kittens is largely paternally determined (Beaver, 1992). More work is needed on any genetic propensities for behavior, but progress has been made recently by McCune (1995). In a controlled experimental study, cats fathered by "friendly" or outgoing cats were more likely to explore unfamiliar people and inanimate objects when tested at 1 year of age. These effects were enhanced by early handling.

SENSORY FUNCTION AND STRUCTURE
Cutaneous Sensation

The cutaneous response is interesting in cats and may account for some of their abnormal and undesirable behaviors. Their cutaneous mechanism is composed of both type 1 SA (slow-adapting) epidermal units, and type 2 SA dermal units. The type 1 SA units are grouped in "touch corpuscles" and terminate in specialized structures called Merkel cells (Iggo, 1966). The resting rate of the discharge is proportional to the amount of the displacement of the hair or the indentation of the skin. Accordingly, cats are very sensitive to stroking. Anyone who has ever stroked a cat has noticed this. The type 2 SA dermal units are far more widely distributed and terminate in Ruffini endings that are very sensitive to touch. Cats have an abundance of both types of units in greater proportion and density than does the rabbit, an animal that has been regarded as extremely sensitive to touch (Iggo, 1982).

The scratch reflex in response to stimulation on particular points of the skin provides a fairly good mapping of the SA units and rapidly adapting mechanoreceptors.

The extent to which the cat's SA type 1 and type 2 receptors may factor into the development of self-mutilation (overgrooming, psychogenic alopecia), and may be one of the mechanisms for this apparent obsessive-compulsive type of disorder is unknown, but the association suggests that further inquiry is needed. There are also SA cells in the soft tissue at the bases of claws that signal the degree of extension and sideways displacement of the claw (Gordon & Jukes, 1964). This feature has been totally ignored when the subject of onchyectomy (declawing) arises, yet certainly the presence of these SA cells could be one of the mechanisms for persistent discomfort or "phantom pain" that some declawed cats appear to have. No population-specific prevalence data exist for this condition.

Cats have sensory hairs (vibrissae) around the head. These are found on the cheeks in the shape of whiskers (mystacials), above the eyes (superciliary vibrissae), and on the side of the face (genal vibrissae). They do not have interramal vibrissae associated with their submandibular glands. This absence may be associated with their pattern of social investigation that contrasts from that seen in dogs: nose-to-nose, neck-to-flank, then anal sniffing (Leyhausen, 1979). All vibrissae are supplied with rapidly adapting (RA) mechanoreceptors and SA units. These signal the central nervous system about the amplitude, direction, and rate of the displacement of the vibrissae. Cats possess short, stiff hairs around the base of the lips that have similar receptors. Cats are preeminently adapted to be predators. They have laterally compressed canines, rooted in mechanoreceptors, that hold food and permit them to dislocate the vertebrae of prey in one bite (Bradshaw, 1992a). In combination with the mechanoreceptors at the base of the canines, these vibrissae allow exquisite control over adjustment of position in the predatory strike. Carpal hairs on the ventrum of the carpus have both SA and RA receptors and vibration-detecting Pacinian corpuscles (Burgess & Perl, 1973). These can function in both the pawing motions that are seen in play and the pouncing motions that are seen in predatory behavior. Cats are extremely manually dexterous. They are particularly sensitive to touch around the muzzle and have a somatosensory area larger than that of a dog (Bradshaw, 1992). The scratch response is a "complete reflex"—one that requires no feedback from the forebrain. The characteristic postures for urination and defecation, as well as burying behavior, are also complete reflexes and may be associated with some of the limited scratch behaviors.

It is certainly not uncommon to see cats scratch in the air (Bradshaw, 1992a). Mating and estrus behaviors are also considered reflexive, as are the reflexive components of rubbing, rolling, calling, crouching, treading with the hindlegs, and the afterattack (Bard & Macht, 1958).

Biting in cats has been studied as a corollary of studies of agonistic and predatory behaviors (Ademec, 1975; Ademec et al., 1980a, b, c). One of the classic feline bites has been characterized as the "quiet biting attack" (Bernston & Leibowitz, 1973). This is controlled by groups of neurons in the hypothalamus and midbrain that mediate the effects of learned behavior (Bernston et al., 1976a, b; c, Kolgan, 1989 Egger & Flynn, 1963; Hutchinson & Renfew, 1966; Levinson & Flynn, 1965). This type of bite involves trigger zones around the face, lips, and mouth, and the tactile stimuli of the guard hairs in the forepaw. It is apparent how the RA and SA receptors in the vibrissae interact to facilitate this. Again, this may be one of the reasons that cats with self-mutilation disorders do more chewing while dogs tend to do more licking. The extent to which these neurological responses are responsible for self-mutilation behaviors and potential obsessive-compulsive disorders is not currently explored. Persistent biting in cats requires the stimulus of the trigeminal receptors around the mouth, plus all the touch receptors already discussed (Siegal & Potts, 1988). This association could also function in grooming abnormalities and potential obsessive-compulsive disorders.

Olfactory Sensory Epithelium

Feline olfactory epithelium is relatively extensive. Domestic pet felines have 20 cm^2 of olfactory epithelium compared with 2 to 4 cm^2 in humans. This elaboration does not quite approach that of the maxilloturbinal development seen in the dog, where rapid respirations during exercise bring more air over the olfactory apparatus. The difference between the canine carnivore and the feline carnivore in the extent of olfactory epithelium could be an adaptation to differences in hunting styles (Radinsky, 1975). Canids tend to take down prey much larger than themselves; canids as a group follow the prey over an extensive period of time. Most cats are solitary hunters, and hunt and consume prey that requires a burst of, but not sustained, activity. It is possible that the development of the olfactory apparatus is an adaptation to, or a corollary of, these differences in hunting styles. It is known that dogs can detect some compounds at concentrations 1000 times lower than humans could detect them (Davis, 1973). It is likely that cats are similar in their ability to do this.

Cats, unlike dogs, exhibit a true gape/Flehmen response. They possess a vomeronasal organ (VNO)/fluid pump. Fluid is expelled into the canal (as far as the roof of the mouth) and is drawn back into the VNO along with accompanying chemical signals (Hart, 1983; Hart & Leedy, 1987). The equivalent apparatus is nonfunctional in dogs, and no chemoreceptors are found in the sacs (Ewer, 1973).

COMMUNICATION

There are three main modes of communication that are used by cats:

1. Vocal and auditory communicatory mechanisms that are largely exploited by animals that are separated in space over long distances
2. Vision, which is most useful for animals that are close to each other
3. Olfaction, which is useful for animals separated not only in time, but also in space

Olfactory Communication

The cat has sebaceous glands on the tail (the caudal glands), the forehead (temporal glands), the lips (perioral glands), the chin, the pads (pedal glands), and associated with the whiskers. Rubbing of the tail and lips is more common on inanimate objects (Fox, 1975). Rubbing may make it easier to pick up a scent rather than function to deposit one (Hart & Haugen, 1971; Rieger, 1979). Cheeks, ears, and flanks may also produce odorous secretions (Wolski, 1982). Cats that rub on people are said to be *bunting*. This is associated with scent deposition. It is also associated with objects that inspire a gape or Flehmen response—urine as old as 3 days can elicit it (Verberne & deBoer, 1976). Bunting may be a display of social status or social dominance. Rubbing with cheek glands is more commonly exhibited by a dominant animal toward a subordinate (Macdonald et al., 1987). The form of head rubbing depends in part on topography (Verbene & deBoer, 1976). Cats that rub at the level of the cheek usually form a line from the corner of the mouth to the ear; if the cat is rubbing a higher object, he or she usually rubs the under surface of the object using his or her forehead and ears followed by the side of the throat. Inanimate objects are rubbed by the flanks and tail. Males do not appear to rub more than females, but they may have more active sebaceous glands (Verbene & deBoer, 1976).

If no other cats are present when a new cat is introduced into the environment, the new cat will sniff the room and rub with the submandibular gland. If other cats are present, this sequence is omitted. If two cats are introduced into a room, the one that is familiar with the room initially becomes the dominant animal and may follow the new cat, attempting to smell his or her anal region. Rebuff usually takes the form of swatting and hissing. Such observations are particularly relevant for the introduction of new cats into established households and support observations that cats can share time and space (Bernstein & Strack, 1993).

The role of olfaction cannot be overestimated in the deposition of urine and feces, including spraying and nonspraying marking. The rate of scent marking has been noted to correlate with dominance status or rank (Ralls, 1971). There has been some evidence that dominant male cats may scent-mark more by rubbing their cheeks than do more subordinate males. Spraying is a complex feline behavior; it has been postulated that males frustrated in rubbing and other social interactions might spray as a displacement activity (Ralls, 1971). Lower status males could also spray as a passive status signal rather than engaging in an active one involving physical conflict.

The interaction between status and the deposition of urine or feces, regardless of the form of the urine, is complicated and poorly investigated. It is not unusual for cats to mark the edges of their range with urine. If a new male or female comes into an area, the first approach is often to mark with urine. Females tend to mark by spraying only when they enter a hunting range, and then intermittently while foraging (Fox, 1975). Estrous females spray more frequently than do nonestrous females, regardless of whether they are hunting (Macdonald et al., 1987). Both sexes exhibit a Flehmen response to unfamiliar urine. DeBoer (1977a) estimated that urine loses most of its attraction after 24 hours. In free-ranging cats, feces are usually covered in core areas of farms, but are not often covered on pathways (peripheral areas) (Macdonald et al., 1987).

The extent to which anal sacs are involved in olfactory communication or scent marking is underexplored. Urine that is sprayed may be more oily and viscous than urine that is eliminated in a squatting manner, and may contain anal sac secretions (Wolski, 1982). Feral cats spend more time sniffing sprayed urine when compared with excreted urine of unknown cats, suggesting that the urine produced may be qualitatively different (Natoli, 1985). In experimental situations, cats can distinguish between urine that has been deposited by spraying and squatting (Passanisi & Macdonald, 1990).

The ability to respond to catnip is genetic (Hart and Leedy, 1985; Tucker & Tucker, 1988; Wolski, 1982). *Cis*-trans-neptalactone-monoterpene can be detected in concentrations as low as one part in 10 to 10 (Waller et al., 1969). Cats that respond to catnip experience an intense combination of both face rubbing and body rolling and may lick, chew, or eat the catnip, shake their heads, gape, roll, rub, and twitch (Hatch, 1972; Palen & Goddard, 1966; Todd, 1962). These behaviors are done in a context and style that sets them totally apart from those associated with sex or hunting behaviors and are not unlike obsessive-compulsive behaviors. This suite of behavioral responses to catnip and the mechanism for them have not been clearly elucidated.

Visual Communication

Cats have acute visual capabilities. Although they can discriminate elimination at $1/5$ the threshold of humans, their resolution is only $1/10$ that of humans (Ewer, 1973). Siamese cats appear to have decreased stereoscopic vision compared with other feline breeds (Packwood & Gordon, 1975). Felines, like astronauts, arctic explorers, and seafarers, may experience an environmental training effect on their vision: free-ranging cats are hypermetropic, whereas caged cats are myopic (Belkin et al., 1977). Cats are capable of color discrimination (Sechzer & Brown, 1964). The extent to which this ability factors into intraspecific signaling is unexplored. The contrast between the color of pupil and iris must be apparent to cats. Much of their immediate intent in fearful and agonistic situations is communicated by pupil size and shape. Round pupils are associated with fear, oblong pupils with aggression, and slightly off-round pupils with a relaxed state. Size of pupil correlates with intensity of underlying state.

Visual communication in domestic pet felines involves the use of the eyes, ears, mouth, tail, and coat (pelage) (Wolski, 1982). Facial signals change far more quickly than do postural signals and may in fact contain the most up-to-date contextual information based on the response of the receiver of the signal. Postures that also convey information include the body posture, the head carriage, the back position (arched or level posture), and leg positioning. Leyhausen (1979) has illustrated sequential variation in all of these postures and signals in a classic set of illustrations (Fig. 4-1). Although Leyhausen's interpretations are possibly more static than is currently believed to be representative, they do outline the range of feline communication. Veterinarians and clients should understand the signals that the cats are giving to them and to other individuals in the household; should it be necessary, this will permit intervention that can prevent an undesirable event, or that corrects the cat in a manner. To this end, the Leyhausen pictures (Figs. 4-1 and 4-2) can be very useful for both veterinarians and clients in helping to describe and identify the postures.

Ears are fluid and move quickly in domestic pet felines. Erect ears are apparent when the cat is alert and focusing on a stimulus. Slightly relaxed ears are indicative of a cat that is not focusing on any stimulus, but could focus instantly; such a cat is relaxing and not intimately involved with any other interaction in the environment. Ears that are swiveled, displaying the inner pinnae sideways, are indicative of increased passive aggression or of offensive or actively assertive activity. Ears that are swiveled downward and sideways, or that are rotated downward, are associated with defensive, deferential, or more submissive signaling. Ears that are pulled all the way down and to the rear so that the inner pinnae are not at all visible, while the outer pinnae are flattened in a masklike molding against the head, are indicative of extreme defense postures or the potential aggression when all other choices have failed. However, if the inner pinna is visible and flat against the head again as if sculpted in a mask, this is indicative of extremely offensive behavior and the potential for actual aggression should avoidance fail.

The pupil is the most instructive and least ambigu-

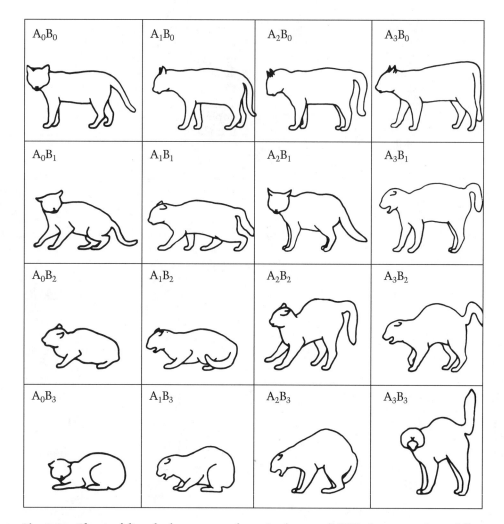

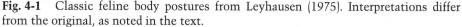

Fig. 4-1 Classic feline body postures from Leyhausen (1975). Interpretations differ from the original, as noted in the text.

A_0B_0 represents the basic relaxed, copacetic cat that is monitoring the environment.

As one moves from A_0B_0 to A_3B_0 (across the X-axis), the cat is becoming more assertive, more confident, and more offensively aggressive. Note that even offensive aggression here is passive and is related more to eliciting deferential behavior than about actual combat. Factors to note include the fully extended hind legs, the elevated rump and piloerected tail, the set of the head and neck, and the ears that are slightly pulled back.

Moving from A_0B_0 to A_0B_3 (down the Y-axis), the cat is becoming more withdrawn, more avoidant of interaction, potentially more fearful, and more defensively aggressive. Aggression will ensue only when this cat can no longer escape.

The cat represented in A_3B_3 is exhibiting mixed signals and is in an extremely heightened state of reactivity. The tail is elevated, indicating that interaction is a possibility. The back is arched in a classic fearful posture (note that the back is also arched in A_0B_3, but the cat is lying down). The neck is tucked and the underside of the neck and all teeth are exposed. Full disclosure is a signal that is used to diffuse an undesirable situation. This cat is signaling that he will stand his ground but will not overtly seek aggression unless pursued. It would be inappropriate to call either this posture or that portrayed in A_0B_3 as fearful aggression: whereas the latter precludes withdrawal, withdrawal and avoidance are the first choices of the former. Note that the cat portrayed in A_3B_3 is not confident like the cat in A_3B_0. The cat in A_3B_0 will back down any challengers and will pursue them if they do not back down; the cat in A_2B_3 would neither seek nor choose to interact with a challenger, given the choice.

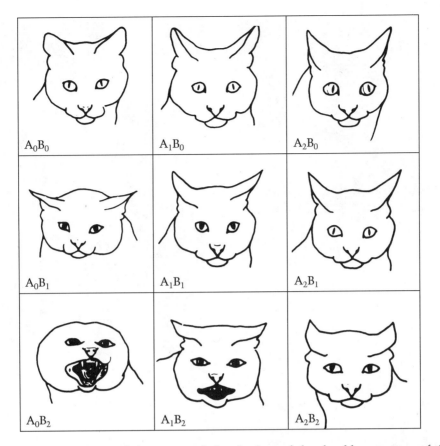

Fig. 4-2 The position of the ears, neck, head, plane of the shoulders, posture of the mouth and nares, and shape and size of the pupils are all important in feline communication.

A_0B_0 represents the relaxed cat who is monitoring the environment.

A_2B_2 represents a cat that is more offensively and assertively aggressive as represented by body posture A_3B_0 (see Fig. 4-1). Note the set neck and shoulders, slightly lowered head, movement of the pinnae, dilation of the nares, and clamping of mouth. This is a very confident and serious cat.

A_2B_0 represents that cat that is fearful and attempting to withdraw. This cat will avoid interactions if possible. Note the positioning of the eyes and the oblique (non-direct) gaze. The cat's ears are back, but up, and his neck and head are more withdrawn than set and pushed forward as in A_2B_2. This is the facial expression of the cat in A_0B_3 in Fig. 4-1.

A_0B_2 represents a cat that will pursue aggression, but only as the last resort. Note that the neck, inside of the throat, and the teeth are all exposed, in contrast to A_2B_2. Note also that the pinnae are totally swiveled and everted. This is the facial expression of the cat in A_3B_3 in Fig. 4-1. (Classic feline facial expressions from Leyhausen [1975]. Interpretations differ from the original, as noted in the text.)

ous source of feline signals. Unfortunately, people may not be able to see the pupillary changes in time to help them to avoid damage. Cats read cat behavior better than people read cat behavior. Miotic pupils are correlated with autonomic parasympathetic responses. Mydriatic pupils are correlated with sympathetic, fight-or-flight response. It is important to evaluate pupil size in conjunction with ambient light conditions because many pupils could dilate even in a relaxed cat if the room is dark. Regardless, a direct stare is a challenge or threat in cats and is usually exhibited by high-ranking, confident cats. The lower ranking cat usually withdraws in response (see Fig. 4-2).

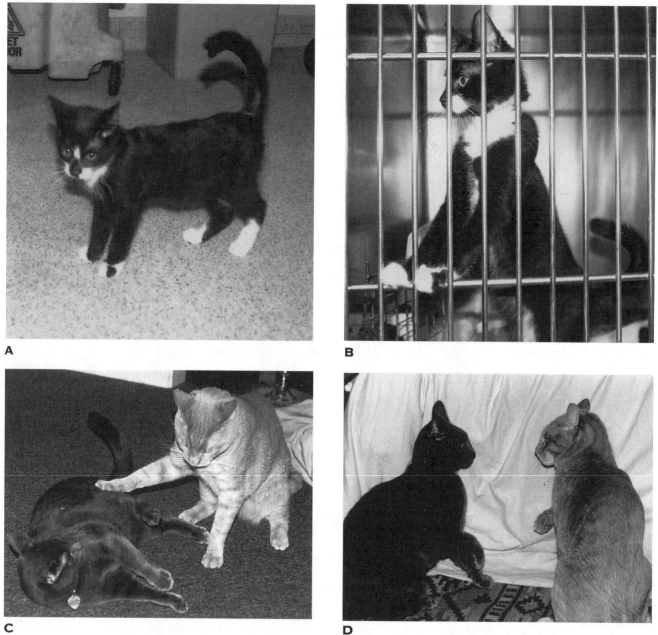

Caro (1981b) noted that as cats age, social, play patterns become associated with approaches, pawing, and bites, instead of the behaviors associated with kittenhood—arches, rears, and chases. **A,** Young kitten demonstrating arch of tail and slight arch of back and rump. **B,** Young kitten demonstrating rearing behavior while caged. **C, D,** Rearing behavior shifts into pawing behavior as the kitten ages. *Continued.*

The tail is a very useful signaling device. Tails that are kept out and behind usually signal that the cat is alert, confident, relaxed, and friendly—the basic copacetic, willing-to-explore-the-environment state. Tails that are erect, but slightly curled, can also indicate a relaxed and friendly cat, but a cat that is very outgoing and would volitionally solicit interaction. Cats that are walking or trotting often hold their tails at 40-degree angles to the horizon of the back; the tail lowers as the pace increases (Kiley-Worthington, 1976, 1984). Their changed posture may be primarily functional, not communicatory. Offensive postures use tails that are straight down or that are held perpendicular to the ground. Erect, bristled tails are associated with a combination of offensive (passive) and defensive (active) behaviors. Any animal with an erect, bristled tail is in a heightened state of reactivity and will react in a context that is indicated by its facial signals.

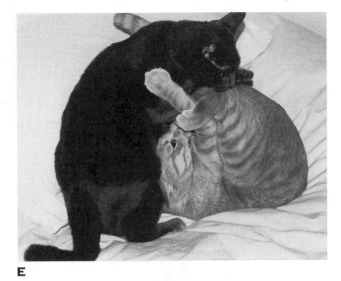

E

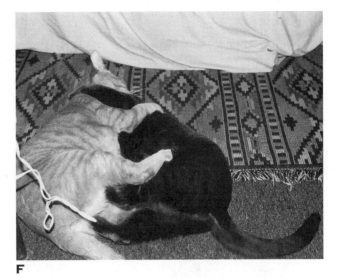

F

E, F, Chase behavior metamorphoses into bite behavior. (Photos by K.L. Overall and Liz Krug.)

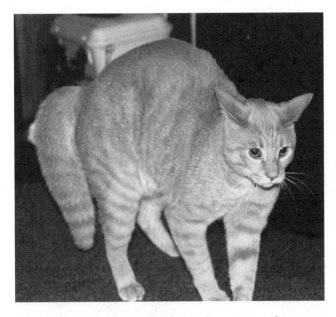

Cat exhibiting behavior similar to that portrayed in A_3B_2, Fig. 4-1. Note the mixed signals of trepidation about further interaction coupled with an unwillingness to back down. This cat has a broad hind limb stance, providing him with a good pivot zone, and arched, elevated, and piloerected tail. His neck and shoulders are set, but his mouth is clamped shut and his neck is not exposed. Notice that he has begun to elevate one front paw. The extent to which paw signals and strikes factor into integration of further aggressive behaviors has not been studied. (Photo by Liz Krug.)

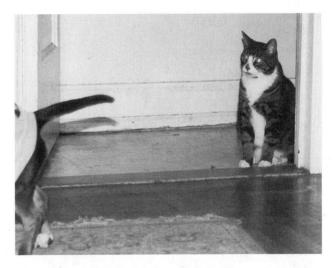

This cat is confident and alert and merely monitoring the rest of his social environment. Note the erect ears. (Photo by Emily Elliot and Nirit Rosenberg.)

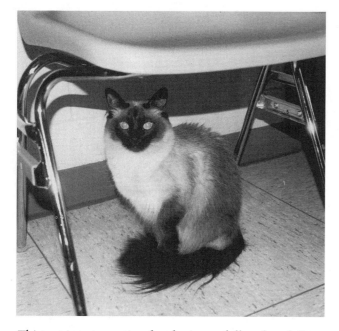

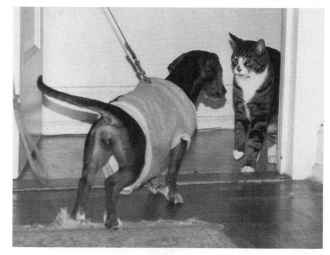

This cat is not reactive, but he is not fully relaxed. Note that the fur on his back is slightly spiky. He is not completely at ease in the surroundings. He is also relatively withdrawn: his tail is wrapped around his feet, indicating a decreased propensity for interaction. Notice how the long fur could affect signaling behavior. (Photo by K.L. Overall.)

The cat in the last photo on p. 61 has risen to a standing posture and picked up one paw as he stares at the dog. The stare is a threat or warning that will, if necessary, be reinforced by the paw. The cat does not want to interact and is very confident. (Photo by Emily Elliot and Nirit Rosenberg.)

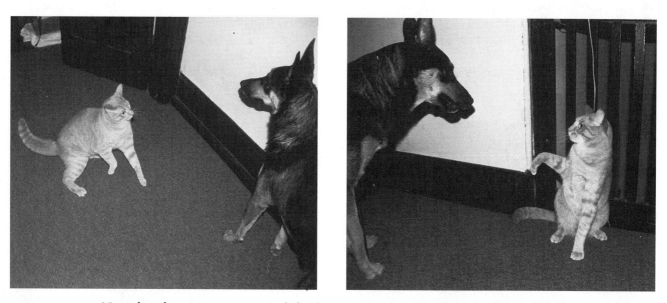

Note that the cat's ears are swiveled sideways in an increasingly extreme manner as the distance between the cat and dog decreases and as the cat is unable to get away. He is sitting and warning the dog, but his ears are cocked, his jaw and neck are set, and he is staring at the dog, who is actually not making direct eye contact. (Photo by Liz Krug.)

In the second photo, this cat swivels his ears as the puppy approaches. Note the curled tail and the withdrawn stance. (Photo by Emily Elliot and Nirit Rosenberg.)

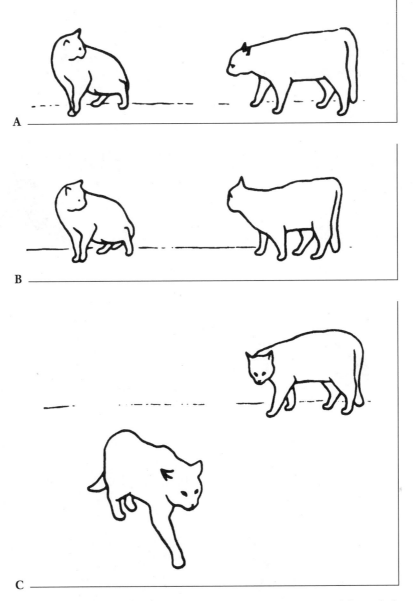

Fig. 4-3 This sequence represents an overt, assertive confident challenge. **A,** Note the stare and rump humped posture from the cat on the right. The recipient of the challenge has picked up one forepaw in an intention signal, has tucked its tail and lowered its hindquarters (a deferential gesture) and has tucked its neck while flattening its ears. **B,** The challenger then looks away and the recipient of the challenge intensifies its behaviors. **C,** The response to the challenge is withdrawal. Notice that the challenger continues to stare. (From Leyhausen, 1979.)

Bradshaw (1992a) has adapted the classic tail signaling as described by Leyhausen (1979), in combination with data from Kiley-Worthington (1976) and unpublished data from Brown, and classified tail positions as vertical, half-raised, horizontal, concave, lower, and between legs. The vertical tail position has been associated in Bradshaw's classification with greeting, where the animal could be walking, trotting, or standing, or engaging in social play or object play, and sexual approaches by females. The half-raised tail appears to be solely associated with sexual approaches by females. Horizontally held tails can indicate an amica-

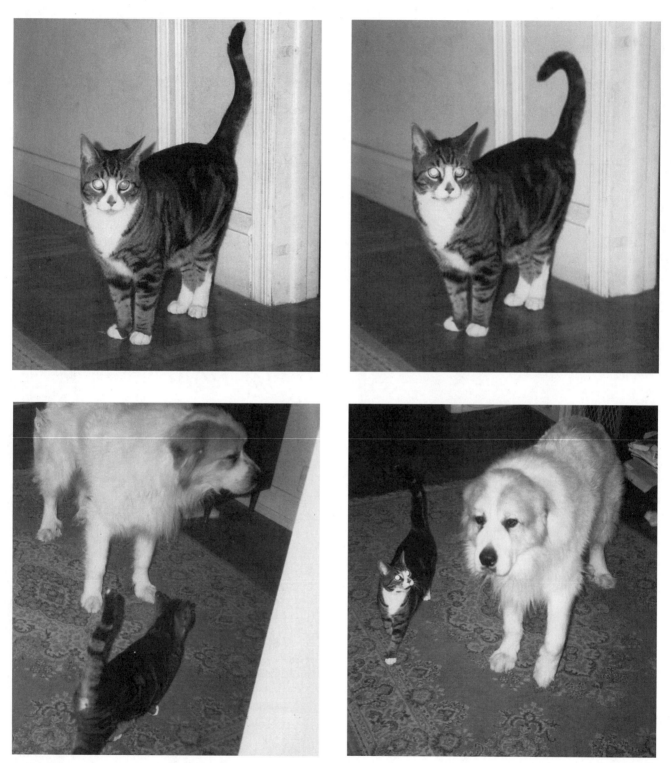

For legend see opposite page.

Continued.

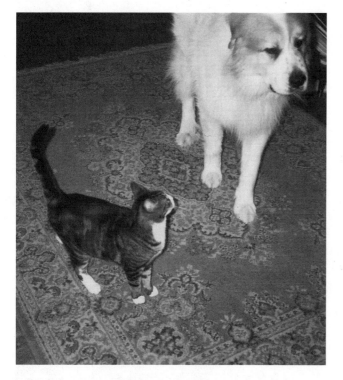

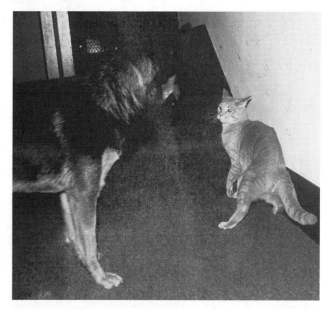

All of these poses show cats with erect tails. The tails can be curved or straight but all indicate volitional solicitation of interaction. Interaction can be good or bad, a challenge or a deferential behavior. Context and the recipient's response is important. The dog in the photo above is not meeting the stare (challenge) of the cat. This is a very pushy cat who has solicited and then pummeled the dogs. (Photos by Emily Elliot and Nirit Rosenberg.)

ble approach or a sexual approach by the female. Concave tails are indicative of defensive aggression, whereas lowered tails are indicative of offensive aggression. Tails found between the legs are indicative of submission. These tail signals and other body postures are summarized in Table 4-5.

Not all concave tail postures fit this classification. Some cats, particularly young cats, often carry their tails in U-shaped, concave position. If the tail is concave in a U over the dorsum, the cat usually changes the distance between itself and another animal by inactive means. It may chase the other cat and decrease the distance simply because it will run the other cat down. This signal can also serve as a distance-increasing measure if the cat is able to chase an intruder away, emphasizing the role of context and timing in the understanding of any signal function. Tails that are concave away from the back in an inverted U shape usually are associated with animals that are willing to interact (an interaction may be aggressive or not), but that are a little unsure about taking the lead. This posture is often accompanied by sitting on the hind feet. Individuals displaying these postures generally decrease the distance between themselves and an-

Offensive tail postures include those that are held between straight down and perpendicular to the ground. The rest of the cat's signals and posture indicate an offensive tack. (Photo by Liz Krug)

TABLE 4-5 FELINE TAIL POSTURES

Posture	Interpretation of Signal
Vertical	Play
	Greeting, often with motion
	Sexual approaches by females
	Frustration (if whipped)
Half-raised	Sexual approaches by females
Horizontal	Amicable approach
	Sexual approach by females
Concave	Defensive behavior
Lower	Offensive aggression (if rigid and flicking)
	Defensive aggression (if more flaccid)
	Relaxed and surveying environment if tail still or langorously moving and possessed of tone
Between the legs	Submission
	Fear

Adapted from Bradshaw, 1992.

other individual, but do so by soliciting the other individual to play the active role in decreasing the distance.

More recent work by Bernstein (Bernstein & Strack, 1993) has identified a five-posture tail classification that is a variant of that already discussed. In positions 1 to 3, respectively, the tail is slightly down and behind the cat; curved above the horizon of the back, with or without movement, or high above the back

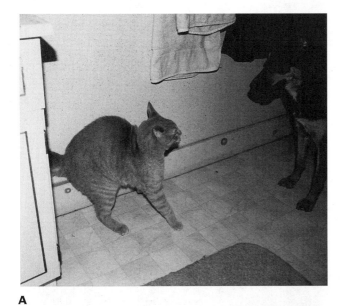

A

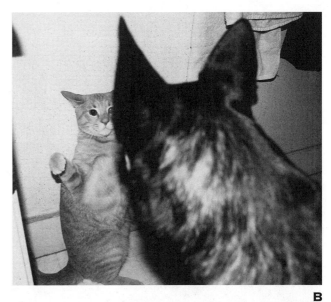

B

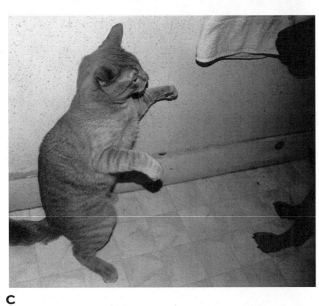

C

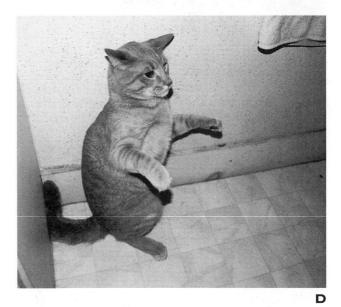

D

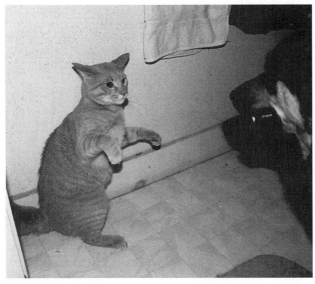

E

The cat portrayed here is confident, assertive, and trapped. Notice that his tail is bristled as he is rebuffing the encroaching dog. Ear postures are those for offensive, not defensive aggression as indicated in Fig. 4-2, A_2B_2. Notice that the cat's first response is to box, not to bite. Given the context, this is an expected sequence. Cats with inappropriate aggressions will bite without preparatory behaviors. This cat's pupils are dilated, his jaw and neck are set, and he continues to stare at the dog, who is actually just being a pest. In the first photo the cat is demonstrating posture A_2B_2 from Fig. 4-1. Once the dog does not back down, the cat switches to full assertive mode. (Photos by Liz Krug.)

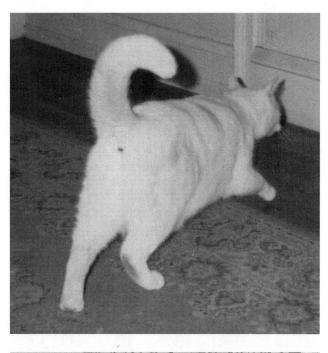

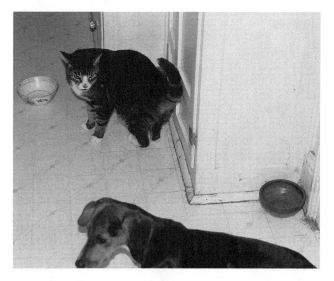

Concave tails can act as distance increasing measures. In this case the cat is successfully discouraging the dog from approaching his dish. Eye and ear signals are also important. (Photo by Emily Elliot and Nirit Rosenberg.)

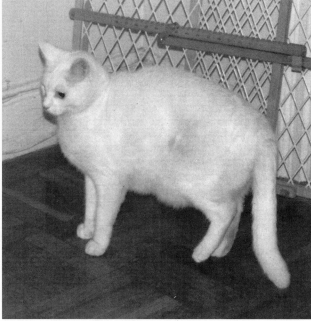

Concave tails (U shaped tails over the dorsum) are associated with defensive aggression, avoidance, and distance increasing measures. This cat is avoiding a dog. When the dog continues to pursue, the cat switches his tail posture to a lowered tail, which is associated with more offensive aggression. (Photo by Emily Elliot and Nirit Rosenberg.)

with the tip slightly back and curved or up. These positions are associated, respectively, with information gathering, monitoring approaches, and beginning a non-aggressive interaction. In position 4, the tail is curved down, and between the legs. This is a defen-

sive posture that indicates that escape is a possible option. In position 5 the entire tail is whipped. This is associated with an incipient and active aggressive behavior (biting and scratching) or is a precursor to active, defensive escape. It has also been associated with unattainable prey (birds outside a window); if the cat is really frustrated, the teeth also chatter and the cat may meow.

It has been suggested that some of these tail postures, particularly in very aggressive or defensive situations, are less apparent because of the risk of potential injury to the tail. Most clients are tacitly aware of the extent to which cats communicate with tails, but few understand that in a grassland environment (one presumptive ancestral environment) a tail can be an excellent long-distance signal. Some signaling may have been derived from the adaptation to deflect tails during situations in which they may be injured.

Discussions of body posture should include the position of the head, the back, and the legs, usually in combination with each other.

Head up: A head-up, back-straight posture, accompanied by a tail that is out and behind, is generally indicative of a relaxed, alert cat.

Straight legs; rump hump: Straight legs, particularly if they are accompanied by elevated hindquarters, are indicative of an offensive posture. This posture is simple for the cat to execute because the cat's hind legs are slightly longer than are the front legs. This creates the classic appearance where the rump is humped so that the base of the tail and the rump become very apparent. The fur on the tail may be piloerected, but the tail is held down. An elevated rump is visible from a distance; almost invariably, if there is an agonistic interaction, the animal that successfully exhibits the elevated rump posture first is the animal that controls the interaction.

Sternal crouch: A posture that involves a sternal crouch is defensive; this usually is accompanied by a tail that is on the ground and tucked to one side. Once again, it may be true that it is extremely important to protect the tail because it is so involved in signaling.

Belly-up: The belly-up display involves the ventrum and is the classic posture seen in play in kittens. It is also seen in some fights. The common interpretation of this display usually includes commentary that play and aggression can often be part of the same reactive, interactive suites of motivation. It might be more appropriate to view this display in the same context that similar behaviors in rodents have been reviewed (Ferris et al., 1995). A belly-up display could indicate an unwillingness to pursue a more overt, direct, agonistic behavior. When a cat displays its underbelly it indicates, by exposing one of its most vulnerable areas, that it is exhibiting deferential behavior, much in the same way that canids do when they display the side of their neck to the individual with whom they are interacting. This is a signal that indicates that one is not willing to initiate and pursue an overtly aggressive act. Cats that display the belly-up posture in a protective, defensive context also tend to bring their back feet up, with their claws unsheathed, to protect the softest, most vulnerable area of their abdomen; they are still giving the same signals about an unwillingness to initiate the aggression. In such cases, if the aggressor backs off, the cat that is displaying the protective belly-up posture will not pursue the aggression. Hence, it is appropriate to interpret this as a deferential behavior. There has been a substantial amount of work conducted in the fields of evolutionary biology and behavioral ecology about signals that function to indicate when one will or will not engage in pursuit. Such signals are valuable because they permit the avoidance of conflict. Much signaling and posturing is intended to avoid actual battle. Such signals also allow the signaler to conserve the energy that would otherwise be used in a fight. The belly-up display must be interpreted in the context in which it is occurring: part of that context is the positioning of the hind feet.

Arched back: The classic "Halloween cat" is the final body posture with which most clients are familiar. This is another posture that indicates a high degree of reactivity. Reactivity can be directed in either an offensive or a defensive manner. Cats exhibiting this posture are not conflicted about those behaviors, but instead are informing the individual with whom the interaction is occurring that, depending on that individual's behavior, the cat is prepared to act in either modality, although they would not seek active aggression. Such signals provide all of the participants with the option of stopping the interaction.

Overt fights are far more likely if there is no difference in social stature between the individuals and if the cats view each other as equals (Wolski, 1982). Cats with high status, or dominant or high-ranking cats may decline to actively fight their antagonist; instead they will often just walk away from the individual that is perceived to have "lost" the fight, and then sit, groom, and look away. Only a very confident, high-ranking cat (i.e., a cat who could elicit deference) would be able to do this. Some high-ranking cats will leave and abandon the situation. This indicates that they are sufficiently confident that they do not even feel the need to maintain an enforcement presence. These cats can spray in a victory display; spraying is a very overt, long-lasting challenge.

The classic definition of dominance emphasizes both the minimization of fighting and that a truly "dominant" animal can aggress against another with impunity (Immelmann & Beer, 1989). Dominant animals seldom actually aggress against others, although they engage in much posturing and signaling behavior that encourages the other animal, or the recipient, to initiate a deferential behavior. This signaling or posturing can be very subtle, and can be as simple as standing and blocking access to an entryway or to a desired area. Examples of this interpretation are found in the classic feline display postures. In some superb studies done by Feldman (1993, 1994), juvenile males roll over preferentially for older males, and older males were the recipients of most of the "belly-up" displays. Dominant cats stay in litter boxes longer than lower ranking cats, control access to them, and use them first (Bernstein & Strack, 1993). These observations indicate that it is important to evaluate these displays in the context in which they occur. Play and deference do share some aspects in common with regard to underlying motivational states and information about intent that is conveyed. Telling these apart is challenging.

Finally, a note about vibrissae position: whiskers rotate forward with aggression.

Vocal Communication

Cat vocalizations have been described by a variety of authors, but the first to do so in a systematic manner was Moelk (1979, 1944). Moelk's classification of vocal communication involved five categories of vocal display: the purr, the chirr, the call, the meow, and the growl/snarl/hiss.

Adults. *The purr:* The purr is the classic feline sound that is recognized as being associated with a contented cat. It is given by nursing kittens and, occasionally, by older cats when they are slightly anxious. Very little sonographic information is available about cat calls (see McKinley, 1982), but it is conceivable that the purr that is elicited in the slightly anxious situation is considerably different from one elicited in others, and that it communicates different information than does the purr that is elicited in very relaxed situations.

The chirr: The chirr sound is very much like a meow that has been rolled on the tongue; it is given by a queen when she is calling the kittens out of the nest. Often, if cats are friendly with each other, the chirr is a sound that one might make in eliciting the approach of another.

The call: The call is a very loud murmur that is produced with the mouth closed. It is primarily associated with a female who is solicitous of mating. The same signal has been reported to occur in males who are fighting with each other (Wolski, 1982).

The meow: The meow is probably the most variable of the feline communicatory signals, although without sonographic analysis it would be inappropriate to make too many conjectures about it. The meow is the classic signal heard when cats are announcing their presence, are soliciting attention from any other living thing (epimeletic), or are thwarted in their ability to attain something that they would like.

The growl: The growl/snarl/hiss sounds are all open-mouthed calls that are given in both offensive and defensive agonistic situations. They may function to warn about subsequent behaviors, should the aggressor pursue the interaction. There may also be a component of intimidation to these sounds that is associated with sex and body size (although no one has studied this aspect for domestic pet cats). An element of vocal surprise may accompany these signals, which could be beneficial in an agonistic situation.

Chatter: Kiley-Worthington (1984) also noted that cats also chatter their teeth when watching unattainable play; this was termed displacement activity, although it may be indicative of a form of underlying anxiety.

Using Moelk's (1944) basic categories, McKinley (1982) performed sonographic analysis of feline vocalizations and classified them into two broad groups on the basis of spectral characteristics: homogeneous, or pure, calls and complex calls involving two or more pure types. Pure calls include murmurs, growls, squeaks, shrieks, hisses, spits, and chatters. Complex calls include mews, moans, and meows. A summary of this classification is found in Table 4-6. Elaborations of the basic interpretations discussed previously are included where relevant.

Kittens. Kittens can recognize a familiar voice by 4 weeks, but do not generally take special notice of each other's vocalizations until 9 weeks (Moelk, 1944). Brown et al. (1978) describe a variety of cries given by kittens. Their type A cry often is given by kittens that awaken and are hungry, cold, or trapped (Haskins, 1979). Kittens have been reported by Moelk (1979) to purr and tread while suckling. The interpretations he attributed to the treading is that it stimulates milk letdown. Purring starts as early as 2 days (Frazer-Sisson et al., 1991; Remmer & Gautier, 1972; Stogdale & Delack, 1985). Grunts are common at birth, but disap-

TABLE 4-6   Interpretation of Feline Vocalizations

Call	Description and Interpretation
Murmur	Rhythmically pulsed vocalization; exhalation; social interactions, solicitation, nonthreatening; possibly related to dyssynchronous contraction of muscles in larynx and diaphragm (Remmers & Gautier, 1972)
Growl	Low-pitched, harsh; lengthy; agonistic (Bushnell, 1963)
Squeak	High-pitched, raspy; associated with anticipation of feeding; given by females after copulation
Shriek	Loud, high-pitched; pain, fear, aggression
Hiss	Agonistic, mouth open, teeth visible; offensively defensive (avoids frank aggression)
Spit	Short sound before or after hiss
Chatter	Anticipation, frustration
Purr	Contentment, nursing, mild conflicting anxiety
Chirr	Queen's call to kittens
Mew	High-pitched, medium amplitude; mother-kitten interaction for location, identification, encouragement
Moan	Low frequency, long duration; epimeletic; regurgitation, solicitation
Meow	Greeting, epimeletic, willingness to interact

Data from Moelk (1944) and McKinley (1982).

pear at maturity unless the cat is engaged in a particularly difficult task. Moelk also describes an "acknowledgment" vocalization that starts at about 12 weeks of age and occurs when the kitten visualizes something he or she is about the receive. Mothers approach kittens with a variety of the chirr call that has been called a "brrp" or a "mhrn" (Moelk, 1979); this call is probably equivalent to the "chirp." These calls may function to stimulate kittens to nurse or to urinate or defecate. Very young kittens give an ultrasonic call if they are distressed so that their mother can locate them.

By 3 weeks of age, calls of deaf kittens were *louder* and lower pitched than normal (Romand & Ehret, 1984). This may be part of the reason that they may appear abnormal to others. It is not clear whether these kittens are shunned early and may have abnormal social development in part because of that.

Integration of Behavioral Cues

Friendly behaviors may integrate many of the olfactory and facial cues, cues attained from body postures, and vocal cues already discussed. Leyhausen (1979) classified friendly behaviors into six groups:

1. Sleeping together
2. Grooming

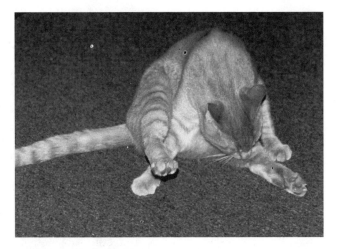

Grooming may distribute some glandular secretions and may be important for feline olfactory communication. (Photo by Liz Krug.)

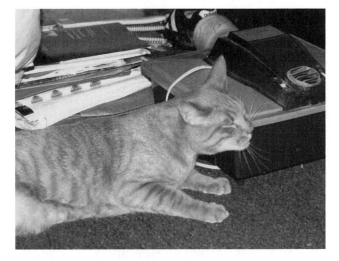

Cats can rub substrates to acquire and to leave odors. This cat is exhibiting marking behavior and may be delimiting his turf. The facial region is rich in vibrissae and glands. (Photo by Liz Krug.)

3. Rubbing against each other and sharing olfactory marks (this has been postulated to be very important in group situations and may be one of the factors that irritates other cats in the household when one cat has visited the veterinarian)
4. Friendly greeting after a prolonged absence (although "friendly" is left undefined)
5. Running beside each other and purring, while rubbing with the tail raised
6. Play behavior

These are not unambiguous behaviors that would allow evaluation of the extent to which they were used in cats that know each other well compared with those that do not. Quantification of these behavioral categories *could* provide that information.

Moelk's (1944) friendly approach categories include murmuring (a variable dependent on both the respiratory rate and response of the other individual involved), purring, rubbing, and rolling. Behaviors like rubbing and rolling are visual, but may communicate olfactory information. Given the glandular distribution of cats, any rub deposits odor on a substrate or on an individual. Cats that rub acquire odor from an individual or substrate. Individual cats that live in a group situation may rub together frequently and create a colony odor; this is a much faster way of recognizing whether an individual is an intruder than identification and recognition of each individual odor. Rubbing, or allorubbing, is a key behavior that acts as social cement. If animals are well known to each other, they may rub bodies more frequently than do animals that are not known. Allorubbing can include rubbing of foreheads, cheeks, flanks, and tails. If two animals that are known to each other approach and raise their tails, it may mean that they intend to rub (Bradshaw, 1992a). The tail itself could specify the form of rubbing, depending on the response. If a second cat raises

its tail, the cats might simultaneously rub each other; if the second cat does *not* raise its tail, the recipient may rub after the initiator has rubbed, or the recipient may not rub (Bradshaw, 1992a). The interaction in the series just described also signals information about confidence and status: the animal who is able to elicit the *first* rub is the higher status animal. Clients can use such information to understand social relationships in their own household.

Head rubbing can also be understood with regard to humans. Many individual cats head rub both their owners and strangers (Bradshaw, 1992a; Mertens & Turner, 1988). If this is the first behavior that the individual cat exhibits on approaching a stranger, *and* if it is followed by the animal stepping back and looking at the individual, the head rubbing may be indicative of a hierarchical challenge. Individuals that can force another animal (including humans) to sustain rubbing are generally the more confident animals.

Laboratory cat colonies of cats often provide an opportunity to observe cats that are relatively nonaggressive to each other in a confined, controlled situation. Podberscek and colleagues (1991b) studied a colony of cats that was composed of seven male castrated cats and one male intact cat. Thirty-six percent of the behaviors observed in laboratory cats were maintenance behaviors, which included resting, sitting, eating, defecating, and urinating. Comfort behaviors included grooming, scratching, sneezing, coughing, head shaking, stretching, and yawning, and made up 30% of the observed behaviors. Locomotor behaviors included walking, running, jumping, and jumping to and from ledges, and composed 24% of the behaviors noted. Agonistic behaviors made up *less than 1%* of the total interactions; this is remarkable, given that all of the individuals were male and one was intact, but it indicates how rare such behaviors are in situations when the social "rules" are apparent. Marking and investigational behaviors, including clawing, scratching at a scratching post, rubbing, anal sniffing, body sniffing, and wall and floor licking composed 4% of the observed behaviors. Play behaviors and vocalization behaviors each made up 2% of the observed behaviors.

These data reveal several important points. First, they act as a baseline for setting a frequency for agonistic behaviors. If agonistic behavior occurs less than 1% of the time in a colony that is small and comprises same-sex cats, this indicates that agonistic behavior is not the normal mode of behavior in the animals. Although Podberscek and colleagues (1991b) did not look at the signaling components of any of these behaviors, yawning may also be a passive challenge and not just a comfort behavior. Second, the comfort behaviors (30% of time allocation) are ones that are largely associated with ritualistic or stereotypic behaviors that may be part of an obsessive-compulsive disorder (Overall, 1992c,d,e; Luescher, 1991). This has been reported in a variety of species, including primate species.

These findings are consistent with those reported by Hart (1980) for six to eight intact males kept in a colony situation. He found that the most frequent mode of conflict resolution was withdrawal in response to a threat. Again, it is critical to pry people from the belief that the main mode of conflict resolution is combat. The main mode of conflict resolution is *not* combat; it is *avoidance* of it, or it is *deference*. Situations that result in outright combat may be the abnormal ones. Almost without exception, reports of laboratory cats have noted that fights are the exception.

In a study of only female laboratory cats, Hurni and Rossbach (1987) found that all the cats would sleep together and were quite companionable.

Although Podberscek and co-workers (1991b) grouped scratching and clawing behaviors under marking and investigational behaviors, occurring only 4% of the time, it is important to realize that such a low incidence of these behaviors may not be representative of the incidence in feral domestic cat populations. Turner (1988) noted that feral cats performed claw sharpening more often in the presence of conspecifics than when alone. Functional behaviors can also have signal value. The sole function of scratching is not to just remove sheaths, although excess sheath material may increase the frequency of actual scratching. Kittens cannot completely withdraw their claws until approximately 4 weeks and scratch on available substrates by 5 weeks; however, they will do this even if declawed just after birth before they have any experience with scratching (Hart, 1972). Scratching is not only a visual signal that may convey information about status and is long-lasting, but it is also potentially an olfactory signal, given the deposition of glands around the pads. Cats scratch new or old objects; the longer the object is scratched, the more significant it is to the cat. The best signals have tandem modes to communicate their intent. An olfactory signal that lasts anywhere from 24 to 48 hours, accompanied by a visual signal that will last longer, conveys information not only about the individual, but when the last time that individual visited the area was. Such approaches are undervalued in veterinary behavioral medicine.

Finally, a short discussion of the postures used by a female with her kittens is warranted. Clients need to be aware of normal behavior patterns, and when, if they have a queen with kittens, those behaviors deviate from normal. The postures that have been elucidated for females caring for their young include sit, sit-nurse, half-sit, on-side-lie, half-sit and on-side-lie, crouch, lie, crouch and lie, and shift. On-side-lie, half-sit, and the shift posture all occur very early in the caretaking of kittens. Sit-nurse peaks at about 4 weeks, concomitant with the beginning of weaning. Sit, crouch, and lie are all behaviors that are seen later in the weaning period more frequently than earlier. With the exception of the half-sit, all of these behaviors are influenced by both the mother and the stage of the development. The half-sit (Lawrence, 1981, cited in Deag et al., 1988) was not a significant function of age.

SOCIAL RELATIONSHIPS IN CATS
Overview

Linear hierarchical relationships have been emphasized in most commentaries on cat sociality. Discussions of the sociality of cats has been couched in the dominance-submission terminology (Fonberg, 1985). It behooves us to question whether this approach is valid.

Some early work by Winslow (1938, 1944) found that cats forced to share a room developed a linear hierarchical relationship with an identifiable alpha male; this relationship was independent of food resources. Dominance relationships were estimated by using mounting behavior as an indication of status: individuals that permitted themselves to be mounted were of lower status, whereas those that did the most mounting were of higher status. Winslow then ascertained that if you removed the most aggressive animal, the "next most aggressive" took over. In Winslow's system, the highest ranking animal mounted all newcomers regardless of their sex. No other study has demonstrated this type of linear dominance hierarchy.

Masserman and Siever (1944) and Baerends et al. (1957) examined social relationships between cats and found that stable dominance hierarchies were apparent if the group size was limited to four *and* if the measurement of hierarchy was taken at a feeding station. If the animals were forced to be anxious, less

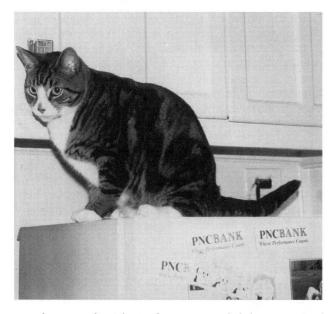

Height can indirectly confer status, and ability to control access to perch sites can be an important determinant of status. Height also allows monitoring of the social environment without direct involvement. The extent to which the choice not to interact is involved in status determinations has probably been underestimated. (Photo by Emily Elliot and Nirit Rosenberg.)

anxious animals became higher ranking. This probably has some applications for levels of anxiety in animals in social situations where they demonstrate inappropriate, out-of-context aggression. It makes sense that animals that are less anxious are more able to interact normally in an appropriate social context; this could facilitate higher ranking. These studies also demonstrated that stability of the social grouping affected motivational levels for feeding and other activities; however, use of feeding stations to assess overall social hierarchies is flawed. This is particularly true for cats that are fed periodically: these cats are less cooperative and more aggressive than are cats fed ad libitum (Finco et al., 1986).

Dominance hierarchies also have been found *not* to be influenced by changes in hunger motivational status (Cole & Schafer, 1966). As motivational level (assayed by desire for food) increases, aggression increases, and frequency of submissive activity increases, but aggression was not the controlling factor in attaining dominance status in this study. Instead, *the response of the challenged cat* determined the hierarchical relationship. It is unclear whether the individuals had higher status in this system because they made the required response, or because they were capable of making other animals respond to them. The latter appears likely; this may be among the first studies to demonstrate that threat behavior, rather than outright aggression, is more common in higher ranking animals.

Clear, linear dominance hierarchies appear to be artifacts of provisioning (Baerends et al., 1957), and such hierarchies appear stable over time *only* in experiments that are driven by food. Stable hierarchies are postulated only on the basis of a lack of agonistic behavior; few studies emphasize specific behaviors. Only studies that do so could provide information about the rules for any complex social affiliation.

The top cat in a captive colony may display the most agonistic behavior (Podberscek et al., 1991b), but interpretation of this observation is confounded by the lack of receipt of any agonistic behavior and the lack of interaction with the other cats in the contexts of rest, play, and grooming. "Dominant" animals may be able to announce or enforce their status by occupying specific spaces (Bernstein & Strack, 1993; Strack & Bernstein, 1993). In this colony study (Podberscek et al., 1991b), dominant animals favored shelf areas (occupied by the dominant animal 48% of the time) and sleeping boxes (occupied by the dominant animal 25% of the time).

The animals most likely to induce deferential behavior in any social group are often older animals; they are also often the largest or heaviest. Such factors should be considered in any study of hierarchical relationship. In the aforementioned situation there was no association between age and mass. These issues are potentially complex because of competing allocation decisions (e.g., eating or mating), but should be carefully examined in any study purporting to dismiss or rely on them. This concern is a valid one for cats, because it is known that females vary less than males in proportion of day spent hunting (26% to 46% for females; 5% to 34% for males) (Turner & Meister, 1988). Podberscek et al. (1991b) also report that top cats were black, but it is unclear whether this is either true or important. The manner in which cats respond to people may not affect feline hierarchies, although many of the behaviors that a dominant cat demonstrates to other cats can be demonstrated to people (Podberscek et al., 1988). In this study, the cat identified as the dominant cat performed the fewest noncontact attention behaviors and the most no-attention behaviors (resting, eating, jumping to a shelf, self-grooming, rubbing the wall, and walking away) and would make contact with a stranger immediately on the first day of an experiment, but not pay any attention to the stranger again. It should be noted that there is a tremendous amount of individual variation in attentiveness to people in experimental situations (Mertens, 1991; Mertens & Shär, 1988; Mertens & Turner, 1988). Evaluation of this type of variation is important before generalizing the results of a small study.

The study by Podberscek and colleagues (1991b) is interesting because all of the cats were 2 to 3 years of age. Cats mature socially somewhere in this age range, with most cats maturing between 2.5 to 3.5 or 4 years of age; sexual maturity can occur by 6 months of age. It would be interesting to know how and if animals maintained in a colony alter the hierarchical relationships as they all attain social maturity.

Hierarchical relationships can be influenced by colony shape. Laboratory cats with free access to food eat several small meals a day (7 to 16 meals) randomly without developing a hierarchical relationship and, when given the opportunity, will sleep alone (Thorne, 1985). Given that most laboratory cats sleep more in the day than during the night (Kuwabara et al., 1986), it would be interesting to know if most of the observations would change throughout a diel cycle.

Complex Relationships

Some of the best work on free-ranging cat social systems has been done by Natoli and de Vito (1991). They describe shifting linear dominance hierarchies that are based on the outcome of agonistic encounters. Their linear hierarchical relationships are *not* associated with any measure of copulatory success, suggesting that there are structured and functional social groups, separate from those formed during mating and feeding opportunities (Macdonald et al., 1987). This finding is substantiated in other studies (Fitzgerald & Karl, 1986; Izawa et al., 1982; Natoli, 1985, 1990) in which

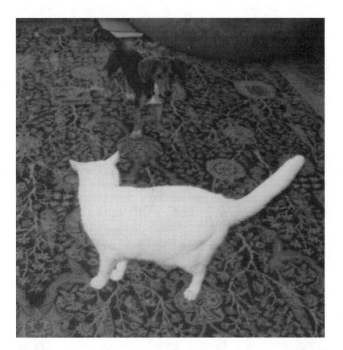

Deference systems are usually based on expectations of known individuals, like this dog and cat. Note that the cat has control of the area by virtue of occupation of the central region and that the dog is averting his gaze and not directly facing the cat. (Photo by Emily Elliot and Nirit Rosenberg.)

cat densities range from less than 1 cat/km^2 to 2350 cats/km^2. Early theories about cat behavior postulated that cats are essentially solitary (de Boer, 1977), form groups composed of nonstructured aggregations around food (Laundré, 1977), or are social only when they are in estrus or exhibit estruslike behaviors including vocalization; rubbing of the head, chin, and neck on vertical objects; rolling on the ground; and crouching, after the exhibition of which males' efforts to copulate were met with complete acceptance (Michael, 1961; Beaver, 1977). It is now clear that the main focus of cat social behavior should not be as a vehicle to attain successful mating.

Fighting and threats are rare, and the differences in these between individual males in a large, unmanipulated colony are not significant (Natoli & de Vito, 1991). All of the males in this study marked regularly, but there is no difference between the type and frequency of marking in which any individual male engages; this suggests that linear dominance hierarchies are not the rule in this colony. Agonistic behavior between males includes the following behaviors:

1. Threats, including striking with a paw, assuming a threatening posture, hissing, and flattening the ears
2. Interference of copulation by blocking a male from mounting another female or by mounting the male himself
3. Ritualized vocal threats
4. Submissive postures, including crouching, fleeing, leaving, and territorial marking, including chin rubs and spraying

Leyhausen (1979) discusses the concepts of relative dominance and location dominance with regard to free-ranging cat populations. Individual animals defer to others by sitting, moving to the side, or looking away. Deference systems based on knowledge of individual animals in the group are one characteristic of sociality. Normal, friendly cat approaches include nose-to-nose approaches, head-rubbing, and ear-licking, followed by flank rubbing and mutual perianal sniffing (Wolski, 1982). Less friendly approaches stop at nasal sniffing. Allomarking includes cheek and perioral rubbing, and rubbing of the dorsal surface of the tail down the cheek and under the chin of the recipient (Macdonald et al., 1987). Such behaviors are postulated to help structure social relationships. Behaviors indicative of more "submissive" status present a much clearer picture of social dominance or hierarchical ranking than do agonistic, aggressive behaviors (Natoli & de Vito, 1991).

The Role of Scent

Data from other studies indicate that the role of marking (feces, urine, or both) can be important in the maintenance of complex, social hierarchies. Unless such subtle communicatory signals are noticed, one could assert that the social system is maintained by a far simpler mechanism such as linear dominance. For instance, Wolski (1982) and Macdonald and colleagues (1987) noted that the edges of ranges are often marked with urine. Usually, if a new male enters and his scent is not one of the scents that is common for the group, a female will not let him approach within 4 to 5 m without exhibiting a defensive posture; however, the avoidance of conflict was correlated with urine marks and ability to induce withdrawal of intruders (de Boer, 1977a).

Social distance may affect the type and intensity of signaling behavior. Common ethological categories of distances include, from the largest to the smallest area affected:

1. Flight distance—the distance at which one will flee a potentially threatening situation
2. Home range—the area in which one spends the most time (95% of all activities occur here), daily or seasonally
3. Territory—an actively defended area (*sensu* Burt, 1943)
4. Critical distance—the interpersonal area in the center of use of the territory's core area
5. Social distance
6. Personal distance (Hinde, 1970)

In free-ranging situations, females most commonly spray only when entering a hunting range and intermittently while foraging, unlike males who spray as they patrol edges of a range (Fox, 1975). Both sexes exhibit a Flehmen response. Urine loses it attractiveness after 24 hours, and estrous females then spray more frequently (de Boer, 1977b). Feces are covered when deposited in core areas of farms, but may not be if deposited on pathways (Macdonald et al., 1987; Panaman, 1981). Feces can accumulate on elevated sites and on rabbit trails if not buried; some of the subordinates may cover their feces more frequently than do the more dominant animals (Panaman, 1981), as is known for wolves (Peters & Mech, 1975). This hypothesis has not been tested, but data from Bernstein and Strack (1993) suggest that more dominant animals control access to and use of preferred elimination areas. The findings of Natoli and de Vito (1991) corroborate this theory.

Natoli (1985) reported that adult cats of both sexes could distinguish the urine of strange males from familiar males, and males would investigate odors for longer than did females. Cats spray once every 5.4 minutes at rabbit burroughs when traveling (Corbett, 1979). Spraying also varies by sex and frequency when animals travel. Nonbreeding males sprayed 12.9 times per hour during travel, whereas breeding males sprayed almost twice that, 22 times per hour (Liberg, 1980; Liberg & Sandell, 1988). Hunting females spray once every 16.7 minutes or every 70 meters (Panneman, 1981). In general, males spray more frequently than females (62.6 times per hour compared with 6 times per hour) (Apps, 1986). Urine marking is less

commonly exhibited by transient males; only five of nine "occasional" males urine mark (Natoli & de Vito, 1991). For regular (nontransient) males, urine spraying is positively correlated, not with the threats they give, but with the threats they receive ($r = 0.568$; $p < 0.05$). The amount of interference with copulation one receives ($r = 0.692$; $p < 0.01$), rubbing of the chin ($r = 0.533$; $p < 0.05$), and vocal threats ($r = 0.656$; $p < 0.02$) also correlate with the frequency of urine spraying. Urine spraying is *not* correlated with threats given ($r = 0.0145$), with the act of interfering with copulation ($r = -0.043$), or with the action of participating in true or false mounts ($r = -0.201$) (all data from Natoli & de Vito, 1991). For occasional or transient males, spraying correlates with their rubbing behavior ($r = 0.95$; $p < 0.01$), but chin rubbing does not differ among regular males. Chin rubbing is correlated with both giving and receiving threats and vocal duets ($r = 0.648$, $p < 0.02$; $r = 0.870$, $p < 0.01$; $r = 0.692$, $p < 0.01$, respectively).

It is worthwhile to note that this study reflects the situation with problems with marking in the house. There is a correlation between the number of cats in a household and the probability of at least one spraying (Jemmett & Skerritt, 1979, cited in Mertens & Shär, 1988). Borchelt and Voith (1982) report that only 25% of cats in single-cat households spray, but that there is a 100% probability of spraying in households containing 10 or more cats. Spraying is often a passive, rather than an active, form of aggression and may be more frequently exhibited by animals with less, not more, control over the environment. These are some of the best data that might allow us to assess social problems in households, but they have been largely ignored in the veterinary literature.

Finally, the concept that spraying is probably socially mediated and can be an indicator of lower social status or decreased ability to control an interaction is supported by Wolski (1982). He indicates that as late as 13 to 18 months of age, young males may only squat to urinate. This suggests a strong social component to elimination posture. It is rare for free-ranging males to show urine-marking in paternal areas. Housecats that are not interacting in the complex feline social environments previously outlined usually stop squatting at about 8 to 10 months of age, suggesting some release from social interaction.

The Role of Location: Spatial Structure

Much of the research on hierarchical positions and spatial use focuses on who gets to meet with whom. Within a population, central locations may differ from peripheral ones. In one study involving the roles of central versus peripheral position, toms mate sequentially with the same female, regardless of core use location, rather than monopolizing her (Liberg, 1983). Multiple males are frequently reported to be in attendance of one estrous female (Dards, 1983), and it may be the case that under certain demographic situations there is no competition for females because the females are unlikely to reject *known* males. This concept requires further testing. Dr. Sharon Crowell-Davis (1994) has an interesting series of slides that demonstrate a group of male barnyard cats waiting, in turn and without apparent aggression, to copulate with a very compliant female. Whether the individual males in these groups are more related to each other than they would be to the average male is also unknown, but genetic relation may not be required to allow this system to work. The argument can be a purely demographic one. Copulation guarantees neither paternity nor live offspring.

Central and peripheral individuals may not have the same success in reproduction. When the number of kittens produced per female per year is examined with regard to location in colony (peripheral versus central), more litters fail per year in the periphery of large colonies than in small and medium colonies, but central areas of small colonies have failure rates greater than those of the periphery (Kerby & Macdonald, 1988; Macdonald et al., 1987). These data are summarized in Table 4-7. There is an interaction between colony size and reproductive parameters, and between colony size and location of breeding individuals in the colony. Female cats with peripheral locations in colonies have a greater distance between their den and food sites; after 7 years, these individuals have no surviving descendants (Kerby & Macdonald, 1988). This suggests that rank and environment interact. More males disperse during their second or third year (correlated with the attainment of social maturity), if they are not protected by harassment by conspecifics. The extent of colony size on this buffer effect is unclear but merits further study. These findings have a direct application for individuals who allow their pet cats to roam outdoors. One of the most commonly given reasons for the loss of pet cats is that the cat "left"; lack of refugia in a complex social system that the people do not understand can contribute to feline emigration, particularly if disappearance occurs at social maturity.

Population Dynamics: Density and Social Dynamics

In free-ranging situations cat population densities range from 0.9 to 2350/km^2; colony sizes range from 1 to 52 cats (Jones & Coman, 1988; Rees, 1981), and home-range size is equally as variable. Densities of greater than 100 cats/km^2 are associated with plentiful resources, and densities of fewer than 5 cats/km^2 are associated with scarce, dispersed resources (Liberg & Sandell, 1988). Social relationships should be complex.

Groups of adult females with young comprise 2 to 7 to 15 to 20 individuals (Izawa et al., 1982; Liberg, 1980). It has been postulated that female home ranges largely center on food and shelter, and that male distributions center on those of females. This is the classic resource defense polygyny postulated by Emlen and Oring (1977), but one area can fulfill a variety of functions without the implication of mechanism. The integration of the demographic, resource, predation, and physiological and biophysical environments defines the types of interactions that occur and the frequency with which they take place (Dunham et al., 1989).

Regardless of colony size, most amicable social relationships occur between females at the rate of 0.5 to 0.9 interactions per hour (Macdonald et al., 1987). Most aggressive social interactions occur toward intruders. Cats in dense populations (23.5 cats/ha*) have separate memberships in feeding groups that do not reflect their other interactions (Izawa et al., 1982). That multiple factors may be acting is substantiated by a study by Jones and Coman (1982): home ranges for both males and females (male home range 620 ha, females 170 ha) overlap minimally, but there is a greater overlap under patchy resource conditions. In one study of cats in a dockyard that has been enclosed by a high wall since it was built in 1711, family groups range from 2 to 11 individuals ($\overline{X}$ = 4.5) (Dards, 1983). All adult females are related. Mature males have freely overlapping home ranges that average 8.4 ha. Other males and females share group home ranges, ranging in size from 0.03 to 4.2 ha. Male home ranges can be two to four times larger than those of females and juveniles, and males can travel 4 km per night in the course of monitoring these (Wolski, 1982). In one of the rare studies that reports time budgets and activities (Kerby & Macdonald, 1988), a relationship between colony size and activity, including time spent associating with another cat, is noted. Male interactions with females are most common in small

TABLE 4-7 ASSOCIATION OF COLONY SIZE, NUMBER OF KITTENS PER FEMALE PER YEAR, AND LITTER FAILURE RATES

Rank*	Colony Description	Litters Failing (%)
1.56	Large, central	53.0
1.40	Medium, central	50.0
1.20	Small, peripheral	30.0
1.14	Medium, peripheral	62.5
0.90	Small, central	50.0
0.42	Large, peripheral	82.0

Data from Kerby & Apps, 1988.
*Based on number of kittens per female per year.

*1 ha = 1 × 10^{-6} km^2 or 1 × 10^4 m^2 = 10,000m.

colonies, but male interactions with males are most common in medium colonies. Female interactions with females are most common in medium-sized colonies; in these colonies, females spend 40% of their time with another cat, usually touching it. Groupings of cats are nonrandom; social groups are highly structured. In small colonies, males spend 31% of their time in the area that is the focus of most activities, whereas females spend 65% to 85% of their time in this area.

Home-range size is affected by social and physiological factors, such as queens in estrus. Males range farther than usual at such times. In one cited example, a 0.25 km^2 area in Manchester, UK, contained 2 of 70 females that had not been spayed, and 19 tom cats. The largest male home range was 0.061 km^2, but the mean male home range was 0.009 km^2. When the 2 unspayed females came into estrus, they attracted 8 to 10 males that traveled outside their normal ranges (Bradshaw, 1992a).

Males in free-ranging groups usually have home ranges that are 3.5 times larger than those of females, and they range up to 10 km^2 (Liberg & Sandell, 1988). Two- to 4-year-old males may challenge resident males, but they are not able to succeed in these challenges until they are approximately 3 to 5 years of age and have attained adult mass. Female home ranges overlap with those of males, but the breeding lives of most females are short and do not last more than 6 years. The social system has some effect on breeding and may, in fact, control access to breeding for both males and females. Under normal free-ranging conditions, domestic felines may be similar to lions (Bertram, 1975) and not bear their first litter until they are socially mature, at approximately 2 to 3 years of age (Wolski, 1982).

Most of the previously discussed studies focus on *free-ranging* domestic cats. Very few data are available for pet cats in smaller groups that are confined. Early data from longitudinal studies on domestic cats indicate that most people are able to identify a "dominant cat" and that they do so on the basis of responses that that cat *receives* from other cats in the household (Bernstein & Strack, 1993). Frank aggression is exceptional. Hierarchies appear to be associated with groups into which the cats assert themselves and with the locations in which cats are found. Accordingly, one cat might elicit deference in one group situation, whereas another elicits deference in a more solitary situation involving a perch site. Data such as these are essential to understanding the complexity and elegance of the social behavior of the domestic cat.

Why Know About Normal Cat Behavior?

One of the reasons further study is critical is that only one third of all pet cats remain in the same household in the United States for their entire life; each year 25% of adult cats leave their households (Rowan & Williams, 1987). The complaints by clients about cats include spraying, other indoor marking, "loss of house training," nervous urination, a nervous condition (such as fear of visitors), aggression to other cats, aggression to people, self-mutilation, and other miscellaneous complaints (Neville & Bradshaw, 1991). Feral cat complaints can also factor into how people perceive their relationships with cats. In a study that surveyed people's concerns about neighborhood cats, Ablett (1981) found that fouling of areas was the primary complaint. Nocturnal fighting, with caterwauling, was also important. Less important but still significant were complaints about finding corpses of cats who had died, attacks on people and pets, entering homes uninvited, fleas, health risks posed to humans, killing of birds and fish, and digging of gardens. Cats are found dead for a variety of reasons; however, mortality increases with exposure to potentially injurious situations such as moving vehicles and aggressive dogs. Free-ranging cats have higher mortality in urban areas than do indoor cats (Childs & Ross, 1986; Comfort, 1956; Hamilton et al., 1969). Between 1972 and 1983 euthanasia in U.S. shelters declined from more than 20% of cats taken in to 10%. If this trend is to continue, and if cats are to be kept in households longer, understanding of normal behavior is critical (Gerber et al.,1973; Overall, 1992a). Many of the complaints noted by clients reflect undesirable but normal behaviors that occur because of artificial social situations in which we force cats to live. This does not imply that clients should be encouraged to live with the problem simply because a cat is a cat; it does imply that clients must appreciate the extent to which cat social systems have been neglected in the understanding of cat behavioral disorders. Treatment of problems must address the social system—either behaviorally, environmentally, or pharmacologically.

5 ····· Taking the Behavioral History

The tendency for those who are pressed for time will be to skip this chapter and to just use the history sheets. Please resist this temptation and read the entire text.

The key to most diagnostic skill is history-taking ability. This is especially so for behavioral medicine. Behavioral histories can be more difficult to take than many medical histories because clients may perceive no tangible signs of the developing problem. A dog in behavioral extremis is almost always thought by the clients to have a sudden onset; a dog in physical extremis may have been noticeably ill before collapse. This dichotomy is related to ignorance both on the part of the client and, often, the veterinarian who has been caring for the pet. Veterinarians and clients need to be able to recognize when a pet's behavior deviates from what is normal and acceptable for that pet. This judgment cannot be made without an understanding of the range of normal behaviors. If veterinarians are unsure of this range of behaviors or are blinded by their own prejudices, what are they to convey to their clients? The topic of normal behavior is covered in Chapters 3 and 4. This chapter focuses on obtaining an accurate portrait of the pet's behavior.

Clients feel profound guilt and responsibility for any improper or undesirable behaviors that their pets exhibit. No one would expect their own or their child's behavior to be purely the outcome of the environment, but such expectations are not unusual for pets. Clients in the Behavior Clinic at the Veterinary Hospital at the University of Pennsylvania (VHUP) frequently state that their trainer, their veterinarian, or a friend told them that this was all their fault. This is an oft repeated experience among behaviorists. Such impressions are further reinforced by even the best books on puppy raising (such as *The Art of Raising a Puppy* by The Monks of New Skete, 1991) that directly or implicitly state that if you do everything correctly, you will have the perfect pet. This is simply not true and is the biggest myth perpetuated about aggression, the most dangerous behavioral problem.

As is true for human psychiatric medicine, behavioral medicine is plagued by guilt and fault. Clients' preconceptions of these can interfere with obtaining an accurate and truthful behavioral history. Behavioral history taking often requires longer than standard physical history taking: a session of 2 or more hours is common. Behavioral histories can require lengthy and detailed note taking and questioning, must have the cooperation of the clients, and must respect confidentiality (refer to the most recent American Veterinary Medical Association (AVMA) Directory for guidelines). As with any history, there are some facets that cannot be known. Thorough questioning of everyone who routinely interacts with the pet and close observation of the animal minimize the unknown. This is one reason why telephone consultations with clients, especially for cases involving aggression, are *not* recommended. Clients' descriptions of their pets' behaviors are not a substitute for seeing the actual behavior.

Even people who understand dogs and who raise them kindly and consistently can have a dog or cat that behaves normally until social maturity (18 to 36 months and 24 to 36 months, respectively); at that time aggression can appear regardless of early experience. Certainly, early, good interaction and attention to acceptable *and* nonacceptable behavior should favorably slant the odds. However, there are no sufficient data that demonstrate the extent to which this is the case. If behavioral problems in pets are influenced by genetics, hormones, and neuroendocrine pathways, as is becoming clear for humans, doing everything "right" will not be sufficient to abort the behavioral problem. Regardless, by doing everything involved in early training and rearing as well as possible, any developing problems can be spotted early, before the inappropriate behavior becomes self-reinforcing. Early work with dogs not only sets standards for the dog, but gives clients the kind of relationship with their pet that will allow them to notice questionable behaviors when they begin to appear as abnormal. In the Behavior Clinic at VHUP, clients who have close relationships with their pets are also excellent observers of the pet's behavior.

Early intervention is an area in which veterinarians can excel during first puppy or kitten visits or during annual appointments. The use of the first puppy appointment to attempt to create an atmosphere where behavioral problems are minimized is discussed in Chapter 14. Early intervention alone will not be able to obviate some behavioral problems but will render them more tractable by virtue of treating an inappropriate behavior that has not been reinforced by years of repetition.

At the outset of the appointment it may be wise to disabuse clients of the notion that most of the problems were caused by them. The clients may have made the problems worse through ignorance or inattention, but in truth the clients are not at the root cause of most behavioral disorders. Certainly, there are pet and client personality mismatches, just as some pets' needs cannot be met by the household. To blame one side for this is unkind and fruitless. Should the behavioral history elicit these dyssynchronous personalities or expectations and the interaction not be malleable, placement of the pet may be the best option. Expectations and prognoses should be discussed when the diagnoses are postulated and treatment formulated. If there is blame for the problem, as in abuse, it can be laid at that time. This is another area in which help from social workers can be invaluable (see Chapter 16). The history-taking procedure needs to start as a nonjudgmental partnership, with the clients' fears allayed.

The steps for history taking discussed below are compiled from a variety of sources (Beaver, 1992; Danneman & Chodrow, 1982; Hart & Hart, 1985a). Because most specialists in behavioral medicine are at teaching/referral hospitals, their caseloads may contain more complex cases than does that of the average practice. Practitioners are encouraged to adapt the following history-taking procedures to their needs given the rationale provided.

GENERAL COMMENTS

Signalment is important because some behavioral conditions are affected by age, sex, and reproductive status. Clients may also believe that breed affects behavioral problems. Because this belief can affect their judgment and facilitate justification of the animal's behavior, it is important to tell clients that breed is usually less central to the problem than is commonly believed. The issue of breed is discussed in Chapter 3.

It is important to estimate the animal's age as accurately as possible because of concomitant medical problems that may make the behavioral case more difficult to treat. Furthermore, it is unwise and unsound medical practice to dispense psychotropic medication to animals that are older and may be physiologically compromised without first adequately evaluating the animal physiologically. Interpretation of the evaluation may depend in part on the pet's age (e.g., puppies have different baseline cholesterol values than adult dogs).

Some conditions are more common in one sex than the other; this does *not* mean that every animal of that sex will develop the condition, or that the condition is normal or acceptable; it *does* mean that the animal may be more at risk for the problem. The age of neutering has received scant attention in domestic dogs and cats with regard to the development of behavioral problems compared with reproductive status itself (O'Farrell & Peachey, 1990). Both may be important factors, but interpretations of the latter may be confounded by variance in the former. For example, if one contends that spayed females are more likely to become aggressive than unspayed females, one cannot know without the type of controlled experiment done by O'Farrell and Peachey what proportion of those females that were spayed would have eventually become aggressive anyway. Replicates in time are impossible to create; thus these studies require careful attention to experimental detail and statistical analysis and interpretation. It is important to take a behavioral history without any of the biases to which these issues are subject.

COMPONENTS OF A SPECIFIC HISTORY

Sample history-taking sheets are provided in Appendix A. Their format follows that of the discussion below. Box 5-3 provides an outline of the critical topics to be discussed in a behavioral history.

A good behavioral history should contain the following information.

1. Why Seek Advice for this Pet?

Discover at the outset why the clients have sought advice and what they expect to get from it. They may not actually want to fix the problem. You need to know this. Clients should be asked to describe the two factors important in their decision to deal with the behavioral aspect: (1) what do they perceive the problems are, and (2) what caused them to seek help? The problem may be growling when strange dogs approach, but the clients are seeking help because they are being sued—they did not consider the growling a problem until their dog bit, and even then, they believe it justified. The scenario just described is a complex one. No amount of assertion on the veterinarian's part that the dog does have a problem will convince the clients; however, through thorough history taking and questioning, the clients may begin to see the pattern of the problem and may be more willing to address it.

A corollary of this is to discover why the clients obtained the pet. Ask why they obtained that particular breed *and* that particular individual. Identify the clients' expectations about the breed in general and about their individual dog in particular. The clients' perceptions of the problem may be affected by acceptance of myths about breed or by unrealistic expectations. For example, consider the following anecdote: one client actually reported that they obtained their breed because "macho husband needed macho dog." A large, "hot" breed of dog may not be the appropriate choice for an individual with back problems or for a household with children when no one has experience with dogs.

Ask if the clients have ever owned any kind of pet before and especially if they have ever owned the patient's type. If the clients have always had cats and birds but now have their first dog, they need to learn about pets with a different social system than those to which they are accustomed. Lack of knowledge is a potentially dangerous thing. If your clients have never owned dogs and chose a 5-month-old, previously owned (recycled) male, intact Neapolitan mastiff because they wanted a large dog and they loved the color, there may be trouble brewing.

Your first job is to explain normal behavior and to address expectations; your second job is to address the pet's problems. You and the client will then have to decide whether the pet's problems can be addressed within the context of what is normal for that species, age, sex, and so on, and, given that, if the clients' expectations can be met. This is certainly a case in which the client's misinformation or lack of information can cause problems or worsen any preexisting behavioral problems. This approach does not presuppose breed-specific tendencies for behavioral problems; it does assume potentials for differences in energy levels and traits (pointing, herding) associated with breed. Medical conditions associated with breed, size, pelage, and so forth should also be addressed. The main factor in the example of the Neapolitan mastiff involves relative strength, size, and concomitant potential for control.

2. Guilt

Determine whether the clients feel guilty about the problem or believe that they have caused it. If the clients *do* feel guilty, discover why, and if possible, reassure them. Clients often deny in writing on a questionnaire that they feel guilty, but orally express guilt and remorse in an interview. Believe the latter. If they feel guilty, rightly or wrongly, they may be unwilling to share with you all the relevant behavioral information about their pet.

3. Primary Caretaker Responsibility

Remember that one person can supply most of the love and play, and another provides more visceral sustenance. Determine the primary caretaker of the pet and the pet's relationship with various household members.

The entire family and anyone who routinely deals with the dog (e.g., the housekeeper, the law clerk in chambers, the bookkeeper at the office) needs to be present during the behavioral examination. That "Fifi" bites the youngest daughter may not be understandable without input from the older son, who eventually owns up to putting rubber bands on "Fifi's" tail, knowing she will redirect her aggression to the child less able to fight back. Furthermore, not all of the people in the household may be having the same problems. It is not unusual for a dominantly aggressive dog to behave in a manner that may be, and is considered by one owner to be, acceptable: the dog truly does not try to aggressively control that person as it does all others in the household. Every problem with every individual in the household must be noted and ultimately addressed.

4. Activity Patterns and Space Considerations

Get an idea of the pet's normal routine, its social interactions with people and other animals, and the daily expectations it has regarding people, and those they have regarding the pet.

In what kind of an environment does this dog or cat live? Does it have free range on a farm where it is never leashed, or is it living in a small, urban, high-rise apartment? Does it spend all day alone, or does it accompany one owner to the office or stay home with a rotating crew?

Are there other pets with whom the patient lives, and do they interact? How? Remember: aggression is an interaction.

How frequently, and for how long, is the pet exercised by running, leash-walking, or aerobic play? Cats and dogs can have lots of toys, but may not play with them by themselves. Is this pet really getting enough exercise? Most clients overestimate the amount of exercise their pets get; the nonsedentary evolutionary history of canids must be considered, with the realization that two 20-minute walks per day is not equivalent to 40 minutes of Frisbee playing.

How frequently, what, where, and when is the pet fed? Does it eat well or is it a picky eater? "Picky" eaters may be beaten out of their food by a more aggressive eater, or may have trained their people to "bribe" them with tempting morsels that come to replace the standard diet. A pet who is fed canned or homemade food twice a day, plus midday biscuits, and the milk from the breakfast cereal is probably being better observed than the one that is self-fed kibble from a dispenser in the basement that is filled once a week. This can be a clue as to expectations of client and pet and as to the accuracy or detail of the client's information.

How frequently does the animal urinate and defecate, and where? This, again, allows you to evaluate attention to daily routine and may provide information germane to the problem. If the client maintains that the puppy is exercised by running on a leash three times a day, but is still overactive, it might be because those same three times a day are its bathroom breaks and last only 5 minutes each, or until the animal eliminates, whichever comes first. If the cat is confined indoors, in a multicat household with seven other cats and one litter box and the client does not have any idea how often the cat defecates, you may have a clue about the elimination problem. There is no method other than taking a history that specifically asks for frequency and details of events to uncover such confounding information.

Determine whether there are other pets in the household, and ask how the patient interacts with them. Find out whether any of the behaviors about which you are being consulted occurs in the presence or absence of the other pets or during particular activities involving them.

Find out what the pet does when left alone. Is there hair on the sofa, or are the curtains ripped down? These are clues. If nothing is destroyed, but the carpet by the door is soaked by saliva, the pet may still be having attacks of separation anxiety.

Is the pet ever crated or isolated, and when, why, and how? One should not assume that the animal has a problem just because he or she is crated or has restricted access in the house. Some people crate their dogs as a management style, not because they have problems. Some people do not like cats in their bedrooms and isolate them. Still, there may be a reason associated with the problem that is the cause of this modification, and the reason should be known. Given the crate or confinement style, the pet's behavior, and the people's needs, you need to learn whether the confinement style is being used appropriately. Crates used for punishment become unsavory locations for pets; furthermore, crates should not be used to warehouse pets for extended periods. Also, it may not be possible to evaluate the full range of behaviors exhibited if the animal is confined. For example, the dog's separation anxiety may be controlled phenotypically by crating, but undiminished at the neurochemical level. Efficacy of drug treatment will be hard to evaluate in the presence of constant confinement.

How big is the area where the client lives and to how much of it does the pet have access? This will tell you about both exercise and exposure for the pet.

How do the clients say good-bye to the pet, and how do they greet it when they come home? This provides information on attachment, attentiveness to detail, and on interaction. Attachment does not cause problems; however, it may influence the client's willingness to address them.

Where does the pet sleep? Again, depending on the answer to this question, the client may have more or less opportunity to observe the pet. If there has been a change, find out why. This could be a factor in the behavioral problem or the result of it.

Is there a yard, is it fenced, and does the pet have access to it? If so, how does the pet behave when in the yard and how does this compare with its behavior in the house? You may find that the dog lunges at strangers when in the house and within the confines of the fenced yard but never did this before the yard was fenced and is fine on the street. That is a clue to the "problem."

Some of these questions can be better answered if the client draws a map that is grossly to scale. Maps are particularly useful for problems involving cats. Any objects, accessories, or contested areas should be noted on the map. For example, if the complaint is that the cat will not use her litterbox, the map could indicate locations of doors and windows, location of litter boxes, favorite perch sites for all household cats, areas where cats are fed, locations of tile versus carpeted floor, and so forth. Be forewarned: if you provide clients with the opportunity to draw maps before the appointment, you could get very detailed, color-coded versions. This is a great detail, but it is not a substitute for the rest of the history.

5. Medical Considerations

Get a good medical history. There may not be an association with the behavioral problem, but the medical history is important in providing comprehensive care.

How often does the animal have fecal examinations and get vaccinations; which ones does it receive, and when was the last vaccine? If your client does not know why pets need to be vaccinated or that some immunizations are annual, what else do they not know about responsible pet ownership?

If you are in a rabies-endemic area, obtain an excellent vaccination and exposure history. Is this pet, and anyone who has interacted with it, at risk?

Does this animal, or any pet in the household, have any atopic conditions? If so, how are these managed, and is the behavioral problem particularly apparent or associated with the outbreaks or therapy? Corticosteroids can render behavior more labile and potentiate aggression.

Has this pet, or any other in the household, had a transfusion history? Why, and are there any untoward reactions? You may need to know this if this animal repeatedly sustains major trauma and blood loss.

Is this pet, or any other, subject to known food hypersensitivity, and how does this manifest itself? This information can contribute to explaining elimination or self-mutilation disorders; it may not, but the history should be complete.

Is this pet, or any other in the household, being treated for chronic illness (lupus, diabetes, Cushing's disease)? Any illness and some therapies can alter a pet's behavior.

Has this pet, or any other in the household, had any infectious, parasitic, or toxic conditions in its lifetime? How were they resolved? Were there any long-lasting effects? Did any of the behavioral problems begin or alter at those times? If the patient is a young animal and exhibits stereotypic or ritualistic behaviors that could be related to nervous system deficits, consider any infectious conditions that might have been present in utero. What are the other puppies or kittens like?

When was the last time this pet had laboratory analysis of blood samples, and were the results unremarkable? This is an important question. If you may need to use drugs, baseline blood work (complete blood cell count [CBC], serum biochemistry profile) must be performed first. If blood tests have not been done within the last few months, or the clients do not know and cannot get the results, repeat the tests. Unlike humans, pets cannot articulate complaints attendant with early physical signs of disease or illness. Without frequent blood work, the veterinarian has no clue when the value in question became egregiously high, or the extent to which it was altered by behavioral drugs. It is generally a good idea for any client, even those whose pets do not have behavioral problems, to have annual blood profiles performed once the pet is middle aged (3 to 5 years for dogs; 5 to 7 years for cats). Clearly, laboratory examination is also indicated in any illness. This comprehensive plan provides a baseline from which future deviations can be gauged.

Has this pet had any surgeries (including castration or spaying)? Were there any complications? Is there any association between the surgery and the onset of or alteration in the behavioral problem?

If the pet has not been castrated or spayed, why not? Is this a breeding animal? Has this pet been bred? If so, how many times and with what results? Were the heats "normal," and were there any behavioral changes in the periestrus period? These questions provide information about nuances of behavioral changes that may be attributable to hormones.

Is the pet currently receiving *any* medication, including heartworm prophylaxis? Not only will this information provide some idea of the client's awareness, but you must be vigilant about drug interactions if use of behavioral drugs is contemplated. A cautionary note is warranted: ask this question in a variety of manners including use of the words drugs, medication, treatment, pills, solutions, and so on. Once, after taking the history on what was purported to be a particularly aggressive cat, I was very impressed with the cat's mellow mood and commented on it. The owner replied, "Yeah, isn't it great what 'tranqs' can do?" We had used all the other words above and received a negative reply to each.

6. Behavioral Descriptions

Get a good description of the problem behavior. Do animal imitations and impressions if necessary. Imitate the difference between a bark and a growl; demonstrate the difference between a play posture (play bow) and submissive roll. Make sure that what you *think* you understand is what the clients are describing. Ask about the position and demeanor of the animal's tail, ears, and facial/neck hair. Use pictures to help you (see Chapters 3 and 4). Ask about body postures and vocalizations (Boxes 5-1 and 5-2). Ask about actual behaviors: does the growl go from low to high, or high to low, and during the growl is the pet approaching or backing up? Interpretation of these behaviors is covered in Chapters 3 and 4. If the clients are unsure of your meaning and you do not understand their description, ask them to videotape the behavior. Start a collection of videotapes; then you can show the client another animal doing the behavior

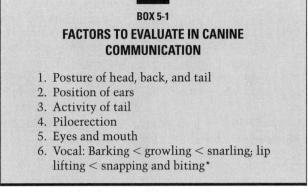

BOX 5-1

FACTORS TO EVALUATE IN CANINE COMMUNICATION

1. Posture of head, back, and tail
2. Position of ears
3. Activity of tail
4. Piloerection
5. Eyes and mouth
6. Vocal: Barking < growling < snarling; lip lifting < snapping and biting*

*This could be an orderly progression; but it need not be; in profound cases it will not be and need not be progressive.

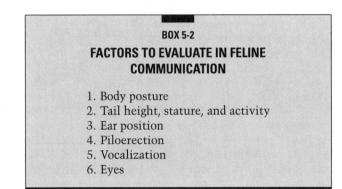

BOX 5-2

FACTORS TO EVALUATE IN FELINE COMMUNICATION

1. Body posture
2. Tail height, stature, and activity
3. Ear position
4. Piloerection
5. Vocalization
6. Eyes

and ask, "Is it like this?" The use of videotapes can also be invaluable if you wish to consult a specialist.

7. Daily Schedule

Obtain a good 24-hour history of an average day in the life of the pet. Start in the morning when the owner wakes up. Where is the pet? What does it do? Who gets up first? Take the client step by step through the day, even though he or she may not know exactly what the pet does when no one is home. Find out who (the dog or the person) goes to bed first, at what time, and where. This provides you with a true window into the social milieu of the pet. You are further able to evaluate how accurate and detailed the client's recitations and interpretations may be. Also, you can evaluate which therapies might have the best chance of success and which have none, given the scheduling situation.

8. Recent Problematic Incidents

Ask the clients to describe, in detail, the three or four most recent events when the behavioral problem has occurred. Remember that the most recent incident may have occurred in your office or as you greeted the client. You need to know exactly what happened: who was there, what happened, which behaviors preceded the inappropriate behavior and which followed it, what body postures and signals everyone used, how the situation was resolved, and the pet's response.

Distance can be important and informative: did the dog start to growl as the individual entered the room, or did he start when the individual reached down to pet him? Did someone have to look at the dog before he began to growl? Was the dog backing up when he growled? Did the cat hiss first, or just tense her back before the bite? Was the patient lying down, sitting, or standing immediately before the aggressive event? Did the cat go into the litter box and poke around before eliminating next to it, or did she just perch on the side and never touch the litter? The clients may not know all of this information, but you can be sure they will watch carefully in the future. You have just educated them. Make sure you detail every single behavior you want them to watch. This includes tail position, hair position, body posture, orientation of ears, pupil shape, mouth shape, vocalization nature and frequency, whisker movements, tail movements, and so on. *Be explicit and write everything down in the discharge instructions.* Make a standardized discharge sheet where all the behaviors you want the clients to watch can be noted. Now you have the data to interpret the actual problem, rather than relying on the client's interpretation of it. Furthermore, once the clients begin to try to accurately describe and order the events, not only are they able to provide more detail and more information on variation in the behavior or outcome depending on who is present, but also they are apt to remember more incidents of the inappropriate or undesirable behavior. This is the first step in getting them to cooperate with treatment.

9. Frequency, Duration, Intensity, and Percentage of Occurrence

Ask the clients two questions regarding frequency of the inappropriate or undesirable behavior:
1. How frequently does this happen: multiple times per day, daily, weekly, monthly?
2. What percentage of the time that the pet is exposed to the circumstance does the inappropriate behavior occur?

These questions pertain to very different issues. The dog may only lunge at strangers monthly, but it happens 100% of the time he sees a stranger: the clients have learned to restrict the dog's access. The first question asks about the control, access, and expression; the second asks about the pet's reactivity. You need to know both.

10. Ownership History

Find out whether this pet has lived with previous owners and why. Recycled pets may be at more risk for behavioral problems, although as with most issues

in behavior, data are scant. If the pet has lived with other people, realize that much information is going to be skewed, missing, or incorrect. This is particularly true for questions regarding age of onset, frequency, and response to correction and previous therapies.

11. Previous Treatment

Ask what treatments or therapies have been tried to date, and their outcomes. Prompt the clients if they say "none." Surely someone must have yelled at the pet; what did it do? If the dog is walked on a leash, what type of collar is used? Did the clients ever try to leash-correct the dog either by pulling on the collar or hitting the dog with the leash? What was the dog's response? Make sure that the clients know that you do not presume that they are dog abusers; rather, you are trying to obtain a comprehensive and accurate portrait of the range of the dog's behaviors. Knowing what may have worked and what did not during past events or occurrences can be beneficial in framing a treatment protocol. Furthermore, the response to correction can make a critical difference in how you decide to rank your differential diagnoses.

Disabuse clients of the notion that obedience school is a substitute for behavioral therapy; it is not. It *is* a terrific idea, but six group lessons are hardly adequate to help the neophyte dog owner who has a pet with behavioral problems. This issue is more fully discussed in Chapter 12.

Determine whether the client has used private trainers. Why? Was this a convenience for them, or is there a reason they did not want the dog in public? Did the trainer help or render the situation worse? What specific techniques were used? How did the client feel about previous training? If clients cannot execute the techniques of that particular trainer, they will not do them. If they are hesitant in doing them, they will not accomplish what the trainer suggested. Both circumstances are potentially very dangerous and need to be addressed. As with any therapy for a medical condition, the ability to comply is critical.

12. Age at Onset and Duration of Condition

Ask when the clients thought the inappropriate or undesirable behavior started and how long it has been ongoing. You may have a different view after in-depth questioning, and both answers should be recorded. For example, the clients may truly believe that their 5-year-old spayed female dog was never aggressive until the bite that occurred during the previous week. The bite occurred when the son saw the dog chewing a rawhide on his bed and tried to remove it. Close questioning about whether the dog allows people to pick up her food dish when it is full or empty and whether the clients can take a biscuit or a real bone from the dog elicits the response that they always leave the dog alone while she is eating. This may strike you as good courtesy and common sense, but wouldn't you like to know *why* the clients always leave the dog undisturbed in this context? In this case, you would discover that the clients do so because, as a puppy, the dog always growled at them when she had food and they have "learned" to leave her alone. This is a dog who has been aggressive around food for 5 years, but has only just recently bitten.

13. Changes in Pattern

Ask whether the undesirable behavior has increased in intensity, frequency, or duration since starting and record the pattern. Are there any correlational events or factors associated with any changes (e.g., moving to a new house, the addition or death of a pet or human family member, an illness)? An undesirable behavior that is increasing under all these conditions has a worse prognosis than one that is decreasing. Also, any decrease in problematic behavior may be a clue as to what might work in the final resolution.

14. Familial History of Behavioral Problems

Find out how many littermates of each sex there were, and whether any littermates or relatives have or had similar problems. Some behavioral problems appear to run in family lines. Not only might this be early warning for owners of pups, but also it might be a contraindication to breeding. Certainly, this information is the only way to understand any behavioral problems that have a heritable component.

15. Placement and Euthanasia

Ask whether the client has thought about placing or euthanizing the pet. Do not do this in a pejorative manner or make it sound like you recommend it a priori. It is best to find out before the appointment; this can be done with the preappointment questionnaire. You may wish to reassure the client at the start of the appointment that, although you know that this is a concern of theirs, decisions to place or euthanize animals should be made after the diagnosis is known, and after some thought is given to what implementing the therapy will mean. Getting the issues out in the open and reassuring the clients that no decisions have to be made immediately may help you to get a better history. I tell clients who are obviously concerned that I almost never recommend euthanasia on the first appointment; often they burst into tears after I tell them this, so convinced were they that I would automatically recommend getting rid of the pet instead of helping it. It is important that the clients view the behavioral appointment as a time to establish a diagnosis and get help; otherwise you will not get an accurate history. Accurate histories lead to realistic prognoses. Certain conditions must be met to improve any pet's behavior; these conditions may place constraints on the clients that they find untenable. If these conditions cannot be met safely, ethics mandate an honest evaluation. The clients must act on that. Euthanasia and placement are dealt with fully in Chapter 12.

16. Client Behavior and Interaction

Observe the interaction between the clients, the clients and the pet, you and your staff and the pet, and you and your staff and the clients. If the pet, or children in the family, are so disruptive that you cannot hear the clients, then they cannot hear you. Put the disruptive individual in another room; dogs can be returned for observation of their behavior when all energies can be devoted to observation. I have even pressed veterinary students into service as babysitters. This time is too important to waste, and you and the clients need to attend to each other. These socially awkward situations are to be controlled, not avoided. If you had not seen the disruptive manner in which the children interacted with the dog, how would you have known that you had to address it?

If the clients are combative about their interpretations of their pet's behavior or about their descriptions of the pet's behavior, it is time to call your local social worker. You will need help in dealing with the familial dynamics in the process of treating the pet.

If the dog yaps throughout the examination and jumps on the clients until they pick him up, you have some idea of the problem. Clients virtually never recognize attention-seeking behavior, yet it is among the most common canine diagnoses. One of the functions of the clinician in this situation is to act as a mirror for the clients: they cannot actually see what is going on in the situation because they are in it. If you can observe and behave differently to the pet, they will be able to see the difference. At the Behavior Clinic at VHUP we have a room with one-way glass; this glass is mirrored. Clients frequently catch themselves in the mirror interacting with their pet in a way they did not heretofore perceive. They are momentarily startled to realize that they are doing something they did not realize, and the experience is invaluable. Most practices cannot justify the expense of one-way glass, but ordinary mirrors, videotapes, and human "mirrors" all help.

17. Anything Left Unsaid

Finally, ask the clients if they have anything else they wish to tell you or ask you. You might be surprised.

This is a lot of information. In the interest of efficiency, many of these questions can be combined on a questionnaire that the clients can complete and return before their appointment (see Appendix A). You can then use this to make a plan, and appointments then can be scheduled according to the amount of time needed and billed by the hour. During the actual appointment, use an additional questionnaire form; *do not ad lib* (see Appendix A). First, if you ad lib you will miss something. Second, like anything else, this takes practice. After a few behavioral examinations you will begin to see patterns. You cannot attain this if you subscribe to the helter skelter approach. Third, written documentation is always an excellent idea. Not only does it have the potential to protect you legally, but it is the correct and thorough way to collect information. No Nobel prize–winning scientist relies on his or her memory for data retrieval. Why would you?

If you need to think about your diagnosis, you can have the client come back for a second appointment during which the treatment plan and diagnosis will be discussed and the treatment implemented. In fact, if the client and the pet are wearing down, this may be the best approach. Long examinations are difficult for everyone. Clients are receptive to this idea. As veterinarians we already practice this strategy for medical appointments; when we say we will call someone back pending results of blood studies, we are also giving ourselves some time to think. Clients can be trained to understand that if we are to do the best job possible we need to think, observe, and modify as needed. Ideally, clients and patients should then be reexamined at 2- to 4-week intervals until improvement is maximal or complete (see Appendix A). Even if all family members could not come to the first appointment, they must be present at the reexaminations. This is where all the desensitization/counterconditioning regarding specific behaviors and evaluation of change will take place. Everyone needs to participate. This is more fully discussed in Chapter 12. Important points for taking a good behavioral history are outlined in Box 5-3 and highlighted in Box 5-4.

SPECIALIZED ADDITIONAL QUESTIONS FOR SPECIFIC PROBLEMS

This section deals with specific questions that expand the focus of the forms in Appendix A. Because an important part of treatment is to prevent continuation of the inappropriate behavior, it is important to obtain very context-specific responses about the problems. This section concentrates on three topics for which more specific answers are desirable: feline elimination disorders, canine aggression, and stereotypic behaviors (obsessive-compulsive disorders).

Feline Elimination Disorders (Appendix A):

Questions about specific components of elimination behavior (number of litter boxes, style of box, location of box) can be dealt with, in part, through the preappointment questionnaire. The focus of the appointment during the consultation should focus on descriptions of actual behaviors. If the client had tried liners or covered boxes, why do they not use them now—what actual behaviors changed? Has there ever been any change in whether or not the cat covers its urine or feces; if so, is any of that variation associated with another cat?

Questions such as these allow correlations to be made between the appropriate and inappropriate be-

---

BOX 5-3

CRITICAL TOPICS TO BE DISCUSSED DURING A BEHAVIORAL HISTORY

1. Signalment—breed- or sex-specific risks
2. Client's complaint
3. Reason for seeking help
   a. Client's perception of problem(s)
   b. Causal reason for appointment
4. Client's perception of guilt and responsibility for problem and reasons for this
5. Primary caretaker responsibility for pet
6. Activity pattern of pet
   a. Daily schedule
   b. Weekend and holiday deviations
   c. Housing and exercise environment of pet
7. Medical considerations
   a. Medical history
   b. Current medical problems
   c. Medication taken
8. Actual descriptions of problem behavior
   a. Facial cues
   b. Body postures
   c. Vocal cues
9. Listing of problematic incidents
   a. Most recent three or four incidents
   b. Historical problems
   c. Initial event
   d. Changes with progression, season, corrections, and so on
10. Pattern of problem behaviors
    a. Frequency of incidents
    b. Duration of average bout
    c. Percentage of occurrence of problem if exposed to elicitor
11. Client/owner
    a. Number of previous owners for pet
    b. Reason for client having any pet
    c. Reason for having this particular pet
12. Previous treatments
13. Age at onset and duration of condition
14. Any familial history of this or related problems
15. Changes in pattern of problem
16. Familial behavioral history
17. Considerations for placement/euthanasia
18. Patterns of interclient interaction and interaction with pet
19. What has been left unsaid?

---

haviors and the environments. *Correlation is not causality*, but correlation will provide you and the client with the opportunity to then formulate hypotheses and test them. For example, if the cat always uses the litter immediately after you clean and change it, and only at such times does it dig in the litter (at all others it hangs on the side of the box and digs on

---

BOX 5-4

OVERVIEW OF HISTORY TAKING

1. Signalment
2. Client's complaint
3. Reason client is seeking help
4. Specific description of behaviors about which the client is concerned:
   a. Most recent three or four events
   b. Initial event
   c. Changes with progression, season, corrections, and so on
5. Any familial history, *with* descriptions
6. Age at which problem or related behaviors started
7. Frequency of undesirable behavior
8. Probability of behavior happening
9. Corrections tried and responses
10. Client's schedule—daily, weekly, seasonal changes
11. Any medical, nutritional, or pharmacological associations (spaying?)
12. Record of bites and legal documentation
13. Reason for client having any pet *and* this particular animal
14. Good description of pet's physical and behavioral environment
15. Ask what client's goals are

---

the floor), you have data suggestive of an ultrafastidious cat or one that may be controlling access to a valuable resource.

Test your hypothesis. Get multiple new, litter boxes (ones that have no scent), give the cat a choice of a couple of litters, including a clumpable litter, confine the cat with the boxes, keep all scrupulously clean, and see how the cat behaves. If the cat gets in the box and digs away while consistently using it for a period of weeks, you have verified your hypothesis about cleanliness and have also seen in which litter the cat uses the most enthusiastic elimination behaviors. If you maintain this degree of rigor in maintenance of the elimination environment yet changes occur when the patient is reintroduced to the feline household, consider the *social* environment.

A complete list of suggestions for the step-wise diagnosis and treatment of feline elimination disorders and a diagnostic/treatment flow chart is found in Chapter 8.

Canine Aggression (Appendix A)

The following discussion refers generally to both feline and canine aggression, but focuses primarily on the latter. Although more than $25 million dollars in health care costs are incurred each year in the United States as a result of cat scratches, dog bites more fre-

quently cause profound debility and death. It should be noted that there have been no rigorous studies that examine canine aggression in a prospective way, and the data collection on dog bites and their outcome are largely felicitous.

Aggression cases require some special questioning because it is important to understand the behaviors that the animal exhibits before the bite. Perception and comprehension of these behaviors will allow the client to minimize risk while using behavior modification to prevent further events.

In any case in which the complaint is aggression, you need to know who was present when the aggression occurred. If no one was present, it will be difficult to piece together a correlational scenario. In such cases you are reduced to relying on interpolation from the epidemiological aggression literature. Although this may be your only choice, you should realize that you cannot have the same faith in your diagnosis as you would were you able to obtain an excellent description. This means that the situation might be riskier because you cannot suggest specific scenarios, events, or behaviors that might trigger the aggression. Hence clients do not have knowledge of specifics of circumstances to avoid. The more incomplete the information surrounding the bite, the lower your *likelihood* (a measure of relative support among different hypotheses) of accurate diagnosis and intervention.

If the individual who was attacked is not a young child, another animal, or dead, you can ask him or her about the circumstances leading up to and following the aggressive event. Otherwise, if someone else was present when the aggression occurred, you can ask specific questions that might allow you to understand the behaviors that are indicators of aggression. This will both allow you to form testable hypotheses about factors that predispose the animal to act inappropriately and to apply principles of sequential hypotheses testing and risk assessment in avoiding or aborting future aggressive events. This sounds cold and technical when potential danger is involved; however, it is what is done whenever we work with a problem animal. Since we are functionally doing the experiment anyway, we might as well collect the information (data) within the construct of a logical system.

For example, one can ask where everyone was when the aggressive event occurred. In addition, one would like to know where the animal was with regard to the individual attacked. Did the animal streak across the room growling and grab the "victim" by the neck, or did the "victim" walk over the animal while he or she was sleeping and receive a bite that was not preceded by any vocalization? If you can instruct clients to begin looking for the first signals of aggression such as dilated pupils, piloerection, flexion of the toes, change in posture from lying down to sitting or standing, muscle tension, vocalizations such as hisses or growls, head lowering, teeth display, and approach, you can teach them to interrupt the behavioral process that progresses into the aggressive event. In other words, because behavior is a process, clients can learn to flag the individual behaviors that occur at the beginning of the time sequence that leads to aggression and to interrupt them. Interruption of the behavior at such times is most valuable because correction and punishment need to occur no later than the first 30 to 60 seconds after the *onset* of the behavior to be effective. This concept is fully covered in the Chapter 12.

When a client is able to interrupt the behavior early in the temporal sequence there are multiple benefits. First, this is when correction is most potent. Second, the patient does not have the experience of self-reinforcement that would emanate from being allowed to complete the sequence; therefore the component of learning the aggression has been diminished and the aspect of learning that such behavioral sequences are not completed is enhanced. Third, the client has minimized the likelihood of risk.

Look for patterns: do the inappropriate behaviors occur only in one section of the house, only when certain individuals are present, only when certain interactions are occurring (petting the cat, playing ball with the puppy), only when the animal is disturbed from rest, or only when kids between the age of 18 and 36 months are present? Are the bites always preceded by vocalization or never, and do all the bites come from behind, or are they precipitated by staring at the animal? Unless you are rigorous in your questioning techniques, you cannot expect to determine a pattern even when one is present. Animals are excellent at recognizing patterns; that is why we are so successful at training them. We must at least match their observational skills if we are to fix behavioral problems.

In addition to obtaining information about the locations of the victim and the aggressor and the behaviors preceding the aggressive event, it is critical to know what happens after the event. How does the event end? How is it terminated? For example, does the dog inflict one bite and back off, or does the dog continue to bite until the victim can drag herself to another room and pry the dog off with a door? Does the animal terminate the aggressive event (the cat that bites while being petted and then leaves), or does the client terminate the aggressive event (separating the dogs with brooms and dragging each of them to separate rooms)? What are the behaviors exhibited by the animal after the event? Do not allow the clients to tell you that the animal "didn't mean it" or that she looked contrite and sorry after the event. It is difficult enough to investigate our own underlying motivation for our behaviors without attributing to our pets underlying emotional states that cannot be independently assessed. The dog may "look sorry," not because he just ate your kitten, but because he is responding to vocal and nonverbal cues you are giving in what now is a separate behavioral sequence that may not be associated with the aggressive event. The

risk of the latter increases as time between the events increases; hence the emphasis on early interruption.

How have the clients tried to prevent the problem, and how have they tried to interrupt the problem? These are two different questions and both must be answered. Much information about diagnosis and prognosis can be obtained by observing and noting responses to any deformation of the extant behavioral system. Again, pattern is critical.

Find out what scares the clients. They may not have the words to describe the behavior, but they generally know when they are frightened. If there is an identifiable circumstance that makes them fearful, ask what about the animal's posture concerns them. They will probably say that they do not know. Start to ask about specific postures; ask if it is the way the eyes look. If they say yes, push the client to tell you what it is about the eyes. If they still do not know, give them some choices. Were the eyes very dark? This could indicate pupil dilation. There is a fine line between leading the clients to say what you want to hear and encouraging them to describe what they know. To accomplish the latter task, your choices must be exhaustive and the final patterns should be fairly consistent with your own observations of the animal. Clients observe much more than they realize, but the age of television has limited their descriptive skills.

Any aggression situation is potentially dangerous; hence this may be the stuff of which lawsuits are made. Know this beforehand. Ask whether any legal action has been considered or taken as a result of the event. This will not change anything you do or say; however, you will be quite sure to take exhaustive notes. Furthermore, if you perceive there *might* be legal complications (any reported bite or scratch, any bite or scratch outside the immediate family, any bite or scratch when the animal was at large, any fatal event, even in the family), *get a witness!* I personally prefer never to talk to clients unless a student or one of my assistants is present. Clients do not always hear what I intend to say, and even when they do hear what I am saying they may not understand what I was trying to convey. Get help. If you have no witness, ask the clients if you can use a tape recorder to help you maintain and transcribe notes. The Nixon era made many of us shy of recording devices and I am not suggesting *any* covert behavior; however, you need to protect yourself and still do the best job possible. In addition, write everything down. All instructions to clients should be in writing. If there are addenda, send them by certified mail and keep a copy in your files. If the case is really horrendous, have the copy notarized. (NOTE: If the case is this difficult, refer it to a specialist; it is likely that you could be overreaching the standard of competence to which you should be held.)

In a bite case, ask how many bites broke the skin as opposed to dented the skin. This might provide an idea of the extent to which the animal inhibited following through. Ask if the bites were reported and to whom. If the case necessitated treatment in the emergency department, do not assume that the personnel there reported the bite. Urban emergency departments may be too busy to do this. These data could be factors in your prognosis. A dog whose bite was reported absolutely *must not* have another such incident, and the clients must understand this. Ideally, all dog bite cases should be regarded this way, but a reported bite might provide the extra edge you need to convince the client to treat or kill the dog. Use every tool you have.

Use a preformulated set of behaviors that are associated with certain aggression as an aid in assessing pattern. The Aggression Screen used in the Behavior Clinic at VHUP for dogs is provided in Appendix A. Obtain an actual response for each category of aggression. The screening tool divides these responses into broad categories. If the aggressive response happens to only one person, note this. You can incorporate the frequency of the behavior and the individual to whom it was directed into this questionnaire. This degree of specificity is important because it sets minimum aggression standards for that dog *and* helps in formulating a prognosis. The dog that growls only at one particular visitor while effusively greeting all others is very different from the one who growls at *everyone* who is not a family member.

Ask about progression: if the dog snaps and bites in a specific situation (taking a rawhide), does the dog growl first? If so, is the growl prolonged or very brief? All of this information is essential for ascertainment of risk. This type of disciplined approach will ensure that you have noted the most prominent correlates of the behavioral diagnosis and will allow you to compare these between cases. Such comparisons will form your clinical impression.

Finally, particularly during a behavioral history in an aggression case, minimize outside disturbance. A quiet room is essential; others must be instructed to knock and wait for your approval before entering. Disconnect the telephone or use the answering machine. Do not make sudden movements or gestures. Do not pet or smooch with the patient. Do not reach toward the patient unless it is restrained. Do not stare directly at the patient, but do not take your eyes from its vicinity. Before doing anything to the patient, have it gently restrained and have one of your assistants always watch its face and eyes; that will be your first cue to any untoward behavior. If the clients feel more comfortable keeping the animal on a leash or crated, let them. You can then release the animal for observation in an extremely controlled context. Never turn your back on the animal. Leave the room only when the animal is restrained, and then back out. These cautions may sound excessive; they are not.

Stereotypic/Ritualistic Behaviors (Obsessive-Compulsive Disorders) (Appendix F)

Histories for stereotypies should include all of the previously mentioned information and must also detail specific information about the abnormal behaviors. The frequency of the bouts should be augmented by the average duration of the bouts and the range of duration of the bouts. Furthermore, it is critical to understand what terminates the bouts. Quite frequently the terminating factor is exhaustion. Ask the clients if calm restraint can stop the event. Be critical; the clients can evaluate whether physical restraint stops the event but not the motivation. If the animal still desires to pursue the behavior, the behavior is *not* stopped by restraint, although the physical ramifications might be.

It is absolutely critical to obtain accurate and detailed daily patterns for these behaviors. Some behaviors can appear ritualistic yet be more closely affiliated with anxiety. The presentation of the behavior is the same, but the cause is different. Because anxiety is not treated in the same manner as a behavior representative of an obsessive-compulsive disorder, these distinctions are critical. A separate sheet for augmented histories for these types of cases is included in Appendix A.

• • •

Sample questionnaires for clients and interviewing are in Appendix A. The first questionnaire provides basic health and maintenance information about the pet and should be given to the client before the visit. Providing the client with adequate time to complete these forms allows better information gathering and allows all family members to have the chance to contribute. These questionnaires also contain questions that are designed to allow clients to tell the practitioner what they perceive the problems to be and what they want to fix (not always the same thing), and sections on how they feel about both the pet and the problem. *Do not let the client diagnose the problem for you;* that is your job. Thus if they list *aggression* as the problem, you need to know what they mean by that term. Client questionnaires allow the interviewer to then formulate specific questions that address any special needs in addition to a general history questionnaire. It is useful if you have the first questionnaire before the appointment. Clients can either return it at your office before the visit or mail it.

Remember that the history is your chance to collect data with which you will formulate a hypothesis (diagnosis). The response to your questions plus the animal's observed behaviors make up the data. Treatment is a test of your hypothesis, and the response to therapy, good or poor, provides more data. Use the reexamination questionnaire and the aggression screen (both in Appendix A) to collect data about behavioral changes. This type of structured thought process is essential if we are to give behavioral medicine the rigor it deserves.

6 ····· Canine Aggression

···

Up to about 1970, many studies contained the unstated assumption that aggression is a unitary phenomenon that can be "measured" by recording a single feature of agonistic behavior such as the frequency of attack or even as contrived a response as biting an inanimate object (Azrin et al., 1965). This assumption underlies a sizable scientific literature representing a highly simplistic approach to the subject. This approach has been attacked repeatedly for nearly two decades and cannot but die; however, the corpse seems reluctant to lie down.

Fraser and Rushen, 1987, p. 285

*C*anine aggression is the most common behavioral problem in dogs seen at behavioral practices and is the most dangerous one seen in pet dogs (Beaver, 1990, 1993a,b; Borchelt, 1983; Landsberg, 1990a, 1991a; Voith, 1981d, 1983a,b, 1984a; Wright, 1991; Wright & Nesselrote, 1987). Diagnosis and treatment of canine aggression are volatile, controversial issues. Much is unknown about this condition; however, it would be criminal if, because of this, the focus on available knowledge, extant therapy, and response to available therapy were blurred. This chapter covers the following subjects:

1. The epidemiology and outcome of dog bites
2. A review of the arguments surrounding breed predispositions for aggression
3. A discussion of prevention and early intervention
4. A section on myth, misunderstanding, and issues yet to be resolved
5. Categorization and diagnostics of canine aggression
6. Treatment of aggressive dogs
7. Case reports illustrative of the aggressions discussed

Before any discussion of factors mitigating aggression, it is critical to define aggression and to again review the factors in human and canine social systems that facilitated domestication and the social situation involving pets today.

DEFINING THE ISSUE

Aggression is best defined within a given context as an appropriate or inappropriate threat or challenge that is ultimately resolved by combat or deference. This broad definition encompasses the standard definition of agonistic behavior and is consistent with those for hierarchical terms that focus on the ability to control access to any resources (Immelmann & Beer, 1989).

It is important to realize that aggression can be an appropriate response in certain contexts. Defense *may* be an appropriate form of aggression. A dog that attacks visiting friends as they hug their hosts is responding inappropriately and out of context. Dogs that aggressively defend their people from rape, theft, attack, or attempted murder are considered heroes regardless of whether they do so by merely being present, by inflicting an element of fear and surprise regardless of their behavior, by growling, by baring their teeth, or by biting. In such circumstances I would classify the aggression as *appropriate*, and *in context*. The form of the aggression might not matter to me were I the rape victim, but I would firmly support the concept that if a threat sufficed, I would prefer that the dog not bite, and that if it did bite, that it not maim or kill. The latter distinctions emphasize the dog's ability to make fine, contextual decisions.

The issue of whether a behavior was contextually appropriate is seldom raised when one perceives that one's life was saved, but we should strive to remove emotion from the situation so that we can understand the behavioral sequence and evaluate possible problem areas. Some believe that regardless of circumstances, a dog should *never* bite. Police and guard dogs are useless (and dangerous) if their first recourse in any situation is to bite. They are trained to withhold their teeth and act in a contextually appropriate, coordinated manner with their human partners. This scenario is an example of learned aggression. These dogs are taught to exhibit aggressive behaviors in response to patterns of provocative events. They are reinforced to inhibit themselves, and biting is the exception. But if dogs are never to bite people, *without exception*, does this mean that they should not bite in defense, even if all other levels of aggression fail as a deterrent? Does it mean that no matter to what extent a human tortures a dog, that dog cannot bite, even if it means its life? And if one wavers on the last issue, given the interspecific communicatory problem, how would a dog convey to a human (particularly a young one) that the dog perceives its life to be at risk? These are ethical issues that should be discussed and argued in forums free from myth if we are to understand canine aggression and decrease risk from it.

The term *provocation* must be discussed in the context of a dog known to be aggressive in certain circumstances compared with a dog that has never reacted in those circumstances. If a dog is known to have a propensity to behave inappropriately in certain contexts (i.e., petting or reaching over its head), it may be "unintentionally provoked" (*sensu* Podberscek & Blackshaw, 1991a) by what would otherwise be considered a normal gesture. For *abnormal* animals, *normal* gestures will not be perceived as such; this is part of the symptomatology that can be understood and treated. It is important to realize that dogs exhibiting inappropriate, out-of-context aggressions are not misbehaved or poorly behaved—they are clinically abnormal and must be regarded as such. When one acknowledges that the dog is abnormal and is *not* misbehaving, many problematic issues, such as aggressive responses to corrections, make sense. A corollary of this point is that a normal, nonthreatening, nonprovoking human behavior may be perceived by the dog as provocative. For the dog's behavior to improve it is *critical* that the dog not be "provoked." To do so, even unintentionally, only reinforces the inappropriate, undesirable, and perhaps dangerous behavior.

For all dogs that are aggressive in *any* circumstances, it is important to determine the following aspects of the behavior:

1. Whether the behavior was appropriate
2. In what context the behavior occurred
3. Whether the behavior involved threats, combat, or deference
4. The ultimate resolution

Inherent in this assessment is an understanding of the extent to which the dog inhibited its own aggression in response to a *changing* context. Social situations are not static; they are a continuous interplay between signal and response. A problem pet may have more difficulty responding to this changing situation than would a nonproblem dog.

Although a dog that barks or growls can potentially be as dangerous as one that bites, some idea of the extent to which the dog has been able to inhibit itself can be obtained from the dog's reactions (Boxes 6-1 and 6-2). A dog that *never* reacts in a given context probably does not have a problem with it. This does not mean that some problem may not develop in the future, especially given that "dominance" or hierarchical standing is a social phenomenon. Dominance

---

BOX 6-1

FACTORS TO EVALUATE IN CANINE COMMUNICATION

1. Posture of head, back, and tail
2. Position of ears
3. Activity of tail
4. Piloerection
5. Eyes and mouth
6. Vocal: Barking < growling < snarling/lip lifting < snapping and biting*

*Could be orderly progression; in profound cases will not be and need not be progressive.

BOX 6-2

CONSIDERATIONS FOR INTENSITY OF AGGRESSION

1. Position on continuum: Barking < growling < snarling/lip lifting < snapping and biting
2. Physical signals congruent?
3. Warning given?
4. Can behavior be interrupted?
5. Can behavior be inhibited?
6. Can behavior be redirected with activity?

---

aggression (see Appendix F for the necessary and sufficient diagnostic conditions) develops at social maturity (18 to 24 months), and these dogs may well have been nonaggressive before the onset of social maturity (Borchelt & Voith, 1986a). A dog that barks in the same context is more reactive, whereas snarling or lip lifting (usually silent), growling, and snapping or biting represent increasing levels of aggression (see Fig. 3-3). Body posture during these events is revealing: lying down is a less reactive posture than is sitting, which is a less reactive posture than standing. This does not mean that a dog that is lying down cannot bite. It *does* mean that the dog that is lying down must proceed through more behavioral sequences before it is in the position to bite, giving another individual more time to react or to anticipate a problem. Dog owners must not be misled by the myth of the "tail-wagging dog"; a wagging tail is only an indication of willingness to interact. A dog that is standing rigid, hair up, ears back, barking, growling, baring its teeth, and wagging its tail will be very willing to interact in an extremely aggressive manner, given the appropriate cue or stimulus (see Fig. 3-2). If the dog has an aggression diagnosis, staring at or reaching for the dog may be sufficient to trigger further agonistic behavior and frank aggression.

By definition, a *first bite* means that the dog has never bitten before; it does not mean that there have been no aggressive events, as conveyed by the signals described previously. The dog could have been inhibiting appropriate or inappropriate behavior either out of good judgment or because of fear, insecurity, or lack of opportunity. In the case of phenomenon related to social maturity (e.g., dominance aggression), the condition experienced by the dog has actually been changing because of changes in the interactive social environment. Most aggressive dogs are clinically behaviorally *ab*normal, but the abnormality is usually progressive and is influenced by the social environment; the signs perceived by the client and clinician have been changing. Clients may not attend to the changes until the aggression is profound, so data on effects of early intervention and the extent to which behavioral trajectories can be modified are lacking. We can easily understand such progressive changes in infectious and noninfectious disease; why are we so unwilling to accept them in conditions that manifest as behavioral illness?

Finally, aggressive dogs should *not* be described as vicious. Viciousness connotes an underlying emotional state that may not correlate well with canine behavior and is impossible to evaluate in dogs. These dogs can be described as aggressive or dangerous, but *vicious* is an inappropriate term.

EPIDEMIOLOGY OF DOG BITES

A brief review of the basic epidemiology of dog bites leads one to the conclusions that biting dogs do *not* fit the stereotypes of rabid, prowling, stray, untrained animals, and that dog bites are more common than visits to behavioral specialists might lead one to believe.

In the United States, more than 1 million people per year *report* dog bites (August, 1988; Beck et al., 1975; Harris et al., 1974); many bites result in death (Borchelt et al., 1983b; Winkler, 1977). One study estimated that 10 people die in the United States each year as a result of dog bites (Young, 1988a). Fifty percent of dog bites leave scars, and 30% result in time lost from work or school (Bergen & De Hoff, 1974; Pickney & Kennedy, 1982).

Most dog bites in the United States are inflicted by pet animals (Pickney & Kennedy, 1982); the same is true in Australia (Podberscek & Blackshaw, 1991). The family dog is involved in the bite 25% to 33% of the time (Podberscek & Blackshaw, 1991). Free-ranging pet dogs may be more aggressive than strays when approached, and may be more aggressive when closer to home (Bikash & Bikash, 1990; Rubin & Beck, 1982; Wright, 1985, 1990b). An apparently high proportion of *stray* dogs (37%) identified as pit bulls are implicated in dog bite–related fatalities (Sacks et al., 1989).

Estimates indicate that by the age of 11 years the majority of children have been bitten by a dog, generally one known to them; 2% to 15% of U.S. children 5 to 9 years of age are bitten annually (Beck, 1981; Borchelt et al., 1983b; Kizer, 1979). In one study involving 3200 children 4 to 18 years of age, 45% reported being bitten in their lifetime (Jones & Beck, 1984). Animal bites have been estimated to be the fourth leading cause of death in children (Rice et al., 1956; Undermann, 1987). Because of children's height, bites commonly occur in the upper extremities, shoulders, head, and neck regions (Podberscek & Blackshaw, 1991). In one study 67% of bites to children 4 years of age and younger and 56% of those to children 5 to 9 years of age involved the face and neck (Chun, 1987; Kizer, 1979).

Although not explicitly discussed in reports of dog bites in the literature, it is implicit that a bite of the same force, administered by the same jaw configuration, could potentially be more injurious when delivered to the victim's head and neck than when delivered to the torso or extremities. Furthermore, a dog that is lunging for the head of an adult or one that is chasing any individual may become airborne in the leap immediately preceding the bite. Leaping animals hit their victims with more force, and potentially inflict more shearing damage, than does a dog that bites from a grounded posture. This scenario of interrelated factors explains why the majority of fatalities occur in the two age-groups of victims least able to defend themselves: the very young, and the old and debilitated. Seventy percent of dog bite–related fatalities occur in children younger than age 10, and 10.2% occur in individuals older than 69 years of age. The death rate for neonates is 370 times that of adults 30 to 49 years of age (Sacks et al., 1989). Unfortunately, the converse information—the proportion of individuals of each age who are bitten—is not available because poor records are kept on dog bites.

Of 96 cases of dog bites reported in *The Veterinary Record* (1991), 85% occurred in the owner's home, 62% represented adults bitten by their own animal, 75% of bites to children occurred when they visited neighbors or friends, 54% involved bites in which the victim was younger than 15 years of age, and male dogs were responsible for most bites. Sustained attacks were more commonly reported for large-breed dogs such as German shepherds, Dobermans, or Staffordshire bull terriers. However, rottweilers and Dobermans were responsible for only a small percentage of injuries that required plastic surgery. Clearly, breed-specific characterizations should be viewed with caution.

At least one study indicates that bites inflicted by strays (50.3%) are more likely to be examined by a physician than are bites from family pets (29.1%) (Jones & Beck, 1984). These percentages are still frighteningly low. Underreporting and underexamination of dog bites is unfortunately a reality even when mandated by law and when the bites are treated at emergency services (Beck & Jones, 1984; Moss &

Wright, 1987). Busy, urban emergency departments that fit the demographic profile for a potentially large number of dog bite–related visits have the least discretionary time with which to pursue the epidemiology of these. The emergency department at the Hospital of the University of Pennsylvania (Philadelphia) admits to treating nonmajor dog bite wounds without reporting them. When solicited for a collaborative study on the demographics of dog bites in urban areas, it became apparent that no one on the staff had the time or inclination to do so, despite the findings of the Delta Society, the Humane Society of the United States, the American Humane Association, and others (Felthous, 1980; Felthous & Kellert, 1987; Rigdon & Tapia, 1977; Tapia, 1971) that some classes of dog bites can be good indicators of child abuse. When resources are stretched thin, it is the scientific method and pursuit of solid data that most suffer. The child abuse/animal abuse association deserves more attention. The American Veterinary Medical Association (AVMA) is taking steps to ensure that this happens.

Most dog bites, particularly to children, occur in the summer, most bites occur on weekends, and the diurnal peak in bite activity is in the late afternoon and early evening (Kizer, 1979). Not only is the dog's basic behavior the cause of the bite, but the environment in which the bite occurred also plays a role. More children and dogs are outdoors and active during these periods (Clifford et al., 1983a,b). Greater contact, alone, could be a factor contributing to the pattern of dog bites; however, were this the sole reason, one would expect that the incidence of dog bites would scale with increased opportunities to bite. There is no valid evidence for or against this view; no one has studied this factor.

Examination of individual bites leads to the hypothesis that although increased contact is important, it may not be the sole cause of these patterns. The greater the number of both children and dogs, the greater the potential reactivity of each group. Again, there are no objective measures of this, but empirical evidence from pack or crowd situations in both dogs (Borchelt et al., 1983a,b) and people (mobs at soccer games, and so on) indicates that the more excited any participant, the less stable and predictable the situation. Such circumstances are ideal for unilateral or joint misinterpretation by the participants of any signaling behavior. Proximity facilitates violence, rather than retreat, as a response in such conflicts.

In the case of canine aggression toward children, there are two participants with similar evolutionary social histories, and enough overlap in patterns of sociality that it is possible to misunderstand the extent to which the same signal has two different messages and meanings (Smith, 1965; 1977). When the human participants are children, they may be uncoordinated and appear unpredictable because of their sudden shifts in postures and vocal range when excited. Some

behaviors and some intensities of behaviors in young children can frighten dogs and make them feel threatened. Other behaviors, like shrill squealing, could be misinterpreted by the dog as sounds and signals given by a prey item. Repeat bites, which are a function of the carnivory and shake-and-kill behaviors, that dogs can display in such circumstances may be a clue that they are confused about signals and context. In any excitable state the participants might be less aware of shifts of motivational state or willingness to participate than they would be under calmer circumstances. This description is particularly apt for children. The potential for bilateral misunderstanding and inappropriate reaction with concomitant disastrous circumstances is great. In such cases it is possible that the dogs are normally well behaved and not exhibiting any untoward signs of inappropriate behavior, including out-of-context aggression. Children can be unpredictable, dogs can be unpredictable, and the interaction can be toxic. This is a conclusion that is totally compatible with the epidemiological data on dog bites, but wholly incompatible, as are the epidemiological data, with the concept of breed-determined aggressive propensity. The latter topic warrants extensive explication.

THE ROLE OF ENVIRONMENT, GENETICS, AND BREED

Although much is asserted about breed differences and behavioral expectations, there are few data on this and even fewer on individual behavioral variation.

All behavior has environmental and genetic components. The variation in the genetic component is sufficient to produce a wide array of individual behavioral phenotypes in the absence of any specific breed. Hence, not all mixed breed dogs look alike or demonstrate identical behaviors in response to similar situations. (See data from Scott & Fuller, 1965, as presented in Chapter 3.) This is true within and among litters. Evolutionary biologists since and including Darwin have recognized these differences. The extent to which behavioral plasticity is a function of genetics is a hotly debated issue in the fields of behavioral ecology and evolution. Some recent experimental evidence on desert toads living in highly variable environments indicates that selection may be operating to maintain developmental and concomitant behavioral plasticity, rather than selecting one or a few modes, each of which would persevere under alternate conditions (Newman, 1989). These issues are important and relevant in discussing the issue of breeds.

Humans, as the agents of selective breeding, may have removed some of the advantages of plasticity through domestication while selecting for traits that have little adaptive or survival value (e.g., coat colors, particularly those associated with defects; white boxers are usually deaf). Selective breeding is particularly interesting with regard to behavioral medicine because breeding for temperament is still less popular than breeding for physical or vanity traits. The American Kennel Club (AKC) provides a decision-making graphic that tells clients whether to breed their dog. Temperament is further along in the process than are looks and the number of championships within the line (see Fig. 14-1). I prefer temperament as one of the first decision points, because fewer people might then be tempted to rationalize poor behavior to breed champions.

One function of establishing and maintaining a breed is to canalize some of the overall genetic variation within the species (and within the breed). Although domestic canine breeds have a relative body size that spans two orders of magnitude, such variation in size is absent in wild canids. The process of domestication itself relieved many of the pressures for which wild canid body size was a response, allowing the underlying genetic variation to respond to artificial selection. In the process of selecting for certain physical and behavioral traits within any breed, one has also selected for some variation in that trait. Accordingly, caution is urged in discussions of breed-specific behaviors.

Selection, natural or artificial, cannot act if there is no underlying genetic variation. Some variation (termed *additive genetic variance* by quantitative geneticists) must be present for a trait to be developed. This is easy to visualize in considering a physical trait such as coat color. It is less easy to see in selecting for a behavioral trait such as protectiveness. Protectiveness is actually a constellation of behaviors; breeding for this constellation produces a continuum of protective behaviors, some of which will not be what the selector desired. In fact, some of these behaviors will be inappropriate because they are not complete or force-

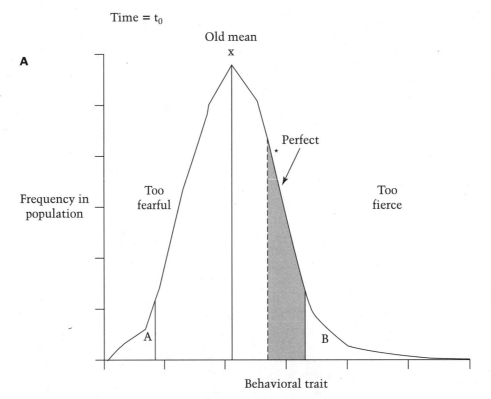

Fig. 6-1 Theoretical distribution of suites of behavioral characteristics before (**A**) and after (**B**) selection based on paradigms from population genetics (actual simulation; selection coefficient not specified) using the gestalt of herding/guarding behaviors.

Time t_0 = present

Time t_0 + 20 = 20 generations of selection (part **B**)

A, Area under the curve, or proportion of dogs that are too fearful to perform herding or guarding tasks. *B,* Area under the curve or proportion of dogs that are too aggressive to perform herding or guarding tasks; they injure or kill those they were to protect.

X, Old mean of population (normal distribution assumed).

*Desired profile of behaviors on which selection is practiced; stippled area indicates that a range of behaviors are considered good. *Continued.*

ful enough, and some will be unacceptable because they are too forceful and out of context. Under natural, rather than artificial, selection these behaviors would have been selected against at their extremes; however, it would be an error to regard the wild environment as producing absolute phenotypes. The demographic and local climatic environments act in concert to determine what scope of the continuum of variation will survive. In a very good year even the most inept hunter might live to reproduce and contribute genes to the next generation. This is the source of the additive genetic variance. That such genetic variance exists is demonstrated by the extent to which artificial selection has developed so many and such varied breeds in a few hundred years, whereas thousands of years of natural selection have not developed that degree of canine variability, although the initial stock should have been similar (Clutton-Brock, 1987; Serpell, 1987).

Accordingly, if one has developed a breed for certain specific behaviors (rather than overall ability to survive, as in the wild situation), one should expect

that there will be variation around that behavior and that some of this variation will result in inappropriate, out-of-context behavior. It is in this light that charges made about breed predilections should be viewed. This means that if one has selected a breed for protectiveness or guarding, some of the individuals in that breed may inappropriately protect or guard against objects that pose no threat (Green & Woodruff, 1988).

Consider a simple, theoretical example. If one starts with a normal distribution (Fig. 6-1) of individuals exhibiting variations of the trait for which one is attempting to breed—here, protective ability—some animals will be very friendly, but too shy, unmotivated, or fearful to protect (Fig. 6-1, A). Others will protect against anything, even when no protection is warranted (Fig. 6-1, B). This population of animals will have a mean (X; Fig. 6-1) for the distribution of the protective behaviors. The mean, in this example, does not represent the behavior that one desires; rather, the desired behavior is just to the right of the mean at the asterisk (*). Individuals clustered around

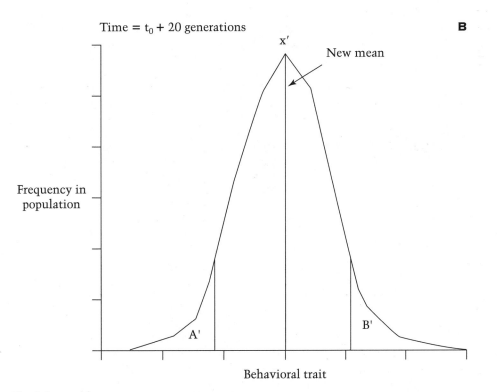

Fig. 6-1, cont'd.
NOTE: The boundaries for A and B are independent of the population distribution. They reflect a determination of whether the behavioral suite is desired or not. Only the area under the curve can increase or decrease with regard to the position of these. The position of these, in this model, does not change. This may not be what actually happens. What actually happens is that we become tolerant of undesirable behaviors and move these boundaries.

X', New mean after 20 generations of selection.

the mean, the desired behavior, are now bred (Fig. 6-1, stippling). Twenty generations of breeding with the same criteria produce the *same* distribution, but that distribution is now shifted to the right. Now, the mean (X') matches the desired suite of behaviors, and fewer of the dogs in the population are shy, fearful, or unmotivated, but a substantial proportion of the population is composed of dogs that protect when there is no need—in other words, those that are aggressive inappropriately, out of context. This is what happens in breeding for only one trait without a knowledge of population genetics. This represents precisely what happens when breeds get "hot" and are carelessly bred. Witness the incidence of hip dysplasia found in German shepherd dogs.

A specific example illustrates these points. Canine herding behavior was probably developed from the first phases of stalking behavior associated with predatory behavior. It is conceivable that unless selection were extremely discrete, sufficient variation should exist so that the occasional herding animal exhibits inappropriate predatory behavior toward the individuals that it is supposed to be protecting or herding. This is a common phenomenon recognized by sheep ranchers (Green & Woodruff, 1988).

Concepts regarding genetic variability in the development of behaviors are difficult, but given the amount of misinformation regarding some breeds and prejudice toward others, the issue should be addressed by both veterinarians and breeders. It should also be realized that cultural differences and biases of the *breeders* can affect the traits exhibited by the breed. Members of Asian societies may choose or are perceived to display less emotion in public than do those of Western societies, and it has been postulated that Akitas can be tough to "read" for people unfamiliar with them. "Apparency" in signal behavior *may* be culturally affected by the tendencies of those doing the artificial selection, but no one has studied whether this is an actual anthropological phenomenon or a bias.

Hart (1979a), Hart and Hart (1984, 1985b), Hart and Miller (1985) and Hart et al. (1983) have attempted to group breeds of dogs according to certain constellations of behavioral attributes. Although their classifications are based on subjective opinions (which can invoke prejudice and folklore) rather than objective classifications of individual behaviors, and their categories confound discrete behaviors and behavioral diagnoses, some overall patterns of behaviors correlated with breeds are apparent. Cluster analysis grouped animals according to reactivity, trainability, and aggression. It is no surprise that high trainability characterized most working and guard dogs, but this may be a teleological result. Still, it is intuitive: before selecting for any specific *other* behavior, the ability to work with and be trained by people would have to be elaborated. Less reliable are the characterizations of aggres-

sion and reactivity, because these are both diagnoses and descriptions of amalgam behaviors. More recent studies have attempted to focus on specific behaviors (e.g., growling when disturbed while sleeping, stalking small animals, barking at approaching strange people). This is important because there is scant documentation of the frequency, duration, intensity, and pattern of occurrence of the actual behaviors that are involved in behavioral problems. It is only in such contexts that fair evaluations of breed-related behaviors should be made.

Because so little is known about normal behavior and behavioral precursors of serious problems, early signs of problems are often not recognized. A survey of the faculty and senior students that I conducted at the Veterinary Hospital of the University of Pennsylvania (VHUP) and local practitioners revealed the following: (1) virtually all individuals thought that there were more and less aggressive breeds and could rank these; (2) the ranks of the three survey groups were different within and among groups with no rank being statistically significant; and (3) with the exception of the majority of the students, few individuals in the other two survey groups could, when provided with a list of discrete behaviors, accurately identify those that were outright aggressive or precursors of future agonistic behavior. Interestingly, rottweilers were ranked among *both* the least and most aggressive of the breeds. Given the failure to accurately identify behaviors that were outrightly aggressive or were precursors to future agonistic behavior, no faith should be placed in the breed-specific rankings. Such rankings often reflect individual preferences. They may be more indicative of the relative popularity of a breed within the practitioner's hospital population, or of the animal with whom one has had the most recent difficult experience, than of a breed propensity for aggression.

In the most recent data complied from the VHUP patient pool, a comparison of the behavior clinic breed population with that of the hospital revealed only four breeds that were "overrepresented" in the behavior clinic population. These were chows (G statistic; G_{adj} = 4.830; $p < 0.05$, but *one* dog made the statistical difference), cocker spaniels (G statistic; G_{adj} = 8.739; $p < 0.05$), dalmatians (G statistic; G_{adj} = 6.537; $p < 0.05$), and English springer spaniels (G statistic; G_{adj} = 76.315; $p < 0.05$). This distribution might not represent the breeds seen 5 years ago. In 1993 the five top breeds registered by the AKC were, in order, Labrador retrievers, rottweilers, German shepherds, cocker spaniels, and golden retrievers. Close questioning of the clients revealed another aspect that has been ignored in discussions of breed prevalence: for example, clients with English springer spaniels at VHUP appear to be quicker to seek help than do clients with other breeds because it has been well known for more than two decades in the United

States that springer spaniels have problems with aggression. Borchelt (1983a) found that purebred dogs were overrepresented when compared with mixed breeds only for one form of aggression: dominance aggression ($G_{adj} = 12.92$, $p \leq 0.05$ [my analysis]). One could hypothesize that the statistically significant overrepresentation of purebred dogs within this diagnostic category is due to the covariation of behaviors and temperaments associated with aggression that result from selection for confident, assertive, and flashy presentation in a conformation ring (e.g., head held high and forward, rostral posture, stance of forelegs and shoulders). *Any* discussion of breed–specific aggressive propensities *must* be viewed in a critical light that includes such considerations in combination with the abovementioned problem of the "apparency" of popular breeds.

Because of the previous emphasis on dog bites and dog bite–related fatalities, a brief note regarding breed associations with these is in order. Various authors have reported that in cases for which the data are available, bites from dogs are most frequently administered by mixed breeds, German shepherds, German shepherd crosses, pit bull terriers, and pit bull crosses (Kizer, 1979; Pickney & Kennedy, 1982; Sacks et al., 1989; Wright, 1991). The latter four groups are most frequently implicated in fatalities. (Pickney & Kennedy, 1982; Sacks et al., 1989). A careful reading of the literature indicates three findings:

1. The breeds most represented in the dog bite data change rank with time; this may indicate changes in breed preference by owners, rather than changes in breed-specific aggressive tendencies per se.

2. The breeds most frequently represented are *popular* ones, and *no one breed* may be represented in the bite data in disproportion to its occurrence in the population. Good data on population size of each breed and mixed breeds are unavailable.

3. The term *pit bull* is widely applied, often without biological basis, to a range of dog types, regardless of the underlying genetic stock (Lockwood & Rindy, 1987; Sacks et al., 1989; Segrest & Clifford, 1986a, b). This latter problem is probably magnified in areas that have already experienced one publicized "pit bull"–related attack.

Even in studies designed to elucidate heritable components of breed-specific performance traits, the results are not definitive. Tracking and scenting ability in German wire-haired pointers appears moderately heritable (having high additive genetic variance) and so should respond rapidly to selection (Geiger, 1972, cited in Willis, 1989). It should be noted that attempts to breed for high-performance with these parameters and absolute lack of gun noises failed (Fält, 1984). That these two suites of behaviors could not be simultaneously "optimized" is a clue. For a more complex behavioral suite, such as sheep herding, the mode of inheritance and the extent to which any of the behaviors comprising the style of approach and instinct are heritable is arguable and complex (Burns & Fraser, 1966). Investigations of unpredictable aggression have produced no firm results regarding heritability (Reinhard, 1978; Van der Velden et al., 1976; Willis, 1989). Shyness or lack of exploratory behavior has been investigated in pointers (Murphree, 1973; Murphree et al., 1977); although these behaviors appear in family lines, environmental factors could not be eliminated. A fearful, shy line of mixed-breed dogs, sired by a Siberian husky, has been produced under conditions designed to minimize environmental influences. In this particular example, the tendency to fearful behavior appears to be inherited in a simple mendelian dominant mode (Overall & Acland, unpublished data, 1996). Some evidence exists to link temperament and the probability of development of hip dysplasia in German shepherds (MacKenzie et al., 1985, 1986); however, this assessment involved a scored system for rating temperament that may have obscured individual behaviors. The genetics of normal and abnormal behaviors is another area that still requires intensive work.

Finally, many factors that are correlated with breed attributes are associated with damage and potential to cause damage. Evaluation of the role of these factors, separate from a breed appellation, in injury would greatly assist in dispelling myths about canine aggression. Physical factors that may affect the amount of damage caused by an aggressive dog include size (both mass and height), age (younger dogs are more energetic and less constrained by physical disability), jaw structure (tenacity of purchase as for mastiffs and rottweilers), and physique (distribution of muscle mass and relative strength). Rottweilers and Doberman pinschers, dogs with nasty reputations, are responsible for a small percentage of injuries requiring plastic surgery, whereas *sustained* attacks are most common in German shepherds, Doberman pinschers, and Staffordshire bull terriers (*Vet Rec*, 1991). These associations illustrate the interplay between physical and behavioral factors. Behavioral factors that may be correlated with damage include age at onset of aggression, duration of aggressive behavior, intensity of aggressive bout, frequency of aggression, and response to correction and other contextual information. These behavioral factors emphasize the roles of learning and context-appropriate behavior. Unfortunately, they are often ignored in behavioral evaluations.

Of course, any dog breeder or client who accepts the occurrence of inappropriate aggression or who believes that such aggression is "normal" for their breed (an oft-heard statement from people with some popular breeds) or not dangerous because the dog is small, contributes to the problem. One client actually told me, "Well, of course, if he was a rottweiler I'd be concerned, but he's just a Westie and he can't do any harm." The dog had already caused nerve damage and loss of the use of her husband's hand. No one should tolerate, excuse, rationalize, or accept as unimprovable any out-of-context aggression.

In summary, caution is urged regarding any generalizations about inappropriate breed-based behaviors. It is best to view selection for specific behaviors as a *risk assessment analysis.* Breeds that have been selected for one or a few particular and specific behaviors may be more at risk for developing undesirable variation for those behaviors. This does *not* mean that dogs selected for protective behaviors are more aggressive than dogs for which this selective pressure was absent. It *does* mean that that particular breed may be more at risk for developing a disproportionate number of dogs who exhibit inappropriate, out-of-context protective aggression given the selection/breeding conditions outlined previously. Inherent in this concept is that any dog, regardless of breed, can also exhibit the inappropriate behavior. A further corollary is that dogs that are selected for tenacity and jaw strength in their in-context work (bull terriers, rottweilers, Rhodesian ridgebacks), will, when they respond inappropriately or out of context in another behavioral setting, exhibit this same tenacity. Coupled with the physical traits attendant with such selection (large jaws, heavy musculature), they can and will cause extensive damage

on a first strike. These factors, rather than increased breed-specific aggression, are the cause of the severity of wounds, when inflicted. More research about all of these factors is desperately needed.

ROLE OF HORMONAL FACILITATION

The role of hormones in canine aggression has been discussed largely on the basis of correlational data. Most dominantly aggressive dogs are male (Borchelt, 1983; Borchelt & Voith, 1986; Voith, 1981b). Most dogs involved in dog bites are male (see Wright, 1991, for review). Although the dog bite data often do not indicate whether the dog is intact or neutered, the data for dominantly aggressive dogs seem to indicate that neutering status has little effect on whether a dog's behavior is diagnosed as dominantly aggressive. Studies defining *aggression* alone indicate that intact male dogs are more often implicated in aggression than are castrated ones (Borchelt, 1983; Wright & Nesselrote, 1987). Testosterone acts as a behavior modulator that makes dogs react more intensely. When an intact dog decides to react to something, he reacts more quickly, with greater intensity, and for a longer period of time. If the dog is reacting to a strange person or another dog, he will be quicker to bark, growl, or bite, and will continue for longer than a neutered dog (Fig.

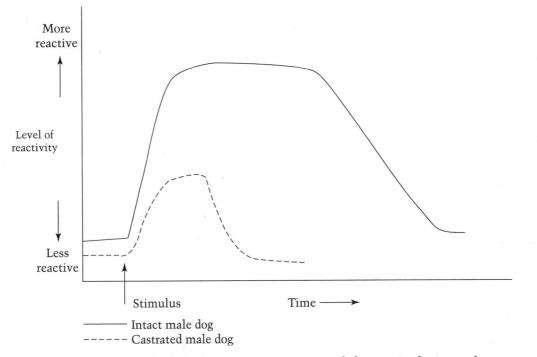

Fig. 6-2 Hypothetical effect of castration on "reactive" behaviors In the intact dog, baseline level of reactivity is higher, reaction to stimulus is quicker (greater slope), reaction reaches higher level of intensity, reaction remains elevated for a longer time, and cool-down or denouement phase is slow. The dog may not return to baseline.

In the castrated dog, baseline level of reactivity is lower, reaction to stimulus is slower (lesser slope), reaction reaches lower level of intensity, reaction remains elevated for a shorter time, and cool-down or denouement phase is relatively quick.

6-2). This point is discussed in depth later in the chapter. Castration decreases aggression to other dogs in 62% of the cases (Hopkins et al., 1976); however, few data exist on the decrease in aggression seen within each type of aggression. Male dimorphic aggressions may be disproportionately represented in such studies.

Data for unspecified aggression in intact female dogs indicate that they are less frequently implicated in aggression than are neutered females, the reverse of the pattern seen in males (Borchelt, 1983; O'Farrell & Peachey, 1990; Wright & Nesselrote, 1987).

A reanalysis of Borchelt's (1983) data indicates that the only statistically significant findings are as follows for all pairwise comparisons of sex and reproductive status within aggressive diagnosis:

- Dominance aggression: Intact males represented more frequently than neutered males or females ($G_{adj} = 6.51$, $p \leq 0.05$; $G_{adj} = 23.38$, $p \leq 0.05$; respectively).
- Fear aggression: Intact females represented more commonly than intact males ($G_{adj} = 7.58$, $p \leq 0.05$).
- Protective aggression: Neutered males represented more commonly than neutered females ($G_{adj} = 5.22$, $p \leq 0.05$).
- Possessive aggression: Intact males represented more frequently than intact females, neutered females represented more frequently than intact females, and castrated males represented more frequently than intact females ($G_{adj} = 3.90$, $p \leq 0.05$; $G_{adj} = 38.23$, $p \leq 0.05$; $G_{adj} = 6.42$, $p \leq 0.05$; respectively). There were no statistically significant differences for any pairwise comparison for predatory aggression—a situation that clients frequently blame on the dog's "testosterone kicking in."

There are few reliable data available for either males or females that investigate whether the age at neutering and the age at which aggression was first apparent are associated; this type of study is essential for any conclusions regarding hormonal facilitation and environmental interactions. Actual and specific behaviors that lead to the diagnosis of aggression are seldom described sufficiently to allow comparison between age and reproductive status categories of either sex.

An exception is a study by O'Farrell and Peachey (1990) that has made a good first attempt to quantify behavioral influences of early neutering for dogs both with and without a history of behavioral problems. In a preliminary study examining the effects of neutering on the behavior of dogs younger than 6 months of age and 12 months of age or older, one group stood out. Females younger than 6 months of age who were *already* showing signs of dominance aggression became more aggressive after ovariohysterectomy ($G_{adj} = 5.95$, $p \leq 0.05$ [my analysis] (Overall, 1995c). All other statistical comparisons indicated that aggression either did not change, or decreased with age, regardless of hormonal status, although a slight trend toward increasing aggression was noted for bitches as they be-

came socially mature. This makes sense. The number of dogs in this study was small, and many of the aggressive determinations are based on client descriptions. Regardless, these data suggest that the interaction between aggression and hormones is complex. Some of this complexity is apparent in the extent to which the organization of the neural system can be sex dependent (Compaan et al., 1993). It is postulated that hormonal facilitation in males and lack of it in females predisposes to aggressive acts, suggesting an androgen basis for the aggression. If this is so, the aggression should be related to different mechanisms; the following discussion shows why such logic does not apply. Progestins have been used (mostly inappropriately and excessively) to treat male aggression (Hart, 1974a, 1979b, 1981c), yet progestin levels are *seasonally* higher in intact female dogs. *Intra*sexual aggression is commonly associated with the breeding (i.e., periods of progestin) season in rodents that have estrous cycles and are, hence, seasonal breeders (Floody, 1983; Harding, 1983; Musi et al., 1993; Villars, 1983). High levels of aggression in hamsters are associated with the presence of progesterone, and many females show increases in attack behavior toward their own and other species in the periparturient period (i.e., high progesterone environments) (Moyer, 1968). Estrogen and ovarian implants can increase aggression in hamsters (Vandenbergh, 1971). It is during this period of elevated progestins, not the period of low progestin levels, that intact females are *more* prone to intrasexual interdog aggression. Furthermore, there are no data to support the contention that they are more prone to other aggression at these times. It would be inconsistent to reason that progestin-induced "feminization" of male dogs is homologous or analogous. Furthermore, prepubertal castration appears to have no effect on the development of canine aggression in males (Le Boeuf, 1970). These data are in agreement with more recent data (O'Farrell & Peachey, 1990).

Data from VHUP indicate that androgens may be implicated in dominance aggression in females. Although less common in males than in females, when dominance aggression *does* occur in females, the patients tend to be very young (younger than 6 months of age compared with 18 to 24 months of age for males), present with profound aggression that gets rapidly worse, and may have delayed heat cycles (Overall, 1995c). This leads to the question of whether the puppies have been androgenized in utero as happens in cows and rodents (Vom Saal, 1981, 1989). Although dogs (zonary chorioallantoic) do not share the same kind of placenta as cows (cotyledonary chorioallantoic) or rodents (discoid chorioallantoic), embryos can be exposed to substances in the blood of neighboring embryos via the mother. Intersex cows are the result of in utero hormonal contamination; these cows have inappropriate reproductive behaviors. Reports on rats, mice, and hamsters have all indicated that fe-

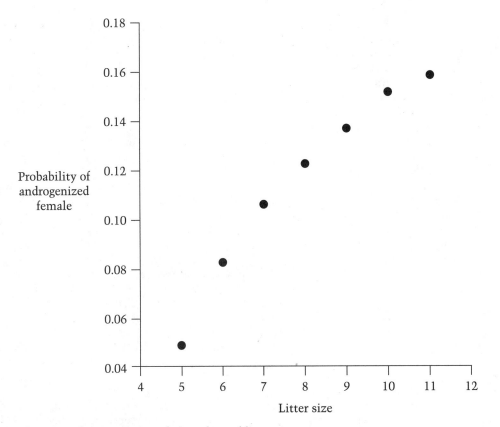

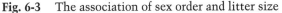

Fig. 6-3 The association of sex order and litter size

Y-axis, Probability of in utero androgenization given a bicornuate uterus and assuming an independence in ova fertilization, with each zygote having a 50% probability of being female.

• Probability of a female fetus being nestled between two male fetuses.

X-axis, Number of individuals in a litter.

males holding uterine positions between two males are more aggressive than are other females, and more closely resemble males than females in their conflict behavior (Brain & Haug, 1992; Vom Saal, 1984, 1989). Intrauterine position also appears to affect mating success in rams (Vom Saal, 1989). Birth order is something that can be ascertained in dogs, yet a survey of the literature and of reproductive specialists located at veterinary schools revealed that no one has considered this issue. It may merit further investigation. The probability that a female puppy rests between two males in utero is affected both by the bicornuate condition and by the number of puppies in the litter. The probability of such positioning, which could provide the conditions under which androgenization could occur, increases with litter size, but approaches an asymptote at less than 0.20 (or 20%) (Fig. 6-3). It will be very interesting to know whether this represents or approximates the proportion of bitches in the overall population that display early-onset dominance aggression. Female pups treated with testosterone after birth and *in utero* were more successful at competing for a bone than were normal females, but less successful than males (Beach et al., 1982), suggesting that testos-

terone may at least be a factor in the early development of some very specific manifestation of an artificially induced aggression.

As a test of the androgenization hypothesis, I asked clients to delay ovariohysterectomy for the few dogs for which it was an option. Female dominantly aggressive dogs that were not spayed experienced delayed or absent heat cycles. No hormonal assays or vaginal swabs were taken; therefore it is possible that the heats were "silent." That, in itself, would be interesting. Still, these anecdotal data illustrate the need for further research in the area of female canines and aggression. This form of dominance aggression may not be the same phenotypically or neurochemically as dominance aggression that appears at social maturity, or may not have the same catalog of behaviors seen in dominance aggression that appears at social maturity. Early spaying precludes knowledge about the latter in most cases. In adult male and female dogs the social rather than the sexual stage appears to be the major factor in the development of dominance aggression. Any differences in the pattern of the aggression exhibited by dogs that become aggressive at social maturity compared with those that exhibit it early in puppyhood suggest multiple underlying mechanisms for dominance aggression. This is true, although one form might be quite rare. The concept of multifactorial causality has only recently begun to be accepted in medicine. This is another area that warrants better description of the symptomatology, more specific diagnoses, and more experimental research.

PREVENTION OF AGGRESSIVE DISORDERS

Traumatic experiences early in life appear to have a less defined role in the behavioral difficulties of dogs than for humans. Dogs experience developmental periods during which they are most plastic in terms of responses to certain stimuli. These periods are best defined as sensitive periods (Bateson, 1979; Clark et al., 1951; Denenberg, 1968; Fox, 1965b; Scott & Fuller, 1965) and should be cautiously interpreted in light of risk assessment. If the animal is not exposed to the appropriate stimuli during these periods, it may never develop the appropriate or desired repertoire of behavioral responses. These periods have been well defined for dogs. See Chapter 3 for a complete description of early developmental periods.

Stray bitches that give birth on the streets may raise puppies that are well adjusted to the varied novel circumstances of street life and are well socialized to other dogs. These pups may still be fearful of people. They can be brought into a household, but the amount of effort required to make them good pets can be enormous. They generally retain some of their initial shyness, fear, and inappropriate greeting and play behaviors. Their problematic behavior could manifest as hiding, trembling, urination, or aggression. It appears that fewer people are willing to try to rehabilitate these pups compared with the number of people who are interested in trying to rehabilitate wild cats. In the past 2 years at the Behavior Clinic at VHUP, we have seen only one of the former, but half a dozen of the latter. One wonders if this is because people believe that dogs with limited early exposure to humans can be more aggressive and dangerous than cats with the same experience.

Pups that are hand-reared are at risk for developing inappropriate social behavior regarding other canids. If they live in isolation from other dogs during this period (rare) this is possible, but in very few of the cases of interdog aggression that I have seen could this be suspected. Regardless, it sometimes cannot be ruled out.

Pups that stay with breeders for extended periods of time (until 3 to 4 months of age) without exposure to novel circumstances and individuals may respond inappropriately. If they are exposed to only a few people during this period, this behavior could be generalized to all strangers. The situation that appears to be more common is that kenneled pups, when adopted, exhibit fear of all new, nonkennel environments. This fear can be so crippling that these dogs are unable to enter and leave the house or walk on the street. These dogs can improve with behavior modification and pharmacological intervention but are probably never normal.

Gene × environment interactions have been reported with respect to early environmental influences on the development of aggression. Increased aggression has been reported in male mice isolated from their peers (Denenberg, 1973). Male mice raised only with females have increased aggression in adulthood (Namikas & Wehmer, 1978). These effects are thought to be related in part to the inhibitory role of interaction with other males in the development of social learning. Increased aggression is reported in rhesus monkeys that are isolated (Bernstein, 1981). Mice cross-fostered from nonaggressive individuals to aggressive ones become aggressive (Southwick, 1967, 1968), but this effect may depend on species. Grasshopper mice (aggressive) that are fostered by white-footed mice (passive) become less aggressive, but the reverse does not occur (McCarty & Southwick, 1979). Pfaffenberger and Scott (1959) maintain that pups kept in kennels beyond 14 weeks of age are never normal, exhibiting timidity and a lack of confidence. Pups that are brought home at 8 weeks of age and kept inside with only one person or a few people may also find it difficult to make the transition to other environments.

It is clear from the above that the best time to recommend that a client adopt a pup is between 7½ and 8½ weeks of age. At this time pups are ready to be housebroken and are optimally poised to benefit from exposure to all socialization environments. There are two caveats to this rule of thumb. A later age for adoption is acceptable if the dog is going to be exposed to many different people, instead of just one person, at the breeder's. Remembering that pups learn from novel experiences at this time, the adoption process should not be scary, painful, or associated with horrific circumstances such as traumatic shipping, mutilation, tattooing, or severe punishment. Although observance and understanding of the appropriate periods is no guarantee that future problems will not develop, the client will be able to minimize the risk that future problems are the result of lack of exposure during these periods.

It is important to appreciate that some of the effects of developmental or sensitive periods may be mitigated by the personality of the individual puppy and by the intensity of attention that the animal receives. The extent to which mitigation of lack of exposure is possible is unclear. Early experience may affect brain development; the extent to which early exposure structures cognitive development is under-explored in dogs.

EARLY INTERVENTION AND THE CONCEPT OF TREATMENT

Given the previously cited conditions, there are a few problems that can be prevented outright, but there are some that can be greatly diminished by early intervention.

Aggression, like diabetes, is not curable, but it *may be controllable* in the majority of cases. In a retrospective analysis of prognosticators of aggressive cases seen at VHUP client compliance and extent of effort was the single best determinant of success. When both the behavioral specialist and the clients believe the dog is greatly improved and the clients are comfortable *and* content to live with the dog, the case is considered a success. Because of the potential danger and liability involved, everyone involved in treating *any* aggressive animal must have realistic expectations of the dog's behavior, and what the clients want and can handle. Requirements vary from one household to the next. A dog that could live safely and nonaggressively in a childless household may not be able to do so safely in one with children. It would be unfair and perhaps dangerous to guarantee absolute reliability in *any* dog, including those treated for aggression. A dog could appear "cured" but could relapse if clients cease to reinforce the dog's appropriate behaviors. In the case of dominantly aggressive dogs, such reinforcement may mean *never* letting the dog succeed with subtle, nonaggressive signs of control, such as pushing.

Until clients can seek qualified help, they should avoid circumstances known to precipitate the specific aggression. Any time the animal executes an inappropriate behavioral response, it learns from that response. It is critical that the dog *not* be allowed any reinforcement. Reinforcement allows learning of inappropriate behaviors. With therapy it is usually possible to desensitize the dog to circumstances to which it reacts aggressively, but avoidance is key and the first step in minimizing danger.

Treatment of canine aggression is both rewarding and frustrating. The Behavior Clinic at VHUP has a very high success rate, with improvement in more than 85% of all aggressive animals, and improvement sufficient that the animals appear unremarkable in 75%. "Improvement" means that there are fewer active and passive aggressive events, they are less intense, they are easier to interrupt, and these changes are associated with an increase in the dog's solicitous and friendly behaviors. Fewer than 10% of these patients are euthanized 1 year after diagnosis. *Temporary relapses* are not uncommon in households with clients who believe that after behavior modification, their animals are cured and hence normal. Euthanasia is a last resort, but it is preferable to "dumping" a dangerous animal on someone else. One study that investigated factors contributing to euthanasia of aggressive dogs found that people were more likely to euthanize their dog if they believed that the dog was "unpredictable" (Reisner et al., 1994). This finding *strongly* suggests that accurate diagnosis and client understanding of canine behavior and signaling are crucial for treatment success. With early intervention and improved client education, euthanasia for behavioral problems may become the exception rather than the rule.

Early warning signs of most aggressions are recognizable if the client learns what to look for early in the relationship with the dog. It is easier to set a pattern of good behavioral interaction than to break a bad one. In order for correction (punishment) to best succeed, it has to occur preferably in 1 second, but generally within the first 30 to 60 seconds, of the *onset* of the inappropriate behavior (Voith & Marder, 1988). Behavior is a sequence, not just an event. Startling the animal within the first 1 or 2 seconds of the onset of the behavior is optimal; however, the earlier in the behavioral sequence that *any* correction or startle occurs, the better the learning potential for the animal. For example, a dog that habitually steals items from countertops does not just spontaneously jump and take the item when in the vicinity. More likely, the dog enters the room with the counter, looks and sniffs around, moves to the edge of the counter, explores it, gets up, and steals. Startling the dog as soon as it looked and sniffed around the counter would abort the sequence of behavior before the dog learned it could get up and take something. Any punishment should preferably startle the animal sufficiently to interrupt the behavior and abort any attempt at immediate resumption (Borchelt & Voith, 1985; Domjan & Burkhard, 1985; Voith, 1986). The purpose of punishment as a correction is to decrease the probability of the behavior occurring in the same context in the future. This has a chance of occurring only if the behavior is thoroughly aborted by the correction. The pup can then be taught a more appropriate behavior, such as sitting and staying (Hart, 1978a; Voith, 1982a,b). Sitting and staying are natural dog behaviors that correspond to lower positions in the social hierarchy in the context discussed here. This serves as a time-out, teaches that the client is the leader in the situation and is deserving of deferential behavior, and that the pup must take all cues as to the appropriateness of his or her behavior from the client. This is important because at the crux of aggressive problems is the fact that these dogs are abnormal; they are incapable of making appropriate, in-context distinctions. These dogs exhibit inappropriate, out-of-context behavior. Early intervention must be aimed at achieving excellent voice control and teaching the dog to make better context distinctions by taking cues from the client.

Food-related aggression is an example of a relatively common aggressive situation that benefits greatly from early intervention. Food-related aggression is often a precursor of dominance aggression, but it *can* occur in the absence of any other aggression. For this reason it is best to consider it a separate diagnosis rather than to group it with dominance aggression (Beaver, 1983; Borchelt & Voith, 1982a; Voith and Marder, 1988). (See Appendix F for necessary and sufficient conditions for individual aggressive diagnoses.) Dogs that are aggressive around their food are also usually aggressive with table scraps, rawhide bones, and real bones. The latter two are excellent elicitors of this type of aggressive behavior. In general, food-related aggression is very difficult to treat; it is usually far simpler and safer to preclude treats, bones, and rawhides and to feed the dog in isolation. But what should the client do at the first signs of such aggression, before it becomes an intractable problem?

STARTING OUT

All pups should be taught to sit and stay for verbal praise or food treats; no pup older than 7 weeks of age is too young to learn this (Voith, 1982a,b,c). Clients should then routinely practice making the pup sit and wait to be fed and taking the dish away. The first signs of any aggression can be corrected with a sharp "no" and removal of the pup from the situation; he or she must then earn return of the food by sitting and staying. The crux of this type of instruction is that the dog perceives the client as the one from whom she or he must take the cues about the appropriateness of the behavior. Should the pup continue to threaten, it is already time to seek professional help. Should the pup learn to relinquish his or her dish to the client, the potential for dominance aggression later in life should be discussed.

Although dominance aggression commonly develops at social maturity, usually between 18 and 24 months of age (range, 12 to 36 months) (Voith & Borchelt, 1982a; Voith, 1981), early intervention can be critical. Dogs exhibiting this behavioral syndrome challenge and threaten clients or other humans for control by staring, barking, or growling when given commands, leaning on the clients, growling or biting when disturbed while sleeping or when stepped over, or frequently have to have the "last word" when verbally corrected, and when physically punished, including hanging from a choke collar, become more aggressive. The condition is treatable and controllable with proper therapy, but it can be recognized before any biting has occurred if the clients are attuned to the previously mentioned signs. As soon as clients recognize *any* of these early behaviors, they need to start a program or schedule of behaviors that compels the dog to yield to the client for everything he or she wants. This can be as simple as sitting and staying for all attention, food, play, egress or ingress, grooming, and so forth (Voith, 1982). The dog must learn to take all the cues about whether behavior is appropriate from the client. Absolutely no physical punishment should be used; to do so is to risk allowing the dog to intensify its aggression to the client, thus putting the client in a risky situation. Early intervention can prevent this situation from becoming dangerous and injurious. It should be emphasized to clients that behavioral problems involving aggression are controlled, not cured, and that the dog will have to live with that level of discipline forever.

Treatment principles are discussed in Chapter 12. Comments on treatment of specific aggressive disorders follow the discussion of aggression below, but presuppose familiarity with the concepts in Chapter 12.

THE ROLE OF TRAINING: WHAT IT WILL AND WILL NOT HELP

Obedience training, puppy kindergarten, and individual training all have their roles. They function best to help recognize early signs of possible behavioral problems rather than to prevent them. Certainly for some dogs, particularly those with limited opportunities to interact with other dogs, or those who have people with little knowledge of dogs, they can be extremely worthwhile. They are invaluable from the standpoint of getting the dog and the client to interact and to teach the client directly or indirectly about variation in dog behavior and response to training. Once a problem develops, such measures are an *inappropriate* substitute for intervention from a behavioral specialist (Overall, 1994g). Most dogs with behavioral problems are *not* just misbehaving, they are *not normal*, and to treat them as normal, but misbehaving, animals and expect normal responses to ever-intensifying corrections is dangerous to the pet and client alike. The negative effect of inappropriate training, particularly regarding the use of physical punishment, is finally being addressed by those in the field (Myles, 1991). It is *never* appropriate to recommend to a client to hang a dog from a choke collar to subdue aggression. If the client cannot back the dog down, and this may take a fight to the death, the client risks being injured. Furthermore, the dog is at risk for injured ocular vessels, tracheal and esophageal damage, and recurrent laryngeal nerve paralysis. In the few cases of laryngeal nerve paralysis caused by hanging by a choker seen at VHUP, all dogs have died despite therapy that included a ventilator.

CATEGORIZATION, DIAGNOSIS, AND TREATMENT

Early discussions of aggression focused on "motivation" and its postulated neural organization using rodent models (Blanchard, 1984; Blanchard & Blanchard, 1977, 1981, 1984a,b; Blanchard et al., 1984a,b,c). The rat, mouse, and hamster display clear behavioral and motivational distinctions between offensive (dorsal biting by territory holder) and defensive (upright boxing in response to intruder or shock) forms of attack. Hinde (1956) and Tinbergen (1957) postulate that there are two components to the motivational basis of territorial aggression: site attachment and hostility. This thought process is consistent with that of the Blanchards and is interesting in the absence of early neural evidence to support distinctions between intermale aggression, territorial aggression, and maternal aggression. Reis (1974) used the term *nonaffective aggression* to indicate aggression without autonomic activation (play, maternal, predatory, and sex-related aggressions and those associated with an underlying organic cause). Affective aggression is categorized as that involving an intense, patterned autonomic activation associated with sympathetic and adrenal stimulation (intrasexual, pain, fear, competitive, dominance, protective, learned, and redirected aggressions). Although they provide a model for the cellular and neurochemical basis of aggression, such approaches are not intuitively useful for the diagnosis and treatment of problem aggressions. In a broader social context, aggression can be viewed as a range of solutions to certain problems (Archer, 1988); hence, functional and causal groupings of aggressions can be based on contextual behaviors (Brain, 1981). This approach does not conflict with earlier approaches; aggression that is protective in a functional sense can be offensive or defensive on the basis of form, motivation, or physiology (Archer, 1988). For the purposes of understanding the "normal" range of aggressive behaviors and addressing the abnormal, functional classifications (level 1; see Box 1-1 on p. 3) are very useful (Moyer, 1968; Brain, 1981; Brain & Haug, 1992). Caution is urged in assuming that these represent any solitary mapping to underlying mechanistic levels of causality (levels 2 to 5; see Box 1-1 and Appendix F for distinctions).

In the Behavior Clinic at VHUP, the following categories of aggression are recognized (Young, 1988a, after Borchelt and Voith, 1982a, based on Moyer, 1968): maternal aggression, territorial and protective aggression (both split and lumped), interdog aggression, redirected aggression, food-related aggression, possessive aggression, predatory aggression, idiopathic aggression, dominance aggression, pain aggression, fear aggression, and play aggression. Other authors use similar to widely differing categories (Beaver, 1983; Blackshaw, 1991; Hart, 1985b; Hart & Hart, 1985a; Houpt, 1979, 1991b; Mugford, 1984b; O'Farrell, 1986, 1990; Wright, 1991). Categories that are poorly defined

(e.g., irritable aggression *sensu* Young, 1988; Houpt & Reisner, 1995; competitive aggression *sensu* Hart, 1985b) are not included in this classification, and their signs are usually nonspecific and subsumed by other categories. The aggressions discussed here are all diagnoses: none of the aggressions represent normal, appropriate, in-context behaviors. Hence, learned aggression of the form exhibited by highly trained attack dogs is excluded from discussion. Any inappropriate or abnormal behavior can be enhanced by learning (e.g., conditioned aggression, *sensu* Thompson, 1969). Arguments have been made that terminology in behavioral medicine should conform to that in human psychiatry (Walker, 1993); however, the human classifications of aggression (dyssocial, felonious, emo-

---

BOX 6-3

RANK ORDER OF AGGRESSIVE DIAGNOSES IN PATIENTS AT THE BEHAVIOR CLINIC AT VHUP (1987-PRESENT)

1. Dominance aggression (1)
2. Fear aggression (3)
3. Interdog aggression
4. Protective aggression (2—tie)
5. Predatory aggression (6)
6. Territorial aggression (2—tie)
7. Food-related aggression
8. Possessive aggression (10)
9. Redirected aggression
10. Play aggression
11. Idiopathic aggression (18)
12. Maternal aggression

NOTE: These ranks may change over time as new data are added. The rank of animals euthanized included those for all behavioral diagnoses, including those not involving aggression.

Parenthetical numbers indicate the rank order for euthanasia for all behavior diagnoses, including those not involving aggression.

BOX 6-4

GOOD PROGNOSTICATORS

1. Later onset
   • Less time for learning inappropriate behavior
   • Suggests that at one point dog knew an appropriate behavior
2. Ongoing only a short time
   • **Prognosticators 1 and 2 emphasize the critical role that early intervention and prevention can play.**
3. Infrequent bouts
4. Bouts of short duration
5. Aggression directed to only one or a few people (less generalized)
6. Fewer aggressive diagnoses
7. Highly motivated family who can and will comply and who is realistic about risk assessment

---

BOX 6-5

POOR PROGNOSTICATORS

1. Early onset if left untreated*
2. Long duration*
3. Aggressions becoming more frequent*
4. Aggressive bouts becoming longer in duration*
5. Aggression exhibited more frequently*
   • More contexts
   • Directed toward more individuals (more generalized)
6. Multiple aggressive diagnoses
   • Role of learning is critical
7. Client unwilling or unable to respond to instructions

NOTE: This is the only factor that does not depend on the dog.

*Caution: Client who absolutely needs to be able to favorably trust dog.

tional, and instrumental violence) are difficult to define and may not relate directly to the behavior, or are not applicable to dogs. It is likely that most inappropriate canine aggressions are related to anxiety, as discussed later (Overall, 1993b-d, 1994c, 1995a,b).

The most common forms of aggression in patients at the Behavior Clinic at VHUP are dominance (nearly 20% of all aggressive cases at VHUP since 1987) and fear (10% of all aggressive cases at VHUP since 1987) (Box 6-3). Most aggressive dogs seen at the Behavior Clinic at VHUP have two or more forms of aggression; the modal number of aggressive diagnoses is four. Severe cases can show more than four types of aggression; the record is nine. In general, the more types of aggression the animal exhibits, the earlier the age at onset, the longer the duration, and the more intense or frequent the bouts of aggression, especially if intensity or frequency increases with time, the worse the prognosis (Boxes 6-4 and 6-5). Examples of cases with

good and poor prognosticators are found in Boxes 6-6 and 6-7.

The attributes of the above classes of aggression are discussed next. A summary of hallmark features of each class of aggression is found in Table 6-1. An aggression screen, developed for diagnostic purposes, is found in Table 6-3 and the questionnaire blank for this is in Chapter 5. In the treatment section of each aggressive diagnosis, two to three tiers of behavior modification programs are discussed. These programs are found in Appendix B. The necessary and sufficient conditions for making these diagnoses are found in Appendix F.

Maternal Aggression

Diagnostic Profile. Maternal aggression occurs during pregnancy or pseudocyesis, proximate to whelping, or postpartum (puerperal aggression) (Allen, 1986; Freak, 1968). The mother dog may correctly or incorrectly perceive a threat, and may show the full range of aggressive actions such as growling, snarling, snapping, or biting.

BOX 6-6
EXAMPLE OF A CASE WITH A GOOD PROGNOSIS

Signalment: 3-year-old, female spayed Jack Russell terrier

Problems/diagnoses

- Jumps
- Barks for attention
- Growls at daughter and wife if they correct her
- Growls at daughter and wife if they disturb her while she is sleeping
- Growls at anyone who takes a rawhide (since 8 weeks of age)
- Only husband can move her dinner dish
- If wife tries to put on leash or groom, dog growls
- Started about 4 months ago, is getting worse, but fewer incidents since wife refuses to interact with dog
- Diagnoses:
  Food-related aggression
  Dominance aggression
  Attention-seeking behavior

Considerations

- Husband "loves dog to death" and realizes she is "manipulative wench"
- Wife is not taking this personally; is willing to work with dog if some reasonable measure of safety is possible
- Willing to use Promise system head halter
- Willing to increase amount of exercise
- Dog improved with daughter and husband doing exercises during first visit
- All people read the signals well
- Willing to avoid rawhides and use baby gates
- Clients understand that if they let up, dog may relapse

BOX 6-7
EXAMPLE OF A CASE WITH POOR PROGNOSIS

Signalment: 8-month-old, male, Old English sheepdog

Problems/diagnoses

- Will not lift leg when urinating
- Thrown out of obedience and handling classes (client wants show dog)
- Interdog aggression that is getting worse after three visits
- Dominance aggression—formerly to female client, now to both
- Theft of objects
- Jumping
- Pulls on leash
- Never stops
- After three visits, mugs clients for rewards for behavior modification programs—will do something only if client shows food now

Considerations

- Client wants show dog
- Client will not castrate
- Client will not use head halter
- Client bribes to get dog into crate
- Client takes dog back home as soon as he growls at another dog
- Client will not do any more behavior modification, says it does not work
- Early onset, worsening in frequency, duration, and scope
- Dog has almost doubled in size since initial appointment

TABLE 6-1 Classification of Canine Aggression: Sentinel Symptoms (See Appendix F for Necessary and Sufficient Diagnostic Criteria and Conditions)

Diagnosis	Symptoms
Maternal aggression	• Protects toys, bedding from people or dogs • Long-distance vocalization if puppies present • May nip if pup taken, usually vocal • If constantly threatened, may eat toy or pup • Dependent on hormonal state; passes with change in hormones
Play aggression	• Barking, growling, snapping while playing, usually with people or other dogs (not in solo play) • May start out with play vocalizations and change to serious growling in response to rougher play • Usually puppies or younger dogs • Dog may have never learned to play (early orphaned or rough play as a puppy); plays roughly and uses actual growls, rather than play growls, with other dogs • Uses teeth to grab people's hands, legs, clothing • Even when playing tug with a toy will grab arm
Fear aggression	• May bark, growl, or snarl while backing up • May shake and tremble during and after aggression • May bite from behind and then run away • May be associated with painful medical treatment or abuse • Can be induced by inappropriate punishment • Recipient can be canine or human • Dog will cower, and look for escape route; becomes dangerous if cornered
Pain aggression	• Usually in response to being manipulated, or before manipulation of something the dog has learned is painful • Does not necessarily back up—will grab hands with its teeth in an attempt to stop pain or anticipated pain • May be in response to rough play from children or other dogs, particularly if recipient is old and arthritic • Can progress to fear aggression
Territorial aggression	• Protects property by barking, growling, snarling, biting • Property can be stationary (house) or mobile (car) • Protects regardless of who is present • Made worse by any kind of fence or confinement (can tell exactly where boundaries are) • Aggression intensifies as approach distance decreases • Unaggressive in the absence of the territory, *but* may quickly redefine a territory (e.g., a kennel run) • May be part of the control complex that includes dominance aggression
Protective aggression	• Protects people from other people or dogs • May single out one person to protect • Stands between person being protected and others • Barks, growls, snarls, bites, with likelihood for more aggressive behaviors to occur the closer the person is • May be stimulated to react by quick moves, embraces • Unaggressive in the absence of its people
Interdog aggression	• Commonly male-male; female-female and related to social hierarchies • Can be a form of sexual competition (may be worse if female dog in heat is present with intact male dogs) • Usually starts at social maturity (18 to 24 months of age) • Challenges may start as stares, bumps, mounting, or exclusion by lateral body blocks from food, play, or attention • May be generalized or may occur only in specific singular control/contest situations (e.g., access to a bed, access to doors, in a certain room) • May be made worse by endogenous hormones, but is *social* and usually occurs in households with neutered pets; can occur between early-neutered pets • Related to *actual* or *perceived* hierarchical relationships • Older or weaker dog may be victimized (**caution** for temporarily ill dogs that have frequently been challenged as above)
Redirected aggression	• In response to a correction or thwarting of a desire • Correction could be physical or verbal • May be a growl or involve active inhibition of the person or animal doing the correction or thwarting (biting of hand or wrist); biting of a third dog that intervenes in a dog fight

TABLE 6-1 Classification of Canine Aggression: Sentinel Symptoms (See Appendix F for Necessary and Sufficient Diagnostic Criteria and Conditions)—cont'd

Diagnosis	Symptoms
	• May be more common with social maturity (18 to 24 months of age)
	• Individual victimized (human or animal) was not part of original social interaction
	• Part of the control complex that includes dominance aggression
Food-related aggression	• Growling when eating if approached or in sight of other dogs or people
	• Involves tremendously long approach distances
	• Will bite if perceives threat (real or imagined) to food
	• Either turns and actively guards food or continues to eat in uncoordinated manner while growling, often dropping food
	• May be nonaggressive with dog food, but aggression escalates with rawhides, real bones, food scraps, or treats
	• Part of the control complex that involves dominance aggression
	• Single best early indicator that dominance aggression may develop
Possessive aggression	• Will not relinquish toys or stolen objects; can be objects stolen in play from another (human or dog)
	• May present objects for play and then growl if someone tries to take them
	• May protect an object that dog has been watching from across the room
	• Part of the control complex involving dominance aggression
Predatory aggression	• Silently stalks small animals, birds
	• May also stalk infants or stare at them silently, drooling
	• May track and stalk bicyclists or skateboarders
	• Pattern of high-pitched sounds, uncoordinated motion, and sudden silences may provoke aggression
	• Dangerous
Dominance aggression	• See Boxes 6-8 through 6-10
	• 90% of those diagnosed are male
	• Occurs at social maturity (18 to 36 months of age)
	• If female, may occur in very young puppy
	• Worsens with punishment (hallmark)
	• May run in family lines
Idiopathic aggression	• Atypical, toggle switch aggression
	• No contextual association identifiable
	• Most commonly reported in dogs 1 to 3 years of age
	• Usually is misdiagnosed dominance aggression

Some dogs show maternal aggression when a toy is taken from them. This can be especially common during false pregnancies. Maternal defense of the toy becomes important to the dog, although it is not an appropriate response in the eyes of the client.

Maternally aggressive dogs generally guard their pups, toys, or both from very long distances—across the room or in another part of the house. They will usually warn with a growl and will not bite unless the toy or the puppy is taken. If pressured by continued approach, they may eat their toy, as a disturbed bitch might eat her puppies. When the pups are weaned, or when the pseudocyetic event is over (as long as 2 months), the aggressive behavior usually abates. Animals displaying pseudocyesis once are at risk for repeat events. Ovariohysterectomy should take place after the signs of pseudocyesis have abated.

Treatment. Treatment of maternal aggression relies on time and avoidance. Unless the bitch is savagely aggressive and poses a threat to her pups or to humans, it is best to let her be. Calling her away from her nest site and rewarding her for being calm and good can help ease her anxiety. Under no condition should she be teased either with her puppies or toys. If she will accept having her leash put on for walks, she can be walked while the bedding is changed and the pups handled and checked. Between weeks 3 and 5 the pups will start being more mobile. If the bitch consents to interacting favorably with people, then this provides an opportunity to practice some relaxation exercises when she can be rewarded for allowing the pups to roam. Practicing some behavior modification exercises before the pregnancy or pseudocyetic event may help in diminishing future anxieties. There are no data to support or reject this, but being able to rely on a pattern of favorable behavior may help. Nest boxes can be put in out-of-the-way places, with food provided at distances that increase a little every day. False pregnancies tend to recur; therefore it is propitious to spay the dog after the initial pseudocyetic event (Voith, 1980b,c). Bitches that kill their pups may be at risk to repeat this behavior, and the tendency may run in the family lines (Mugford, 1984b). Ovariohysterectomy is recommended.

Play Aggression

Diagnostic Profile. Play aggression involves barking, growling, or snapping while playing. Some growls may change in pitch and volume on response to the amount of attention the pup receives, as a result of increased stimulation, or in response to increased rough play by people. In the latter case the aggression may be reinforced by social feedback. A play growl can be distinguished from a serious one, and clients should be taught to discriminate. Play growls are usually high-pitched, short, and repeated frequently. True aggressive growls are lower pitched and prolonged. Change in the tone of the growl may not always be present. Changes in the pitch of the growl can happen too abruptly to safely detect. Some dogs give other signals that they are becoming aggressive during play: the hair on the neck may go up, the ears may flatten, and the pupils may dilate. Some dogs exhibiting play aggression never learned to play appropriately. This may be the result of abandonment, lack of interaction in humane shelter or kennel situations, or restricted access to other dogs in normal play situations. Also, the dog may never have learned to play appropriately because the clients encouraged rough play. No puppy or dog should ever be slapped about the face and head in the course of play or be offered a hand or arm to grab in play. All play should take place only with toys. Play aggression is frequently self-sustaining: the dog becomes more aggressive to elicit any response from the client (Voith, 1980f,g). It is important to teach clients to play with the dog only in a manner that encourages the client to always control the intensity of the interaction and that teaches the dog to take the cues as to the appropriateness of his or her behavior from the client.

Puppies that have not been exposed to other dogs often play inappropriately with them. If play aggression continues after repeated exposure, avoidance may be best because the nature of normal dog play can lead an abnormal dog to perceive threats where there are none.

Treatment. As stated, rough play with the dog is to be avoided at all costs. Play should occur only with toys and only on the clients' terms. If people want to play tug with the pup, they can do so with a soft, large toy around which the dog can get its jaws. The people, not the dog, should always determine when play begins and ends. This is accomplished by having the dog sit and offering the toy coupled with the command "take it." Once the dog takes the toy, it is acceptable to play tug if and only if the following rules are adhered to: (1) the dog can mouth *only* the toy; (2) at the first instance of any part of the dog connecting with the client's arm, the game stops and the client acts horrified—the dog must then sit; (3) the dog can relinquish the toy in exchange for the command "drop it";

(4) the *client*, not the dog, is the one who determines when the game is over, and the game always ends with the dog sitting or lying down and dropping the toy at the client's request. These guidelines will allow excellent, safe aerobic play and teach the dog to be more compliant to the owner's wishes. A copy of these rules is found as a client handout in Appendix B. It is a fallacy that if you play roughly with young puppies, particularly if you tap them about the face and head so that they snap, they will be more protective. This type of play only teaches the dog to play inappropriately and aggressively. Rough play blurs contextual boundaries for any dog and may be particularly dangerous for a dog that is already having difficulty ascertaining whether the behavior is contextually appropriate.

Any dog that continues to solicit rough play or grabs at the client's feet, hands, or clothing, or that pounces on clients as they come around corners, needs to be corrected. *Do not* hit the dog—this will simply encourage more aggressive play. Instead, all people who interact with the dog should carry a water pistol, fog, horn, or air canister and blast the dog at the first signs associated with the approach of a play aggression bout. Use the minimum stimulus necessary to get the dog to stop the aggressive play. (If, when you startle the dog, it barks hysterically, you are encouraging another set of problems.) Then *immediately* request that the dog perform a more appropriate behavior and reward this. Put a bell on the dog's collar so that he or she can be monitored. After the dog has aborted its aggressive charge, ask the dog to sit and stay and relax. Reward with praise and a treat. Later, petting can be used as a reward, but care must be taken so that the dog does not interpret petting as another opportunity to mouth. If the dog does this, the client must freeze and say "no." If a verbal command does not work, the dog again should be startled with any of the devices listed previously and corrected. A Gentle Leader/Promise System Canine Head Halter (Premier Products, Richmond, Va.) can also help in these instances because it provides clients with a safe, gentle, humane way to close the dog's mouth and extricate themselves. These collars are fully discussed in the "Gizmos" section of Chapter 12. The client handout, "Protocol for Teaching Children (and Adults) to Play With Dogs and Cats," is found in Appendix B.

Fear Aggression

Diagnostic Profile. Fear aggression is a response to people. It is the second most frequent type of aggression (first is dominance aggression) seen at the Behavior Clinic at VHUP and represents 10% of the total number of canine behavior cases. Borchelt (1983a) maintains that of 365 cases of canine aggression, fear aggression was the most common diagnosis. This assertion does not hold up to statistical analysis; a re-analysis of the data indicates no statistically significant differences among fear, dominance, possessive, and protective aggressions. This is another demonstra-

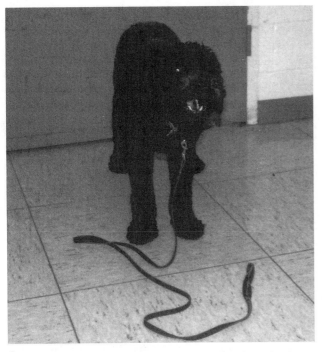

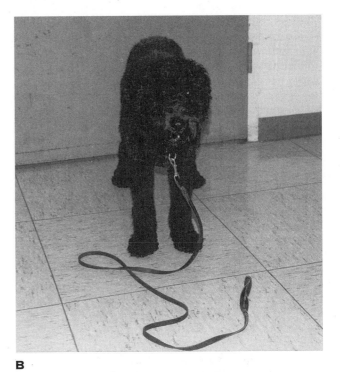

A   **B**

This dog was diagnosed with fearful aggression. Notice the broad-based hind leg stance, the mouth that is agape, showing teeth, and the tucked tail (**A**). The dog also—of its own volition—backed against the wall and door away from the clients, staff, students, and clinician. **B,** The clinician approached and the dog's head and neck become more rigid, the mouth closes, and the dog stares. These behaviors and the changes in overall behavior are correlated with an increased propensity toward active aggression rather than threat. If pursued, this dog would have bitten. The situation was rendered safer by the presence of a head collar (which is the same color as the dog). (Photos by K.L. Overall)

tion of the dangers of substituting a comparison of percentages for statistical rigor. In a study involving 86 fearfully aggressive dogs, 15% (13) developed fear aggression by 3 months of age (Borchelt, 1984b), and reanalysis of the data indicates that it was apparent in 50% of the dogs by 46 months of age. These data suggest that social maturation and the behavioral and neurochemical changes that occur then are factors in the development of fears and attendant aggression.

Signs of fear aggression include initial behaviors of snapping, growling, and escape attempts (Voith, 1976a,b, 1980a; Young, 1982). Subsequent behaviors may involve changes in pitch and volume of vocalizations, snapping and biting if the stimulus continues, and possibly urination, defecation, or anal sac expression. Body postures associated with fear aggression include a lowering of head and body, tucking of the tail, piloerection, ears moved back, wrinkled muzzles, horizontal and then vertical lip retraction, and snarling. Clients can learn to recognize the contexts in which these behaviors occur.

Fear aggression occurs when the dog is scared, regardless of whether an event has occurred that scared the dog. A dog that is afraid of an unknown person who is walking on the same street is not normal. If this dog responds by growling, this is a sign of fearful aggression. Some situations in which fear aggression commonly occurs include situations in which no threat is apparent, such as when a person reaches for the dog, when the dog is approached by a person on the street, when the dog is in the veterinarian's office, or when the dog is yelled at. Dogs with fear aggression growl, snap, or bite when afraid. In a pairwise comparison of fear aggression/dominance aggression, fear aggression/possessive aggression, and fear aggression/protective aggression that examined specific behaviors (barking, growling, baring teeth, snapping, biting, and staring) (Borchelt, 1984b), a reanalysis showed that the only behavior in any comparison that was exhibited more frequently in fear aggression was barking ($G_{adj} = 13.17$, $p \leq 0.05$; $G_{adj} = 41.92$; difference not significant; respectively). Fearfully aggressive dogs try to avoid the situation by backing up. Many dogs with fear aggression growl until they are cornered, then they bite. These behaviors are in contrast to those of the normal dog who puts his tail between his legs, cowers, and hides when afraid, but who shows no vocal or physical signs of aggression.

Dogs that undergo prolonged, painful medical treatment may develop fear aggression and respond to the approach of the veterinarian. Inappropriate punishment may result in a fearfully aggressive animal; these pets associate the approach of the person with the punishment experience, rather than associating the punishment with the inappropriate act. Fear aggression can be induced by abuse. It is important to remember that abused dogs have learned to be fearful. Although fear aggression is an inappropriate response, it may be the one that they learned. Data from VHUP, the Humane Society of the United States, the American Humane Association, and the Delta Society indicate that dogs that have been abused may act as a flag for child abuse or the potential for child abuse. *People who abuse dogs are at risk for abusing children. Abused children are at risk for abusing dogs.* Social services agencies are becoming more receptive to alerts from veterinarians about potential abuse situations. Veterinarians should also inform clients about the pet abuse/child abuse link (see the Alpha Affiliates reference in Appendix C).

Dogs can also become fearfully aggressive toward other dogs. Check for histories of dog fights (and pain aggression) or personality mismatches (e.g., young, exuberant, large puppy and small, old Yorkie who's in pain).

Treatment. Every time a fearfully aggressive dog experiences an event that causes it to react inappropriately, regardless of whether the event is—to all outward appearances—nonprovoking, that dog learns to be more fearfully aggressive. All situations in which the dog exhibits fear aggression *must* be avoided until the dog can be desensitized to the stimulus. This means that if the dog shies away, growling, whenever it meets another dog, dogs must be avoided until the behavior modification program is well under way. Since barking is a statistically significant feature of fear aggression, citronella bark collars (Aboistop, Quebec, Canada; ABS system, ImmunoVet, Tampa, Fl.) may be useful adjuvants to treatment. They mist the dog with citronella, which startles the dog and permits interruption of the behavior. They can be used in conjunction with a head collar. Clients should note that if the barking is due to anxiety or profound fear rather than functioning as a warning in the aggressive sequence, these collars are unlikely to help. During the first phase of any behavior modification program the dog must learn to sit or lie down and relax while people it trusts move around, talk to people who do not exist, and leave the room. Throughout the process the dog is rewarded with food treats for being calm, happy, and nonreactive while it sits or lies down and stays. Future iterations of the program use a more unpredictable reward schedule. When this program can be executed in a protective, nonreactive environment repeatedly, with no problems, the dog is ready for the second phase of the behavior modification programs. The second phase is designed to desensitize the dog to the stimuli to which it reacts. These programs and treatments are more fully discussed in Appendix B and in Chapter 12. Any behavior modification program must be executed carefully and, generally, slowly. It can take 2 to 4 months before the dog learns to react more appropriately to approaches from strange dogs. In the interim, the dog must not be allowed to have an aggressive experience.

Flooding has sometimes been recommended as a treatment for fearful dogs, including those that are fearfully aggressive (Young, 1982). The flooding technique requires that the dog be exposed to the type of situation that causes the inappropriate response, at the level of stimulus that provokes the response. (This is in contrast to the often coupled counterconditioning and desensitization. In the latter, the dog is exposed to the stimulus at a level below that at which it will react. In counterconditioning, the approach is the same, but the dog is taught to instead engage in a behavior that competitively inhibits the performance of the undesirable behavior. The new behavior should be fun and be rewarded with a treat when the dog does not respond inappropriately as desensitization continues.) The dog is kept in the flooding situation and is restrained gently on a leash and head collar, until his fear has decreased considerably, generally by 50% per session. Flooding can be a risky technique, and one that is easy to practice inhumanely. If it is executed incorrectly, the dog's behavior can worsen. Generally, flooding works best for dogs that have recently begun to exhibit fear or fear aggression, and for fears and aggressions that are situation specific, rather than global. Flooding also is generally recommended as a treatment for only those dogs that are not afraid of their people, that have not been fearful from birth (they have more of an environmental than genetic or developmental component to their fear), and for dogs that have some knowledge of commands and will work with the client and the veterinarian.

Sometimes aggressive events cannot be avoided because we are not omniscient. Fitting any aggressive dog with a Gentle Leader/Promise System Canine Head Halter can help. This is particularly true for a fearfully aggressive dog. The halter can be used to correct the dog and turn it away from the stimulus at the first sign of any aggressive event. The dog can then be requested to sit, stay, and relax. If the dog cannot do this, the halter can be used to lead the dog away from the situation in as gentle and nonaggressive a manner as possible.

Never physically discipline an aggressive dog. Fearfully aggressive dogs become worse and may have no recourse except to bite.

Never corner a fearfully aggressive dog. Although the dog may have backed up while growling, once cornered it will have no choice but to bite if further frightened. If the patient is fearfully aggressive to other dogs, do not let another dog approach uncontrolled.

Dogs with fear aggression should not be reassured

that it is "all right." It is *not* all right, and to calmly, reassuringly tell them this while petting them reinforces their inappropriate behavior.

Many dogs with fear aggression respond to antianxiety medications. It would be inappropriate to prescribe a benzodiazepine that might inadvertently release any inhibitions that the dog is exhibiting, but tricyclic antidepressants such as amitriptyline, or some of the newer anxiolytics (e.g., fluoxetine or buspirone) can be efficacious and excellent adjuvants to behavioral therapy. These are discussed in Chapter 13.

Further client instructions are included in "Protocol for Dogs with Fear Aggression" in Appendix B.

Pain Aggression

Diagnostic Profile. Aggression can be an appropriate or inappropriate response to pain (Ulrich, 1966). An injured dog may growl, snap, or bite when moved because it hurts. Although these dogs may warn first, do not count on it. If they are in excruciating pain, such as from a broken bone, a bite may be the dog's perception of its only recourse. Most bites at VHUP occur in the emergency service or orthopedic service sections where dogs can be in great pain. Arthritis can also stimulate pain aggression. A push on the shoulders or the rump, or a small child's landing on a dog with arthritis or dysplasia may cause pain and could cause pain aggression. Children in the 18- to 36-month-old age-group are frequently implicated in this type of aggression because of their tendency to play roughly, coupled with their lack of coordination and judgment. Children and dogs both can exhibit some unpredictable behaviors; therefore it is critical to teach young children appropriate ways to interact with dogs.

It is important to remember that other dogs can also cause pain aggression. Dog fights result in painful wounds; these lacerations and punctures can teach the recipient to be fearful or fearfully aggressive to the aggressors. In profound cases, the recipient may generalize its fear or fearful aggression to all dogs, or to all large, dark dogs, for example. Puppies, like small children, can inadvertently traumatize an older, arthritic dog, leading to avoidance, fear, or fearful aggression on the part of the older dog.

Pain aggression at the slightest touch is inappropriate. Biting should be the *last* resort in canine communication, not the first.

Treatment. If pain aggression is associated with necessary medical care, it can be difficult to treat and avoid. This argues for a stronger use of analgesic medication for hospitalized animals (Hansen & Hardie, 1993). Such a view is becoming common, and the Morris Animal Foundation has funded research on pain control in pets. Minimal restraint may be better than extreme physical restraint, because then the animal has options other than biting. Muzzles and head collars can help prevent a bite. The muzzle does not *prevent* an aggressive event; it just limits the damage ensuing from one. A Gentle Leader/Promise halter can alter the course of the aggressive event and help the dog to learn a more appropriate behavior. It is underused in such situations.

Abuse is also implicated in pain aggression, and practitioners should be aware that dogs that have been roughly handled may first display painful aggression and then fearful aggression.

In the case of an older, arthritic animal that must contend with small children, behavior modification programs should focus on teaching the dog to relax in the presence of the children and on teaching the children to handle the dog gently. It is not unreasonable to work with children as young as 18 months of age to teach them a safe way to approach the dog. Regardless, children and dogs should be physically separated when unsupervised.

Territorial and Protective Aggression

Diagnostic Profile. Most social animals are territorial to some extent. Territories can be floating, transient, or seasonal, or more permanent. Territorial aggression results when a dog protects an inappropriate location as its territory, or when a dog protects appropriate locations but in an inappropriate context. Dogs may exhibit territorial aggression toward only humans, toward only other dogs, toward any animals, or any combination of these. Dogs that defend an area can begin to defend property on that area. If they wander or roam, this area enlarges.

Some dogs become territorial around their crates or the places they sleep. Others have an individual approach distance that they protect. In this sense they have a mobile territory—the space around them—and become aggressive toward anyone who invades that space. Confined spaces, such as cars, crates, or restrictive chains, may intensify this behavior. This is what occurs when a dog is in the car at a gas station or toll booth and barks or growls at people who approach.

Territorial aggression is most obvious when the dog is in the yard and a person or a dog passes, or when the dog is inside and a stranger knocks on the door or enters the room. Most or all dogs will bark to warn or announce the visitor. This is a normal first step in the sequence of behavior characterizing protection. The problem occurs when the dog refuses to stop barking on command or becomes so defensive and aggressive that he may not allow the visitor to enter. In territorial aggression the dog persists in the behavior despite cues indicating a contradictory context.

The hallmark of territorial aggression is that the dog is not aggressive when he is removed from the territory. A dog who protects the area around his food dish might not protect his personal space when he is lying in the living room. A corollary of this is that chained or enclosed animals may have a heightened sense of a territory to defend; hence, no dog with territorial or protective aggression should be left unat-

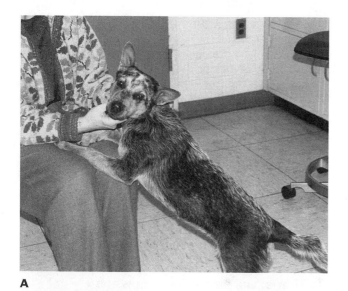

A

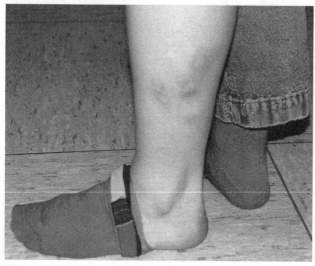

B

A, This Australian cattle dog was diagnosed with an odd form of territorial and protective behavior that manifests in profound herding behavior. The aggression included nipping, pushing, and herding (**B**) but occurred only when the dog was off-lead. The signal to the dog that she did not need to protect apparently was a leash. The dog had been rescued and was obtained to be a pet and to help with the family's sheep. The dog was absolutely perfect with the sheep, but she herded her people and anyone else in an inappropriate, out-of-context, protective and territorial manner. (Photo by K.L. Overall)

tended in a fenced area. Fences, including those that are electric, remove any ambiguity about territorial boundaries, and will render a dog more secure and confident in its inappropriate aggression.

Protective aggression occurs when the dog perceives that the client is threatened and there is no actual threat. This may occur when the stranger is at the door or entering, or when the dog is in a car and the car is approached by someone, or when another dog approaches the person. The dog may show protective aggressiveness when someone raises his or her voice to the client, or if the client is hugged or touched in the presence of the dog. These dogs must be distinguished from dogs who are watchful and make good decisions about when to react. In each case, the dog often positions itself between the possible threat and its person. True protective aggression occurs when there is no real threat and the dog reacts inappropriately and out of context. Instead of maintaining distance, the dog lunges, nips, herds, growls, or bites. Appropriately behaved dogs monitor the newcomer's activities quietly, with their back turned only to their person. In situations involving movement they may preserve these relative postures by maintaining a separation between their person and the newcomer. It is acceptable to be vigilant; it is unacceptable to respond in a manner that contradicts the contextual significance of any cues. Furthermore, any vigilance, even if it merely involves intense watching of strangers, must be receptive to countermanding by the client.

Controlling access to areas associated with resources or resource acquisition is one characteristic of dominance in animals (which is not the same as dominance aggression) (Immelmann & Beer, 1989). Accordingly, territorial and protective aggressions are often listed as attributes of dominance aggression. This is an inappropriate characterization. Protective and territorial aggression can occur independently of dominance aggression, or in concert with it, as part of a control complex. Dominance aggression is a behaviorally varied and complex diagnosis. Not all assertive behaviors are predictors of it.

Treatment. Dogs with territorial aggression should never be left alone, outside, confined, or in a patrolling mode, unsupervised, because they may pose a risk to any individual (human or animal) unable to perceive where the dog believes its territory to be. This is the problem with fences, particularly electronic fences, for dogs with territorial aggression. A fence allows the dog to know exactly the boundary of his or her territory and to patrol and protect it. Instead of becoming less aggressive, territorially aggressive dogs are often more aggressive when fenced. Because there are no outward signs of an electronic fence, intruders do not recognize the boundary and may cross it. It should also be noted that a highly motivated dog will endure a shock to cross an electronic fence in pursuit of territorial defense. Whether shocking a dog makes it more aggressive is hotly debated. Dogs "trained" with manually operated shock collars often do become more aggressive because of problems both with timing of the shock and with problems of human motivation. The same circumstances do *not* apply with stationary electronic fences.

Similarly, dogs with protective aggression must not be put in situations in which they believe that they have to protect. This means that before the door is opened to a visitor (canine or human) the dog is placed in a crate or behind the closed door of another room. If the owner expects visitors, this can be done well in advance of their arrival so that the arrivals are not associated with being locked up. Until the dog responds flawlessly to the first phase of the behavior modification programs, designed to achieve excellent voice control of the dog and to teach it to take all the cues as to the appropriateness of its behavior from the client, strangers and circumstances that induce the protective aggression are to be avoided. Only when the dog is perfect in a protected context for everyone it knows, can it gradually start the second phase of the programs. The second tier of behavior modification is designed to teach the dog to not react to situations in which it had previously been aggressive. Again, a Gentle Leader/Promise System Canine Head Halter helps. It not only helps the clients to abort any inappropriate behaviors early enough in the sequence so that the dog can learn from them, but it also renders the dog safe for strangers for the phase of therapy that requires gradual exposure to them. In some cases, antianxiety medication may be a useful adjuvant to therapy.

Appendix B contains the client handouts "Protocol for Dogs with Protective and/or Territorial Aggression."

Interdog Aggression

Diagnostic Profile. Interdog aggression is common between same-sex dogs (male/male, female/female) and, hence, is a situation in which early neutering or spaying can make a difference (Voith, 1980e; Hart, 1981a). The aggression is a manifestation of canid hierarchical conflicts. Most abnormal aggression is a manifestation of underlying anxiety. In this case, the dog is uncertain—regardless of the signals other animals are giving—of its role in the hierarchy. Only one dog needs to be abnormal for interdog aggression to be a problem. Furthermore, it is not necessary for any challenge to be present for the problem dog to perceive a hierarchical conflict.

In canine social systems, there is usually a top-ranking female and a top-ranking male within the group. These are invariably the older or more vigorous animals, but they may also have been descended from older or more vigorous animals. The role of "culturally inherited" status is underestimated in domestic dogs; however, high-ranking dogs often successfully intervene on behalf of lower ranking ones. Their presence, posturing, and status can be sufficient to prevent outbursts of interdog aggression.

There are two broad categories of interdog aggression: that directed toward dogs outside the household, or unknown dogs, and that directed toward known dogs, generally those in the household. Do not assume that aggression between unknown dogs is de facto interdog aggression; it may be fear or territorial aggression. O'Farrell (1986) supports the idea that these types of aggression can be difficult to distinguish, but finds that in her populations of dogs that territorial ag-

gression is *not* preceded by preliminary threat rituals. Because treatment is rooted in desensitizing the dog to the underlying situations in which it reacts, an accurate diagnosis is critical. Only a careful, context-specific history can provide this.

Aggression to unknown dogs may still be related to status; invariably, the aggressive dog perceives the presence of any dog that crosses his or her path as a challenge. This is true regardless of whether the approaching dog is signaling any threat or challenge. The aggression is an irrational one and occurs regardless of context. Again, this is a good demonstration that the dogs exhibiting these behaviors are not misbehaving or behaving inappropriately. They are behaving out of context, and their responses must be considered abnormal.

Dogs that are aggressive to all strange dogs in the context of interdog aggression may well *not* have a problem with other dogs in the household. This is because they have established hierarchical rules and are existing in a known hierarchy. It is the underlying anxiety about unknown relationships that may contribute to interdog aggression in the case of unknown dogs. Accordingly, many of these dogs respond very well to treatment that consists of a combination of behavior modification and pharmacological intervention (antianxiety medication).

The form of interdog aggression that is more commonly seen at the Behavior Clinic at VHUP is within-household interdog aggression to a known dog. This form of interdog aggression usually manifests in one of two ways. The most common involves two dogs of similar age or stature that contest for status. Occasionally, these dogs are the same or similar ages and thus reach social maturity at approximately the same time. The more common scenario involves an older and younger dog that were nonproblematic until the younger dog attained social maturity. At that time the younger dog contests the status of the older dog, or the older dog perceives subtle, passive status-related changes in the younger dog and responds to quash these. In this situation, the younger dog may never actively challenge the older; the older simply will not tolerate the normal passive changes attendant with social maturity. Challenges may be active and involve food, rawhides, toys, attention, or access to any of the aforementioned, or passive and involve posturing and the ability to manipulate the trajectory and behaviors of the other dog (see Chapter 3 for a discussion of these behaviors). If the older dog capitulates, the situation usually resolves. If the older dog refuses to give way, or if either dog cannot maintain sufficient status to fully vanquish the other dog, interdog aggression results.

The more uncommon form of interdog aggression between known dogs involves an aggressor (which may be either the younger or the older dog) and the recipient of the aggression. In this instance, capitulation of the recipient is *not* sufficient to truncate further aggression. In fact, full submission (roll on back, expose belly and neck) by the recipient can result in a move in for the kill by the aggressor. Of all the forms of interdog aggression, this is the most frightening scenario. The extent to which these aggressive dogs are abnormal is indicated by their potentially lethal response to normal canine behaviors designed to signal nonengagement and to thwart further aggression. The best solution to this latter problem may be eventually to find another home for the less aggressive dog. This is not to say that behavioral, environmental, and pharmacological treatment should not be tried; however, the clients need to have a keen grasp of the potential danger involved and be willing to separate the dogs when they are not supervised.

Finally, regardless of the form of interdog aggression, clients need to understand that it can be generalized or specific. Conflict can result in *all* contexts involving hierarchy and deference, or only in specific situations (access to food, doors, sleeping areas) without *any* generalized propensities.

Interdog aggression generally becomes apparent at social maturity (18 to 24 months of age) when challenges to status first become apparent. Sex hormones act as further facilitators and promoters. A dramatic change of a 62% reduction in aggression to other dogs may even be seen if an older dog that has been fighting with other males is neutered (Hopkins et al., 1976). The effects are most pronounced for dogs with fearful aggression and territorial aggression to other dogs, but may still be apparent for dogs that are aggressive because of real or perceived hierarchical conflicts. Veterinarians should caution clients, however, that if the aggression has been ongoing for a long period, much of the behavior has been learned. Castration still might lower the animal's reactivity, but will not obviate the situation for dogs when there is a substantial learned component. Regardless, *castrate* or *spay* the implicated animals. If aggression is one manifestation of an anxiety disorder and if that is heritable (and there is evidence that both of these may be true), these dogs should not be bred; furthermore, removing hormonal fluctuations may make the dogs more amenable to behavior modification.

Treatment. Extensive behavior modification coupled with castration or ovariohysterectomy is the therapy of choice. The first phase of the behavior modification program again focuses on teaching the dog to take all the cues as to the appropriateness of its behavior from the clients. Until all dogs can sit and stay, or lie down and stay in a variety of contexts in protected circumstances, they should not be exposed to dogs to which they react. This is more easily accomplished if they are not aggressive to any dogs in the household.

In the case of dogs that are not aggressive to canine housemates but only to dogs outside the household, behavior modification should focus on desensitizing the dog to the approaches of other dogs after they have successfully completed the first tier of the behavior modification programs (see Appendix B). Regardless of

how well these dogs do, they should never be left off-lead to play with dogs unknown to them or left loose in a yard into which another dog might stray. Therefore invisible fences are inappropriate for these dogs. If the other dog challenges them, they *will* respond. People should *never* get in the middle of a dog fight—this is one of the most common ways in which people are injured. Instead they should throw water on the dogs, slip cardboard or a broom between them, or throw blankets over them, then restrain and lead them away. If the clients know that their dogs have a history of aggression, those dogs should be walked on the Gentle Leader/Promise System Canine Head Collars or other well-fitting head halters. Not only will these allow clients to prevent dog bites, but they also permit the clients to intervene sufficiently early in the behavioral sequence so that the dog learns from the correction.

In the case of interdog aggression occurring toward dogs *within* the household, the dogs should be separated whenever they are unsupervised. Try to determine which dog is demanding of and likely to hold status. Unfortunately, these descriptors may not apply to the same dog. If the dog that is the challenger is a young, healthy, strong dog, and the one being challenged is older and arthritic, the general rule is that the younger dog should be reinforced over the older one. The younger is reinforced as the higher ranking dog by making sure she has everything first: food, walks, treats, grooming, toys, play, having her leash put on, being let out the door, and so on. These are all active mechanisms by which its status is reinforced. Passive techniques are often underappreciated but can greatly help. If the dogs each have dog beds, the dog whose status is being reinforced should have the preferred bed in the preferred area. When they are separated when left alone, the dog that is being reinforced as being higher in status should either be locked in the higher quality area (bed or kitchen?) if the other dog is locked in, or the other dog should be incarcerated in a lower quality room (spare bedroom) while the dog whose status is being reinforced has the run of the house. When leash-walking the dogs, the one whose status is being reinforced can have the longer lead, and so be slightly in front. If the older dog is willing to accept a change in status, this will help facilitate the process. As long as the other dog is still willing to coexist with the older dog, everything will eventually work out. Both dogs can be gradually desensitized to each other during the second phase of behavior modification.

Things are not quite so simple if the dog attempting to assert its status is a bully. In this case that dog may not accept capitulation of power from the other dog—he wants the other dog gone. Simply reinforcing the challenger as the dog with higher status is insufficient; that only reinforces his belief that it should dispense with the other dog. In this case it is the older, weaker dog that must be given status so that the younger dog understands that the older dog has a right to survive. In the first case, eventually leaving the dogs alone together may not be problematic; in this case, leaving the dogs alone together will never be an option. If the challenger is still determined to dispense with the other dog, antianxiety medications (amitriptyline, buspirone, or, particularly, fluoxetine) may help, but sometimes the patient is best in a single-dog home.

If the younger dog is less healthy or weaker than the older dog and cannot be expected to maintain its position in the absence of human intervention, it is best to curtail its intent to assert its status. Always make it sit and wait or defer to the other dog for food, love, play, walks, attention, grooming—everything.

Gentle Leader/Promise System Canine Head Halters can be very helpful both with dogs that are aggressive to dogs outside their household and dogs that are aggressive to dogs within the household. In the former case, the halter can be used to correct and abort the first signs of any aggression and to elicit compliance from the dog in leaving the scene. In the situation involving dogs in the same household, the halter can be used to abort any inappropriate behavior and to render the situation safer for both dogs, because their mouths can be closed with the halter. Muzzles can prevent biting, but they do nothing to abort or modify the aggressive event. Furthermore, muzzles do not prevent all injuries, just those caused by biting. The muzzled animal can still seriously physically injure a less able opponent. Medication may help to control the underlying anxiety that renders the aggression more labile. In some cases, all participants benefit from medication.

A complete set of client instructions, "Protocol for Interdog Aggression," is found in Appendix B.

Redirected Aggression

Diagnostic Profile. Redirected aggression is often seen when a dog is yelled at, physically punished, or otherwise thwarted from pursuing another aggressive behavior. Dogs may redirect aggression if interrupted in another aggression (i.e., interdog aggression). These dogs may then turn and threaten or bite another person or another animal. They usually go after the nearest individual who is not involved; this may not be the individual who was aggressive to them. In the absence of the interruption of the threat, these dogs can be nonaggressive. Were the dog consistent in showing aggression to an individual who punished or was aggressive to him, fear and dominance aggression would also have to be considered among the differential diagnoses. Redirected aggression could be part of the "control complex" (described later) for dominance aggression.

When a dog redirects his or her aggression to another animal in the household, the client often thinks that the dog is jealous or being competitive for attention. Few or no data exist to back these assertions. They are dangerous ones to make because they focus attention away from the real problems.

Treatment. Avoidance is key in such situations. Re-

member that redirected aggression follows the thwarting of another inappropriate behavior. *That* behavior must be addressed, diagnosed, and treated. Separating the animals when they are not supervised will greatly help to prevent reinforcing of their poor behavior. Rules for separation are the same as for dogs with interdog aggression. The offending dog can have a bell placed around its neck so that it can be monitored from a distance when supervised. It can also wear a Gentle Leader/Promise System Canine Head Halter in the house. The combination of these two devices allows the client to acutely monitor the behavior and to correct and interrupt the dog at the first sign of any inappropriate response. Foghorns and water pistols can also be used, but care must be taken not to startle or terrify the victim; that will worsen the problem. Primary therapy needs to be directed toward desensitizing the offending individual to the situation in which he or she reacted inappropriately (e.g., chasing the cat) (see "Protocol for Redirected Aggression" in Appendix B).

Food-Related Aggression

Diagnostic Profile. Dogs with food-related aggression react inappropriately to people by growling, lip lifting, snarling, or lunging and biting when approached while eating, when dog food is reached for or retrieved, when human food that has fallen on the floor is retrieved, or when a bone or biscuit is taken away. Generally, the higher the quality of food (table scraps, real bones, and rawhide), the more pronounced the aggression. Dogs can also exhibit food-related aggression only to other dogs. Data from the Behavior Clinic at VHUP indicate that food-related aggression, when directed at people, may be an excellent early clue that the dog is at risk for developing dominance aggression later in life. This presents an excellent opportunity for the veterinarian to discuss dominance aggression, signs that are indicators of these conditions, the danger and liability attendant to such a disorder, and the importance of early control over the dog's responsiveness. Because food-related aggression is probably tightly coupled to canine evolutionary history, it is not surprising that it is very difficult to successfully treat. Canids are, historically, binge-and-gorge eaters. Protecting food may be an ancestral adaptive behavior. In staged contests, puppies will form hierarchical rankings on the basis of possession of a bone; the effects of this may be modulated by sex (Beach et al., 1982; James, 1949). Also, some dogs from large litters that are fed from one bowl may learn to be aggressive to each other to successfully compete for food. Free-ranging street dogs may get enough food only by successfully fending off competitors.

Treatment. It is much easier to avoid the consequences of food-related aggression than it is to treat it. This is true whether the dog is aggressive only to dogs when fed, or also to people. Dogs with food-related aggression should not be allowed to have rawhides or real bones, and they should be fed or given biscuits or treats only in an environment where they cannot be disturbed (behind a closed or locked door). This is particularly true if young children are present. In such cases, the children should not be permitted to walk around with food in their hands if the dog is present.

If the dog is aggressive only to other dogs, the dogs should be fed either separately or at a distance at which they are not aggressive. Any time a biscuit is given, it must be finished before the dogs are released. Many dogs with food-related aggression hoard or steal biscuits as part of an ongoing social squabble. The biscuit that was hidden in the living room sofa may become the focus of a major battle. Clients must be instructed *not* to dangle body parts between the dogs. Use water, brooms, cardboard, blankets, or a foghorn to separate them. If one of the dogs is nonaggressive around food and the client would like to give it a rawhide, this must be done behind closed doors separate from the other dog.

If the dog is aggressive in the presence of its dog food even if no one tried to manipulate it, some behavior modification can be useful. Clients should teach the dog to sit and stay for very small food treats (see Appendix B, "Protocol for Deference: Basic Program" and "Behavior Modification Tier 1: Relaxation"). The dog should be unaggressive for this. Clients can then ask the dog to sit next to their chair and offer the dog a very small amount of food in a bowl. The clients should then tell the dog to stay while they refill the bowl, tell the dog to wait, and then offer the food bowl. Amounts should be small, but combined, should make up a normal meal. If the dog growls, the client should reduce the meal size. Clients often desire to hand-feed dogs. They should do this *only* if they can hold the bowl first as described. Because movement can stimulate these dogs and make them feel threatened, clients should *not* reach into the bowl. Rather, they should offer food with their open hand. If, and only if, the clients are able to feed both by hand and bowl, they can gradually teach the dog to relinquish his or her bowl, first starting with an empty bowl. The dog should be instructed to sit and wait first, and then have the bowl taken and immediately returned with the food or a treat. Teasing *worsens the situation* and makes such dogs more dangerous. Any client who doubts his or her ability to execute desensitization around food should absolutely avoid it. It is safe to feed the dog in an area that guarantees no disturbance. Although the dog's behavior will not improve, this will not *worsen* the situation because he or she experiences no provocational upset.

Possessive Aggression

Diagnostic Profile. Dogs exhibiting possessive aggression do not relinquish toys or objects to clients; these objects may be stolen possessions of the clients. If the client tries to take the object, the dog growls, snarls, snaps, or bites. Frequently these dogs present the object for play at the owner's feet and strike if the owner reaches for the object. The dog with possessive

aggression can quickly cycle through behaviors associated with solicitation of attention and then respond to the attention with a challenge. A reanalysis of data collected by Borchelt (1984b) indicated that 50% of dogs diagnosed with possessive aggression exhibited it by 7 to 12 months of age, and 25% (16/65) exhibited it by 3 months of age.

Treatment. These dogs can be counterconditioned to relinquish objects. However, they must have performed superbly on the first tier of the behavior modification program. Then they can gradually be desensitized to the object that they present and guard. Until then it is safer not to meet the challenge. The aspect of challenge in this behavior may act as a risk factor for developing dominance aggression. This is another behavior that can be part of a "control complex" as discussed later.

The "Behavior Modification Tier 2: Teaching Desensitizing and Counterconditioning Dogs to Relinquish Objects" is found in Appendix B.

Predatory Aggression

Diagnostic Profile. Two classes of culprits and behaviors are generally uncritically lumped within the diagnosis of predatory aggression: dogs that stalk, stare at, or silently pursue small animals, including birds, squirrels, cats, other dogs, and sometimes infants; and those that chase moving objects such as bicycles or skateboards. The latter can incite the dog to react in the same manner, but some dogs that chase individuals may be exhibiting territorial aggression. If the dog openly bounds after a bicyclist, barking, and stops the chase when the cyclist is out of bounds, check for other evidence of territorial aggression. Open advertisement of intention within prescribed territorial confines is not a characteristic of predatory aggression. If predatory aggression can truly include responses to moving objects, it is likely that an analysis of the actual behaviors involved would reveal differences that distinguish this form from that involving living individuals. No such analysis has been done to date. Dogs that bark and bound after either moving objects or people are potentially far less dangerous than those that silently stalk them. Stealth is an ingredient of hunting behavior, and the stealthy dog could make incorrect decisions about what or whom is prey (Polsky, 1975a,b). Often the animal is not eaten, but either killed and left or dragged about. In addition to the problems attendant with a pet dog preying on the neighborhood pet, bird, and squirrel populations, predatory aggression toward small animals may be a predictor of the same type of behavior toward human infants. Not all dogs that prey on small animals will demonstrate the same behavior to infants, but the few data available strongly suggest that dogs that behave in such a manner to infants had previously behaved predatorially to small animals, thus indicating risk.

Young infants unintentionally act in a manner similar to wounded prey. They are uncoordinated, they have abrupt sleep and wake cycles, and they scream suddenly in high-pitched tones. Generally, once infants can sit up on their own, they no longer elicit predatory responses from the dog. No dog should ever be left alone with an infant. This is particularly true for dogs with predatory aggression.

Treatment. Until the infant can sit up and maneuver *and* the dog ceases its attentive behavior, dogs with predatory aggressive tendencies should never be with an infant unless restrained with a leash or harness. Predatory tendencies or behaviors to small animals do not guarantee that the dog will react inappropriately with infants; such behaviors may indicate that these dogs are at greater risk for such problems. Predatory tendencies do not forbode other problem aggressions, nor do they preclude the dog from doing well with the child as the child ages. Considerations of risk analysis and assessment allow for safe, rational approaches in an area fraught with emotionalism. Do not delude yourself or your clients into believing that this problem can be successfully treated. It is not worth the risk. If the clients are unwilling to adhere to the standards set forth in the handout "Protocol for Introducing a New Baby and a Pet" (see Appendix B), everyone would be better off with the dog placed in an infant-free home. These dogs can go to other homes and do not need to be euthanized.

Dogs that are predatory to other animals should *never* be off lead, unsupervised, at large, or confined in a fence that other animals might cross (i.e., invisible fences). No unprovoked killing of any other species should be excused or tolerated.

Dominance Aggression

Diagnostic Profile. Before discussing dominance aggression, a brief discussion of the concept of *dominance* would be useful. Dominance is a concept found in traditional ethology that pertains to an individual's ability, generally under controlled conditions, to maintain or regulate access to some resource (Hinde, 1967, 1970; Landau, 1951; Rowell, 1974). It is a description of the regularities of winning or losing staged contests over those resources (Archer, 1988). It is *not* to be confused with status and, in fact, does not need to confer priority of access to resources (Archer, 1988). In situations in which the concept has been used with regard to status, it is important to realize that it is *not* defined as aggression on the part of the "dominant" animal but rather as the withdrawal of the "subordinate" (Gartlan, 1968; Rowell, 1972, 1974). The behavior of the *lower* status individuals, *not* the higher ranking one, is what determines the relative hierarchical rank. Rank itself is contextually relative. Truly high-ranking animals are tolerant of lower ranking ones (Barrette, 1993; Boyd & Silk, 1983; Kaufmann, 1967). Dominance displays infrequently lead to actual combat. Instead, combat ensues when they are *not* effective (Walther, 1977). The concept of dominance was originally developed for use in describing territorial interactions in birds (Hinde, 1957), and

since then the concepts of both dominance and linear hierarchies have been grossly misunderstood and misapplied (Archer, 1988; Beaver, 1987f; Gartlan, 1968; Rowell, 1974).

Although dominance is a concept that must be cautiously used, it is *not* the same as dominance aggression. The latter is an abnormal, inappropriate, out-of-context aggression that is manifested by dogs toward people when the "resource" is *access* to control (see Appendix F). It is likely that dominance aggression, like most other diagnoses of aggression, are manifestations of an underlying anxiety disorder. When a dog is pathologically anxious (i.e., the anxiety is not induced by the environment or by abuse) about its relative role in the social environment, the default rule is either to take control or test the social environment to determine whether the dog can challenge control. When this behavior pattern is associated with people, it is called dominance aggression; when it is associated with dogs, it represents one manifestation of interdog (interanimal) aggression. The role for anxiety in aggression—particularly in dominance aggression—is further substantiated by the physiological findings discussed later in the chapter.

Dominance aggression is the most commonly seen form of aggression in the Behavior Clinic at VHUP and is a diagnosis in 20% of the canine behavior cases handled from 1987 to the present.

A reanalysis of specific behaviors (barking, growling, baring teeth, snapping, biting, and staring) occurring in pairwise comparisons of fear aggression/dominance aggression, possessive aggression/dominance aggression, and protective aggression/dominance aggression reveals some interesting patterns. In the comparison between behaviors exhibited in dominance versus fear aggression, growling, baring teeth, biting, and staring occurred statistically more frequently in dominance aggression (G_{adj} = 18.62, 4.67, 11.22, 18.18, respectively; all $p \leq 0.05$).

The comparison of behaviors exhibited in dominance versus possessive aggression revealed that barking, growling, biting, and staring were all statistically more common in dominance aggression (G_{adj} = 9.41, 4.82, 9.65, and 14.08, respectively; all $p \leq 0.05$). This substantiates that possessive and dominance aggression may co-occur (Voith & Borchelt, 1982b), but that the former is not a symptom of the latter. This casts some doubt on the validity of the use of possession of a bone as an assay for dominance in puppies (James, 1949; Pawlowski & Scott, 1956; Scott & Fuller, 1965).

The comparison between protective and dominance aggression indicates that barking, as expected given its warning function, is more commonly exhibited in protective aggression (G_{adj} = 16.50, $p \leq 0.05$). Growling, baring teeth, biting, and staring are all more commonly exhibited in dominance aggression (G_{adj} = 17.17, 12.69, 16.96, 14.08, respectively; all $p \leq 0.05$). In no pairwise comparison was snapping statistically more frequently represented. This suggests that biting

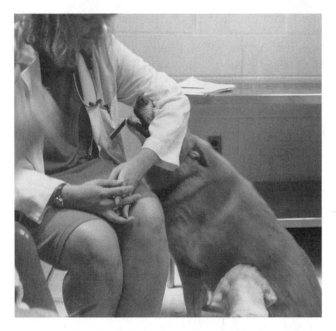

Pushy or dominant behaviors can include leaning on, pawing at, pushing, blocking access, and putting a head in a lap. "Dominant" behaviors can be associated with attention-seeking behavior, as in this photo, but do not have to be associated with dominance aggression. The dog pictured accompanied the patient and had no aggressive tendencies but was extremely pushy and attention seeking.

(which was *always* more common in dominance aggression) and snapping may not be tightly coupled.

Dominance aggression is also the most complex of the aggressions and warrants further study. Much has been written on the structure of the canine hierarchy, with the client as the alpha or dominant dog, at the top. This is dangerously simplistic. Dominance aggression is about the concept of control, not about overt challenges (a bone) or ambiguous challenges (access to a sofa), as has been maintained in recent literature (Reisner et al., 1994).

Canine and human social systems are quite similar and have fluid social hierarchies that are largely maintained by deference; challenges to deference structures can be decided by aggression, as defined previously. Most dogs innately defer to people (Netto et al., 1992). This behavior is further reinforced by some forms of training. Some dogs will challenge this leadership role and cannot accept that they are not dominant. A dominant or pushy dog may not be aggressive—it may just never have learned to defer, or worse, it may have learned that the only way to get any attention was to be pushy (see the section on Attention-Seeking Behavior). Any aggressive problems, including dominance aggression, are actually the dog's problems and are generally *not caused by the response of the client*, although the client could inadvertently encourage the

inappropriate behavior to develop. If the client chooses to use forceful physical restraint or physical punishment, the situation could worsen. The dog is faced with a challenge about control in any punishment situation; hence, the term *punishment-elicited aggression* (Borchelt & Voith, 1982a) is uninformative. For a dog that already challenges a leadership role, the only choice is to return any challenge in kind. Unless the client is able to sufficiently rebuff the dog so that the dog is convinced it cannot win a battle predicated on frank aggression, the situation will worsen with the use of force. Few clients are willing to fight their dogs to the death. Unless they can absolutely quell the challenge so that the dog capitulates and defers of its own volition, the dog will respond with more aggressive behaviors. The more likely scenario is the one in which the client backs down and, inadvertently, defers to the dog. This behavior also provides the anxious dog with a set of rules. Future interactions with the dog will continue to be controlled by the dog's demands and aggressions. Because there is still no generalizable set of rules that can relieve the dog's anxiety, the dog will continue to deform the social system through active and passive challenge. These challenges may continue to change in form and may vary depending on the individual's involvement. Although punishment provides a "rule," the rule does not treat the problem anxiety, which is the dog's management of his or her relative role in the social environment. Physical punishment contradicts the tenet on which canine and human social systems are based: deference (see Chapter 3). The dog with dominance aggression forces the suspecting or fearful client to defer to him by force. Any rational treatment requires a mechanism that causes the dog to defer to the client.

The client could also inadvertently reinforce the inappropriate behavior by deferring to the dog in the initial stages of the challenge. Clients may not recognize their own behaviors as deferential, nor may they recognize the dog's behavior as anything but loving. As a result, they may inadvertently reinforce anxiety-related behaviors. This is why it is so critical that clients understand normal dog behaviors and signals. Because clients defer to the initial challenges that they perceive to be nonaggressive, such as the pressing of paws on the client's shoulders, frequently interpreted as a "hug," the appearance of aggression is then viewed as having a "sudden onset."

Clients need to learn to recognize that all of these behaviors are used by dogs to test the status of other dogs and may be being used in the same way with them. Do not let the clients overreact. If the dog pushes on them and groans when they shove him off the couch, but goes happily, anyway, they may have no cause for concern. If that same dog begins to push harder and resist being physically moved, and starts growling and grabbing with his jaw, the clients *do* have cause for concern. The former dog may just be a little pushy or dominant. The latter may be dominantly aggressive. It is underappreciated that a dog can be dominant without being *dominantly aggressive.* Some clients like the cocky, assertive natures of dominant dogs; these are also traits that can make these excellent show or working dogs. The critical distinction must be made between the forceful, personable dog and the one that aggressively manipulates the client in contexts associated with dominance.

Dominance aggression correlates with social maturity (age at onset is 18 to 24 months). This is also the developmental age at which phobias, separation anxiety, obsessive-compulsive disorder, and other anxiety-based problems become apparent. Social maturity is the developmental phase during which many mental illnesses begin in humans, also. It may be displayed if the client approaches or disturbs a dog while he is eating, playing with toys, or sleeping. A dominantly aggressive dog may react aggressively if stepped over, pushed from the bed or couch, reached toward, put on the leash, or pushed on the shoulders or rump. These dogs may react aggressively when their paws are toweled off or when stared at. Some dogs react aggressively to being rolled on their back. Others react aggressively to being yelled at or leash corrected. A dominant aggressive dog may stand over the client, or the perceived challenger, or press or lean on them

physically. Such dogs get the last word and may growl or lift a lip if stared at. Aggressive reactions can include any or all of the following: growling, snarling, lip-lifting, and snapping and biting. It is a hallmark of dominantly aggressive dogs that they become more aggressive if punished. These scenarios are all united by issues of control that are not necessarily hierarchical. Behaviors associated with dominance aggression are outlined in Boxes 6-8 and 6-9.

This is the generalized view of dominance aggression. Because of its relationship to anxiety, dominance aggression is extremely variable, ranging from very definite aggressive behavior associated with unambiguously asserting control, to very subtle, nonvocal behaviors. Discussions of dominance aggression tend to deal only with dogs that exhibit an unrelenting tendency to control the household social hierarchy. This is simplistic and misleading.

Dominance aggression is a description for a complex of multifactorial disorders. It is affected by social contexts and the extent to which the dog is affected by anxiety. Dogs demonstrating dominance aggression can be divided into two broad groups: (1) those that have no doubt that they are in control and can compel their clients to do their bidding (Masters of the Universe), and (2) those that are unsure of their social role

---

BOX 6-8

HUMAN BEHAVIORS THAT MAY ELICIT BEHAVIORS THAT ARE PART OF DOMINANCE AGGRESSION

1. Staring at the dog
2. Toweling head, neck, back
3. Toweling or handling feet*
4. Leaning on, or pushing on back, neck, or head
5. Handling head, muzzle
6. Reaching over head (including to put on leash)
7. Pushing on rump
8. Stepping over
9. Disturbing while sleeping
10. Pushing from bed or sofa
11. Verbal correction
12. Leash correction
13. Any physical punishment *including* alpha rolls and dominance downs

*Excluding having toenails cut, if the only sign that the dog is exhibiting is fear or aggression during nail clipping and no other signs are added with time, the dog is probably *not* dominantly aggressive. Many dogs are anxious about nail clipping; one cut is sufficient to teach them to be forever concerned. It must be very painful but the reaction is not sufficient by itself to make the determination of dominance aggression. If the dog has *never* been injured during nail cutting and starts to growl or show other aggressive behavior, caution is urged; this could be a sign of incipient dominance aggression, and clients should be warned to watch for other signs.

BOX 6-9

CANINE BEHAVIORS THAT ARE PART OF DOMINANCE AGGRESSION

1. Snarling, growling, or biting in any of the contexts listed in Box 6-8
2. Pushing on people
3. Placing paws/head on people's shoulders, head, back
4. Straddling people with or without mounting
5. Blocking access, particularly in doorways
6. Blocking correctional possibilities (holding the leash or the person's wrist)
7. Staring, particularly if accompanied by pupil dilation
8. "Talking back"
9. Leaning on people's feet/legs, particularly with paws or back
10. "Hugs," "kisses" (particularly if all over face), "talking"
11. "Bill pops" (the smacking together of the upper and lower jaws or lips, combined with one lick of one side of the mouth) when asked to comply
12. Snorting when asked to comply
13. Stamping feet when asked to comply

NOTE: In the absence of number 1 above, all of these behaviors could be associated with "dominance" without accompanying aggression.

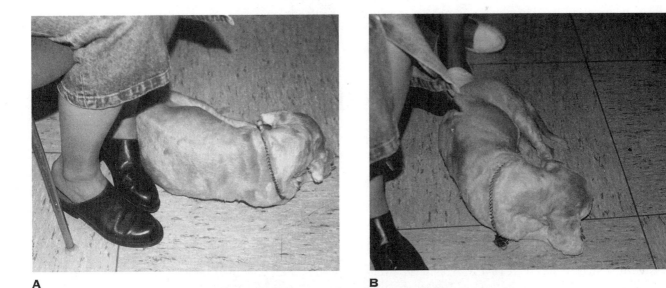

A

B

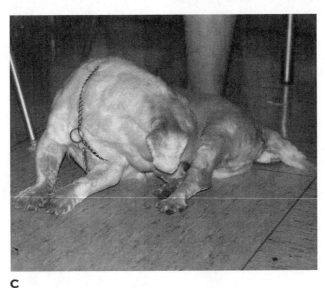

C

Dominant or pushy behaviors can be extremely passive. When associated with inappropriate, out-of-context aggression, they are usually part of dominance aggression. **A,** The dog pictured was extremely dominantly aggressive. He is lying on the student's feet and has turned his back to her. Turning the back to another can be a challenge, or it may indicate either passive avoidance or normally confident behavior. Context is important. The confident dog will not be distressed if prohibited from lying on a foot or leaning against someone who withdraws. That was not the case for this dog. **B,** The dog has moved to passively challenge someone else after the student withdrew her leg. Dominance aggression, like other aggressions, is probably rooted in anxiety. This dog is exhibiting two other signs of anxiety: he is resisting letting his head relax on the floor although he is exhausted by the long appointment and manipulations, and he has lick granulomas, albeit mild, on all carpi and tarsi (**C**). Notice that he is leaning on yet a third person's foot in this photograph. (Photos by K.L. Overall)

and use the aggressive behaviors to deform the social system to get much needed information about what is expected of them. They define their social and behavioral boundaries using the response to their aggression. This is analogous to teenage children with behavioral disorders who are disruptive and sometimes aggressive. These dogs appear to be less sure of their relative hierarchical status and to express more ambiguity in their vocal and physical responses about the intensity of their aggression. The aggression is not applied equally to all humans in the second class of dominance aggression because the dog responds to the

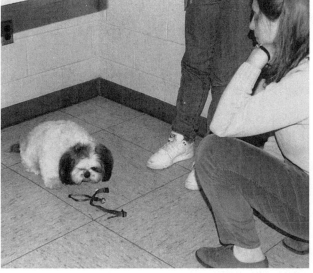 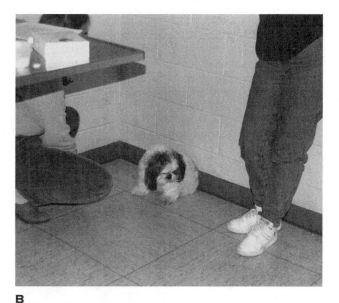

A   **B**

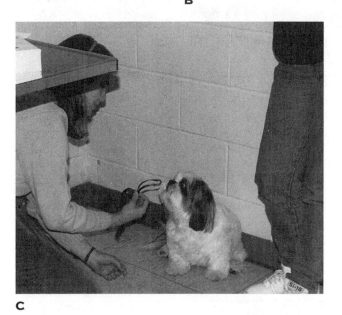

C

A, The dog in this photo is extremely dominantly aggressive and demonstrates both active and passive challenges to control (the attempted placement of a head collar). The student lets the dog sniff the head collar without trying to put it on. Note that the dog is still in an exploratory mode and in the center of the room. **B,** As the student gets more active in attempting to place the head collar the dog moves away and averts his head. **C,** As the student attempts to slip the head collar over the dog's nose, the dog sets his head and neck, brings his ears forward, stares at the student, shows his incisors and canines, and growls. After an hour the dog was still without a head collar and the client and clinician decided that it might be too dangerous, given the dog's response, for her to fit the head collar. Notice that throughout the client stayed against a wall, out of the way, and with her hands in her pockets. We had requested this and she was happy to comply. (Photos by K.L. Overall)

social environment in a differential manner on the basis of individual social interactions. A retrospective analysis of the dominantly aggressive dogs seen at the Behavior Clinic at VHUP since 1987 revealed that the majority of these dogs also exhibited attention-seeking behavior. These are dogs that are very needy and are constantly setting people up to defer to them, not simply because they have an abnormal urge to control, but also because this is their only mechanism for receiving information about their role in the social environment. It should be implicit that this need for information about their role in the environment has less to do with that dog's particular social environment than it has to do with an inherent abnormality. Consistent, generalizable rules and expectations (benign doggie boot camp) work well for these dogs; they work less well for dogs in the first group. Dogs in the first group are very dangerous because they have no doubt that they are in control. Response to antianxiety medication supports this categorization. Dogs in the second group do well with ancillary anxiolytics (e.g., amitriptyline) to help with their behavior modification; dogs in the first group often behave more poorly when given the same drugs because the drugs may relieve any inhibiting anxiety that was preventing the dog from being more aggressive. These two behavioral profiles also help to explain the different human groups that may be victimized by dogs exhibiting these different forms of dominance aggression. This stratification is outlined in Box 6-10.

Interestingly, about 90% of the dogs with dominance aggression problems are males (Borchelt & Voith, 1986a, Line & Voith, 1986; Voith and Borchelt, 1982a). Unfortunately, castration is *not* a treatment or preventative for dominance aggression, but it *may* be a useful adjuvant in a complete treatment program. It is important to realize that aggressive behavior is learned and reinforced during each aggressive event. Because of this, neutering an aggressive dog later in life may not have as profound an effect as it would have earlier in life. Testosterone acts as a behavioral modulator. Dogs that are exposed to testosterone and who have an inappropriate, out-of-context behavior (1) may be more reactive at any given time and may react more quickly to a stimulus, (2) may react to a more intense level, (3) may stay reactive for a longer period of time, (4) may have a longer and more protracted de-

nouement phase, and (5) may stabilize at their prereaction levels only after a delayed time (Fig. 6-2). Although castration may provide an edge by decreasing the chemical motivation toward aggression, it does nothing to diminish the learned component. Most of the testosterone is out of the system within 6 hours after castration, with the bulk decreasing within 72 hours of castration (Hopkins et al., 1976). Removal of one chemical component of the reaction can be beneficial and should be done, but the learned component of the behavior must still be addressed with treatment.

That dominance aggression is a complex disorder that is "organic" in nature and one based in or closely related to underlying anxiety disorders is demonstrated by a study at VHUP (Overall, Jezyk, Giger, unpublished data, 1996). Urine of canine patients at the Behavior Clinic at VHUP was screened for abnormal metabolites (Giger & Jezyk, 1992). The results of the overall survey are found in Table 6-2. Aggressive dogs more frequently have abnormal metabolic screens, in the absence of any metabolic disease, statistically more frequently than do dogs with a nonaggressive diagnosis (e.g., separation anxiety, incomplete housebreaking, thunderstorm phobia). The three most common metabolic abnormalities were excessive amounts of glutamine, taurine, and alanine. Glutamine and taurine are excitatory neurotransmitters (Fonnum, 1984). Glutamine anomalies have been reported to occur in familial aggregations of human aggression (Brunner et al., 1993; Cases et al., 1995; Coyle & Puttfarcken, 1993; Geer et al., 1971, 1989; Smirnova, 1993a,b) and are associated with neuronal death and excitotoxicity (Olney, 1994). The mechanism for this may be associated with the toxic effect of nitric oxide (Dawson et al., 1991, 1992; Nelson et al., 1995; Snyder, 1995). When dogs with only dominance aggression were examined, only 17/139 dogs screened had normal metabolic screens; 122 of the results were abnormal, and the most frequent abnormality was increased amounts of urinary glutamine. The data are not yet completely analyzed, but it appears that these abnormal metabolites may be present in some cases before the aggressive symptomatology. Many puppies with abnormal levels of glutamine in their metabolic screens later developed dominance aggression at social maturity. Further research may indicate that metabolic screens are useful tools in the diagnosis of canine aggression. The current findings further support a mechanistic hypothesis for canine aggression, and provide a tentative mechanism for the favorable response

---

BOX 6-10

RECIPIENTS OF DOMINANCE AGGRESSION BY STRATIFICATION

Compliant client (2; occasionally 1)
Confident, demanding client (1)
Children aged 3 to 8 years (2)
Children aged 8 to 11 years (2; sometimes 1)
Children aged 11 to 14 years (1; sometimes 2)

Key
1. Truly dominant dog that must control environment; no anxiety about position; "master of universe" type; potentially very aggressive
2. Dog that is uncertain of its role in the hierarchy; uses dominance challenges to deform the system and obtain information; potentially dangerous, but imminently treatable.

TABLE 6-2 METABOLIC SCREEN RESULTS

Behavior Clinic Diagnosis	Abnormal	Normal
Aggressive	185	25
Nonaggressive	65	19

Log likelihood ratio test, $p \leq 0.05$.

to antianxiety medications noted for these patients (Overall, 1994a-c, 1995a,b).

Many authors report that dominantly aggressive dogs are also territorial (Hart & Hart, 1985b; Houpt, 1991; Landsberg, 1990). Food-related aggression, possessive aggression, territorial/protective aggression, dominance aggression, and, to a lesser extent, redirected aggression, are all part of a *complex related to the issue of control.* It is important to realize that any one of these diagnoses can occur independently, without being part of the larger control complex; however, the presence of any one of these should flag the potential for the existence or development of any of the others (Box 6-11). Multiple diagnoses may be more dangerous and more difficult to treat because of interactive effects.

Treatment. As with all aggressions, the first line of treatment for dominance aggression involves avoiding the circumstances that elicit the aggressions or any inappropriate, noncompliant behaviors. This means that the dog should not be reached for, pushed on, stared at, or handled if these are things that prompt aggression or bad behavior. Table 6-3 displays the aggression screen from Appendix A with the classes of aggression that may be implicated by these signs noted. *Anything* to which the dog reacts must be avoided. This may mean that the dog can no longer sleep on the bed. This will upset some people; therefore it is important to emphasize to them that these omissions will be more difficult for them than for the dog. If people want the best chance at being safe and achieving better behavior, compliance is critical. These dogs are difficult at best, but the people who work the hardest achieve the best results, regardless of the prognosis.

Again, the focus of treatment is in teaching the dog to relax and comply in benign contexts and then gradually desensitizing the dog to situations in which it reacts inappropriately (Overall, 1993e,f). The programs for this process are in Appendix B, as is the "Protocol for Dogs With Dominance Aggression."

Because the root of dominance aggression appears to be based in anxiety, behavior modification designed to consistently reinforce the dog's status and expecta-

tions to him or her affects great changes in the patient's behavior. Treatment for these dogs focuses on soliciting deferential behavior from them in *all* interactions. These dogs must sit and wait until they are told it is acceptable to get up or until they are invited to participate in another activity whenever they are interacting with a person. This means that they must sit and wait for walks, treats, food, grooming, play, having the leash put on, and any form of attention. Even if they cut their foot, they must sit or lie down so that it can be examined. If these dogs butt clients with their heads while the clients watch TV, it is *not* acceptable to simply reach out and pet them. They must first be asked to sit and wait; then they can be briefly petted. They are to be expected to stay unless they are released.

It is not necessary to reinforce a prolonged period of waiting and staying; the dog's rump must touch the ground and it must wait at least a few seconds so that he or she knows that the person, not the dog, will direct the course of any activities. Remember that sitting and lying down are deferential behaviors in the context of canine nonvocal communication. It is important to use the canine social and communicatory systems in the process of getting the dog to cooperate.

Clients are concerned that this protocol means that they cannot give their dogs any attention. This is untrue. They can give their dogs as much attention as the dogs *earn* by being calm, not anxious, and happy while performing deferential behaviors. This protocol provides the dogs with an unambiguous set of rules whereby they can be guaranteed attention. If the dog brings a toy, the client is permitted to play with the dog *only after* the dog has been requested to sit, stay, and drop the toy, and the game can be controlled and terminated by the client. People are still allowed to have dogs on their laps *if and only if* they can ask the dog to sit and wait, and then invite him or her up, *and* the person can verbally order the dog down and the dog complies. If this is not possible, it is too risky and dangerous to have the dog on the client's lap. Under no circumstances are the people to push the dog down or use physical punishment. This will only worsen the behavior and put the person at risk. If the dog does not comply with the person's first set of commands, they can be repeated once. If the dog still refuses to sit and wait, the person should *leave the room.* These dogs are so desperate for attention and interaction, albeit in a controlling manner, that they will follow the person. The request should then be repeated. If after one chance for correction the dog refuses to comply, the person should again leave the room. This process must be repeated until the dog complies. Until then, the dog will receive no attention and interaction. Sooner or later the dog will want food or a walk; because the dog can have neither without sitting for them, it will eventually comply.

Clients are often concerned that by doing this, and by *not* using physical force, *they* are actually being

---

BOX 6-11

DIAGNOSES ASSOCIATED WITH A CANINE CONTROL COMPLEX

1. Food-related aggression
2. Possessive aggression
3. Territorial aggression
4. Protective aggression
5. Dominance aggression
6. Redirected aggression

TABLE 6-3 DIAGNOSTIC CORRELATES OF AGGRESSIVE SIGNS

Aggression Screen

Note whether the reaction is consistent or applies to only one person or in one circumstance. Also note if the dog's behavior has been worsening in one category. (See Appendix A for expanded screens with more detailed instructions.)

Action	Reaction					Aggression Diagnosis
	No reaction	Snarl	Bark/growl	Snap/bite	Not applicable	
1. Take dog's food dish with food						Food
2. Take dog's empty food dish						Food Possessive
3. Take dog's water dish						Food Possessive
4. Take food (human) that falls on floor						Food
5. Take rawhide						Food
6. Take real bone						Food
7. Take biscuit						Food
8. Take toy						Possessive
9. Human approaches dog while eating						Food
10. Dog approaches dog while eating						Food
11. Human approaches dog while playing with toys						Play Possessive
12. Dog approaches dog while playing with toys						Interdog Redirected
13. Human approaches/disturbs dog while sleeping						Dominance Territorial
14. Dog approaches/disturbs dog while sleeping						Interdog
15. Human steps over dog						Dominance
16. Push dog off bed/couch						Dominance
17. Reach toward dog						Dominance
18. Reach over dog's head						Dominance
19. Put on leash						Dominance
20. Human pushes on dog's shoulders						Dominance Pain
21. Dog mounts, pushes on shoulders						Interdog
22. Human pushes on rump						Dominance Pain
23. Dog mounts, pushes on rump						Interdog

24. Towel feet when wet						Dominance Fear
25. Bathe dog						Dominance Fear Pain
26. Groom dog's head						Dominance
27. Groom dog's body						Dominance Pain
28. Human stares at dog						Dominance
29. Dog stares at dog						Interdog
30. Take muzzle in hands and shake						Dominance Fear
31. Push dog over onto back						Dominance Pain Fear
32. Stranger knocks on door						Territorial Protective
33. Stranger enters room						Protective Territorial
34. Dog in car at toll booth						Protective Territorial
35. Dog in car at gas station						Protective Territorial
36. Dog on leash approached by dog on street						Interdog Territorial
37. Dog on leash approached by person on street						Protective
38. Dog in yard—person passes						Protective Territorial Fear
39. Dog in yard—dog passes						Interdog Territorial
40. Dog in veterinarian's office						Fear Pain Dominance
41. Dog in boarding kennel						Fear Territorial
42. Dog at groomer						Fear Pain
43. Dog yelled at						Fear Dominance Redirected

Continued

TABLE 6-3 DIAGNOSTIC CORRELATES OF AGGRESSIVE SIGNS—cont'd

Action	Reaction					Aggression Diagnosis
	No reaction	Snarl	Bark/growl	Snap/bite	Not applicable	
44. Dog corrected with leash						Dominance Fear Redirected
45. Dog physically punished—hit						Dominance Fear
46. Someone raised voice to client in presence of dog						Protective
47. Someone hugs/touches client in presence of dog						Protective
48. Squirrel, cat, small animal approaches						Predatory
49. Bicycle, skateboard nearby						Predatory Territorial Fear
50. Crying infant						Predatory
51. Playing with 2-year-old children						Dominance Pain Fear Territorial
52. Playing with 5- to 7-year-old children						Dominance Fear
53. Playing with 8- to 11-year-old children						Dominance
54. Playing with 12- to 16-year-old children						Dominance

controlled by the dog's behaviors. To the extent that any of us are controlled or affected by social systems in which we are involved, this is true, but the people are *in no way* yielding ("caving in") to the dog on this program, if the program is executed correctly. The clients have taken a very strict, disciplined approach to shaping the dog's inappropriate behavior. The problem arises because many training books encourage people to confuse discipline and violence.

For any dog that jumps and resists control, and especially those for whom a stare or a restraining gesture is a threat, Gentle Leader/Promise System Canine Head Halters are invaluable. They can be worn in the house with the indoor lead and provide a margin of safety in working with very aggressive dogs. The dog can be prevented from biting and growling and can be prohibited from lunging. Better yet, as soon as the dog threatens, it can be interrupted immediately

in a manner that uses the same physical signals that another dog would use: when pulled forward, the halter puts a small amount of pressure on the dog's neck, a dominant gesture in itself. The instant correction allows the dog to learn that it cannot threaten, and thus the dog is not inadvertently reinforced in its aggression by a client who is too fearful to otherwise deal with it.

Both groups of dominantly aggressive dogs, the masters of the universe and those seeking active definition of where they fit in, respond well to an environment in which the rules of deference are clear and are consistently enforced. Dogs in the latter group, however, may respond very well to adjuvant therapy with antianxiety medication (amitriptyline 1-2 mg/kg orally every 12 hours; imipramine 1-2 mg/kg orally every 12 hours; fluoxetine 1.0 mg/kg orally every 24 hours) because relieving their anxiety allows them to

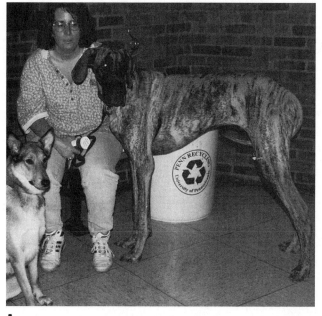

A

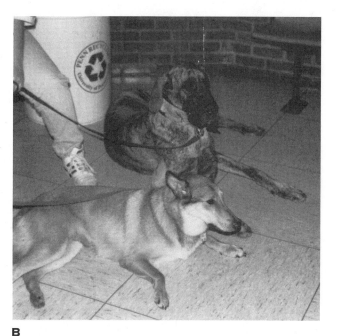

B

The great Dane was diagnosed with profound dominance aggression when he was only a few months of age. He also has other anxiety-related problems including manifestations of obsessive-compulsive disorder. He is 14 months of age in the photo and is wonderfully improved. The following aspects factored into his improvement: (1) a realistic client and great breeder (both came to the appointment, and the client is holding his lead), (2) perfect compliance with the behavior modification programs, (3) a Gentle Leader/Promise Canine Head Collar, (4) continued use of antianxiety medication (relapses occur when these are withdrawn—they will be used all his life, and he continues to have bi-annual laboratory testing done), and (5) another dog. The second dog in the photo was a rescue picked especially for her calm temperament and tendency to "mother." The Dane has learned to take his cues, in part, from her and is noticeably distressed when she is not with him. He had improved by more than 75% before we discussed the addition of another dog (the breeder's idea since he exhibited many fewer of his anxiety-related behaviors when with his sister). The addition resulted in further improvement. (Photos by K.L. Overall)

interact more appropriately in their social environment (Overall, 1992a, 1994a,b). Dogs in the first group may be inhibiting their aggressions because of training or anxiety; treatment with antianxiety medication tends to increase aggression.

That such medications are useful in treating this condition makes sense; the drugs all affect serotonin metabolism, and, hence, glutamate. Serotonin has been postulated to decrease aggression in cats (Katz & Thomas, 1976) and humans (Linnoila & Virkkunen, 1992), whereas norepinephrine has been postulated to facilitate it (Eichelmann, 1977a,b; Reis, 1971; Reis 1974; Yudofsky et al., 1986, 1987). Serenics, or specific 5-hydroxytryptamine (serotonin) agonists, have been shown to cause an experimental dose-dependent decrease in aggression in the standard rat model (Mos & Olivier, 1989; Mos et al., 1990). Arginine vasopressin

antagonists experimentally decrease offensive aggression in the rat model (Ferris & Polegal, 1988; Ferris et al., 1995), possibly through enhancement of the neural network controlling agonistic behavior that is normally restricted by serotonin. All these data link aggression, anxiety, and the serotonin/glutamate complexes.

Idiopathic Aggression

Diagnostic Profile. In this last category of aggression, the dog's aggressive behavior is unprovoked, unpredictable, violent, and uncontrolled. It is as though someone threw the switch, turning on the aggression and the violence. Some clients say their dog gets "a possessed look." This look could be the result of a sympathetic nervous system reaction that enhances tapetal reflection and should not be a criterion. A dog

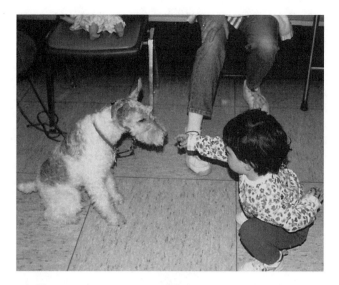

Children as young as 18 months of age (the age of this child) can learn to do the behavior modification programs. Portrayed here is "kid sit, dog sit!" This dog has dominance aggression directed primarily towards the child (See Box 6-10). The child has been taught not to reach over the dog's head, not to stare at the dog, and not to wave her arms and yell. The dog had previously learned the relaxation techniques by working with the parents—a prerequisite step before working with children. Note that the dog is waiting until the child gives him the treat—and that he is wearing a head collar. The head collar is what makes the behavior modification safe to execute. Note the presence of the parents: one is watching the child, while the other is watching the dog. (Photo by K.L. Overall)

TABLE 6-4 NECESSARY CONDITIONS FOR "SEIZURE" ACTIVITY TO BE CAUSAL FOR AGGRESSION

	Abnormal EEG	Normal EEG
"Seizure" present	A*	B
"Behavioral" diagnosis	C	D

EEG, Electroencephalogram.
A = Probably accurate representation.
B = False-negative; might rule out seizure when it is present.
C = False-negative; would miss all seizure activity if EEG was not obtained.
D = Assumption for most behavioral conditions.
*Only situation for which any certainty exists.

in the midst of a bout with idiopathic aggression may be foaming at the mouth and twitching; therefore it is critical to rule out primary epileptiform seizures (Andermann & Andermann, 1988; Mosh et al., 1988). This may not be easy. The extent to which "behavioral" and "neurological" diagnoses overlap and can be difficult to discern is illustrated in Table 6-4. The extent to which preictal, prodromal, or premonitory behaviors occur and can be recognized by clients has not been sufficiently or consistently documented

(Abel & McCandless, 1992; Elliott, 1978; Gedye, 1989; Gilbert, 1992). The afflicted dog may violently attack people or objects, including furniture.

Idiopathic aggression seems to appear most often in dogs 1 to 3 years of age, which may be a confounding factor in distinguishing it from dominance aggression. This is also, unfortunately, the age at which most idiopathic epilepsy develops. It is interesting that these are such critical years for the development of behavioral and neurological problems. It cannot be behaviorally induced in a clinical setting. Thus it is more difficult to study than a category such as food aggression, during which the dog can be given food and observed when the food is removed.

Idiopathic aggression is similar to other noted behavioral disorders: rage or spaniel rage syndrome (Campbell, 1992), mental lapse aggression syndrome (Beaver, 1980), idiopathic viciousness (Hart, 1977; Hart & Hart, 1985a), stimulus responsive psychomotor epilepsy (Crowell-Davis et al., 1989), and episodic dyscontrol (Dodman et al., 1992; Gedye, 1989a,b; Geier et al., 1977; Ounsted, 1967; Waterman et al., 1987). Beaver (1980) characterized mental lapse aggression as occurring in 1.5- to 2-year-old dogs (see Dominance Aggression section) with low-voltage, fast activity electroencephalograms (EEGs). Dodman et al. (1992) have identified the occasional dogs that have abnormal EEGs comprising moderate amplitude (20 to 30 μV) spike discharges at 2 to 3 Hz, from tracings on left hemispheric and transfrontal channels. Other researchers have not published consistent findings. One of three dogs in the study by Dodman and co-workers responded to phenobarbital. This is not a sufficient base to argue that such aggressions are rooted in epileptic disorders, and caution is urged about cavalier interpretations. Problems inherent in this approach include the lack of repeatable EEG tracings for dogs with established seizure disorders, and sampling paradigms. Psychomotor epilepsy characterized by bouts of rage in dogs has always been thought to be rare (McGrath, 1960). Sporadic anomalies should not cause repeated, frequent aggression, yet it is unknown how such spike phenomena are distributed in time or space. Many of the suppositions about aggression and neurological abnormalities stem from the findings that lesions of the amygdala decrease aggression and that lesions of the ventromedial hypothalamus increase aggression (Zagrodzka & Fonberg, 1977). Primary control over aggression seems to occur through the hypothalamus and is modulated by cortical limbic structures and thalamic pathways (Bandler & Flynn, 1974; Siegal & Pott, 1988; Siegal et al., 1977).

Treatment. There are no effective treatments for idiopathic aggression, largely because hypotheses about underlying causality have been poorly or incompletely formulated. Furthermore, because by definition the aggressive outbursts are unpredictable, results of the aggression screen (see Appendix A) will *truly* be negative, and it is very difficult to avoid the circumstances that provoke the aggressive events. This unpredictability makes dogs with this condition very difficult to keep.

It is possible that the constellation of aggressions in this last group of aggression may be obsessive-compulsive disorders, unipolar disorders, or other abnormalities of the limbic system (Overall, 1992f, 1994d). The number of cases that do not respond to phenobarbital therapy is *underreported.* It is important to be able to clearly distinguish the sedative effect from the therapeutic effect when using phenobarbital or any other drug.

Some success in treating dogs that are exhibiting idiopathic or extremely aggravated dominance aggression has been achieved with lithium (Reisner, 1994); however, the expense of frequent monitoring for toxicity made this a difficult drug to prescribe. It cannot be prescribed in the absence of blood monitoring because therapeutic and toxic dosage levels overlap.

SPECIFIC TREATMENT OF AGGRESSION

Specific modalities for dealing with each of the aggressive diagnoses discussed were outlined earlier. The rationale of behavioral therapy is outlined in Chapter 12. Concepts pertaining to behavioral modification are difficult to implement without practice (Voith, 1979a,b, 1980h, 1981a, 1986). Understanding its principles will allow the diligent practitioner to construct the appropriate therapeutic regimen for each patient. Examples of a stepwise approach to aggression and a diagnostic example are found in Boxes 6-12 and 6-13. Clients should understand that, regardless, the first step in treating any aggressive condition is to avoid the circumstances associated with its expression. Any time an animal is successful in expressing any inappropriate behavior, the behavior is reinforced (Azrin, 1965; Potegal, 1979). Interruption and correction of aggression are not as safe or successful, at the outset, as is avoidance. Punishment, in the absence of other behavior modification, could render any aggressive dog more dangerous and successful in its aggression. Abuse will always render an animal more dangerous and less predictable.

Role of the Endogenous Hormonal Environment

Much attention has been directed to the role of hormones, primarily those that are sexually dimorphic, and their potential effects on undesirable behavior. Although 90% of all dominantly aggressive dogs may be male (Voith & Borchelt, 1982a), testosterone does not cause dominance aggression. Instead, it would be more appropriate to view testosterone as a behavioral modulator that may facilitate the attainment and escalation of the aggressive state. As discussed, if a dog is already aggressive, the difference between being neutered and unneutered is one of degree (See Fig. 6-2). Other dimorphic behaviors associated with the presence of testosterone include urine marking with lifted leg, roaming, and some types of mounting. Mounting is an unclear issue because it is a challenge and control behavior as well as a sexual one; little work has been done to determine whether the nuances of the mounting behavior are identical in both situations. Hopkins and colleagues (1976) determined that castration resulted in an androgen decrease within 6 hours of castration and that the bulk of the hormonal decrease was complete in 72 hours. There was a 90% decrease in roaming in male dogs that roamed before castration, a 62% reduction in male-male aggression, a minimal 50% reduction in urine marking, and an 80% reduction in mounting. Marking, mounting, and, to a lesser extent because of the modulator effect discussed above, fighting, are complex behaviors not wholly controlled by hormones alone. There is a large learned component in these that many people neglect. If marking has been ongoing, castration alone will not ablate it, but it may decrease it. This is because of the learning component; the same logic holds for mounting.

As a final cautionary word about overemphasis of the endogenous pharmacological environment in the etiology and causality of behavioral problems, it is important to note that most aggression is a social, not a hormonal, condition. Certainly hormones can act as modulators. Accordingly, work continues on the effects of thyroid hormones and those associated with the hypothalamic-pituitary-adrenal axis. Expect elegant complexity, not single-factor quick fixes. In the absence of a specific diagnosis consistent with all clinical signs and evaluations, uncritical treatment or supplementation with any medication is not encouraged.

BOX 6-12

STEPWISE APPROACH OUTLINE FOR IMPLEMENTING TREATMENT IN CASES INVOLVING AGGRESSION

1. Accurately assess aggressive propensities (correct diagnosis critical, *consider referral to a specialist*)
2. Caution client
3. Design plan appropriate for patient and household:
   - Role of neutering
   - Environmental modification
   - Behavioral modification
   - Gizmos
4. Premedication blood studies and diagnostic workup
5. Recall client in a week
   - Assess progress
   - Answer questions
   - Question about specific responses
   - Use responses to confirm or reject diagnosis
   - Modify plan
   - Schedule reexamination

BOX 6-13

STEPWISE APPROACH OUTLINE FOR DIAGNOSIS WITH SPECIAL REFERENCE TO CASES INVOLVING AGGRESSION

I. Diagnosis

1. Consider diagnosis as a hypothesis to be rejected or confirmed.
2. Consider response to treatment as data to confirm or reject hypothesis.
3. Realize that specific behaviors associated with the diagnosis are only correlations; therefore it is not necessary for the dog to exhibit every behavior associated with dominance aggression with everyone to be dominantly aggressive.
4. Make a problem list.
5. Make a frequency/circumstance/likelihood list.
6. List diagnoses and/or problems.
7. Use "cost of error" minimization (diagnosis as a hypothesis).
8. Offer to call a specialist or refer to one.

II. Caution

1. *Any* dog that is aggressive for *any* reason can potentially be dangerous, even if you think that the aggression is *appropriate, in-context behavior.*
2. Caution client about aggression, aggressive propensities, and availability of laws (different from dispensing legal advice).
3. Suggest use of a "Dog on Premises" sign.
4. Warn friends, neighbors, and any relevant municipal authorities
   - Referral letters
   - Enlist help in treatment of dog
5. Suggest catastrophic insurance policies.
6. Define treatment objectives
   - Teamwork
   - Stop point
   - Disabuse client of potential for outright "cure"
7. Offer second (specialist) opinion.
8. Use *extreme caution* about recommending eu-

thanasia, especially as a "treatment" of first choice.
9. Maintain impeccable records.

Diagnosis Example

Signalment: 2-year-old, castrated male, 34 kg, random-bred

Problem List: Growls at strangers when they approach the dog while leashed on the street; tries to run away. Growls and barks at anyone setting foot on the property; very confident when inside house. Growls at client when she tries to take rawhides, but not food dish. Pulls on the leash. Jumps on visitors. Jumps up on counters to see what's on top. Pushes against and bats client when she uses telephone or reads.

Diagnoses: Food-related aggression; territorial aggression (may be appropriate); fearful aggression when approached by strangers; attention-seeking behavior; poor manners in general.

Logic: Rawhides are special—perhaps should be removed from diet or given when isolated. Jumping could injure someone, but may not be malicious. If forced to interact with a stranger may become more aggressive—need to treat this and discover if dog is fearful of strangers or fearful of being outside. Is propensity to protect territory appropriate, and can client control dog? How much of this is associated with either endogenous anxiety or just a lack of rules? Caution about social maturity and association with food-related aggression. Use passive and active behavior modification and confirm or reject hypotheses (diagnoses) based on findings. Will require assessment at follow-up visit and perhaps further treatment.

Factors Affecting the Success of Treatment

Assessment of improvement is usually subjective (Beaver, 1983; Houpt, 1983; Line & Voith, 1984). At the Behavior Clinic at VHUP, direct measures are also taken to assess the actual behaviors and any changes in them. This allows us to ascertain when the behaviors change, rather than relying on the clients' perception of them.

Five main factors contribute to the success of treatment: client compliance, age of onset, predictability of outbursts, duration of the condition, and the pattern of the behavioral changes in response to environmental, behavioral, and pharmacological intervention. Client perception that aggressive outbursts are unpredictable has been associated with increased euthana-

sia rates (Reisner et al., 1994). Of these factors, client compliance may be the most critical. As veterinarians we rely on clients to administer treatments as we have best learned to prescribe them, and to report hopeful or worrisome changes. Therefore clients must pay attention. Emphasize this to the clients from the beginning. Then if the behavioral therapy fails, clients will not carry the burden of guilt for the failure if they truly complied. The remaining factors are related. The younger the animal was when the problem started, the less predictable the outbursts, the longer the condition has been present, and the more frequent and intense the rate and extent of the outbursts, the worse the prognosis. Part of the reason for this is that the degree to which the inappropriate behavior has been learned increases with the changes stated for these parameters. The ability of the client to recognize the potential for the aggressive event and to abort it before it happens cannot be overemphasized. Clients sincerely committed to treatment can learn this, as demonstrated by the high proportion of improved dogs (90% considerably, 75% substantially) seen at the Behavior Clinic at VHUP.

Issues Yet to Be Resolved

1. No population level data are available on the population of children who are bitten versus exposure to dogs, or on the percentage of dogs in any population that bite. Ideally, the latter should be collected with reference to the behavioral and environmental circumstance in which the bite occurred.

2. No data exist on the extent to which specific situations or social groupings modify or prevent aggressive behaviors. For example, if there is a very appropriately behaved, high-ranking dog in the household, to what extent does the example of and the control exerted by this dog ameliorate problems? We tend to think of behavioral problems as having single factor causality, but this is seldom the case.

3. There are no credible studies that quantify and qualify specific suites of behaviors and the extent to which they are associated with specific breeds. If there *is* a heritable component of any behavior (and it appears there is), this association should be studied. Unfortunately, more so than for almost any other topic, science has been replaced by myth and publications by lay people.

4. If aggressions have begun to appear in puppyhood, they may be worsened by early spaying. The data to substantiate this are preliminary, but given the American Veterinary Medical Association (AVMA) emphasis on early neutering as an adjuvant for pet overpopulation control, further explicit work is warranted.

5. Few data exist that quantify actual behaviors that occur as a precursor to and substantive part of any category of aggression. Such quantification is necessary to understanding the ontogeny of the actual aggressions. It will also render us safer.

CASE 1

Signalment: "Snow," a 7-year-old, spayed female, 48 kg, Great Pyrenees

Presenting Problem: Aggression toward client and a smaller dog in household

History: The clients adopted this dog 5 months ago from Great Pyrenees rescue. Until then she had apparently lived on the same farm for all of her life. The lady who owned the farm died, and the dog was included in the farm auction. The people who bought the farm at auction decided, after a few months, that they did not want the dog, and she was turned over to Great Pyrenees rescue. No information about her behavior before coming into this household is available.

Snow was fine for the first 3 months in the clients' household. Shortly thereafter she began to be aggressive to one of the other dogs (8-year-old, sprayed female, 18 kg, mixed breed). Snow does not seem to have many problems with the other dog in the household, a 2-year-old spayed female Great Pyrenees. The incidents with the smaller dog have involved food, sleeping locations, and just the presence of the other dog. Snow once bit the smaller dog seriously enough that it needed sutures. During the examination at VHUP, Snow stared frequently at the smaller dog, who cowered and tried to hide behind the female client whenever she met Snow's stare. The last time these two had an aggressive interaction, the small dog fought back (at first), and the clients noticed that Snow became more aggressive in response. They are terrified for the safety of the small dog.

Within the past few weeks Snow has also begun to show aggression to the clients, particularly the woman. The contexts in which the aggression occurs first involved food: taking Snow's dish or approaching her while she was eating. At such times she growls. The dog has also begun to growl at strangers when they knock, when they enter a room, or when they pass in the yard. She has also growled at dogs on walks and those that pass while she is in the yard.

During the appointment Snow continually solicited the male client for attention, draping herself across his lap and feet, pawing at him, barking at him, placing her head on his chest, and standing on his lap. He continually gave her love in the forms of verbal reassurance and pats and hugs when she behaved this way.

The female client is fearful because Snow was the most aggressive she has ever been when she was approached while eating 2 weeks ago. She perceives that the aggression is getting worse and is worried about potential risks to their friends and her smaller dog, who is becoming more withdrawn. The male client believes that this is a dog with a traumatized past who just needs love.

Physical Examination: The physical examination revealed no abnormalities, except for a profound flea infestation.

Laboratory Evaluation: All parameters of the complete blood cell count and serum biochemical profile were within the laboratory's limits, except for the eosinophil count (13%, corrected 1352).

Diagnoses: (1) Attention-seeking behavior, (2) food-related aggression, (3) dominance aggression (mild), (4) interdog aggression, (5) external parasitism (flea infestation)

The dominance aggression manifests itself only when the clients try to correct the dog, and is very subtle and passive. Hence, the male client is most victimized by this. I finally convinced him that most of what he considered to be the dog's "loving" behaviors were actually subtle challenges. It is not unusual for a rescued dog to behave perfectly in the new house for 3 months. That period allows them to be sufficiently comfortable that they can learn who will be a good victim. It is impossible to know if the dog's early or later experiences on the farm contributed to either the interdog aggression or to her food-related aggression, but it is a possibility in both cases. The interdog aggression was directed toward only the smaller, less confident dog, indicating that it was associated with anxiety about the new dog's place in the social hierarchy. Snow had to control someone, in the absence of a rule structure that told her where she ranked with regard to this dog. The indifference and confidence of the other Great Pyrenees provided information about her relative rank with regard to her.

Treatment: We used the basic behavior modification programs designed to teach Snow to take all the cues as to the appropriateness of her behavior from her people and to defer to them. As in most cases, physically contesting her challenges, or punishing her, would be a terrible idea, invariably making her behavior worse and putting the clients at risk. It was difficult to convince the male client that he was actually contributing to her problems until it was explained to him that most aggressions, particularly the ones that manifest themselves in this time frame in rescued dogs, are the result of anxiety, and that he was worsening hers when he sought to reassure her that it was "okay" when it truly was not. Had his reassurance worked, it would have been correlated with a decrease in her inappropriate behavior, not an *increase,* as was the case. Furthermore, I reassured him that I thought that this dog needed a committed household and that Snow could not be passed around anymore. Because they are committed to keeping her into old age, he was happy to hear this and was willing to work with her. His love and empathy were blinding him to some of her problems and to his wife's fears. I recommended that all dogs sit and stay for everything that they want. The smaller dog was to have first choice at anything: walks, love, attention, food. We practiced the programs with both dogs and emphasized that after the dog's behavior was perfect with the foundation program for behavior modification, we could start counterconditioning and desensitizing her to other dogs and to situations in which she responds inappropriately. The clients were to start this at home by starting to practice the programs with both dogs, together, after they were perfect separately.

In addition, the dogs were to be separated when not supervised, with Snow being placed in the less desired location. This is a passive way to reinforce relative status. When the dogs were together, Snow was to wear a bell so that they could always monitor her location.

The dogs are to be fed separately, but preferably at a distance where they can see each other, but not react. If this distance can be found, their dishes can be moved closer together at the rate of 1 inch every few days if there are no problems. There will be no bones or rawhides in the house, and biscuits will be fed to the dogs when they are separated.

Snow was fitted with a Gentle Leader/Promise System Canine Head Halter for leash walks and for use in the house when she is together with the smaller dog, and when greeting people at the door.

Finally, because the dog was so anxious and constantly in need of attention and reinforcement, therapy with 50 mg amitriptyline orally every 12 hours was prescribed.

We also gave specific recommendations for flea treatment and provided a handout on the subject. Because fleas can make a dog more irritable, that dog may be more unpredictable.

Follow-up: The clients reported that the first week was awful. Snow was far more aggressive to the smaller dog once the clients implemented the plan of rewarding the smaller dog first. During the second week Snow became a different dog. She is less tense, solicits the clients by sitting and being quiet, and if she starts to challenge the smaller dog about a ball, the clients can just verbally tell her to stop and she will. Snow has begun to demonstrate previously unseen "submissive" behaviors, including rolling over while being groomed. The clients were not using the halter in the house, and it was explained that this would help facilitate the avoidance of aggression and correction of the first signs of inappropriate behavior that Snow exhibits toward the smaller dog. It was also explained to the clients that dogs that have been without rules frequently get worse before they get better. It is likely that the antianxiety medication facilitated the change in the dog's behavior in the second week. The second phase of the behavior modification programs focused

CASE 1–cont'd

on desensitization to behaviors that trigger the dominance and interdog aggressions.

Note: This was a difficult case because of the clients' preconceptions and desire to believe a more sympathetic view. The male client was only convinced once he understood normal dog behavior and signaling, and thus could appreciate deviations from that. He later called us and explained that he now fully understood what we were saying; it was only when he saw Snow "happy" (his word) that he could appreciate her anxious state. Also, it was important to treat the entire dog, including her fleas. This is a specialty discipline in *medicine.*

CASE 2

Signalment: "Chopper," a 4-year-old, male, 41 kg, Rottweiler/Siberian husky mixed breed

Presenting Problem: Aggression to clients, licking of rough surfaces and feet, and snapping and licking at air

History: This dog was acquired at 4 months of age after having one other owner. For the past 3 years the dog has bitten at the air and licked at rough surfaces (sweaters, carpeting) until physically interrupted. The licking and biting at the air preceded the licking rough surfaces by about 6 months. When licking at and biting the air, the dog often wanders until he ends up in a corner. Both of these behaviors happened a few times a month at first, but are now daily occurrences. Within the past year Chopper has also begun to lick his paws on a daily basis. The paw licking seems to have coincided with an attempt on the clients' parts to decrease the other behaviors. The dog can be called away from any of the behaviors, recognizes the clients during them, and will come to the clients if they call when interrupting the dog.

In the past few months the dog has become aggressive in situations when the clients try to correct his unruly leash behavior, or when they try to get him to go somewhere they do not think he wants to go. Careful questioning revealed that Chopper had always been a little pushy, and was far worse for the woman than the man. The woman is fearful of his aggression. Two weeks before the visit to the VHUP Behavior Clinic, the dog growled and snarled at her when she told him to sit so she could take his leash off after a walk, during which he had dragged her down the street. He has always been "fussy" about having his leash removed, but has recently started snarling and snapping when his leash is taken off. Chopper will let the clients reach toward and over him, but he snarls if he is pushed from furniture. This, too, is a relatively recent development. The clients are unable to push on his shoulders or hips without eliciting a growl, and cannot take biscuits or human food from him. They stopped giving him rawhides and real bones when he was a puppy because they were frightened by the look on the dog's face when they came into the room. Recently the clients have had trouble getting him to relinquish toys when they are playing, and Chopper has begun to growl at them in these contexts.

The dog has always barked when strangers enter the house, knock, or approach the car or yard if he is present. In the past year the dog has become far more aggressive in these situations, snapping and growling when people approach. He appears to exhibit these behaviors primarily when his people are present. He is fine if he is on a leash and people approach him.

Finally, when Chopper is interrupted during his air-snapping behaviors, he has begun to redirect his aggression to the person closest to him.

As an aside, the clients commented that Chopper is getting very little exercise, because neither of them can really control him on a leash. Since Chopper began to be aggressive, the clients are fearful about their lack of control in public places, although he has never had a problem or aggressive incident under those circumstances.

Physical Examination: Physical examination was nonremarkable. The dog is intact.

Laboratory Evaluation: The intent had been to obtain blood samples for a complete blood cell count and serum biochemical profile, but the dog was too aggressive to manipulate for this.

Diagnoses: (1) Food-related aggression, (2) dominance aggression, (3) possessive aggression, (4) protective aggression, (5) redirected aggression, (6) obsessive-compulsive/stereotypic behavior

Treatment: Chopper was too aggressive to handle for blood work, so the following measures were taken. I recommended that he be castrated. First, we do not need to perpetuate these genes. Second, because testosterone is a behavioral modulator, its presence can facilitate aggression in aggressive dogs. Compared with dogs that are neutered, dogs that are intact tend to react more quickly to a given stimulus, tend to reach a higher level of reactivity, tend to stay reactive for a longer time, and tend to be more difficult and take longer to calm. The clients did not have a veterinarian whom they liked, so I suggested that the castration be performed at VHUP on a day when I could help the surgical team. When the dog arrived, we would give him a little sedation, obtain the blood for tests, anesthetize and neuter him, and send him home with subcuticular sutures, a Gentle Leader/Promise System Canine Head Halter, and antianxiety medication if the laboratory results were not worrisome.

Meanwhile, the clients were to start on behavior modification programs designed to teach Chopper to take all the cues as to the appropriateness of his behavior from them. He was to sit and stay for everything and anything he wanted. Only then could he earn what he wanted while being relaxed and quiet. The clients were to use the same technique to interrupt the stereotypic behavior. The first tier of the behavior modification program was demonstrated to the clients and it was emphasized that the point of desensitization and counterconditioning was to teach the dog to not react and to relax while stimuli were gradually introduced that caused him to react. Every time he exhibited an appropriate response for a minute task, he was praised and got a food reward. The clients had been bribing him; we explained the difference between a salary and a bribe. The dog was superb practicing the exercises at VHUP. We emphasized that these dogs with abnormal, out-of-context behavior, particularly those that are anxious, need some kind of a consistent rule structure (benign doggie boot camp).

Follow-up: Two weeks later the dog was neutered at VHUP. The woman had been working intensely with him and believed he was greatly improved—and he was. He sat, was quiet when she told him to be, and responded to

leash corrections. The surgical staff, despite his bad press, had no problems with him, but used only subcuticular sutures, just in case. All of the laboratory test results were within the laboratory reference limits; therefore he was sent home, with 50 mg of amitriptyline to be given every 12 hours. Clients were instructed to continue to avoid all situations associated with aggressive incidents and to continue to call him away from any stereotypic behaviors, using a substitute exercise for which he would be rewarded if he relaxed. Finally, we fit Chopper with a Gentle Leader/Promise System Canine Head Halter that the clients were to use for walks and some behavior modification in the house. Clients were also to increase his exercise by leash-walking.

Two weeks after castration the clients believed that they were doing terrifically. They had had *no* aggressive events, the stereotypic behavior had almost stopped, and the dog sought them out for friendly interactions. They still are having trouble with the part of the exercises that require them to go to the door and knock, but are working on this. We planned to see them for a reexamination in a few weeks.

Note: In this case, the stereotypic behavior may have been a derivative of displacement activity, and associated with anxiety about appropriate social behaviors. It would have been fruitless to focus only on that aspect of his problem. Furthermore, a low-tech, inexpensive antianxiety medication worked well in combination with behavior modification. Had this *not* been the case, more exotic medications (fluoxetine [Prozac]) may have helped, but could cost $5 per day for a dog this size.

Finally, for dogs that can easily get (or already have) bad press, names like Chopper may not be the best idea. If I had a Rottie, I'd call her "Fluffy."

CASE 3

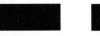

Signalment: "Edward," 1½-year-old, castrated male, 34 kg, Old English sheepdog

Presenting Problem: Aggressive behavior with strangers

History: Approximately 1 year ago the dog reacted aggressively for the first time when a stranger approached him in his yard. At that time he barked and growled; his people told him it was okay, and he calmed down. Recently, Edward was tied on his pulley run outside at a garden party. He had a radius of mobility of about 2 m. A very tall, older lady in complete garden party attire (long,

flowing dress and huge hat), who previously professed to be fearful of dogs, swooped down on him with a sandwich in her hand. He bit her on the hand. The lady fell backward, shrieking. The only injury anyone could find was the scratch on her hand, and when she swooned and screamed, the dog ignored her. When everyone came running he ignored them, also. He did not resist being put in the house.

The clients have had Edward since he was 2½ months of age and recalled that before this event, he had an occasion of growling when he stole a loaf of French bread that had been sitting on the counter. The clients tried (unsuccessfully) to take it away from him and he ate the entire loaf. He was not ill afterward. He does not resent having his food taken away, and the client can hold a rawhide while he is chewing it. The clients can take toys from him, but he has a long history of stealing objects like bread or socks. When he recently stole a sock and the client grabbed him to try to make him give it back, he growled at her and swallowed the sock. He was not ill after this episode either.

The clients noted that the dog has always had problems with people approaching his yard, ringing the doorbell or knocking at the door, or approaching the car while he was in it. During such instances he started to bark and growl when he was about 6 months of age; he has recently become worse. Edward also growls at other dogs as they pass his yard and has become aggressive to some, but not all, dogs on the street, at the boarding kennel, and at the veterinarian's office.

This dog does not like to have his feet handled and will occasionally snap at the client, but it is difficult to know whether this is anticipatory for grooming: he dislikes being clipped ever since tangles were roughly pulled out. He will let the family members rub his belly, but probably no one else, and while at VHUP he growled at two people when they stared at him. The client says that he has occasionally done that to strangers recently.

The dog responds to being yelled at and forceful, physical corrections with cowering and agitation. He participated in an obedience class when he was 6 months of age where the trainer hung and beat him the first time he resisted a leash correction. The client was horrified and never went back. The client *does* say that when he is highly motivated to growl (a person or a dog near his fence), he responds to virtually no corrections.

While at VHUP the dog consistently whined at the clients and batted at them for attention, which he invariably obtained.

Physical Examination: No abnormalities were detected on physical examination.

Diagnoses: (1) Attention-seeking behavior, (2) dominance aggression, (3) protective/territorial aggression, (4) mild possessive aggression

Treatment: The clients were advised to avoid circumstances that would trigger the aggression. They were to put away objects that Edward might have a penchant for stealing (including bread) and not leave him tied or alone in the yard. The presence of a fence or a chain leaves no

ambiguity in the dog's mind about where his turf begins and ends; accordingly, such situations render dogs that are territorially aggressive more aggressive. It was not clear from the history or his behavior if he was also protecting the people in the household, so we also talked about early recognition of precursor behaviors that indicate that the dog may perceive a threat (regardless of whether one exists). The clients are to interrupt these behaviors by either taking the dog out of the system or by asking him to sit, stay, and relax. If he can relax under such circumstances, instead of becoming agitated, the clients are not to continue with their activity until they have enforced his relaxation.

Edward was fitted with a Gentle Leader/Promise System Canine Head Halter so that he could be walked and exercised while supervised and corrected, if needed. In addition, the dog was to sit for all attention and was to be ignored unless he was quiet, calm, and willing. The clients were to inform their neighbors that they were working with the dog and were instructed to post a "Dog on Premises" sign.

The first tier of the behavior modification programs is aimed at teaching the dog to relax in a series of benign situations. The second tier concentrates on desensitizing him to situations in which he reacts and is the focus of a reexamination visit.

The trainer did us no favors—Edward is a highly anxious dog. We discussed that it might be easier to practice some of the modification in public if the dog was taking antianxiety medication. The clients wanted to work as hard as possible at the outset. A complete blood cell count and serum biochemical profile revealed some grossly abnormal values: serum alkaline phosphatase (248 U/L; reference range 35 to 169 U/L) and cholesterol (260 mg/dl; reference range 150 to 260 mg/dl). The cholesterol is only mildly elevated; statistically, one abnormal test result is not unusual when this many tests are run (see Romatowski, 1994). Taken in conjunction with the other abnormal finding, though, this could be evidence of a liver disorder, incipient Cushing's disease, or an iatrogenic response to medication. In the absence of any clinical symptoms, it is very difficult to be overly concerned about these results. The client assures us that the dog has taken no medication, other than heartworm prophylaxis, and that he has no clinical signs of any problem. The clients still wanted to try the antianxiety medication and were willing to closely monitor the dog. A regimen of amitriptyline, 50 mg orally every 12 hours, was started.

Follow-up: The clients are ecstatic. The dog is a charm to walk on the Promise halter, and is much calmer and

CASE 3—cont'd

more responsive than he has ever been. They are all working very hard with him, and they and he are enjoying the work. They commented that he is actually getting more attention now, but in a structured context. We pointed out to them that this is part of the point and that anxious dogs do best when they have fair, clear, rules. They have had fewer problems with him being aggressive to strangers and are able to verbally correct him now. Edward has not had the chance to steal anything since the first appointment. He has had no untoward responses to the antianxiety medication. His reexamination focused on desensitization to strangers and other triggers. Should he continue to take antianxiety medication, the serum biochemical profile will be repeated annually or as indicated by clinical signs.

Note: One of the reasons that the clients were anxious about seeking help was their horrible experience with the trainer a year before the behavior consultation. First, it is *never* acceptable to abuse an animal (human or otherwise) if the goal is to modify their behavior. Second, the trainer did more harm than good for the discipline: not only did he give the clients the wrong impression about behavioral therapy *and* obedience training, he actively delayed their ability to seek competent help.

CASE 4

Signalment: "Dobie," 5-year-old, castrated male doberman

Presenting Problem: The clients are being sued by their next door neighbor because the dog bit one of the neighbors' children. The dog was on the clients' property at the time. The bite did not require sutures. People who saw the event say that the dog actually held the child's arm and that the child pulled away vehemently. The lesions are consistent with pressure in response to pulling.

History: The dog lives on 5 acres that abut a road where there is a rural school bus stop. Every morning the dog walks the clients' children to the bus. He usually waits for them in the afternoon if he is not following the client and her horse. There is a leash law in the township and the dog has never been "at large." Although he is seldom leashed, the dog has never left the property to the best of the clients' knowledge. The client has warned the neighbor children before about throwing stones and sticks at her horses and her dogs. When the dog greeted her children one day, the neighbor children were also walking back along the shared lane; they started to throw stones, some of which hit the dog. The dog began to growl, and the clients' children told the neighbor children to stop. The neighbor's child then picked up a branch and started to threaten the clients' child. The dog growled. The neighbor's child then started to beat the dog, whereupon the dog growled louder and tried to push the child out of the way. The child began to kick the dog in the abdomen and face while hitting him, and the dog grabbed the arm with the stick, growling. The child screamed and pulled away, the dog let go and did not chase the child, nor did he snap again. The clients' children called Dobie and he came.

Diagnosis: Aggression in context—normal dog behavior; inhibited, provoked bite. No aggressive propensities

Follow-up: The suit was dropped (after written opinions by experts), and the dog was not declared a "vicious" dog, as the neighbor wanted (which would have resulted in the dog's death), but the township required the owners of the dog to post a "Beware of Dog" sign and leash or otherwise restrain their dog when within 10 feet of a public accessway.

CASE 5: REEXAMINATION EXAMPLE*

Signalment: "Nick," 1½-year-old, castrated male, 21 kg, Dalmatian

Presenting Problem: Avoidance of and aggression toward people outside of the family, particularly on the street, and elimination in the house

History: The clients obtained this dog at 3 to 4 months of age. He had always been a little leery of strangers, but had recently begun to bark and growl frantically, while pulling away from any person, or strange sound, on the street. By the time they came to the Behavior Clinic for the first examination, the clients had virtually ceased to take the dog out during normal hours. Any people and any unexpected machine sounds startled him. The clients would try to take him out in the yard for elimination, but while outside he would not eliminate. As soon as they brought him in, the dog would eliminate in the house. In his struggles to back up, growling, when he was approached by anything, he was dragging the clients and choking. There appear to have been no predisposing events for this behavior.

Physical Examination: No abnormalities were detected on physical examination; although the dog was muzzled, he was growling and shaking sufficiently to render a superb physical examination impossible.

Diagnoses: Fear aggression and inappropriate elimination related to anxiety

Treatment: At the first visit the dog was started on the first tier of the behavior modification program. The foundation program is designed to teach the dog to lie down or sit and stay while relaxing in a variety of circumstances. Dogs are to take their cues as to the appropriateness of their behaviors from the client. Nick was able to perform the first of the exercises well at the clinic. The clients were encouraged to avoid all circumstances that triggered the undesirable, inappropriate behavior and to work intensively with the first phase of the program. Once Nick's performance was perfect, they could start to walk him in areas where he would see people only at a distance. If he started to become anxious or fearful (ears back, stiffening, trembling, pupils dilated), they were to ask him to sit. If Nick was still upset, they were to turn him around and take him away from the situation. To facilitate this, he was fitted with a Gentle Leader/Promise System Canine Head Halter. He was instantly calmer with this while at VHUP.

In addition, the clients were to take him out to eliminate frequently, and praise and reward him for outdoor elimination. It was emphasized that they were rewarding the timing and location of the elimination—the act itself is self-rewarding. They were to try to stay out long enough so that he would eliminate, but were to bring him in if he became anxious. When unsupervised in the house he was to be restricted to one area. The clients were to clean all affected areas with a good odor eliminator.

We discussed that antianxiety medication is often useful for such dogs. The clients expressed an interest in trying the behavior modification alone, first.

Follow-up: A phone call a few weeks later revealed that the clients loved the Gentle Leader/Promise System and were able to walk the dog in low-traffic areas. He had begun to react less to some people, and the clients continued to practice the program. If anyone approached him, he still had a full-blown problem, and there had been no attenuation of the elimination problem. At this point the clients asked if they could start the antianxiety medication for the dog. After a discussion with their veterinarian, the dog received 25 mg amitriptyline orally every 12 hours when his complete blood cell count and serum biochemical profile (performed by the referring veterinarian) revealed no abnormalities.

The clients came for a reexamination after a few weeks of amitriptyline treatment. They reported that after the first week with the mediation, the dog would willingly go for walks and always eliminated outside, and when people approached he did not growl. They took advantage of this change in behavior and gradually introduced him to people, first outside, and had him sit and relax while they approached, talked to, and then briefly petted him. Unlike at his first visit, when he growled, snarled, and backed into a corner, he was totally calm at the reexamination appointment, allowing everyone to pet him, wagging his tail, and responding to all commands. The clients are to maintain the antianxiety medication regimen for at least another 2 months. If they do decide to have a trial of his behavior without it, they are to wean him from it, not stop suddenly. We will be talking between now and then. The clients understand that the antianxiety medication facilitated his ability to overcome his fears about the outdoors. Because he had been housebroken previously, he was willing to eliminate outside once he could manage his fear. He may also have benefitted from the side effects that are associated with tricyclic antidepressant use: anticholinergic action and increased urinary sphincter tone.

Note: This case illustrates the importance of follow-up and client compliance. These were great clients; they were highly motivated and superb observers.

*This case is discussed from the aspect of the elimination problem in Chapter 9.

CASE 6: REEXAMINATION EXAMPLE

Signalment: "Molly," 3-year-old, spayed female, 19.5 kg, Australian shepherd

Presenting Problem: Aggression toward children not in the household

History: The dog and the child in the family are approximately the same age. About 6 to 8 months ago, the dog began to nip at the heels of friends of the clients' daughter when they were playing. The dog has continued to intensify this behavior, always putting her body between the daughter's and her friends. There have been two close calls when children have reached out to pet Molly while she was "guarding" the daughter and she has snapped. She has never bitten anyone. She does not growl, except immediately before the snap, but her body postures, which these young children are incapable of interpreting, are consistent with agonistic behavior (ears back, pupils dilated, teeth bared, hair up, and the classic "eye" posture of herding dogs). During the first appointment Molly positioned herself between the students and clinician and daughter, and exhibited the above behaviors in a close circumstance. When the daughter ran up and down the hall, shrieking, the dog became anxious, panting and exhibiting vigilance and scanning. If the daughter shrieked when the dog could not see her the dog became fearful. During the appointment, the dog paced and solicited attention from the female client frequently by nudging her, pushing against her, pawing and looking at her, and by "talking." This behavior intensified when the client would tell her not to exhibit anxious behaviors when people entered the room or when her daughter shrieked. The client petted the dog during these times, which resulted in an intensification of these behaviors. When requested to stop petting the dog, the client found that the dog would sit quietly and look at her, at which point she could calmly love the dog.

Physical Examination: The dog was easy to examine and no abnormalities were detected on physical examination.

Diagnoses: (1) Attention-seeking behavior, (2) inappropriate herding behavior associated with protective aggression, and (3) fearful behavior around small, rambunctious children

Treatment: Both behavior modification and the use of antianxiety medication were discussed with the client. The client wanted to try behavior modification without medication at first. The dog started the foundation behavior modification program with instructions to avoid children (by placing the dog in another room when they come) and teaching the dog to relax and use vocal cues in benign contexts. The second tier of the program would desensitize the dog to the behaviors of small children. It was explained to the client that the dog was trying to herd these children away from her child, but, regardless, this behavior was potentially very dangerous. All children and parents were to be told not to reach for the dog and that the dog was undergoing treatment for a behavioral problem. The dog was fitted for a Gentle Leader/Promise System Canine Head Halter so that the clients could correct her at the first signs of any inappropriate herding and protective behavior when on walks.

During the first reexamination, the clients worked on the parts of the foundation program with which they had had difficulty: knocking at the door and entering rooms. Corrections in timing were suggested, and the use of antianxiety medication was again discussed in response to the clients' queries. At that time they decided to decline the use of antianxiety medication.

During the second reexamination, the dog was much improved with regard to hospital personnel and the clients thought that she was less anxious overall and much better on her walks. They walked her only on her halter, and when children came to visit, she could sit and watch them (warily) without herding them. However, they had had a close call the previous week. The husband had been taking the daughter and the dog for a walk, and the dog was behaving well. A child and her parent approached and the mother asked if the child could pet the dog. The husband (through some lapse of sanity) said "yes," without asking Molly to sit first. As the child, who was about 3 and a little uncoordinated, burbled and reached for Molly, Molly snapped. Molly *did* inhibit the bite and the husband pulled her away, but the clients are seriously concerned and think that Molly has been more anxious since then.

During the latest reexamination, Molly was clearly anxious whenever the daughter shrieked. Whenever the daughter was out of sight, the dog was also anxious. This reexamination concentrated on introducing the dog to strange adult humans and strange noises in a gradual manner designed to effect desensitization and counterconditioning. The client was not reading the dog's nonverbal cues well and we worked with that and her timing for more than an hour. By the time we stopped, Molly was ignoring sounds, was happy, tuned out the daughter, and could be quickly approached by adults. The client also wanted to try antianxiety medication in an attempt to both facilitate the behavior modification and with the intent of decreasing the dog's anxiety about the quick actions and sharp noises associated with children. A serum biochemistry profile and a complete blood cell count were both within laboratory reference limits; therefore a regimen of amitriptyline, 25 mg orally every 12 hours, was started. Other drugs that were discussed include clomipramine and fluoxetine, but they are both expensive.

It was also emphasized that *no one* should reach for this dog and that she should be in another room when children visit. The plan for the next reexamination was to desensitize her to children using the friends' children (and parents).

After 10 days the client reported that she was not sure if the drugs were working. The effect was not dramatic. They had had a large adult party and had put the dog in the back bedroom until everyone was in. Once in the house, two people opened the door to say hello to the dog and she greeted them in a friendly manner. They let her out and she made the rounds, sitting and begging, and allowing everyone to pet her. The night was totally without incident and the dog slept through part of the evening. All people were able to leave without being herded. The next day, children were visiting and the daughter let Molly out. She was fine until one child chased her, at which point she exhibited herding behaviors, but no snapping. Molly was then put on the screened-in porch. A toddler (18 months) went to the porch and pounded on the screen door, shrieking. Molly hit the door growling and snarling, but did not go out or through the door. She was agitated for a long time after the child was removed. The clients are concerned about what they perceive to be contradictory or incomplete responses.

We discussed increasing the dosage of amitriptyline, changing to another drug, or placing the dog in a home without children. The female client does not want to do this, but her in-laws are telling her that Molly will kill someone and that they will be sued. This is not necessarily the biological reality, but the decisions in this case will probably be made on the basis of family interactions, not the dog's behavior. Because of his parents' views, the husband is not working as intensely with the dog as possible, and Molly is not experiencing the full benefit of the behavior modification. The clients, after pressure from the mother-in-law, decided to place this dog in another home. Because of family pressures, they could not make any progress with the dog because of lack of a consistent plan within the family.

The dog went to a home with no children, but two cats. She loves the cats, but for one of them the feeling is not mutual and her nose is well scored. She has never snapped at or shown any other aggressions to the cats. The person who adopted her is familiar with dogs and the Promise halter. She uses it for all walks and all introductions. Molly must sit before anyone approaches on the street. She has stopped reacting inappropriately to strangers in public. She still has some problems when people visit. Now she is put in another room and, when calm, is let out after everyone arrives. Visitors are instructed to ignore her until she comes to them. She does this, shyly, wagging her tail, and with her ears back. She will growl if they reach toward her suddenly, so they are asked to tell her to sit and talk to her. The second time she approaches them, they are to ask her to sit and wait, and to give her their hand, outstretched, to sniff. If she is sweet (as she is 95% of the time), they can give her a piece of biscuit. She continues to improve and continues to take anxiety medication a while longer. Everyone who meets this dog loves her.

Two-year follow-up indicated a wonderful relationship with all the cats (including an additional "rescue" kitten that Molly found in the woods and helped nurse back to health). Molly's new family (and both of their families) adore Molly. She is good with the young children in the family, but the people have continued to be very cautious with unknown children.

Note: This case illustrates the dual importance of client compliance and familial pressures that can affect it. The latter are discussed in Chapter 16. Also note that after each aggressive event this dog was subdued and withdrawn. This is common; the dog may be depressed, appalled, or confused by a horrific situation; it is difficult to know. However, this phenomenon illustrates that we need to be concerned about more than the dog's ability to learn from and enhance her aggression with subsequent bouts; we need to have humane concerns for the dog.

7 ····· Feline Aggression

···

EPIDEMIOLOGY OF CAT BITES

Problem aggression is second only to problem elimination in common complaints about cat behavior. Feline aggression and feline elimination disorders are frequently interrelated. Given the multifaceted role played by scent in feline social systems, this is not surprising. Unfortunately, the extent to which the interaction between feline aggression and elimination disorders is involved in difficult aggression or elimination problems is underappreciated.

In a survey of 100 cats with behavior problems, 25% (25) of them involved aggression (Olm & Houpt, 1988). Beaver (1989c,d) found that 35.75% (64/179) of feline cases did not involve elimination, and 13% of visits involved aggressive cats. Borchelt and Voith (1982b, 1987) found that 29% of telephone calls about cats involved aggression. Twenty-seven million households in the United States (30%) have at least one cat (Troutman, 1988). Feline aggression is emerging as a common and worrisome problem, especially when its potential to cause serious illness in people is considered.

CAT SCRATCH DISEASE

A total of 22,000 cases (1.8–10 cases/100,000 people) of cat-scratch disease (CSD) are reported each year in the United States, and 2200 people are hospitalized annually (Jackson et al., 1993). The presumptive agent in CSD is the rickettsial organism, *Bartonella* (formerly *Rochalimaea*) *hensalae,* and a contributory role has been postulated for the bacteria, *Afipia felis.* Of 45 human patients with CSD, 38 had titers of at least 1:64 for *B. hensalae.* CSD is most commonly seen in the late summer and fall and coincides with seasonality in births of kittens (spring) and the entry of these kittens into the house in the winter. Flea infestations may be associated with a higher incidence of CSD; most human patients with CSD have at least one kitten that has fleas (Zangwill et al., 1993). Patients with CSD are more likely to have a kitten a year of age or younger, or to have been scratched by a kitten, than are non patients (Zangwill et al., 1993). Although human patients with CSD living in kitten-owning households are more likely to have been scratched or bitten than patients with CSD living in households without kittens, there appears to be no association, other than age, with patients' cats and those of controls when indoor/outdoor status, litter box use, and hunting behaviors are examined (Zangwill et al., 1993).

Cats transmitting CSD appear healthy, although they may have long-lasting, active *B. hensalae* infections (Regnery et al., 1992). People with CSD tend to have localized skin lesions and regional lymph node involvement 3 weeks after exposure. Lymph nodes remain enlarged for several months. Systemic illness is rare, but fever, headache, splenomegaly, and malaise are common. These symptoms are usually self-resolving; however, arthritis, neuroretinitis, pleurisy, pneumonia, osteolytic lesions, granulomatous hepatitis, and encephalitis with coma and seizure can be unusual sequelae (Tompkins & Steigbigel, 1993). Individuals with acquired immunodeficiency syndrome (AIDS) or those immunosuppressed for other reasons are at risk for more severe disease, including bacillary angiomatosis (Hughes & Faragher, 1994; Koehler et al., 1994).

Treatment of human patients with CSD is also financially costly: the cost of treatment for ambulatory patients averages $5.2 million per year in the United States. The cost of treatment for hospitalized patients exceeds $6.9 million per year (Jackson et al., 1993).

Feline aggression should be treated as soon as it is recognized. This is a prudent public health approach and is the humane approach for the cat.

AGGRESSIVE BEHAVIORS

Survey studies indicate that, during their life span, 80% of cats hiss at each other, 85% swat at each other, 70% fight with each other occasionally, 25% hiss or growl at people, and 60% scratch or bite people occasionally (Borchelt & Voith, 1987). Of the pet cats that were studied, 53.6% exhibited hissing sometimes (1 time per month) or frequently (1 or more times per week), 63.1% exhibited swatting sometimes or frequently, and 44.5% exhibited fighting sometimes or frequently (Borchelt & Voith, 1987).

Statistical examination of data collected by Borchelt and Voith (1987) indicate that cats are more often aggressive to other cats than they are to people in situations involving defensive and territorial aggression ($p < 0.05$; $G_{adj} = 32.627$ and 11.442, respectively), but they are more often aggressive to people than they are to cats in circumstances involving play aggression ($P < 0.05$; $G_{adj} = 25.091$). This study did not evaluate a baseline of normal behaviors (perhaps cats are not involved in play aggression often with cats because they are corrected by the other cats sufficiently early in the sequence of play to avoid frank aggression), but it suggests situations in which people might be at risk.

Feline aggressive behavior may not manifest itself in the same manner toward all people. Careful examination of data published by Borchelt and Voith (1987) indicates that for cats that are deemed "frequently" aggressive, there is no difference between the frequency of growling or hissing that is directed toward strangers compared with that directed toward family members (NS; G_{adj} = 0.209). Family members are stated to be more frequently subjected to swatting, scratching, and biting without breaking the skin, and bites that break the skin ($p < 0.05$; G_{adj} = 21.197, 30.014, and 9.554, respectively). Closer statistical investigation reveals that family members are more frequently victimized than are strangers by cats that break the skin, and only by cats that have inflicted three, four, or more than eight bites ($p < 0.05$; G_{adj} = 3.874, 4.179, 22.311, respectively) (my analysis of data from Borchelt & Voith, 1987).

UNDERLYING NEUROANATOMICAL BASIS OF FELINE AGGRESSION

Cats have been used as models for studies of aggression that have concentrated on affective defense and predatory responses. Maeda (1978) established that excitation of the ventromedial hypothalamus (VMH) led to a defensive response in cats. Adamec (1990a,b,c) and Adamec and co-workers (1980a,b,c), found that both the amygdala and the VMH have a role in the defensive response to threats in felines. The amygdala has a central position in a variety of limbic circuits: it has monosynaptic, efferent projections to the ventrolateral aspects of the VMH, where stimulation leads to aggressive behavior (Kruk et al., 1983), and to the bed nucleus of the stria terminalis (BNST). The amygdala also has entorhinal cortical inputs to the ventral hippocampus (VHP) (Krettek & Price, 1978). The medial amygdaloid nucleus (AME) is involved in (1) social behavior, including intraspecific aggression (Vochteloo & Koolhaas, 1987), (2) avoidance (Bolhuis et al., 1984; Luiten et al., 1985), and (3) sexual behavior (Harris & Sachs, 1975; Lehman & Winans, 1980). Testosterone-binding sites in the AME may interact with vasopressinergic neurons within the amygdala (Roselli et al., 1989). This is potentially important because sexual differentiation in vasopressinergic innervation of the lateral septum is dependent on perinatal testosterone (vasopressin disappears after castration) (DeVries et al., 1983). Even the role played by the different regions within the amygdala is complex. Stimulation of the lateral amygdala facilitates predatory attack and defensiveness in cats (Adamec et al., 1980b,c, 1983; Siegal & Pott, 1988; Siegal et al., 1977), but stimulation of the lateral amygdala using high intensity also recruited the VHP in these behaviors.

These associations between neuroanatomical stimulation and aggressive behavior have implications for the underlying mechanisms of normal and abnormal cat behavior. Cats that are more defensive exhibit less predatory aggression than do less defensive cats (Adamec, 1975b; Adamec et al., 1980a,c; Anand & Brobeck, 1951). These behavioral differences between more and less aggressive cats are stable over a year, but it is unclear if the social pattern is a reflection of neural functioning or of the influence of neural function on the social pattern. Adamec (1975b) established that threatening stimuli recruit a larger population of cells in the amygdala of defensive cats than in those of less defensive cats. VMH cells are more responsive in defensive cats (Adamec, 1990b).

The interaction between neural substrate and behavior is complex. This is substantiated by studies of rats (Koolhaas et al., 1990). In rats that were recently castrated and in those that had been castrated long term, a single, local microinjection of arginine vasopressin (AVP) into the medial amygdala resulted in an increase in offensive behavior. This response levels off over time in both groups. Testosterone modulates the expression of AVP messenger ribonucleic acid (mRNA), but both AVP and testosterone have independent actions on behavior (Koolhaas et al., 1990). The extent to which the amygdala modifies social behavior can be predicated on previous social experience (Luiten et al., 1985; Sarter & Markowitsch, 1985).

The amygdala is also implicated in mating, and its activity may account for associations between aggression and mating behavior (Hart, 1970a; Hart et al., 1973; Hart & Voith, 1978; Maes, 1939; Sutin & Michael, 1970; Sutin et al., 1974). Activity in the amygdaloid nuclei and pyriform cortex is correlated with the estrous behaviors of rolling and vocalization. It has been postulated that the electroencephalographic (EEG) changes noted in the amygdala during postcoital reactions are involved in ovulation (Hart, 1974g; Hart & Leedy, 1983; Hart & Voith, 1978). Lesions of the lateral amygdala or lateral midbrain induce the copulatory cry and afterreaction, although queens with such lesions still tolerate mounting (Kling et al., 1960).

Brain areas other than the VMH have been implicated in aggressive activity in cats. Leyhausen (1979) described what he called *affective defense behavior* associated with affective signs: piloerection, retraction of ears, arching of back, pupillary dilation, vocalization, unsheathing of claws, and hissing (Shaikh et al., 1990). These behaviors can be produced by physical/electric or chemical stimulation of the medial hypothalamus or brainstem periaqueductal gray matter (PAG). Leyhausen's (1979) quiet biting attack was elicited by electrical or chemical stimulation of the lateral perifornical hypothalamus, the ventral aspect of the midbrain PAG, or lower brainstem tegmentum (i.e., the region of BNST) (Bernston & Leibowitz, 1973; Bernston et al., 1976a,b; Shaikh et al., 1990).

One of the chemical mechanisms for modulating feline aggression was suggested by Shaikh et al. (1990); they hypothesized that several regions of the limbic mid-brain (including the mid-brain PAG, BNST, nucleus accumbens) were key structures where opioids interact with receptors to modulate affective defense behavior. These investigators found that naloxone caused a dose-dependent and time-dependent decrease in affective defense thresholds (as defined previously) and an increase in the predatory response threshold. Opioid peptide systems act as a selective and potent modulator of affective defense systems in cats; they suppress affective defense behavior by acting at synaptic regions within the limbic mid-brain (Shaikh et al., 1990). The ramifications of this for both the treatment of some feline aggressions and for the treatment of self-directed or mutilatory behaviors are clear. Although the role of central nervous system (CNS) serotonin has been less investigated in cats than it has in dogs, it has been postulated that serotonin acts to inhibit aggression in cats (Katz & Thomas, 1976). It is in this context that low-protein diets have been suggested as part of the treatment for feline aggression. Diets lower in protein should allow more tryptophan (a serotonin precursor) to traverse the blood-brain barrier, but the effect, if any, in dogs does not appear to be this simple (Crowell-Davis et al., 1994; Dodman et al., 1996).

Cats have been a model for the study of neural substrate and its role in aggression. The neuroanatomical and neurochemical associations discussed should be borne in mind when considering the form feline aggression takes and its treatment.

CATEGORIES OF FELINE AGGRESSION

Feline aggression has been broadly classified into offensive, defensive, and protective aggression. Protective aggression involves the use of claws and feet in a first-time attack. The diagnostic categorization of feline aggression follows that of Moyer (1968) and is adapted from this terminology. Moyer listed eight different kinds of aggression based on studies in laboratory animals:

1. Predatory aggression: in response to a natural object of prey
2. Intermale aggression: in response to the proximity of an unfamiliar male
3. Fear-induced aggression: shown by a confined or cornered animal and preceded by escape attempts
4. Irritable aggression: in response to a broad range of external circumstances, such as pain, frustration, or deprivation that is shown toward inanimate and animate objects
5. Territorial aggression/defense: in response to an intruder into an area in which the individual has established itself
6. Maternal aggression: in response to an intruder into an area where the queen is sequestered with her kittens
7. Instrumental aggression: a learned response to obtain reinforcement
8. Sex-related aggression: in response to competition for a mate

Within the purview of laboratory studies, these can be useful categories, but it should be noted that the original criteria for classifying the types of aggression were inconsistently applied (Archer, 1988). This is a problem for medical diagnosis in general but is particularly problematic when part of the treatment goal when using a phenomenological or functional approach is to avoid circumstances in which problems arise. Archer (1988) has also pointed out that predatory aggression (in context) is probably hardwired for a predator. This should be especially true for cats, who are virtually obligate carnivores. As is true for dogs, predatory aggression that is not directed toward humans is very difficult to alter; predatory aggression is also difficult to alter when directed toward people, but people learn to conscientiously avoid eliciting it (unless the people are infants).

Moyer's (1968) categories form a descriptive catalog of aggressions that can be adaptive (*sensu* Hinde, 1956; Mayr, 1982; Tinbergen, 1957). He emphasized that aggression leads to, or appeared to lead to, the damage or destruction of a target or goal. In behavioral medicine, we tend to use such categorizations to identify when the behavior deviates from appropriate goals and becomes maladaptive or abnormal. The determination of the latter rests in the context in which the suite of signals and behaviors occur. Agonistic behavior can involve threat, withdrawal, and attack; arousal is required, but contact and combat are not (Immelmann & Beer, 1989). Referring to the definition of aggression found in the chapter on canine aggression, the following relevant facets are emphasized: aggression can be appropriate (largely the basis of Moyer's [1968] classification), inappropriate, in context, or out of context. This definition specifies a particular case of agonistic behavior.

Phenomenological categories of diagnosis can be useful because (1) they allow us to avoid specific events that might provoke the aggression and, hence, decrease the probability that the animal that is behaving inappropriately will have his or her behavior reinforced through the event, (2) they allow us to shape the inappropriate behavior to one more appropriate with behavior modification, and (3) they are independent of the underlying neurophysiological and genetic basis of the behavior. This last point is important because it acknowledges that numerous underlying mechanisms, whether genetic or cellular, can produce a similar, and possibly indistinguishable, constellation of signs. Archer (1988) criticizes Moyer's classification on the basis of this, stating that it does not allow one to distinguish between the categories on a neural basis. This is true based on the previously mentioned laboratory work on the neuroanatomical basis of feline aggression, but the latter is complex and probably does not represent a singular mapping. Furthermore, gene × environment effects are notoriously difficult to evaluate for heterogenous, multifactorial behaviors that are quantitative and polygenic. For our purposes, a modification of a phenomenological/functional terminology can provide enough information to work at a level where we can intervene: the actual behaviors.

In her classification of feline aggression, Beaver (1989c, 1976) acknowledged that some aggressions could be normal and potentially adaptive:

1. Aggression to people or regarding personal space (normal)
2. Aggression associated with dispersion (normal)
3. Aggression associated with dispersion (atypical)
4. Aggression associated with epilepsy
5. Fear-induced aggression (potentially normal)
6. Intermale aggression (potentially normal)
7. Irritable aggression (potentially normal)
8. Maternal aggression (potentially normal)
9. Aggression associated with pariahs
10. Play aggression
11. Redirected aggression
12. Territorial aggression
13. Aggression caused by unknown sources

Beaver (1989) points out that dispersion from families occurs naturally at about 8 months of age in cats, although, depending on the structure of the social group, this can be as late as 2 years of age (Macdonald et al., 1987). Although cats shift from social play to social fighting at about 14 weeks of age (Caro, 1980a, c; Karsh & Turner, 1988), Beaver comments that another phase of fighting might occur at dispersion. This is true and fits nicely with the intercat aggression categorization used in this chapter.

Voith (1984a, 1983b) cited four categories of feline aggression based on Moyer's (1968) terminology:

1. Intermale aggression
2. Territorial aggression
3. Fear or fear-induced (defensive) aggression
4. Aggressive behavior toward people

This has been subsequently expanded (Chapman, 1991; Voith & Marder, 1988) to include the following categories:

5. Predatory aggression
6. Play aggression
7. Redirected aggression
8. Maternal aggression

The terminology of Young (1988a) and Houpt and Reisner (1995) follows that of Voith (1984a), Voith and Marder (1988), and Chapman (1991), but Houpt and Reisner include idiopathic aggression, as discussed by Borchelt and Voith (1987). The terminology in this chapter is derived from those listed previously and has been expanded to include aggressions that are being recognized as the complexity of the feline social system begins to be appreciated.

RELATIONSHIP OF AGGRESSION TO SOCIAL SYSTEMS

Feline social systems differ from those of dogs primarily in the extent to which solitary versus social daily activities are prevalent. Cats are primarily solitary hunters, ingesting prey that is smaller than they are, whereas most wild canids work in groups to obtain prey larger than themselves (Clutton-Brock, 1987). These forces act to shape social relationships within groups. Most aggression in cats appears to occur in contexts involving territory and social rank that are complexly interrelated in cats (Young, 1988a). It is not surprising that the types of inappropriate aggression witnessed by clients differ from those that are perceived in dogs or that they are understandable given the evolutionary context of feline social systems and the developmental context of sensitive periods.

Attention has been focused on the extent to which feline aggression is covert rather than overt (Wolski, 1982) and defensive rather than offensive (Young, 1988a). These distinctions can be useful in understanding and intervening in the interactions between cats and other individuals involved in aggressive circumstances. Clients must learn to read the signs of these behaviors to correctly interpret the ongoing interaction and to help us treat the problem appropriately. Offensive aggression generally involves components that decrease the distance between the individuals. These behaviors can include approach (as a threat with subsequent flight of the other individual) and attack. Regardless, the *aggressor* controls the interaction through the use of threat or the escalation of violence (Young, 1988a). Defensive aggression involves passive behaviors designed to encourage avoidance and withdrawal. The *recipient* or *respondent* controls the aggression in this case. This serves to remove the stimulus for further aggression (Young, 1988a). Spraying can act as a defensively aggressive behavior when it serves this purpose.

Clients often have trouble recognizing aggression in their feline household because they are only aware of overt forms of aggression. It helps to emphasize that *cats are not small dogs:* the most common form of aggression in cats is subtle, covert aggression that involves posturing on the part of the aggressor and deference on the part of the recipient of the aggression. Unfortunate and misguided assertions that cats are not social have interfered with our ability to understand these types of aggressions both when they occur between cats and when they are directed by the cat to people (assertion or status-related aggression). Cats generally exhibit overt aggression when they perceive each other as equal rivals and neither cat defers to the other (Wolski, 1982). This situation is more common in crowded situations such as laboratory colonies, households with too many cats, or urban, stray groupings. Overt aggression also occurs in situations where cats in a household contest for status when one reaches social maturity. Covert aggression is more likely to occur if cats know each other well and if all cats involved either agree that they do not see each other as equals, or if some cat is not sufficiently confident to overtly challenge another cat. The latter can include situations involving the introduction of new cats to the household. Spraying and nonspraying marking can play a role in both of these circumstances.

The categorization of feline aggression used is similar to that of canine aggression and is derived from the aforementioned sources; differences in the manifestation of the aggressions may be attributable to differences in mating behaviors and differences in social hierarchies (Overall, 1994j, 1994l). Categories of feline aggression are listed in Box 7-1.

The following diagnoses are behavioral, functional, phenomenological classifications of aggression. It should be noted that cats, like dogs, can be aggressive because of or as a sequela to underlying organic disease. Medical conditions associated with feline aggression include toxoplasmosis, hepatoencephalopathy, feline ischemic encephalopathy, meningioma (primarily older cats), lead poisoning, hyperthyroidism, epilepsy, and rabies (Beaver, 1989a; de Lahunta, 1983; Houpt, 1991b; Parker, 1989; Parker et al., 1983). To the extent that pain aggression is sometimes associated with illness, disease should act as a flag for a possible underlying condition that should be ruled out before further intervention; however, in the sense that the term is used here, the *aggression* is the result of the *pain*, not of the underlying condition.

When organizing an approach to feline aggression, it can be useful to use an algorithm that first sorts the aggressions by whether the recipient is a person, another cat, or another animal. This does not add a heuristic level to the diagnosis but can help practi-

---

BOX 7-1

CATEGORIES OF FELINE AGGRESSION

1. Aggression as a result of lack of socialization
2. Play aggression
3. Fear aggression
4. Pain aggression
5. Intercat aggression: most commonly male-male
6. Maternal aggression
7. Predatory aggression
8. Territorial aggression
9. Redirected aggression
10. Assertion of status-related aggression
11. Idiopathic aggression (includes that associated with obsessive-compulsive behavior)

BOX 7-2

TARGETS OF FELINE AGGRESSION

To cats only	To people only	To cats, people, and other animals
Intercat aggression	Assertion or status-related aggression	Aggression as a result of lack of socialization* Play aggression* Fearful aggression Maternal aggression* Predatory aggression† Territorial aggression Redirected aggression Idiopathic aggression‡

*Primarily directed toward people.
†Usually directed toward people when considered inappropriate, rather than undesirable.
‡May be "victimless" or self-directed.

---

tioners rule out some diagnoses. Box 7-2 categorizes the aggressions by recipient.

Aggression as a Result of Lack of Socialization

Diagnostic Profile. The effect of exposure during sensitive or developmental periods in young animals has been debated. In the 1950s Scott and Fuller (1965) investigated the role of developmental periods within the first few months of dogs' lives for their effects on the development of appropriate social behaviors. Although these periods, called *sensitive* periods by Bateson (1979), exist, they are best viewed in the context of risk assessment. Animals for whom all sensitive period requirements are met can still have problems, and animals who miss "socialization" for or exposure to the relevant periods can do well; however, the *risk* of having problems attendant with the respective sensitive period increases if exposure during that period is missed.

For example, cats who have not had contact with humans before 3 months of age have missed sensitive periods important for the development of normal approach responses to people. Karsh (1983, 1984), Karsh and Turner (1988), and McCune (1995) have examined the extent to which the social environment experienced by cats affected their ability to interact with people. Among their findings, which are more fully discussed in Chapter 4, were that cats that were not handled until 14 weeks of age were fearful and aggressive to people, regardless of the circumstances. These cats would not volitionally approach humans and were aggressive if they could not escape. In contrast, cats handled for as little as 5 minutes per day from the day they were born until they were 7 weeks of age were quicker to approach and solicit people for interaction and gentle play, were quicker to approach inanimate objects, and were quicker to play with toys. This suggests that there are complex, far-reaching consequences of early interaction with people. Lack of such social interaction with other cats may result in the same lack of normal inquisitive response to other cats.

Negative responses can be augmented by suboptimal nutritional conditions for the pregnant queen. Kittens born to such queens generally have delayed developmental skills in addition to a decreased ability to learn, an increased (and usually inappropriate) reactivity to novel situations and stimuli, and an inappropriate response to other cats (more fully discussed in Chapter 4). The chance that such cats will respond normally to most situations involving any interaction is diminishingly small. Furthermore, total isolation from other cats can have negative consequences for future interaction with humans. This constellation of deprivation scenarios may be contributory to many of the aggressions seen in urban, feral cats. Abnormal cats and those with genetic tendencies toward decreased friendliness may be overrepresented in the feral cat population. These cats are aggressive at an early age and may be "dumped into" or returned to the stray population before neutering. In fact, it is possible that they are aggressive, in part, because of in utero androgenization. Models predict that this should be rare and affect no more than 20% of the population (see Fig. 6-3). The concept of in utero androgenization is fully discussed in Chapter 6. No one has investigated this possibility.

Treatment. These cats will never be normal, cuddly pets, although they may attach to one person or to a small group of people over a period of time. If forced into a situation involving restraint, confinement, or intimate contact, these animals may become extremely aggressive. This is very similar to the "pariah" situation discussed by Beaver (1992). Avoidance of the aggression is best. Gestures that would be considered solicitous by normal cats may be considered provocative by these cats. Passive attention should be encouraged through the provision of food and shelter and the use of kind words.

Play Aggression

Diagnostic Profile. Cats that were weaned early and then hand-raised by humans may never have learned to temper their play responses. Social play in cats peaks early and is replaced by more predatory activities by weeks 10 to 12 and by social fighting by week 14. Cats that never learned to modulate their responses as kittens may play too aggressively with clients. These cats may not have learned to sheathe their claws (which is possible by 4 weeks of age [Beaver, 1995]) or to inhibit their bite. Of 27 cats studied by Chapman and Voith (1990b) 7 had a diagnosis of play aggression. The frequency of this aggression is likely to be directly related to the demographic environment of the cat community; urban practices may have more cats with a history consistent with the development of play aggression.

It is unclear if there is an oral response component associated with play aggression and bottle-feeding by clients. Were the kitten to nurse too hard on the queen or to hurt her in play, the queen would have swiftly corrected the kitten. She may also have interacted with the kitten during lactation in a manner that would encourage other, more desirable behavioral responses. Few studies exist on the development of behavior in these discrete circumstances. Clients playing the nursing role correct cats less frequently and are unable to provide the other species-specific behaviors attendant with nursing. Injuring the kitten during a correction is a valid concern; however, if clients mimic feline behaviors such as neck bites and growls or hisses, the kitten learns to respond by inhibiting his or her fierce mouthing and inappropriate play behavior and play aggression may not develop.

Treatment. Should these problems still ensue, they are treatable with behavior modification that interrupts the inappropriate behavior and replaces it with a more appropriate one. For example, the kitten that is playing roughly can be surprised with a water pistol, or a compressed air canister can be used at close range. The point is to startle the kitten so that the inappropriate behavior stops immediately. This goal is best accomplished if the startle occurs as the cat is commencing the inappropriate behavior. Then, when the cat seeks out the client's company, the client can stroke, massage, and provide the cat with food treats whenever it is acting calm. It is very easy for clients to forget to reward good, calm behaviors. This is unfortunate because by doing so, the clients may accomplish more than they will with correction. Clients must be vigilant for the first signs of any inappropriate behavior (pupils dilating, claws unsheathed, ears back, legs and shoulders stiffening, tail twitching) and correct the cat with a correction designed to startle the cat as early in the sequence as possible. The startle technique, whether it involves blowing in the face or use of a water pistol or air canister, should be humane. This means that the *lowest level* of stimulus that achieves the desired effect of aborting the behavior and moving to another is the one that should be used. Tapping on the nose or head could encourage the kitten to tap back. Techniques that do not involve interactive behaviors work the best. It should be remembered that cats have exquisitely sensitive pressure receptors at the base of their canines. It is unlikely that a female cat, behaving appropriately, will injure a kitten. Humans do not have the same degree of control and should avoid forceful corrections whenever possible.

Fearful, Fear, or Fear-Induced Aggression

Diagnostic Profile. Fearfully aggressive cats will hiss, spit, arch their backs, and piloerect if flight is not possible (Beaver, 1992; Manteca, 1995; Young, 1988a).

Fearful aggression usually involves a combination of offensive and defensive postures and overt and covert aggressive behaviors (Leyhausen, 1979). Flight, a defensive activity, is virtually always a component of fearful aggression in cats. As they are pursued with increasingly fewer escape opportunities, cats will stop, draw their head in, crouch, growl, roll on their back when approached (this is *not* a "submissive" behavior in cats; it is an overt, defensive behavior), and paw at the approacher (Young, 1988). If the approacher continues his or her pursuit, the fearfully aggressive cat will try to strike at him or her and follow the strike by holding the approacher, using the forepaws, while kicking with the back feet and biting around the neck (Young, 1988a). Most people who have seen or experienced rough play from cats are also familiar with this sequence of behaviors. When fearful aggression involves other cats, the cats that are fearfully aggressive generally do not seek out the other cat for aggressive interactions (Beaver, 1992; Borchelt & Voith, 1987).

Only 5 of 27 cats studied by Chapman and Voith (1990b) had a diagnosis of fear aggression; however, it is the most commonly diagnosed aggression between cats that undergo a change in the feline household (Borchelt & Voith, 1987).

There are genetically friendly cats and genetically shy cats. It is unclear the extent to which shy cats have the potential to become fearfully aggressive, but there are cats that, despite the best "socialization" possible, become aggressive whenever fearful. These cats also may become fearful without an apparent stimulus. Regardless, if threatened, any cat will defend itself. Depending on the outcome of the threat, any cat can learn to become fearfully aggressive. This phenomenon is particularly important when small children are involved because they may not know how to appropriately respond to a cat that is crouching. Any animal that is cornered and cannot escape has the potential to attack. It is imperative that the cat not learn that its only recourse is aggression because this could lead to aggression in response to any approach.

Treatment. Behavior modification can be very effective early in the development of fear aggression. Protocols are found in Appendix B. Emphasis should be placed on desensitization and counterconditioning for the fear-inducing circumstances. Clients should remember that cats can remain reactive for quite long periods of time after an aggressive event. Caution may be urged for clients seeking to provide solace. Cats should be neither rewarded nor told that "it's okay" for anxious or fearful behaviors. Clients are seeking to calm the cat, but are instead reinforcing the inappropriate behavior. Cats that are calm enough to accept a food treat can be helped with behavior modification. Pharmacological intervention designed to decrease the fear and facilitate the behavior modification can be a useful adjuvant. It is unclear whether any intervention can be successful if the condition has a genetic basis.

Pain Aggression

Diagnostic Profile. As is true for dogs, cats that are in pain, either because of an injury or as a sequela to an underlying medical condition, can be in pain on manipulation. Practitioners can often induce this type of aggression in injured or arthritic and dysplastic cats. Pain aggression can often become fearful aggression if the cat is subjected to long-term painful treatment. Pain aggression is a defensive aggression and responds to measures that alleviate the pain and minimize the potential to be exposed to it. Companion animal analgesia is finally receiving the attention it deserves (Hansen & Hardie, 1993; Werner & Taboda, 1994). Appropriate use of such analgesia can minimize painful aggression in any animal.

Cats that have had their tails caught in doors are often very aggressive whenever anyone attempts to touch their tail. Some of this aggressive response could be related to fear, but even when restrained, these cats appear to become aggressive during manipulation. It is possible that they have some long-standing damage (e.g., a neuroma) that is not apparent in medical and neurological examinations. Behavior modification designed to teach the cats to relax and tolerate touching can be useful as can antianxiety medication. The same phenomenon of apparent pain in the absence of abnormal physical findings is infrequently reported for cats that have undergone declawing and that now will not use their feet. When their feet are manipulated, these cats apparently are painfully aggressive. Full examinations, including radiography, usually reveal no detectable abnormality, leading to discussions of "phantom" pain. Pain is a complex issue and probably underappreciated in such circumstances. These cats also often respond well to behavior modification designed to teach them to relax and to antianxiety medication, but this phenomenon argues strongly against automatically encouraging prophylactic or therapeutic onychectomy.

If there has been no painful medical intervention and the cat appears to exhibit pain aggression, abuse should be considered. Cats, particularly strays, are good victims for torture and may indicate that untoward events are occurring in a household where there are children.

The role of pain aggression in cat-cat interactions has been underexplored. When cats are mismatched by size, health status, or temperament, pain aggression is probably not a trivial problem. This would be particularly true for cats that have already been in fights and may have painful abscesses—any physical contact by another cat may cause them to react defensively in an aggressive manner.

Treatment. Treatment should focus on the following.

1. Not rewarding the cat for the aggression, even though the client is sympathetic
2. Avoiding provocative circumstances, particularly in chronic conditions like arthritis
3. Alleviating the pain

4. Alleviating the anxiety associated with the anticipation of pain

The latter can be accomplished through behavioral modification and pharmacological intervention. (See Chapters 12 and 13.)

Intercat Aggression

Diagnostic Profile. Intercat aggression can involve male-male aggression that is associated with access to mates, or it can be more complex, involving hierarchical status within the feline social group. The situation involving access to mates is a special case of the social hierarchical situation and is a result of the evolutionary history of cats. This does not mean that other sex combinations of cats cannot also have hierarchical problems with intercat aggression. Even in households where cats have lived peacefully, problems may erupt, regardless of sex composition, when one or the other cat reaches social maturity (estimated at 2 to 4 years of age).

Intercat aggression is thought to be most common between toms seeking mates; hence the nomenclature of male-male aggression (Beaver, 1992). In most wild, feline social systems, few males mate with most of the females. The skewed sex ratio in the breeding population is induced and maintained by vigilance and aggression on the part of the males. This evolutionary history is probably responsible for the finding that male cats are more likely to spray and fight in households with female cats than with other male cats (Hart & Barrett, 1973; Hart & Cooper, 1984). There is an additional olfactory component of spraying and nonspraying marking that contributes to the frank aggression.

Male-male aggression is classic and involves flattened ears, howling, hissing, piloerection, and threats using eyes, teeth, and claws in combat. Early neutering (before 12 months of age) decreases or prevents fighting by 88% and spraying by 87% possibly because it decreases roaming by 92% (Hart & Cooper, 1984). The proportion by which these problems are reduced is the same if castration is postpubertal (Hart & Barrett, 1973). These data suggest that testosterone acts as a modulator of social positioning and that learning might be less important than physically placing oneself in a social situation that could encourage a fight. It is unclear whether very early spaying and neutering programs would further reduce the development of aggression, but given the early onset of the hormonal facilitation of the aggression and the extent to which learning could still be a component, this hypothesis could be true.

It would be unfortunate if more complex forms of intercat aggression were eclipsed by intercat aggression that occurs between toms. The latter does not reflect the average situation for indoor cats, yet such

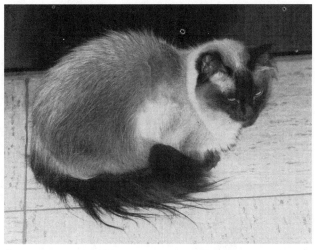

A

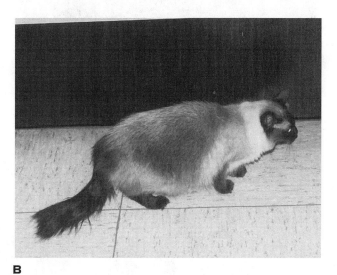

B

Intercat aggression—particularly between known household members who are approximately the same chronological age and who have entered social maturity—can be covert and difficult to assess. The cats in this series of photos were deemed by the client to get along well and to be nonaggressive. **A,** This cat is the aggressor and chose to be outside of the cat carrier for the entire appointment. While he is controlling movement in much of the room, his tail and body postures indicate that he is not open to interaction. Note that his dorsal hair is just slightly spiky and that he is not really focusing on anyone or anything. **B,** There is a second cat in the carrier in front of the aggressor. As that cat made an attempt to exit, the aggressor's response was photographed. Notice the lowered body posture, the stare, the cocked ears, and the tail posture that is slightly raised, but out behind. The postures are discussed in Chapter 4. (Photos by K.L. Overall).

Continued.

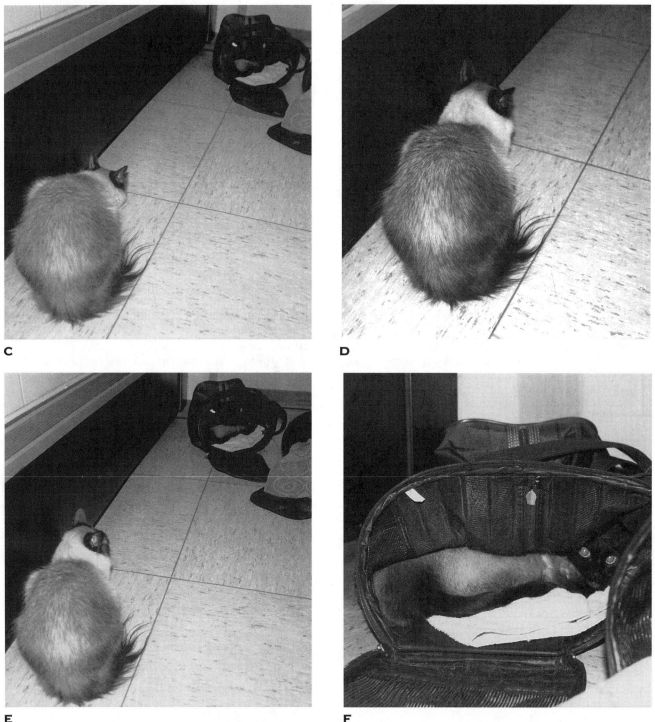

C to **E**, The aggressor approached the cat still within the carrier and stopped 1.5 m from him, assuming the hunched posture. Note the stare and the flattened ears. This is an extremely assertive, confident, and aggressive cat. In these photos it is possible to see that the second cat has withdrawn to the extent allowed by the carrier and will not make direct eye contact with the aggressor. **F**, The cat in the carrier is the victim of the aggression and has developed anxiety-related disorders including self-mutilation. Notice the classic avoidance postures (see Chapter 4). These cats were raised together and are the same age (almost 3 years at the time of the appointment). Based on the history, the passive aggression had probably been ongoing for about a year. (Photos by K.L. Overall).

households often experience intercat aggression that is not primarily or initially related to fear aggression or territorial aggression. Intercat aggression can also occur between females or between males and females and can be associated with social hierarchical status in the household. Assertions that competitive aggression does not occur between cats because they lack a social order (Beaver, 1992) grossly underestimate the social complexity that commonly occurs in feline households.

Treatment. Treatment of intercat aggression that involves a cat that is not in the household can be difficult if access is not controlled. The household cat should be prevented from seeing (blinds, curtains), smelling (odor eliminators), or interacting with the other cat (kept in) if at all possible. Sometimes, if the household cat is allowed to go outside to mark and display, the situation can be resolved. Caution is urged in areas where there are cars, in areas where marauding dogs roam, or if the household cat cannot or will not defend itself. The ultimate solution should be banishment of the intruding cat. Community compliance is helpful for this, and some communities have laws about problem cats. Clients can also make their property unappealing to other cats by patrolling it, scaring them, or booby-trapping areas of ingress using partially sprung mousetraps under newspapers, tack boards, sticky paper (sticky side up), water hazards, and remote control devices. Fences can be fitted with electronically controlled gates that only allow the collared resident cat entry. This solution does not address intruders who enter by more aerial routes. It is important that clients realize that some of these measures can entail a risk for wildlife and nice animals. They *must* minimize that risk.

Aggression between cats in the household is far more difficult to manage. First, the participating cats must be separated when not supervised. The aggressor should be enclosed in a less desirable space (e.g., a spare room), and the victim should either have free range or access to the more desirable space (the living room window, the client's bedroom, the kitchen) (Overall, 1994l,m). Any time any cat is isolated, the cat must have its own water and litter box.

When the cats are together, they should be belled by placing the loudest bell available (on a breakaway collar) so that their clients can monitor the cats' activity. If more than one cat is belled, the bells should sound different. The cats are not to be together unless the clients are willing to be vigilant. At the first sign of any aggression, the aggressor is to be startled. If the cats can remain quietly together, they should be rewarded with food treats. If the client finds that the cats can be in the same room but will not approach each other, they can facilitate their proximity with harnesses, leashes, and food.

For milder aggressions, feeding the cats at a distance where they can see each other but do not react can help. If this distance is attainable, the food dishes can be moved closer together at a slow rate of 1 to 2 cm per day only if the cats do not become distressed. More complex instructions for this particular problem are found in Appendix B.

Maternal Aggression

Diagnostic Profile. Maternal aggression, as in canines, may occur in the periparturient period. Queens may protect nesting areas and kittens, but the aggression is usually in the form of threats with long approach distances, rather than attack. Such threats are usually directed toward unfamiliar individuals, but inappropriate aggression can be directed toward known individuals. Avoidance is the strategy of choice because a cornered queen can attack. As the kittens mature, the aggression resolves. It is unknown whether the kittens learn any aggressive behaviors as a result of the mother's aggression. One would hypothesize that for strays in particular, this could be the case. Because male cats have been reported to practice infanticide in free-ranging situations (Macdonald et al., 1987), it is not unusual for females to exhibit maternal aggression if in the presence of male cats, even those that are familiar.

Treatment. Queens and litters need to be protected by separation, if necessary, from the potential for infanticide. Queens with kittens should be left relatively unmolested. If avoidance doesn't decrease the level of the queen's aggression, she should be spayed.

Predatory Aggression

Diagnostic Profile. Predatory behavior and predatory aggression imply different behavioral circumstances in cats. The quintessential work on the development of predatory behavior was done by Leyhausen (1979). "Normal" predatory behavior may be exhibited by free-ranging cats; field voles, house mice, and birds at bird feeders can be victims of predation. This behavior can occur even if the cats are well fed, although it is apparently more common if cats are to fend for themselves. Cats that are well fed may kill and only behead their prey without eating them. Clients are often concerned about this behavior and want to stop it. Although it may be impossible to fully stop, it is *not* true that there is nothing that can be done.

Predatory aggression in felines is similar to that in canines. Hallmarks of this aggression include stealth, silence, heightened attentiveness, body postures associated with hunting (slinking, head lowering, tail twitching, and pounce postures in cats), and lunging or springing at a prey item that exhibits sudden movement after a period of quiescence.

There is considerable variability in feline temperament regarding predatory inclinations. Some cats have no interest in hunting, whereas other cats make inappropriate context distinctions about prey items. The latter situations become a concern if the prey item is the client's foot or hand or a young infant. Any cat that exhibits the prepounce behaviors described previously in these contexts may be at risk for inappropriate predatory aggression. This is another good reason to never leave young infants alone and unattended when pets are present. The cat that regards infants as prey items usually ceases to do so once the infants have matured sufficiently to demonstrate postural responses. Regardless, this is a potentially dangerous situation, and utmost caution is urged. As a cautionary note it is important to remember that a cat (or dog) does not have to be predatory to injure an infant, toddler, or older child.

Finally, a form of predatory aggression can be seen in free-ranging domestic cats when a new male enters the group. This male may kill all the very young kittens present because their deaths will facilitate the queen coming into season again. It has been postulated that this is the equivalent behavior that Bertram (1975) reported for savannah lions and that it functions to ensure the male cat certainty in paternity for any kittens raised on resources on his territory.

Treatment. The most powerful tactics that people can use to control feline predatory behavior directed toward wild life include corrections or startle (foghorns, airhorns, misters, water pistols, partially sprung mouse traps, and so forth) and avoidance. If the cat preys on birds at the client's feeder, the client can let the cat out only at certain times. During those times the client can signal to the birds that the cat is out by the use of wind chimes or wind sock/decoy owls. If the cat always follows the same path, an electric electronic mat could act as a deterrent, but the cat will usually find a way around it. Invisible electronic fences can be tailored for cats and can restrict the area of their wandering. These can be coupled with a collar and sensor that will allow access to only selected animals. Belling the cat may not be efficacious unless the bell is sufficiently large and loud to always ring—even if the cat springs quickly—or if the ringing of the bell is not coupled by some startle on the part of the client as described previously. The best insurance that outdoor wildlife are not preyed on is to deny the cat access to them. Solitary predatory behavior is developed when kittens are quite young (5 to 7 weeks), and cats can become proficient hunters by 14 weeks of age.

Predatory aggression to humans is best treated by avoidance. Cats that exhibit predatory tendencies to infants should be confined or tethered when in their presence. Like dogs, cats may recognize the infants as non-prey items when the child can sit up, but until then caution is urged. Cats can learn to associate a reward structure with the absence of an inappropriate response to humans by following the instructions outlined in the Protocol for Introducing a New Baby and a Pet (Appendix B).

Adult humans can learn to anticipate predatory aggression directed toward their body parts and avoid activities that stimulate the cat. They can also employ punishment by startling the cat. Placing a bell on the cat will help the client to anticipate the cat's approach. Electronic fences can also be used to restrict indoor access.

Territorial Aggression

Diagnostic Profile. Territorial aggression can be exhibited toward other cats, dogs, or people. Territorially aggressive cats may delineate their turf by patrol, chin rubbing, or spraying or nonspraying marking. Because of the complex, transitive nature of feline social hierarchies, a cat that is aggressive to one housemate may not be aggressive to another. If the cat is defending or marking a turf and the perceived offender crosses into it, threats and a fight may ensue. If part of the struggle involves social hierarchy, cats may lure or seek out their challengers and then attack after the territory has been invaded. Because of the social component, territorial aggression can be difficult to treat, particularly if there is a marking component. Any marking problem should act as a flag for a possible underlying aggressive situation.

Treatment. Environmental modification, behavioral modification (see Appendix B for protocols) and pharmacological intervention are all treatment options; however, aggressions involving strong, underlying social strife are notoriously difficult to treat. Pharmacological intervention can also be useful. Treatment should be aimed at relieving the anxiety associated with the cat's abnormal perception of and challenge in the social interaction. Drugs of choice are tricyclic antidepressants (e.g., amitriptyline, nortriptyline, clomipramine) or selective serotonin reuptake inhibitors (SSRIs; e.g., fluoxetine, paroxetine). Ultimately, one cat may have to be placed in another home or be banished to another region of the property.

Redirected Aggression

Diagnostic Profile. Redirected aggression (equivalent to displaced aggression in the terminology of Houpt and Reisner, 1995) is seen in felines, as well as in canines. However, it can be difficult to recognize and may only be reported as incidental to another form of aggression. Redirected aggression occurs when a motor pattern appropriate for a specific motivational state is redirected to an irrelevant but accessible target because the primary target is unavailable or inaccessible (Bastock et al., 1953). In redirected aggression, any interruption of an aggressive event between two parties by a third party results in redirection of the aggressive behavior to the third party or to another, uninvolved individual. It is important to realize that the interrupted aggressive event may only be a threat, so that the person (or animal) interrupting it may not realize what is occurring. This lack of awareness creates a *very* dangerous situation. Cats appear to remain reactive for an extended period of time after being thwarted in an aggressive interaction (Borchelt &

Voith, 1982b; Young, 1982), and changes in activity in the amygdala during such periods may suggest a basis for this (Adamec, 1975, 1976a). Clients need to realize that this reactivity is occurring and should be aware of the subtleties of feline behavior that communicate intent. Because redirected aggression is often precipitated by another inappropriate behavior, it is important to also treat that behavior.

Feline redirected aggression can be focused on other cats or on people. In their 1990 study, Chapman and Voith reported that redirected aggression to people accounted for 14 of 27 cases of feline aggression involving humans. Unfortunately, because redirected aggression is difficult to diagnose, humans can easily be victimized by these cats and perceive that these attacks are unprovoked and malicious. One exposure of redirected aggression that is focused on another feline household companion is sufficient to induce extreme fearful or fearfully aggressive behavior in the recipient of the aggression. This is probably because the behavior is so unanticipated and so out-of-context that the social bond between the cats is damaged.

Treatment. Treatment involves standard behavior modification techniques. If there is a socially mediated conflict among household cats, some environmental modification may be necessary to decrease the extent to which the involved cats are capable of interacting. Clients should be encouraged to use inanimate objects (battery-operated water pistols, buckets of water, foghorns, compressed air canisters) to intervene between fighting animals. Cat bites and cat scratches are a $25 million-a-year medical industry in the United States. Use of inanimate objects to interrupt fights minimizes danger to the clients and may abort the behavior while teaching the cat that there are consistent, undesirable consequences to the inappropriate behavior.

Assertion or Status-Related Aggression

Diagnostic Profile. Assertion, or status-related, aggression, has been underexplored (Overall, 1994l). This type of aggression has been called the "leave me alone" bite and most frequently occurs during petting. This type of aggression considers the context of the cat's aggression and the cat's prebite signaling. The most similar situation in canines is dominance aggression; however, the divergent evolutionary history of canine and feline social systems argues that these are not homologous situations. Cats exhibiting this form of aggression share with dogs with dominance aggression the similar problem of the need to control most situations. Nothing the client did directly or deliberately provoked the cat; rather, the cat demonstrates a desire or need to control when any attention starts and when it ceases. Some cats do this by biting and leaving, whereas the occasional cat will take the client's hand with its teeth but not bite. Often the cats behave as do dominantly aggressive dogs: they deliberately

block the client's path or solicit attention when the client's guard is down (for example, when the client is talking on the telephone). This form of aggression can be accompanied by territorial aggression.

Treatment. Fortunately, clients can be taught to observe signs of impending aggression (tail flicking, ears flat, staring, pupillary dilation, head hunched, claws possibly unsheathed, stillness or tenseness, low growl) and to interrupt the behavior at the first sign of any of these signals by standing up and letting the cat fall from their lap. Clients can also abandon the cat and refuse to interact until the cat is exhibiting an appropriate behavior. Clients should be discouraged from direct physical correction of the cat because the cat may view this as a challenge and intensify the aggression. If the cat does not respond to passive control or redirects the aggression, it is safer to counter the behavior with a fog horn or a battery-operated water pistol. Corrections must occur within the first 30 to 60 seconds of the onset of the suite of inappropriate behaviors to ensure learning; corrections within the first second are best.

Clients with such cats should be aware that their cats are never going to be very cuddly, although if the client can refrain from petting these cats, they may be willing to sit quietly on the client's lap for extended periods. The extent to which cats exhibiting this form of aggression also exhibit intercat aggression is unknown. Cases seen at the Veterinary Hospital of the University of Pennsylvania (VHUP) indicate no association, but no rigorous studies have been done. There is no association between aggression to people and aggression to dogs for dogs with abnormal responses to social situations. The same might be true for cats because the issue is whether the behavior is appropriate or in context; an abnormal response to people need not mean that a contextually inappropriate response to other cats will occur and vice versa.

Idiopathic Aggression

Diagnostic Profile. By definition, idiopathic aggression is poorly understood, and, often, poorly defined. As is true for dogs, idiopathic aggression in cats is truly unprovoked (and this must take into account that *abnormal behavior* is being discussed and therefore the aggression cannot occur even in abnormal, but predictable circumstances [e.g., territorial aggression]), unpredictable, toggle-switch aggression. It probably does happen but is rarely reported at VHUP. The majority of the cats brought in for aggression represent one of the other 10 categories.

Treatment. Because the characteristics of this aggression, it can be difficult, if not impossible, to treat with standard behavioral and environmental modification techniques. Some of these rare behaviors may represent epileptiform or seizure activity and, accordingly, may respond to sedative or anticonvulsant medication.

UNDERSTANDING THE INTERACTION BETWEEN FELINE AGGRESSION AND ELIMINATION DISORDERS

The most common feline behavioral problems involve inappropriate elimination behavior. This inappropriate behavior can take the following forms: substrate or location aversion; substrate preference for urination, defecation, or both; location preference for urination, defecation, or both; and marking/spraying (see Chapter 8). It is important to remember that feline elimination behaviors do not happen in a social vacuum: domestic and wild cats use scratch marks, scrapes, and elimination products to mark their territory. Any elimination disorder must be considered in the context of the relative social environment. The extent to which elimination disorders and aggression co-occur in cats is grossly underestimated (Box 7-3). Simply cleaning the soiled areas and the litter box is not sufficient to treat elimination disorders with an aggressive component. The aggression *must* be addressed.

OVERVIEW OF ELIMINATION DISORDERS AND THEIR ROLE IN FELINE AGGRESSION

For most preferences for elimination substrates or locations, the social environment is less of a factor than is the cat's endogenous choice. This may not be true for many substrate and location aversions. Social environment is very important for most marking behaviors. Undesirable spraying and marking behaviors are another set of disorders that must be addressed in a multifactorial manner (Overall, 1993a, 1994e).

Spraying and nonspraying marking are commonly seen in outdoor cats and may serve to delineate territories. Unfortunately, the same behaviors can often occur within a household. Bold cats often may announce their presence and status by spraying everywhere. Less confident cats may try to carve out an area of their own by spraying only there or by marking with feces or by squatting. Faced with outright aggression, less confident cats may resort to spraying after the fact because they are not temperamentally suited to direct fighting. All of these social ramifications must be considered before treatment of marking can be successful.

It is critical to realize that both males and females can spray and that animals can spray both because

they feel confident and because they feel insecure. Furthermore, spraying can be an advertisement, a threat, or a response to a threat.

Spraying can be performed by intact or neutered animals (Neville & Remfry, 1984). More intact males spray than do intact females. Of 134 male cats and 152 female cats that were prepubertally gonadectomized, 10% of the males and 5% of the females sprayed later in life (Hart & Cooper, 1984); the difference in the numbers of each set that spray in later life is not statistically significant ($p > 0.05$, $G_{adj} = 2.568$). These proportions are no different than those for animals that were neutered after they started to spray (10% of all males that sprayed before neutering persist in doing do, whereas 5% of all females that sprayed before neutering persist) (Hart & Barrett, 1973). In these studies the decrease in spraying behavior was accompanied by a concomitant decrease in fighting between cats. The age of prepubertal castration appeared to have no influence on the individual cat's propensity to spray or fight later in life (Hart & Cooper, 1984); however, early spaying and castration (at 6 to 8 weeks of age) was not investigated in this study.

This same study indicated that 51% of males and 39% of females sprayed, were aggressive occasionally or frequently, or exhibited both behaviors. Of the males in this hospital population, 9% sprayed frequently, as did 5% of the females (Hart & Cooper, 1984). These data were not dramatically different from those collected through a similar survey on cats owned by students. When the data from both populations are combined, 39 of 134 males and 23 of 152 females spray occasionally or frequently and 59 of 134 males and 46 of 152 females fight occasionally or frequently. Males are statistically significantly more frequently represented in both the spraying and fighting populations ($p \leq 0.05$, $G_{adj} = 8.153$ and $G_{adj} = 5.782$, respectively). Fighting is more commonly reported than spraying ($p \leq 0.05$; $G_{adj} = 15.719$). Hence, although spraying and fighting are to some extent dimorphic behaviors, response to neutering does not appear to depend solely on sex.

Many reports focus on in utero androgenization. It has been postulated that cats show a similar response to this phenomenon as do rodents (Inselman-Temkin & Flynn, 1973). Female rodents that develop between two males in the uterus are masculinized from birth with regard to their aggression. These rodents also develop more like males than females with regard to social aggression when evaluated at social maturity (vom Saal, 1989). The exact uterine order in cats and dogs is seldom known, but it is possible to know the number of each sex of kittens. It is possible that prenatal masculinization of female fetuses is not a factor in predisposing females to spray or fight. Hart and Cooper (1984) found that 40% (18/46) of female cats that fought (46 of 152 fought; 40% = 18) were from all-female litters and hence do not meet the criteria

---

BOX 7-3

TYPES OF AGGRESSION MOST FREQUENTLY ASSOCIATED WITH ELIMINATION DISORDERS

1. Intercat aggression
2. Territorial aggression
3. Fearful aggression
4. Redirected aggression
5. Status-related aggression

for classic androgenization. Thirteen female cats that did not spray or fight came from litters of two or more males, and eight came from litters of three or more males (mean litter size of six), suggesting that the female kitten likely developed next to at least one male kitten.

Without knowing the complete distribution of litter compositions for the 28 cats in this study who fought and were not from all-female litters, it is not possible to compare these results with the theoretical ones predicted in Fig. 6-3. However, it should be noted that with an average litter size of 6 (the mean in this study) the probability of androgenization is only 0.08 (8% chance), a figure wholly compatible with the proportion of cats not exhibiting aggression. The data presently available are inadequate to test hypotheses of the effect of in utero androgenization on aggression.

PSYCHOTROPIC MEDICATION IN THE TREATMENT OF ELIMINATION-ASSOCIATED AGGRESSION: A ROLE FOR STRONG INFERENCE

Regardless of the sex of the individual spraying cat, all spraying is *not* related to the same underlying cause. Spraying is a nonspecific diagnosis that is multifactorial. Distinguishing among feline social interactions can be difficult and frustrating. The extent to which these are involved in spraying is largely underexplored. Understanding this social involvement may be the key to prescribing the appropriate pharmacological intervention. Some clues about probable social motivation can be gleaned from failed drug therapies. Agents that either have specific mechanisms or locations of action can be ideal for testing neurochemical correlates of spraying. Most drugs that are currently available are not this specific.

First, as with any elimination disorder, underlying medical causes (cystitis, lower urinary tract disease, urinary tract infection, obstruction, anatomical abnormalities) must be ruled out. Should there be no apparent medical cause, treatment can proceed with diazepam, buspirone, clomipramine, or other medications (Box 7-4).

Diazepam (1.0 to 3.0 mg [0.2-0.4 mg/kg] every 12 to 24 hours), when used appropriately, can control spraying in 75% to 90% of all cats (Marder, 1991). Generally, cats for whom it is successful will stagger mildly and have impaired depth perception for a few days; staggering should resolve spontaneously by the end of the week. Some cats may require diazepam for a few weeks, some seasonally, some forever. The lowest effective dose should be used. Some cats that do respond to diazepam require a benzodiazepine with a longer half-life. Clorazepate dipotassium (Tranxene) at 0.5 to 1.0 mg/kg orally every 12 to 14 hours as needed can be used; however, if the cat did not respond to increased doses of diazepam, this approach may also be unsuccessful.

Benzodiazepines have global anxiolytic affects.

BOX 7-4	
USEFUL AND COMMONLY USED DRUGS FOR THE TREATMENT OF FELINE ELIMINATION DISORDERS AND FELINE AGGRESSION	
Amitriptyline (tricyclic antidepressant; Elavil)	0.5-1.0 mg/kg orally every 12 to 24 hours
Buspirone (nonspecific anxiolytic/serotonin agonist; BuSpar)	0.5-1.0 mg/kg orally every 12 to 24 hours
Clomipramine (tricyclic antidepressant; Anafranil)	0.5 mg/kg orally every 24 hours
Diazepam (benzodiazepine; Valium)	0.2-0.4 mg/kg orally every 12 to 24 hours
Imipramine (tricyclic antidepressant, Pamolar)	0.5-1.0 mg/kg orally every 12 to 24 hours

From Overall, 1993, 1994e.

They amplify the effects of the inhibitory neurotransmitter, gamma-aminobutyric acid; the mechanism for their facilitation of social interactions may be because attendant anxiety is inhibited. Indeed, clients may note that the cats become excessively friendly while taking benzodiazepines. This social facilitation may be responsible for the cessation of spraying in successful cases. As such, the spraying is related to, or symptomatic of, the social conflict. Benzodiazepines also cause patients to be less reactive to their surroundings and less responsive to provocational stimuli. This appears to be the main effect for their use in the treatment of feline spraying. The mood elevation effects of the benzodiazepine are the result of the effects on the inhibitory neurotransmitter, not because the drug elevates brain chemicals associated with upbeat moods. Such subtleties may play a role in the treatment of complex social phenomenon such as spraying (Overall, 1996). Benzodiazepines interfere with learning and short-term memory and therefore are not the ideal drugs to use in conjunction with intensive behavior modification. In humans they are psychologically and physically addictive; abusable substances should be dispensed with caution because of substance abuse problem with clients (Abruzzese & Swanson, 1965, Chai & Wang, 1966; Colte et al., 1984, Cunningham, 1965). There have been recent reports of atypical hepatotoxicity and sudden death associated with diazepam therapy in cat populations. These idiosyncratic reactions have been reported for both generic and brand-name diazepam and for cats exposed to the drug for variable periods. It is surprising that most reports have been recent, given the decade-long-plus use of benzodiazepines in cats. Insufficient epidemiological data are currently available to infer or suggest tests of etiology; however, cats with large amounts of body fat and for whom no pretreatment hepatic biochemical data are available are overrepresented in the affected population (Center et al., 1996; Hughes et al., 1996).

Buspirone (BuSpar) is a newer nonspecific anxiolytic that appears to act as a partial presynaptic and postsynaptic 5-hydroxytryptamine agonist. It has been suggested that its primary effect may be as a dopamine receptor antagonist, although this modality of action is widely debated. In cases when benzodiazepines, progestins, or both fail, it has been successful (although less so than originally hoped) in controlling spraying, particularly in cats for which spraying is associated with intercat aggression at dosages of 0.5 to 1.0 mg/kg orally every 8-12 hours (Hart et al., 1993). Buspirone takes 4 to 6 weeks to reach safe, steady-state blood levels, and clients should not expect to see an effect for 6 to 8 weeks. The drug has no effects on short-term memory, which makes it superior to diazepam for situations that involve fear and anxiety for which behavior modification might be useful. However, there is no statistically significant difference between the responses to buspirone and diazepam or in their recidivism rate, although some cats respond to one but not the other (Overall, 1994h). This suggests that the population of cats that spray is heterogenous and the condition is multifactorial (Overall, 1994m). This anxiolytic appears to have comparable side effects of many antianxiety drugs, and clients should be warned that potential side effects include inappetence, lethargy, and possible interference with thyroid medication. If the symptoms are not transient, the drug should be withdrawn.

Newer tricyclic antidepressants such as clomipramine (Anafranil) may be useful for treatment of spraying associated with anxiety and aggression (Overall, 1994b, 1996). No published studies are currently available on clomipramine use in cats. Caution is urged against its cavalier use because it may be a potent arrhythmogenic agent in cats. Its use at a dosage of approximately 0.5 mg/kg orally every 24 hours looks promising (Shanley & Overall, 1995) (for further information of this and other tricyclic antidepressants, see Chapter 13). Medications, including the selective serotonin reuptake inhibitors (SSRIs) sertraline (Zoloft), paroxetine (Paxil), and fluoxetine (Prozac) will prove useful for different classes of feline spraying, non-spraying marking, and anxiety-related elimination problems.

For cats that do not respond to other medications, progestins can be used, but they should be used only as a last resort because of potential side effects that include gynecomastia, diabetogenesis, potential implication with mammary neoplasia, and bone marrow suppression (Chastain et al., 1991; Hernandez et al., 1975; Kwochka & Short, 1984; Romatowski, 1989). Progestins should never be used in breeding animals. Of cats that do not respond to diazepam, 50% respond to either megestrol acetate (5 to 10 mg orally every 24 hours for 1 week then decrease dose and frequency to minimum effective dose) or medroxyprogesterone acetate (50 to 100 mg intramuscularly or subcutaneously no more than 3 times per year) (Cooper & Hart, 1992; Marder, 1991). Of the cats that respond to neither diazepam nor one of the progestins, about 50% respond to the other progestin. Progestins are not benign drugs, and under no circumstance should they be dispensed without a baseline complete blood cell count and serum biochemistry profile and follow-up laboratory tests every 6 to 8 weeks. Clients should be warned of all side effects because of liability and they must sign a release form that specifically lists side effects.

Progestins appear to have two modes of action: a calming affect, which may provide a nonspecific anxiolytic benefit, and a feminization effect. At the cellular level progestins inhibit 5-α-steroid reductase neurons in the hypothalamus and the limbic system. If an animal is spraying because of hormonal stimuli (testosterone) or because of dimorphic behavioral stimulation, progestins may ablate the behavior. Accordingly, females may respond less well to progesterone treatment than do males. Certainly, if there is a slight component of anxiety, particularly in an intrasexual, hierarchical situation or one fostered by estrous queens, progestins may be efficacious because of their dual actions. The calming effect of progestins alone is not strong when compared with other anxiolytic medications; this drug should not be chosen because of this effect. Progestins should be prescribed with utmost caution and are contraindicated in patients with glaucoma or thyroid disorders and in any breeding animal. Because of their numerous potential side effects (gynecomastia, adenocarcinoma, diabetogenesis, bone marrow suppression), progestins should be prescribed only after a complete physical examination, including blood studies, and the patient should be closely monitored. If the animal continues progestin therapy, blood studies should be performed every 6 to 12 months (depending on the animal's age and physical condition) to monitor any effects on the renal and hepatic systems.

A decision algorithm for diagnosis and pharmacological intervention of feline elimination disorders is found in Chapter 8.

REASONS FOR TREATMENT FAILURE

A few general precautions should be noted. First, any cat that does not respond to the previously mentioned treatments should have further medical tests. At VHUP, cultures reveal many infections not apparent on regular screening tests. Sometimes two or three urinalyses and one or two cultures are necessary before the complicating medical etiology is revealed. Clients should be informed of this. Furthermore, signs of fluid, feline urologic syndrome, or sterile cystitis can cause the presence of bladder diverticulae to wax and wane. These may be diagnosed by ultrasound or cystoscopy (Osborn et al., 1987, 1995).

Second, any multicat household will have greater problems. If one cat is spraying, chances are that others are, too. With 10 or more cats in the household, the chance of spraying at some point is 100% (Marder, 1991). Clients will deny that other cats are involved, but they should be told anyway that this is usually true; many will call back to tell you they finally saw the third cat spray. Watch out for bullies. The reason the kitten may not use the litter box is because someone else sits on top of or behind it and swats the kitten every time it approaches. Do not get duped into believing that the only cat that needs treatment in the household is the one with the elimination problem. When both aggression and elimination are factors, the behavior of the cat that elicits the aggression may need to be altered. Because of their specific behaviors they could also benefit from antianxiety medication and may require a different drug than the cat originally presented as the "patient."

Finally, accurate and discrete diagnosis is essential. Any diagnosis of any condition must meet the necessary and sufficient diagnostic criteria specified in Appendix F. Feline social systems are complex and signs of aggression or anxiety may be subtle. Repeating the history-taking aspect of the examination and having the client keep a log of actual behaviors and events may suggest a definitive diagnosis. Treatment of nonspecific signs alone is unlikely to meet with success.

DECLAWING

Declawing (onychectomy) is a focus of dispute. The most commonly reported undesirable feline behaviors include jumping on counters and tables, defecation or urination outside the litter box, clawing, and biting (Bennett et al., 1988). The latter two are frequent reasons that clients resort to declaw. In a study of 273 declawed cats, 86% (235) were declawed for scratching, 29% (79) for injury to people, 9% (24) because they were to be kept exclusively indoors, 8% (23) to ensure the safety of the other pets (no information is provided on whether there was an actual risk), and 1% (3) to decrease the need for punishment (Landsberg, 1991b). Some veterinarians report that clients automatically request declawing with new kittens to prevent "accidents" in play with their children (D. Frank, personal communication, 1994). These categories are not mutually exclusive. It is interesting that in Landsberg's study 1990 the most common reason for desiring declawing involved scratching, yet this is a normal cat behavior. Kittens begin to retract their claws at about 4 weeks of age and begin to scratch by day 35 (Beaver, 1992). Hence there is ample time and opportunity to modify this behavior. Automatic declawing should not be encouraged. Instead, cats should be directed to use more appropriate substrates.

Bennett et al. (1988) found that complications from declawing occurred less than 10% of the time and that there was no risk of increasing undesirable, when compared with desirable, behaviors. Landsberg (1990, 1991b) found that most cats recover from declawing within 3 days (67%; 157 of 233) and 96% (223 of 233) of cats are fully recovered within 2 weeks. The most commonly reported complication in these studies was claw regrowth (3%).

One concern is that if cats are deprived of the use of their claws as a deterrent to further approach and interaction, those cats will then escalate their aggression by using their teeth. Data from Bennett et al. (1988) indicate that cats that bite and are subsequently declawed do not bite more frequently than they did before declawing. Landsberg has commented that 4% (10 of 276) of people who declawed their cats reported a possible increase in biting or an intensity in biting after declawing. Clients considered this a less severe problem than scratching.

Borchelt and Voith (1987) studied three categories of bites (one or more, more than eight, and those requiring treatment) for cats that were clawed and declawed and for those bites directed toward strangers or family members. Statistical examination reveals that within the group of cats that bite family members or strangers, there is no difference in the frequency of biting by declawed, or clawed cats, regardless of bite category (all log-likelihood ratio chi-square test; all $p < 0.05$). Bennett and colleagues (1988) and Morgan and Houpt (1990) found that when the behavior of intact and declawed cats was compared, declawing does not appear to lead to a change in behavior or personality.

Clients and practitioners are beginning to be vocal about their ethical concerns for onchyectomy. These concerns are developing at the same time that attitudes are changing in the United States about tail docking and ear cropping. Declawing is a form of elective mutilation, but it is commonly believed to save cats' lives. The extent to which this perception is a function of the manner in which choices for redressing behavioral concerns are presented to clients has not been examined. Landsberg (1990) has noted that anywhere between 10% and 75% of clients who declawed cats in Ontario, Canada indicated that they would not have kept the cats had they not been able to declaw them. Unfortunately, the beliefs driving this attitude are seldom known, and the extent to which more knowledge and early intervention with undesirable behaviors has not received a lot of attention, but this is changing.

Alternatives to declawing exist for clients who wish to modify their cat's behavior but keep the cat's claws. Landsberg (1991b) has been somewhat successful in encouraging clients to use hand-held ultrasonic devices to treat cat scratching. Behavioral and environmental modification, nail trimming, nail capping with plastic sheaths, and flexor tenonectomy (which still requires that the nails be trimmed) can all be suitable alternatives to declawing.

Cats use their claws for a variety of functions. The issue of scratching is more fully discussed in Chapter 11. The American Veterinary Medical Association's policy on onchyectomy indicates that the procedure is justifiable with adherence to appropriate surgical and medical principles when the cat *cannot be trained* to not use its claws destructively but should *not* be performed solely for cosmetic purposes (emphasis added) (Phillips, 1992). Few cats are resistant to reshaping of their scratching behavior if the clients understand that this is a normal component of feline behavior and they redirect it early. The Canadian Veterinary Medical Association's policy, which is slightly more restrictive, indicates that although it may be the only option for cats that will otherwise be placed in shelters or killed, the focus should be on postoperative discomfort, and *only* the forepaws should be subjected to the procedure.

TREATMENT OF FELINE AGGRESSION

The same principles that are used to treat canine aggression can be used to treat feline aggression. Practitioners should refer to Chapter 12 for an explanation of the techniques. Appendix B contains client handouts targeted for the prevention and treatment of specific aggressions.

General principles include the following:

1. Encourage clients to learn to recognize the physical signs of incipient aggression. Teach them to startle the animal, using the minimum startle necessary, to abort the aggression as early in the sequence as possible. Clients should *not* use aggressive behaviors such as smacking the cat or flicking the nose to startle the cat. These behaviors are dangerous and will cause the aggression to intensify. A noise or a burst of air can be sufficient to startle the cat. The client must be aware of and beware of the signs of redirected aggression.
2. Avoid all situations known to facilitate the aggression. Unless the aggression can consistently be interrupted and aborted in such situations, the animals will not learn from these experiences. Instead, they will have learned to reinforce their inappropriate behavior.
3. If the aggression involves specific cats within the household, separate those cats when they are not supervised. Even if there are no overt signs of battle in the client's absence, the cats may be interacting with each other in an inappropriate or aggressive manner (see no. 2 above).
4. Avoid physical punishment. In addition to being

problematic from the operant conditioning standpoint, it is risky to the client, particularly given the incidence of CSD.

5. Counterconditioning and desensitization techniques also work for cats. Teach your clients how to do this cautiously with food rewards, gates, and leashes and harnesses (see Appendix B).
6. Drug therapy can be useful in the treatment of feline aggression. As always, it is an adjuvant to, not a substitute for, behavioral and environmental modification. Rational and judicious use mandates premedication and regular postmedication blood tests, complete disclosure of potential side effects (client consent forms), and a true and good client-practitioner relationship.
7. Consider increased use of three-dimensional space. Cats can share space and time-share (Bernstein & Strack, 1993), and the more area they have in which to do this, the more options they will have. It should be remembered that the size of the average apartment is one to three orders of magnitude smaller than the area that would be traditionally exploited by a free-ranging cat as part of his or her home range.

Issues Yet to be Resolved

1. As with most issues in behavioral medicine, the underlying frequency of age-specific appropriate and inappropriate feline aggressions is unknown. Such information would be useful in understanding the development of problems.
2. When quantitative data exist, they are scant. Further quantification of dimorphic behaviors is warranted.
3. The feline social system is understudied. In particular, the effect of social maturity on aggression deserves more attention.
4. Specific behavioral sequences involved in aggression to people need to be pursued as vigorously as was feline predatory behavior. Signaling is complex in cats and has seldom been addressed.
5. The development of feline aggression and the potential underlying heritable basis needs to be addressed. An acceptable start has been made here, but it needs to be expanded. A particular focus should be exploration of the possibility that stray cats comprise a population distinct from "pet" cats from the standpoint of behavioral genetics. This information will have profound animal welfare consequences.
6. Rather than using invasive means to study the neuroanatomy of induced aggression, a more thorough understanding of naturally occurring aggression using imaging techniques, pharmacology, and genetics is warranted.

CASE 1

Signalment: "Zooey," 1-year-old, 4.8 kg, castrated male Siamese

Initial Problems: Biting the clients and tearing around the house

History: This cat was obtained from a breeder at 12 weeks of age and was castrated and declawed (forepaws) at 7 months of age. Within the first 3 months of his arrival in the household, Zooey began to exhibit thrice daily bouts of enthusiastic, uncontrolled running behavior in the house. The clients reported that he tore from room to room, bouncing off furniture or other objects in his way. If the clients were in the way, he would occasionally swat at them. After he was declawed he would paw at the clients, but not gain purchase.

At about the same time that he started to tear around the house, Zooey also began to attack people's feet and legs when they passed a room or a door where the cat was crouched. Whenever the phone rang, Zooey would wait until the person was talking and then fling himself at them and wrestle, bite, and run away. Until recently Zooey had not hurt anyone, and the family encouraged his behavior by chasing him and wrestling with him. The father in the household has recently had cataract surgery and is virtually blind. He is unable to anticipate the cat and is now startled by these pounces.

Otherwise, everyone adores this cat. They have always played roughly with him, using their hands, but are able to do anything with him. He was wonderful for all of us at VHUP and is very charming, confident, and friendly. If someone stopped petting him, he would gently bat at them. The entire time he was at VHUP, someone had to be giving him attention.

Physical Examination: No abnormalities were detected on physical examination.

Diagnosis: Attention-seeking behavior and play aggression (and normal cat behavior).

Treatment: The energetic coursing is normal; however, this cat needs to learn the boundaries. The clients were instructed to pay attention to him only if he was quiet and not batting them. They were to stop playing aggressively with him and to play only with toys. If he ever touched one of their body parts, they were to shriek as if they were mortally wounded. The clients are able to recognize the anticipatory behaviors that tell them that the cat will spring. They are to startle him with a loud noise, air canister, or foghorn when he exhibits these behaviors, before he attacks. They are to fit him with a breakaway collar with a bell so that the father is not at this cat's mercy. They are also to play aerobically with him and to use grooming and massage to encourage more calm interaction. The possibility of adding a slightly older, energetic kitten to the household was discussed.

Follow-up: Since the examination the clients have had no problems and are implementing the strategies. They will call us if they need us.

CASE 2

Signalment: "Larry," 3-year-old, 4.8 kg, castrated male, Abyssinian cat

Initial Problem: Attacking the clients

History: The aggressive behavior started at about 2 years of age, 1 month after the clients moved from an apartment to a house. The house had not previously had cats in it, and there appear to be no feline visitors. The cat is an indoor cat, except for 1 to 2 hours per weekend when the cat is allowed outside on the patio on a harness when the clients are also there. There appears to be no pattern connecting the aggression to these outings.

The aggression was formerly a rare circumstance, but in the past few months it has become a weekly, and now, a nightly occurrence. The behavior has multiple facets.

The cat will be sitting on the couch in the living room, dozing or just relaxing. As soon as the husband comes home from work and enters the room, the cat begins to hiss, growl, and spit. This used to be an occasional event, but in the past few weeks has occurred daily; the behavior starts as soon as the husband puts his key in the door. If the husband approaches the cat, the cat attacks him, springing from the couch, wrapping his legs around the husband, and biting repeatedly. He does not let go on his own; he must be removed. The husband is able to love and pet the cat once the cat is asleep in the bedroom at night. The cat sleeps on the clients' bed, between them and touching them. The husband can also pet the cat when they both awaken, if he has not yet left the room. If he has left the room and returned, the cat becomes slightly aggressive to the husband, hissing and growling. The bedroom is the room where the cat is best behaved with the husband. The husband can make no associations between events, schedules, and scents that correlate with the development and expression of the cat's behavior.

Furthermore, the cat restricts paths that the husband can take through the house by staring at the husband, by standing in access ways, and by glaring and hissing at the husband. Because of these behaviors the husband has changed his plans about seating locations and traffic patterns within the house. The husband is positive that if he does not respond to the cat's body postures in this manner, he will be attacked.

The cat has also attacked the wife, but only in one circumstance (two instances). In the first instance, the wife was sitting with the cat on her lap or next to her and a new person entered the room. The cat savagely attacked the wife. The other time the wife was bitten involved a loud noise that startled Larry. She was both the person who made the noise and the closest person to the cat, so it is unclear if the cat sought her out or attacked opportunistically.

All bites from this cat are severe, deep punctures.

The clients have recently had a baby. The cat does not seem to react to the baby's crying and, thus far, has sniffed, but largely ignored the baby.

While at VHUP, the cat targeted people to stare at and rub against. If the person did not break the cat's stare, the cat quivered the tip of his tail, which was elevated, rippled the skin on its back, became agitated, and licked, then paced. Finally, the cat began to growl and pace frenetically while his skin rippled to the point of dancing. During this entire time the cat stared at the target individual. The clients reported that this behavior was seen at home, often after a bite.

During the entire 3 hours that the cat was at VHUP, he was very assertive and confident. He jumped from his kennel onto the examination table, looked at anyone who entered in the eye, groomed, settled down, and watched everything from the examination table. The students were able to examine the cat without restraint (this was not true when we obtained blood samples).

Previous Treatment: One month before the visit at the Behavior Clinic the cat was declawed in an attempt to prevent him from attaining purchase to bite. This cat is agile.

The referring veterinarian had previously treated the cat successfully with progestins (Ovaban) (2.5 to 5.0 mg per bout) for three treatments, but the cat was beginning to require the medication more frequently. The referring veterinarian then attempted treatment with amitriptyline (5 mg orally every 12 hours), but the clients could not get the cat to take the pills. The referring veterinarian submitted no laboratory evaluations. The clients had been successful in aborting the attacks with a water pistol; a squirt bottle worked at VHUP.

Physical Examination: The physical examination revealed no abnormalities.

Laboratory Evaluation: A complete blood cell count and serum biochemical profile were submitted and were within laboratory reference limits.

Diagnosis: Redirected aggression and status-related aggression

Both incidents of aggression involving the wife occurred when the cat was startled and unable to anticipate the source of his startle. The attacks on the wife appear sudden, frenzied, and unpremeditated. This is classic in cases of redirected aggression.

The aggression involving the husband, while ferocious, was not unpremeditated. The cat anticipates the husband's presence and behaviors and works to control the husband. The fact that the cat passively controls access to parts of the house and paths that the husband must take by posturing and positioning himself in those areas demonstrates the extent to which the cat will go to manipulate the situation. The cat positions himself on the couch before the front door before the husband comes home and threatens him when he enters.

The same assertive postures and challenges are exhibited by the cat in situations involving strangers. This cat is constantly surveying the social environment to see what he can manipulate and control. Any sign of resistance is met with aggression. Once the cat realizes that he can back someone down, he continues to victimize the person. This is classic behavior in situations involving status-related aggression.

Status-related aggression is an analogous condition to canine dominance aggression. It revolves around control of the social environment involving people and is an abnormal social response to uncertain social circumstances. Instead of waiting to decipher the social patterns, cats demonstrating this behavioral pattern must challenge every human individual in their environment. The responses received help the cat to decide whom to manipulate. As with dominantly aggressive dogs, cats with status-related aggression do not have to be equally aggressive to all individuals in the household.

CASE 2—cont'd

Treatment: The clients were instructed to watch for the anticipatory signs of any agonistic behaviors: staring, ears pulled back or flicking, tail held vertical with quick flicking at the tip, rippling of the skin on the back, elevation of the hindquarters accompanied by a strut, and tail flicks, growling, and hissing. At the first hint of any of these signs the clients are to blast the cat with a water pistol with a 5% to 10% vinegar and lemon juice solution (a foghorn would have been preferable, but having a newborn in the house precluded this). Clients are to carry water pistols at all times as a form of correction and to interrupt the behavior.

Most of the counterconditioning and desensitization focuses on the cat's interaction with the husband. The only time the cat has ever had catnip, he was calm, friendly, and ecstatic and continuously solicited the husband. If the husband is willing to try to interact with the cat with a catnip mouse, he can start this in the bedroom, where the cat is less reactive. The husband should build up from just being with the cat when he plays with the mouse to playing with and petting him.

The cat is to be put in another room before the husband comes home. He is to be let out to be fed by the husband, and the husband is to use the water pistol as described, if needed. The husband is also to feed the cat (which he does frequently anyway).

The clients can talk to the cat, but they cannot fuss over him physically. If they want to do this, they must control all affection and withdraw it before the cat is really ready to have it withdrawn. As time progresses, the clients will give more attention, accompanied by food treats or the catnip mouse (if it works), always watching for any signs of incipient challenge from the cat.

Finally, because this cat is so intense in his behavior and because the sequence of behaviors after and preceding

his aggressive events is stereotypic and worsening, clomipramine treatment was started (0.5 mg/kg orally every 24 hours). Most aggressions have a basis in anxiety about the animal's perceived or defined role in the social environment. Accordingly, many aggressive animals proceed more quickly with behavior modification once they are treated with an antianxiety medication. Because this cat is anxious in unanticipated circumstances, medication also might be useful in raising his threshold for reactivity in situations where redirected aggression has developed. This cat needs all the help he can get. It is either a better cat or a dead cat, and the clients have a very clear perception of this and of the potential damage the cat can do.

Follow-up: Within 10 days of starting Larry on the clomipramine, the clients reported that the cat was more loving and purred and sought them out for attention more often. There have been no incidents of hissing, and the cat is actually trying to play with them and inanimate objects (they had forgotten how long it had been since they had seen the cat play). The cat is eating more and is a little less active, overall, because he is no longer pacing and exhibiting many of the anxious and stereotypic behaviors seen at the Behavior Clinic and reported during the appointment. The clients are keeping the water pistols with them, although they have not had to use them recently. They have not yet obtained a catnip mouse because they wanted to first assess the drugs and behavior modification program, but the husband has been complying with the other suggestions and is happy with the cat's progress to date. The clients have been instructed to call the Behavior Clinic *minimally* every 3 weeks for the first few months of treatment so that questions about behavioral changes can be addressed as they occur.

CASE 3

Signalment: "Fred" and "Woody," 14-year-old, 4.4 kg, male castrated, declawed, short-hair cat and 5-year-old, 6.4 kg, male castrated, declawed, short-hair cat

Initial Problems: Urine spraying and squatting to urinate outside the box by Woody, and aggression by Fred toward Woody.

History: The client acquired Woody at 3 months of age and Fred at 6 months of age. Both cats were castrated and

declawed at approximately 6 months of age. No other animals have lived in the household. Until the elimination problem was first noticed 18 month ago, there had been no behavioral or medical problems with either cat. Neither cat had ever been extremely friendly with or groomed the other.

Eighteen months ago, the client noticed a puddle of urine in the living room. The client began to find urine in the living room on a weekly basis. Woody had been seen to spray urine: he would stand vertically, quiver his erect tail, knead his feet, and spray. The most recent spraying had occurred the week before the appointment when Woody sprayed the area above the pilot light on the stove while the client stood directly in front of him. The client had also seen Woody squat and leave a puddle. She estimated that equivalent amounts of urine were produced by both postures. The client had found urine on walls in the dining room and kitchen, on the basement and living room stairs, on the stepdaughters' bedroom doors, and on the side of the kitchen trash can. Woody had sprayed or squatted in these areas every other day for the 6 months before the appointment. The first overt aggression between the cats occurred during this 6-month period.

In the year preceding the appearance of the overt aggression, the client had noticed a behavior that she called "squaring off": Fred would approach Woody and block Woody's access to a perch or a doorway. There would be no hissing, growling, shrieking, piloerection, spitting, or postural body and tail changes, but the cats would stare at each other. If Woody attempted to move past Fred, Fred repositioned himself in front of Woody and stared; Woody always left. Six months ago the squaring off became a daily event. In the 4 months before the appointment, actual fighting occurred three times per week as a sequela to the squaring-off behavior. Fred was the aggressor. He growled, shrieked, flattened his ears, lowered his head, and arched just before he batted Woody. Fred would then pounce on Woody, sinking his teeth into Woody's scruff.

Woody only attacked Fred when Fred was asleep; after the attack Woody always fled.

If the client held Woody on her lap and Fred entered the room, Fred would approach them. Approximately 50% of the time, Fred's approach was followed by a bout of squaring off. If the client held Fred on her lap and Woody entered the room, Woody would immediately leave. At the time of the appointment, the client believed that the cats squared off about 25% of the time that they saw each other and that they fought almost as often if she did not intervene with a water pistol.

The cats had two uncovered litter boxes, both filled with unscented clay litter. The client scooped the urine and feces from the boxes frequently, replaced the litter daily, and washed the boxes weekly. The client reported that Woody had never covered his feces, but that he energetically scratched outside the box after eliminating.

During the appointment Woody was allowed to roam, but Fred was kept in a cat carrier at the clinician's request. When Fred was released from his carrier he strode from the box with his head up, tail held vertically, and ears pricked and approached all unfamiliar individuals. He then turned, tread and kneaded with all four feet and quivered his tail. He did not spray. After he had done this to all unfamiliar people in the room, he rubbed all surfaces that were at cat height with his chin and head ("bunting"). Woody huddled in a corner and stared at Fred.

An attempt to pick up Woody, who, until then, had been favorably responsive to handling, was rebuffed by hissing. Physical examination revealed that Woody's heart rate had increased from the previously measured rate of 178 beats/min to well over 300 beats/min. This increase in heart rate was accompanied by panting. As soon as Woody was placed on the table, Fred immediately approached the individuals handling Woody and began to energetically rub them, vocalizing with mews and miaows. When Woody was replaced on the floor, he retreated to his corner, continuing to hiss, while Fred stared at him.

Physical and laboratory examination: Physical and laboratory examination revealed no abnormalities except a slight tartar accumulation and gingivitis for both cats.

Diagnosis: Woody had a diagnosis of spraying and urine marking (squatting associated with passive aggression) and intercat aggression (victim), and Fred's diagnosis was intercat aggression, as the aggressor. Although Woody did not cover his feces and performed most of his postelimination scratching outside the box, his behaviors were not consistent with an aversion or with a substrate or location preference.

Treatment: The client was asked to thoroughly clean all marked areas with a good odor neutralizer and to restrict the cats' access to these areas. The client was to add a covered litter box to provide an option for marking that had not previously existed. The client was to continue with her rigorous litter box cleaning routine. Both cats were to be separated when they were unsupervised so that they did not have the chance for subtle challenges. The client was to preferentially give Woody attention. If Fred entered the room and stared at Woody, she was to squirt Fred with a water pistol. If Fred persisted, she was to banish him to an undesirable area of the house. Both cats were to be fed in sight of each other and to have their dishes moved closer together at the rate of 3 to 5 mm every few days only if they ignored each other so that food was used as a reward for being calm in each other's presence (desensitization and counterconditioning). The client was to put both cats on leashes to prevent injury and to reward them with food treats when they either ignored each other or exhibited none of the

CASE 3—cont'd

signs of aggression discussed previously while in each other's presence (counterconditioning). If Fred showed any signs of aggression to Woody, he was to be sprayed with a water pistol. If he persisted he was to be banished. If Woody showed any signs of aggression to Fred, Fred was to be rewarded with a food treat if he looked away.

Woody was treated with buspirone (5 mg orally every 24 hours) with the hope that it would make Woody less anxious about both his previous marking and Fred's aggression and make Woody more assertive. Fred was treated with diazepam (1 mg orally every 12 hours) in an attempt to decrease his reactivity to Woody and to render Fred friendlier.

Follow-up: Two weeks after the initial appointment, there had been no spraying or marking. Within 1½ months the cats were tolerating each other when in each other's presence and there had been no spraying. After 2 months of problem-free behavior the client began to decrease both cats' drug doses. Fred was given 1 mg of diazepam every 24 hours for 1 week. Attempts to lower that dose resulted in a resurgence of an attenuated form of the original challenges. Woody began to pace and scan if given less than 2.5 mg of buspirone daily; therefore this was the maintenance dose. Six months later the clients report that they were able to discontinue Fred's diazepam and are able to control the occasional posturing events with the water pistol. The cats now tolerate each other and frequently sit side by side in the same window or on the same sofa. Woody has become more assertive and does not run from Fred, and Fred seldom threatens Woody. Woody's buspirone therapy will continue; he will have a serum biochemistry panel performed every 6 to 12 months or as warranted by clinical signs.

8 ····· Feline Elimination Disorders

···

*F*eline elimination disorders are the most common behavioral complaints of clients with cats. It has been estimated that between 40% and 75% of all cats with behavioral symptoms have an elimination disorder (Beaver, 1989, 1992; Blackshaw, 1988, 1992; Borchelt, 1991; Borchelt & Voith, 1986b; Halip, 1994; Olm & Houpt, 1988; Overall, 1993a). Olm and Houpt (1988) report that spraying and urination outside the litter box are equally common and are the most often reported feline elimination problems, followed by defecation and a combination of urination and defecation, respectively. Factors contributing to feline elimination disorders include those associated with environmental or social stresses, idiosyncratic preferences or changes in preferences, and medical problems, primarily feline urological symptoms (FUS) (Osborne et al., 1995; Ross, 1992). Because any number of urinary tract disease symptomologies are classified as FUS, newer terminology suggests that this acronym be used to mean feline urological *signs*, a concept encompassed in the more comprehensive label *feline lower urinary tract disease* (FLUTD) (Osborne et al., 1995). Although stressors associated with the social and physical environments are most frequently implicated in feline elimination disorders, associations with medical problems warrant some discussion.

In their study, Olm and Houpt (1988) reported that the overall lifetime incidence of FUS/FLUTD for the 59 cats studied was 30%, or 20 cats (5 of 19 sprayed; 7 of 19 urinated outside their box; 3 of 11 both urinated and defecated outside the box). The annual incidence rate in the United States and Great Britain of FUS/FLUTD (hematuria, dysuria, or urethral obstruction) is considered to be less than 1% (Lawler, 1985; Willeberg, 1984). The apparent disparity between the two figures suggests that medical problems may contribute to or cause feline behavioral problems involving elimination. In fact, the clinical signs of hematuria and frequent elimination of urine are the most common components of FUS and FLUTD, including cystitis, urethritis, and urethral blockage. The medical profile also fits many cats with behavioral elimination disorders: 2- to 4-year-old, male, castrated, overweight, indoor cats who eat primarily dry food (Buffington et al., 1994; Osborne et al., 1989). Accordingly, inappropriate urination is frequently cited as an initial sign for FUS and/or FLUTD (Barsanti & Finco, 1983; Green & Scott, 1983). A case-control study by Halip (1994) found that the presence of FUS or cystitis was a significant factor ($p \leq 0.0001$), but not necessarily causal, for cats with elimination disorders (85 cases) but not for controls (249 healthy cats with no discernible underlying pathologic condition). The latter study did not ask what percentage of the population of cats with medical urological symptoms have behavioral disorders as the cause of the symptoms. Invariably, this is the part of the scenario that is unexplored. Neurogenic inflammation has been implicated as a mediator in FLUTD. Unfortunately, the same constellation of chemical signals that cause pain is confounded with those that cause anxiety. Any animal in pain can learn to be anxious about the causes of pain.

Cats that have profound sterile cystitis may chew or lick at their abdomens (Buffington et al., 1993). Barbered patches or ulcerations that are found only in these areas may provide a clue to the underlying medical condition. It is critical that a cat brought for any elimination problem have a complete medical examination and rigorous follow-up.

A careful analysis of data collected from the Veterinary Hospital of University of Pennsylvania (VHUP) patient pool indicates that most behavioral disorders focusing on feline elimination are *not* caused by an underlying medical condition, but they may be associated with them (Beebe & Overall, 1997). Of 264 cases divided between those with behavioral problems and those with a medical (urinary tract) problem, 85% of the medical cases had no litter box problem, whereas 15% did. Of the behavioral cases, 63% had no concomitant medical problem, but 37% did (Fig. 8-1). Of cats whose main problem was behavioral, 45 had FLUTD; of 165 cats whose problem was medical, only 25 had a recorded history of an associated behavioral disorder (Fig. 8-2). These highly significant ($p < 0.001$) data suggest that the populations of patients with medically and behaviorally based elimination disorders are *not* the same, although cats that concomitantly experience both may form a third population. These data also suggest that urinary tract disease does not predispose a cat to a behavioral elimination problem. The definitive tests of the extent to which FLUTD is involved in behavioral problems would require that cystoscopy and ultrasound be done on all patients with behavioral signs and that all patients with medical signs be subject to behavioral history and observation.

Medical examinations should minimally include an excellent physical examination, including palpation of

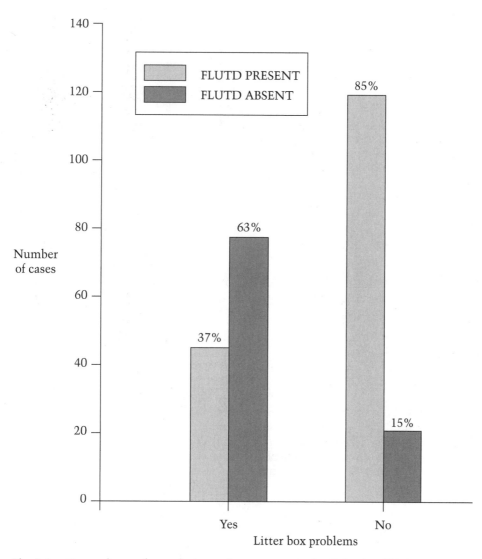

Fig. 8-1 Comparison of populations of cats seen at the Behavior Clinic at VHUP. "Yes" represents those with primary behavioral problems, "No" represents those with primary medical problems. Most of the patients with primary medical complaints that had some form of FLUTD did not have concomitant behavioral complaints. Approximately one third of patients with primary behavioral complaints had had a history of FLUTD at some point in their lifetime. Behavior Clinic data from Clinic patient population 1990-1994; medical population ($n = 264$) from survey of patients in 1994. (Beebe, unpublished, 1994.)

the kidneys and bladder, and a urinalysis or a fecal examination depending on the initial problem (Bernstein, 1977). If the cat is middle-aged or older (5 to 6 years of age or older), it might be advisable to perform a complete blood cell count, a serum biochemistry panel, and any viral titers deemed necessary on the basis of the cat's exposure. It is always advisable to perform at least annual blood studies on a middle-aged animal and annual to semiannual blood tests for an older animal because animals cannot tell us when they begin to feel ill. Clients should be encouraged to practice good preventative medicine. Performing an

annual prophylactic blood screening is an excellent idea that can solidify the veterinarian-client bond. When behavioral drugs might be used, it is especially critical to understand baseline values of serum biochemical profiles. Pending the results of the urinalysis, fecal examination, complete blood cell count, serum biochemistry panel, and any viral titers that may have been submitted, it may be advisable to perform ultrasonography, cystoscopy, or contrast radiography. Before rushing to perform all of these tests, it is important to remember that these cases are the exceptions; most feline elimination disorders are truly be-

Urinary tract disease

Litter box problems		Yes	No	TOTAL
	Yes	45	78	123
	No	120	21	141
	TOTAL	165	99	264

Statistic	Difference	Probability
Chi-square	1	0.000
Likelihood ratio chi-square	1	0.000
Continuity adjusted chi-square	1	0.000

Fig. 8-2 Chi-square table and statistics for numerical data presented in Fig. 8-1, indicating that the patient populations for behavioral versus medical complaints are different ($p < 0.001$) and that it would be imprudent to assume a causal association between the two. (Beebe, unpublished, 1994; Beebe and Overall, 1997.)

havioral. However, we would be remiss if we did not realize that complications from the disease can also complicate any elimination problem. Use of the "History Questionnaire for Cats with Elimination Disorders" (see Chapter 5) will aid greatly in organizing the clinician's thinking.

Finally, knowing when there is a problem or which cat is responsible for the problem can be difficult. For cats that are known to have medical conditions in which urine pH may play a role, diagnostic cat litter is available. MONIpHOR (Animal Resources, WestPort, Conn.) litter changes color to indicate pH in the range of 5.0 to 8.0. It can be mixed with other litters. Identification of the culprit in urine spraying or squatting can be more difficult. Fluorescein can be administered subcutaneously (0.3 ml at 100 mg fluorescein/ml = 10%) in the evening and will mark morning urine, or it can be administered in the same concentration orally (0.5 ml or distillate from 6 fluorescein strips in capsules) (Hart & Leedy, 1982; Koroffsky, 1987).

The first part of this chapter focuses on a description of the elimination disorders commonly experienced by cats. The second part of the chapter focuses on therapies for these elimination disorders. Box 8-1 lists the basic categories of behaviorally mediated inappropriate elimination, and Table 8-1 lists the relative frequency of the diagnosis based on the experience of the Behavior Clinic at VHUP.

AVERSIONS

Aversions to substrates or location can be difficult to distinguish from preferences and may invariably lead the cat to choose another location or substrate for elimination as a sequela to the aversion. It may never be clear why the cat developed an aversion to one location or to one substrate. When this occurs the aversion becomes apparent because of the cat's total avoidance of the offending area or surface. Cats can develop aversions quickly, as a result of horrific experience, or slowly, because of persistent, undesirable experiences. In the first case the cat could learn to avoid the litter box because something startled it when it was in the box. This is a problem for individuals who keep the

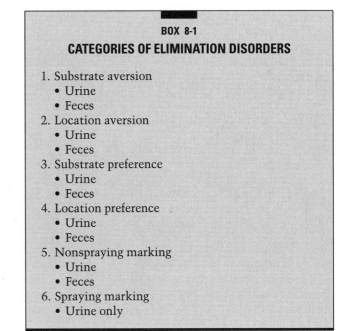

BOX 8-1
CATEGORIES OF ELIMINATION DISORDERS

1. Substrate aversion
   - Urine
   - Feces
2. Location aversion
   - Urine
   - Feces
3. Substrate preference
   - Urine
   - Feces
4. Location preference
   - Urine
   - Feces
5. Nonspraying marking
   - Urine
   - Feces
6. Spraying marking
   - Urine only

TABLE 8-1 FREQUENCY OF CAT DIAGNOSES ASSOCIATED WITH ELIMINATION DISORDERS AS A PROPORTION OF TOTAL DIAGNOSES

Behavioral Diagnosis	% of All Diagnoses
Substrate preference for urination	25
Spraying	14
Substrate preference for defecation	12
Nonspraying marking	4
Location preference for defecation	3

NOTE: 58% of all feline behavioral problems involve elimination

Data from Behavior Clinic, Veterinary Hospital of University of Pennsylvania, 1987 to 1994.

litter boxes near pieces of equipment that are attached to timers (e.g., televisions) or that cycle (e.g., washing machines).

In the second case the cat may decide that it dislikes the area or the substrate because it has had difficulty with it over a period of time. This is the more common situation if an animal has been frequently teased, abused, or victimized either by another cat, dog, or human while it is in the litter box or as it is either entering or exiting the litter box. Occasionally, in cases that involve aversions that have developed quickly in response to a horrific experience, clients report that the animal will hiss, growl, slink, or piloerect when found in proximity to either the substrate or the area.

Location Aversions

Aversions to locations are uncommon, but they certainly can be associated with the presence of any undesirable individual (Box 8-2). The undesirable individuals could include a person, a large dog, or a cat that torments the patient. An aversion to a location can also be associated with an object or a circumstance that the cat finds objectionable, such as a litter box that is placed in a busy access way or one placed by a noisy piece of equipment. Regardless, these circumstances should be rare, and the presence of litter boxes in laundry rooms, hallways, or closets was not significantly correlated with elimination disorders ($p \le 0.0612$, 0.0496, and 0.1094, respectively) in Halip's study (1994). Location aversions are best tested and addressed by environmental modification. Usually if the cat likes the litter, it is sufficient to identify what the cat dislikes about the area and to alter it. If it is impossible to alter the area after confirming a location aversion as a diagnosis, it may be best to find a new area to place the litter box. If the cat's aversion is purely to the location and not to the substrate, moving the box to an area that does not resemble the location postulated to be at the root of the aversion will help to be diagnostic. If the cat then uses the same box and same litter substrate, the client can be relatively sure that it is the *area* that the cat dislikes. If

the clients have multiple cats in their household, this is the time for them to ensure that there are no ongoing aggression problems with the cats that use that area. The association with feline aggression must be addressed. If the cat will use the relocated litter box and the client is willing to leave it in that area, this can be sufficient treatment for a location aversion.

Extreme caution is urged when the object of the dislike is mobile: a cat that torments another is unlikely to do so only in one location. If a cat is absolutely avoiding a specific area or a substrate for elimination, it will find another area until suitable options are presented. Regardless, clients should be aware that even in an aversion, there is a sampling and learning component to any elimination behavior.

Substrate Aversions

Substrate aversions are more common than location aversions. Cats can learn to dislike their litter because they associate it in a causal or noncausal manner with pain. For example, severe cystitis, a bad bout of colitis, or an experience with hard gravel after onychectomy (declawing) can all cause cats to associate their unfortunate experiences with the litter. It is also true that substrate aversions can be caused by a dislike of the sensory ramifications of the litter. In Halip's study (1994), lack of litter box use was significantly statistically correlated with sensory stimuli such as liners and litter type ($p \le 0.03$ for each). Sensory ramifications may include tactile and olfactory components such as filth, moisture, sticky litter, increased deodorants, a strong smell (e.g., aroma of cedar wood chips), litter box or litter odor, the odor of an ill animal that shares the box, hard or large gravel size, noises, or extraneous smells. Any tactile sensation associated with the litter itself, such as the fizzing of baking soda in boxes where the client adds baking soda to the gravel, may affect the cat's perception of the litter or litter box.

There are few solid, experimental data that evaluate the extent to which *any* of these factors are in-

---

BOX 8-2

PATTERNS OF CHANGES IN LOCATION OF ELIMINATION INVOLVING AGGRESSION

1. Location aversion
   - Scent of other cats
   - Physical exclusion by other cats
   - Victimization by other cats
   - Victimization by people, pets, or objects
2. Secondary location preference
   - Away from other cats
   - Away from noise
   - Away from activity
   - Other behaviors that correlate with an anxious, avoidant cat

volved in a multifactorial way in elimination disorders, but single-factor data from Halip (1994) indicate that there is no association between the incidence of disorders and incidence of scented litter, depth of litter, frequency of scooping out the litter box, or the addition of baking soda. The problem arises in such studies because multivariate data are treated in a bivariate (e.g., scented versus nonscented) form. Such treatments underevaluate any interactions and fail to identify subpopulations of cats that might cluster along constellations of correlated covarying factors. The assumptions are that all cats examined are from the same population and that behaviors within that population are normally distributed. Neither of these may be the case. The issues warrant further investigation.

If possible, it is important to identify and eliminate the putative offending substance and to offer the cat a wide choice of other substrates in a variety of depths and presentations. As with location aversion, clients can test whether the aversion is to a substrate by changing aspects of the substrate while leaving the box in the same area. If the cat returns to full use of the litter box, they know that the cat was developing a substrate aversion.

In any case involving an aversion, the cat develops a secondary substrate or location preference if the aversive situation is the cat's only other choice. It is critical to treat aversions as soon as they start to happen. Clues that the cat may dislike its litter or the area in which the litter is placed, but has not yet developed another preference, all involve attempts by the cat to exhibit appropriate elimination behaviors. In such situations the cat will often stand on the edge of the box and scratch outside it, but will not put its paws in the box. Cats can aim urine or feces in the general direction of the box while clinging to the edges so that they do not have to touch the litter. The cat can eliminate in an area adjacent to the litter box but not get in the box. If, after the advent of a new pet, the cat suddenly switches to one location where it tries to exhibit normal elimination behaviors but cannot (e.g., the back of a closet), a location in which the box might be placed is suggested (the closet) while hinting that the animal is having a problem with the present location. These are hypotheses that can be tested by altering first one and then the other of the potentially aversive options.

In some cases involving aversion, the cat, if forced to use that area, or if concerned about not being able to find a suitable area that is appropriate, will vocalize. Unfortunately, vocalization is a nonspecific symptom and may also be associated with an illness such as a urinary tract infection. If the cat does vocalize or seems to be distressed before elimination and either seems to be looking for an area similar to the one that it has used or seems to be moving around the box but not touching the substrate itself, this suggests that the source of the aversion is the box, the substrate, or the location.

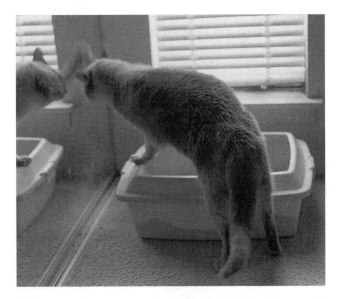

This cat does not have a clinical behavioral problem with elimination but does not like to stand in the box to eliminate. The box is next to a mirror, which the cat sniffs. It is likely that he recognizes himself, but if marking along the mirror were a problem one possibility would be whether he considered the reflection a challenge. When the cat finally does eliminate he does so with his back to the mirror (significance unknown), and perched only on the edge of the box. He could have perched on the side of the box, but then would have been turned slightly toward the mirror. This cat usually covers his urine, but does not always cover his feces. The clients keep the box fastidiously clean but report that the cat has never liked to walk in the litter. Dislike of the litter can be associated with a preference for something else. (Photo by Jesse F. Griffin.)

PREFERENCES
Substrate Preferences

Cats can develop preferences without developing a complete aversion. In such cases, they usually prefer soft substrates (Borchelt, 1991). Although Halip's study (1994) found no correlation between breed and elimination disorders, long-haired cats appear to be overrepresented in the population of cats with substrate preferences. One must question the extent to which long, fine hair is implicated in a desire for a clean, soft substrate. The usual presentation for a substrate preference is a cat that likes a consistent class of other substrates such as fabrics, bedding, towels, bath mats, and plastic trash bags but may use the litter box much of the time—particularly if excluded from other substrates that it prefers more.

Cats can prefer one aspect of a substrate, so it behooves the client to be a good observer. Some cats prefer open, reflective surfaces such as linoleum, wood floors, tiles, and bathtubs. The ancestral and wild condition for elimination in felines actually resembles the latter. It has been postulated that one reason for such a preference is visual and olfactory marking of a territory. It is also possible that leaving feces exposed is one way of reducing parasite load and recontamination by gastrointestinal parasites. Many cats that do not have elimination disorders never cover their feces; this can be a variant of normal. However, in Halip's case-control study (1994), cats that rarely or never cover their feces are overrepresented in the problem population ($G_{adj} = 15.90$, $p \leq 0.05$) and those that always do are underrepresented ($G_{adj} = 5.55$, $p \leq 0.05$) (statistics by author). These data suggest that these cats are exhibiting a suite of elimination behaviors, including those associated with normal marking behaviors, that predispose them to develop what people perceive as problems. No one has examined specific behavioral differences in cats that never covered their urine or feces and then stopped using their box and those that did cover but still stopped using the box, but there should be a difference in behaviors between these two groups. The variability in covering behavior is further inferential evidence that we do not "train" or "retrain" cats either to boxes or to specific elimination behaviors.

Any substrate preference or elimination can develop spontaneously or can be induced by a preexisting aversion. Many clients report a problem after an extended vacation when someone fed their cat but would not change the litter. In this case, an aversion is involved, but it is not an idiopathic aversion to an event that had remained constant. In this case, the aversion is iatrogenic: the cat is repulsed by the filthy litter and seeks another area from desperation. In the process of seeking another area, it learns about other substrates and may learn to prefer them. Iatrogenic aversions and preferences may well be neurochemically different than idiopathic ones (see Box 1-1 on p. 3).

Illness can also be implicated in the development of a preference. Any cat with cystitis or diarrhea may be unable to reach the litter box in time to eliminate in the appropriate area. In the process of eliminating in an inappropriate area, the cat could discover that it likes carpeting, for example. Inherent in these two descriptions of a secondary substrate preference compounded by either illness or iatrogenic effects is the concept of learning. Early intervention should occur before having the cat learn that it likes a variety of substrates and before a complete shift in preference occurs. If cats do shift preference, the shift is possible to treat but is harder to address the longer it has occurred. When clients first obtain cats, they should be made aware that elimination disorders are the single most common behavior complaint in cats. Clients who know this can observe and define "normal" for their cat and seek help early in the history of undesirable behaviors. In many cases involving substrate preferences for elimination, the preferences are subtle or have been occurring for years. These cases are difficult, and an alert, educated client is the best ally.

A substrate preference for urination is far more common than that for defecation. Some cats will defecate in the litter box, but look elsewhere for an area or substrate to urinate. Any time a cat behaves in this manner, it is a hint that the ultimate resolution might require separate litter boxes for urination and defecation. If clients are able to observe the cat's behavior both inside the litter box and when using the inappropriate substrate, they can learn whether the cat exhibits behaviors associated with like or dislike of their substrate. A cat that will not get inside the litter box but stands on the edge and digs outside the box might not like the feel of the substrate. If the same cat then circles, digs, and covers the urine or feces aggressively when using the client's sheets, a change of substrate is indicated. The newer, fine-grained, silaceous, disposable kitty litters have been a real boon to cats with substrate preferences (see photo below). In a study conducted on naive cats that were having no inappropriate elimination behaviors (Borchelt, 1991), most cats in humane shelters would switch to the clumpable litters if given the choice of plain kitty litter, which they had formerly used without incident, and the soft, silaceous, recyclable, clumpable litters. This is an important finding because these are animals that never had a problem. This result hints at an innate preference for a softer substrate that is similar to substrates experienced by ancestral cats. No data are available to indicate whether *Felis libycus* would choose a gravel substrate over a sandy one, but strong inference based on the evolutionary history of the cats may give some clues as to why they behave the way they do. The drawback to the newer silicate, clumpable litters is that they are quite fine, and clients often complain about sand being dragged through the house (but there are newer less soft, nontrackable formulations). A jute mat placed around the

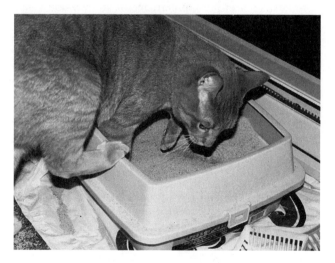

Cat digging in clumpable, silaceous litter. This cat likes digging in this box and he does not have a problem. Notice evidence of energetic digging in litter scooped outside. Note that box and litter are clean (see scoops at lower right). (Photo by Liz Krug.)

outside of a litter box can help, as can a soft, terry bath mat. If the cat truly likes soft toweling far more than it likes any soft litter, the client will learn this quickly because the cat will prefer to use the terry bath mat. In such cases it will not be possible to use a soft mat to catch the sand from the litter box.

The other issue that has not been examined in depth is the extent to which long-haired cats could potentially like the softness of these litters or dislike them because of the fineness of their fur. Soft, fine substrates catch in soft, fine fur. Fur texture in cats and preferences for substrates for litter and for resting spots have not been well examined. There may be more of an interaction than any data currently suggest. It is interesting to note that an autosomal dominant form of polycystic kidney disease is recognized in Persians (Biller et al., 1990). Affected cats can show signs as early as 6 to 8 weeks. The extent to which such conditions are a factor for cats that "were never litter box trained" is unknown.

Location Preferences

No aversion or preference is developed in a vacuum: social situations and individual personality traits must be considered (Box 8-2). In addition to a new litter, a shy cat might prefer a covered litter box. A cat that feels vulnerable to other cats in the household might prefer a litter box in a closet or one behind a kitty door. With patience and attention to what the cat is trying to "tell" the client, these situations can be resolved. In severe cases involving social ramifications, an indoor, electronic fence can be fitted to cats to keep them out of other cats' boundaries. Electronic eyes can be adapted to cat flaps or closet doors so that only the cat wearing a coded collar can enter the litter box. Although these solutions are more complicated than most, they are still preferable to euthanizing a cat because of either a preference or an aversion based on profound social ramifications.

Location preferences develop more frequently because of a social situation or because the cat prefers another spot of access, smell, or view. Location preferences are often difficult to understand but are easy to treat if the client is patient. Whereas treatment for a substrate preference involves offering the animal a variety of substrates, sequentially, to identify preferences, treatment for location preferences involves placing the litter box with the same substrate in it in the area the animal is using for elimination. If the cat then eliminates next to the box, the client has a hint that the problem is either a mixed substrate-location preference or a substrate preference. Location preferences usually are restricted to one or a few spots, which facilitates placement of the litter box in that particular area. In a true location preference, the cat chooses one or a few locations for urination or defecation; these usually exclude the current area of the litter box. Again, if a litter box is placed in this area and the cat starts to use it, the diagnosis of a location preference for elimination has been confirmed.

If the cat either shifts to another area or has generally a few areas that it uses, some clients have been successful in counterconditioning the cat not to use that area. This can be done by either placing food or water dishes in one of the areas that the cat has used while placing the litter box in the other. If the animal eliminates right next to the food or water dishes, the concept of feeding stations to countercondition the cat will not be successful.

If the cat starts to use the litter box in any of the areas where it has been placed, the box can be moved 1 to 2 inches a day until it is in a more appropriate place. The mistake that clients make in modifying the cat's choice of a location is that they move the box too quickly. Once the cat starts to use the box in the area where it has already soiled the underlying substrate, that box must be left there for a week or two until the cat has demonstrated that it is not going to choose other areas. Then, and only then, should the client gradually start to move the box. Moving the litter box 1 to 2 inches a day is not a large distance by clients' standards, but it is a huge distance by cats' standards. Practitioners need to caution clients that if they expand the rate at which the box is moved, it will be apparent to the cat that it has a choice of disparate areas and the cat may relapse.

Marking

Marking most commonly involves spraying; however, nonspraying marking is a serious problem in cats and can be difficult to differentiate from a location preference.

Nonspraying Marking. Marking can involve spraying or marking with urine or feces. Large, wild cats frequently mark the boundaries of their territories in all of these manners. Domestic cats can mark in one location or in a variety of locations. Marking problems are not resolved without understanding the underlying social system of the cat. If feline visitors come to one door and that is the only place where feces or a pool of urine is found, nonspraying marking is probably the diagnosis. Spraying can certainly occur in the same circumstances, but nonspraying marking is underrecognized and underdiagnosed in veterinary medicine. In many cases, nonspraying marking is inappropriately diagnosed as an intractable or refractory substrate or location preference. If relationships between cats in the household have changed or the client has noted a change in nonhousehold feline visitation, nonspraying marking should be at the top of the list of differential diagnoses. Hypotheses that the problem is one of a location or substrate preference can be tested with the previously described manipulations. If these manipulations do not address the problem, some data about the social environment will convince the clinician to consider a diagnosis of nonspraying marking.

Nonspraying marking with urine is one presentation of the ancestral condition in cats, as is marking with feces. There is no evidence that we have exerted any selective pressure to eliminate the tendency to squat and mark in the domestic cat.

Spraying. Spraying is part of a normal, feline behavioral repertoire in free-ranging situations. Domestic cats spray as part of normal elimination behavior and as part of a normal social system. Spraying is a dimorphic behavior; more males spray than do females. This dimorphism may be related to the skewed sex ratio for mating that is noted for lions (Bertram, 1975; Macdonald, 1983) and free-ranging and domestic cats (Beaver, 1981d; Hart, 1975; Macdonald & Apps, 1978). After neutering, 10% of all males that sprayed before neutering persist in spraying, whereas 5% of all females that sprayed before neutering persist (Cooper & Hart, 1992; Hart & Barrett, 1973; Hart & Cooper, 1984); however, when raw data are compared statistically, neutering does not decrease spraying more for one sex than the other ($p > 0.05$, $G_{adj} = 2.568$). These data suggest that spraying is not solely modulated by sexual influences. In fact, despite the fact that it is a dimorphic behavior, spraying is less a sexual problem than it is a social problem. The extent to which this sexually dimorphic behavior reflects the social system of felines has been underappreciated in veterinary medicine.

Domestic cats can mark in one location or in a variety of locations. Marking problems are not solved without addressing any relevant social situations (Hart & Cooper, 1984; Hart et al., 1993). Indoor cats that are visited by outdoor cats might start to spray the windows or sliding doors where outdoor cats are visible, particularly if the visiting cats spray.

Such situations can also occur within a household. Bold cats can often announce their presence or status by spraying everywhere. Less confident cats may try to carve out their own niche by spraying there, by marking with feces, or by squatting. Faced with outright aggression, less confident cats may resort to spraying after the fact because they are not temperamentally suited to direct fighting. The extent to which spraying and nonspraying marking occur in various social situations has never been carefully documented. Theoretically, spraying should occur less frequently in situations in which cats feel confident; however, there is a documented role in wild cats for advertising displays involving both the visual and olfactory components of spraying. The situation is likely to be more complex in domestic cats that are confined. All social ramifications must be considered before the treatment of any marking can be successful. Because both males and females can spray, it is important to realize that either sex can experience anxiety associated with the social system. Anxiety is often indicated by autonomic hyperreactivity (tachycardia, mydriasis when in the presence of another cat), by increased motor activity (fleeing, pacing) when approached by or within view of another cat, or by vigilance and scanning of the environment. Furthermore, either sex can spray as an advertisement, a threat, or a response to a threat. The manner in which the inappropriate behavior is manifest largely depends on the social system in the household.

Clients often confuse spraying with urination. Clients should be encouraged to describe the cats' postures and to note locations. If they are able to see the cat and they note that it is standing and wiggling its tail with a blissful or a silly look on its face, then it is spraying. Clients should know that cats, particularly those that are confident, can exhibit the behaviors associated with the visual display of spraying without excreting any urine. Cats often knead with their feet while they spray; it has been postulated that when they do this, they are also marking the area with interdigital sebaceous gland secretions. Sprayed urine usually hits vertical surfaces and drips down. It is important that clients examine backs of chairs, backs of couches, and walls above the baseboards. It is preferable if clients are willing to get down on their hands and knees in their stocking feet and both sniff and feel any areas they might believe implicated. The fact that the urine is not found on a vertical surface does *not* mean that the animal is not spraying. Cats can stand in the middle of a horizontal surface, such as a bed, and spray. In these situations they leave a long, thin, wet area, rather than a circular puddle. It is important that clients crawl over every inch of carpet. If there is a urine puddle in the middle but nowhere else, it is unlikely that the cat is spraying.

THE ROLE OF FELINE AGGRESSION IN FELINE ELIMINATION DISORDERS

The extent to which elimination is associated with feline aggression is discussed in Chapter 7. Behavioral factors underlying the elimination and their potential associations with aggression are discussed here.

Because most common feline behavioral problems involve inappropriate elimination, it is critical to evaluate the extent to which an aversion, preference, or marking situation can be involved in a social problem. Feline elimination behaviors do not happen in a social vacuum: domestic and wild cats use both scrapes and elimination products to mark their territory. Cats are motivated to respond to olfactory cues in their environment, and cats are well equipped with a variety of devices, including glandular secretions, by which they can lay their scent in the area. When cats rub against someone and knead or mark with their head, chin, or cheek whiskers, they are leaving behind sebaceous gland secretions that can be detected by another cat. Cats have a superb sense of smell. It has been estimated that the size of the olfactory epithelium in cats can be up to 20 cm; this contrasts dramatically with the 2 to 4 cm of olfactory epithelium estimated for humans (Bradshaw, 1992a). It has been postulated that cats' olfactory abilities run on a parallel order with those of dogs, and dogs can detect compounds of thresholds a thousand times lower than those detectable for humans (Davis, 1973). Given this fact, it is not surprising that feline social systems are mediated in part by olfactory mechanisms and that these in turn may be a factor in elimination disorders. Accordingly, it is important to characterize patterns of spraying and nonspraying marking that are involved in feline aggression.

Patterns of spraying that are involved in feline aggression include the following (Box 8-3): (1) active aggression, (2) passive aggression, and (3) status-related spraying. Active aggression usually involves a confident cat spraying. Confident cats can spray because of sexual advertisement in competition, advertisement unassociated with sex, or after aggression or as a victory display. Advertisement unassociated with sex may actually avoid future physical aggression. Postaggression victory signals may decrease the probability of future aggressive events. Victory displays have been postulated to function in any situation involving allocation of resources, including time. Any time that can be spent defusing an aggressive situation, particularly if it is a hopeless one, can be better used for other behaviors (Sebeok, 1977).

It has been underappreciated that passively aggressive cats can spray. Cats that are exhibiting a passive, rather than an active, physical aggression are usually less confident than other cats. They can use spraying as (1) a passive threat, (2) a response to a preceding physical threat from an animal with which they do not feel they can adequately contest, (3) a response to an olfactory cue from another animal that may be higher or lower on the hierarchy but still is not a viable target for a physical contest, or (4) an anxious or fearful response to uncertain circumstances. The latter has been underappreciated as a form of passive aggression. Animals that are less than confident may, when a social system changes by the addition or absence of another animal, learn to deform that social system further by spraying. This is a form of advertisement that could provide information that otherwise would not be available. Depending on the response to their spraying, they are able to

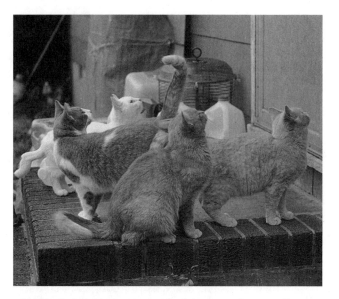

This multi-cat situation is ideal for complex social interactions that may include aggression and marking. The postures of the cats indicate that the order and placement of the cats at the door is not random. (Photo by Jesse F. Griffin.)

ascertain information that they cannot get in a direct manner.

The extent to which cats are exhibiting spraying because of their social status has been underappreciated. This type of status-related spraying could also involve marking with urine or feces, but it could be a purely behavioral rather than a behavioral and olfactory display. The postures that accompany spraying are stereotypic and would be recognized by another feline as associated with assertion of status, the claim to territory, or both. In many cases cats of high status will be defining a "mine" versus a "not-mine" situation. The objects they may be claiming could be locations, inanimate objects, or people. In this case the spraying is less related to the rest of the underlying social interactions; it acts to preempt status for them. In status-related spraying, the presence or absence of other cats in the social system is relatively less important than the overall statement of assertion of position by the individual spraying cat.

It is also important to address patterns of nonspraying marking that are involved in aggression (Box 8-4). Nonspraying marking can also involve cats that are active aggressors, passive aggressors, and individuals that alternate between the two strategies. In nonspraying marking, the active aggressor tends to be a confident cat. The cat is usually (1) marking a new territory, (2) conducting a preemptive strike against a newcomer or a potential newcomer, (3) exhibiting and demonstrating differences between core and use areas for its territory, or (4) making a social statement without any form of sexual statement. There are insufficient data to ascertain the sex ratio of cats that engage

---

BOX 8-3

ELIMINATION DISORDERS MOST FREQUENTLY ASSOCIATED WITH AGGRESSION

1. Spraying
   - Victim
   - Aggressor
2. Nonspraying marking
   - Victim
   - Aggressor
3. Location aversion and second preference
   - Victim

BOX 8-4

**PATTERNS OF NONSPRAYING MARKING
INVOLVING AGGRESSION**

1. Active aggression—confident cat (aggressor)
   - New territory
   - Preemptive strike
   - Differences between core and use areas
   - Social without being sexual
2. Passive aggression—less confident cat (victim)
   - Attempt to claim turf
   - Response to socially thwarted challenge
3. Passive and active aggression
   - Response to physically thwarted challenge (visual or olfactory cue out of range)

---

in nonspraying marking. Without such data, it is fruitless to compare the extent to which this behavior is dimorphic with the extent to which spraying is dimorphic. There are also insufficient data to determine the extent to which nonspraying marking is prevalent in the aforementioned behavioral circumstances.

In passive aggression associated with nonspraying marking, the less confident cat or the victim in the aggressive event may attempt to either claim turf by using urine or feces in a nonspraying fashion or respond to a socially thwarted challenge by using nonspraying marking. One can postulate that nonspraying marking may be a component of the behaviors in these passive or victimized cats because the behaviors associated with spraying convey information separate from that conveyed by olfactory cues. These victimized cats may be unable to risk the social consequences of such an overt behavioral display. For nonspraying marking associated with victims, the victims do not have to risk giving behavioral information that they may be unable to back up physically.

Finally, some cats switch between passive and active aggression by nonspraying marking. In these cases they are usually responding to a physically thwarted challenge in which the cue is out of range but is either visual or olfactory. They then act as the aggressor; however, if the other individual responds, they become passive again until the individual is out of sight. There are few data on such cats, but in-depth histories from clients indicate that they appear to exist.

Data collected on free-ranging domestic cats have shed some light on the importance of the social system in both feline elimination disorders and the potential for feline elimination disorders involved with aggression. Macdonald and Apps (1978) studied free-ranging cats living under farm conditions in Great Britain. They measured both the core areas and the home-range use areas for these cats over the course of a year. Not surprisingly, male cats ranged farther than

female cats; the average home-range size of males extended from 0.4 ha to 990 ha. The home-range size for females ranged from 0.02 ha to 170 ha. The average range, overall, was between 0.1 ha and 0.45 ha. The average apartment is anywhere from one to three orders of magnitude smaller than that range. Is it any wonder that when multiple cats converge in small territories, there may be some social jockeying?

Hierarchical systems based on deference are usually a mechanism for avoiding conflict in households (Bernstein & Strack, 1993). The study of feline social systems in wild cats, such as lions has focused on females as family units (Bertram, 1975; Packer & Pusey, 1983). In such situations the females in the group are usually related and the males are unrelated to the females. One male controls access to breeding of many females. Few younger males ever have any reproductive success. In evolutionary systems involving high variance in reproductive success, contest for position is common. Selection over evolutionary time may have reinforced social systems that facilitated such competition. Such social systems would be maintained in the absence of sexual overtones. This is exactly what happens in domestic cat situations involving neutered animals. Even within the free-ranging, wild felid social hierarchies, females have an independent hierarchy that is largely based on age but that is also influenced by other social characteristics and physical characteristics such as strength. Bernstein and Strack (1993) have noted that most individuals with more than one house cat are able to rank their cats according to some deference-based or conflict-based hierarchy and to articulate reasons pertaining to specific behaviors for why they think one cat is more highly ranked than the other.

If elimination disorders and their social ramifications are to be addressed fully, it is important that these newer findings be heeded. An outline for using behavioral and environmental modification in these situations is found in Box 8-5.

TREATMENT OF FELINE ELIMINATION DISORDERS

Any potential underlying medical cause must be ruled out for problem elimination in cats, even if not generally implicated. Such causes include various gastrointestinal diseases, endoparasitemia, bacterial disease; inflammatory disease; anatomical abnormalities; partial or complete obstructions; inflammatory bowel disease; nutritional disorders such as maldigestion and malabsorption syndromes; metabolic disease, including liver and kidney disease; food allergies, or debilitating conditions that would preclude easy access to appropriate elimination areas, such as arthritis. Urinary incontinence caused by ureteral ectopia or incompetence of the urethral sphincter mechanism is more rare in cats than in dogs (Barsanti & Downey, 1984). Urine leakage associated with sphincter incompetence is seen only in female cats and is more common when they are recumbent or asleep. Urinary tract

---

BOX 8-5

BEHAVIORAL AND ENVIRONMENTAL MODIFICATION FOR ELIMINATION DISORDERS ASSOCIATED WITH AGGRESSION

1. Reduce stressors and anxiety-provoking event
   - Separate animals when not supervised
   - Provide additional three-dimensional turf
   - Cover windows
   - In cases of status-related aggression or active aggression, banish aggressor to less desirable turf
2. Countercondition and desensitize animals to each other's presence
   - Feeding arenas
   - Treats with leashes
   - Crates/gates
   - Games/pleasurable experiences (grooming)
3. Correction/punishment
   - Bell—spy on animals
   - Correct within first 30 to 60 seconds of **onset** of behavioral process
   - Use banishment
4. Reward structure
   - Reward if pet responds to correction *and* will exhibit a better behavior
   - Reward when calm and quiet
   - Reward in small increments
   - Provide quality time for each pet
5. Environmental modification
   - Barriers
   - Exclusion
   - Clean and odor neutralization
   - Gradual reintroductions

---

infections are more common in cats with ureteral ectopia (Holt & Gibbs, 1992).

Although prevalence rates are unknown, constipation, anal sac impaction, and pain have been listed as reasons that cats will not use the litter box (Houpt, 1991b). Only after these potential underlying physical and physiological causes have been ruled out should the practitioner proceed with the premise that the elimination disorder is rooted in behavior. Generally, this step can be quickly and effectively completed.

The second step in treating any aversion, preference, or marking situation is to interfere with the olfactory component. All affected areas must be cleaned with a good odor eliminator. All layers involved must be cleaned. This means that if the client has wall-to-wall carpeting over a subfloor, the wall-to-wall carpet, the pad underneath it, and the subfloor all must be cleaned, or replaced. When replacement is not possible, the client can seal the connecting areas with either heavy-gauge plastic, physical moisture/vapor barriers, or chemical moisture barriers that can be painted on the subfloor. In some cases floorboards

or tiles must be replaced. Odor eliminators that have been relatively successful include The Equalizer,* KOE,† ElimOdor,‡ Anti-Icky Poo (AIP).§ Comparative studies (Beaver, 1989b; Melese, 1994a,b) indicated that clients report the best success with AIP. Information on where to obtain odor eliminators is provided in Appendix C. No odor eliminator can be expected to undo years of repeated assaults. Accordingly, clients should be told of the importance of early treatment for elimination disorders, just as they are provided with advice about prophylactic vaccinations. Behavior kills more cats annually than does viral disease.

After cleaning the affected areas, clients should cover the areas with heavy-gauge insulating plastic to both change the tactile sensation for the cat and to prevent penetration in the event of further elimination. While this step is ongoing, it is preferable to isolate the cat to an area with controlled access to litter boxes and different substrates. It is critical to break the olfactory cycle.

The next procedures are more suited to treatment of aversions or preferences but can also be helpful for spraying and nonspraying marking (Beaver, 1981e; Hart & Cooper, 1984).

Substrates

Encourage the client to get multiple litter boxes, generally one more than there are cats, unless the clients are inundated with cats. Large numbers of cats may render work to inhibit response to a stimulus ineffective. Anyone with large numbers of cats can expect that they will not have the response that they would have if they had fewer cats. If individuals have 10 or more cats, they have a 100% probability that at some point one of those cats will spray (Hart & Cooper, 1984; Marder, 1991). Again, this refers back to the importance of the social system in the hierarchy. Because litter boxes can be implicated as turf in socially mediated conflicts, it is critical to apportion the litter box turf in a manner that will convince the cats to use them appropriately. Litter boxes should be placed in a variety of locations and should be of a variety of styles (open, covered, deep, shallow, big, small); they should *not* all be placed in one area.

Although Halip's (1994) study showed a nonsignificant association with litter box cleaning frequency, his study did not test for specific populations of cats that were more affected by this than others. Data from VHUP indicate that this population of cats exists and that instantaneous use of a clean litter box can be re-

---

*Enzymatically degrades urine (EVSCO, Buena, NJ).
†Prevents aerosolization of volatile compounds (AOE, Thornell Corp., Penfield, NY).
‡Prevents aerosolization of volatile compounds (Beecham, West Chester, PA).
§Both enzymatic degradation of urine and prevention of aerolization of volatile compounds (Bug-A-Boo Chemicals, Lakeside, CA).

lated to hierarchy. Preemptive use of newly cleaned litter boxes has also been reported by Bernstein and Strack (1993).

Litter should be scooped daily, and most litter should be dumped totally every other day. The exception to this is the clumpable, recyclable litters and the litter boxes that involve stones and pads that absorb moisture. In the latter case the pad is discarded daily. In the former case the soiled litter will clump up and the rest of it remains relatively uncontaminated. Regardless, even clumpable litters must be dumped minimally every couple of weeks (consider more frequent dumping). The cat will tell the client when the litter needs to be dumped. The stones in the apparatus involving pads must be washed weekly. Without exception, boxes should be washed weekly. Halip's (1994) study found that heavy use of disinfectants caused cats to use boxes less. Some old boxes may be so permeated with scent and so scratched that they prevent elimination of scent by cleaning, and they should be discarded.

A variety of litters should be offered to the cat in a variety of boxes. Unfortunately, it is impossible to set up a controlled experimental design for cats. Still, the clients can gauge how successful they might be by using substances resembling the substances the cat has chosen to use. If the cat is using soft substrates such as bedding, towels, or laundry, consider softer litters. Number 3 blasting sand and fine-grade playground sand are inexpensive and extremely soft to the touch. They do not absorb either moisture or smell as well as some of the commercial litters, but they can be dumped multiple times a day at little expense. Shredded newspaper or paper toweling are also relatively inexpensive and soft. Again, neither absorb moisture or scent as well as traditional litters. Yesterday's News (Moncton, NB) is a newer litter made from recycled newspapers. It has been formulated to absorb moisture well, but it still does not absorb some odors as well as some other litters. Many cats are fussy about touching soft substrates and will use this litter in the absence of any others. Sawdust or wood chips that are not from strong smelling substances (i.e., not cedar) can be useful as adjuvants for litter boxes. Saw mills may allow clients to have these for free or for a small charge. Some of the newer clay litters have pine chips added to provide the softening aspect. The most successful results appear to be obtained by using recyclable, clumpable litters (Borchelt, 1991). The client must be observant and creative. Clients are usually cooperative because they are being provided with an opportunity to do something.

Locations

If the elimination problem involves a location preference or aversion, a litter box with a litter that the cat likes can be placed in the area. If the cat starts to use it, a location preference or aversion is indicated. If the cat does not use it, the client will have to use the sampling procedure outlined here.

Counterconditioning can work for some disorders involving locations. Food dishes can be placed in the effective area. Generally, cats will not eliminate where they are fed; some will. If the number of locations is great, this approach will not work, but if the number of locations is small, a location preference is not indicated. If it is possible to rearrange furniture or move a large plant so that the cat's favorite spot is covered, this should be done. Sometimes the cat shifts its spot. If this happens, it may be that the location was not sufficiently altered or it may be suggestive of a mixed substrate/location preference.

Scat Mats (Contech Electronics, Saanichton, BC) and other aversive devices are often suggested as part of the treatment for elimination disorders. A Scat Mat (see Appendix C) works electronically by emitting a shock whenever the cat stands on it. Of course, any other animal in the household not exhibiting the problem will also have the same experience if it touches the mat. Because such devices do not change the perception of the regional environment, cats often shift their elimination pattern so that they are eliminating next to the device, but not on it. It would be inappropriate to recommend these devices unless one specific area is to be avoided, and there are no social impediments involved in the problem. Almost without exception, this is never true.

Cats are not trained to litter boxes. It is a myth that cats are retrained to use them. In the absence of human intervention, cats develop a substrate preference. At 3 to 5 weeks of age, cats begin to explore open substrates and, if presented with a litter box, a kitten might lie in it. Between 5 and 7 weeks of age the cat might start to eliminate in the litter box and may, or may not, cover the feces. Covering of the feces occurs at about 7 weeks of age when the olfactory system and the neuromuscular system are more developed. It is not abnormal if cats do not cover their urine or feces. As discussed previously, not covering urine or feces may be the ancestral state. Accordingly, cats with an elimination problem cannot be retrained to use a litter box; however, they can be encouraged to make their own preferred associations in ways clients find acceptable. This can be done by taking the cat to the litter box frequently and waiting with it. If it uses the box, it should be praised. Some clients are also able to associate the appropriate elimination behaviors, such as scratching in the box, with giving the cat a food treat. Anything that can be done to encourage the cat to use its litter box should be done. No cat should be disturbed or frightened while it is in the litter box.

If the cat is seen to squat outside the box, the only type of punishment that should be executed is punishment that is geared to startling the cat so that it aborts the inappropriate behavior and is able to be placed in a situation in which a more appropriate behavior can be encouraged. It is best if the startle or correction takes place within the first few seconds of the onset of the behavior. Within the first 30 to 60 seconds of the complete behavioral sequence, which includes sniffing, turning, and scratching, if startled, the cat will be able to couple the startle behavior with learning. If the cat has been digging and has already eliminated, it is fruitless to startle or correct the cat. Psychologists have demonstrated that individuals learn best if they are interrupted in the act of doing something inappropriate. The interruption must come within the first few seconds of the onset of the behavior but no later than 30 to 60 seconds after the onset of the suite of behaviors associated with the problem behavior. It is important to remember that clients will be able to identify behaviors associated as precursors to elimination, including facial expressions in some cats. If the cat is startled after it has finished eliminating and is digging in the carpet, the clients might simply need to teach the cat to become more secretive and/or to abort the last phase of the elimination behaviors. The startle must be sufficient to make the cat abort the behavior and leave but cannot be so horrific that the cat becomes fearful. This means that the amount of stimulus necessary to startle the animal will vary from cat to cat. Obviously, a foghorn should not be used on a timid animal that is already eliminating in an out-of-the-way place because of problematic social interactions. Similarly, a foghorn should not be used if there is another fearful animal or a human infant in the house. Foghorns are usually inappropriate in apartments, but water pistols, whistles, squeakers, compressed air canisters, perfume atomizers, and tins of pennies all work with some cats. Usually, the softer the stimulus (tins of pennies), the more easily the cat habituates to it. Clients usually derive a great deal of pleasure from any apparatus that allows them to participate in correcting the cat. Because this is true, it really must be emphasized that physical punishment, including rubbing the cat's nose in the soiled area or flicking the cat's nose with a finger, is absolutely useless and should be avoided. Physical punishment, especially if it is painful or scary, often has the reverse effect, particularly in elimination disorders associated with social problems. It is easier for clients to spy on cats and correct them within the first few seconds of the onset of the inappropriate behaviors if they know where the cat is. This can be accomplished by placing a bell on the cat's collar. The preferred collar type is a feline breakaway collar. No animal should be left confined with a collar on which it might strangle. (NOTE: This also means that leaving a dog with a choker on in the house is absolutely inappropriate.) Because cats are prone to squeeze themselves through strange spaces, even regular, flat buckle collars can pose a danger to them. Any cat that wears a collar should wear a breakaway collar.

In some cases if the problem has been ongoing for an extended period of time, it is optimal to separate the cat from everyone in the household and confine it. At this point the clients must realize that the confined cat needs the same amount of attention it would have received had it not been confined. This means that they should be willing to go into the room and spend time with the cat and groom it, play with it, and make sure that it is getting appropriate nutrition. The cat should be placed in a room that has not been previously soiled and should be offered food, water, and a choice of litter box styles and litters. Litters can vary in type and in depth, and boxes can vary in size and attribute (covered vs. not covered). It is impossible for clients to be able to do a complete factorial design that would unambiguously provide a significant result about which attributes that cat prefers, but based on the history, educated guesses can be made about the types of substrates, locations, or litter box styles the cat might prefer. Examples of these are given in the case histories.

If there is a problem in the social hierarchy in the household, it will influence where the cat is incarcerated. If a high-ranking cat is spraying and it is being medicated for spraying (discussed below), even if it does not have problems generally with the choice of litter boxes, it may be encouraged to spray against the back of a covered box. Regardless, while adjusting to therapeutic levels of the medication suggested for controlling the spraying, it is critical that the aggressor be isolated. It would be inappropriate to isolate the aggressor in a high-quality area that the aggressor prefers. Such areas may include kitchens, bedrooms, or rooms with big picture windows that are commonly used as perch sites. In this case the aggressor has to accept that other animals are allowed to live in the household, and one of the ways to passively reinforce that is to place this animal in a neutral or lower quality room. "Lower quality" is determined by social attributes, not physical ones. It would be inappropriate to enclose the animal in a dank garage or a damp basement. If possible, it is desirable to give cats perch sites at all times. If the individual cat with the elimination problem is a lower-ranking animal and you suspect that part of the problem is related to its inability to assert itself in the social hierarchy, it is best to isolate that animal in an area of high status. If the cats sleep with the client, the cat should be kept in a bedroom all day long. The cat does not know where the other cats are, but they will be able to tell that this animal has been allowed to occupy the "high-quality" area. When there are two equally matched aggressive animals, it is best to either separate them into neutral areas or to alternate between the high-quality and neutral or low-quality area. Regardless, it is critical to monitor their elimination behaviors while they are in these rooms because if they either start to spray or continue not to use the litter box, it is important that additional substrates not be soiled. Once the animals are using the appropriate substrate for elimination, they can be released from the confined area gradually. This means that they are to be belled, again using a breakaway collar, and for increasing periods of time over a few weeks gradually reintroduced to small sections of the house only when they are supervised. If after a few weeks the clients have had no problems with either the other cats in the household or with elimination in any other area, they can build up the amount of time that the cat is allowed to range free during the next week until the cat again has free range.

Clients should be warned that relapse can be problematic in cases of feline elimination disorders. A complete "Protocol for Cats With Elimination Disorders" in client handout form is found in Appendix B.

Pharmacological Approaches

The environmental and behavioral modifications necessary to treat feline elimination disorders were discussed before the pharmacological ones because it is important to not proceed directly to a pharmacological approach, thereby skipping the behavioral and environmental modifications. Clients who proceed only with pharmacological measures often maintain that the medication does not work. Medication used to treat behavioral disorders does not work in a vacuum—it works in the context of the environmental and behavioral environments. It would be wholly inappropriate to treat a behavioral disorder pharmacologically without pursuing these other avenues either before pharmacological intervention or simultaneously with it. In many cases, such as location aversions or preferences for defecation in cats, pharmacological intervention is virtually never necessary. If the aversion is strong or it is impossible to get the cat to favor an appropriate substrate and there is an aversion component to its behavior, antianxiety medications may be beneficial. Medications commonly used include benzodiazepines, tricyclic antidepressants (TCAs), nonspecific anxiolytics, and progestins (Box 8-6).

In any situation involving a strong preference or aversion, the medication of choice is either a TCA or a nonspecific anxiolytic. It would be totally inappropriate to use a benzodiazepine such as diazepam in these cases. Diazepam, the most frequently used benzodiazepine used in cats, is a nonspecific, antianxiety agent that has global gamma-aminobutyric acid enhancement effects. Unfortunately, cats can also inhibit *appropriate* behaviors when so treated. If the cat truly disliked the litter but was trying to overcome that dislike because it was repulsed by using a nonlitter substrate, it may actually use the litter box more frequently than it wants. This is classically seen in cats that are balancing on the edge of litter boxes but do not want to touch their feet to the substrate. Giving such a cat a benzodiazepine causes a global release of their innate inhibition. In such a situation, it is not unusual to see the elimination behavior worsen. If fact, many clients have complained that the cat then eliminated right in front of them. This is because the cat was already attempting to inhibit an inappropriate behavior and its behavior worsens with release from that inhibition. Unfortunately, cats can learn from

BOX 8-6

PHARMACOLOGICAL TREATMENT FOR ELIMINATION DISORDERS

1. Benzodiazepines (diazepam, clorazepate)
2. Tricyclic antidepressants (amitriptyline, nortriptyline, clomipramine)
3. Nonspecific anxiolytics (buspirone) and selective serotonin reuptake inhibitors
4. Progestins (as a *last* resort)

such instances; every time they experience an inappropriate or undesirable behavior, it acts to shape their future behavior by acting as a reinforcer. Hence, it is absolutely critical to not do anything to make the situation worse. If the practitioner is not sure and chooses to use a benzodiazepine, the response can be diagnostic; however, this approach is not without risk.

The more appropriate drug in this case would be a TCA such as amitriptyline (Elavil). A dose of approximately 1 mg/kg orally every 12 to 24 hours can relieve the anxieties associated with specific stimuli, such as litters or litter boxes, but unlike the benzodiazepines, amitriptyline will not interfere with learning involved in behavior modification. The use of tricyclic antidepressants, benzodiazepines, and nonspecific anxiolytics is more fully discussed in Chapter 13. Amitriptyline is a TCA that acts as a serotonin reuptake inhibitor. It probably also has presynaptic and postsynaptic effects and may affect other neuroendocrine systems. Accordingly, the cat experiences a relief from anxiety and may be considerably more amenable to working with either new litters or new substrates. In the clinical experience of the Behavioral Clinic at VHUP, approximately 50% of all cats given amitriptyline exhibit symptomatic emesis at some point in their lives. The reported frequency of emesis ranges from occasional to daily. Decreasing the dose may stop the vomiting, but generally by the time the dose is decreased to a level that does not cause side effects, it is also not efficacious.

Cats do not accommodate drugs as well as dogs. The glucuronic acid metabolic pathway is the primary pathway that is used in the metabolism of TCAs and most other anxiolytics. Cats do not make as efficient use of this pathway as do dogs, so it is not surprising that cats experience more side effects with behavioral drugs. In many cases decreasing the frequency of the dose to every 24 hours from every 12 hours is sufficient to maintain the therapeutic effects without causing side effects. Alternatively, changing medication from amitriptyline to nortriptyline at the same dose may minimize side effects while maintaining efficacy. Nortriptyline is the active intermediate metabolite of amitriptyline. The extent to which it may be responsible for the therapeutic, antianxiety effects is unknown; however, because of vagaries of the metabolic pathway, intermediate metabolites may have greatly extended half-lives in cats. This tendency may be more pronounced in overweight or obese animals.

If the cat cannot tolerate amitriptyline or nortriptyline, there is some evidence (Hart et al., 1993) that some cats respond to buspirone (Buspar) as a treatment for preferences or aversions associated with the litter box. For patients treated with either amitriptyline or buspirone, it may be impossible to withdraw the medication and still have the cats maintain appropriate litter box habits. This finding suggests that the cats have some underlying, ongoing, endogenous anxiety about some condition associated with the box.

In case of successful weaning from medication for treatment of litter box aversion or preferences, the clients aggressively manipulated the behavioral environment and the physical environment. Clients should continue to give the medication until a minimum of 3 to 4 weeks have passed during which no inappropriate elimination has occurred. At this time, the medication should carefully be weaned. If the cat has been given medication every 12 hours, it should now either be given half the dose every 12 hours for a week, or it should be given the same dose every 24 hours for a week. Clients can again halve the dose for the following week. During the third week clients can use an every-other-day schedule. By week 4 they can stop giving the drug altogether. If clients abruptly discontinue medications, it is unclear to what extent the cats experience a rebound phenomena associated with increased anxiety because of the sudden absence of the antianxiety agent. There are no data to test this effect for drugs that are not thought to be physiologically addictive. It would be terrific to know to what extent such relapses occur and whether these relapses correlate with either blood or central nervous system levels of the active ingredients of any antianxiety agent. Regardless, should the cat require some minimal level to maintain its appropriate behavior, clients will be able to determine the necessary level by gradual withdrawal. Gradual withdrawal has the additional hidden advantage of requiring that the clients still work with the cat and monitor it. These are essential factors in therapeutic success.

Spraying

Most spraying is best treated by addressing problems in the *social* environment. Environmental, behavioral, and pharmacological modification are all generally required. Unless the spraying has commenced only recently and is not yet habitual, treatment of the behavioral and physical environments alone are not sufficient to abort the spraying. If the spraying has been an occasional occurrence or has just started and the client is able to identify the stimulus that precipitated its start, it may be appropriate to modify only the physical and behavioral environments. If such an approach does not work within the first week, pharmacological intervention must be initiated as quickly as possible. The reasons for this are twofold. First, olfactory cues are important to cats, and every time a cat sprays, that cat is reinforcing an olfactory cue. Second, cats learn from these behaviors—ignoring the problem could be potentiating further social havoc.

The primary drugs used to treat feline spraying and nonspraying marking include TCAs such as amitriptyline (Elavil), nortriptyline (Pamelor), and clomipramine (Anafranil); benzodiazepines such as diazepam (Valium); and nonspecific anxiolytics such as buspirone (BuSpar). Currently there are no good data to determine whether other nonspecific, antianxiety agents (fluoxetine [Prozac]) are efficacious in some situations, but based on their performance in other canine and feline behavioral disorders (Overall, 1995), it would not be surprising if these drugs were to have bright futures for some feline elimination disorders. The drug of choice has traditionally been diazepam. Diazepam has been used for more than a decade with varying degrees of success to treat spraying.

Diazepam (1.0 to 3.0 mg per cat orally every 12 to 24 hours [Houpt, 1991b; Marder, 1991]; 2 to 4 mg per cat orally every 12 hours for spraying [Cooper & Hart, 1992]; 1.25 to 2.5 mg per cat orally every 12 to 24 hours for skeletal muscle relaxation in FLUTD [Osborne et al., 1987]), when used correctly, controls spraying in 75% to 90% of all cats (Marder, 1991). Generally, cats for whom diazepam is successful will stagger mildly, with impaired depth perception for a few days; staggering should resolve spontaneously by the end of the week. Some cats may need to take diazepam for a few weeks, some seasonally, some forever. The lowest effective dose should be used. Some cats that respond to diazepam require a benzodiazepine with a longer halflife. Clorazepate dipotassium (Tranxene-SD) at 0.5 to 1.0 mg/kg orally every 12 to 14 hours or 0.55 to 2.2 mg/kg orally as needed, can be used; however, if the cat did not respond to diazepam therapy, it may not respond to this regimen.

It is important to realize that all spraying is not related to the same underlying cause. This has been emphasized previously and is emphasized here again. Failures of pharmacological intervention may suggest testable hypotheses about underlying behavioral causes of the spraying and may suggest a possible mechanism by which the behavioral cause is neurochemically mediated. Elucidation of feline social interactions can be difficult and frustrating. Understanding social involvement may be the key to prescribing the appropriate pharmacological intervention, but a failed response can also provide critical information. This reemphasizes the importance of taking an excellent behavioral history; the information about why the chosen drug did not cause the cat to respond is found in the behavioral history. It is only by pursuing a course on the basis of hypothesis testing and strong inference that some progress will be made in the field of behavioral medicine.

It has become popular not to use benzodiazepines

and instead to use buspirone to treat spraying. Buspirone is useful for treatment of spraying in some cats. A critical review of data from various studies (Hart et al., 1993; Marder, 1991) indicates that it is no more successful overall than diazepam and is substantially more expensive. Whereas the dose of diazepam is generally 1 to 2 mg (0.2 to 0.4 mg/kg) orally every 12 to 24 hours (starting dose = 1 mg/every 12 hours), the dose for buspirone is generally 5 mg orally every 12 to 24 hours (starting dose = 5 mg orally every 24 hours); hence, the cost of buspirone may be a factor if prolonged therapy of 6 to 12 months, as is often recommended, is instituted. This cost might not be a problem overall were this the more efficacious drug, but careful, statistical reanalysis of the data indicates that this is not so.

Marder (1991) presented data that indicated that 43% of cats treated with diazepam for spraying ceased spraying totally. The sample size is small (23; 43% = 10 of 23). Of the cats, 74% (17 of 23) that were treated for spraying with diazepam experienced a 75% or better reduction in spraying. These data are slightly more favorable than those presented by Cooper and Hart (1992), who indicated that 55% (11 of 20) experienced a reduction in spraying. Each study relied on a small sample size (23 and 20, respectively). Treatment with buspirone resulted in a 75% or better reduction in spraying (Hart et al., 1993) in 55% (32 of 62) of cats studied. Of the cats that responded, 21 of 32 experienced a complete cessation of spraying. When the data from these studies are statistically compared, they are not different with regard to the number of patients experiencing at least a 75% reduction in spraying ($G_{adj} = 3.47$; $p \geq 0.05$; log-likelihood ratio χ^2 test = G test). The data presented by Hart et al. (1993) are also not statistically significantly different than the previous data reported for diazepam (Marder, 1991) when the number of patients ceasing to spray are compared ($G_{adj} = 2.60$; $p \geq 0.05$). Accordingly, buspirone is no more effective than diazepam overall in treating feline spraying or in affecting the proportion of the population that cease spraying altogether.

More work is needed in these areas. Sample sizes are small, and these statistics hint that significance may be coupled to sample size. An expanded study, particularly one that notes behavioral aspects of animals that responded and those that did not respond, may produce a more informative result, especially for the proportion of cases in which spraying ceases. Unfortunately, in neither of these studies is the role of the social environment explored or discussed. Of cats from multicat households, 58% (32 of 55) responded to buspirone, whereas none from single-cat households did (Hart et al., 1993), although the number of single cats studied was small. This strongly suggests that the social environment is critical in determining the cause of the underlying spraying and in suggesting a pharmacological agent that will help that underlying cause. Various workers in the field have noted that buspirone-responsive cats may become more assertive

to other cats or that buspirone-responsive cats may become more willing to interact in general. These instances suggest that data gleaned from social changes may provide clues about how both drugs act and why the spraying occurred. Evaluation of and intervention in the social environment is important when treating complex, multifactorial problems such as spraying.

In practice, relapses are not uncommon on cessation of treatment with diazepam. Invariably, subsequent retreatment with diazepam requires a higher dose than previously used to treat the spraying. Occasionally the cat becomes refractory to further treatment. There are no good, large population sample data either on the extent to which cats become refractory or on the extent to which ancillary dosing requires an increase of dose. This is another area that requires additional study. Such a response is likely to be related to physiological dependence (File, 1990).

Psychological addiction does not appear to be a problem in animals, perhaps because they are not permitted or able to self-medicate. Benzodiazepines are humanly abusable substances, and clients should be warned when using them for their pets that this is the case. Because many animals receive maintenance medication for spraying for a prolonged period, it is inadvisable for the veterinarian to dispense a large amount of any benzodiazepine at one time. It is far preferable to repeatedly renew a prescription or to dispense a new prescription monthly or bimonthly after seeing the patient. This also provides the practitioner with the opportunity for updates on the behavioral condition of the cats.

Recidivism rates for animals that spray are notoriously high. This may be in part related to the lack of appreciation of the interacting social environment. Marder (1991) and Hart et al. (1993) differ dramatically with regard to recidivism rates for cats that were treated for spraying with diazepam. The latter (based on Cooper & Hart, 1992) reported that 95% (10 of 11) resumed spraying when diazepam was discontinued, and Marder (1991) reported that 75% (13 of 17) reverted at some time. For buspirone, the recidivism rate was 53% (17 of 32) when the drug was totally withdrawn after 8 weeks. These results (13 of 17 versus 17 of 32) are not statistically significantly different ($G_{adj} = 2.56$; $p \geq 0.05$). Hart et al. (1993) did not note the time frame over which the withdrawal was done or the attendant dosage schedule.

Time frame and dosage schedules are important because the data discussed refer to an 8-week time period; hence the recidivism rate for buspirone may be underestimated. This is especially true because, in humans and dogs, 2 to 4 weeks may be needed for blood levels of buspirone to reach therapeutic levels (Marder, 1991; Robinson et al., 1989). Clearance time may also be prolonged in such cases, making assessments for recidivism rates that are computed for times close to drug cessation unreliable. Hence it is unclear if treatment with either drug differentially affects relapse rates. However, because buspirone does not interfere with short-term memory as does diazepam and because of the postulated effects of buspirone on serotonin and dopamine, it could facilitate social interactions that would decrease the probability of agonistic spraying.

It is appropriate to consider the modes of action of all medications used for cats with nonspraying marking or spraying disorders. Drugs with certain modalities of action may be more appropriate than others for cats with particular sets of behaviors.

All benzodiazepines have global, anxiolytic effects. They amplify the effects of the inhibitory neurotransmitter, gamma-aminobutyric acid (GABA); the mechanism for their facilitation of social interaction may be because attendant anxiety is inhibited (Bertilsson et al., 1990; Jaeken et al., 1990; Paul & Skolnick, 1982). Indeed, clients with cats may report that some cats become excessively friendly while taking benzodiazepines. This social facilitation may be responsible for the cessation of spraying in successful cases. As such, the spraying is secondary to, or symptomatic of, the social conflict. Benzodiazepines cause patients to be less reactive to their surroundings and less responsive to provocative stimuli. This appears to be the main effect for their use in the treatment of feline spraying. The mood elevation effects of the benzodiazepines are the result of their effects on the inhibitory neurotransmitter; they are not associated with elevation of brain chemicals, such as serotonin, that are associated with upbeat moods (Jaeken et al., 1990). Such subtleties may play a role in the treatment of complex social phenomena such as spraying.

Diazepam has a notoriously short half-life in cats, so it is likely that the intermediate metabolite, desmethyldiazepam, is acting as the efficacious, therapeutic compound. It has been reported (Marder, 1991; Overall, 1992b) that although therapeutic levels are being attained, cats often act uncoordinated and may stagger. This lack of coordination, or sleepiness, is transient in nature if the cat receives an appropriate dose and is not given a sufficient dose to cause sedation. A general rule of thumb is that the incoordination should resolve within 3 to 4 days, which, presumably, if human models are exemplary, is associated with the intermediate metabolite reaching steady-state levels. Should the incoordination not resolve within 4 to 7 days, the cat may be receiving too high a dose of diazepam for that cat's particular metabolism. Invariably, decreasing the dose results in cessation of the incoordination without the loss of the therapeutic effects in situations involving spraying. If the cat never staggered or acted uncoordinated, it is possible that it never received a high enough dose of the intermediate metabolite. It has been noted that cats that never experience the transient incoordination do not stop spraying. This suggests that if the intermediate metabolite hypothesis is correct, increasing the dose might provide the cat with a therapeutic level of the drug. In many cases, this appears to occur. In some cases the cats never act incoordinated but progress to being immediately drugged. Obviously, benzodiazepines are not appropriate treatment for these cats.

One appealing reason for the use of buspirone to treat spraying cats is because in the past 5 or 6 years there have been incidental, often anecdotal, reports of spraying of cats treated with low doses of diazepam experiencing sudden hepatic failure and death (Center et al., 1996; Hughes et al., 1996). The doses reportedly have been as low as 1 mg per cat, and the findings have been reported for cats receiving generic diazepam and those receiving the brand-name drug (Valium). Unfortunately, no excellent population level epidemiological data exist to suggest an underlying cause for this event. Recent work involving reanalysis of cats' responses to diazepam and reanalysis of necropsy data on cats exposed to diazepam (Hughes et al., 1996) indicate that sudden death associated with diazepam may be an idiosyncratic reaction when considered in the context of overall population risk. Obese cats appear to be overrepresented in the population of cats experiencing sudden death, indicating that accumulation of active intermediate metabolites may be important (Center et al., 1996). Accordingly, although it is wise to caution clients that there have been some untoward effects, the untoward effects appear no more common than idiosyncratic reactions to phenobarbital in dogs. The best prophylaxis would be a thorough medical examination, including a complete blood cell count and a serum biochemistry panel, before any dispensation of medication. It is unclear whether some of these idiosyncratic reactions are either gene × environment interactions or virus × drug interactions or perhaps indicate the development of an immune-mediated hepatic response. Because only the rare cat that died had any premedication blood studies, it is impossible to rule out underlying, preexisting disease.

Buspirone is a nonspecific anxiolytic that appears to act as a partial 5-hydroxytryptamine (5-HT) agonist, both presynaptically and postsynaptically (Coop & McNaughton, 1991; Lucey et al., 1992; Robinson et al., 1989). It has been suggested that buspirone's primary effect may even be as a dopamine receptor agonist (Lucey et al., 1992). Any effects on serotonin, dopamine, or both agents could potentially render the patient less concerned about perceived threats attendant with the social situation while increasing its capability to interact appropriately in a social manner. The extent to which spraying is a signal or an aggressive act in such circumstances would influence the extent to which the drug decreased the behavior. Aggression (and spraying can be an aggressive act [Overall, 1994e,k,l,m]) is behaviorally complex; it is not surprising that different pharmacological compounds effect a variety of therapeutic responses. An effort should be made to explore the efficacy of all relative compounds.

TCAs have shown promise for the treatment of fears, phobias, and social anxieties (Rang et al., 1995).

The TCA group is diverse, but most drugs within the group act through presynaptic or postsynaptic central nervous system enhancement of serotonin function. Short-acting, older TCAs such as amitriptyline can be useful in the treatment of aversions and preferences. They have seldom been used to treat spraying or non-spraying marking, although amitriptyline, at least, is available in an easy-to-administer liquid formulation. If the anxiety associated with the social situation is low level or of recent onset, "low-tech" TCAs may be efficacious in marking situations. Amitriptyline is currently the recommended treatment of choice for FLUTD, FUS, or sterile cystitis (Buffington et al., 1993; Eschalier, 1990; Fromm et al., 1991; Hanno et al., 1989). It is used because of its effects on norepinephrine (NE) and norepinephrine's role in treating neurogenic inflammation; however, it is impossible to rule out the extent to which it may relieve anxiety that is secondary to pain.

Clomipramine, a relatively specific 5-HT reuptake inhibitor, has only recently been used to treat spraying and extensive response data are lacking. It appears to be equally efficacious in situations involving one or multiple cats and in situations that involve anxiety but are refractory to other medications. There is no information about the efficacy of clomipramine in cases involving marking associated with sexual advertisement. Although it can take as long as 4 to 6 weeks of treatment to attain therapeutic levels of clomipramine in dogs and humans, cats appear to respond more quickly and generally start to show a response within the first week. As with most medications, cats may be more susceptible to side effects than are dogs or humans. Newer medications such as clomipramine have many fewer side effects than do most other drugs, but the definitive toxicity data are currently unavailable.

For cats that do not respond to any of the previously mentioned drugs, progestins can be used (Beaver, 1992c; Chesney, 1976; Hart, 1980a) but should never be a first choice because of potential side effects that include gynecomastia, diabetogenesis, potential implication with mammary neoplasia, and bone marrow suppression. Progestins should never be used in breeding animals. Under no circumstance should they be dispensed without a baseline complete blood cell count/serum biochemistry panel and follow up laboratory studies every 6 to 8 weeks. Clients should be warned of all side effects because of the risk of liability. Consider use of an informed consent or release statement. Disclosure of all known risks of any drug should be done without exception.

How does one choose one medication over another?

Diazepam and progestins may affect spraying behavior through two separate underlying neural substrates. Progestins are bound by cytosolic androgen receptors with direct inhibiting effects on steroid 5α-reductase neurons in the hypothalamus and limbic system (Gupta et al., 1979; Henik et al., 1985). Diazepam is bound by specific benzodiazepine receptor sites throughout the neural axis. It induces depression of neural activity through the enhancement of GABA (Haefely et al., 1981). Such effects on underlying neural substrate may account for the observation that, in contrast to the response to diazepam, response to progestins is greater for single-cat than for multicat households (Cooper & Hart, 1992).

In a comparison of buspirone and diazepam, the following points can be made. Diazepam works well for situations in which aggression and the resultant elimination disorder is secondary to an anxiety regarding the social system or to a perceived change in the social system. Accordingly, it works well in (1) passive aggression with spraying or nonspraying marking; (2) active aggression with spraying and nonspraying marking, particularly if it is in response to a perceived change in the environment (review the data from Hart et al., [1993]) on cats in single-cat households; these will often respond to diazepam but do not respond to buspirone; (3) a location aversion associated with aggression; there must be a strong, fearful, and anxiety component to this so that the location aversion is secondary. (If this is not the case and the location aversion has not been caused by the fearful and aggressive component, treatment with diazepam will invariably make the situation worse.) Diazepam is useful if a quick response is needed because invariably within a week the client should be able to detect some change in the behavior of the animal. Diazepam can be used if it has worked in the past, although the clients may need to expect to use a higher dosage. Again, some small percentage of animals may be refractory to the drug; although the percentage is not currently known and further work needs to be done in this area. Regardless, if the cat experiences a relapse because of the same social stimuli that provoked it before and diazepam worked then, it may well work the following time. Diazepam is probably the drug of choice if expense is an issue. No drug should be recommended solely on the basis of cost; however, clients may be more willing to try a more expensive drug after treatment with the less expensive drug has failed.

Buspirone works well for situations in which aggression may be primary, in which the cat is very confident, or in cases in which the cats are unable to make themselves sufficiently assertive within the social system. This is because it facilitates social interactions and alterations in hierarchical relationships. Buspirone is useful in the following situations: (1) active but fairly covert aggression with spraying or nonspraying marking; (2) status-related aggression associated with spraying; in this case it facilitates more appropriate social hierarchical relationships and diminishes the status of outright aggression; and (3) passive aggression marking if the clients understand that the cat could become more assertive. This feature can be useful in a readjustment of the social grouping. Buspirone is useful when a longer half-life is required and expense is not an issue. If the cat is expected to require maintenance therapy, buspirone is better than diazepam because of physiological tolerance that occurs with the latter. Also, buspirone is not a substance abusable by humans. Buspirone can be used if TCAs and benzodiazepines have failed or if they have made the cat ill. It can be used first if aggression is a major concern, but the type of aggression is important, and the extent to which the aggression is overt or covert may be important to evaluate. Buspirone can be used in all of these situations but it might render more assertive and overtly interactive a cat that had been showing more covert threats. If managed correctly using behavior modification and controlled interactions, this can be a desirable effect. Examples that illustrate these choices follow (Box 8-7).

If there are two cats involved in the aggressive event and one has become absolutely terrified, treating the cat that is absolutely terrified with diazepam may both impede its short-term memory of horrific events and make the cat friendlier. Buspirone, given to the aggressor, then may also facilitate the appropriate social interaction between the two because it relieves the anxiety associated with the aggression. It is important in this situation that the aggressor has maintained the anxiety, despite all information received from the victim that the latter poses no threat and that the aggression is the result of anxiety. Concomitantly, it is also important that the diazepam alleviates the fear exhibited by the other cat.

Hart et al. (1993) noted that many cats treated with buspirone become more assertive; it is unclear in what context such an assertion was a problem. The logic here is complex. If the cat is inhibiting any of its aggression and is confident, it may be inhibiting aggression because it has learned that the aggression is inappropriate for other reasons (i.e., the clients have punished the cat). Diazepam is *not* the appropriate drug of choice in this circumstance because it can relieve inhibitions, including those that are appropriate. This is the one situation in which the confident, actively aggressive cat that is not demonstrating the full extent of its aggressive propensities may fare better with buspirone than diazepam.

If the cat is anxious about its relative status and is overtly aggressive regardless of response, as a way to constantly proclaim its status, diazepam may be the better drug. Buspirone could augment the extant aggression, whereas diazepam renders such individuals friendlier and relieves anxieties so that the cat can start to resolve social conflicts. Clomipramine may also work well in these contexts. The recipient of the aggression in this situation may benefit from buspirone because it might increase assertiveness. It is important to emphasize that the drugs are being used not only to treat underlying anxiety, but also to facilitate concomitant behavioral modification.

Finally, a confident bully should not be treated with buspirone because this drug is likely to render

---

BOX 8-7

WHEN TO USE DIAZEPAM VERSUS BUSPIRONE

Diazepam

Works well for situations when aggression (and the resultant elimination disorder) is the result of anxiety or a perceived challenge

1. Passive or covert aggression associated with fear or anxiety and with spraying or nonspraying marking
2. Active or overt aggression with spraying or nonspraying marking if the cat is *not* inhibiting any aggression (otherwise it will worsen) and if the goal is to make the cat friendlier
3. Location aversion associated with aggression (must have strong, fearful, and anxiety components)
4. Use if fast response is needed
5. Use if drug has worked in the past (although expect to need a higher dose)
6. Use if expense is a factor

Buspirone

Works well for situations when aggression may be primary (response to confident cats) because it facilitates social interaction and alterations in hierarchical relationships

1. Active or passive aggression with spraying or nonspraying marking, if based on anxiety (could make a confident cat with overt aggression more assertive)
2. Status-related aggression toward humans associated with spraying
3. Longer half-life and expense may be prohibitive for some clients
4. Use if client expects to maintain cat on drug
5. Use if tricyclic antidepressants and benzodiazepines have failed or make cat ill
6. Use first if aggression is a major concern

---

the cat *more* assertive. If the recipient of the aggression is withdrawn and terrified, this could become a particularly horrendous situation. In this case the bully should be treated with an agent that renders it friendlier (diazepam), and the recipient is treated with an agent that relieves its anxiety and facilitates its reintroduction to the social system. Because of its tendency to encourage assertion, buspirone may be preferable here, but diazepam and clomipramine could work equally well.

There are no data that evaluate whether the mild, transient ataxia attendant with diazepam treatment facilitates reestablishment of a social order, but such factors cannot be ruled out.

Surgical Approaches

Because of the effects of hormonal facilitation, all animals that spray should be castrated or subject to ovariohysterectomy (Bali & Hormeyer, 1986; Bovée et al., 1985). Other surgical procedures that have been suggested for the treatment of spraying include olfactory tractotomy (Hart, 1981b, 1982) and ischiocavernosus myectomy (Hauptman & Komtebedde, 1989; Komtebedde & Hauptman, 1990). Although the former procedure does not appear to adversely affect the cat's ability to feed, it appears to be no more effective than pharmacological intervention and is repugnant to clients. The latter was efficacious in reducing urine spraying and urine puddling (behavioral diagnosis unknown) in 7 of 10 male castrated cats older than 6 months that had previously been unsuccessfully treated with progestins or diazepam.

• • •

In summary, the primary drugs of choice for treating feline spraying and nonspraying marking are diazepam, buspirone, amitriptyline, and, potentially, clomipramine, and selective serotonin reuptake inhibitors (SSRIs) paroxefine, fluoxetine, and sertraline. All of these agents can potentially affect renal and hepatic function, and the TCAs can affect cardiac function. Premedication screening and evaluation are warranted. Schematics for when to use each drug are found in Boxes 8-8 to 8-11. An overall plan for outlining the behavioral and environmental modifications

---

BOX 8-9
TRICYCLIC ANTIDEPRESSANTS

Mode of Action/Effects

1. Augments serotonin (consider use of newer SSRIs such as fluoxetine, sertraline, and paroxetine)
2. Relieves association-specific anxiety
3. Does not affect short-term memory
4. Facilitates social interaction and normal social functioning and response
5. May increase appetite and thirst

Indications

1. First drug of choice in thwarted situations that produce anxiety (nonspraying marking, second location preference)
2. Status-related spraying: facilitates normal social interaction with people and behavior modification
3. First or second drug of choice for passive aggression associated with spraying that's a response to active (overt or covert) aggression; facilitates normal social interaction and relieves anxiety
4. Drug of first or second choice in active (covert or overt) aggression when recipient of aggression has not directly elicited response (e.g., recipient reached social maturity and this is a problem for the aggressor)

BOX 8-8
BENZODIAZEPINES

Mode of Action/Effects

1. GABAminergic
2. Increases appetite in healthy cat
3. Renders cat more friendly
4. Interferes with short-term memory
5. Renders cat less concerned about social environment

Indications

1. Great for passive aggression associated with spraying and nonspraying marking
2. First drug of choice in active aggression associated with spraying if cat is not inhibiting any aggressions
3. Caution in status-related situations; may release cat's own inhibitions (inhibit inhibition via GABA)
4. May be helpful in location aversion–associated aggression, but use caution; may facilitate second substrate or location preference

---

BOX 8-10
NONSPECIFIC ANXIOLYTICS (BUSPIRONE)

Mode of Action/Effects

1. Augments serotonin and, possibly, dopamine
2. May have "proactive" effect because of effects on dopamine
3. Facilitates normal social interaction, possibly because of effect as partial $5HT_{1a}$ agonist
4. Relieves nonspecific, nonsituation-associated anxiety

Indications

1. Drug of first or second choice in active (overt or covert) aggression associated with spraying
2. Useful in passive aggression associated with nonspraying marking
3. Useful in passive or covert aggression that is a response to active aggression (may make the cat more assertive and so could facilitate social interaction)
4. Useful in all situations in which tricyclic antidepressants give some, but not a complete effect

---

BOX 8-11

PROGESTINS

Mode of Action/Effects

1. Acts via central hormone receptors
2. Affects dimorphic behaviors
3. May produce calming effect

Indications

1. Side effects are too numerous to count; may be drug of last resort in active aggression situations that are related to the following:
   - Sexual advertisement and competition
   - Intrasexual hierarchical social systems

---

for elimination disorders associated with aggression is found in Box 8-1. Specific aggressions are discussed in Chapter 7. A decision-making algorithm for all elimination behaviors is shown in Fig. 8-3. Appendix B contains a protocol for the treatment of feline elimination disorders. This protocol is for clients; the salient steps in the process are outlined in Box 8-12. Dosages of drugs that are useful for treating feline aggression and elimination behaviors associated with feline aggression are found in Box 8-13.

Options are limited if none of these medications and modifications alter the cat's behavior or if the client does not wish to try drug therapy. Often, allowing the cats to become indoor and outdoor cats helps. Even if the cat is declawed, this may be an option if the client otherwise plans euthanasia.

A few general cautionary statements are needed. First, any cat that does respond to the above treat-

---

BOX 8-12

PROTOCOL FOR MANAGEMENT OF LITTER BOX ENVIRONMENT IN THE TREATMENT OF FELINE ELIMINATION DISORDERS

1. All affected areas must be cleaned with an odor eliminator. All layers must be cleaned. If the problem has been ongoing for some time the odor has soaked through the floor. In some cases floor boards need to be replaced, as does carpeting and padding. This is especially true if subfloors are involved.
2. After cleaning, cover affected areas with heavy-gauge plastic (consider vapor barriers if subfloor involved) to both change the tactile sensation for the cat and to prevent further penetration in the event of elimination.
3. Encourage the client to get multiple litter boxes, generally one more than there are cats, unless there are more than 5 cats; large numbers of cats may render the stimulus too strong. These litter boxes should be placed in a variety of locations and be of a variety of styles (open, covered, deep, shallow, big, small).
4. Litter should be scooped daily, and most litters should be dumped totally every other day. The exception to this is the clumpable litter; this does not have to be discarded, but does need to be topped up. Many cats differ in their preference for litter depth. Boxes should be washed weekly. Some old boxes may be so permeated with scent that they should be discarded.
5. A variety of litters should be offered to the cat in a variety of boxes. If the cat is using soft substances consider softer litters: number 3 blasting sand, playground sand, shredded newspaper or toweling,

sawdust, wood chips (*not* cedar). Encourage the clients to be observant and creative; they are usually extremely cooperative because you are providing them with the opportunity to do something.
6. Cats are not trained to litter boxes; this is a behavior that develops in kittenhood in the absence of human intervention. Accordingly, we do not "train" cats with an elimination problem to use a litter box; however, they can be encouraged to make owner-preferred associations if taken to the litter box frequently, waited for, and praised whenever they use the box.
7. If the cat is seen to squat outside the box, negative reinforcement will work if the cat is scared in the first 30 to 60 seconds of the onset of the behavior (that includes circling, facial expressions, and digging) and if the scare is sufficient to make the cat abort the behavior and leave, without causing undue panic or inducing fear associated with the litter box or area. Foghorns, water pistols, whistles, and tins of pennies all work with some cats. Foghorns are usually inappropriate in apartments, although owners get a great deal of satisfaction from their use. Regardless, physical punishment, including rubbing the cat's nose in the soiled area, is useless after the fact.
8. Some cats may need to be confined to a restricted area at first. Their access to the rest of the house can be expanded once they are using litter appropriately in the confined area and are then closely watched as their access is slowly expanded.

<table>
<tr><td colspan="2" style="text-align:center">

BOX 8-13

USEFUL AND COMMONLY USED DRUGS FOR THE TREATMENT OF FELINE ELIMINATION DISORDERS AND FELINE AGGRESSION

</td></tr>
<tr><td>Amitriptyline (TCA; Elavil)</td><td>0.5 to 1.0 mg/kg orally every 12-24 hours</td></tr>
<tr><td>Nortriptyline (TCA; Pamelor)</td><td>0.5 to 1.0 mg/kg orally every 12-24 hours</td></tr>
<tr><td>Buspirone (NSA; BuSpar)</td><td>0.5 to 2.0 mg/kg orally every 8-24 hours ($\bar{x}$ = 1.0 mg/kg)</td></tr>
<tr><td>Clomipramine (TCA; Anafranil)</td><td>0.5 mg/kg orally every 24 hours</td></tr>
<tr><td>Diazepam (BZ; Valium)</td><td>0.2 to 0.4 mg/kg orally every 12-24 hours</td></tr>
</table>

TCA, Tricyclic antidepressant; *NSA,* nonspecific anxiolytic; *BZ,* benzodiazepine. Some rounding of dosages may be necessary to use standard size dosages.

ments should have additional medical examinations. At VHUP cultures reveal many infections not apparent on regular screening. Sometimes two or three urinalyses and one or two cultures are necessary before the complicating medical cause is revealed. Clients should be informed of this. Second, any multicat household will have greater problems. If one cat is spraying, chances are the others are, too. If there are 10 or more cats in the household, the chance of a cat spraying at some point is 100% (see Marder, 1991). Clients will deny it, but they should be told this anyway; many will call back to tell you they finally saw the third cat spray. Finally, watch out for bullies. The reason the kitten may not use the litter box is because someone else sits on top of or behind it and swats the kitten every time it approaches.

A Note on Cleaning Up

In any substrate aversion or preference or marking situation it is implicit that the cat is soiling an inappropriate substrate. It is critical that that substrate be thoroughly cleaned with an odor eliminator. Vinegar and ammonia should be absolutely avoided because they can smell like urine and the latter is a urine metabolite. Although manufacturers of odor eliminators are loathe to discuss their contents or mode of action, most odor eliminators act by preventing aerosolization of volatile compounds by enzymatically or bacterially degrading urine or by some combination of these. Some odor eliminators that rely on degradation may be rendered ineffective if the cat is being treated with antibiotics. All affected substrates and locations must be aggressively treated. It is not sufficient to merely deodorize a carpet: cats have much keener senses of smell than do humans and appear to be able to still detect previously used areas and return to them. Odor eliminators are a useful step in breaking this cycle. All layers of carpeting must be cleaned. If a subfloor is present, this must also be cleaned. If deeply impregnated, all layers, including flooring, may need to be replaced. Covering the substrate or location with heavy-grade plastic can be useful in both interrupting the sensation of the substrate and in preventing further assaults from compounding the olfactory problem. Also, if clients find it easier to clean indiscretions, they may be more willing to work with the cat.

Issues Yet to be Resolved

1. The feline social system is still misunderstood or poorly understood. Its role in specific categories of elimination disorders still needs to be elucidated.
2. Quantitative and qualitative analysis of normal feline elimination behaviors has not been done.
3. The range of feline elimination behaviors that clients will tolerate or consider to be normal, compared with those that clients will not tolerate or consider abnormal or undesirable, has not been elucidated. This would be useful data to estimate the actual prevalence of problems and to determine where intervention would best help.
4. The underlying neurochemical basis for feline anxiety has not been elucidated, but is probably heterogeneous. Understanding this, and coupling it to actual behaviors, facilitates drug treatment. Conversely, responses to drug treatment may confirm or reject neuroanatomical hypotheses about feline behavior.

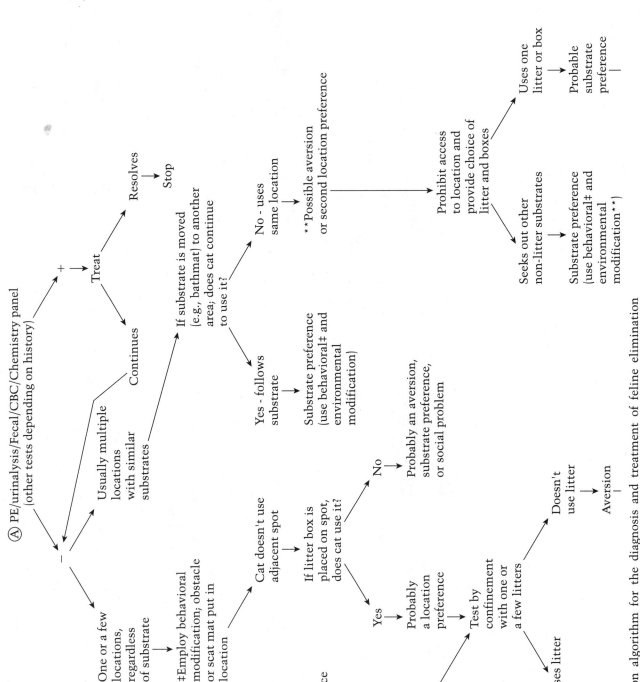

Fig. 8-3 Decision algorithm for the diagnosis and treatment of feline elimination disorders that do not involve spraying. As we learn more about discrete feline behaviors and better pharmacologic agents are developed, modes are likely to be modified.

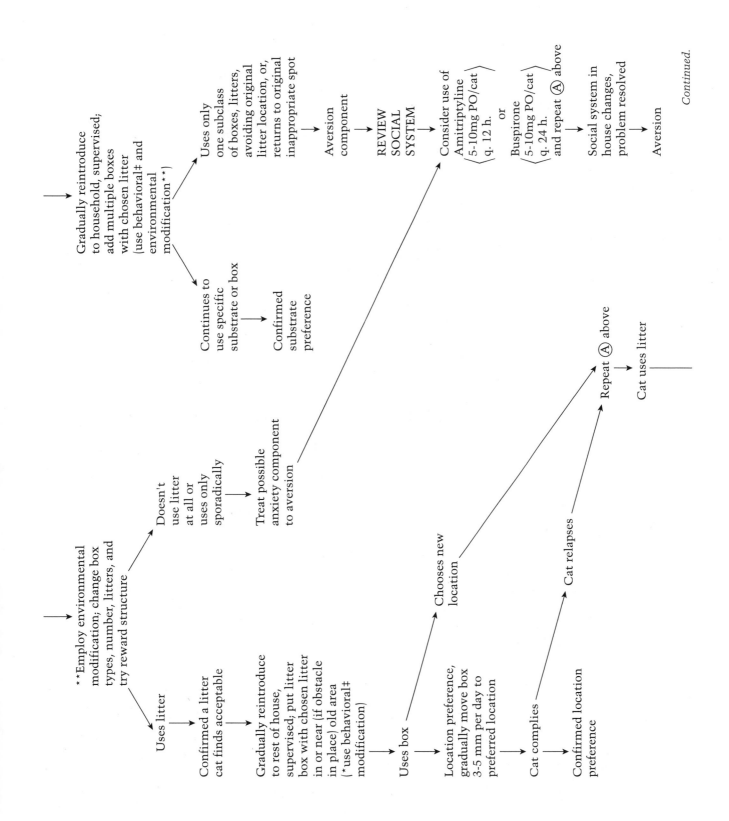

Continued.

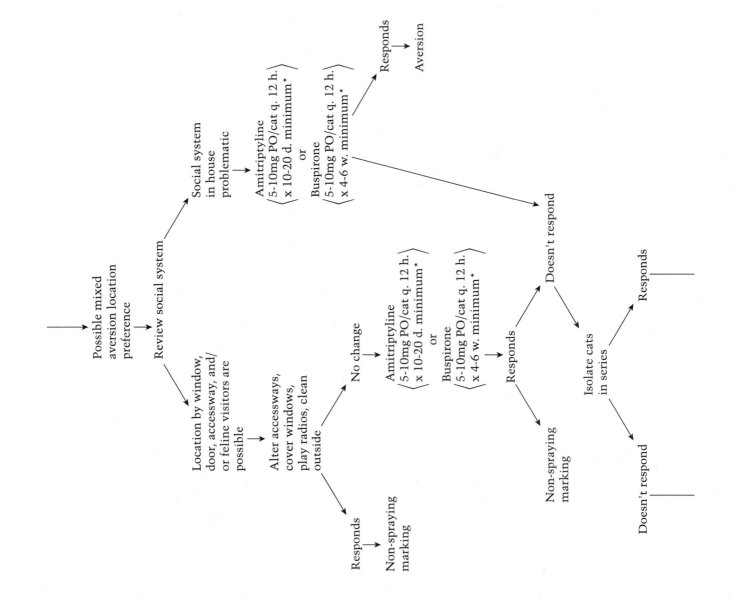

Aggression (may be a variant of non-spraying marking) compounding aversion

Review above— if still no change, atypical—isolate this cat with litter or make into indoor/ outdoor cat

*Unless shows side effects.
‡Behavioral modification includes:
1) Belling cat and spying on it
2) Using water pistols, whistles, fog horns, air horns to startle cat in act and abort behavior. Remember—the object is *not* to make the cat fearful.
3) Putting food in area
4) Putting a noxious substrate in area (tacky paper, tack boards, rubber runners)

**Environmental modification includes:
1) Cleaning with odor eliminators
2) Covering and/or lining affected areas with heavy plastic
3) Changing the number of litter boxes
4) Changing style of litter boxes (covered v. uncovered; small v. large; liners v. unlined)
5) Changing the location of litter boxes
6) Changing the amount of litter
7) Changing types of litter
8) Changing scooping, dumping, and washing schedules for boxes and litter

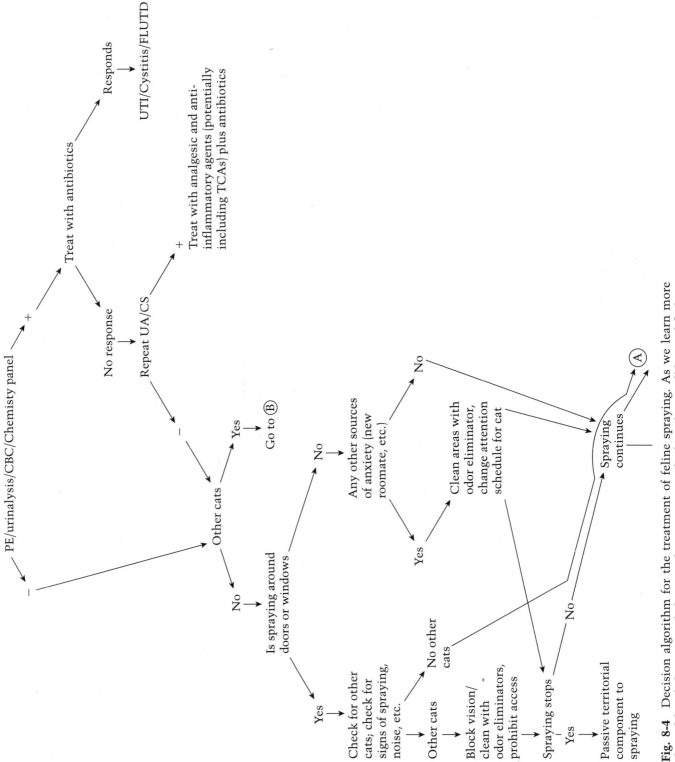

Fig. 8-4 Decision algorithm for the treatment of feline spraying. As we learn more about feline behaviors and pharmacologic agents, such algorithms will be modified.

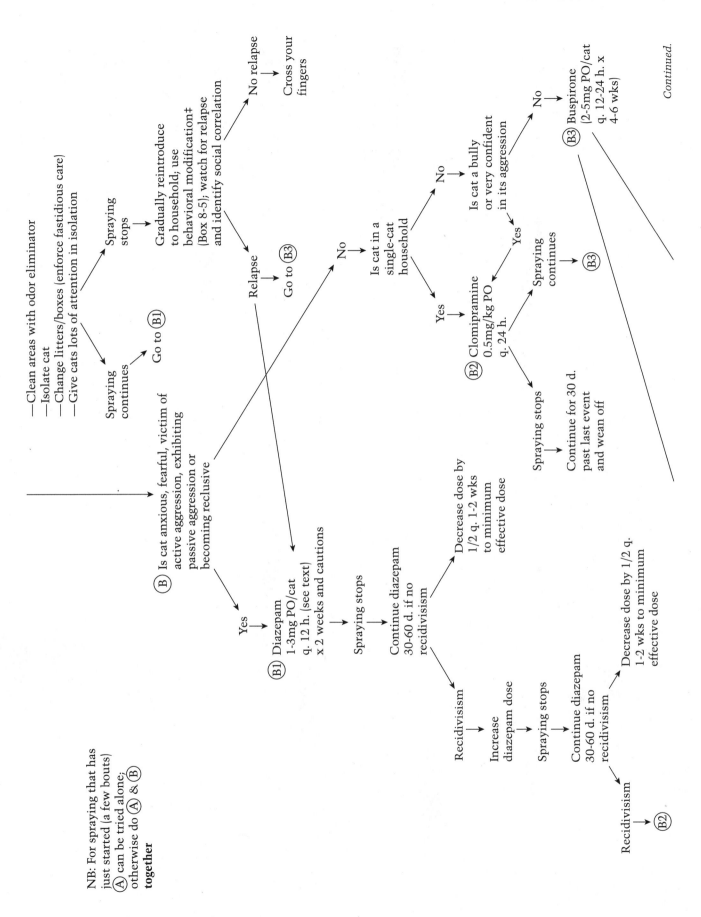

NB: For spraying that has just started (a few bouts) Ⓐ can be tried alone; otherwise do Ⓐ & Ⓑ **together**

—Clean areas with odor eliminator
—Isolate cat
—Change litters/boxes (enforce fastidious care)
—Give cats lots of attention in isolation

Spraying stops → Gradually reintroduce to household; use behavioral modification‡ (Box 8-5); watch for relapse and identify social correlation

No relapse → Cross your fingers

Relapse → Go to Ⓑ3

Spraying continues → Go to Ⓑ1

Ⓑ Is cat anxious, fearful, victim of active aggression, exhibiting passive aggression or becoming reclusive

Yes

Ⓑ1 Diazepam 1-3mg PO/cat q. 12 h. (see text) x 2 weeks and cautions

Spraying stops → Continue diazepam 30-60 d. if no recidivism

Decrease dose by 1/2 q. 1-2 wks to minimum effective dose

Recidivism → Increase diazepam dose → Spraying stops → Continue diazepam 30-60 d. if no recidivism

Decrease dose by 1/2 q. 1-2 wks to minimum effective dose

Recidivism → Ⓑ2

No → Is cat in a single-cat household

No → Is cat a bully or very confident in its aggression

No → Ⓑ3 Buspirone (2-5mg PO/cat q. 12-24 h. x 4-6 wks)

Yes → Ⓑ2 Clomipramine 0.5mg/kg PO q. 24 h.

Yes

Spraying continues → Ⓑ3

Spraying stops → Continue for 30 d. past last event and wean off

Continued.

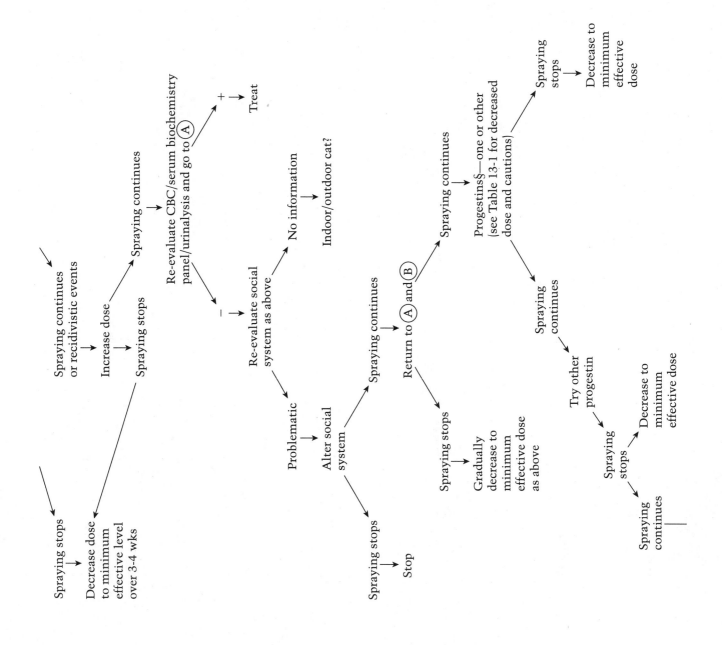

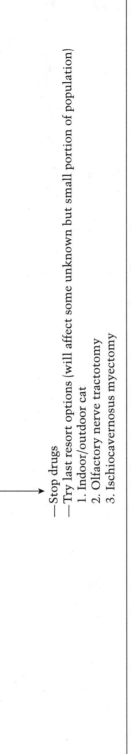

—Stop drugs
—Try last resort options (will affect some unknown but small portion of population)
1. Indoor/outdoor cat
2. Olfactory nerve tractotomy
3. Ischiocavernosus myectomy

§If you reach this point, either you have missed something, you have not fully understood the social ramifications affecting the situation, or you have a very rare patient.

CASE 8-1

Signalment: "Pansy," 8-month-old female Himalayan kitten

Initial problem: Not using litter box

History: This kitten was obtained by the fiancé from a pet store 4 months previously. Since coming to this house, Pansy has, with increasing frequency, defecated outside the litter box. The pattern of defecation is not consistent with substrate; if the client isolates the cat, sometimes the cat still does not defecate in the litter box. Whenever the client is able to observe Pansy, it appears that the cat heads toward the litter box and, part way there, squats and defecates.

Physical examination findings relevant to history: Pansy has been treated for *Coccidia* infections three times. The cat does not scratch or circle before defecation. The cat cries before elimination. Pansy defecates four to six times a day. Even with additional litter boxes, the cat often just misses the litter box.

Diagnosis: This is a medical problem; it was unclear if Pansy had chronic parasitemia, a food allergy (she has no dermatological manifestations of this), or colitis. She was developing a substrate aversion subsequent to the medical problem because the feces were often loose and created a messy situation for the cat.

Treatment: Pansy was referred to medicine for colonoscopy. Meanwhile, she was to be confined and given more small, low litter boxes. These were to be filled with clumpable litter or shredded newspaper. All areas where she eliminated were to be cleaned with an odor eliminator.

Follow-up: The cat's behavior improved with medical treatment for colitis. Clients addressed the aversion using multiple easy-access litter boxes filled with clumpable litter while the cat was being treated medically. The clients understand that the cat may be prone to relapse.

CASE 8-2

Signalment: "Sam," 4-year-old, castrated male Siamese cat

Initial problem: Urine spraying

History: Sam is one of four cats in the household; he has been spraying for at least 4 to 5 months. The clients are not certain about the duration of the spraying because they did not realize what was happening for a while; they smelled urine, but they did not realize that there was urine on the sofas and in the corner of the living room until they got down on their hands and knees. The back of the sofa has what looks like old urine stains. The problem appears to have developed subsequent to the addition of the fourth cat, a confident, very outgoing and playful 2 year-old, spayed female domestic short hair. When the new cat first came into the household, Sam hissed and tried to chase it out of the house; the new cat ignored him and continually solicited play, which he rebuffed. As Sam rebuffed the new cat more energetically, she growled at him and began to preempt him aggressively. The spraying cat, Sam, always got along with the other two original cats (both spayed females and both 3 years old) and was always found in the company of the black female; he would groom her and sleep with her. The clients have pictures of the living room where Sam and the black cat are curled up on the couch and the original third cat is seen in other pictures as parts of both duos and triads. Since the arrival of the new cat, the black cat has played with her all the time and now sleeps with and grooms her. Since the new cat's arrival, Sam seldom emerges from the basement and the pictures the client now has taken show Sam on a shelf or in a corner, when the other three cats are congregating in a pile on the couch. If the new cat comes into the living room and looks at Sam, he flees. The patient, Sam, is never seen spraying, but the sprayed areas are always found after he has been in the living room.

Physical Examination: Nonremarkable; normal urinalysis

Diagnosis: Spraying associated with anxiety and passive intercat aggression

Treatment: Gradual introductions using food dishes as encouragement were recommended. Sam is to be isolated in an area that is neutral to help change his status. He must learn to tolerate the presence of the new cat, but he shouldn't have to retreat to the basement. Both cats are to be belled so that the clients can hear when they are together. The clients are to startle them at the onset of any aggression. Additional covered litter boxes were recommended. All soiled areas were to be cleaned with odor eliminators, and heavy gauge plastic was to be placed over those areas. Diazepam was prescribed for Sam, and amitriptyline was prescribed for the passive aggressor (the new cat). The flooding technique may be another treatment option.

Follow-up: Amitriptyline was the efficacious treatment for the passive aggressor. After 3 months of rigorous work, the clients had succeeded in greatly decreasing the aggression and getting the cats to tolerate each other. Spraying still occurred occasionally (once every 2 to 4 months). Diazepam was withdrawn, but amitriptyline was continued at a low, maintenance level. The clients believe that the black cat has never been totally happy since the introduction of the fourth cat.

Signalment: "Marnie," 6-year-old, spayed female, 6.3 kg, domestic long hair cat

Initial problem: Urinating outside litter box

History: This cat was adopted off the street at approximately 2 years of age. She was pregnant when adopted. She subsequently had two kittens, for which the client found homes. The cat was then spayed.

When first adopted, the cat was very suspicious of people. The client reported that it took 2 to 3 months before she could even pet the cat. After the cat accepted the client, she became friendly with other people, although the client believes that most strangers would not find her to be "cuddly."

The client had a baby 2½ years ago and stopped having a lot of time for the cat, on whom she had previously doted. When the client's son began to crawl, about 2 years ago, the cat began to urinate around the perimeter of the dining room and in spots in the living room where the child's playpens were kept. When the client set up a play area for the child in the living room, she found an area in the center of the play area that looked like the cat had stood in the middle and circled, spraying. This is the only area in the living room that the cat has soiled.

The cat uses the litter box for all defecation. She also urinates in the box two or three times per day; the client has never seen the cat spray while in her box. The cat has one uncovered box with guards on the rim. The box is in the corner of the kitchen, not a high-traffic area. The client has always used a clumpable litter, although she thinks that she may have recently tried a scented version. The cat does not scratch much in her litter box and often stands with her feet on the edge, particularly if defecating. During the past 2 years urination outside the box has increased from occurring occasionally to daily.

The cat is never aggressive to anyone in the house, and she largely ignores the baby.

The client reports that the only time she gets any time to herself is at 11 PM when she sits on the couch to relax. The cat instantly jumps on her lap, purring and rubbing. This is now the only attention the cat receives during the day.

The client is desperate and may want to place or euthanize the cat. They have decided to sell their house and do not want to take this cat to a new house if her problem will continue. They are also concerned about their ability to sell this house given the condition of the dining room.

Previous Treatment: All urinalyses performed by the referring veterinarian have been nonremarkable. The referring veterinarian prescribed diazepam (1 to 2.5 mg orally every 12 hours) for the cat, but the client admits that she administered the medication inconsistently and missed doses. The referring veterinarian also prescribed methionine (dosage unknown) without a favorable response. The client has had the rugs steam-cleaned multiple times but has been inconsistent in her use of good odor eliminators. Placing bars of deodorant soap in corners of the dining room has been associated with the cat avoiding those corners.

Physical Examination: No abnormalities were detected during the physical examination.

Laboratory Evaluation: Blood samples for a complete blood cell count and serum biochemistry profile were submitted; all values were within laboratory reference limits.

Diagnosis: Urine marking associated with anxiety and a possible secondary substrate aversion

CASE 8-3—cont'd

Treatment: The client was instructed to remove the cat from the rooms it soils and place it in a room that it likes with two litter boxes (one covered) and with food, water, and bedding. The boxes were to be kept scrupulously clean. The client was to play with the cat, love her, groom her, and so on for 5 to 10 minutes 3 to 5 times per day. Meanwhile, she was to treat all affected areas, including padding, wall-to-wall carpet, and subfloors with a good odor eliminator (AIP, Elimin-odor, KOE, The Equalizer). Space between subfloors and padding and the padding and carpet were to be sealed with a plastic vapor barrier. The client was also to give the cat amitriptyline (5 mg orally every 12 hours) with the intent of decreasing the cat's anxiety about the baby and the decreased attention the cat has gotten since his arrival so that when the area was cleaned, the client could execute a successful reintroduction. Once the cat had been isolated for about 2 to 3 weeks and the areas were clean, the cat was to be introduced to the rest of the house in small increments, during which time she was to be supervised. The clients were to bell her so that she could not sneak off and were to monitor her, squirting her with a water pistol if she even smelled the carpet in these areas. In addition, the clients were to sit with her and the baby, giving her lots of love when she was calm and encouraging the baby to give her love. It was explained to the client that marking is a component of normal feline communicatory behavior and was the only way this cat could communicate her feelings about the attention deprivation to which she had been subjected since the baby began to crawl. It was also explained that there was an anxious component to the cat's behavior and that a trial of a variety of medications might be needed before one was found that both worked and did not produce side effects. Amitriptyline was chosen, in part, because of the client's sense of urgency; it is fast acting compared with buspirone, clomipramine (another excellent choice), and fluoxetine. Finally, the client was told that although it was her company the cat craved, a slightly older kitten that would play with and dote on the cat might help.

Follow-up: After a week the client had still not instituted the isolation and cleaning recommendations and had not tried any of the environmental suggestions (second box). The client admitted she does not really want to try—she just wants to get rid of the cat. Two weeks later she had not changed her mind and was being erratic in giving the cat its medication. She still had not implemented most of the suggestions. We said that we would try to find a home for this cat (because she is friendly and gorgeous) where she would get lots of attention. Her new people will need to know all of her problems and be able to work with them, including, possibly, the option of continuing to medicate her.

CASE 8-4

Signalment: Ralph, 6-year-old, castrated male domestic short hair cat

Initial problem: Defecation outside litter box

History: Ralph has an 8-month history, since being moved to a new apartment, of defecating on the carpet next to the sliding glass terrace doors. The cat did not have any problems for the first month that the people lived in the new apartment. Ralph has been and is an only pet. There were never any problems in the old apartment, although the cat has never covered its feces after defecation. The clients have had the cat since 3 months of age without any problems; the cat still uses the litter box for urination. The clients have checked the walls and woodwork for signs of urine staining or scent and found none. When this problem first started, it was of sudden onset and for a couple of weeks all defecation took place by the door. After onset the pattern became more sporadic, but in the past month Ralph is defecating outside the litter box virtually all the time and is now using all of the living room carpet.

Physical Examination: Non-remarkable—fecal study results were negative.

Diagnosis: Marking with feces; subsequent development of substrate preference for defecation

Discussion: The sudden, frenetic onset by a sliding glass door (or picture window) indicates that there may have been an intruder and that Ralph was responding to that; the sporadic pattern supports this. The clients' search for spraying is good, but it is not the only type of marking that can occur. The clients were asked to census their apartment complex for other cats and discovered that there was a cat that they had seen before; in fact, when

that cat would stand in the parking lot and spray the bushes, they discovered that this was visible from their doors. When they watched their cat during such episodes, he became agitated. The problem had been ongoing long enough that their cat had learned that he liked the carpet for defecation. This is consistent with a cat that does not cover its feces (but not required).

Treatment: The client was requested to confine the cat in a small room in which he had not defecated previously. They were to provide him with multiple litter boxes and litters, including one of the clumpable ones. They were also asked to try covered versus uncovered and deep versus shallow litter boxes. During such time, if he was let out of the room he should be on a harness. They were to put lace curtains over the windows and plants outside on the balcony to interrupt the cat's view. They were to make sure that Ralph had lots of attention while confined. Once he began to use his litter box reliably and would do so for a month, they were to gradually reintroduce him to the rest of the apartment in a free-range manner. To do this they were to put a bell on his collar so that they always knew where he was, and they were to supervise him. He was to be startled with a water pistol if he started to sniff and circle. If he still patrolled the door, we discussed a course of diazepam for him. This was the drug of choice because of the GABAminergic effects that would inhibit his anxiety about the "intruder" and would make him care less about that perceived threat.

Follow-up: The cat responded to the behavioral and environmental modification without recourse to pharmacological intervention. The clients realize that any future "visitation" could put this cat at risk for relapse and that he might then require medication.

9 ····· Canine Elimination Disorders

*F*ortunately, prevention, diagnosis, and treatment of elimination disorders for dogs is far easier than it is for cats. Many canine elimination disorders are truly management related (Voith & Borchelt, 1982b, 1985). Elimination disorders associated with abnormal behaviors that are not related to an underlying medical cause, to mismanagement (including early learning), or to social stimuli (a normal behavior in undesirable circumstances) are rare. Given this background, most of the diagnoses that make up canine elimination problems are probably not technically "disorders."

NORMAL ELIMINATION BEHAVIORS

The first step in the evaluation of elimination problems requires an understanding of age-specific, normal behavior. Puppies that are adopted at 8 weeks of age can urinate hourly while awake (and once or twice during the night when young) and defecate four times per day and be considered normal. Puppies may complete housebreaking easily if given the opportunity to eliminate in the desired spot on a schedule that mimics this one. If clients are not able to take the pup out during the night, confinement on absorbent surfaces may be required for a period of time after the pup has ceased to have accidents indoors during the daytime. In an older dog, the need for such frequent elimination would be a cause for concern. By the time most dogs are 6 months of age they usually defecate once or twice a day and urinate three or four times per day. Females may need to eliminate more frequently than males; females may not develop full sphincter tone until they have had a heat cycle. Frequent opportunities to eliminate prevent a full bladder and decrease the probability of accidents. This is particularly true for dogs that urinate when they are excited or afraid. Adult dogs can urinate as infrequently as twice a day and defecate once a day, if this is the schedule with which they are provided access for elimination. Dogs will be more comfortable if they are given at least three opportunities to eliminate per day, preferably ones that are also coupled with the opportunity to exercise.

Most dogs will eliminate frequently if given the opportunity. They do not eliminate only because of physiological stimuli and do not actually require, although they may enjoy, frequent access for elimination. Much of the additional elimination may have a social and communication component. Social facilitation occurs concomitant with estrous cycles, strange dogs, changes in social hierarchies within the household, the onset of social maturity, and so on. Changes in diet, environmental conditions, or water consumption can also alter elimination frequency without rendering it "abnormal."

Some breeds, generally those that have been selected to have a particularly keen sense of smell (e.g., beagles) can be difficult to housebreak not because they are stupid, but because they scent any previously soiled area and return to it. This tendency was substantiated by survey studies (Beaver, 1982a; Hart & Hart, 1985b; Hart & Miller, 1985). The same studies classified Yorkshire terriers, not renowned for their tracking abilities, as very difficult to housebreak. One has to wonder if clients are less motivated to comply with the exigencies of housebreaking for a dog for whom it is easy to clean up, owing to size of the error, when compared with one for whom the cost of the error is greater. No good data have ever been collected on this issue.

Some clients are concerned that their dogs eliminate in the "right" postures. The classic work of Sprague and Anisko (1973) indicates that virtually any elimination posture can be considered "normal" (see Fig. 3-1). Standing to urinate and leg lifting are affected by testosterone (Berg, 1944), and males generally use other positions only about 3% of the time. Borchelt (1984a) demonstrated that by 2 years of age, most male dogs elevate one or the other of their hind legs to urinate regardless of reproductive status. This indicates, to a large extent, that the posture is influenced by the social milieu. These same influences operate on females, although less attention has been paid to them. Most females squat most of the time (68%, Berg [1944]), but elevated elimination can be within the bounds of normal. That it occurs often in kennel situations hints at the social underpinnings. Posture, alone, is insufficient reason to postulate an elimination disorder unless it represents a change in the animal's behavior.

GENERAL CLASSIFICATION OF CANINE ELIMINATION DISORDERS

Differential diagnoses for inappropriate canine urination and defecation are as follows (Fig. 9-1).
1. Medical conditions (including urogenital and gastrointestinal disease, related illnesses, geriatric conditions, neurological conditions, and anatomical anomalies)

2. Incomplete housebreaking
3. Insufficient access
4. Substrate preference
5. Anxiety, primarily separation anxiety
6. Marking behavior
7. Submissive urination
8. Excitement urination
9. Elimination associated with fear
10. Attention-seeking behavior
11. Geriatric incontinence or estrogen-dependent incontinence

As is true for most other behavioral conditions, few good numerical or epidemiological data exist for canine elimination disorders. Incomplete housebreaking, separation anxiety, marking behavior, and substrate preferences are the most common diagnoses in the Behavior Clinic at the Veterinary Hospital at the University of Pennsylvania (VHUP).

Medical Conditions

As with any behavioral problem, ruling out any affiliated or causal medical problem is a prudent first step. This is particularly true for problems involving elimination because inappropriate urination and defecation can be nonspecific signs. The most common canine elimination-related disorders that are primarily medical include urinary tract (including renal) disease; congenital or anatomical malformation; endocrine disorders (e.g., adrenal disease); neurological abnormalities including reflex dyssynergia and lissencephaly; and polydipsia unrelated to disease (Blackwell, 1993; Crawford et al., 1984; Fenner, 1995; Lulich et al., 1995; Meric, 1995; Moreau & Lees, 1995).

Polydipsia is not uncommon in young puppies, and in the absence of other congruent signs, it usually signals no underlying abnormality, despite the copious production of dilute urine. Often young pups drink water because they are playing with it and with the shadows caused when the water moves. Although this is not a medical problem, ruling out concomitant disease is important because some cautious water restriction might be desirable. A chronically full bladder hinders the success of the most dedicated housebreaking program. Providing the puppy with small but frequent drinks can safely modulate intake. Ice cubes or chipped ice can also slow the rate of intake. Giving pups appropriate toys and encouraging their use will minimize the extent to which they play at the water dish.

Elimination problems involving defecation may be attributable to an underlying medical condition including gastrointestinal parasitemia, gastrointestinal bacteremia (e.g., *Campylobacter, Salmonella*), viral conditions (e.g., parvo), foreign bodies or gastrointestinal obstruction, anal sac disease, toxicosis (e.g., lead [plumbism] or garbage), food allergies, rapid dietary shifts, and gastrointestinal transit time alterations associated with age, condition, treatment regimens, or activity level. Changes in gastrointestinal motility warrant particular attention because they are often not considered.

Any dog that has pain in the hips or back may be reluctant to fully squat to eliminate. As dogs age, stool softeners such as bran, lactulose, and psyllium hydrophilic muciloid (Metamucil) derivatives may render defecation easier. If defecation is easier and not painful, the chances of a dog being able to complete defecation in one bout increase. Straining can be accompanied by elimination in inappropriate places and may be a sequela to constipation associated with pain. Older dogs, like older people, undergo changes in gastrointestinal tract physiology and mobility. They may require a more digestible diet or one that has a higher biological value. Fortunately, such diets are usually compatible with those recommended as part of the management protocols for renal and cardiac disease. Increases in frequency of defecation, the presence of straining, changes in consistency (generally, but not always, hardening), and changes in flatulence or comfort may all be clues that transit time/motility alterations are occurring. Changes in diet and exercise, increases in water content of food, and the addition of substances that act to osmotically enhance the water content of the stool at stimulus can be boons for older animals. Agents need not be expensive. Unprocessed bran is cheap and readily available in grocery stores. Addition of small amounts of bran and water to food can help older dogs to defecate more easily. If possible, increases in nonstressful, low-impact exercise or the addition of gentle massage can also aid in addressing altered gastrointestinal tract motility and pain. Some older dogs may just need to be walked more frequently to feel comfortable, regardless of whether they eliminate. Well-housebroken, fastidious dogs may be concerned about changes in their elimination behaviors that are attendant with age. In such situations, anything that can be done to decrease the dog's anxiety will prevent or ameliorate problems.

Treatments involving narcotic agents can cause constipation. The previous suggestions can help to prevent elimination problems in such situations.

Medical problems that are often heralded by a behavioral complaint are more fully covered in Appendix E.

Incomplete Housebreaking

The first step in diagnosing a presumptive behavioral problem involving elimination should be to ensure that the dog is actually fully housebroken. If the dog is older than 6 months of age and has always occasionally eliminated in the house, he or she is not fully housebroken. Care should be taken to define "occasionally": dogs that are frequently left for 12 to 15 hours without egress for elimination or those that have a bladder infection or bout of diarrhea and eliminate in the house *only* as such times may be fully housebroken. Dogs that are incompletely housebroken will eliminate in the house regardless of changes in the client's schedule and regardless of the presence or absence of the client. A diagnosis of incomplete housebreaking can be made only if the dog never had a prolonged period (at least a month) during which no elimination in the house occurred, regardless of household activity. Dogs that are not housebroken fall into three broad categories: those that show a disregard for substrate, those that prefer the substrate of their puppyhood (e.g., newspapers), and those that prefer a substrate that they have learned to like because it is where they have had a lot of accidents and is now impregnated with a stimulating scent (e.g., carpet).

Clients often assume that adult dogs adopted from the streets or from a humane shelter will be housebroken because of their age. This is a faulty assumption. Dogs that have been allowed free range do not know that they are to eliminate outside: they eliminate outside without inhibition because this is where they are. When brought inside they exhibit the same lack of inhibition about substrate, although they may not soil their sleeping areas. These dogs are not stupid, spiteful, or malicious, although the clients often believe that they are. Adopted, formerly free-ranging, or rehomed adult incompletely housebroken dogs will require work on the client's part to shift their substrate preference to a more appropriate one, or to help them develop a suitable substrate preference. They may never prefer a particular substrate such as grass, sawdust, or cement, but can learn that there are substrates to be avoided. Clients requiring that their new dog already be housebroken may do better by adopting an animal from a shelter that can provide an accurate history, a person they know who wishes to relocate a dog with known propensities, or from a rescue group where the dogs had lived with a reliable foster family.

Puppies are best able to develop a substrate preference for elimination at about 8½ weeks of age. Their gastrocolic reflex is well developed by 3 to 5 weeks of age (Fox, 1971a), and they do not require maternal stimulation to eliminate. Beginning at about 3 weeks of age puppies are capable of passing urine and feces without stimulation but have little regard for either the locale in which these are deposited or for any clues that the events are impending. These develop as the pup's neurological development proceeds. By about 8½ weeks of age, pups have sufficiently developed senses of smell and physical coordination that they can begin to learn to use a preferred substrate. If the clients do not offer them such a substrate, they will develop a preference to substrates that they are forced to choose. Hence, pet store puppies that are not adopted at 7½ to 9 weeks of age may come to their new homes with a preference for the substrate on which they were housed. This is often shredded newspaper or newsprint. The clients will have to shift this substrate preference to a more appropriate one. Clients who "paper train" their puppies because they are absent from them for long hours will face the same dilemma and attendant delays in full and consistent use of a preferred substrate. These problems are not insurmountable, but they should be brought to the attention of clients before they make the choice of where they obtain their pet and at what age that pet is obtained.

Dogs will develop their own substrate preference if denied access to one that the clients prefer. If the puppy is not supervised and not encouraged to eliminate in a specified spot, that dog will learn to eliminate in the area that it used most frequently as a youngster. Preferred areas for elimination are considered inaccessible if the dog is too ill or is developmentally delayed and cannot get there, if the animal is not provided access within a schedule that meets its physiological needs and not the client's desires, or if it is physically prohibited from reaching the area (e.g., inadvertently closed doors or snow drifts in front of dog doors). Clients should not automatically assume that their puppy is no longer having accidents in the house unless the pup is fully supervised. Like cats, dogs can ruin carpets without the clients ever having witnessed an elimination event. Not all dogs develop at the same rate, and clients need to make allowances for this variability even if they have had the same breed or obtained the dog from the same breeder and lines. One of my own Australian shepherds was born with physical defects and not fully housebroken until 8 months of age although she had good supervision, an older dog to mimic, and a huge yard—all attributes that my older Australian shepherd, who was housebroken in 1 day at 8½ weeks of age, lacked as a puppy. The breeder was the same for both dogs.

Protocols for housebreaking puppies and older dogs are found in Appendix B. General guidelines for housebreaking a dog include the following rules:

- Take the dog out frequently—generally immediately after awakening (even from a nap), playing, or within 15 to 30 minutes of eating
- Dogs should *not* be allowed to play and socialize first—they should be allowed to do this *after* they eliminate
- Choose a few restricted areas at first, and return to those
- If the dog is leash-walked, shorten the leash to encourage walking in a small area to mimic elimination behavior
- If the dog is not leash-walked, the client should stand relatively still and not stroll or play with the dog until he or she has eliminated
- Permit cautious sniffing
- Praise the dog as soon as it squats (this means that the client has to be there even if the dog is not leash-walked)
- Do not physically punish dogs that eliminate in undesirable areas—this could induce fear—instead startle the dog *only* if caught actually in the act and then only use enough startle to get the dog to attend to you and cease elimination—then take the dog out

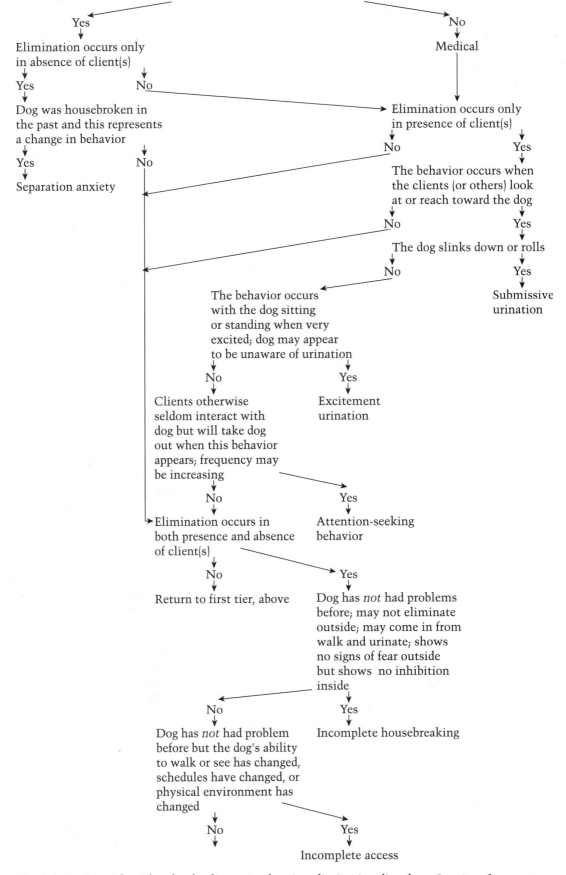

Fig. 9-1 Decision algorithm for the diagnosis of canine elimination disorders. *Continued on next page.*

Dog seeks out one specific
substrate; may eliminate
outside, but regardless of
schedule and exercise
returns to one or a few
locations of same type;
urinations are full-fledged,
not small amounts

No → Yes

Urine is deposited in   Substrate preference
numerous small amounts,
on more than one substrate,
and dog may also
experience full-fledged
urination and defecation
outside

No → Yes

Dog will not eliminate in   Marking behavior
certain circumstances that
may be numerous but are
identifiable and may
include presence of traffic
or strangers or in open
environments,
              AND
the dog exhibits concomitant
physical signs of fear (decreased
interaction, shaking, increased
heart and respiratory rates,
and cringing) when outside

No → Yes

Change is associated with   Elimination associated
age or change in hormonal   with fear
status (may be months
after ovariohysterectomy)

No → Yes

Something was missed   Geriatric incontinence or
                              estrogen-dependent
                              incontinence or canine
                              cognitive dysfunction

- Praise the dog when it eliminates in the appropriate place; you are not rewarding the act (this is self-rewarding), you are reinforcing the location
- Remember that female puppies may take a little longer to housebreak than do males and may need to go out more frequently
- If the pup has to go down stairs to eliminate, carry him or her; it may even be necessary to press a towel to the crotch area, the act of being placed on the floor can stimulate puppies to eliminate—do not worry that the pup will never learn to go outside on its own—you are helping the pup to form a substrate preference, not teaching it to walk
- Confine the pup when not supervised
- Bell the dog or use an "umbilical cord" leash to aid in supervision
- Watching an older dog can help a puppy
- Be consistent
- Be patient
- Restrict access
- Use good odor eliminators

Insufficient Access

Dogs that have been completely housebroken may still eliminate in the house if the client's schedule changes in a manner that prohibits either access to the areas in which they usually have eliminated in the past or maintenance of a schedule in which they eliminated. This is a particular risk for older dogs when switched to a more restrictive schedule. As dogs' abilities change they may require concomitant environmental changes. The extremely arthritic or dysplastic dog, or the one recovering from back surgery, is denied access if these special needs are not met just as is a dog that is locked in a room for 24 hours. If the portion of the yard where the dog eliminates becomes covered in ice during a bad winter (and snow that is walked on can go through more frequent freeze-thaw cycles, rendering conditions treacherous), few dogs will be willing to brave an unstable environment if there are other choices.

Social conditions can also be involved. Dogs that are timid in the absence of other specific pets may be unwilling to eliminate in their absence. Dogs that are afraid of certain people or animals, or dogs that are concerned about noises, including traffic, will not eliminate if they are anxious. This is a purely autonomic response and a normal sympathetic (fight-or-flight) reaction. Forcing such dogs to be exposed to the stimuli that they consider worrisome, in the absence of any other treatment, is liable to compound any elimination problem and worsen or create other fear-related problems.

The important fact to remember about insufficient access is that the dogs will, of necessity, eliminate elsewhere. Sampling and use of an alternate substrate is the first step in learning to seek that substrate. This is particularly true for substrates that absorb odor well and for dogs that are highly motivated by their sense of smell. Problems involving insufficient access usually lead to those involving substrate preferences. Prevention is paramount. If there are problems, address the initiating factor (e.g., the fear of street noises rather than the elimination problem, which is secondary).

Substrate Preference

Dogs start to develop substrate preferences for elimination between 7½ and 8½ weeks of age. Before this age they avoid soiling their sleeping areas but are otherwise relatively nondiscriminating. Clients can encourage the development of an appropriate or desirable substrate preference by avoiding mistakes and regarding successes as described previously and in the detailed protocol in Appendix B. Dogs can learn to discriminate globally between appropriate and inappropriate substrates, or can learn a very specific preference (the occasional show dog is taught to eliminate only on sawdust). They can also learn to eliminate opportunistically when the appropriate substrate is available, or to eliminate only on command (most po-

lice dogs). The clients need to choose which option will best suit their needs; if a restrictive option is called for, the earlier they start reinforcing it, the better. If the dog will be required to travel to and eliminate in a variety of locations and on a variety of substrates, early exposure is best, but lack of it does not doom the dog. As is true for all behaviors, the longer and more consistently the behavior has been ongoing, the more work that will be necessary to alter it. Show dogs, in particular, should be exposed to a variety of substrates early and learn to eliminate on command. I have seen dogs at shows that are not permitted to leave the premises make themselves ill because they will not eliminate in the conditions provided. Some show veterinarians and stewards will not temporarily excuse these dogs so that they can eliminate outside. Country dogs that will have to go to the city may go through a period of adjustment in asphalt and concrete jungles, and vice versa.

The development of a substrate preference usually requires some work on the part of the dog-client team but will generally occur unless something horrific happens. Most problems with substrate preferences involve situations in which dogs use what the client considers an undesirable substrate either because of having an "emergency" need and learning to like the new substrate (see the previous discussion on insufficient access), or because of a substrate preference that was in place before adoption that is not considered appropriate. The most common of the latter situations involve either dogs that were kept in a kennel in a concrete run and now will use the concrete basement floor, or puppies that were raised in kennel situations on something like newspaper. When no newspaper is available, these puppies are amenable to learning a new substrate, but even temporary placement of that day's newspaper on the floor can trigger a response that will enforce their first substrate. Preferences can be shifted by (1) monitoring the dog through the use of crates, gates, a leash tied to the client, or a bell (check on the dog if the bell stops making noise after dog moves away), (2) startling the dog with the minimum amount of startle necessary to get the elimination behavior to cease and while convincing the dog to attend to the client (i.e., do not use a fog horn if "oh-oh" suffices), and (3) taking the dog to the area where the client wishes him to eliminate and rewarding with praise, play, and possibly a treat when the dog eliminates appropriately. There are no rigorously collected data that support a reinforcing role of treats in the formation of a substrate preference. Elimination is a self-rewarding behavior and the fuller the bladder the greater the reward. Praise given at the instant of the squat can reinforce the choice of substrate. A food treat may more readily reinforce the combination of the squatting behavior on the desired substrate. Anecdotally, when I first had my first Australian shepherd, "Maggie," I carried treats and rewarded her every time she squatted. After a few days I noticed that she had begun to squat multiple times during walks. Being concerned for the development of a urinary tract infection, I then reached under her the next time she squatted to find . . . no urine. She had learned (at 9 weeks of age) that every time she exhibited a squat posture outdoors, but not indoors, I would give her a treat. She also eliminated only outside and had no accidents indoors. Smart dog.

Dogs that have never had to inhibit themselves (stray, roaming dogs; research kennel dogs) may have no preference and no inhibition. The keys to treating this problem are twofold: (1) Disabuse the clients of the impression that dogs "know" where to eliminate; in fact, a choice of location or timing has never mattered to them before. How are they to know these are important factors? (2) Take them to the preferred space often, focus on any quick response or apparent preference to a new area or substrate, and reinforce that. Development of a substrate preference can be more easily accomplished in older dogs because they can practice volitional inhibition; the client's task then focuses on encouraging this. Appendix B contains a protocol for housebreaking an older dog that will be useful in these cases.

Anxiety/Separation Anxiety

The most commonly diagnosed anxiety in dogs is separation anxiety. This is discussed more fully in Chapter 10; only the elimination component of this problem is addressed here. Dogs with separation anxiety become distressed when one or more of their people leave them (Borchelt, 1983b; Borchelt & Voith, 1982d; Voith & Borchelt, 1985d). Symptoms of separation anxiety can include destruction, particularly around windows or doors, elimination, and vocalizations. If the presumptive diagnosis is elimination as a consequences of separation anxiety, the following conditions *must* be met: (1) the dog eliminates in the house *only* when the clients are not home or *only* when a particular and consistent individual in the household is not home (in truly extreme, and rare, cases visual separation is sufficient to trigger the response); (2) the dog *never* eliminates in the house when the client or clients are home, regardless of whether the schedule is the same or the intervals between elimination opportunities are lengthened; (3) everyone, including the veterinarian, is certain that at some point the dog has been housebroken (separation anxiety is more common at social maturity and beyond); (4) there are *no* detectable medical conditions correlated with the change in elimination behavior; and (5) changes in schedule are less important than presence or absence of the client or clients. Correlated behaviors may include destruction and vocalization, but a diagnosis of separation anxiety can be made if only elimination is present if these other criteria are met. The treatment of this form of elimination disorder hinges on treating the underlying problem—the separation anxiety. Counterconditioning, desensitization, making the dog

feel safe (which can entail measures from crates to babysitters), frequent walks so that the size of the urine or fecal pools is smaller, and hence less likely to act as an olfactory and behaviorally reinforcing stimulus, and the use of antianxiety medication can all help. These treatments are more fully discussed in Chapter 10. If the problem has been ongoing long enough, the dog may have developed a new substrate preference. This can be addressed as discussed above.

Marking Behavior

The type of marking behavior that receives the most attention is male urine marking that is a result of leg lifting or cocking. This is both a social and hormonally facilitated behavior (Dunbar & Buehler, 1980; Dunbar et al., 1980, 1981; Gerber, 1973; Hart, 1974d, f). It is most common in intact males, and castration will prevent or decrease the frequency of the behavior by about two thirds (Hart, 1968, 1974b, c, 1979c; Hopkins et al., 1976). The fact that castration neither prevents nor ablates the behavior suggests that the social component can be complex and that learning is involved. In fact, although few quantitative data exist, the dogs that appear to respond to castration with the greatest decrease in the behavior may be those for whom the behavior has not been ongoing a long time. The removal of the hormonal facilitation is sufficient to decrease their interest and prevent the potentiation of the behavior through repeat performance.

It is less commonly appreciated that females can mark by squatting and urinating, and that both males and females can mark by defecating. To some extent, female urine marking, whether by squatting or elevation, is affected by endogenous gonadal hormones (Beach, 1974, 1975). Females in proestrus or estrus will urinate more frequently and pass smaller amounts of urine when they do urinate. They may squat in the presence of other females or in the presence of males, regardless of the male's reproductive status. This marking behavior can be associated with other postural displays that may reflect patterns in the social hierarchy. Although social and sexual maturity are widely separated in time and relatively independent of each other, social hierarchies may be affected by hormonal influences. In free-ranging canid groups one male-female mated pair may do most, if not all, of the reproducing. This is modulated through social interactions that include marking on the part of the female. In households with multiple breeding females, marking and posturing are not uncommon. In fact, these behaviors often increase concomitantly with the stress of social challenges associated with the presence or absence of young and the age of those young. Even in the relative absence of hormone surges, marking can reflect relative social rank in female dogs. In households of spayed dogs it may be possible to ascertain relative hierarchical rank partly by using marking pattern: very confident females can choose (or not) to cover other animals' urine (male and female, but the pattern may be intrasexually exaggerated), but when they do cover another's urine, theirs will then not be covered. Females can change in their response to other females: younger pup's urine may be smelled, but not covered, until they reach social maturity sometime between 18 and 36 months of age. If the younger dog tries to eliminate over the older or higher ranking dog's urine, the latter will again cover the urine of the upstart. Such marking is often accompanied by physical challenges such as butting, rolling, T-challenges, parallel posturing, scruffing, vocalizing, and presenting the corner of the mouth for sniffing or licking.

Fecal marking can occur in the same contexts as urine marking, but has not been well investigated. It is not a sexually dimorphic behavior and may be a form of marking that is more apparent in social situations that involve frustration or those that are becoming newly established, or in situations where there is no established, interactive social hierarchy, but where turf is being delineated (property boundaries). Feces decay at a much slower rate than does urine and present a visual (and probably olfactory) stimulus for a period of time that far exceeds the visual or olfactory stimulus for urine. Little work has been done on this, but for dogs that appear to be anxious about their canine neighbors, appear to be less confident themselves, or for those who are leaving feces in accessways or visual pathways, fecal marking as a correlate of passive aggression or anxiety should be considered.

It is clear from the previous discussion that the underlying motivating factor for the marking behavior should be addressed. General guidelines for treating marking behavior must include obtaining an excellent behavioral history that accounts for all social interactions, including those that may be transient, occasional, or not well established in anything but a passive mode. This is the only way to determine how social interactions can be adjusted. The dog that lifts his leg on the couch every time the client's new boyfriend visits can interact with the boyfriend in a positive manner. Once the dog feels more comfortable with the relationship, he should stop marking.

Marking can act as advertisement, and very confident dogs can mark. This is occasionally (again, no specific incidence is reported for the population as a whole) associated with other assertive behaviors, such as dominance aggression. The associated and underlying conditions must be treated concomitantly.

Confining the dogs when unsupervised so that they do not repeatedly mark (and enhance the stimulus) a certain area can be helpful in the treatment of canine marking. When supervised, the dog's behavior should be monitored. Putting a bell on the dog's collar or using a lead can help. Some clients have used a series of mirrors, remote video devices, and remote sound devices to help them follow the dog's movements. As soon as the dog begins to display behaviors that precede the marking (i.e., leg lifting), the clients startle the dog at a sufficient level that they abort the behav-

ior, but not at such a level that the dog becomes fearful. Remote punishment devices can be used, but sneaking up on the dog and blasting him with a water pistol, whistle, or foghorn, providing that no one else suffers for this, may be equally efficacious. If the timing is correct, the dog will associate the startle with the initiation of the behavior, and not the client's presence.

Dogs that mark as a consequence of feeling anxious or unsure can also benefit from antianxiety medication, if behavior modification alone is ineffective. The least expensive and quickest-acting drug in such situations is the tricyclic antidepressant amitriptyline (Elavil) (1 to 2 mg/kg orally every 12 hours to start). Other tricyclic antidepressants and nonspecific anxiolytics have also been used with some success. Although they are generally less efficacious and more risky than these newer drugs, progestins have been used to control marking, particularly in situations when there is a sexually dimorphic component or a frank sexual one. Progestins are no longer the drug of choice to control marking behavior. Benefits, modes of action, guidelines for use, and side effects of all of these agents are discussed in Chapter 13.

Submissive Urination

Submissive urination is more commonly a problem of young pups, younger female dogs, and dogs that have been repeatedly corrected or kept in a dependent situation. The latter could range from kennel dogs to those that have been truly abused; dogs with clients who have corrected too frequently in too inappropriate a manner fall somewhere in between. The hallmark of submissive urination is that as the dog is approached or reached toward, or as an arm is moved over the dog, the dog assumes a more submissive posture and urinates. The submissive posture can range from sitting, hanging the head, and exposing the groin to a full-fledged grovel, with rolling on the back, tucking the tail, retracting the flexed forelimbs, turning the head, and salivating and urinating. Dogs do not have to have been beaten to assume this extreme posture.

Submissive urination is a normal canine behavior when it occurs in the context of an older dog nudging a puppy and sniffing his or her inguinal region. Humans have selected for "submissive" types of behaviors in dogs in general. These are frequently recommended in training manuals as a way to control a dog. Not all dogs are the same: forcing a submissive posture can elicit responses that range from attack of the client—in the case of a seriously dominantly aggressive dog—to copious urination. Because a dog's social system is actually based on deference and not on submission, clients would fare better by using other methods that require that the dog defer to them and to take their cues as to the appropriateness of their behavior from the client. As a corollary of this, submissive urination is best treated by not responding to submissive behavior. This does not mean that the clients should encourage the dog to run roughshod over them. It means that deferential behaviors that are not submissive (e.g., sitting and looking at the client rather than rolling, to get attention) are the only passive circumstances in which the dogs will get attention. If the dog can play, be fed, or do obedience exercises without displaying submissive urination, those should be encouraged. Any behaviors that reflect the dog's acknowledgment of its more dependent status must be passive and not active. Accordingly, clients will not be able to reach toward the dog to put on a leash if that action induces active submission and urination. Instead the clients will have to let the dog out to an enclosed area to eliminate, without reaching toward it, or lasso the dog, and then talk calmly to and praise the dog after elimination. Some very sensitive dogs cannot directly meet the client's eyes, even if that gesture is not truly a stare, without urinating. In such cases the clients will have to be more patient and more clever in their interactions with the dog. They will not be able to look directly into the dog's eyes, even if they do so adoringly, unless the dog is relaxed and not concerned about displays of status. If the dog likes to play ball, the clients can look at the dog then, and follow this by passively holding the ball and looking at the dog for short intervals without play. The ball will act as a bridging stimulus that will reassure the dog and allow it to learn about more affirmative social interactions.

Most clients are able to teach the dogs not to exhibit submissive urination by a desensitization/counterconditioning process that involves food treats. First, the dog should start with an empty bladder. The dog is then asked to sit while the food is held over its head and moved backward over the head; the dog will then sit as it tracks the food, but the dog doesn't meet the eyes of the client. As soon as the dog's rump touches the ground without any leakage, the treat is released. Clearly, if the dog rolls, grovels, or leaks, it does not get the food. The client can gently say "no," and move away. Once the dog has returned to a less concerned state, the client tries again. Sooner or later the dog will be without residual urine and will be able to get the treat. The treat has to be released quickly, and another treat instituted. The protocols in Appendix B provide more detailed instructions for this process.

Some dogs truly cannot initially overcome the stimulus of being reached toward or over even if a treat is involved. These dogs must first learn that the treat, itself, is associated with good things. These dogs can be encouraged if the client will ignore them while casually holding a treat dangling in the hand. Once they have repeatedly approached the client this way, the client can begin to alter his or her body posture until sitting, then facing the dog, then giving the signal to sit, and so on. Patience is of paramount importance. Verbal reassurance can accompany the good behavior, but some of these submissively urinating dogs will cringe and leak at very loud and exuberant words, even if they are positive. Clients must be alert to full manifestations of the dog's excessively deferential behavior and avoid providing any of the cues that could provoke it. As the dog's behavior improves, the clients can gradually add all the behaviors that provoke the elimination, but must do so in a manner that does not elicit relapse. This means that they must proceed slowly and pay attention to the dog's signals. Punishment has absolutely *no* role and will worsen the situation. It is important to eliminate odor because many dogs with these behaviors are young and may not be fully housebroken. The addition of a reinforcing olfactory stimulus will slow the latter process.

Ancillary treatment suggestions that may help include diapering the dog (it is physically more difficult to assume the submissive squat with the diapers on) and the use of a mild antianxiety agent if the dog is overly submissive in all social situations *and* the behavior modification alone either has not helped or is impossible to execute. The role of the drugs should be to augment the response obtained through behavior modification, not to substitute for it. Tranquilizing agents are undesirable, but tricyclic antidepressants can be useful, particularly because they have secondary anticholinergic effects and may result in increased bladder and sphincter tone.

Excitement Urination

Excitement urination is particularly common among young, exuberant dogs that do not have complete neuromuscular control. It may be worse if the dogs are awakened or startled and then become very excited. These dogs do not have to squat and may urinate while walking, standing, or jumping up and down. The dogs often outgrow this behavior. Keys to controlling it include (1) frequent walks so that the bladder is always as empty as possible, (2) teaching the dog to relax and to ignore excitable circumstances (see the protocols in Appendix B), and (3) once the clients are sure that the dog is housebroken and does have neuromuscular control, verbally correcting the dog by saying "no," and not interacting with the dog when it exhibits excitement urination. The latter should be followed by requiring the dog to perform an activity that is incompatible with the excitement (lying down with the neck and chin fully extended). Treating the excitability is the key to treating the urination. Very excitable, exuberant dogs often need more daily aerobic exercise. This can be provided by playing with Frisbees, agility training, high-jumping, or running with other dogs off lead in a safe, protected environment.

Elimination Associated With Fear

Fearful dogs can experience a reflex contraction of their bladder and colon muscles (encopresis) (Beaver, 1995). This is generally considered an extreme fear response. It is not clear if this response is an extended or more exaggerated version of submissive urination.

Dogs with elimination associated with fear show other autonomic signs of and physical postures associated with fear. These can include tachypnea, tachycardia, mydriasis, piloerection, shivering, salivation, distal limb contraction, avoidance, and catatonia. The urination and defecation exhibited in fear-provoking circumstances tend to be more explosive and involve a single bout; the urination exhibited in submissive urination may involve multiple bouts and may be dribbled. A dog that is urinating submissively may also exhibit signs of wanting to please or interact, but does not feel in a sufficient social position to do so. Accordingly, these dogs may wag their tails, may "grin," and may lick people's hands. Dogs that are fearful do not exhibit these behaviors. Just reaching toward a fearful dog in the context of putting on a leash may not be sufficient to elicit the elimination; however, loud voices, shouts, agonistic or aggressive approaches, and rapid raising of arms will elicit the full-blown fear response and the elimination. The difference in the behavioral patterns exhibited by dogs with submissive urination and those exhibited by dogs with elimination associated with fear may be one of degree, but it is necessary that other signs of fear be exhibited to diagnose the latter.

In this situation, treatment of the elimination behavior is directly related to treatment of the fear. All eliciting stimuli and events should be avoided if possible. No punishment is to be used. Only positive reinforcement designed to teach the dog to learn how to earn affection (see Protocols in Appendix B) should be used. Drugs may be necessary and ones that have proved useful include buspirone, amitriptyline, fluoxetine, clomipramine, and some of the newer benzodiazepines. Any concomitant aggressions must be identified because some of these agents can worsen aggression. Use of pharmacological agents in the treatment of fear and aggression is more fully discussed in Chapters 6, 10, and 13.

Attention-seeking Behavior

Attention-seeking behavior is more fully discussed elsewhere; however, clients and clinicians must remember that dogs that do not get sufficient attention by acceptable means will resort to unacceptable ones. Some dogs do a very good job of "training" their people to rush them outside by squatting inside. Such elimination is generally done only in the client's direct presence, and once the dog gets outside it is happy and playful, and may not eliminate. This helps to distinguish the dog that is too afraid of the outside conditions to eliminate outside. Clients can induce this behavior by hovering over the dog and always rushing her out, but never otherwise giving her access to play or enjoy the outdoors. Increasing outdoor exercise on a regular schedule, following the "Protocol for Treating and Preventing Attention-Seeking Behavior" (Appendix B), and learning to confine or ignore the dog once the client is sure that the dog does not have to eliminate can all help. Treatment of the primary problem is necessary.

Geriatric Incontinence/Estrogen-deficient Urination/Canine Cognitive Dysfunction

Female dogs that have been spayed later in life or older dogs may experience leakage of urine when asleep or relaxed. Except for keeping their bladder as empty as possible, behavioral modification techniques will have little use here; punishment has even less use. Diapering the older dog can help (there are dog diapers available, but they are hard to find; britches for bitches in season can be substituted, or a homemade, custom version can be created from disposable baby diapers and surgical tape or moleskin). The key to controlling these behaviors is to find a drug that effectively increases urinary sphincter tone without other excessive anticholinergic side effects. These are listed in Table 13-1 in Chapter 13. In general, the best agents are those with the fewest side effects. These include tricyclic antidepressants because of the mild anticholinergic effects, decongestants (phenylpropanolamine) because of the mild anticholinergic effects, and drugs designed specifically to treat geriatric cognitive dysfunction (L-deprenyl). In the latter condition, dogs urinate indiscriminately, hypothetically because of senility changes (Brandeis et al., 1991; Milgram et al., 1993; Ruehl et al., 1994a, b). Phenylpropanolamine should be viewed as the first drug of choice because it is inexpensive, has few side effects, has a wide therapeutic range, and often works quickly. Other drugs can later be tried if this fails.

CASE 1

Signalment: "Collieflower," an 11-year-old, spayed female, rough-coated collie

Initial Problem: Defecation in the house

History: The clients report a gradual change in the dog's defecation behavior during the last 6 to 8 months. Until then, Collieflower eliminated outside 100% of the time. In fact, she was astonishingly easy to housebreak and is very fastidious. Beginning about 6 to 8 months ago the clients began to find feces in the house. At first these events were occasional, but in the last month they have become daily, and rarely have occurred multiple times a day. The dog appears to be depressed and hides from the clients on days when feces are found in the house, although they have never punished her or yelled at her. Over the past year the dog has become more arthritic and less active. Because of this the clients tend to walk her less frequently and less intensively than they used to. The clients think that days without feces might be associated with longer walks, but they do not know for sure. The clients are seeking help as a last resort; they are seriously considering euthanasia because the dog has all the signs of rapid deterioration and appears miserable. She still likes her biscuits and has a good appetite. She has been fed a premium adult dog food since puppyhood.

Physical and Laboratory Examinations: All laboratory tests were within reference range, and physical examination revealed no abnormalities, except for arthritis in the hips and shoulders. This is not crippling but does appear to be aggravating.

Diagnosis and Discussion: Gastrointestinal transit time/motility changes associated with age. The feces that the clients describe and the sample that they presented appear well formed, a little firm, and seem to be deposited in smaller, but more numerous clumps than one would expect for a dog this size. It is possible that the dog is no longer benefitting as much as she could from an adult diet, and is unable, because of her arthritis, to pass large volumes of feces in one bout. She was also not being exercised regularly and may not be getting enough exercise to stimulate full digestion of an adult diet.

Treatment and Outcome: Collieflower's diet was switched to a geriatric diet that was more digestible, and she was walked more frequently, but regularly and on grass (to minimize impact). Within 2 weeks her stools were smaller, softer, and more easily passed, defecation in the house had ceased, the dog was happier and more playful, and the clients were once again smothering her with love, now that they were not so fearful that her death was imminent. We discussed the occasional and cautious use of buffered aspirin to help relieve the periodic stiffness and hip pain. The clients reported that a few months later they had used one buffered, coated aspirin, given in food fewer than six times, but that this seemed to encourage the dog to want to continue with her exercise program. The clients were also instructed to carefully monitor stool texture; if stool became hard, they were to add a small amount of bran (1 tsp) with water to the dog's food daily. They did this as needed (which seemed to be associated with cooler temperatures [decreased water consumption] and decreased exercise) with good results. (NOTE: Since this patient was seen, newer agents have been developed for the treatment of canine arthritis).

Signalment: "Nick," a 1½-year-old, 21 kg, castrated male Dalmatian

Presenting Complaint: The clients brought Nick to the Behavior Clinic at VHUP because of his avoidance of and aggression toward people outside the family, particularly on the street, and his elimination in the house.

History: The clients obtained this dog at 3 to 4 months of age. He had always been a little leery of strangers, but he had recently begun to bark and growl frantically, while pulling away from any person, or strange sound, on the street. By the time they came to the Behavior Clinic for the first examination, the clients had virtually ceased to take the dog out during normal hours. Any people and any unexpected machine sounds startled him. The clients would try to take Nick out in the yard for elimination, but while outside he would not eliminate, regardless of how long he was left outside. Instead, he would become more anxious and agitated and more difficult to control if someone outside the family approached him. As soon as the clients brought him inside, he would eliminate in the house. In his struggles to back up while growling when he was approached by strangers, Nick was choking on his collar and dragging the clients during his walk. The clients could identify no predisposing events that correlated with this behavior.

Physical Examination: No abnormalities were detected on physical examination. Urinalysis was unremarkable.

Diagnoses: The diagnoses were fearful aggression and inappropriate elimination related to anxiety. The clues were as follow. First, Nick invariably backed up while growling and often shook while aggressive. His tail was never wholly vertical and flagged, but was often tucked below the line of his back. Although he lunged in confined situations, he also retreated after the lunge. These are behaviors consistent with a diagnosis of fearful aggression. In the absence of unfamiliar people or objects, he was still nervous when out of the house. The clients reported that he tucked his tail, exhibited constant vigilance and scanning, and was "jumpy." These behaviors started as he approached social maturity (18 to 36 months of age in dogs; range 12 to 48 months). This is also the age at which many fearful behaviors and early signs of mental illness appear in another social animal, human beings. He had never been all that outgoing with strangers, but had not become aggressive until recently, and the aggression was worsening. "Nick" had been fully housebroken as a pup and had no problems sleeping through the night without eliminating despite his propensity to eliminate in the house in the daytime. The onset of the elimination problem coincided with the worsening of the aggression.

Treatment: At the first visit Nick was placed on the first tier of the behavior modification program. The foundation program is designed to teach the dog to lie down or sit and stay while relaxing in a a variety of circumstances. Dogs are to take their cues as to the appropriateness of their behaviors from the client. This is not an obedience exercise; it is one involving relaxation and desensitization. It is critical that clients realize this and reward the physical signs that the dog is relaxing and is becoming less reactive to external stimuli. Nick was able to perform the first of the exercises well at the clinic. The clients were encouraged to avoid all circumstances that triggered the undesirable, inappropriate behavior and to work intensively with the first phase of the program. Once he performed perfectly on that phase, they could start to walk him in areas where he would only see people at a distance. If he started to become anxious or fearful (ears back, stiffening, trembling, pupils dilated) they were to ask him to sit. If he was still upset, they were to turn him around and take him away from the situation. To facilitate this, he was fitted with a Gentle Leader/Promise System Canine Head Collar (Premier Pet Products, Richmond, Va). He was instantly calmer with this while at VHUP.

In addition, the clients were to take him out to eliminate frequently and praise and reward him for outdoor elimination. It was emphasized that they were rewarding the timing and location of the elimination—the act, itself, is self-rewarding. They were to try to stay out long enough so that he would eliminate, but were to bring him in if he became anxious. When unsupervised in the house he was to be restricted to one area. The clients were to clean all affected areas with a good odor eliminator.

We discussed that antianxiety medication is often useful for such dogs. The clients expressed an interest in trying the behavior modification, alone, first.

Follow-up: A phone call a few weeks later revealed that the clients loved the head collar and were able to walk the dog in low-traffic areas. He had begun to react less to some people, and the clients continued to practice the program. If anyone approached him he still had a full-blown problem, and there had been no attenuation of the elimination problem. At this point the clients asked if they could start an antianxiety medication regimen. After a discussion with their veterinarian, the dog started to take 25 mg amitriptyline orally every 12 hours after the complete blood cell count and serum biochemical profile revealed no abnormalities.

The clients brought Nick for a reexamination after a few weeks of amitriptyline treatment. They reported that after the first week with the medication, the dog would willingly go for walks and always eliminated outside, and when people approached he did not growl. They took advantage of this change in behavior and gradually introduced him to people, first outside, and had him sit and relax while they approached, talked to, and then briefly petted him. Unlike at his first visit, when he growled, snarled, and backed into a corner, he was totally calm at the reexamination appointment, allowing everyone to pet him, wagging his tail, and responding to all commands. The clients are to maintain the antianxiety medication for at least another 2 months. If they do decide to see if he can sustain this behavior without it, they are to wean him from it gradually, not stop suddenly. The clients also realize that Nick may need antianxiety medication for life.

The antianxiety medication facilitated Nick's ability to overcome his fears about the outdoors. Because he had been housebroken previously, he was willing to eliminate outside once he could manage his fear. He may also have benefitted from the side effects that are associated with tricyclic antidepressant (TCA) use: anticholinergic action and increased urinary sphincter tone. It is worthwhile to note that (1) a physical examination and blood tests were performed before administering medication, and (2) the first drug of choice was a low-tech one. Amitriptyline is one of the oldest TCAs available. It is inexpensive, acts quickly, and has relatively few side effects (gastrointestinal upset, inappetence, regular tachycardia and concomitant panting, lethargy) for which the clients were instructed to watch. This is a good example of a rational approach to pharmacological intervention for behavioral problems. Such cautions are warranted because few psychotropic medications are licensed for use in domestic animals (hence, all use is extra-label), and pets cannot tell us that they are experiencing side effects—clients have to help us watch for these.

This case is discussed from the aspect of the aggression problem in Chapter 6.

Signalment: "Sasha," 10-month-old spayed female beagle

Initial Problem: Eliminates, usually feces, in house

History: The pup was adopted by the client's husband 2 months ago as a surprise; the client has never had a dog. The dog came from a pet store, but had one other client, a student, who could not keep her and advertised for adoption. The client has a 3-year-old-son.

The dog is walked three times a day and usually urinates on the walks but does not defecate every day on the walks. The dog is very anxious to meet other dogs on walks and pulls on the leash. The client wants the dog to be able to use the fire escape/terrace for elimination in bad weather; she puts the dog out there first thing every morning. The dog will usually urinate out on the terrace, especially if there is newspaper there, but usually is found to have defecated within 20 minutes of coming back in. The client does not see the dog defecate. If the husband puts his newspaper on the floor after reading it, it is often found later covered with urine.

The clients are feeding the dog Puppy Chow (Ralston Purina, St. Louis, Mo.) three times a day; she seldom finishes each dish of food. Feces are usually found once daily in the house, but often twice a day. Each of the above walks last 15 minutes, and the dog is put out on the terrace three or four additional times per day.

The pup follows the son and shares all his snacks; the pup never steals from the child, but always waits until food is offered. If the son steps on the pup, the pup yelps but has never shown any signs of aggression. Whenever the dog is alone, there is no destruction, but sometimes the client finds feces. Whenever the client finds feces, she drags the puppy over to the pile and yells at her, then swats her with a newspaper. While here, the dog jumped on everyone and did not know how to sit on command.

Physical Examination: Results of physical examination were within normal limits. The pup was spayed last week and the incision is healing nicely.

Diagnosis: Attention-seeking behavior and inappropriate housebreaking

Treatment: The dog is to be crated when not directly observed by the client. The placement of a bell on the dog's collar will help the client notice when the dog disappears when out of the crate. If this happens the client is to sneak up on the dog and squirt her with a water pistol if the dog begins to eliminate or if she shows any of the behaviors associated with an intention to eliminate.

The client is also to increase the dog's aerobic exercise through increased play indoors and by increased walks and runs outdoors. The dog is to be walked on a Gentle Leader/Promise Canine Head Collar so that the client can reinforce good behaviors and correct inappropriate ones. In addition, if the client is not struggling with the dog during the walk, she will be willing to take the dog on leash walks more often. The leash walks, while increasing in frequency and duration, are to be on a regular schedule to help entrain the dog's elimination behaviors. During the first part of each walk no play or interaction is allowed; the focus is elimination. The dog is rewarded for elimination by praise and a more extensive, interactive walk. The client was cautioned not to rush the dog into the house immediately after elimination.

Feeding times are also to be regular and predictable and coupled to walk schedules. The dog is to be walked 30 to 45 minutes after each meal or any treats. This means the son will have to either modify his snack schedule or exercise the dog more. He's a bit young to do these without parental help.

If the client is determined to break the dog from newspaper use, no newspapers can be placed, even temporarily, on the floor. Otherwise, a large, short litter box can be equipped with newspaper and placed by the door. This doesn't excuse the client from having to perform the other modifications.

Finally, the client is to follow the Protocol for Treating and Preventing Attention-Seeking Behavior, Protocol for Deference: Basic Program, and Protocol for Relaxation: Behavior Modification Tier I (Appendix B). This dog needs to learn to attend to the client for clues as to the appropriateness of her behavior. These programs will help teach the pup basic manners. The client also knows that indoor use of the head collar may help expedite these changes.

10 ····· Fears, Anxieties, and Stereotypies

···

*D*iagnoses are not diseases; correlation is not causality. Conditions for which there is putative etiologic and pathophysiologic heterogencity (multifactorial disorders) are complex, and nowhere is this more true than for the topic of fears, phobias, and anxieties. By definition, diagnosis and treatment of these conditions is complex. Fears, phobias, anxieties, and stereotypies (obsessive-compulsive disorder [OCD]) are among the most difficult behavioral problems to diagnose and treat. There is probably no other area in behavioral medicine that is fraught with so much confusion and opinion. Fear and anxiety are probably closely related but may not be identical at the neurophysiological level. It is worth remembering that a diagnosis of a problem as related to fear or anxiety is at the level of the phenotypic or functional diagnosis, but that when psychotropic medication is used, such conditions are treated at the neurophysiological level (Box 1-1). Phenotypic (functional, phenomenological) diagnoses are open to various mechanistic bases of all subsequent levels. Some of these more reductionistic levels can be tested with treatment (specific pharmacologic agents), but few phenotypic diagnoses can be specifically tested with behavior modification. Regardless, the logic for using very specific phenomenological diagnoses related to fear and anxiety is to (1) enumerate and identify the particular behavioral manifestation that needs to be altered or assessed, and (2) to identify areas where specific behavioral intervention can be useful.

DEFINITIONS

This is one subject where cautious and discrete use of terminology will lead to clear thinking. With that in mind, a list of accepted definitions follows. Although these definitions are clear, the conditions for which they are relevant may be multifactorial and heterogeneous. Diagnosis may not be as simple or clear-cut as a definition. We do not understand the manner in which the levels cited in Box 1-1 (p. 3) interact to produce the problem—we can only evaluate the phenotypic form in which interactions occur. Clear use of terminology can help to make apparent the parts of these phenotypic diagnoses that are consistent, so that we can understand and separate them from those that are more complex.

Abnormal Behavior. Activities that show dysfunction in action and behavior (Fraser, 1980)

Mental Disorder. "Clinically significant behavior of psychological syndrome or pattern that occurs in an individual and that is associated with present distress (e.g., a painful symptom) or disability (i.e., impairment in one or more areas of functioning) or with a significantly increased risk of suffering death, pain, disability, or a loss of freedom" (American Psychological Association [APA], 1995). Regardless of cause, the disorder is a "manifestation of a behavioral, psychological, or biological dysfunction in the individual" (APA, 1995). The most prevalent disorders in the human mental health arena are anxiety disorders: panic disorder, phobias, OCD, generalized anxiety, and posttraumatic stress syndrome.

Fear. A feeling of apprehension associated with the presence or proximity of an object, individual, social situation, or class of the above. Fear is part of normal behavior and can be an adaptive response. The determination of whether the fear or fearful response is abnormal or inappropriate must be determined by context. For example, fire is a useful tool, but fear of being consumed by it if the house is on fire is an adaptive response. If the house is not on fire, such fear would be irrational, and, if the fear is constant or recurrent, probably maladaptive. Normal and abnormal fears are usually manifest as graded responses, with the intensity of the response proportional to the proximity (or the perception of the proximity) of the stimulus. A sudden, all-or-nothing, profound, abnormal response that results in extremely fearful behaviors (catatonia, panic) is usually called a phobia.

Phobia. Most fear reactions are learned and can be unlearned with gradual exposure. Phobias are defined as profound and quickly developed fear reactions that do *not* extinguish with gradual exposure to the object, or with exposure (as fears will) over time. Phobias involve sudden, all-or-nothing, profound, abnormal responses that result in very fearful behaviors (catatonia, panic). An immediate, excessive anxiety response is characteristic of phobias. Phobias develop quickly, with little change in their presentation between bouts. Fears may develop more gradually, and within a bout of fearful behavior, there may be more variation in response than would be seen in a phobic event. It has been postulated that once a phobic event has been experienced, any event associated with it or the memory of it is sufficient to generate the response. In fact, without reinforcement (exposure to a shock collar) these phobias can remain at or exceed their former high level for years. Usually the genesis for such events was either very scary and traumatic, or the dog has profound problems with fear, internally, and the fear (conditioned response [CR]) itself acts as a reinforcer (an unconditioned stimulus [UCS]). Phobic situations are avoided at all costs or, if unavoidable, are endured with intense anxiety or distress.

Anxiety. Anxiety is the apprehensive anticipation of future danger or misfortune accompanied by a feeling of dysphoria (in humans) and/or somatic symptoms of tension (vigilance and scanning, autonomic hyperactivity, increased motor activity and tension). The focus of the anxiety can be internal or external.

Separation Anxiety. When animals exhibit symptoms of anxiety or excessive distress when they are left alone, the condition is called separation anxiety; however, the most commonly exhibited behaviors (elimination, destruction, excessive vocalization) are only the most visible signs of anxiety. Drooling, panting, and cognitive signs of anxiety may not be diagnosed but probably occur.

Vacuum Activity. An activity involving an instinctive, unconscious, or response behavior in the absence of the stimulus that would elicit that behavior. Such activity seemingly has no apparent, contextual, useful purpose.

Displacement Activity. An activity that is performed out of context, or "displaced," because the animal is "frustrated" in its attempt to execute another activity or otherwise occupy itself. This is considerably less specific than redirected activity, which implies a substitution of behavior "in kind," but toward another target. In cases of displacement activity, the activity may not be "in kind."

Redirected Activity. Direction of an activity away from the principal target and toward another, less appropriate target. This is usually best identified when the recognized activity is interrupted by the less appropriate target or by a third party, and, in contrast to displacement activity, redirected activity appears to be a substitution "in kind" of the interrupted behavior.

Stereotypy. A repetitive, relatively unvaried sequence of movements that have no obvious purpose or function, but that are usually derived from contextually normal maintenance behaviors (e.g., grooming, eating, walking) (Luescher et al., 1991; Mason, 1991). Inherent in the classification of dysfunction is that the behavior interferes with normal behavioral functioning (Overall, 1994d).

Obsessive-Compulsive Disorder. This APA classification includes abnormal behaviors that have as characteristics recurrent, frequent thoughts or actions that are out of context to the situations in which they occur. These behaviors can involve cognitive or physical rituals and are deemed excessive (given the context) in duration, frequency, and intensity of the behavior. One of the hallmarks of this condition that distinguishes it from motor tics, and other signs is that

behaviors associated with OCD follow a set of rules created by the patient. The condition in domestic animals is probably similar and analogous. The neurophysiological basis of OCD may be homologous by descent (Overall, 1972c-e). OCD includes stereotypies, self-directed behaviors, and so forth. The behavior must be sufficiently pronounced to interfere with normal functioning.

Frustration. A motivational state that arises when an animal is engaged in a sequence of behaviors that it is unable to complete because of physical or psychological obstacles in the environment (Hinde, 1970).

Conflict. A motivational state in which tendencies to perform more than one type of activity are simultaneously present (Hinde, 1970).

Psychosis. A group of mental disorders (manic depression, schizophrenia) that are related to an inherent malfunction of the brain (a term best reserved for human psychiatry). This term has been used to describe dogs that do not respond to alerting stimuli because they are too anxious to do so, dogs that overreact to sounds, and dogs that are "hyperkinetic" (Campbell, 1992). Caution is urged for any nondiscrete use of the terms *psychosis* or *hyperkinetic.*

Neurosis. Neuroses are a group of affiliated anxiety states or phobias that are regarded as abnormal reactions to external circumstances. This term has an accepted colloquial meaning and may be best reserved for human psychiatry.

THE ROLE OF STRESS AND STRESSORS IN THE DEVELOPMENT OF FEARS, PHOBIAS, AND ANXIETIES

The perception and measurement of stress can be difficult to achieve in any nonverbal species. Stress is generally assessed through behavioral correlates of underlying physiological states that are known to change in stress-related situations. Well-being is defined for domestic animals as the absence of stress (Houpt, 1991a,b; Wolfe, 1987). It is interesting that the roles of fear, loneliness, and boredom—very complex, endogenous phenomena—are potentially more important for the assessment of well-being in laboratory animals than is pain (Wolfe, 1987, 1990). If this is also true for domestic pet animals—and there is no reason to expect that it is not—simplistic approaches that seek to alter only immediate and visible environmental stimuli will fail in the treatment of any anxiety-related problem.

Recognizing that stressful phenomena and responses are complex and sometimes adaptive, Breazile (1987) discussed three behavioral categories of stress and their behavioral guidelines. *Eustress* is used to signify a good stress associated with an intricate response that is beneficial to comfort, survival, and reproduction. *Neutral stress* is neither harmful nor hurtful over the long term. *Distress* is not harmful itself, but the response to it may interfere with the animal's well-being, comfort, and ability to reproduce. Behavioral guides that are associated with these types of stress include normal behaviors such as mating and feeding. Acute stress stimulates feeding (consider studying for an upcoming examination); chronic stress inhibits feeding. The responses are modulated through altered cholecystokinin (CCK), opioid, and dopaminergic mechanisms.

In a laboratory situation we might note the presence of distress earlier than we would in pet animals because we would note an alteration in reproduction, but laboratory-induced fears are *very* different from naturally occurring fears in humans and animals (Marks, 1970; Seligman, 1971; Seligman & Minoka, 1971). The other criteria associated with well-being or discomfort can be more difficult to recognize and may remain unrecognized longer in pets than in laboratory animals because we assume that our pets are all right if they are not in pain. Anxiety-related disorders are probably the most common class of disorders in pet animals and humans. The longer that these conditions are unrecognized and untreated, the more complex they become. We must change the manner in which we view well-being and discomfort in pets and humans to include the nontangible. This is difficult, but it is an attainable goal.

Physiological measurements that have been used to evaluate the presence of stress include (1) catecholamine levels and the extent of resultant bradycardia or tachycardias, (2) corticosteroids resulting from stimulation of the pituitary adrenal axis, (3) neutrophil/lymphocyte ratios, and (4) response to adrenocorticotropic hormone (ACTH) stimulation. These, too, are complex.

Increases in catecholamines can result in tachycardia as an initial response to stress, but bradycardia is a long-term response. These responses are the result of the interaction of the parasympathetic and sympathetic branches of the nervous system.

Corticosteroid levels have been noted to increase in situations involving crowding, isolation, and transport. The extent to which levels are altered as a result of crowding and isolation would be expected to vary depending on the extent to which the species is social and, under undisturbed situations, would seek close contact from conspecifics. Accordingly, primates may be more affected by isolation, whereas naked mole rats might be more affected by crowding. As a secondary effect of increase in corticosteroid levels, neutrophil/lymphocyte ratios decrease, an occurrence that might predispose to infectious diseases. This association may be a factor in multicat households that experience coronavirus and calcivirus outbreaks. Under prolonged and profound stress conditions associated with adrenal exhaustion, poor stimulation responses are obtained after administering ACTH.

Changes in glucocorticoid function that occur under conditions of stress include metabolic alteration, inflammation, changes in immune functions, and gastrointestinal (GI) alteration. Glucocorticoids effect these changes through two major interactions: (1) they elicit the production of the peptide hormones lipocortins by affected cells, which then decrease the production of prostaglandin, thromboxanes, and leukotrienes; and (2) they facilitate a neutrophilia that results in the release of marginated neutrophils into the circulation.

Responses to exogenous or endogenous stress can also be central. Vasopressin (ADH) is produced in the paraventricular neurohypophysis in response to diminished extracellular fluid volume, plasma hyperosmolarity, or distress. The presence of ADH changes the permeability of the nephron's collecting duct, resulting in the production of decreased urine in acutely stressful situations.

In humans, the perception of stress leads to changes in the pattern of neuroendocrine activation. An easily handled challenge leads to norepinephrine release and increases in testosterone with success. With anxiety, epinephrine, prolactin, renin, and fatty acids increase. Cortisol increases with distress (Henry, 1993).

Other substances that may be affected by stress include β-endorphins; production and release of substance P from the sympathetic terminals is also affected. The latter affects small intestine muscular contractility, arteriolar vasodilation, and salivary gland secretions. The effects on substance P provide one hypothetical mechanism for many of the behavioral effects that we see in animals that are "stressed" (drooling, flushing, GI distress).

The behavioral correlates of these physiological signs are generally based on comparisons (e.g., comparison of the types, style, and frequency of behaviors in captivity with those in the wild [for nondomestic animals]); choice experiments for behavioral, social, or affiliative situations; or operant-conditioning experiments that indicate the extent to which the animal will work for a given reward. The latter helps to assign a value to the reward and, in the presence of alteration of response in an experimental or "treatment" situation, can be an indirect measure of the extent to which the "treatment" is stressful. These behavioral criteria work best for experimental animals, but the concept of using a *change in behavioral parameters* to gauge the extent to which a *change in situation* might be disruptive or stressful can be adapted to pet situations where stress is purported to play a role.

NEUROANATOMY OF FEAR, ANXIETY, AND OBSESSIVE-COMPULSIVE DISORDER

The extent to which learning and memory play roles in fear, anxiety, phobias, and OCD has been poorly studied because it is difficult to do so given the complexity of the neurochemical systems involved. However, the following facts *are* known: (1) a functioning amygdala and long-term potentiation (LTP) are required to learn fear, (2) a functioning forebrain is required to unlearn fear (i.e., to effect habituation), and (3) many human fears appear to be the result of the inability to inhibit a fear response. Accordingly, it has been hypothesized (Rolls, 1990) that fear is related, in part, to chronic amygdala overreaction, failure of the amygdala to turn off after the threat has passed, or both. The specific neuroanatomy of a fear response involves the locus ceruleus (LC), the principal norepinephrinergic (noradrenergic) nucleus in the brain. Dysregulation of the LC appears to lead to panic and phobias in humans (Charney & Heninger, 1986; Charney et al., 1990). The LC directly supplies the limbic systems and may be responsible for many correlated "limbic" signs. Patients with true panic and phobic responses are more sensitive to pharmacological stimulation and suppression of the LC than are control subjects (Charney & Heninger, 1984; Heninger, 1986; Ko et al., 1983; Pyke & Greenberg, 1986).

Imaging techniques have been useful to study fears, anxieties, and phobias, although they are currently of limited therapeutic and diagnostic use. Positron emission tomography (PET) scans have been used to study regional brain flow as a measure of neuroanatomical correlates of emotion. In these studies painful electric shock has been applied before, during, and after anticipation of it. Increases in blood flow in bilateral temporal poles during anticipatory anxiety have been noted. These same neuroanatomical regions are implicated in lactate-induced anxiety attacks in panic disorders (Reiman et al., 1989), suggesting a mechanism for the development of panic in humans. The lactate test is an accepted test to provoke (and diagnose) panic attacks in people, but it has not been evaluated in pets. In human lactate-responsive/susceptible patients, parahippocampal blood flow (a marker of neuronal activity), blood volume, and oxygen metabolism are asymmetrical when evaluated by PET scans under resting, nonpanic conditions. This suggests that the abnormality is both biochemical and structural. The biochemical abnormality is postulated to be the result of an increase in norepinephrine output from the LC, which, in turn, stimulates parahippocampal "overresponsiveness."

PET studies to evaluate cerebral glucose metabolism in childhood-onset OCD after 1 year of pharmacotherapy indicated that there is a decrease in the orbitofrontal regional cerebral glucose metabolism bilaterally that correlated with two measures of OCD improvement (Swedo et al., 1992). Changes in caudate nucleus metabolism have also been detected (Baxter et al., 1992; Insel, 1992). Use of neurophysiological indicator variables associated with conditions suggests that these regions at least deserve further study (Coon et al., 1993). Changes in ventricle/brain ratios have been noted in comparisons between psychotic depressed and nondepressed patients (Rothschild et al., 1989).

FEARS AND PHOBIAS

Fear is usually indicated by flight, escape responses, expressive facial and body signals, and concomitant physiological responses including increased heart rate, increased respiratory rate, muscle tremors, urination, defecation (encopresis), and, in dogs and cats, anal sac expression (Archer, 1979). Physiological components of this fearful response involve those related to both the autonomic and neuroendocrine systems. The pattern of the physiological response can be affected by individual genetic variation, individual historical effects (entrained nervous systems), sex, intensity and duration of the response, and the extent to which any response could be adaptive in that situation (Mayes, 1979). Profoundly fearful responses may include immobility or freezing (Archer, 1979).

Stimuli that are usually associated with fear include predators, intense physical environmental stimuli, and a conspecific (same species) threat signal (Russell, 1979). These stimuli demonstrate that fear, in context, can be an adaptive response. Maturation and experience with certain situations can play a role in the development of a specific fear (Salzen, 1979). Experience and developmental stage can have an effect on the development of fear if the animal is not sufficiently exposed to the relevant stimulus during a sensitive period (Elliot & Scott, 1961; Freedman et al., 1961), or they can act to enhance a fear if exposure is too severe (Clarke et al., 1951; Fox, 1968; Stur, 1987). The rate of eating as an adult can be based on infantile food deprivation in puppies, but faster eating puppies do not eat more than nondeprived animals (Elliot & King, 1960). Syndromes related to lack of exposure that have been identified include isolated syndrome, in which one has limited exposure, and Kaspar Hauser syndrome, in which one is kept only under severely restricted and deprived conditions (Beaver, 1995). Specific patterns of fearful behavior and their intensity are determined by multiple, interacting factors including genetic makeup, previous experience, the class of stimuli (which, in turn, depends on evolutionary effects—i.e., cats and dogs may not respond in the same manner to the same stimuli), intensity of stimuli, and the relevance of the social system (Hinde, 1970; Russell, 1979).

The evolutionary and domestication histories of any animal may reflect the extent to which any fearful response has, and is perceived to have, an "emotional" component, in addition to behavioral and physiological ones (Shull-Selcer & Stagg, 1991). Early studies indicated that general activity level could be used as a sign of "emotional" level (Ader, 1965; James, 1951). The extent to which animals "know" that they are acting in a bizarre or abnormal matter has been the subject of much debate (Griffin, 1992). Subjective awareness, an important component of the emotional response, can be difficult to evaluate in dogs and cats, although it probably does change their behavior. Because we cannot ask dogs and cats what they are thinking or feeling when they exhibit a response that is "fearful" (judged by behavioral and physiological measures), it is difficult to separate the subjective awareness or emotional component of the fearful response from the stimulus (Rachman, 1974). Humans

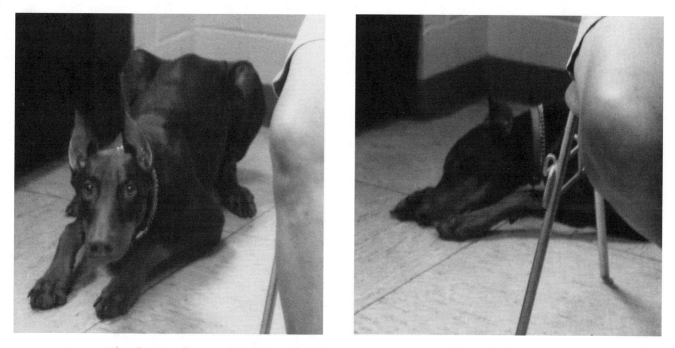

This dog was diagnosed with fear of approaches by strangers. He was not aggressive. In the first photo he is backed into the corner of the room and while he is lying down, he is tense and alert and showing parasympathetic signs associated with fear. In the second photo he is exhausted. He moved further behind the client and cannot fully relax; his nose is flush against the floor and holding up his head. This posture is associated with alert behavior. (Photos by K.L. Overall)

can describe actual secondary or emotional effects that are associated with their fearful behavior; these secondary or emotional effects can then act as the stimulus for a subsequent response. The same pattern of response is seen in dogs and cats, so we can infer that they, too, should experience "emotionality" or subjective awareness of abnormal fearful responses.

Behaviors that are usually associated with fear in dogs and cats include lowering and tucking of the tail, piloerection, and flattening of the ears. None of these signals, alone and unqualified, is sufficient to indicate a fearful animal. Sighthounds frequently carry their tails lower than do other dogs, and a tucked tail can be "normal" for them.

Darwin (1865) believed that although dogs may cower, the hair does not come up unless some anger is involved. Canine signaling is slightly more complex than this, but Darwin's early observations demonstrated both the separation and the interaction of systems that govern aggression and fear. Piloerection itself indicates a dog that is reactive: raised hair along the entire dorsum is usually associated with more assertive aggression, whereas raised hair along the dorsal shoulders and hips is more closely aligned with fear and fear aggression. Ears can be flattened when the animal is unsure of whether it will have to flee or behave offensively, and the extent to which flattening is noted may depend on the breed. This may be particu-

larly true for breeds like Scottish fold cats. Behaviors associated with anxiety include panting, pupil dilation, ears back and down, pacing, drooling, hiding, shaking, exfoliation, shedding, whining, and destruction. Urination and defecation, when present, can be explosive, and lack of control or awareness might be indicated by dribbling with locomotion. As is true for any other physical evaluation of communication, signals should be congruent, and interpretation should depend on evaluation of more than one system.

Individual differences in breed and parental differences appear to be important determinants of fear in dogs (Scott & Fuller, 1965) and rodents (Corson & Corson, 1976). Genetic factors have been identified for lines of mice (Balk, et al., 1995; Cases et al., 1995; Tsirka et al., 1995) and dogs (Acland, Aguirre, & Overall, unpublished 1995; Humphrey & Warner, 1934; Murphree, 1973; Murphree et al., 1967). In these examples—and in fact, in most clinical cases involving fear—the response cannot be generalized to a specific conditioning event (Hottersall & Tuber, 1979).

The extent to which breed is involved in the development of fear and anxiety responses is important. Dogs may be fantastic models for human psychiatric conditions because dog breeds and breeding practices within breeds (line-breeding) serve to canalize overall genetic variation. If advances are made in the study of the genetics of anxiety, understanding homologous and analogous conditions in dogs could be critical. For example, 19% of more than 600 puppies (German shepherds, golden retrievers, and Labrador retrievers) in the guide dog program were frightened by loud noises (Scott & Biefelt, 1976). Eleven percent of German shepherds in a breeding program had what the evaluators considered to be increased auditory sensitivity (Tuber et al., 1982). For such fears the age of onset is typically after 1 year (Shull-Selcer & Stagg, 1991).

Breed also appears to canalize behaviors involved in shaping the manifestation of a response to stress. If wire-haired fox terriers and beagles are placed in total isolation during the first 4 months of life, they exhibit extreme fear in response to the stress of a novel environment. This response involves the assumption of bizarre postures, protracted freezing, and withdrawal. The manner in which the breeds diverge in their response is interesting: beagles become even less active in response to a stimulus, whereas terriers become more frenzied (Scott & Fuller, 1965). Scottish terriers that are reared in a 3 foot × 6 foot cage with little contact with people freeze and flatten against the floor, front legs extended and ears back when later tested at 7.5 months of age with new people or in an unfamiliar room (Clark et al., 1951). When these dogs were evaluated after 6 months of work designed to countercondition this response, there was little evidence of fear. Subtle behaviors are not usually subject to evaluation, but such data indicate that not all categorical responses are solely attributable to the environment. The extent to which genetics is involved is difficult to assess, especially if the ability to recover from early deprivation covaries with the ability to exhibit the response. A very brief period of handling attenuated the stress of a novel environment of puppies (Fuller & Clark, 1966). The effects of this may be modulated by genetic predispositions toward plasticity (Newman, 1989).

Phobias are probably quantitatively and qualitatively different from fears, but they are so closely related that they are often considered together. Counterconditioning experiments that induced fear in cats provide the basis for some of the first work on human phobics (Wolpe, 1967).

In one study about prevalence of fears, anxieties, and phobia in patients at a behavior clinic at Ohio State University separation anxiety (68% [81/118]), fear of loud noises (20% [24/118]), and fear of strangers or strange environments (8%, [9/18]) were all considered fearful conditions (Tuber et al., 1982). Phobic dogs comprise 8% of a patient population (160 patients) seen at the behavior clinic at the University of Tennessee College of Veterinary Medicine (UTCVM) (Shull, 1994).

There are multiple forms of responses to phobias. The most common include startle and fear reactions to sudden or loud noises (traffic, dropped objects) indoors or outdoors, hiding in the house or garden, fear-

ful reactions to some types of people (e.g., men with hats). These reactions commonly wax and wane with time. Risk factors appear to include belonging to a "reactive" breed (border collies, German shepherds) and having less than optimal exposure and experience during the first few months of life (e.g., illness, isolation, stressful shelter conditions) (O'Farrell, 1986). In such situations the phobic stimulus may appear to keep shifting despite application of what is basically counterconditioning by the client. One has to question the extent to which the clients may be actually reinforcing specific anxiety responses that appear in a variety of circumstances in their attempt to reassure the dog (e.g., telling the dog that it is "okay" when the dog is demonstrating the physical signs that correlate with the underlying physiological states of stress). In such cases it may be inappropriate to talk about "reactive" breeds without specifying the criteria used to make this determination, and without evaluating those criteria at a baseline and at exposure to client-administered counterconditioning.

Although phobias are distinct from anxieties and discernible from fears, they are probably related at the neurochemical level. The hallmark of a phobic response is the rapid rate at which the full-blown response develops (fears can develop more slowly and intensify with exposure) and the appearance of fully developed phobias with only one exposure to the stimulus (fears can develop with one exposure, but are subject to change in character with repeated exposure). The extent to which phobias develop from fears is unknown. The extent to which animals with fears or anxieties may be at risk for phobias is also unknown. It would not be unreasonable to postulate that these conditions are somehow related and might worsen each other. It also would not be unreasonable to assume that two animals with identical symptoms of fear differ at some mechanistic level if one has a phobia and one does not. Fears are difficult to treat; phobias are even more difficult.

Laboratory data are not as useful in understanding these differences as one would wish. Unlike laboratory fears and phobias, those that occur naturally or endogenously are often fully developed after one trial. This difference may reflect the extent to which the animal perceived the experience as horrific. Furthermore, natural or endogenous fearful and phobic responses are enhanced by, rather than diminished (and eventually extinguished) by repeated exposure as is true for the laboratory situation. The same stimulus appears to have very different facilatory roles (Marks, 1970; Seligman, 1971). This finding does not refute the fact that learning is involved in the development of fear or phobia because learning reinforces both classes of responses (Gray, 1971; Marks, 1970; Marks & Gelder, 1966).

Clients often seek help for phobic responses, but delay seeking help for fearful responses, particularly those that they deem minor. The dog or cat may not perceive the response as minor, but we have no way to evaluate the extent to which they perceive that they are distressed. This lack of early treatment further compounds the issue when the clients ask about situations that may have led to the phobic response. Client reports associated with phobias include running away, aggression (nonspecific descriptive category, *not* a diagnosis), trembling, hiding, vocalizing, elimination, self-trauma, and property damage (Shull, 1994). Of 49 phobic dogs examined at the behavior clinic at UTCVM, 44 (90%) reacted to thunderstorms and percussive sounds, 4 (8%) to vacuum cleaners, and 7 (14%) to miscellaneous stimuli (e.g., toilets flushing, windshield wipers) (Shull, 1994). The overall prevalence of phobic patients in this clinic was 8%. This number is interesting because it is considerably lower than the 19% reported for more than 600 guide dogs in a training program (Tuber et al., 1982).

THE ROLES OF AROUSAL AND REACTIVITY

Some dogs respond either more quickly or more intensely to a given stimulus than other dogs. At some level this "hyperreactivity" is probably truly pathological and represents yet another phenotypical manifestation of some neurochemical heterogeneity associated with anxiety. These dogs are truly different, and it can be very difficult or impossible to interrupt them once they reach that level where they "fire" indiscriminantly. Anticipation of behaviors that signal early concern is critical for the treatment of these individuals to be at all successful.

Other animals react with a higher level of intensity but may still be workable. Behaviors that can be used to ascertain levels of reactivity or arousal include alertness (hypervigilance), restlessness (motor activity), vocalization, systemic effects (emesis, urination, or defecation), displacement or stereotypic behaviors, and changes in content or quantity of solicitous behaviors. Dogs with the previously described truly pathological hyperreactivity do not generally evince these signs.

ANXIETY

Anxiety, fears, phobias, panic disorders, and obsessive compulsive disorder are neurochemically related, although they probably are not driven by identical mechanisms. Signs of generalized anxiety include increased vigilance and scanning, autonomic hyperactivity, and increased motor activity (APA, 1995). The use of the term *generalized anxiety* should be restricted to a specific diagnosis (see Appendix F for necessary and sufficient criteria). Most animals with behavior problems can be generally anxious, especially in novel situations, but for the diagnosis of anxiety or generalized anxiety to be made, the previous criteria must be met, and the circumstances must be general and unrelated to the immediate changes in the behavioral or physical environment.

Dogs and cats that are anxious can exhibit hesitant behavior that differs from that of fear through the intensity of the withdrawal, the uncertainty of the commitment to the next step in the behavioral sequence, and by the constancy of the environmental censusing. This constant level of anxiety is abnormal and out of context. Treatment involves teaching the dog a set of rules whereby he can guarantee relaxation and a contextually appropriate response (e.g., sitting and waiting—while showing all signs of physical and physiological relaxation—and being rewarded by a treat or love). Part of the anxiety disorder involves an abnormal response to the rules determined by the social environment. For anxious animals, the default rule structure hinges on the assumption that there is a need for vigilance and scanning, autonomic hyperactivity, and increased motor activity. This abnormal rule structure prohibits the animals from gleaning from their social or physical environment the range of behaviorally appropriate responses.

Clients need to understand this because they often maintain that the dog does not always exhibit the problem behavior and, hence, "knows better." That's true, but the animal's innate response, when removed from an absolutely reliable rule structure over which the animal has control, is to "assume" the anxious behaviors described. Anxiety-related conditions can include separation anxiety, noise phobias, aggressions—particularly some forms of dominance and inter-animal aggression—and some forms of elimination associated with fear. The hallmark of the anxiety-component of these problems is the animal's apparent inability to wait until there is a problem before reacting to the stimulus. For example, nothing tragic (except the self-induced damage) happens to the dog with separation anxiety when left alone; the anxiety is induced, out of context, by the action. The dog with dominance aggression may be fine with people who ask her to sit and give her good, consistent signals, but her responses to all others suggest that for each new person she must provoke the environment and formulate her behaviors based on their contextual response.

Because these animals cannot generalize the good and relaxed aspects of the social and physical environmental structure, the anxious part of their behaviors can become self-rewarding. The neuroanatomical, neurochemical, and molecular and genetic mechanisms of the broad phenotypic category termed anxiety should be highly variable.

SEPARATION ANXIETY

In human medicine, separation anxiety is seen as an important antecedent or current affect in panic disorder. Separation anxiety is prevalent as an undercurrent in the dreams of patients with panic disorder (Free et al., 1993). This suggests that in humans, as in pets, separation anxiety can occur separately from panic disorder, but that when the two cooccur the interac-

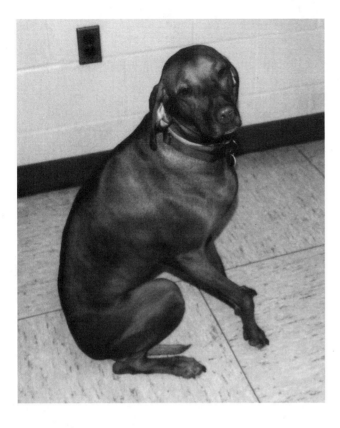 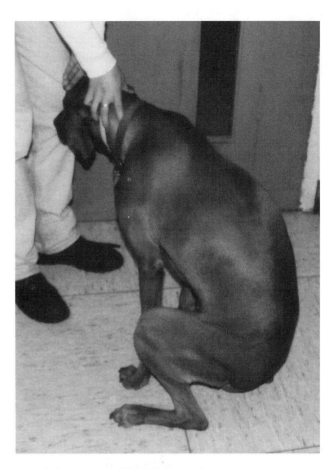

This dog was anxious of all social interactions with humans and had severe submissive urination accompanied by all other signs of anxiety in social situations. The first photo shows how she sits when not actively groveling and trembling while soliciting interaction from people. Note the raised forepaw, an intention movement. This dog wants to interact, but defaults to extremely anxious stereotypic submissive behavior when anyone pays attention to her. The second photo shows her response to being reached for after she solicited the attention: she hunches more tightly, tucks her tail, shakes, puts her ears further back, and dribbles. (Photo by K.L. Overall)

tion is an important factor in the assessment and treatment of either.

Overly fearful human youngsters are at risk for later emotional distress, including anxiety and depression. These individuals also have a higher incidence of allergic conditions. Such observations have suggested that regulation of fearfulness is probably the result of three interconnected parts of the brain: (1) prefrontal cortex, (2) amygdala (and the limbic system in general), and (3) the hypothalamus (hypothalamic-pituitary adrenocortical axis [HPA]).

Studies of monkeys suggest that levels of stress hormones influence how appropriately animals (and people) behave in the face of fear. There appears to be a link between basal cortisol levels and freezing or inhibition (Kalin, 1993).

Elimination, destruction, and vocalization are the commonly reported behaviors involved in separation anxiety (McCrave, 1991; Voith & Borchelt, 1985). Separation anxiety has been postulated to be an outgrowth of a distress response from separation associated with a highly social state (Voith, 1981c; Voith & Borchelt, 1985c). Accordingly, given the modifications that domestication has encouraged in dogs versus cats, one would expect separation anxiety to be more common in the former. Signs of anorexia, depression, and decrease in activity can also accompany some forms of separation anxiety (Voith & Borchelt, 1985c), as can diarrhea, vomiting, and excessive licking. It is interesting to note that the physiological signs seen represent nonspecific neuroendocrine correlates of anxiety. Differential diagnoses for signs should be carefully considered because the complaints of elimination, destruction, and vocalization are nonspecific in origin.

Overactivity associated with greeting can also be a

correlate of separation anxiety, but it is important to recognize that such greeting may be an anxiety response designed to elicit reassurance. Because of the abnormal nature of the condition, the reassurance is seldom sufficient to relieve the signs, but the clients respond as if they are truly attempting to relieve an anxiety. It is important to note that fear is *not* uncorrelated from separation anxiety, and that the interaction between these is poorly understood.

For the signs mentioned previously to be attributable to separation anxiety, they must occur only when the dog is separated or denied access to the client or clients. Differential diagnoses for elimination include separation anxiety, incomplete housebreaking, access to appropriate elimination areas, fear, excitement, submissive elimination, marking, and physical incontinence. Differential diagnoses for destruction include separation anxiety, play, normal puppy behavior, fear, overreaction to arousing stimuli, and overactivity and inanimate play. Differential diagnoses for excessive vocalization include separation anxiety, stimulation by bells, trucks, people talking, social facilitation (other dogs), play, aggression, and fear. Differential diagnoses for salivation are more limited and include thermoregulation, breed-typical behavior, oropharyngeal irritation or pain, nausea, and anticipation of a food reward.

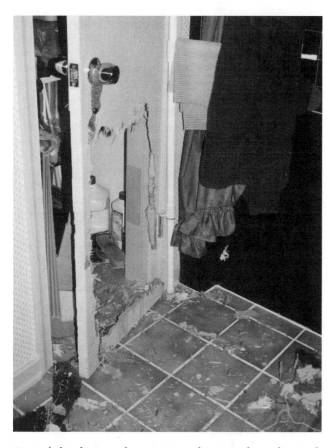

Part of the damage done in one afternoon by a dog with profound separation anxiety. (Photo by John McCann)

Signs of separation anxiety that appear in older dogs may be associated with anticipatory anxiety (Borchelt, 1983b). It is on this observation that the development of the concepts associated with "cognitive dysfunction" in older dogs have been predicated (Ruehl et al., 1994a,b). Failure of function or presence of behaviors associated with anxiety are not uncommon in older dogs. One of the first studies to examine behavioral problems in older dogs (Chapman & Voith, 1990a) found that over a period of 3 years, 10 of 26 dogs 10 years of age or older exhibited destructive behavior, 10 of 26 exhibited inappropriate urination, defecation, or both, and 7 of 26 exhibited excess vocalization. Thirteen of these 26 dogs had a diagnosis of separation anxiety (i.e., the behaviors occurred only in clients' absence), whereas six were attributed to breakdown of house training that did not meet the necessary and sufficient conditions (see Appendix F) for separation anxiety (i.e., "cognitive dysfunction"). The authors emphasize that older dogs have changing physical and emotional needs and that accommodating these needs and treating the dogs with antianxiety medications can help modulate symptoms, although the course of the underlying condition may be inexorable.

Signs of separation anxiety are commonly reported in studies of guide dogs (Scott & Beifelt, 1976); 21% of this population vocalized and 22% were destructive when separated from people. These vocalizing and destructive populations overlap, but few data are provided about specific frequencies and intensities of behaviors of dogs that exhibit both of these problems. Because the dogs were kept continuously with people from the time of weaning, these data have been used as evidence that closeness, attachment to, or "spoiling" by people causes separation anxiety. This is one of the analytical mistakes that is so common in the field of behavioral medicine. The more parsimonious explanation is one involving heritability; this program focused primarily on one breed and on lines within that breed. It is important to realize that these puppies were not unrelated to each other, but the puppy-raisers were. It is far more likely that the similarity that accounts for much of the consistency in the behavioral problems, which are all related to anxiety, is the one associated with relatedness of the dogs, not the behaviors of the people. This logic does not rule out a gene × environment interaction.

In the same study, 700 home-reared dogs experienced nonspecific "shyness." Data collected on fear and shyness in dogs raised for Canine Companions for Independence indicate that these traits appear to run within litters, more frequently than across litters, and that the appearance of problem behaviors does not appear to be affected by early spaying or castration (P. Mundell; unpublished, 1995). The extent to which these findings could be related to the age at which the dogs are fostered (12 weeks) or to any special, restrictive circumstances under which they are inadvertently raised has never been fully investigated. Dogs

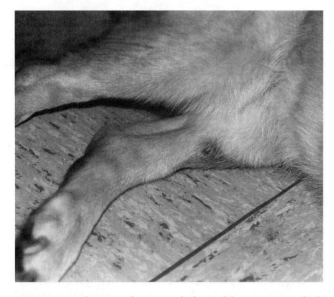

Anxiety can be manifest as subclinical but constant lick lesions. This dog has not been to a dermatologist for its skin lesions and has anxiety-related conditions (separation anxiety and dominance aggression). The extent to which dermatological symptoms correlate with behavioral conditions is unknown and is important. (Photo by K.L. Overall)

in the guide dog program that are transferred to other homes after 14 weeks of age have higher failure rates when they begin training, with the main reason for failure being fear (Pfaffenberger & Scott, 1959).

Studies that have examined client behavior and the development of separation anxiety have demonstrated no association between the former and the development of the latter (Voith & Borchelt, 1985c; Voith et al., 1992). Studies specifically seeking to find causal associations between overall client attachment to their pet and separation anxiety have failed to do so (Jagoe & Serpell, 1996; Serpell, 1987). Clients with little experience with dogs, as well as dogs with little or no training, may be overrepresented in the separation anxiety client/patient population (Serpell & Jagoe, 1995). It is unclear whether this overrepresentation is attributable to a factor already discussed: inappropriate and unintentional reward through reassurance and other patterns of behavior that augment the preexisting or developing anxiety.

For the diagnosis of separation anxiety to be made in humans, three of eight specific behavioral signs have to be present (APA, 1995), and only one of these has to do with any assessment of attachment. The necessary and sufficient conditions for canine separation anxiety do not include the attachment criteria.

This does not mean that some animals with the separation-related (necessary and sufficient) criteria do not also have more problems with being needy and close than do others in the population; however, sleeping with a pet does not cause the problem—the majority of people who do sleep with their pets have no problems. Were this a causal pattern, that could not be true. The issue is illustrated diagrammatically below.

	Separation anxiety	No separation anxiety
Overly attached	A	B
Not overly attached	C	D

For "attachment" to be a necessary condition for the diagnosis of separation anxiety, A would have to be statistically overrepresented compared with C in the population that is composed of A and C. For "attachment" to be a sufficient condition, A would have to be statistically overrepresented when compared with B in the population that is composed of A and B, and D would have to be statistically overrepresented in the population composed of C and D. Neither of these conditions are met, so the point should be moot. There are animals that are needier and may have a more profound or qualitatively different form of separation anxiety. Separation anxiety is a phenomenological diagnosis; much variation in the phenotypic and genetic pools is to be expected.

The standard dogma about separation anxiety includes the admonition that obtaining another pet will not greatly aid the distressed patient because the separation anxiety is focused on a human or humans, not animals (Tuber et al., 1982). However, there are no studies examining whether separation anxiety develops as readily in multidog households or those where the patient has a close and somewhat dependent relationship with another pet. If a dog in a multidog household were predisposed to separation anxiety and at risk, the underlying anxiety could be modulated by the social interactions with the other animals, permitting the potential patient to continue to behave in a socially appropriate manner (i.e., not exhibit separation anxiety). This is *not* the same as treating the separation anxiety with another dog, which should not work because it may actually raise the patient's anxiety level. Relationships with other dogs could provide insight into the development of the problem. In the hypothetical case, were one of the animals that provided the structure to be absent, one would expect an intensification of any signs of anxiety, and were one of these dogs to die, one might postulate that these dogs are at risk for the development of full-blown separation anxiety. It is not known if this scenario occurs.

MISDIAGNOSES

Destruction, if restricted only to bedding material, and post-ovariohysterectomy, may represent a pseudocyetic event. In at least one published case (O'Farrell, 1992) a dog was asserted to have separation anxiety when the few symptoms described would have been consistent with the hormonal ramifications of pseudocyesis (12-year-old bitch with pyometra who was spayed and then destroyed two mattresses, a sofa, and her bed, but apparently nothing else; the destruction was done by digging). In fact, a medical diagnosis would be far more compatible with the outcome of cessation of behavior 3 days after beginning treatment with megestrol acetate than would a diagnosis of separation anxiety. The necessary and sufficient conditions for the presumptive diagnoses must be met. In this case it was unclear what other details were important, but it would be imprudent to overlook the underlying *medical* problem that could be (and probably was) contributory.

PANIC DISORDERS

Anxiety and depression are difficult to differentiate as dimensions in humans. Depression has been attributed to defective serotonergic function (presynaptically or postsynaptically), ineffective compensatory responses to abnormally high serotonergic function, or both (Curzon, 1988). Approximately 20% to 30% of human patients with major depressive disorder have panic attacks. Lifetime incidence of panic attacks in these depressed groups may reach 50% to 60% (Grunhaus et al., 1988). Panic attacks are more easily recognizable in pets than is depression; however, the covariation in humans suggests that we may be missing the extent to which the signs associated with depression are present in animals. It would be interesting to investigate the extent to which dogs with known panic responses had experienced behavioral changes that can be concordant with depression. Currently no data exist.

In human panic disorder, abnormalities detected in the HPA axis appear complex. Some individuals with panic disorder may have increased sensitivity to dexamethasone. Other studies have reported that schizophrenics may be nonsuppressors when evaluated by the dexamethasone suppression test (DST), while schizoaffective and manic patients have blunting of thyroid-stimulating hormone at higher rates than do schizophrenic patients (Kiriike et al., 1988), leading the authors to conclude that the former have a more disturbed HPA. The poor impulse control that is associated with suicide is associated with low central serotonin turnover as indicated by low cerebrospinal fluid (CSF) 5-hydroxyindoleacetic acid (5-HIAA) levels (Roy & Linnoila, 1988).

Panic disorder in humans is usually treated with long-term (at least 18 months) medication. Some of the best results have been obtained with alprazolam and clonazepam, two drugs that are uncommonly used in veterinary medicine (Pollack et al., 1993). It is important to realize that combination drug therapy is the common choice for treatment of these conditions

in humans. Although alprazolam or clonazepam may control the primary symptoms of panic, other medications may be necessary to treat residual symptoms. In cases where there is no improvement, patients may not be receiving enough medication. The mistaken but commonly held view is that patients are getting too *much* medication (Pollack et al., 1993). Combination drug treatment is underexplored in veterinary medicine. More caution is needed than for human patients because our patients cannot tell us about the onset of side effects; however, a rational approach that includes frequent follow-up should modulate most concerns.

OBSESSIVE-COMPULSIVE DISORDER

Ritualistic and stereotypic behaviors have long been recognized in veterinary medicine and in small animals may include tail chasing, flank sucking (particularly in Dobermans), wool chewing (primarily in Oriental breeds of cats), and fly biting; wind sucking and cribbing in horses, and chain rooting and chain chewing in pigs. Most of these behaviors are annoying but relatively benign in terms of damage to clients and patients. Treatment has usually been geared toward physical restraint and control, hence the use of cribbing collars in horses and Elizabethan collars in cats and dogs. Such devices prevent the animal from accomplishing the actual behavior, but do nothing to diminish the desire to commit the behavior, as is demonstrated when the devices are removed. We now believe that this is because the disorder is a behavioral one, rooted in a neurophysiological abnormality.

Parallel examples of stereotypic behaviors are found in human medicine. These include trichotillomania (hair pulling), hand washing, and checking (lights, gas jets, locks) (Perse, 1988). In the past decade much progress has been made in the understanding and treatment of these conditions, which have been grouped in a *Diagnostic and Statistical Manual* (fourth edition) (*DSM-IV*) classification known as obsessive-compulsive disorders (OCDs) (APA, 1995). Obsessive-compulsive disorders in humans frequently appear in adolescence and continue through mid-life (Thyer et al., 1985). Human patients are generally clustered into four major groups: washers, checkers, ruminators, and an indistinct group of primary obsessive slowness (Perse, 1988). Without psychiatric and pharmacological therapy, the conditions rarely resolve. If the medication is discontinued, the patient usually relapses. Symptoms may be more pronounced in stressful or anxiety-producing circumstances.

It is hypothesized that the anatomical focus of the disorder is the limbic system. Studies involving computed tomography (CT) have implicated the basal ganglia, particularly in the region of the caudate nucleus (Baxter et al., 1992; Insel et al., 1983; Luxenberg et al., 1988; Stein et al., 1993). The effects appear to be partially attributable to aberrant serotonin metabolism, although some researchers have postulated a tandem role for abnormal endorphin metabolism (Cronin et al., 1985, 1986; Davis et al., 1982). The basal ganglia and limbic system have also been implicated in animal models of OCD (Pitman, 1989). Excess dopamine in basal ganglia structures has been noted, as has a relative increase in the serotonin metabolite 5-HIAA in the CSF. These patterns are potentially illuminating because serotonin promotes behavioral suppression and extinction of rewarded responses; this effect is opposite to that of dopamine (Soubrie, 1986; Zuckerman, 1986). Neuropharmacological approaches to therapy have sought to address these abnormalities and have suggested possible cellular etiological mechanisms.

Although the underlying cause of these disorders is unclear, the symptomatology and pathophysiology are striking. OCD is characterized by repetitive, ritualistic behaviors, in excess of any required for normal function, the execution of which interferes with normal daily activities and functioning. Inherent in this description is a behavior that is exaggerated in form as well as duration. The behavior can be perceived by the human patient as abnormal and may be controlled to the extent that the behavior is performed only minimally, or not at all, in the presence of others. This is probably also true for domestic animals. Dogs that flank-suck or tail-chase may, after frequent reprimands and corrections, remove themselves from view of the owners and then commit the behavior elsewhere. When the owner approaches, the behavior ceases, to be begun again when no one is watching or when the animal removes himself from view. The presence of a cognitive component is not sufficient to rule out an OCD, but it does suggest that the problem is rooted at a higher level than the behavior alone may indicate (e.g., the Dobie is flank-sucking, but not because anything is wrong with his flank). Not all dogs and cats fit this volitional pattern, instead exhibiting more or less continuous stereotypic and ritualistic behavior regardless of companionship. It is not necessary that the behavior be continuously witnessed for the animal to have an OCD, but it is requisite that the offending behavior substantially interfere with normal functioning in the absence of physical restraint. If the desire to exhibit the behavior is present, despite restraint because of punishment, training, or physical incarceration, the condition is present. The key is that if such control is removed and the animal can commit the behavior, he *will* commit the behavior. This is a crucial point. If it is ignored, many cases of OCD in which the volitional component is present will be undiagnosed and the frequency of OCD in the dog and cat population will be underestimated (Overall, 1992c-e, 1994d).

One could debate whether *obsessive* is a term that should be applied to nonhuman animals. Animals can "obsess" even if we cannot ascertain that they are doing so. Ascertainment of human obsession is made by verbally questioning the human patient. For animal patients that have evolutionary histories exclusive of

speech, obsession is likely to still be a possibility, although its manifestations may be different from those we have learned to expect in people. Given this logic and the otherwise homologous and analogous nature of OCD in humans and animals, there is no reason to discard this terminology. This also suggests that obsessions develop in a more primitive area of the brain than the neopallial cortex, although the latter may influence the form obsessions take.

CONDITIONS THAT COULD INVOLVE SOME DEGREE OF STEREOTYPIC BEHAVIOR

Stereotypic behaviors are found in many conditions that do not meet the diagnostic criteria for OCD (Box 10-1). In humans, startle that occurs in a stereotyped motor pattern (eye blinking, facial grimacing, flexion of head, elevation of shoulders, flexion of elbows, trunk, and knees) indicative of excessive response has been reported as characteristic of three conditions: hyperexplexia, jumping, and startle epilepsy (Andermann & Andermann, 1988). In hyperexplexia the individual is not ataxic but hyperreflexic. Such individuals have an increased and excessive response to visual, auditory, and proprioceptive stimuli, resulting in "stiffman syndrome" if profound. The response is exacerbated by multiple stressors, and some forms appear to be inherited in an autosomal dominant manner. Jumping is associated with violence to the nearest bystander and appears to be inherited in an autosomal dominant manner with variable expressivity. Startle epilepsy connotes an excessive response with a concomitant abnormal electroencephalogram (EEG).

Self-injurious behavior (SIB) is defined as self-inflicted mutilation in the absence of any apparent localized pathologic condition that would stimulate such behavior. SIB is commonly seen in humans with autism, mental retardation, Tourette's syndrome, acute psychosis, organic brain syndrome, borderline personality disorder, and schizophrenia (Buitelaar, 1993; Hellings & Warnock, 1994). Specific behaviors involved in SIB include head-banging, self-hitting, gouging (primarily of the eyes), hair pulling, skin picking, pica, and rectal digging. SIB has been postulated

---

BOX 10-1

POTENTIALLY RELEVANT HUMAN CONDITIONS

1. Autism
2. Self-injurious behavior (SIB)
3. Tourette's syndrome
4. Obsessive-compulsive disorder (OCD)
5. Prader-Willi syndrome (PWS)
6. Lesch-Nyhan syndrome
7. Chronic motor tics

to be related to a variety of neurochemical mechanisms.

The behaviors seen in Prader-Willi syndrome (PWS) include self-injury (compulsive skin picking and gouging) and compulsive eating, hoarding, and explosive outbursts. Behaviors seen in OCD also commonly include skin picking, trichotillomania, and onychophagia (nail biting). (Hellings & Warnock, 1994). The incidence of PWS with SIB is low—1:10,000 to 1:25,000 live births. Infants with the condition fail to thrive, may not suckle, and are hypotonic at birth. After 2 years of age these patients are hyperphagic and obese, and display cognitive and behavioral abnormalities (Hellings & Warnock, 1994). This profile illustrates the importance of understanding developmental patterns in the presentation of the condition and of age-dependent behavioral changes. These data are almost always lacking for animals with OCD.

Conditions that facilitate ritualistic behaviors include behavioral conditions (boredom, attention-seeking behavior, separation anxiety), infectious disease (tick-borne pathogens), neurological abnormalities (psychomotor epilepsy), self-stimulation through endogenous opioid release, and aberrant neuropharmacological activity characteristic of OCD. A logical approach will be suggested that attempts to sequentially rule out each of the above in a manner that further suggests tentative underlying mechanisms for the behavior. Such approaches are undervalued and underutilized in behavioral medicine.

All animals suspected of having OCD should have complete physical and neurological examinations. These examinations should include a metabolic screen, if available, a complete blood cell count (CBC), and serum biochemistry profile, and may include tick titers, distemper and other viral titers, radiographs, and collection of CSF. CT, MRI, PET, or SPECT scan imaging may also prove useful but is expensive and still in its infancy for diagnosis in such conditions.

It is important to obtain an accurate history of the actual behavior the animal is exhibiting (Box 10-2). This includes good descriptions of the behavior itself, even if this means that the clients are required to do animal imitations. An accurate timetable of the pattern of the behavioral events is valuable. Timetables should include frequency and duration of events, any variation in this, percentage of a 24-hour day that the animal engages in the behavior, and the frequency with which the clients believe that the behavior is linked to a precipitating event. Further history must include the age at onset; any changes in the trajectories of the behaviors (better, worse, no change in content of the behavior, but longer individual bouts); any concomitant medical conditions or treatments, even though they may not be causal or implicated; any treatments or punishments and the response; any evidence that any other family member may exhibit the same or similar behaviors; and daily schedule. The latter allows the clinician to assess general household

---

BOX 10-2

HISTORY TAKING

- Sex, breed, and age of animal (breed predispositions)
- Age of onset of condition/problem
- Duration of condition/problem
- Description of actual behavior
- Frequency of condition/behavior (hourly, daily, weekly, monthly)
- Duration of average bout (seconds, minutes, hours)
- Range of duration of bouts
- Any changes in pattern, frequency, intensity, and bout duration
- Any correction measures tried and the response (possibly none)
- Any activities that stop the behavior (e.g., stops only when animal collapses)
- 24-hour schedule of pet and client
- Pet's familial history
- Anything else that the client thinks is relevant

---

patterns that may affect the animal's behavior and provide an estimate of how accurate the client's perceptions are for the behavioral patterns; clients who are not present for 18 of the 24 hours each day may underestimate the frequency of the behavior because they cannot witness it.

BEHAVIORAL CONDITIONS THAT MAY HAVE COMPONENTS OF STEREOTYPIC BEHAVIOR BUT THAT ARE NOT OCD

Behavioral conditions in which stereotypic behavior is displayed may include "boredom," attention-seeking behavior, and anxiety.

Boredom

Boredom is an oft-touted and little demonstrated cause for such behaviors. It is possible that animals that are confined, receive little human attention or canine interaction or have minimal stimulation and decreased exercise spin or chase their tails because they are bored. This occurs in some research and kennel animals; not all of these animals exhibit such behaviors, although the incidence may be higher in these animals than in the population at large. There are no reliable data for either population. It should also be remembered that kenneled animals are often subjected to sleeping and walking on hard substrates that are cleaned with harsh chemicals. These chemicals may cause irritation that predisposes the animal to licking. Should the animal truly be "bored," exposure to human or canine companions, toys, music, increased exercise, or rooms with views to outdoor areas with grass, trees, cars, or other activity should diminish or ablate the behaviors. If this does not occur, the animal was not "bored." Usually a diagnosis of boredom is simplistic and wrong.

Attention-Seeking Behavior

Animals quickly learn that if they are not getting the desired attention from positive, quiet behaviors, they can invariably get it from behaviors the clients find less savory: jumping, barking, howling, swatting at the owner, and so forth. Certainly such attention-seeking behaviors could include spinning, tail chasing, sucking, and fly biting. Because the clients find such behaviors annoying, they yell at or attempt to distract the animal. If the distraction is by good and loving attention such as grooming or play, the animal effects the change it wants and conditions the client. Such a pattern is easily understood. Many clients have difficulty understanding how a behavior could be attention-seeking behavior if physical punishment is involved. If the animal gets very little attention, negative attention is better than no attention. Most of these animals are not abused, and the negative attention takes the form of chasing or yelling. This can be a game for the animal if every time it commits the behavior the client chases it. Attention-seeking behavior is fairly easy to treat or rule out. If the behavior is truly related to attention-seeking, ignoring it and not reacting should greatly diminish it; it is critical to couple this response with calm, loving attention when the animal is quiet. Because the interaction between client and pet has become so stressful the tendency is to ignore the animal when it is finally quiet. If these simple behavior modification techniques do not work, the animal is probably not seeking attention.

Anxiety

Some anxious animals can chase their tail, chew, and suck themselves or fabrics. The anxiety may be in response to a stimulus or may be nonspecific. If animals have had a previous injury to an extremity, they may start chasing that region whenever they become aware of it. This could be whenever they see it or bump it; these animals are often neurologically normal. Anxiety-related responses have been reported in cats. Beaver (1993) reported a seasonal hair loss in a 4½-year-old spayed Burmese; the hair loss occurred only when the cat could see cats outside. Visitation of other cats is, of course, correlated with season.

OBSESSIVE-COMPULSIVE DISORDER—A SUBSET OF ANXIETY-RELATED DISORDERS

In humans OCD is classified as a subset of anxiety-related disorders. Certainly, anxious or uncertain conditions can worsen human OCD. It is unknown to what extent the presence of other anxiety-related disorders may predispose a human or any animal to OCD.

Obsessive-compulsive disorder is probably responsible for some unknown proportion of companion animal behavioral conditions. As we become more aware of the constellation of symptoms associated with this condition, it may become more apparent (see box below). It may be more appropriate to view many of the

	Condition Present	Condition Absent
Behavioral scenario present	A Overrepresented	B Underrepresented
Behavioral scenario absent	C Underrepresented	D Overrepresented

Necessary and sufficient conditions that suggest correlational factors. If A ≫ B **and** D ≪ C are both true, this suggests something about a mechanism to be tested, but you still have only a correlation (i.e., an association of symptoms and social situations). However, you have reason to go forth, and this suggests some hypotheses to test about why this might be true.

conditions that are candidates for OCD status (e.g., some forms of acral lick dermatitis [ALD] or granuloma [ALG]) as symptoms of a multifactorial disorder, of which OCD could be a component. Diagnosis of OCD may be made by successive consideration of more complicated levels of causality for symptoms that appear analogous but may not have homologous underpinnings. Most of the behavioral "conditions" described (ALD, fly biting, wool sucking, flank-sucking, tail-chasing) might be better characterized as "symptoms" of some underlying abnormalities. Viewing these conditions with this perspective provides hope for erasing their intractability and for forging new ways to view behavior and behavioral problems. Given that at least 2% to 3% of the human population is estimated to have OCD, the proportion in the animal population should be greater because genetic variation may already be canalized by the existence of breeds, and within which line breeding and other inbreeding practices are common (Box 10-3) (Robins et al., 1984).

OCD in animals has been, not overly successfully, divided into three groups of behaviors: conflict, vacuum, and stereotypy. Conflict behaviors are associated with restricted, uniform, or impoverished conditions (e.g., cannibalism, urine-sucking, tics, "apathetic" postures) (Wiepkema, 1982; Wiepkema et al., 1980) (Boxes 10-4 and 10-5). Conflict and vacuum behaviors have been considered "disharmonious" and representative of incomplete or nonfulminant forms of stereotypy (Van Putten & Elsof, 1982). Two of the behavior patterns most frequently attributed to conflict and frustration are aggression and displacement activity (Dantzer, 1986; Dantzer & Mormède, 1981, 1982).

BOX 10-3

VHUP BEHAVIOR CLINIC DATA: OCD CASE INCIDENCE STRATIFIED BY YEAR

Year	Dog Hospital Patients	Cat Hospital Patients	Dog Behavior Clinic Patients	Cat Behavior Clinic Patients	Dog OCD Patients	Cat OCD Patients
1992	8951	2880	267	28	11	4
1993	9600	2890	287	52	7	8
1994	9121	3003	272	74	15	7
Total	18,168	8773	826	154	33 (4%)	19 (12.3%)

BOX 10-4

STEREOTYPIES INVOLVING THE PHYSICAL ENVIRONMENT

Behavior	Sudden Environment Change	Tethered/ Restrained	Restricted Rumination	Absence of Bedding
Intersucking			B	
Crib biting/wood eating	D	A, B, D	B	A, B
Self-licking	A, B, C, D	A, B	B	A, B
Licking surrounds	A, B, C	A, B	B	
Weaving	A, D	A, D		
Feather picking	E	E		

A, Pigs; *B*, cattle; *C*, sheep; *D*, horses; *E*, chickens and turkeys.
From Kiley-Worthington (1977).

Both aggression and displacement activity have their roots in anxiety.

Traumatic, cataclysmic events may be associated with the development or suppression of anxiety-related behaviors or OCD (Box 10-6). There is a classic report (Friedberger & Frohner, 1904; cited in Kiley-Worthington, 1977) of the cavalry officer's horse that suppressed his stereotypic crib biting and wind sucking (common in other cavalry horses) after a particularly gruesome battle. Pavlov's dogs also suppressed many of their stereotypic behaviors that resulted from their treatment conditions after the Moscow floods of the 1920s.

The most commonly reported stereotypies are ones of movement. Animals exhibiting these still have a normal component to their movement, and the extent to which the condition is detrimental can be gauged by the relative proportion of these components, in addition to their severity (Fraser, 1975, Fraser & Broom, 1990). The most common movement abnormalities involve changes in the frequency, intensity, or context of movement. Some of these behaviors have been thought to be "coping" behaviors related to the stresses of confinement.

Houpt (1987) noted that ruminants display fewer stereotypies (here explicitly defined as repeated, relative in variate sequences of movements without obvious purpose) than do other large animals, partly because of the action of rumination, a stereotypic behavior, itself. Yet "excessive" drinking (2 to 4 times

---

BOX 10-5

STEREOTYPIES INVOLVING THE SOCIAL ENVIRONMENT

Behavior	Isolation	Group Too Large
Intersucking	A, B, D	A, D
Crib biting/wood eating	A, B, D	
Self-licking	A, B	
Licking surrounds	D	
Weaving		
Feather picking	A	

A, Pigs; *B*, cattle; *C*, sheep; *D*, horses; *E*, chickens and turkeys.
From Kiley-Worthington (1977).

BOX 10-6

STEREOTYPIES NOTED IN LARGE OR FARM ANIMALS

1. Pacing or route tracing (horses, poultry)
2. Rocking, swaying, or weaving (horses, cattle)
3. Rubbing (horses, cattle, pigs)
4. Pawing and stall kicking (horses)
5. Head-shaking or nodding (horses, poultry)
6. Wind sucking (horses)
7. Eye-rolling (calves)
8. Sham chewing (pigs)
9. Tongue rolling (cattle)
10. Licking or crib wetting (horses)
11. Bar biting, tether biting, or crib biting (horses, pigs)
12. Self-mutilation (all)
13. Licking/eating/pulling of hair or feathers (calves, poultry, sheep)
14. Sucking/eating solid objects (horses, cattle)
15. Eating litter or earth (pica), or feces (coprophagia) (horses, cattle, poultry)
16. Overeating (hyperphagia) (horses)
17. Polydipsia (horses, pigs)
18. Anal massage (pigs)
19. Tail-biting (pigs)
20. Belly-nosing (pigs)
21. Intersucking (calves, cattle)

See Kiley-Worthington (1977); Fraser & Broom (1990).

---

normal) has been reported for ruminant species kept in close confinement (sheep), indicating that assessment of OCD must be made, not on the basis of comparisons of relative frequencies of behaviors across species, but from deviations from "normal" within species. It is unclear if the response in sheep is one associated with the absence of social stimulation or if it is associated with interactive stimulation from water that will move. Confined puppies will become polyuric and polydipsic in a manner that closely resembles other signs of OCD, and the same reasons have been postulated.

Chain chewing in pigs leads to a decreased adrenal cortex response to stressful situations (Dantzer & Mormède, 1981). The common stereotypy in heifers is tongue rolling. There is no difference in adrenal response to ACTH in tethered heifers when those that exhibit stereotypies are compared with those that do not; however, tethering heifers after grazing leads to high levels of stereotypy and high output of urine cortisol (Redbo, 1990, 1993). In at least one study, the amount of chain manipulation manifest by pigs was affected by food level (Terlouw & Lawrence, 1993). These observations hint that neither the development of stereotypic behavior nor our interpretations of it should be simple (Mason, 1991).

Some OCD behaviors have been thought to be "coping" behaviors related to the stresses of confinement. Laboratory rats exhibit environmentally induced stereotypies, as have macaques (Goosen, 1974). Some of these stereotypies may be associated with facilitation of social interaction: autogrooming stereotypies are more frequently exhibited by rats that are social subordinates (Raab et al., 1986).

Piglets that have been deprived of suckling and that exhibit stereotypic nibbling have altered brain dopamine levels, and perhaps, metabolism (Sharman et al., 1982). In pigs one sees abnormal chewing, nibbling, and sucking of the ears, tail, preputium, claws and other body parts in early weaned animals (3 to 5 weeks), but not in normally weaned ones (8 to 10 weeks) (Fraser, 1978). Feather-picking and plucking in birds has been associated with an attempt to decrease environmental tension (Delius, 1988). Veal calves that can suck on inanimate objects or tongue roll have a decreased incidence of abomasal ulcers (Van Putten & Elsof, 1982).

Critically viewed, however, these behaviors do not provide true self-medication in the sense that they "fix" the animal; both ulcers and tongue rolling are two abnormal results of distress, neither or which is seen in free-ranging animals. "Self-medication" here involves the substitution of one anxiety-related behavior for another. There is little evidence for either an adaptive function to OCD or for the assertion that OCD allows animals to discharge tension. Instead, positive feedback of sensory stimulation on an underlying control system may result in progressive sensitization of the neurological system (Robins et al., 1984).

Such an explanation would account for the variation in presentation of the signs and history of development of conditions associated with OCD.

OCD in small animals falls generally into the categorization listed previously and has been noted for grooming, hallucinatory, eating and drinking, locomotory, vocalization, and neurotic classes of behaviors (Luescher et al., 1991). Hence, in addition to tail-chasing, fly biting, and flank sucking, the following should be included in any prospectus of potential dog and cat behaviors to evaluate for an OCD component: wool sucking; wool-chewing, with or without ingestion; ingestion of foreign objects such as plastics, other fabrics, or rocks (pica); stereotypic pacing or locomotion; aberrant vocalization, particularly if directed toward the patient, itself, or its food; chewing at hair or air around hair; some unpredictable, toggle-switch aggressions; and lick granulomas (Box 10-7). These are all behaviors that appear to run in family lines, are almost impossible to control, form a major and very peculiar focus of the animal's life, and, in the case of lick granulomas and some ingestion, appear to start sometime during or after the onset of social maturity, as is true for humans.

Obsessive-compulsive disorder has been postulated to serve as self-treatment and to provide an outlet for an animal's anxieties. In fact, there is little evidence for either an adaptive function to OCD or for the assertion that OCD allows animals to discharge tension. Instead, it may be related to positive feedback of sensory stimulation on an underlying control system. This results in progressive sensitization of the neurological system (Dantzer, 1986). Such an explanation would account for the variation in presentation of the signs and history of development of conditions associated with OCD.

It is interesting to note that the conditions to which stereotypic behaviors have been attributed are associated with prevailing thought at the time. Jaw snapping was once attributed to ocular disease, synchysis scintillans (McGrath, 1962); however, a more central focus of mechanism is (whether strictly neurological or OCD) now commonly addressed. Before the development of behavioral medicine as a discipline in veterinary medicine, the common explanation for such behaviors focused largely on the neurological. In one of the first articles to describe jaw snapping in eight dogs, it was noted that five of eight dogs also licked their paws, one of eight licked the floor, and four of eight also had changing locomotor behavior (Cash & Blauch, 1979). These signs, when taken together, provide a wonderful description of behaviors now recognized as part of OCD. It is no accident that treatment with diazepam, phenobarbital, primidone, and diphenylhydantoin was unsuccessful. Tail-chasing that was accompanied by hyperventilation and growling as it increased in intensity has also been reported to be nonresponsive to treatment with anticonvulsants (O'Farrell, 1986). Some medications appear to control the behavior, but they may be suppressing it without effecting long-term change. One case report tells of a cavalier King Charles spaniel that licked at its genitalia (Brown, 1987). The behavior was controlled by megestrol acetate administration, but when the drug was suddenly withdrawn 9 months later the dog exhibited an expanded sequence of stereotypic behavior that included sneezing, head rubbing, and hyperventilation (O'Farrell, 1986), suggesting that the condition had been progressive despite the change in the signs.

Whirling or tail-chasing behavior was first reported in Scottish terriers that had been severely environmentally restricted in early life (Thompson et al., 1956). These animals had spent between 1 and 10 months in isolation cages and would whirl in tight circles, yelp shrilly, and bark or snarl as they chased their tails. The bouts of tail chasing lasted 1 to 10 minutes and were preceded by staring at the tail with a glazed expression and growling. Some of these dogs shared a common ancestry. The authors discretely describe behavioral signs associated with what now appears to be OCD and also note that these behaviors are not similar to true seizures. Tail chasing in Scottish terriers is worsened by restraint (Thompson et al., 1956). If these behaviors are truly anxiety related, the worsening effect of restraint makes sense, because it only hinders access and raises the animal's anxiety level. The restraint does not treat the appropriate level of the condition. This should make us question the use of restraint devices such as Elizabethan collars. As aids to prevent further mutilation and infection, they may have a role, but they are clearly misdirected as the sole form of treatment for any anxiety-related condition or OCD. They do, however, remind me of the devices used (with just as much logic) to restrain women who wished to dissolve their marriages in the 1800s.

BOX 10-7

STEREOTYPIES NOTED IN CATS AND DOGS

1. Circling
2. Tail chasing
3. Fence running
4. Fly biting
5. Self-mutilation (acral lick granuloma, neurotic dermatitis)
6. Hair or air biting
7. Pica
8. Pacing or spinning
9. Staring and vocalizing
10. Some aggressions
11. Self-directed vocalizing
12. Wool sucking or chewing

SPECIFIC CONDITIONS THAT MAY BE PART OF A DIAGNOSIS OF OCD

Many previously described conditions may be driven primarily by OCD or may become a manifestation of OCD when extreme in presentation. These include eating disorders; fabric eating, sucking, chewing in cats; pica; coprophagia; feline hyperesthesia; masturbation; and lick granulomas.

Eating Disorders

OCD could manifest itself as an eating disorder—between 25% and 35% of all pet dogs are overweight (Anderson, 1973). Estrogen inhibits food intake; thus removal of estrogen (i.e., spaying) does stimulate intake and could facilitate weight gain (Houpt et al., 1989). Palatability plays a large role in the amount of food ingested. Drug-induced hyperphagia is also common and corticosteroids, benzodiazepines, and megesterol acetate all stimulate intake. Accordingly, abrupt withdrawal from long-term courses of these could stimulate anorexia. Taste aversions are often associated with illness, although a decrease in appetite alone is more often associated with a preference for certain eating times or foods. True binging and gorging have not been reported for dogs and cats, but this pattern of ingestion can be naturally occurring in wild carnivores.

Fabric Eating, Sucking, and Chewing

Fabric eating, chewing, and sucking may not be associated with any nutritive considerations relevant to eating disorders. These conditions may represent OCD associated with stereotypic chewing or mouth movements. Oriental breeds are among the most common of the breeds in which these conditions are reported. These are also among the more recently derived breeds—a factor that may be important when one considers the extent to which the cat is removed from the ancestral condition. In one study, of 152 fabric-eating cats 55% were Siamese, 28% were Burmese, and 11% were cross-breds (Neville & Bradshaw, 1991). The authors report no sex or reproductive status associations, but note that 93% of these patients started with wool and moved on to other fabrics; 64% ate cotton and 54% ate synthetics. Many cats will also suck or chew plastic or other manmade materials. Some cats exhibit these behaviors only toward plastic and related substances. Wool sucking may be a behavior that is "left over" from the prolonged 6-month suckling period that is common in feral cats (Houpt, 1982), and cats that are particularly early weaned (2 to 4 weeks) seem to be overrepresented in the population of these abnormal cats. No in-depth studies of these cats have been conducted, but some observations may provide the basis for further consideration.

First, cats that chew may be behaviorally and neurochemically different from those that suck. Second, cats that chew fabric and other substances do not do so in the same manner that they eat commercially available cat food. Rather, they exhibit behaviors that are more commonly seen in zoo cats fed hunks of meat, bones, or carcasses, or in cats that hunt, catch, and ingest their own prey. Hence providing these cats with rawhide or bones with residual flesh attached may allow them to redirect their behaviors to a more ancestral focus. This observation is consistent with the available data on the mechanism of persistent biting in cats. Cats require the stimulus of trigeminal receptors around the mouth and types 1 and 2 slow-adapting (SA) dermal units to elicit their entire biting response (Iggo, 1966; Siegel & Potts, 1988). Recent research has hinted that some oral-buccal movements in cats (licking, chewing, biting, or grooming) may promote rapid firing of the dorsal raphe nucleus in the brain stem, one of the most serotonergic regions in the cat brain (Jacobs et al., 1988; Singh et al., 1991). This suggests a mechanism for the grooming, eating and drinking, and neurotic classifications of feline OCDs.

Third, cats that are early weaned appear to be overrepresented in the pool of cats that suck. This is similar to the aforementioned situation for pigs that chew their chains. Is early weaning the cause of these oral behaviors? The role of cautious interpretation of correlation is critical here (see Fig. 10-1). The specific case for this logic is diagrammed below.

	Sucking present	Sucking absent
Early weaned	A	B
Not early weaned	C	D

For early weaning to be a necessary condition for the diagnosis of sucking, A would have to be statistically overrepresented compared with C in the population that is composed of A and C.

For early weaning to be a sufficient condition, A would have to be statistically overrepresented when compared with B in the population that is composed of A and B, *and* D would have to be statistically overrepresented in the population composed of C and D. The data do not currently exist to test these conditions and would need to be collected before any assertions about causality are made. There may be an important association, but good observations only permit one to postulate hypotheses to be tested, not to assert underlying cause.

Wool chewing in cats has been treated with carnassial tooth removal; cats so treated still suck, but cannot chew and ingest. This non-treatment may relieve some of the client's concerns but does nothing to address the underlying condition—namely, the cat's OCD.

Pica

Pica, the ingestion of nonfood items, is more common in puppies, but could be a manifestation of OCD, if the dogs consistently focus on and seek out specific classes of items in the presence of a balanced diet and other available stimuli. Cats that ingest fabric may be exhibiting a form of pica.

Coprohophagia

Coprophagia is not unlike pica. Although a case can be made for the ingestion of feces that might provide additional B vitamins and microbial nutrients (particularly in young ruminants), fecal ingestion is usually an anxiety response in dogs. Primarily pathologic conditions such as pancreatic insufficiency, malabsorption, and starvation should be ruled out. Whether it is associated with overly fastidious maternal behavior is unknown. Certainly feces from other species, particularly if frozen, may be appealing to dogs (Houpt, 1982), but the dogs that force themselves to defecate and ingest their own feces directly from their rectum comprise a discrete population of patients that meet the criteria for OCD.

Feline Hyperesthesia, Overgrooming, and Self-Mutilation

Feline hyperesthesia syndrome has been variously called rolling skin syndrome, neuritis, twitchy cat disease, and atypical neurodermatitis (Shell, 1994). The behaviors demonstrated in this "condition" include (1) those mimicking estrus (e.g., rolling); (2) biting at the tail, flank, anal, or lumbar areas, generally with barbering and/or self-mutilation; (3) skin rippling and muscle spasms or twitching (usually dorsally) often accompanied by vocalization, running/jumping (possibly escape behaviors), hallucinations, and self-directed aggression (ritualistic motor behavior). The feline cutaneous response generated by types 1 and 2 SA epidermal units is characterized by a rate of discharge that is proportional to the amount of displacement of the hair or the indentation of the skin (Iggo, 1966). These SA units interact with rapid-adapting (RA) units in the vibrissae around the face, lips, mouth, and guard hairs to generate the classic biting response that follows vibrissae stimulation in predatory situations (Siegel & Potts, 1988). This sensory response may be one reason that cats chew more frequently than do dogs (who lick) when they experience self-mutilation. Feline postures and head attitude have profound effects on mediation of responses through descending spinal tracts and may augment the duration and intensity of extensor activity (Arshavsky et al., 1978, 1979). Cutaneous and proprioceptive feedback interact to program the relative timing of flexor and extensor activity (Carlson Kuhta & Smith, 1990). Furthermore, not only do many of the behaviors that the cats exhibit during these bouts resemble the classic chewing/aggression mediated by the ventromedial hypothalamus/amygdala, but cholecystokinin B (CCK-B)

BOX 10-8

BEHAVIORS EVINCED AS A RESULT OF FELINE "STRESS"

1. Change in appetite (decrease, pica)
2. Change in grooming
3. Change in elimination (spraying, nonspraying marking)
4. Change in social interaction (rubbing, bunting, challenge, vocal communication)
5. Change in activity (degree and location)

(central brain) receptors are involved in the firing of feline jaw musculature (Singh et al., 1991). All of these pieces of seemingly uncorrelated data could provide a mechanism for a response that is compatible with a diagnosis of OCD.

Of 800 cats with dermatoses, 4.3% (34) had a diagnosis of "psychogenic" dermatoses (Nesbitt & Kedan, 1985). Of the cats with food hypersensitivity, 100% of the cats were pruritic and 64% alopecic. It is unknown what percentage of alopecic cats have food hypersensitivity (White & Sequoia, 1989). Self-licking, biting, and hair loss are nonspecific symptoms. Any conditions, behavioral or dermatological, that enhance these symptoms will render the condition and its treatment more complex.

Fibropruritic nodules in cats are characterized by hyperpigmentation (or depigmentation) or multiple, firm, sessile or pedunculated, alopecic nodules. They are commonly present in the dorsolumbosacral wedge in a bilaterally symmetrical manner that is also consistent with flea infestation (Ihrke, 1995). What is interesting about this condition is that the cats may secondarily suck and chew. At what point do the sucking and chewing behaviors become primary and a sign of OCD (Box 10-8)? See Fig. 10-1 for an algorithm for cats with pica and OCD (based on existing information and subject to change). Cats isolated from other cats for most of the first year of life exhibit a response characterized by galvanic skin responses and disruption of regular sleep rhythms (Konrad & Bagshaw, 1970). Whereas neonatal isolation leads to changes in normal pain response in dogs (Melzack & Scott, 1957), it is correlated with aggression in cats and rats (Guyot et al., 1983).

Masturbation

Masturbation can be for pleasure and may become a manifestation of OCD; 80% of dogs maintain the ability to ejaculate 13 weeks after castration, whereas this is so for 20% of cats (Hart, 1974a). Male animals can mount and masturbate even in the absence of ejaculation. Females may also mount. The extent to which these behaviors are associated with anxiety or scent-marking and social relations is underexplored.

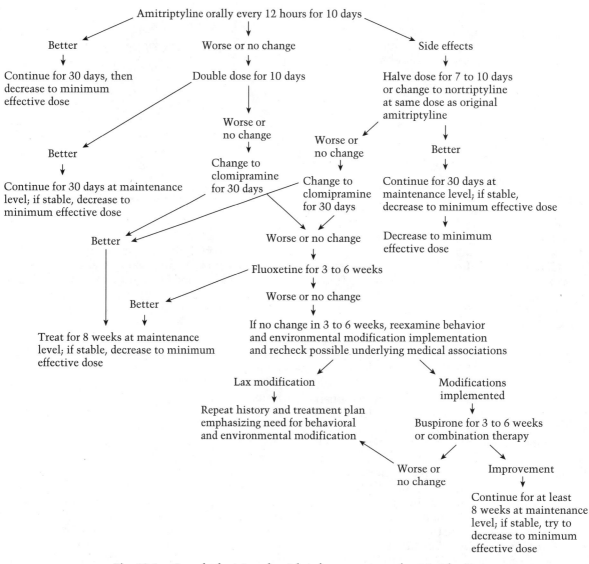

Fig. 10-1 Sample decision algorithm for treatment of cats with pica.

Acral Lick Granuloma/Dermatitis

Many anxious dogs will lick, and closer examination of dogs that have separation anxiety will reveal a high incidence of saliva-stained carpi. Lick granulomas are a good example of multifactorial disorders that may involve, in some but not all cases, either anxiety or OCD (Box 10-9). All lick granulomas should not be related to the same underlying modality because the licking is a relatively nonspecific symptom. The pattern in which the licking occurs hints at the variation in putative underlying mechanisms. Some of this variation is outlined in Fig. 10-2.

The pattern of the *behavioral* development of the lick lesion may be an important clue about the level of underlying dysfunction and which medication may be most effective. For example, lick granulomas in general respond to treatment with anti-OCD medication only about 60% of the time—this is no different than the population average across all treatments (Bul-

lock, 1978; Shanley & Overall, 1992; White, 1990). However, the dogs in the VHUP population that *best* respond to such medications are those whose lesions developed after sudden, violent, continuous, and uninterruptible mutilation (see Fig. 10-2), and those whose lesions worsen concomitant with continuous uninterruptible licking (i.e., a behavior that has become obsessive-compulsive).

Dogs with arthritic joints may lick the affected area and develop a granuloma, and cats with feline lower urinary tract disease (FLUTD) may chew at their distal abdomen. At what point does the anxiety component of the pain associated with these conditions become an entity worth addressing itself? This is not a simple question, but it does illustrate that the criteria for dermatological diagnoses may even be less specific than those for behavioral ones. To assume that *all* chewing is the same neurochemically is fallacious, and such oversimplifications may be the reason why

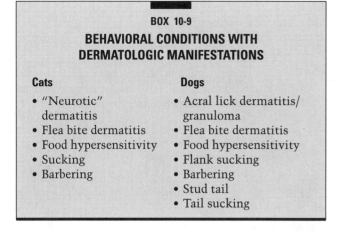

BOX 10-9
BEHAVIORAL CONDITIONS WITH DERMATOLOGIC MANIFESTATIONS

Cats
- "Neurotic" dermatitis
- Flea bite dermatitis
- Food hypersensitivity
- Sucking
- Barbering

Dogs
- Acral lick dermatitis/ granuloma
- Flea bite dermatitis
- Food hypersensitivity
- Flank sucking
- Barbering
- Stud tail
- Tail sucking

rochemical pathologic condition (Level 3). If the stimulus (e.g., shock) engenders fear, the behavior should worsen (Harlow and Harlow, 1971; Hess, 1973). Alternatively, if shock can be self-controlled and used to cue the individual to inhibit the SIB (i.e., operant conditioning), both learning (long-term potentiation [LTP]) and opiate mechanisms are associated with reduction in SIB (Linscheid et al., 1994).

Nerve conduction dysfunction has been implicated in cases of self-mutilation. Even when conduction is impeded, the impediment is bilateral, whereas the mutilation is invariably unilateral. This strongly suggests that the conduction velocity abnormality is not causal. The incidence of conduction velocity abnormalities in the general, nonmutilating population is not known. Furthermore, in animals with acral lick dermatitis and granulomas the amplitude of sensory-evoked potentials is no different in affected versus nonaffected limbs (Van Nes, 1986).

Sensory neuropathies may be more complex. Heritable sensory neuropathy has been noted for a family of pointers (Cunningham et al., 1981, 1983, 1984). Affected dogs multilate and chew off their toes, have loss of nociceptive function, and have reduced substance-P activity. Fine alterations of sensory and substance P-function are seldom examined for patients with ALD/ALG, but such deficits may play a role in

some studies involving very small samples appear to indicate that all drug treatments for lick granuloma are the same, and none is any more efficacious than shock (Eckstein et al., 1994).

Shock, if it increases the anxiety level of the dog, could worsen the behavior if it is based on anxiety or fear. Alternatively, competitive inhibition of one anxiety with another could result in a behavioral or phenotypic (see Box 1-1, p. 3; Level 1) change in the type of behavior exhibited but may not ameliorate the neu-

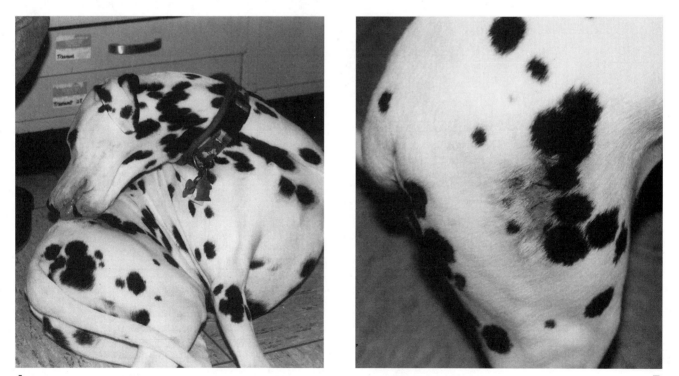

A ... **B**

This dog chewed in a pattern consistent with anxiety and a developing OCD (**A**), but the dog has a metabolic disorder involving uric acid and the lesion appears to be consistent with that diagnosis based on biopsy specimens (**B**). No one debates that the condition also renders the dog more anxious. This dog was not our patient but merely accompanied the patient to the appointment. (Photos by K.L. Overall)

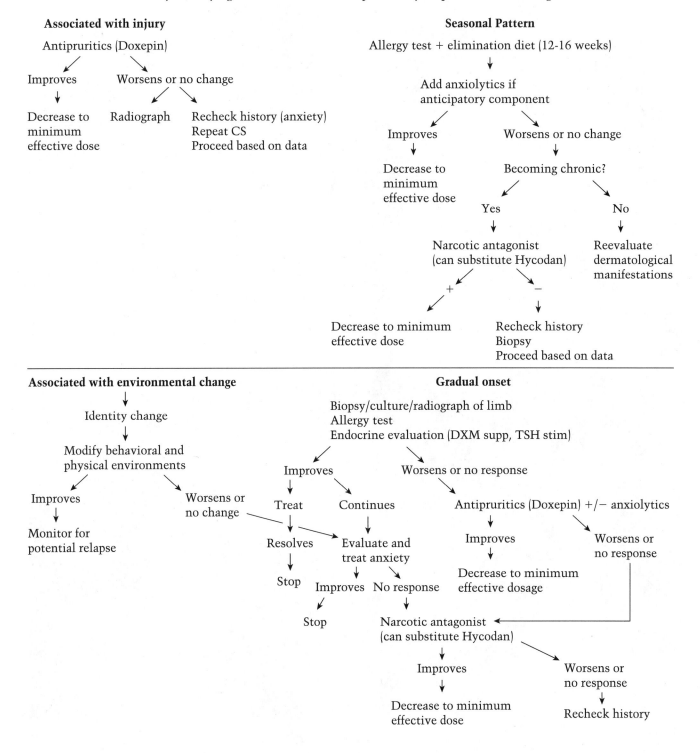

Fig. 10-2 Sample decision algorithm for treatment of behavioral aspects of acral lick dermatitis.

Sudden Onset/Violent Presentation

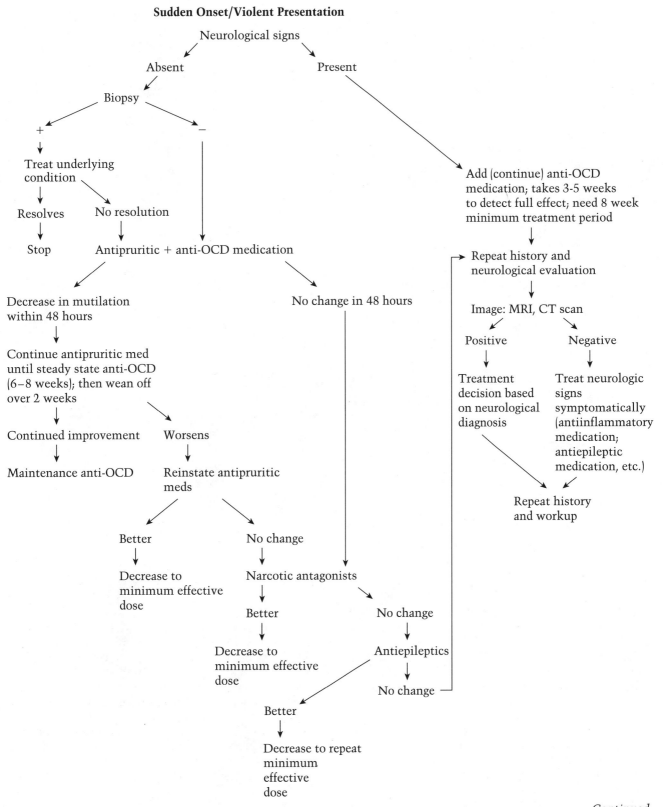

Continued.

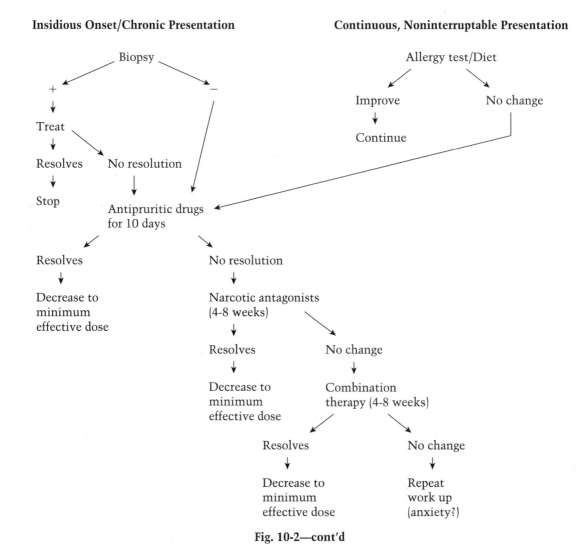

Insidious Onset/Chronic Presentation

Biopsy

+   −

Treat

Resolves   No resolution

Stop

Antipruritic drugs
for 10 days

Resolves   No resolution

Decrease to
minimum
effective dose

Narcotic antagonists
(4-8 weeks)

Resolves   No change

Decrease to
minimum
effective dose

Combination
therapy (4-8 weeks)

Resolves   No change

Decrease to
minimum
effective dose

Repeat
work up
(anxiety?)

Continuous, Noninterruptable Presentation

Allergy test/Diet

Improve   No change

Continue

Fig. 10-2—cont'd

the development of the pathology and facilitate any anxiety associated with it.

Pruritus has been implicated in medical causes of lick granuloma (Shanley & Overall, 1992). Pruritus may have a role in obsessive skin picking (Garney & Tollefson, 1988). Pruritus and anxiety are not unrelated at the biochemical level (Shanley, 1988). Pruritus is best understood as a primary sensory modality, and various types of itching may have a significant role in self-mutilation.

Whatever the basis, lick granuloma appears to fit the OCD profile for increased frequency in families of animals for which another OCD has been diagnosed. Given this, it is not surprising that some breeds appear to be more commonly affected than others. Examination of 98 biopsy samples submitted to the Surgical Pathology Laboratory at the Veterinary School of the University of Pennsylvania during a 17-month period indicated that, when compared with the total in-hospital pool of 44,960 cases seen in this period,

Doberman pinschers and Labrador retrievers were significantly overrepresented in the ALD pool ($p < 0.0001$ and $p < 0.007$, respectively, Cochran Mantel Haenszel chi square [CMH test]) (Shanley & Overall, 1992) (Box 10-10). This strongly supports the possibility of an underlying genetic component to the condition. OCDs are postulated to run in human families and to be heritable. Some proportion of acral lick granuloma/dermatitis (ALG/ALD) cases are likely to be related to an OCD or similar disorder. The potential for developing an animal model of a human psychiatric illness is enormous and would be of great value to any affected breed.

HERITABILITY AND OCD

In a study designed to evaluate the effect of the environmental (e.g., who your neighbor is) versus the genetic components of stereotypic behavior in mink, stereotypic behavior developed on the basis of heritability, regardless of the social environment (Hansen

---

BOX 10-10

BREED PREDILECTIONS FOR ACRAL LICK GRANULOMA/DERMATITIS

Labrador retrievers*
Doberman pinschers†
Akitas‡
Dalmatians‡
English setters‡
Maltese‡
Peke-a-poo‡
Shar-pei‡
Standard schnauzer‡
Weimaraners‡

---

*$p \le 0.007$.
†$p \le 0.001$.
‡Relative risk of at least two.

& Hardie, 1993). The possibility that OCD, or the tendency to develop a stereotypy, is heritable is also hinted at by the reports of tail-chasing in dogs. Bull terriers, Australian cattle dogs, terriers, and German shepherds are overreported in this group when compared with other breeds (Blackshaw et al., 1994; Dodman et al., 1993). Some of these dogs responded temporarily to the opiate antagonist naloxone, although the longest duration of response was only 7 hours—an insufficient amount of control to warrant treatment with injectable medication; however, any response does suggest that at least some of these animals have a component of aberrant central opioid function to their condition. Whether this observation is related to apparency and a few unfortunate genetic lines or whether it is real is currently undetermined; however, five dogs had some brain pathologic condition postmortem that could have been complicit in their behavioral changes (Blackshaw et al., 1994). Does this mean that these dogs did not have OCD? No, but it *does* mean that the neurochemical changes that are associated with OCD may be, in part, driven by neuroanatomical changes. That is not shocking news.

Part of the problem with nomenclature stems from the observation that behaviors associated with OCD can be mild and only vaguely annoying (to the client) to profound and debilitating. Rather than label all of these behaviors with different syndrome or condition names, one of the conventions in human medicine is to rank them on a scale from 0 to 8, with 0 causing no upset and not occurring with normal activities (e.g., onychophagia or nail-biting), and 8 causing severe upset and continually interfering with normal activity (Greenberg & Marks, 1982). Although the more benign representation might be difficult to recognize in pets, the more severe conditions are not, and such a scale is a more rational approach to diagnostic classification than is arguing about conditions whose differences are less remarkable than are their similarities.

DIFFERENTIAL DIAGNOSIS FOR OCD
Infectious and Metabolic Diseases

Diseases that could cause signs of repetitious and stereotypic behavior include, but are not restricted to, those caused by tick-borne pathogens (Lyme disease, ehrlichiosis, Rocky Mountain spotted fever), distemper, or hepatopathies. The practice of good behavioral medicine must include rigorous, routine physical examinations and requisite diagnostic tests. In the absence of any abnormalities in ancillary physical signs, laboratory data, radiographs, and bone marrow biopsies, it is probable that the stereotypic behavior is not the result of an infectious or metabolic disease. Clearly, any relevant clinical signs should be incorporated into the history and if there is any doubt from the first round of blood tests that the condition may be infectious, more invasive procedures are called for (e.g., CSF taps with tick and distemper titers and white blood cell (WBC)/neoplastic cell counts performed on the fluid).

Neurologic Disease

In addition to infectious and metabolic conditions that can impair neurological function, some primary neurological conditions can cause stereotypic behaviors such as circling, chewing, and tail-chasing. Psychomotor epilepsy is a vaguely characterized condition in which animals commit exactly these behaviors; there is apparently no consistent trigger, although anxiety may make the behaviors in the condition appear more frequently. If the behavior responds to therapy with phenobarbital, it is likely that epilepsy was causal. Unfortunately, some of these behaviors occur so infrequently and inconsistently that it is difficult to evaluate the extent to which pharmacological intervention has suppressed them. Regardless, if they are very sporadic they are probably related either to anxiety or to a primary neurological disorder, rather than to an OCD.

Central nervous system neoplastic disease can affect perception and motor coordination and must be ruled out in any ritualistic and stereotypic behavior. If the results of the neurological examination are ambiguous, further study using radiography, computed tomography, and CSF tap examination is warranted. This is particularly true if the behavior is always unilateral.

Disk disease can be extremely variable; a luxated or subluxated disk in the lumbar area could result in tail chasing. The reason the animal chases its tail could actually be related to the manner in which it perceives the neurological deficits. When this behavior is extremely frequent or continuous, should any proprioceptive deficits or other neurological clues be present, the condition should be treated as if it is a disk disorder to see if the behavior changes. Often, short-term administration of prednisolone may be sufficient to reduce the inflammation and alter the behavior. Depending on the duration of the condition, the animal may have developed a fear and anxiety component that would make treatment more complex but not insurmountable.

THE NEUROCHEMICAL BASIS FOR ANXIETY, SELF-MUTILATION, SELF-STIMULATION, STEREOTYPY, AND OCD
Endorphins

A case can be made for ritualistic behaviors being mediated through endogenous opioid receptors (Brown et al., 1987; Cronin et al., 1986; Davis et al., 1982; Dodman et al., 1987, 1988 a,b,c; Terenius et al., 1976). In many people and some animals with mutilatory lesions there may be decreased sensitivity to pain (Davis et al., 1982; Greenberg & Marks, 1982; Pickar et al., 1982). It has been postulated that this may be mediated by endorphin (opiate) receptor sites (Cronin et al., 1986, Davis et al., 1982; Pickar et al., 1982; Terenius et al., 1976). Such patients may have increases in the number, affinity, or activity of endorphin receptor sites.

The endorphin hypothesis of SIB suggests that the injurious behaviors serve to down-regulate the reactivity of the receptors, resulting in an "addiction" to the painful stimuli (Richardson & Zaleskey, 1983). Endogenous opioids are abnormal (metenkephalins increase) in people with self-injurious behavior (Coid et al., 1983), supporting this link.

For some patients the increase in endorphin levels may be present in blood levels, but not in CSF (Davis et al., 1982). If this is the case, morphine, an exogenous narcotic, opioid mimic, should stimulate endorphin receptors, producing an exaggerated response. In contrast, naloxone blocks central endorphin receptors and affords relief from the described stereotypic symptoms. This tandem approach can be used diagnostically, although morphine is not readily available to most clinicians. However, if naloxone does *not* block the response, the etiology of the lesion is not at the level of aberrant endorphin metabolism.

Pure naloxone is available only in injectable form; it must be administered continually or full relapse results. Talwin is a mixed narcotic agonist/antagonist that is an acceptable substitute (Brown et al., 1987). Naltrexone HCl (Trexan), a pure opioid antagonist, has been used (Dodman et al., 1988a). If these drugs do not change the behavior, it is probably not driven by aberrant endorphin metabolism.

A caveat to this logic may be necessary: peripheral and central responses are not equivalent. Foot shock in rats results in a fivefold to sixfold increase in β-endorphin plasma levels and similar increases in ACTH plasma levels, but this physiological increase in β-en-

dorphins induced by stress does not increase brain endorphin levels (Rossier et al., 1977).

The anxiolytics fluoxetine (Prozac) and buspirone (BuSpar) may also be useful in such conditions if they act to ablate the initial stimulus that induces the endorphin cascade (Fontaine & Chouinard, 1989).

Dopamine

Animal models for human OCD exist. Rats that were deprived of social stimuli and developed behaviors associated with OCD experienced restoration of normal function with the administration of the tricyclic anti-depressants (TCAs) amitriptyline or desipramine. Subsequent administration of a dopamine antagonist reversed this response, suggesting a functional increase in activity associated with dopamine synthesis as one mechanism of actions (Sampson et al., 1991).

Dopamine supersensitivity at the D_1 rather than the D_2 receptors has also been postulated to be the cause of SIB in Lesch-Nyhan syndrome (Goldstein et al., 1986), yet some D_2-receptor blocking agents (neuroleptics) have met with variable treatment success. The favorable response to the dopamine antagonists (e.g., sulpiride) suggests that dopaminergic supersensitivity and hypothalamic dysregulation may be one mechanism operating in SIB.

Parkinson's disease (PD) is related to a deficiency of dopamine associated with the loss of neurons in the substantia nigra. Serotonin (5-hydroxytryptamine [5-HT]) may also be involved in some patients to some degree. Schizophrenia is most often thought to be the result of enhanced dopaminergic transmission. Attention-deficit hyperactivity disorder (ADHD) is associated with decreased dopamine in the prefrontal and frontal cortex. The right caudate nucleus is decreased in size in these patients when compared with control subjects. Tourette's syndrome (TS) appears to be associated with increased activity or sensitivity of the dopaminergic system.

Serotonin

Infantile autism has been associated with increased platelet levels of serotonin, decreased levels of aspartic acid, decreased levels of glutamine, decreased levels of glutamic acid, and decreased levels of gamma-aminobutyric acid (Rolf et al., 1993). Serotonin is increased (hyperserotonemia) in 33% of autistic children.

Prader-Willi syndrome is a condition characterized by low CNS serotonin levels. As in other conditions with OCD as a component, some of these patients respond to some of the selective serotonin reuptake inhibitors (SSRIs) (clomipramine [Flament et al., 1985]; fluoxetine [Ricketts et al., 1993]; fluvoxamine [Perse et al., 1987]).

The serotonin hypothesis of SIB focuses on decreased brain serotonin and its precursor 5-hydroxy-L-tryptophan, which temporarily decreases in SIB associated with Lesch-Nyhan syndrome (Eichelmann, 1977a,b).

These associations illustrate how important it is to (1) qualify and quantify the behaviors in question, and (2) to understand that relative amount, location, and direction of change of neurochemicals can all influence the form represented by "abnormal" behaviors. These conditions are not single gene mutations that cause a solitary and unambiguous shift in one neurochemical. These conditions are all complex.

RATIONALE FOR DRUG USE

Specific drugs should be chosen based on specific inclusion and exclusion criteria that are based on a hypothesis of underlying mechanism (Elkin et al., 1988a,b). The actual outcomes of behavioral and pharmacological intervention are likely to be complex. For example, for human agoraphobics most studies indicate that drugs enhance exposure-based treatment (Mavissakalian, 1989; Mavissakalian & Perel, 1992). Animals are unlikely to be different.

The serotonin system is the mediator of fear responses in animals and man (Kahn et al., 1988). The SSRIs commonly used to treat fears include clomipramine, fluoxetine, fluvoxamine, and zimeldine. TCAs and monoamine oxidase inhibitors (MAOIs) decrease the rate of firing of the LC and so decrease norepinephrine (NE) levels (Jann & Kurtz, 1987), although the effects can be regulated through both glutamine and serotonin function. Buspirone increases the rate of firing of the LC (Rickels & Schweizer, 1990), and its effects are mediated through both dopamine and serotonin receptors (Teicher, 1988).

Fluoxetine may not be better than imipramine and other TCAs for some patients (Gram, 1994). Common side effects include nervousness, tremor, anxiety, insomnia, diarrhea, sexual dysfunction, nausea, anorexia, and weight loss. Fluoxetine can interact with MAOIs, causing serotonin syndrome. The metabolism of TCA is inhibited by fluoxetine via inhibition of liver enzyme CYP2D6. Each intermediate metabolite may change the metabolism of another so that excretion of both is prolonged.

Up to 40% to 60% of human patients with OCD do not achieve full relief of symptoms solely from the administration of serotonin reuptake inhibitors (McDougle et al., 1993). Addition of partial $5-HT_{1A}$ agonists do not seem to help, suggesting that multiple modalities of function contribute to the condition. No improvement is seen in most patients with OCD, depressive, or anxiety symptoms with the addition of buspirone to a stable dose of fluoxetine (Grady et al., 1993). Anxiety and depression associated with OCD are secondary to it; treating them in the absence of treating the OCD will fail; they often resolve if the OCD is successfully treated (Montgomery et al., 1991).

TREATMENT PARADIGMS FOR FEARS, ANXIETIES, STEREOTYPIES, AND OCD

The general paradigm for treatment of any anxiety-related disorder should be used for all of these conditions. This paradigm includes the following recommendations:

1. Identification of any actual stressors and manipulative tests of the hypothesis that they are involved.
2. Use of behavior modification to encourage
   (a) Abortion of the inappropriate behavior
   (b) General relaxation that will both be competitive with the undesirable behavior and encourage alterations in neurotransmitters
   (c) Teaching the animal new behaviors that help it to do (a) and (b) above, spontaneously
3. Use of pharmacological intervention as an aid in implementing behavioral modification (Level 1 of "causality") and to address putative pathophysiological basis (Level 3 of "causality") (see Box 1-1 on p. 3). The latter means that the more specific the drug mechanism, the more possible it is to test a hypothesis; even without this, with judicious use of medication and an understanding of its mechanisms, one can choose medications best suited to the particular constellation of symptoms.
4. CBCs and serum biochemistry profiles are the minimum baseline data required before medication. Electrocardiography (ECG) (possibly), and any necessary tests to rule out medical (somatic or organic) conditions should be encouraged. ECG is particularly important if one auscultates any abnormalities and for cats because feline cardiac disease is notoriously occult and many of the recommended medications can cause arrhythmias.

Most behavior modification uses counterconditioning and desensitization. In counterconditioning an animal is taught another behavior that is more enjoyable or pleasant to exhibit in the presence of the stimulus that elicits the abnormal behavior. The animal must first be taught to do this in a benign circumstance before it can be done in a stressful one. The substitute behavior can be as simple as teaching the dog or cat to sit or lie down and look at the client, relaxing and appearing calm and happy, in exchange for a food treat or attention. Some animals will work for play, but this necessitates a more active role on the client's part than does relaxation for food. The period for which the animal is expected to remain calm should be gradually increased, with frequent positive reinforcement, until it lasts for 30 minutes. The animal is then ready to begin to have the trigger event introduced at some attenuated level; this level will gradually be increased to teach the animal to habituate to the stimulus.

For example, if the cat starts to spin and hiss at his tail every time it is touched, the cat should be brushed without touching the tail. The client's hand could then be run over the region of the tail, gradually dropping until it almost touches the fur. Finally, the briefest stroke is given; gradually the client works up to brushing the tail. Throughout the process the animal is rewarded if it is relaxing and looking calm. The animal is not rewarded if it sits still and looks panicked: this teaches nothing and does not decrease the desire to commit the behavior, although the behavior may be controlled.

This behavioral process could take weeks because every time the animal begins to look unhappy or anxious, or gives anything more than a cursory glance to the offending area, the client must back up to a gesture to which the cat did not react.

Antianxiety medication facilitates this entire process. Once the animal's behavior is "normal" (or greatly improved and stable in its improvement), the medication should be continued for an additional 2 to 3 weeks to ensure that no relapses will occur in the absence of constant behavioral modification. This approach means that the animal is treated with medication for at least 30 to 60 days, allowing for attainment of steady-state conditions, interactive effects of the behavior modification, and medication adjustments. The medication can then be gradually decreased during a period of 10 to 14 days, although side effects are seldom reported after abrupt cessation. The primary reason for gradual withdrawal is that some animals require some continual dose of medication to quash the behavior. Gradual withdrawal allows the clinician and client to look for the reappearance of the behavior and medicate accordingly. If an animal must be continuously medicated, renal and hepatic enzyme levels should be monitored at least annually. Before any drug is used, these should be checked in any older animal or one that may have any renal or hepatic damage. The most common side effects of TCAs are a dry mouth (primarily in people, but rare in dogs) and resultant increased thirst and frequency of urination, mild GI distress, constipation, syncope, and arrhythmias, primarily tachycardias. At the high end of the canine dose tachycardias are uncommon but not rare; they may be accompanied by paradoxical excitement. They resolve on decrease or withdrawal of the drug. TCAs should not be used in animals with glaucoma or urinary retention.

If there is no improvement in the animal's behavior by the end of 7 to 10 days of medication and behavioral modification, the drug dosage can be doubled. Should the animal still show no sign of change in the offending behavior, that behavior is probably not related to anxiety. If there is small but not substantial change, other antianxiety medications may prove useful (e.g., buspirone, imipramine, fluoxetine).

Specific protocols for treating fearful behavior, separation anxiety, and attention-seeking behavior are found in Appendix B. Specific information about general treatment of these conditions follows.

TREATING FEARS, PHOBIAS, AND PANIC
Behavior Modification

Treatment of fears, phobias, and anxieties has involved traditional approaches to behavior modification. Desensitization and counterconditioning were introduced in a formal manner in the late 1950s. Programs designed for the specific desensitization of fearful responses were outlined and later expanded (Tuber et al., 1982; Voith, 1982a,b; Young, 1982).

Flooding, synonymous with implosion therapy, has been tried with mixed success for the treatment of fears. Flooding involves placing the patient in the environment in which the fearful stimulus is apparent and keeping him or her there until the fearful response subsides by 50% per session. Flooding is a potentially risky treatment. Clients opting for this method need to understand that (1) there are no guarantees, and (2) that flooding will be effective *only* when *all* of the following conditions are met: fears are generalized to many dimensions, aggressive displays have only recently begun and are low in intensity, the dog does not fear the client, and environmental factors, not genetic ones are the basis of the fear (Young, 1982). Flooding sessions are long, require many people, and can backfire if used inappropriately. In the latter situation the dog becomes more fearful and may become phobic, particularly if the stimulus used in the flooding is of too high an intensity (Levis, 1979; Rachman 1974; Rachman & Levitt, 1988).

One of the problems for which flooding has been used is noise phobias. Noise phobias meet the "phobic" criteria outlined by Tuber and colleagues (1979): (1) the majority of these are limited to a set of sound stimuli, (2) the fear is elaborated by repeated exposure, and (3) one can establish a high intensity of phobia after only one exposure. Noise phobias are best defined as a persistent, excessive fear response to a sound stimulus that results in the dog's attempting to avoid or escape from the sound (Shull, 1994). Of the animals that exhibit phobic responses when presented with noise, 87% respond to thunder, 93% respond to thunder or thunderlike sounds (firecrackers, backfires), and less than 10% react to televisions, stereos, vacuum cleaners, sirens, or motor vehicles (Shull-Selcer & Stagg, 1991). The extent to which animals with an extreme reaction to noise associated with daily activity are overrepresented in this group of noise-phobic animals is unknown. This is another case in which understanding the range of "normal" behaviors would be useful in suggesting hypotheses about deviations from that range. Thunder is a unique stimulus; it involves a high concentration of energy in the low-frequency end of the spectrum and is very percussive (Shull-Selcer &

Stagg, 1991). Some of these animals respond to treatment under flooding conditions; 95% of dogs treated reached the maximum sound intensity (90 db) created under artificial situations by 11 hours of training; however, this response does *not* transfer well to "real" storm situations, suggesting that other facts including changes in atmospheric pressure, changes in illumination, and the presence of olfactory stimuli (e.g., ozone), may be as important or more important than sound.

Unlearning a behavior creates conditions for spontaneous recovery (i.e., the reappearance of the behavior merely with the passage of time and without further work or training). This means that some behaviors must be continuously counterconditioned (Tuber et al., 1982). Stimulus and response generalization mean that after an animal acquires a response (and operant response or a classically conditioned response) to a specific stimulus, the animal tends to engage in a similar response to similar stimuli (Borchelt & Voith, 1985). The quality and intensity of the response are related to the degree to which the stimulus resembles the original.

Caution is urged in using punishment to suppress normal or abnormal fearful responses to stimuli. Across a wide variety of species such use of punishment usually intensifies fear (Harlow & Harlow, 1971 [monkeys]; Hess, 1973 [chicks]; Stanley and Elliott, 1962 [dogs]).

Pharmacological Intervention

Pharmacological intervention has been more successful in controlling a phobic response to noise than has flooding or desensitization. To treat any phobic response it is necessary to treat the fear response. There are three components that must be addressed for this to occur: (1) the behavioral component, (2) the physiological response (autonomic nervous system [ANS]/neuroendocrine response), and (3) the "emotional" response—or the intensity with which the animal perceives the reaction to the stimulus. In any treatment program it is important to distinguish between adaptive and maladaptive fear.

Benzodiazepines act on an inhibitory supramolecular receptor complex that consists of a gamma-amino butyric acid (GABA) receptor, a benzodiazepine receptor, and a Cl^- channel (Mayes, 1979), and they facilitate GABA-induced neuronal inhibition through a decreased rate of firing of the LC. Opiates appear to sensitize pathways associated with affiliative behaviors, whereas benzodiazepines sensitize pathways that respond to an immediate threat. Early studies of neurotic behavior in cats that had been induced to be anxious when exposed to certain experimental stimuli demonstrate the complexity of these interactions (Masserman & Yum, 1944, 1946). Alcohol administered to cats at 0.5 to 2.0 ml/kg results in a disorganized learned adaptive pattern and modified neuroses,

but has no effect on social relationships within hierarchies. Neurotic animals that experience relief of inhibitions and tensions during previous alcoholic intoxications choose milk with 5% alcohol over regular milk. This self-medication disrupts the complex patterns involved in the neurosis that the cats exhibit, and allows the animals to perform simpler, more goal-oriented behavior (seeking food, chasing mice). The correlates of relief follow a dose-response curve over a moderate range.

Dosages of benzodiazepines to treat noise phobias include 0.1 to 0.5 mg/kg diazepam orally as needed, and clorazepate 22.5 mg for large dogs, 11.25 mg for medium-size dogs, and 5.6 mg for small dogs (Schull, 1994). These dosages are based on the available formulations. In a small study on the treatment of noise-phobic dogs Shull (1994) found that four of six dogs treated with alprazolam had a fair, good, or excellent response, three of four treated with clorazepate and two of three treated with acepromazine fared the same, whereas one treated with diazepam had an excellent response. Only one of seven dogs treated with propranolol had a fair response, and only three treated purely with behavior modification had a fair or better response. In all cases the treatment response was better with a mild-moderate problem than with a profound one. Although this study is small, it does suggest that both the range of responses and treatment mode interact in the production of any relief from anxiety. Efficacy in this study was defined by more rigorous criteria than in many other studies: behaviors that phobic dogs demonstrated significantly more frequently than nonphobic dogs (scratching, looking up, vocalizing, hiding, and startling) had to be markedly different before and after treatment to be scored as a favorable response.

Alprazolam has also been useful in treating panic in animals, and it may be a useful adjuvant in the treatment of anxieties that have a panic component. This is certainly a good description of many dogs with separation anxiety.

An extreme form of a fear response is seen in "nervous" pointers from lines that have been bred to maintain profound avoidance of humans (Muphree, 1973). Nervous pointers experience attenuated human avoidance when treated with pimozide (0.3 mg/kg) and chlordiazepoxide (3.5 mg/kg) intravenously every 24 hours. Chlordiazepoxide also decreased the incidence of arrhythmias associated with atrioventricular blocks and nodal escapes in five dogs (Chapin & Newton, 1979). Chronic imipramine treatment did not modulate the behavior of these pointers (Tancer et al., 1990). These dogs also experience hyperresponsiveness to dopaminergic stimulation and increased levels of L-dopa in the cisternal CSF (Angel et al., 1974, 1982). The majority of these nervous dogs are deaf, but hearing dogs do not respond differently than do deaf dogs to a provocative fearful stimulus (Klein et al., 1988).

Beta-blockers have been used to treat the symptoms of fear that are the result of β-adrenergic activity. They have not been overly efficacious in the treatment of fears in humans and other primates (Jann & Kurtz, 1987; Rickels & Schweizer, 1990), although they may be useful in the treatment of very situation-specific performance anxiety.

TREATING SEPARATION ANXIETY
Behavior Modification

Treatments for separation anxiety have involved standard desensitization and counterconditioning to departures, and the use of antianxiety medication (Voith & Borchelt, 1985c). In 125 cases, Mugford (1984b) had an 80% success rate (defined as at least some improvement; no quantification is available) using a bridging stimulus (a recording) that would indicate that the client was returning. This was coupled with not rewarding the dog for its anxiety at the client's departure, rewarding it for being calm on return, and setting up a schedule for regular attention that could be anticipated. These are all factors to consider, although no data are available on correlation of intensity of signs at the outset and extent of improvement. The role of regular, scheduled, and earned attention cannot be underestimated. Rather than attempting to break the attachment between the client and pet (a commonly recommended and arguably inhumane tactic), this provides a set of rules for the pet that permits reasonable expectations and attainment of those. These are the factors that will minimize anxiety without provoking a distressed or depressed response. Anxious dogs are always soliciting attention without obtaining relief from their anxiety. In this context, they can have as much attention as they want, provided they earn it by relaxing. Attention is scheduled regularly enough that the anxiety is not permitted to develop. These are subtle but important modifications. It is absolutely critical that treatment of separation involve *no* punishment; punishment would only increase the patient's anxiety level. Anything that can decrease the animal's anxiety (pet-sitters, baby gates, outdoor pens, radios) should be used.

Pharmacological Intervention

Tricyclic antidepressants are among the most efficacious of the medications available for the treatment of any anxiety-related condition, including separation anxiety. The most readily available and least expensive of these, amitriptyline, has been used at a starting dose of 1 to 2 mg/kg orally every 12 hours (Voith & Borchelt, 1985c). Other TCAs (imipramine, clomipramine) are among the best choices for this condition. Should the separation anxiety have a panic component, combination treatment with alprazolam for the panic and a TCA for long-term maintenance may

achieve the best effects. This is particularly true if the TCA chosen requires a long time to reach steady-state levels at the dosages prescribed (e.g., clomipramine, or fluoxetine, a bicyclic derivative). Combination drug use may aid in faster resolution and may permit the use of lower levels of either medication to control the problem. In the specific example chosen, a small (0.05 mg/kg) dose of alprazolam could be given when the clients awaken so that the dog does not experience the panic associated with the clients' leaving in an hour. Preempting the panic will facilitate the dog's ability to learn, with the help of long-term antianxiety medication and behavior modification, that it can be left alone with no untoward effects. Without interruption of the panic this may not be possible because the panic, and not the client's absence, now is the dog's cue that the anxiety will worsen.

Any extant drug used as part of a treatment plan for separation anxiety must be used continually—these are not drugs that can be given only when the client perceives that the pet might have a problem. The goal of treatment is to lower overall levels of anxiety. One mechanism for this is to increase central levels of serotonin. Hence, pharmacological intervention should be maintained long enough to facilitate all behavioral and environmental modification. Withdrawal of medication should be gradual and may indicate that lifelong maintenance is the best choice. It should go without saying, but it does not, that all animals being treated with any behavioral drug should have complete physical examinations and premedication blood studies, as well as follow-up evaluations as needed.

TREATING OCD
Behavior Modification

A combination of behavioral modification (primarily counterconditioning and habituation) and pharmacological intervention is usually successful if the stereotypic behavior is related to an underlying anxiety. Counterconditioning is usually unsuccessful without antianxiety medication to break the psychological trigger for the cycle (Rachman & Levitt, 1988). Regardless, all behavior modification designed to encourage relaxation and competitive inhibition should be used.

Pharmacological Intervention

One of the newer TCAs, clomipramine (Anafranil), is relatively specific for treatment of OCDs because it lacks antidepressant and antihistaminic properties of other TCAs. This drug is specific for alleviation of obsessive-compulsive effects and has been successful at treating self-mutilatory conditions such as trichotillomania in humans (Flament et al., 1985). Clomipramine also has been successful in treating some lick granulomas (Goldberger & Rapaport, 1991) and motor behavior associated with OCD (Overall, 1994n), as has another SSRI, the bicyclic antidepressant fluoxetine

(Prozac) (Shouldberg, 1990). It is important to realize that conditions such as lick granulomas may represent diffuse syndromes with multiple causality, as discussed previously.

All TCAs act by inhibiting serotonin reuptake. It is postulated that the specific effect of clomipramine is to the localized increase in serotonin in the region of the basal ganglia, particularly the caudate nucleus (Ananth, 1986). Older, less specific TCAs such as amitriptyline are very useful in treating many canine and feline anxiety-related disorders and can be useful as adjuvants for the treatment of OCD. Unlike benzodiazepines, TCAs do not interfere with short-term memory and so are suitable for use with behavior modification. Most nonspecific TCAs have a half-life of about 6 to 8 hours and reach a steady-state blood level within 3 to 4 days. During this period behavior modification can be started.

Clomipramine has many of the same side effects as other TCAs but is a very potent arrhythmogenic agent. Accordingly, all patients should have a cardiac consultation and a rhythm strip should be obtained before the drug is administered. In people, the maximum dose is 200 mg/day or 3 mg/kg, whichever is *less*. For large dogs the dose is probably the same. Because of its potential arrhythmogenicity, it is recommended to start dosages at 1 mg/kg every 12 hours, and over 5 weeks gradually increase to the minimum

effective dose. Should any side effects ensue, the drug should be stopped or decreased to a more tolerable level; it can then be gradually increased again. Treatment must usually last at least 5 weeks to see any effect (Thoren et al., 1980). If clomipramine ablates the behavior, it will have to be continued for life; on withdrawal symptoms relapse, although pharmacological control does render the animal more responsive to behavior modification. Tandem use of clomipramine and behavioral modification may make it possible to use a lower maintenance dose. As is true for buspirone and naltrexone, clomipramine is fairly expensive.

Clearly, it would be foolish to treat the presumed underlying cause of any self-mutilatory condition listed previously without also treating any local lesions. Cultures should be obtained for lesions and the lesions should be treated with appropriate antibiotics.

BOX 10-11

PSYCHOPHARMACOLOGICAL AGENTS THAT MAY BE USEFUL IN THE TREATMENT OF FELINE ANXIETY DISORDERS, INCLUDING OCD AND HYPERESTHESIA

Alprazolam	0.125-0.25 mg/kg orally every 12 hours (start with 0.125 mg/kg)
Amitriptyline	0.5-2.0 mg/kg orally every 12-24 hours (start with 0.5-1.0 mg/kg)
Buspirone	0.5–1.0 mg/kg orally every 8-12 hours
Clomipramine	0.5 mg/kg orally every 24 hours
Diazepam	0.2-0.4 mg/kg orally every 12-24 hours
Fluoxetine	0.5-1.0 mg/kg orally every 24 hours
Hydrocodone	0.25-1.0 mg/kg orally every 8-12 hours
Naltrexone	2.2 mg/kg orally every 24 hours (up to 25-50 mg/cat)
Nortriptyline	0.5-2.0 mg/kg orally every 12-24 hours

BOX 10-12

PSYCHOPHARMACOLOGICAL AGENTS THAT MAY BE USEFUL IN THE TREATMENT OF CANINE ANXIETY DISORDERS, INCLUDING OCD AND ALG

Alprazolam	0.01-0.1 mg/kg orally as needed for panic, not to exceed 4 mg/dog/day. (Start with 1-2 mg for a medium-size dog)
Amitriptyline	1-2 mg/kg orally every 12 hours to start
Buspirone	1 mg/kg orally every 8-24 hours
Clomipramine	1 mg/kg orally every 12 hours for 2 weeks, then 2 mg/kg orally every 12 hours for 2 weeks, then 3 mg/kg orally every 12 hours for 4 weeks (use minimum effective dose; decrease dose if sustained side effects occur)
Doxepin	3-5 mg/kg orally every 8-12 hours
Fluoxetine	1 mg/kg orally every 12-24 hours
Haloperidol	1-4 mg orally every 12 hours
Hydrocodone	1 mg/4 kg orally every 8 hours
Hydroxyzine	2.2 mg/kg orally every 8 hours
Imipramine	1-2 mg/kg orally every 12-24 hours to start
Naloxone	11-22 μg/kg intravenously (subcutaneously, intramuscularly) as needed
Naltrexone	2.2 mg/kg orally every 12-24 hours
Nortriptyline	1-2 mg/kg orally every 12 hours
Thioridazine	1.1-2.2 mg/kg orally every 12-24 hours

BOX 10-13

NEUROCHEMICALS UNDER INVESTIGATION

Acetylcholine
Norepinephrine*
5-Hydroxytryptamine*
Dopamine*
Monoamine oxidase*
Gamma-aminobutyric acid*/Glycine
Cholecystokinin
Excitatory amino acids
Glutamate
N-methyl-D-aspartate receptors
Nitric oxide
Tachykinins
Adenosine triphosphate

---

*Focus for most currently used anxiolytics.

If there is localized itching, the addition of an antipruritic medication is necessary. Another TCA, doxepin (Sinequan), is 880 times more potent an H_1-receptor antagonist than is diphenhydramine HCl, and 67 times more potent than hydroxyzine HCl (Atarax) (Gupta et al., 1987).

If these drugs are used early in the treatment of a self-mutilatory condition, they may abort further stereotypic behavior because the gate control theory of pruritus implicates cells in the dorsal horn of the spinal cord in modulating afferent nerve fibers before stimulation of central transmission cells in the dorsal horn (Shanley & Overall, 1992). Such modulation is affected by central factors, further implicating aberrant sensation in OCDs and related disorders. All TCAs have joint antipruritic and antianxiety components. The extent to which each action is apparent depends on the particular drug formulation. Perhaps this is why amitriptyline HCl has been occasionally successful in treating trichotillomania (Snyder, 1982) and some stereotypies in companion animals.

Other drugs used with mixed results in human medicine may ultimately be useful in some companion animal disorders. These include clozapine (Clozaril, a tricyclic antipsychotic) and carbemazepine (a tricyclic anticonvulsant) (Uhde et al., 1985). Thioridazine, a phenothiazine derivative, has been used successfully to control occasional aberrant motor behavior (Jones, 1987). Treatment of SIB in humans with thioridazine, lithium carbonate, and opiate antagonists (Aman, 1993; Crews et al., 1993)—meets with mixed success. Tryptophan deficiencies may potentiate depression, whereas supplementation of tryptophan (a serotonin precursor) may both potentiate antidepressant action and provide a mechanism for that action. Recent work has indicated that CCK is present in large concentrations in the limbic system of the brain and thus may affect perception and treatment of anxiety. The CCK-B receptor is restricted to the brain and may have anxiolytic effects (Singh et al., 1991)

Combination treatment (Prozac plus BuSpar; BuSpar plus Anafranil) is gaining popularity in human medicine but is underexplored for companion animal behavioral disorders. The fields of behavioral pharmacology and neurophysiology are rapidly growing and should shortly make obsolete much of the present information. Figs. 10-1 and 10-2 contain decision algorithms that will help in treatment. A list of drugs useful in the treatment of fears and anxiety-related conditions is found in Boxes 10-11 and 10-12. These agents are more fully discussed in Chapter 13. Neurochemicals under investigation are listed in Box 10-13.

Issues Yet to be Resolved

1. We actually understand very little about the cause of fears and anxieties. Laboratory-induced fears are not good models for naturally occurring ones. The extent to which the norepinephrine, dopamine, and serotonin systems interact to contribute to phenotypic presentations of fears and anxieties is complex and will be the subject of further study.

2. The role of early experience in the development of fears and anxieties is known only for extreme, artificial situations of early deprivation. Although this sets a lower limit, the pressing questions involve ways in which realistic early experience can make a difference in the development or prevention of a problem. Such studies are correlational, and the data for them are sorely lacking in behavioral medicine.

3. Likewise, the role of genetics for the predisposition to develop a fear has been investigated only in rigid laboratory conditions. It does appear that pathological fears, anxieties (including those underlying aggression and OCD), and phobias may run in family lines of dogs and cats, and, consequently, are more apparent in some breeds (hence the line association) than others.

CASE 1

Signalment: "Sunshine," 4-year-old, 19 kg, female spayed Shetland sheepdog

Initial problem: Shy and fearful

History: This dog was obtained at 3 years of age from the local SPCA. There was no history of why she was turned in, but the clients took her because she was fearful and they were afraid no one else would take her. When they originally adopted her she was very fearful, always slipping out of her collar and running away. The clients decided to keep her totally indoors, restricted to one room, to prevent her from fleeing and to see if having the security of one environment would help her to become less fearful. During a 9-month period she became calmer and gradually gained access to the rest of the house. Her behavior in the house is still not normal. She hides under furniture when possible, and otherwise stays along the periphery of the room. The clients built her a small enclosure with a doggie door through which she can go from the back room. She will go outside but is still anxious. Whenever the clients have company, the dog becomes almost paralytic with fear, hides, and is still hiding, salivating, and shaking after the guests have left.

The clients have one kitten and two other dogs, ages 13½ years and 10½ months. This dog is not shy with the other dogs, but is not close with them either. She will want to be with them, but the puppy is very large and very exuberant, and when he plays too roughly with her she avoids him. If he pushes the interaction she will snarl and growl at him. He backs down.

The clients have made much progress in getting the dog to come out of her shell, but believe that they have stopped making progress. Gentle play, quiet words, and calm interactions have not stopped her from being fearful. During the appointment she spent the entire 3½ hours (except the time during which behavior modification was done) sitting in the client's lap, trying to hide her head. All VHUP personnel were unsuccessful at getting her to look at them or interact with them, even during the behavior modification exercises. Instead of demonstrating the behavior modification, we had to talk the clients through it. If we tried to interact with the dog, she experienced increases in heart and respiratory rates, shook, panted, and tried to hide. Any time there was a noise in the hall, she scanned for the source and then hid her head.

The dog has never been inappropriately aggressive in any context and becomes more fearful when forced to be exposed to situations that scare her.

Physical examination: No abnormalities were detected on physical examination. Her toenails were trimmed without a problem or struggle.

Laboratory evaluation: A complete blood cell count and serum biochemical profile were submitted; all values were within laboratory reference ranges.

Diagnosis: Generalized anxiety and social phobia

This dog exhibited behavioral and physiological signs of anxiety when any interaction was attempted with her or any unexpected stimulus entered her environment. In the 9 months the clients have had her, she bonded with them and has become very friendly, although she did not play. She was most relaxed in "her" room at home, but could and would interact with the dogs and people in the other rooms, although she never stopped exhibiting vigilance and scanning behavior. She could not interact with new people and tried to physically remove herself from them.

These conditions could be genetic, induced by horrible early life experiences (environmental), or (my guess) both. Animals that have a predisposition to social fear certainly become worse if abused or poorly treated. Because there is no available information on Sunshine's early history, there are no specific, horrific events that may have contributed to her behavior against which she can be desensitized.

Treatment: Behavior modification programs designed to teach Sunshine to relax and have fun were started. The clients were to reward any incremental improvement in her behavior, but were not to pay any attention to her or reward her if she was shaking or fearful. After the dog could execute the first phase of the behavior modification programs, happily and consistently, in protected circumstances, the clients were to add other circumstances that upset her slightly to the regimen. She was also (as were the other dogs) to sit and stay for everything she wanted—attention, food, treats, access to other areas, grooming, reassurance. The clients were also encouraged to practice the behavior modification with the puppy because he was unruly, but also because it is possible that Sunshine could use him as a reassuring model. This would also provide her with the ability to mimic him, which can help reassure any anxious social animal.

In addition, treatment with amitriptyline, 20 mg (1 mg/kg) orally every 12 hours, was started. The clients were told that they should see a subtle calming effect, and that Sunshine should be less anxious and more willing to comply with them and the behavior modification within

CASE 1—cont'd

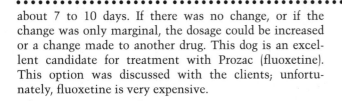

about 7 to 10 days. If there was no change, or if the change was only marginal, the dosage could be increased or a change made to another drug. This dog is an excellent candidate for treatment with Prozac (fluoxetine). This option was discussed with the clients; unfortunately, fluoxetine is very expensive.

Reexamination visits will concentrate on gradually desensitizing Sunshine to circumstances in which she is particularly fearful (approaches from strangers, people entering the room) and attempting to encourage more normal interactions, including play.

Finally, we fit the puppy for a Gentle Leader/Promise System Canine Head Collar (Premier Pet Products, Richmond, Va) so that the clients can walk her and so that they can control her interactions with the patient (and perhaps she can begin to enjoy them).

Follow-up: Ten days after her appointment the clients reported that Sunshine's behavior has improved with the behavior modification: she is not slinking around the house as much, she appears happier to see them when she realizes that they are going to practice the programs, and rests more without scanning. The clients were concerned that the drugs may not be having an effect because they believe they can induce these behaviors just by asking the dog to sit and petting her using deep massage. After an additional 10 days (during which time the dosage was not increased), the clients reported that they think that the dog is responding to the medication. Her behavior is greatly improved from the last week, and Sunshine seeks them out for interaction. She is still fearful when people come to the door, and the clients have noticed no decrement in her fearful behavior at such times. At reexamination, we would concentrate on this situation and decide whether to change the dosage or medication.

Two months after the initial appointment, the clients reported that they believed that the dog had made a lot of progress, but was still anxious and withdrawn. They were concerned about her quality of life and were willing to change medication in an attempt to help her. Repeat complete blood cell counts and serum biochemistry profiles were all within laboratory reference ranges, and the patient was otherwise asymptomatic for disease. The patient's medication was changed to fluoxetine (1 mg/kg orally every 24 hours). Because this medication can take 3 to 5 weeks to produce an effect when used at the recommended dosage, maintenance therapy with amitriptyline, 1 mg/kg every 12 hours, was used for the first week. The dose was decreased to 1 mg/kg every 24 hours during the second week and to 1 mg/kg every other day during the third week, after which it was stopped. Amitriptyline and fluoxetine can interact, potentiating the former and prolonging the half-life of the latter, so the combination can be a potent and beneficial one. A few months later the client reported that the dog had improved slightly in her fear and anxiety, and we concurred; however, the improvement was not to the degree the clients had hoped. The clients elected to continue the medication and to aim for incremental change.

After 7 months of treatment, the dog became ill with vomiting, lethargy, and anorexia. Laboratory examination performed by the referring veterinarian revealed no profound abnormalities. Radiography revealed a slightly enlarged liver and possible mass. Treatment was symptomatic. The patient's disease progressed and the dog was euthanized 1 week later. Necropsy revealed the presence of a hepatic carcinoma.

CASE 2

Signalment: "Annie," 7-year-old, 25.8 kg, spayed female mixed breed

Initial problem: Barking and avoiding younger son in household

History: This dog was adopted from a humane shelter approximately 6 months before the visit. For the past 5 months the dog has barked and acted agitated every time the adult son (37½ years) enters the room. The barking is getting worse in intensity, and the fearful behavior (pacing, slinking, hiding) is becoming more profound. The dog was fine for the first 2 weeks she was in the household. She was relatively shy around everyone, but as she bonded to the parents and other adult son (40 years), the dog became more anxious in the younger son's presence.

While at the Behavior Clinic at VHUP the dog was slightly hesitant about greeting new people, slinking slightly and tucking her tail, but once the people talked softly to her and moved slowly, she approached them,

CASE 2—cont'd

● ●

sniffed and licked their hands, stood to be petted, and rolled over to have her belly rubbed. When the son to whom she reacts came into the room, she barked ferociously while cringing with tail tucked. The longer he stood there, the more agitated she became. She crawled behind the mother's chair and tried to hide in her clothing. The dog occasionally pawed at the mother, whined to her, and tried to crawl onto her lap.

The son is able to play fetch and Frisbee with the dog in the yard and is the member of the household that does this most frequently.

This son has never injured, scared, or abused the dog. He is tremendously distressed and hurt by her behavior, particularly because it was, in part, his idea to rescue her. He is the only member of the family who smokes, wears glasses, and has a beard. If he tries to force himself on the dog, she becomes frantic. She has never bitten or injured anyone.

The clients have noticed that the dog is slightly fearful of some new experiences, but adjusts and does not exhibit this response to anything else. She is very difficult to walk on a leash and is not getting the exercise she needs. The son in question is also willing to leash-walk her, if she would walk for him.

Physical examination: No abnormalities were detected on physical examination.

Diagnosis: (1) Attention-seeking behavior, (2) fear aggression to adult son only, and (3) inappropriate leash behavior

Treatment: Management-related treatments include having the son wear contact lenses, shave his beard, and stop smoking. There is no guarantee that this would change the dog's impression of him, because the dog has had her inappropriate behavior reinforced every time she exhibits it, and has had time to learn to recognize him by other cues. Additionally, he could get his own apartment. This would not correct the problem but would avoid it. The clients want to try to correct the problem.

It is possible that in this dog's past she has been victimized by someone who resembles the son. His overtures to force her to like him have probably made her fearful behavior worse. Although she is becoming both more fearful and more aggressive, she has not bitten, but it was explained to the son that she might do so if she felt she had no other choice. Accordingly, most of the treatment is directed at desensitizing and counterconditioning the dog to the son. The first tier of this is the foundation program designed to teach her to relax in exchange for a food salary in benign contexts (see Appendix B). Once she can do this perfectly for everyone, other than the son, we can start to work with the son during a reexamination. For now he is to perform only passive behaviors: feeding her, giving her dog biscuits, and not forcing her to interact.

The dog was fitted for a Sporn No-Pull Halter (Four Paws Products Ltd., Hauppauge, NY) so that she could be pleasurably walked. If she permits him to do so, the son can walk her. He should play with her in the yard as much as possible and keep his sessions with her short, so that she just enjoys them and does not have the opportunity to become anxious. At such times he should not try to cuddle her; if she starts to make overtures to him, he can respond, but he should be restrained.

The dog's response is sufficiently profound that she would probably benefit from antianxiety medication. In fact, I doubt that she will be able to successfully master behavior modification without it. The clients are not anxious to use drugs. I discussed the pluses and minuses of this approach with them and emphasized that it would be my preference, but conceded that it is something we can always add to treatment. I emphasized that before using any psychotropic medication we would have to perform a complete blood cell count and serum biochemical profile.

Follow-up: The clients had some family disasters and were slow to start the behavior modification. The son is having trouble feeding the dog, largely because he is being too overbearing. We emphasized the importance of short, relaxed interludes and the role of praising the dog when she ignores the son. He does continue to play outside with her. We again emphasized that there are many antianxiety medications available (this dog would do well with fluoxetine or a lower-tech drug) and that we should talk about these when we evaluate her at reexamination.

Signalment: "Aldo," 4-year-old, 41 kg, male rottie/Siberian husky mixed breed

Initial problem: Aggression to clients, licking of rough surfaces and feet, and snapping and licking at air

History: This dog was acquired at 4 months of age after living with one other client. For the past 3 years the dog has bitten at the air and licked at rough surfaces (sweaters, carpeting) until physically interrupted. The licking and biting at the air preceded the licking rough surfaces by about 6 months. When licking at and biting the air, the dog often wanders until he ends up in a corner. Both of these behaviors happened a few times a month at first, but are now daily occurrences. Within the past year the dog has also begun to lick his paws on a daily basis. The paw licking seems to have coincided with an attempt on the clients' parts to decrease the other behaviors. The dog can be called away from any of the behaviors, recognizes the clients during them, and will come to the clients if they call when interrupting the dog.

In the past few months the dog has become aggressive in situations where the clients try to correct his unruly leash behavior, or when they try to get him to go somewhere they do not think he wants to go. Careful questioning revealed that he had always been a little pushy, and his behavior was far worse for the woman than the man. The woman is fearful of his aggression. Two weeks before the visit to the VHUP Behavior Clinic the dog growled and snarled at her when she told him to sit so she could take his leash off after a walk during which he dragged her down the street. He has always been "fussy" about having his leash removed, but has recently started snarling and snapping when his leash is taken off. He will let the clients reach toward and over him, but snarls if he is pushed from furniture. This, too, is a relatively recent development. The clients are unable to push on his shoulders or hips without eliciting a growl, and cannot take biscuits or human food from him. They stopped giving him rawhides and real bones when he was a puppy because they were frightened by the look on the dog's face when they came into the room. Lately, the clients have had trouble getting him to relinquish toys when they are playing, and he has begun to growl at them in these contexts.

The dog has always barked when strangers enter the house, knock, or approach the car or yard if he is present. In the past year the dog has become far more aggressive in these situations, snapping and growling when people approach. He appears to exhibit these behaviors primarily when his people are present. He is fine if he is on a leash and people approach him.

Finally, when he is interrupted while doing his air-snapping behaviors, he has begun to redirect his aggression to the person closest to him.

As an aside, the clients commented that he is getting very little exercise, because neither of them can really control him on a leash. Since he began to get aggressive they are fearful about lack of control in public places, although he has never had a problem or aggressive incident under those circumstances.

Physical examination: The physical examination was unremarkable. The dog is intact.

Laboratory evaluation: The intent had been to draw blood for a complete blood cell count and serum biochemical profile, but the dog was too aggressive to manipulate for this.

Diagnoses: (1) Food-related aggression, (2) dominance aggression, (3) possessive aggression, (4) protective aggression, (5) redirected aggression, (6) obsessive-compulsive/stereotypic behavior

Treatment: The patient was too aggressive to handle for blood work, so we did the following. I recommended that he be castrated. First, we do not need to perpetuate his genes. Second, because testosterone is a behavioral modulator, its presence can facilitate aggression in aggressive dogs. Compared with dogs that are neutered, dogs that are intact tend to react more quickly to a given stimulus, tend to fire to a higher level of reactivity, tend to stay reactive for a longer time, and tend to be more difficult and take longer to calm. The clients did not have a veterinarian that they liked, so I suggested that we do the castration at VHUP on a day when I could help the surgical team. When the dog came in, we would give him a little sedation, obtain the blood for tests, anesthetize and neuter him, and send him home with subcuticular sutures and antianxiety medication if the laboratory results were not worrisome.

Meanwhile, the clients were to start behavior modification programs designed to teach the dog to take all the cues as to the appropriateness of his behavior from them (see Appendix B). He was to sit and stay for everything and anything he wanted. He could only then earn what he wanted by being relaxed and quiet. The clients were to use the same technique to interrupt the stereotypic behavior. The first tier of the behavior modification program was demonstrated to the clients and it was emphasized that the point of desensitization and counterconditioning was to teach the dog to not react and to relax while stimuli were gradually introduced that caused him to react. Every time he exhibited an appropri-

• •

ate response for a minute task, he was praised and got a food reward. The clients had been bribing him; we explained the difference between a salary and a bribe. The dog was superb practicing the exercises at VHUP. We emphasized that dogs with abnormal, out-of-context behavior, particularly those that are anxious, need some kind of a consistent rule structure (benign doggie boot camp).

Follow-up: Two weeks later the dog was neutered at VHUP. He came in on his Gentle Leader/Promise Canine Head Collar (Premier Pet Products, Richmond, Va), and the woman told us how improved his behavior was, and it was improved. He sat, was quiet when she told him to be, and responded to leash corrections. The surgical staff, despite his bad press, had no problems with him, but used subcuticular sutures, just in case. All of his labora-

tory tests were within the reference limits, and he was sent home with amitriptyline, 50 mg to be given every 12 hours. Clients were instructed to continue to avoid all situations associated with aggressive incidents and to continue to call him away from any stereotypic behaviors using a substitute exercise for which he would be rewarded if he relaxed. Clients were also to increase his exercise by leash-walking.

Two weeks after castration the clients thought that they were doing terrifically. They had had no aggressive events, the stereotypic behavior had almost stopped, and the dog sought them out for friendly interactions. They still are having trouble with the part of the exercises that require them to go to the door and knock, but are working on this.

• •

Signalment: "Sidney," 1½-year-old, 21 kg, castrated male Dalmatian

Initial problem: The dog was brought to the Behavior Clinic at VHUP because of his avoidance of and aggression toward people outside the family, particularly on the street, and his elimination in the house.

History: The clients obtained this dog at 3 to 4 months of age. He had always been a little leery of strangers, but he had recently begun to bark and growl frantically, while pulling away from any person or strange sound, on the street. By the time they came to the Behavior Clinic for the first examination, the clients had virtually ceased to take the dog out during normal hours. Any people and any unexpected machine sounds startled him. The clients would try to take him out in the yard for elimination, but while outside he would not eliminate, regardless of how long he was left outside. Instead, he would become more anxious and agitated and more difficult to control if someone outside the family approached him. As soon as the clients brought him inside, he would eliminate in the house. In his struggles to back up while growling when he was approached by strangers, the dog was choking on his collar and dragging the clients during his walk. The clients could identify no predisposing events that correlated with this behavior.

Physical examination: No abnormalities were detected on physical examination.

Diagnoses: The diagnoses were fearful aggression and inappropriate elimination related to anxiety. The clues were as follows: First, the dog invariably backed up while growling and often shook while aggressive. His tail was never wholly vertical and flagged, but was often tucked below the line of his back. Although he lunged in confined situations, he also retreated after the lunge. These are behaviors consistent with a diagnosis of fearful aggression. In the absence of unfamiliar people or objects, he was still nervous when out of the house. The clients reported that he tucked his tail, exhibited constance vigilance and scanning, and was "jumpy." These behaviors started as he approached social maturity (18 to 36 months of age in dogs; range 12 to 48 months). This is also the age at which many fearful behaviors and early signs of mental illness appear in another social animal, human beings. He had never been outgoing with strangers but had not become aggressive until recently, and the aggression was worsening. The patient had been fully housebroken as a pup and had no problems sleeping through the night without eliminating, despite his propensity to eliminate in the house in the daytime. The onset of the elimination problem coincided with the worsening of the aggression.

Treatment: At the first visit the first tier of the behavior modification program was started (see Appendix B). The foundation program is designed to teach the dog to lie down or sit and stay while *relaxing* in a variety of circumstances. Dogs are to take their cues as to the appropriateness of their behaviors from the client. This is not an obedience exercise; it is one involving relaxation and desensitization. It is critical that clients realize this and reward the physical signs that the dog is relaxing and is becoming less reactive to external stimuli. The dog was able to perform the first of the exercises well at the clinic. The clients were encouraged to avoid all circumstances that triggered the undesirable, inappropriate behavior and to work intensively with the first phase of the program. Once he performed perfectly for this phase, they could start to walk him in areas where he would see people only at a distance. If he started to become anxious or fearful (ears back, stiffening, trembling, pupils dilated), they were to ask him to sit. If he was still upset, they were to turn him around and take him away from the situation. To facilitate this, he was fitted with a Gentle Leader/Promise System Canine Head Collar (Premier Pet Products, Richmond, VA). He was instantly calmer with this while at VHUP.

In addition, the clients were to take him out to eliminate frequently and praise and reward him for outdoor elimination. It was emphasized that they were rewarding the timing and location of the elimination—the act, itself, is self-rewarding. They were to try to stay out long enough so that he would eliminate, but were to bring him in if he became anxious. When unsupervised in the house, he was to be restricted to one area. The clients were to clean all affected areas with a good odor eliminator.

We discussed that antianxiety medication is often useful for such dogs. The clients expressed an interest in trying the behavior modification alone first.

Follow-up: A phone call a few weeks later revealed that the clients loved the Gentle Leader/Promise System and were able to walk the dog in low-traffic areas. He had begun to react less to some people, and the clients continued to practice the program. If anyone approached him he still had a full-blown problem, and there had been no attenuation of the elimination problem. At this point the clients asked if they could start an antianxiety medication regimen for the dog. After a discussion with their veterinarian, amitriptyline 25 mg orally every 12 hours, was prescribed after the complete blood cell count and serum biochemical profile revealed no abnormalities.

The clients brought the dog for a reexamination after a few weeks of amitriptyline treatment. They reported that after the first week the dog would willingly go for walks and always eliminated outside, and when people approached he did not growl. They took advantage of this change in behavior and gradually introduced him to people, first outside, and had him sit and relax while they approached, talked to, and then briefly petted him. Unlike at his first visit, when he growled, snarled, and backed into a corner, he was totally calm at the reexamination appointment, allowing everyone to pet him, wagging his tail, and responding to all commands. The clients are to continue the antianxiety medication for at least another 2 months. If they do decide to see if he can sustain this behavior without it, they are to wean him from it, not stop suddenly. The clients also realize that this dog may need antianxiety medication for life.

The antianxiety medication facilitated this patient's ability to overcome his fears about the outdoors. Because he had been housebroken previously, he was willing to eliminate outside once he could manage his fear. He may also have benefited from the side effects that are associated with TCA use: anticholinergic action and increased urinary sphincter tone. It is worthwhile to note that (1) a physical examination and blood studies were performed before administering medication, and (2) the first drug of choice was a low-tech one. Amitriptyline is one of the oldest TCAs available. It is inexpensive, acts quickly, and has relatively few side effects (GI upset, inappetence, regular tachycardia and concomitant panting, lethargy), for which the clients were instructed to watch. This is a good example of a rational approach to pharmacological intervention for behavioral problems. Such cautions are warranted because few psychotropic medications are licensed for use in domestic animals (hence, all use is extra-label), and pets cannot tell us that they are experiencing side effects; clients have to help us watch for these.

CASE 5

Signalment: "Cassanova," 5-year-old, castrated male shar-pei (20 kg)

Initial problem: Destruction of house.

History: This pup was adopted approximately 5 months ago. These people are the dog's third household; the second client had the dog for more than 3 years, but also had five children and could not afford the dog. There are five cats now in the household; one additional cat recently died after an illness. There are no other dogs in the household. The husband and wife are older and both work, although when they first got the dog they were in the middle of an extensive vacation period. When they returned to work, they would come home to find the house destroyed—as time went on, the destruction became worse, not better, and the dog would injure itself. The "last straw" was when they returned home to find the new solarium addition no longer attached to the house by door jambs; in fact, all the door jambs in this house have now been removed for repair. The worst destruction has occurred in the kitchen, where, in addition to damage to the door and window sill, the tile and drywall have been dug through and the wood stained with blood. During the most recent event the dog ripped out almost all of its front toenails. The dog would start to pace before the owners left and is always agitated when they come home. Whenever the people want to go out to dinner or a movie, they take the dog with them; he sleeps quietly in the van. The clients solicited help from a behaviorist with a doctoral degree (not a veterinarian) in their area; this individual recommended a crate and told their veterinarian to start a regimen of amitriptyline (75 mg orally every 24 hours). The dog's behavior became worse when he was in the crate—he chipped his teeth, lacerated his lips and tongue, broke his nails, and avulsed two pads before breaking out of the crate (and destroying it). After 3 days of medication, the dog stopped sleeping, paced and circled the entire house, panted, and exhibited inappetence. In response to the above, the local veterinarian began to give the dog 35 mg of acepromazine every day and insisted that the clients come to VHUP. During the appointment the dog never settled down. He also does not know how to sit on command.

Physical examination: The dog's hair coat was poor, although the clients report that this is much improved since their veterinarian started the dog on a hypoallergenic diet. The referring veterinarian also submitted a triiodothyronine/thyroxine radioimmunoassay to Michigan State University; when the levels were reported to be borderline low, he recommended thyroxine supplementation; this happened concurrent with the diet change. The patient has a history of vomiting every 4 to 6 weeks; this

is not associated with either feeding or fasting, and the patient seldom exhibits food in the vomitus. Abdominal palpation was not remarkable. Fecal studies have been done, with negative results. The dog had signs of recently healed nail beds; the clients say that they are going to cut his nails for the first time next week. There are healed lacerations on the head, nose, around the mouth, and on the pads and forelegs. Some teeth are chipped, but the chips are not stained. Auscultations indicate a normal sinus rhythm without murmurs; pulses are even and synchronous with the heartbeats.

Diagnosis: Separation anxiety, generalized anxiety, possible continuing food allergy or atopic condition

Treatment: The dog was placed on the initial behavior modification programs. After demonstrating these to the client it became clear that the dog had never learned to sit on request. We taught him that and emphasized the importance of relaxation. He was to be baby-sat or confined in an open area (i.e., not a crate). He was to be seen by a dermatologist for further treatment of his skin lesions. I had wanted to withdraw this dog's thyroid medication and acepromazine, but the clients were resistant because they were fearful of another outburst. They agreed to start to decrease the acepromazine gradually over 2 weeks and start amitriptyline at a more appropriate initial dose (25 mg orally every 12 hours for 30 days to start).

Follow up: After 2 weeks the dog was doing better. The clients had left him alone infrequently, but they were able to confine him in the kitchen or in the car. They were working hard with the behavior modification. About 1 month after their initial appointment the clients called me and were distraught. They had left the dog for 6 hours and he had destroyed their kitchen, their bathroom, and their bedroom. They had been packing for vacation and had left the suitcases out. The dog destroyed those. The dog was also severely agitated and shaking.

We hospitalized him the next day. The clients reported that the dog had not slept that night. By the time we saw him he would not or could not focus on us, continued to pace indiscriminately, and was tachycardic and experiencing muscle fasciculations.

Complete blood cell counts were nonremarkable and serum biochemistry panels revealed slightly elevated ALT and ALK. ECG revealed tachycardia but no conduction anomalies (a concern with TCA use), and a T4 level was 4 times the upper limit of the laboratory's reference range. The dog was also vomiting and had profound hemorrhagic diarrhea laced with fiberglass.

Cassanova was placed on fluids by mouth (he ripped IV catheters in his pacing), and fecal smears and cultures were submitted. They were noninformative. When his vomiting stopped he was permitted a bland gruel of a prescription diet and water. As his diarrhea resolved he was switch to a hypoallergenic diet.

He was withdrawn from all medications immediately on admission. After about 3 days of agitation, he finally began to sleep for most of the day. Once he was awake and alert, behavior modification to teach him to be left and relax was started 4 times each day for 15 to 20 minutes at a time. By the end of the week he began to cry when he could not see someone from his run and to destroy his bedding when left alone. He was started on buspirone, 20 mg orally every 24 hours. This drug was chosen for its anxiolytic effect and because of its relative lack of side effects. Behavior modification was intensified, he was walked frequently, and he spent time in different offices, where we worked up to leaving him for up to 15 minutes.

When Cas's people returned from their vacation (after the house was repaired) in 3 weeks he greeted them enthusiastically in the waiting room, but sat on command, walked quietly, entered his run, and lay down when requested.

We cautioned the clients that he may need other medications and that daily behavior modification was important. They could give him as much love as they wanted but couldn't reward his anxiety. We had also noticed that he was calmer when outside and that he spent a lot of time sniffing the air. The clients built him a run with lights, a heat lamp, and a doghouse, where he could spend time with or without them outside. We stressed that the run should not be used in a manner that would be punishment and that he should not be placed in the run only when the clients were leaving. The timing and situation of placement in the run were to be highly variable. Finally, they were to continue the medication and return for a T_3/T_4 and thyroid stimulation test in a month. The thyroid tests, conducted 7 weeks after medication withdrawal, revealed normal thyroid function. The dog's coat looked great, he was maintained on a hypoallergenic diet, and he had no clinical signs of hypothyroidism. Supplementation with thyroxin was wholly inappropriate in this case and was correlated with his presenting signs at hospital admission.

Further response: After about 4 months, the clients had been able to halve the daily dose of buspirone. They have never been really ardent about behavior modification, but became even less so when one of them retired. After another bout of destruction, we reemphasized the importance of behavior modification as a set of rules to provide a reliable, predictable, and relaxing structure to the dog's life. To treat these dogs successfully, one has to shift their rule structure from becoming anxious when they cannot directly monitor their people, to one in which they have rules that tell them it's alright not to be anxious. Medication can help with this. Cas was eventually switched to clomipramine, and the clients, although they fully understand the reasoning of the treatment, prefer to tolerate a lower level of anxiety (now mostly barking, without destruction) coupled with taking him with them. They also obtained a friend for Cas, a 1½ year old beagle, and Cas is happier, calmer, and very attentive to her. The beagle doesn't appear to be an active participant in Cas's setback events. She is as calm 2 years later as she was the day they brought her home.

CASE 6

Signalment: "Jane," 2-year-old female bearded collie, 21 kg

Initial problem: Will not stand for judges

History: This pup is one of a family of beardies that the owner owns and shows. She would really like to get a championship. Starting about 6 months ago the dog started to sit down when the judges examined her. Now she will not even get out of her pen without falling on her belly before she gets to the show ring. Whenever the owner readies the van for the show, the dog hides and will not eat. When she is with the other dogs, she is the same as she has always been—happy and playful. She is fine with the family. With strangers she has become more shy; this was always the pup that lagged back, but would then effusively greet strangers. Now she tries to avoid them and, if this is impossible, she turns her back and tries to hide. Her mother, sister, and aunt are all wonderful; no other sibs have problems. Most of her family members have obedience titles.

Physical examination and laboratory evaluation: No abnormalities were detected.

Diagnosis: Idiopathic fear, possibly similar to overanxious disorder or avoidant disorder of childhood that is described for humans (DSM-IV).

Treatment: The patient was started on the behavior modification programs designed to teach her to relax and to be more relaxed around people. Jane was to be pulled from the show ring and not exposed to such circumstances. The clients were not anxious to use medication at first. When her behavior had altered only slightly, the clients elected to treat her with amitriptyline (20 mg orally every 12 hours for 30 days to start), coupled with the behavior modification. Jane's premedication complete blood cell count and serum biochemistry profile were within the reference range of the laboratory.

Six months later she was sufficiently improved to rejoin her family in obedience work and seemed to really enjoy it. She has done well in competitive events.

CASE 7

Signalment: "Sylvia," 6-month-old female English setter

Initial problem: Flees at loud noises

History: Sylvia was purchased as a hunting dog at 2 months of age. She has been raised in both the house and kennel and seems generally calm. She does well with the other dogs and the people in the house. Adored by the kids, this pup has never *once* even scratched a child during play. She has an extremely soft mouth. Last week Sylvia was taken to the shooting range. While she was sniffing in the grass, a gun went off behind her. She fled through the range, into the parking lot, across the street through traffic, and was eventually found a half mile from home. Since then the owner has tried to fire a gun while she is leashed and she shrieks and tries to get away. The owner wants a hunting dog.

Diagnosis: Noise phobia.

Physical examination and laboratory evaluation: No abnormalities were detected.

Treatment: Do not treat this with the intent of creating a hunting dog; it will not work. This will be a fine pet-quality dog, but if the client won't keep her unless she hunts, the best solution may be to place her in another home. She can be desensitized to some potential noises like firecrackers by using one of the available audiotapes (see Appendix C) or by making a home recording and playing it at gradually increasing volumes. Using maleable foam earplugs made for humans or placing cotton in her ears may help alter her perception of, and change her reaction to, the sound. Before desensitization can occur, she should be taught the basic relaxation programs and then these should be used in conjunction with the sound stimulus. These programs are found in Appendix C. If she continues to become distressed in response to noises, early intervention with antianxiety agents is recommended and was discussed.

CASE 8

Signalment: "Muffin," 4-year-old, spayed female domestic long hair

Initial problem: Chewing on tail

History: About 5 to 6 months ago Muffin's tail was caught in the door. Only the tip was damaged and she was seen by the referring veterinarian, who treated it topically. The tail healed. No changes in grooming were seen. About 1 month ago Muffin began to scream every time she saw her tail. Just before she would scream her back rippled. If the client could hide the tail between her legs, Muffin could calm down, but if the cat saw the tail she would ripple, scream, and try to escape the tail. Two weeks ago she severely mutilated the tip; she continues to bite it if she discovers she cannot get away from it. If we cannot fix this, the owner is going to euthanize this cat because of how nervous the cat has become since starting this problem.

Physical examination: The tip of the tail is bald and scabby, but is dry. No lymph nodes are inflamed. The cat's color is good. Its coat is good (although the owner says she has decreased her grooming frequency since the problem started).

Diagnosis: Self-mutilation/OCD(?)

Laboratory results: Muffin's laboratory work revealed a serum alkaline phosphatase of over 1100 mg/dl. Previous treatment involved phenobarbital.

Treatment: The client was taught to reward Muffin with food treats when she was relaxed and to set up daily grooming and play sessions. These will help provide a rule structure for the cat. She is to be distracted if she even looks at her tail. Grooming will avoid the tail at first and gradually work up to it. The cat will be placed in an Elizabethan collar only if she reinjures the tail. Muffin was prescribed 5 mg amitryptiline every 12 hours after an ECG (no abnormalities detected) and 3 weeks after a second evaluation of SAP, which was still elevated. The cat has blood drawn frequently. Her liver enzyme levels are always elevated, but she shows no clinical signs. The client has maintained the amitriptyline and had been able to interrupt the cat easily. With time, this became more difficult, so after 2 months Muffin was switched to hydrocodone (5 mg orally every 12 hours). The cat's tail has remained unmutilated for more than a year, but she has not lost interest in it. This cat started to mutilate her tail after injury, so it is unclear if the hydrocodone is efficacious because it provides relief of pain.

11 ..... Miscellaneous Behavioral Problems: Emphasis on Management

••

Most of the issues discussed in this chapter involve normal cat and dog behaviors that clients may find undesirable. O'Farrell (1986) estimates that 20% (⅕) of dogs have behaviors or behavioral problems that cause clients inconvenience. Included are normal behaviors that occur in contexts that might be inappropriate and some abnormal behaviors that develop as a consequence of innate, nondomesticated behaviors. The latter become apparent when the animal is constrained to perform in an environment that does not meet innate needs. Many "abnormal" behaviors have a component of "normal" behavior that is directed toward inappropriate stimuli (Beaver, 1989a). This observation may be responsible for the contention that behavior problems are the result of conflicts between excitatory and inhibitory sides of the nervous system (Campbell, 1992). Although useful as a heuristic device, the conflict theory is too general to be useful at a mechanistic level. Only the latter can provide hypotheses that account for profound deviations from the range of normal. It is in the context of these hypotheses that specific treatments are suggested. This discussion *does* illustrate the importance of *context* in which the behaviors occur. This chapter urges practitioners to be sufficiently knowledgeable that they can intervene early and can abort these problems before they worsen. Client handouts for dealing with many of these problems are found in Appendix B.

FELINE PROBLEMS

Feline management problems include the following:
1. Furniture scratching
2. Attention-seeking behavior
3. Inappropriate play behavior
4. Inappropriate consumptive behavior
5. Mounting and masturbation
6. Predatory behavior
7. Tree-climbing behavior
8. Maternal and/or paternal neglect and aggression
9. Reintroduction after hospitalization
10. Travel problems
11. Plant-eating problems
12. Nocturnal activity
13. Vocalization
14. Eating problems

Each of these problems is discussed, with a description of the range of behaviors exhibited and corrections that could be made to prevent the problem from either developing or worsening.

Furniture Scratching

Furniture scratching is widespread but is seldom severe enough for clients to believe that it warrants a visit to a behavioral specialist. In a survey of "normal" cats for which the clients had no behavioral problems, 60% of cats (71/122) scratched furniture (Morgan & Houpt, 1990). Regardless, the scratching of furniture is a common reason for clients bringing their pets to practitioners' offices. Scratching is an innate feline behavior. Modification of any innate behaviors is difficult at best. Cats scratch, in part, to remove the sheath from their claws and will develop a material preference for this (Hart & Hart, 1985a). Because this is the primary reason that cats begin to scratch in inappropriate areas, the very first puppy or kitten visit should include a lesson on nail trimming. Cats whose nails are trimmed regularly, either by use of a nail clipper or an emery board, are easier to handle and experience fewer inappropriate behaviors associated with scratching. Furthermore, if an undesirable behavior begins to develop, the clients will have a chance to see it develop because they will be paying a lot of attention to the cat's feet.

Cats that scratch to mark territory may be more difficult to control than cats that scratch as part of a grooming routine. There are no studies that have investigated the extent to which scratching may be a behavior found concomitantly in households in which cats spray, but Hart and Hart (1985a) indicate that cats frequently scratch near sleeping areas. Regardless, if there are any associated intercat aggressions, seasonal changes in scratching behavior, or associated marking behaviors, the social system warrants investigation.

Scratching is a communication device that helps cats modulate social interactions (Verbene & de Boer, 1976). Cats have interdigital glands; by vigorously scratching they leave both visual markers of their presence in the forms of sheath fragments and claw marks, and olfactory markers. Studies conducted on free-ranging cat populations have demonstrated that the frequency of scratching behavior increases if other cats are present compared with when the scratcher is alone. Accordingly, it is important to address grooming and social aspects in tandem if furniture scratching is to be controlled.

It is important to note whether the cat prefers to scratch on horizontal or vertical objects, or if the cat prefers the dark and privacy or scratches primarily when others are present. Meeting the cat's needs will help, but the chances of successful intervention are greatly increased if the cat can be rewarded when it uses the post appropriately. For an older cat that is scratching for social reasons, placing the post in an area where the cat can scratch to mark can work as a reward. For kittens, rewards take the form of praise when the cat uses the post.

Some cats immediately use a scratching post when it is presented to them; others will disdain it. If the client has a naive cat that does not yet have a problem, the client should be encouraged both to learn how to appropriately clip the claws and to teach the cat how to play with the scratching post. This requires directing and rewarding the appropriate behaviors when the cat does use the scratching post and immediately correcting the cat if the cat scratches on an inappropriate surface. Feline scratching posts can be made from fabric or hemp; many cats prefer just the bark from logs. Use of logs is often not favored by clients because it is messy, but some cats that will use nothing else will use these. Space permitting, a dead tree stump can be used for the cat to scratch. Regardless of the substrate chosen, cats should be taken to the area of choice and allowed to sniff and explore their substrate. If the cat is tractable, clients can move the cat's claws over the surface so that the cat knows that it is acceptable to scratch the chosen surface. As the clients are manipulating the cat's feet and gently scratching the surface with the cat's feet, they can tell the cat that it is good and give it a food treat. This does not teach the cat to scratch; the cat already knows how to scratch—it is an innate behavior. This *rewards* the cat for exhibiting the scratching behavior on an acceptable substrate or in an acceptable area. The rest is up to the cat—some cats will scratch, others will not.

Cats also should be corrected when they scratch in an inappropriate place. Cats should be belled, so that the clients are always aware of their location. Any bells on cats should be carefully sewn to breakaway collars. Even a plain buckle collar can strangle a cat. As soon as the client hears the bell jingling in association with the cat starting to scratch in an inappropriate area, the client should startle the cat, preferably within the first few seconds of the beginning of the scratching, or within the first 30 to 60 seconds of the *onset* of the suite of the behaviors that lead up to the scratching. The startle must be sufficient that the cat stops the behavior, but not so intense that the cat becomes terrified. Clients should *not* follow this action

with trimming of the claws; the cat might learn to associate claw trimming with punishment. Instead, the client should wait until the cat is calm or is soliciting affection and then trim the cat's claws while praising, petting, and massaging the cat or offering food treats. If the cat has been raised with these techniques since it was a young kitten, this should be relatively easy to do. Caution is urged for many cats with status-related or other aggressions. Caution is particularly urged for cats that have been feral. Handling cats in such a manner could be injurious to the client for cats with those problems. These problems are more fully discussed in Chapter 7.

The problem is slightly different if the cat already has expressed a preference for a type of scratching object. First, the clients should note the type of substrate the cat is using to scratch. If it is a specific type of fabric, they can cover a scratching post with that fabric and use the reward/correction system outlined above. If the cat prefers to scratch on a horizontal rather than a vertical object, the scratching post can be made into a horizontal object. Some cats like to mount horizontal objects and scratch them; in this case, a log may be a real boon. If the cat seems to prefer a nubby fabric, hemp or a log can be used. Clients are concerned that if they cover a scratching post with fabric similar to the fabric that the cat likes, the cat will generalize its scratching preferences to everything in the environment. Although there are no reliable data on this subject, this does not seem to be the case, because many scratching posts are covered with carpeting. These cats do not appear to scratch indiscriminately on carpeting. Scratching is more than just a grooming behavior.

Cats scratch not to just remove their sheaths, but also as a visual display. The act of scratching itself is a confident display that indicates that the cat is willing to be seen physically marking an area. Scratching is also an olfactory display, because not only do cats leave behind parts of their sheaths, but they leave behind the scent from their interdigital glands. In many cases, scratching can be coupled with spraying.

The second visual display that results from scratching is the damage or mark left by the scratching. This type of visual display is longer lasting than that given by the act of scratching. In a free-ranging situation, one or two trees may be used as scratching areas for the majority of the cats.

When creating a desirable scratching area and substrate, it is important to identify the physical attributes that the cat finds appealing (Hart, 1980b). These include height, position (horizontal vs. vertical), and extent to which the area is enclosed. If the client can mimic these qualities with an appropriate substrate and use the positive reinforcements and corrections outlined above, the cat will switch to the appropriate scratching area.

If the client was unable to stop the scratching, the appropriate correction must be administered within the first 30 to 60 seconds of the onset of the suite of behaviors that include scratching. The best results are achieved by interruption of the scratching within one to two seconds of its onset. To do this, the client must continually monitor the cat; placing a bell on the collar can help. If the cat does not react to a voice, water pistols, air horns, air canisters, or fog horns can all be used to startle the cat and stop the event (Hart, 1978b). It is important to use the lowest level of stimulus that achieves the appropriate response. The appropriate response involves getting the cat to abort the scratching while still leaving the cat receptive to another behavior. It is critical that correction is not the client's only interaction with the cat. Otherwise the cat will learn to associate correction with the sight of the client, not with the act of scratching. It is best if clients can startle the cat without being seen, although this is difficult.

If the client is not home, it can be very difficult to reinforce an appropriate area for scratching. There are two ways to do this. If the cat returns repeatedly to one area, the easiest solution is to exclude the cat from that area. Unfortunately, many modern houses have fairly open floor plans, making it difficult to block off an area by closing a door. Stackable baby gates can be used to keep cats from rooms, and screen doors have been successfully installed in houses to keep cats from specific areas. Indoor electronic fences can restrict access. If these modifications are not possible and the area that the cat scratches is a smaller, restricted area, there are other booby traps that the owners can use. Pull-string firecrackers from novelty stores can be hung from the object where the cat is scratching. If the cat scratches one of these, it will be sprayed with confetti and startled by a "pop," but it could learn to ignore the area. Small balloons affixed to the same surface can have the same effect. When the cat pops the balloon, it is startled sufficiently to abort the behavior. Caution is urged if the cat is likely to ingest any dangling parts or residues. These types of aversive stimuli are only successful if the stimuli dissuade scratching every single time the animal approaches that area and starts to scratch. Because the objectionable behavior is an established one, we must realize that there is a danger of "resistance to extinction." When animals become resistant to extinction, they usually do so because they learn that sometimes the aversive stimulus is present and sometimes it is not. If the cat is sufficiently motivated to scratch at the object, the cat will test to see whether the stimulus is present. In fact, the lack of continuous reinforcement can backfire because it may make the animal more willing to explore the area to see if it can identify a pattern of when the aversive stimulus is present.

If the client has kittens or a newly acquired cat that does not yet have a problem, they can teach the cat to retract its claws. As part of this process, clients should

not encourage cats to follow them and jump on any dragging clothing, shoelaces, skirts, or pant legs. The rules should be fairly consistent.

The controversy about the treatment of scratching involves the issue of declawing (onychectomy). This surgery is a form of elective mutilation and should *not* be used prophylactically. There is no reason accepted by the CVMA or AVMA to declaw any animal at 3 or 6 months of age in the absence of an established medical or behavioral problem. However, it is certainly preferable to declaw an animal than to kill it because of its destructive behavior, or to break up a relationship because of its destructive behavior. I think that it would be unfortunate if clients were misled into believing that declawing was a fancy claw trim. They should realize that an entire joint of every digit is being removed. They need to know this because (1) they should make an informed decision, and (2) there are complications with such procedures. The most common surgical complications are rare but include the risks attendant with anesthesia and hemostasis. The secondary risks are the behavioral ones. Cats that have been declawed and reintroduced to litter too early, particularly if it is hard gravel litter, may develop a substrate aversion. This problem can be obviated by avoiding reintroduction to inappropriate litters too early or using soft litters (shredded paper towels, the recycled newspaper kitty litter [Yesterday's News Cat Litter, Moncton, NB]). The other behavioral problem that may become apparent after declawing is a fear of having the feet manipulated or unwillingness to bear weight on the feet. These complications are rare, but the cats act as if there is pain present. It is currently impossible to assess phantom pain in animals. Radiographic studies, physical examination, and blood chemistry analyses usually reveal no anomalies, but these cats change their entire locomotive and interactive behaviors.

Clients are often concerned that if a cat's claws are removed, the animal will become more aggressive and persistent with its teeth. First, cats that are declawed can and will still scratch, although now they can do little damage. If they are scratching for purposes of social marking, declawing has not influenced this. Second, furniture scratching is not an agonistic behavior associated with aggressive action; it is a grooming and communication behavior. Cats that were not aggressive in the use of their teeth before declawing do not become aggressive in the use of their teeth afterward (Bennett et al., 1988). Clients should be cautioned that their perceptions might change; if they used to pay more attention to the cat's scratching before declawing, they may not have realized the extent to which the cat used its teeth in play and other instances. Furthermore, if a large part of cat-client relationship was based on the client chasing the cat when it scratched, the cat might receive less attention after declawing and hence will devise other ways to get this attention.

Practitioners should reassure clients that the data do not support a transfer of activity from claws to aggressive oral activity.

Clients who believe that declawing their cats will prevent them from preying on birds are incorrect in their assumption.

Clients should not be allowed to assume that onychectomy is something that is just "done" to cats. If there are no physical problems attendant with the claws, if the clients do not realize that the cat will lose phalanges, or if clients do not understand the associated surgical risk, onychectomy should not be performed. There are also no data to support the contention that prophylactic onychectomy will save the life of a cat that would otherwise be euthanized later when it begins to scratch. Such data would change the tone of the debate. It would be preferable to substitute client education about cats' needs for the automatic perception that declawing cats is "normal." If the clients do not wish to try any of the behavioral methods before declawing, I always find myself hoping that the cat never requires any other time-consuming help from the client; if the required help is not easy to implement, it may not get done. If the cat has other behavioral problems or the client wishes to make the cat into an indoor/outdoor cat for some other reason, declawed cats can survive in the wild. If declawing is performed, it is certainly preferable that the hind feet be left intact. This makes it easier for cats that climb trees to do so. Quite a few cats that are excellent tree climbers can climb them with no claws at all. It is less desirable to let cats run loose because the average life expectancy of a cat that is free-ranging is slightly more than 3 years, whereas the average life expectancy of a cat that is wholly an indoor cat can be up to 20 years.

If clients have tried all of the environmental and behavioral modification suggestions and have not succeeded in getting the cat to stop scratching, but do not wish to declaw the cat, many of the new plastic nail sheaths (Soft Paws Smart Practice, Phoenix, AZ) can be a boon. Plastic nail sheaths are applied with a permanent glue and they require replacing every 6 to 12 weeks as the cat's nails grow. Some cats and clients may have an adverse reaction to the adhesive. The cats still scratch, but unless the fabric is very fine, the plastic-tipped claws cannot cause any damage. Clients also can have fun with this because the nail coverings are available in a variety of colors. The nail coverings are probably best applied at the veterinarian's office first and then the client can certainly apply them at home. These are *not* suitable for cats that are intractable.

Attention-Seeking Behavior

Attention-seeking behavior is most common in young animals in a single-cat household. Young animals have a lot of energy and cannot be left alone 12 to 16 hours a day without getting restless. Cats often sleep in the absence of stimulation. No matter how sophisticated the kitty toy, few cats will play back to the extent that a client or another cat can. Young cats routinely knock objects off tables, or awaken the clients by patting them in the face at 2:00 a.m. They may tear around the house and greet the client inappropriately, using teeth and claws, and follow the client from room to room trying to grab whatever the client is dangling. If the client is sitting quietly, the cat may pounce on the client's feet. If the client is sitting at a desk, trying to work, it is not unusual for the cat to jump up on the desk and drape its body gracefully over the area exactly where the work is occurring. Some cats have become very adept at draping themselves over computer monitors, which would be perfectly acceptable if they could learn to type.

These are annoying behaviors, but they are not dangerous and seldom become more problematic. The key to teaching these cats not to be bothersome lies in *not* shoving them away. In the absence of play, shoving a cat away acts as a form of attention. Any attention is better than no attention for young cats. These are young cats, and they need more stimulation than they are getting. If the cat is young, it will probably not respond to being ignored. It is far more appropriate to shape or redirect behaviors to a more appropriate outlet.

For instance, cats can be taught to play "fetch." Instead of bounding all over the sofa and the client's lap while the client is trying to read, the client could teach the cat to "fetch" a paper or plastic ball. When the cat brings it back and drops it, the cat gets a food treat. This still involves active client participation. If the cat dashes around the house or the apartment and grabs everything it sees, the client can start to play with the cat passively by attaching a cat toy to an elastic or spring cord around the client's waist. The cat toy need be no fancier than a kitty mouse, ball of string, or a plastic sparkler. The cat will then be able to chase this and follow the client everywhere in the house.

Some people have been very successful in teaching the cat to run on a small treadmill (the means to build these so that they accommodate a cat's weight is beyond most people's capabilities), or teaching the cats to play with an interactive toy. Interactive toys can be balls that hang in perpetual motion devices or balls that go through a series of circles, dishes, or tubes where the cat can bat them around. Some cats do quite well if they have a very complex kitty condo system that resembles an agility course for dogs. It provides them a safe way to tear around in enclosed and exposed areas, and it gives them the ability to safely leap from position to position.

Clients should be encouraged to ensure that none of the cat's toys are potentially injurious to the cat.

String foreign bodies are very common in young cats, and can lead to high surgery bills, and/or death.

It is problematic that the clients work 12 to 14 hours a day and the cat sleeps during that time, so that the clients want to sleep when the cat wants to play. Regardless, the clients should absolutely, positively not get up and feed the cat to convince the cat to let them sleep. By doing this, the clients discover that the cat gradually pushes back its mealtime to increasingly earlier hours of the day. Clients should ignore the cat. If this does not work, clients should keep a water pistol or an air canister by the bed and blast the cat. If it takes more than two bursts from a compressed air canister to quell the cat's urges, the client's timing is incorrect (see Chapter 12). Clients should be reminded that the goal is not to produce a terrified or phobic cat; the goal is to couple an aversive stimulus with inappropriate attention-seeking behavior.

The easiest mechanism for remedying this situation is to get the cat a playmate. If the cat in question already plays roughly, it might be more appropriate to get a slightly older kitten. Evenly aged cats often entertain each other and relieve the clients of part of this burden. All of the same caveats discussed for inappropriate behavior in one cat certainly apply to both. It is important to try to match the personalities of the cats. If one cat is a bit of a bully, a second bully certainly is undesirable. Virtually all other combinations will work if the cats like other cats and are friendly or "social." Clients should be forewarned that cats do not reach social maturity until 2 to 4 years of age and *may* experience some interaction conflict at that time. Cats that are quite old seldom have the desire or inclination to interact with a young, feisty kitten, but they can still live in the same house without undue upheaval.

Finally, if the client is unwilling to get another cat, the cat could be turned into an indoor/outdoor cat. The cat *will* continue to exhibit these behaviors around the neighborhood and could be a good victim for intercat aggression or the neighbor's wrath. The incidence of injury, fighting, and fatality is high for outdoor cats, particularly those in urban areas.

If the clients are unsuccessful in the implementation of behavior modification techniques, some cats respond to 2 to 4 mg chlorpheniramine before bedtime. More sophisticated drugs should not be used to treat what is essentially normal behavior. There are both ethical and physiological problems with such an approach. No studies have been done on the use of melatonin to induce sleep in cats. If the situation is severe enough that the clients cannot sleep, they may also wish to change the feeding time so that the cat is fed just before it goes to bed.

If the client is unwilling to take any of these measures, the cat will outgrow most of the rambunctious behaviors, but this can take 3 to 4 years.

If there is an increase in attention-seeking behaviors despite following these recommendations, and if the attention-seeking behaviors occur *in tandem* with other behavioral changes, underlying medical complications (e.g., pain) should be explored (Beaver, 1989). Cats with hyperthyroid can resemble those with attention-seeking behavior, although the former are frenetic. When there is uncertainty, physical and laboratory examinations are recommended.

Inappropriate Play Behavior

Inappropriate play behavior is most commonly seen in kittens who are orphaned early, many of whom were bottle fed and who never learned to control the intensity of their play. Mother cats will whack kittens who play too roughly. Clients are (rightfully) afraid of injuring a young kitten by physical discipline; however, kittens who greet with flying leaps and attach themselves to body parts are a menace. Inappropriate play behavior can develop into play aggression if left untreated. Cats who play aggressively can do serious damage. It should be remembered that cat bites are a $25,000,000 per year human medical industry in the United States currently, and that cat-scratch fever is a problem that is becoming a more visible human health concern.

Using a device designed to dissuade the cat from its exuberant behavior (e.g., water pistols, air horns, fog horns) as the animal first begins to show the signs of the inappropriate play will stop the behavior. In both inappropriate play behavior and attention-seeking behavior, it is critical to couple the averse stimulus with a positive one. This is the concept that clients most frequently misunderstand. When any cat that usually exhibits inappropriate play behavior acts wonderfully, very few clients reward the good behavior. When the cat is behaving as the clients wish, even if the cat is asleep, tell the cat that it is wonderful, and gently stroke and massage it. If the cat is asleep, as long as it is not startled, this rewarding behavior will fit in perfectly with the plan to reward those types of relaxing behaviors. Furthermore, any time the cat plays appropriately (claws retracted and teeth not exposed), it should be rewarded with praise, love, attention, appropriate play, and kitty treats.

Clients should *not* play aggressively with these cats using their hands. Aggressive corrections should also be discouraged. People should not flick kittens on the nose to correct them. Although queens will bat kittens on the nose to control mouthing (Beaver, 1992), they do so *only* after they have received no response to a growl. Humans do not mimic this entire behavioral sequence in their correction, and hence often worsen the kitten's aggression or rough play. The kitten should not be taught to follow the client's hand and to pounce on it. Encouraging the cat to stalk human body parts will only increase the rate at which the cat begins to exhibit predatory behavior (see Chapter 4). Clients should be told that early orphaned cats

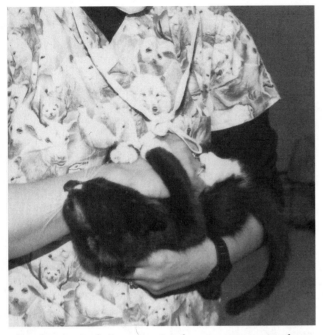

This kitten is being permitted—even encouraged—to mouth and play inappropriately. His claws are retracted, which is good, but it would be better if he directed his mouthing and biting to a toy. He's a pushy kitten, and the risk, which the client fully appreciates, exists that he will exhibit aggression later in life. The client helped set the kitten up for this picture and usually discourages this behavior, now that the kitten is getting big, by blowing in his face or making a sharp noise. (Photo by K.L. Overall.)

are already at risk for developing earlier predatory behavior. Evidence indicates that *appropriate* play behavior is the best precursor to subsequent appropriate social behavior both to cats and people. Accordingly, any time a cat accidentally scratches or bites an individual, the individual should act horrified and withdraw. There is no need to physically punish the cat. If the cat is young, blowing in its nose can be sufficient to startle it. The cat can be taught that it is acceptable to play roughly with toys, but not with people. This can be done by dragging a toy along and letting the cat play with it. When the cat does play appropriately with a toy, it should be told that it is very sweet and very good. The toy is usually a sufficient reward for this behavior; a food treat is not necessary. However, if the cat is being stroked gently and is not reacting, a food treat can facilitate the shaping of that relaxed behavior as an appropriate response to human hand gestures.

Inappropriate Consumptive Behaviors

Inappropriate consumptive behaviors may be superb models for human compulsions. These are one of the classes of problems that may start as management sit-uations and quickly escalate to anxiety-related, stereotypic behaviors. These behaviors may be more common than is usually realized; cats with prolonged (2 to 12 months) sucking behavior comprised 14.1% (9/64 patients) in one behavior service (Beaver, 1989a). Inappropriate consumptive behaviors, including wool sucking, are further discussed in Chapter 10. A brief reintroduction is appropriate because in some cases (and there are no good data on which cases these are, or how common they are), early intervention and redirection of the behavior may be useful. The most common of the consumptions is wool sucking in Siamese cats. Very often, material is not ingested, just mutilated. If ingested, gastrointestinal (GI) upset and intestinal obstruction can occur. Clients should be warned to watch for signs of these disorders. There have been no well-documented cases of dietary deficiencies or early weaning behaviors as causal of this behavior, although early weaned cats appear overrepresented in this group. The situation is complicated by the fact that domestic cats are weaned earlier than free-ranging ones. Both social and developmental (teething) factors then become concerns. Cats fed poor diets or generic cat food often seek other sources for nutrition and may go through a sampling process of chewing on a variety of things. This clearly does not describe most of the Siamese cats and wool sucking. Cats that are weaned early may nuzzle and suckle on their clients and on their clients' clothing. In such cases, the sucking may be directed toward a variety of fabrics, but usually occurs in the clients' presence (on a bed) or on the clients themselves. In these cases, the fabrics are not generally chewed or ingested. This all may be part of a long descriptive continuum of related behaviors, but there are not currently sufficient data to know.

To control these behaviors and prevent them from worsening once it becomes apparent this might be a problem, any items that the cat regularly ingests should be removed. It may be easier to confine the cat. Whenever the cats are allowed free, they should be belled with a breakaway collar and spied on by clients. The clients can then use the aversive devices discussed previously (fog horns, water pistols, air canisters) to correct the cat as it approaches the inappropriate substrate. Occasionally, if a cat restricts its chewing to one small class of objects (socks), an aversive taste stimulus might be helpful. Such tactics do not tend to be overly successful, but they are easy to try. If an aversive taste does not instantly dissuade the cat and cause the cat to remove itself from that situation, this approach will not succeed.

Objects such as pull-string firecrackers or balloons can help if the areas that the cat chooses are in one or a couple of predicable locations. Clients also have had some success in limiting access to the areas by using partially sprung mousetraps under newspaper. The traps go off when the cat approaches to pull or chew at the material.

If the chewing and sucking have not just started, treatment invariably involves antianxiety medication. Treatments for this condition are further discussed elsewhere, but most focus on the use of tricyclic antidepressants or nonspecific anxiolytics. There are other experimental treatments available. Perseverance will probably be rewarded with a response to at least one drug. Clients should be advised that treatment is aimed at changing the cat's desire to pursue the object, not at drugging the cat so that it cannot suck or chew.

Clients can also attempt to redirect the sucking/chewing behaviors to more appropriate substrates such as sterilized bones, vegetables, rawhides, and suitable plants grown and tied in bundles. There have been anecdotal reports that increased access to dry foods can decrease the frequency of sucking or chewing. Changing the diet probably would not be efficacious in long-standing cases.

The extent to which early weaning is a risk factor for inappropriate consumptive behaviors that progress to stereotypic behaviors is interesting and underexplored and should be of interest neurochemically. There have been reports that mechanical jaw activity stimulates cholecystokinin-B(CCK-B) in cats (Singh et al., 1991). It is possible that aberrant numbers of or metabolism of these receptors acts as a factor in the stereotypic chewing behaviors of these cats.

Nonspecific licking that was refractory to treatment has once been reported to be associated with feline leukemia virus–positive status (Beaver, 1989a).

Mounting and Masturbation

Clients occasionally report that their cat will mount or masturbate on stuffed toys, heaps of clothing, pillows, or articles of furniture. Cats that do this are perfectly normal. They can be intact or neutered males or females. If the cat is mounting another cat, the behavior could either be social, because mounting and grabbing by the neck or pressing on the upper body is a form of control behavior in cats, or it could be sexual. Some male cats very low in a hierarchy will allow intact males to mount them. It is unclear if intromission occurs in these cases, but there have been reports of ejaculation. The more frequent scenario is a cat that has been castrated or spayed that exhibits this mounting behavior. It is possible that some small amount of ejaculate could be produced even by a neutered male.

The mounting behavior could manifest itself when the cat is under stressful situations. Masturbation might serve as a relief for anxiety, or it could be a very pleasurable circumstance. I know of at least one cat that probably has been inadvertently reinforced in this behavior because the veterinary student to whom the cat belonged thought that it was so interesting that every time that the cat started to do it, the student invited people to watch. Eventually, whenever there were guests, the cat came into the living room, mounted a pillow or somebody's leg, and masturbated and then licked its penis. For the most part, this is a harmless, although in some circles, socially unacceptable behavior.

Do not punish the cat for mounting or masturbating. Unless the cat is becoming obsessed with a specific stuffed animal or a pillow, this is not a behavior amenable to pharmacological intervention. Only two situations associated with anxiety-related disorders and stereotypic behaviors are amenable to pharmacological intervention: (1) if the cat masturbates only when upset and the clients can identify all the situations that lead to the upset, or (2) if the cat cannot stop masturbating. Cats that masturbate while compulsively sucking or chewing are interesting. In this situation, a very strong case can be made for the masturbation as part of an anxiety disorder. Corrections usually do not stop the behavior but may encourage the cat to masturbate out of sight of the client. That may be enough of a help for the client.

It is appropriate to reassure the clients that animals who masturbate were not incorrectly neutered, and that it is not necessary for the animal to have experienced a sexual encounter to masturbate later in life.

Predatory Behavior

Some forms of predatory behavior are management related. Predatory aggression, an aggression in which predatory tendencies are inappropriately directed toward people, is covered in Chapter 7. Cats learn to exhibit predatory behaviors with their mother's help. Early orphaning causes cats to truncate their period of play and to replace it with predatory behavior. Early orphaning also correlates with less complete play behavior as a precursor to predatory behavior.

Even if cats are well fed, they often will hunt. Some indoor cats vocalize and pounce at windows if they see a bird in flight. They may stalk birds or rodents that are pets in the house. The precursor behaviors to a pouncing cat usually include acute attention involving a stare, alert eyes, gaping, and quick, anxious meows. As the cat becomes more intent on the predatory event, it becomes silent, wiggles onto the feet, and may flick the tip of the tail. Just before pouncing, the cat will ball up its body and push off with the hind feet. Any of these behaviors that are exhibited in the context of a human moving its hands or feet must be aborted as early in the sequence as possible. The best way to abort these behaviors is to startle the cat with a stimulus that is sufficient to abort the behavior without terrifying the cat. Under no circumstances should cats be reassured or teased into inappropriate play that would allow them to pounce in these circumstances. Cats will learn to direct inappropriate predatory behavior to human body parts if people encourage such behaviors. People should never encourage cats to exhibit predatory behavior toward humans.

The second suite of situations in which predatory behaviors are seen involves neighborhood wildlife. I have a personal, conservation-based interest in seeing cats confined; as more species of birds are constrained to use ever-shrinking flyways, the sprawl of "civilization" continues. Free-ranging cats are potent forces of ecological destruction on some rare and neighborhood bird species. It is impossible to prevent these cats from exhibiting these behaviors if they are allowed free range. Cats can be dissuaded from exhibiting predatory behavior through a variety of techniques. First, the cats can be belled with a fairly large and loud bell, using a breakaway collar. This will give the birds some help in getting away. Tiny little jingle bells will not even make a sound before really good hunters have a bird. Invisible electric fences can keep cats from areas where birds commonly are fed. Individuals can separate bird feeding and cat outdoor excursions in time. If clients do this, they need a signal that will tell the birds when the cat is out. Hanging loud wind chimes or displaying wind socks when the cat is out and removing them when the cat is in can help. A trolley or a harness system can be used for the cat when it is outside. This restricts access to birds, but caution should be urged to ensure that the cat does not strangle or otherwise become entrapped.

Not all cats will hunt. Early learning, generally from the queen, will influence whether cats hunt and determine their prey preference. Keeping cats well fed is not sufficient to abort hunting behavior; cats often will not eat what they have killed. This "denning" or "provisioning" behavior is probably a remnant of ancestral wild feline behavior that has been conserved evolutionarily; parts of the behavioral sequence have not been extinguished by the limited domestication to which cats have been exposed.

Finally, people can keep their cats indoors. Unless people live far from vehicular traffic and away from unkind humans who might poison their animals, this is the best solution. Indoor cats can still be leash-walked, but they will live longer and be healthier. Cats that are "outdoor" live an average of 3 years, whereas "indoor" cats live an average of 12 years; the difference is largely related to mortality caused by cars (Childs & Ross, 1986; Kolata et al., 1974).

Tree-Climbing Behavior

Although most cats can climb trees, most also appear to prefer not to do so if the trees are beyond a certain height. Tree climbing can be perfectly normal behavior, and cats will choose elevated perches. Unless cats are panicked into climbing higher than they otherwise would by some provocative event (being chased by a dog or child), most cats can descend from trees into which they have hoisted themselves. Motivation can be an important factor: a cat that is timid or arthritic but was lured into a tree by the promise of a group of birds may find it more difficult to descend than to ascend. The longer they avoid descent the more anxious

they may get. Clients should use caution in extracting cats from trees. Not only do people have to thrust their faces and hands forward to reach the cat, but the cats may be terrified. These combined circumstances are potentially injurious to clients.

Declawed cats can climb trees if they could do so before onychectomy. Some declawed cats seem to have more trouble descending than ascending, possibly because of lack of purchase, but no data exist to confirm or refute this impression.

Maternal and Paternal Neglect and Aggression

Left to their own devices even feral female cats may den communally, with each female having three to five kittens (Beaver, 1992; Bradshaw, 1992a). Queens tend to be good mothers—72% to 87% of kittens are raised to weaning (Beaver, 1992)—unless they are repeatedly threatened. A poor plane of nutrition may make the queen more susceptible to disruption, especially if she, herself, was malnourished as a kitten. Although it is known that kittens that experience a poor nutritional environment in utero are more reactive and less able to learn from their social environment, the extent to which this influences their future ability to mother is not known. It is possible that these cats are less able to teach their kittens appropriate hunting behaviors, but this might only influence preference of food, rather than ultimate ability to acquire it (see Chapter 4). Regardless, cats that have problems learning as kittens may be overrepresented in the wild or feral pool; it might be expected that their early experiences could make them more susceptible to abandoning their kittens if disturbed. Cats that have kittens should be left relatively unmolested until the kittens themselves are venturing from the nest independently.

Because cats are induced ovulators, infanticide may be practiced by males who relocated near queens with kittens. The addition of a tomcat or other cycling queen to a group of female cats is sufficient to induce estrus in hours to days, as can relocation of a colony (Wildt, 1980). Valeric acid has been postulated to modulate this stimulation (Beaver, 1992). Queens and their kittens should be protected from interference by foreign toms. Even resident toms bear close watching. Very young kittens should not be left unsupervised when toms are present. On the other hand, some male cats do a superb job of providing for, succoring, and caring for young. There are numerous anecdotal reports of male cats "nursing" orphaned kittens that are being bottle-fed.

Pseudocyetic events are rare in cats, but they *do* occur. Cats can become protective of toys and beds and aggressive when approached by strangers. The same recommendations useful in dogs are useful here.

Reintroduction After Hospitalization

Cats have acute senses of smell and are generously supplied with sebaceous glands. The extent to which odor plays a role in social interactions has already been covered in Chapters 4 and 8. Because one of the functions of allogrooming may be to create a group odor, it should not be surprising that cats can react strongly to the reintroduction of one of their housemates after an absence. Scents of hospitals or other cats may be foreign, and the returning cat can be greeted with behaviors normally reserved for an intruder. It is also possible that hospital scents are coupled by the cat with its own unpleasant, fearful, or painful past experiences. It is not known to what extent this response occurs, or the extent to which the response could be mitigated by grooming the cat with a cloth used on its housemate before reintroduction. Any actions that encourage the maintenance of group scent should minimize problematic reintroductions.

Cats that become ill, incapacitated, or experience a debilitating treatment for any condition can be scary for other resident cats. Clients can minimize the effect of this by not encouraging fearful or aggressive behaviors (i.e., do not try to reason with the other cats and tell them that it is "okay"—they do not think it is okay). If a cat returns home in a seriously debilitated state and requires special care, clients must also make time for the other cats. They should reward calm behaviors using attention, grooming, or food treats. Finally, if the client is always frantic and tearful, the other cats can learn to make an association with the object of the client's fear, pain, or grief. Cats usually avoid outright conflict and could shun the ill cat or disappear altogether in such circumstances.

Travel Problems

Anyone who has suffered through a car trip with a yowling cat understands the need to prevent or control such behaviors. Starting in kittenhood cats should become accustomed to riding safely and comfortably in cars. This means that they are either on a harness and seat belt or are in a carrier. If cats are taken for rides often enough they will often even eat or use a litter box in the car. Taking a cat that is distressed by travel on a long trip can be painful for the client, but it may be cruel to the cat. Cats can become carsick like dogs, but more frequently their distress is made clear by continuous, ritualized pacing and vocalization. If it is absolutely necessary to travel with a cat that is this distressed, sedation with low dosages of benzodiazepines or of phenobarbital (the one legitimate behavioral use for this drug) may help. Clients need to check on sedated cats frequently, should not enclose them where they cannot see them, should not put them on an airplane sedated, and should not try to feed or offer them water until they are fully awake.

In summary, clients should accustom their kittens to travel early and often, but should consider the more humane approach of a cat sitter for cats that become distressed by travel.

Plant Eating

Cats are the quintessential carnivores, but can be phytophagous, too (Beaver, 1982c). Fifty-one of 122 cats that were not considered by the clients to have behavior problems ate houseplants regularly (Morgan & Houpt, 1990). Clients can grow herbs or grass specifically for their cat to eat. This protects the cats from pesticides in the environment. Any plants grown for cat consumption should be sufficiently dissimilar to other houseplants that the cats are not encouraged to generalize. Many houseplants are toxic to cats in quite small amounts. Lilies are particularly deadly. Until the client is sure that the cat will not randomly forage on *all* houseplants, the cat and the plants should be kept separate when the cat is unsupervised. Clients should not expect their cat to be a better botanist than they are, particularly if the cat is enclosed in a relatively small area without a lot of stimulation.

Emesis can be a common sequela to plant eating. Unless the plant is toxic or the cat appears distressed, vomiting after ingesting some plant material may be a normal behavior. The extent to which cats consume specific plants as anthelmintics has not been explored.

Nocturnal Activity

Some cats, particularly those that are young or have slept all day, are active at night. By nature, cats are crepuscular creatures, so nocturnal activity is a variant of normal. Unless the cat is totally crazed at night (and some cats do appear to experience terrifying "hallucinations" in shadows), most of this activity is attention-seeking behavior or inappropriate play behavior. True *behavioral* hyperactivity should not be associated with diel cycle, and has seldom, if ever, been accurately reported for cats. Hyperactivity associated with hyperthyroidism *is* common in cats and is further discussed in Appendix E.

Vocalization

Excessive feline vocalization can be associated with mating, conflicts in the social system, hyperthyroidism, pain, attention-seeking behavior, or true anxiety. Treatment of the primary diagnosis greatly resolves the undesirable vocalization.

Eating Problems

Eating problems in cats that are unrelated to plants or inappropriate consumption behaviors are usually associated with anorexia. Many anorectic cats respond to treatment with diazepam (Brown et al., 1976; Wise & Dawson, 1974), but it is unclear to what extent this response is related to a central appetite stimulant effect or to a secondary, antianxiety effect. Any cat that has an overeating or undereating problem that represents a changed behavior should be pursued medically.

Marder (1992) has reported on five cases of diet-related problems that range from marking associated with palatable foods and anxiety about access to these to tail chasing associated with a food allergy. Clients infrequently report that their cats act crazed after eating a particular food. Removal of the food from the cat's diet should resolve the behavioral problem. Even in the absence of dermatological lesions usually associated with feline food allergies, such reactions can occur.

CANINE PROBLEMS

Canine management problems include the following:
1. Attention-seeking behavior
2. Destruction
3. Barking/howling/speaking
4. Roaming
5. Fence running/fence fighting
6. Digging/escaping/fence jumping
7. Mouthing
8. Coprophagia
9. Rolling in scents
10. Mounting and masturbation
11. Maternal neglect/aggression/infanticide/cannibalism
12. Excessive water consumption
13. Plant eating
14. Pica/stone chewing
15. Reintroduction after hospitalization
16. Carsickness
17. Chasing bicycles/skateboards/rollerbladers/cars
18. Hyperactivity
19. Diet problems
20. Postulated breed-specific problems

Attention-Seeking Behavior

Attention-seeking behavior is probably the most common undesirable behavior that dogs exhibit. Dogs are far more active in their display of attention-seeking behavior than are cats. In its extreme manifestation, attention-seeking behavior is symptomatic of profound anxiety. In most cases behaviors involved in attention-seeking behavior have been learned by the dog through constant deliberate and accidental reinforcement by the client.

Dogs that exhibit attention-seeking behaviors can bark, whine, or "talk" to the client to get attention, or they can use physical behaviors like rooting, pawing, pushing, leaning, jumping, scratching, or mouthing. The hallmark of attention-seeking behavior is that it can be passive (leaning against) or active (jumping), but it elicits from the client some attentive response. The response may be yelling or shoving, but the dog still controlled the interaction, and for the second that the client needed to respond to the dog, the dog was the focus of the response. Dogs have done a very good job of conditioning their people; in true attention-seeking behavior, the response to the dog's signal is almost instantaneous. This is one reason why the problem is so insidious to manage. A "Protocol for

Treating and Preventing Attention-Seeking Behavior" is found in Appendix B. The main principles include the following: (1) teaching the dog from the outset that it must defer to the client to receive *any* attention; (2) avoiding responding to solicitous canine behaviors unless the dog is exhibiting deferential behaviors; (3) practicing passive withdrawal from the situation by leaving and sloughing the dog off, rather than by pushing it down; and (4) giving the dog attention only when the dog earns it. Once the dog is calm, it can have any type of attention or interaction the client wishes.

Clients usually do not see their own culpability in creating the creature that they now consider a pest. This is one condition for which the onus is truly on the clients. If they do not wish to be bothered by the dog in certain situations, they should not respond to it in those (e.g., if the clients do not wish the dog to beg from the table, they should not feed it there). If the clients do not want the dog to paw at them for attention, they must teach the dog suitable behaviors that will get the dog's attention. And if the clients are not willing to do the latter, they should not have a dog.

Destruction

Destructive behavior can be directed toward people's clothing as a manifestation of attention-seeking behavior, or toward objects as manifestations of attention-seeking behavior, inappropriate play behavior, hunger, teething (in puppies), fears/phobias, or separation anxiety. The underlying cause must be addressed if the behavior is to be stopped.

Dogs that are desirous of attention go to extreme lengths to get it. Unfortunately, their unsavory behavior, combined with client response, quickly leads to worsening behavior. Dogs that have been abandoned and rescued, puppies (particularly those that are teething), and high-energy dogs that are not having their aerobic requirements met, may jump at client's clothing, using their teeth or nails. If the client responds by pushing the dog down, the dog continues the cycle. Dogs, like children who do not get sufficient appropriate attention, will accept and solicit inappropriate or negative attention. Furthermore, by pushing the dog down, rather than by passively sloughing it off, the client is responding with a gesture that can be viewed as a challenge or solicitation by the dog. Clients with such dogs frequently are too exhausted or discouraged to appropriately play, exercise, and interact with the dog, compounding the problem. Matters are further made worse because people with these problems are unwilling to interact with the dog when it is quiet or resting for fear that the dog will again harass them. Unfortunately, this also deprives the dog of the opportunity to be favorably rewarded for desirable, calm behavior. The same scenario arises with dogs that seek attention by stealing personal objects that the client is using and chewing on these.

Clients invariably give chase, encouraging the theft and destructive behavior.

Dogs that have little interactive play with dogs or people and toys will seek out objects in the house that "play back." This may be particularly pronounced in young, curious dogs and is worsened by teething. These are the dogs that characteristically shake and shred cushions and pillows, unroll toilet paper, shred telephone books, unravel tapestries, and so on. Pups that are teething may not be able to comfortably chew on a very hard bone but find the spine of a book suitable to their needs.

For these dogs it is critical to ensure that the dogs are (1) getting the needed exercise; (2) appropriately rewarded with love and massage for calm behaviors; (3) appropriately dissuaded from inappropriate behaviors by passive sloughing, ignoring the dog unless it sits or lies down and relaxes first and by removing temptation, even if this means puppy-proofing a room or using a crate; (4) taught early that they can mouth only toys; (5) provided with appropriate alternative stimuli; and (6) for puppies, provided with objects suitable for teething and easily recognized as such (frozen washcloths, teething rings).

Separation anxiety is a far more complex problem than are the forms of destruction listed previously. Rather than being poorly behaved or misbehaved, these dogs are abnormal and deeply distressed. Often these patients have had a history of early deprivation or are older animals that idiopathically develop separation anxiety as their needs change. When left alone, these dogs are capable of digging through wire crates, flooring, drywall, and mortar, even at the price of self-mutilation. Rather than improving with exposure to the solitary condition, the behavior of these dogs worsens. Canine or feline companionship usually does not help. Behavior modification techniques coupled with antianxiety medication are often efficacious in treating destruction associated with separation anxiety.

Dogs with destruction related to fears and phobias must receive treatment for the primary condition. If a specific stimulus for the fearful or phobic response exists, it is usually identifiable. The destruction is the result of the panic that results from the inability to escape from or deal with the fearful or phobic stimulus regardless of whether this is "rational." Early treatment with behavioral and pharmacological intervention is recommended and discussed elsewhere.

A subset of this type of anxiety-related behavior may be represented by what Houpt (1991b) calls "barrier-frustration." Dogs that experience this respond to enclosure in a crate or a room by destruction of the "barrier." It is unlikely that such antipathy toward an enclosure developed in a vacuum, and other anxiety-associated behaviors should be explored.

Barking/Howling/Speaking

Barking and howling are behaviors that have been exaggerated in pet dogs through artificial selection. To a large extent, their expression is breed dependent; terriers bark easily and with a high-pitched tone, hounds bay with little provocation and will join in group vocalizations (Hart & Hart, 1985b; Hart & Miller, 1985). Well-mannered dogs should not bark unduly in their people's absence and should be quiet when requested to cease vocalization. These dogs are rare.

Most dogs that are considered problem barkers are not behaving abnormally—they are responding to environmental stimuli and exhibiting alerting behavior. However, truly pathological or "abnormal" (contrasted with undesirable) barking probably does exist.

Some dogs that bark do so because they are distressed to be left alone (i.e., they have separation anxiety). These dogs often exhibit a less controlled, more ritualistic bark that changes to a higher pitch as the dog becomes more upset. Some dogs may bark as part of an obsessive-compulsive disorder (OCD). Their barks may occur in the absence of any stimulation, and these dogs may remove themselves from any social situations before commencing an atonal, ritualistic vocalization. There may be a third category of truly abnormal vocalization. Some clients complain about the intensity of their dog's response in approaching either a visitor to the door or another dog on the street. These dogs are highly excitable, but there is another element to their problem. The character of their bark changes from a relatively normal frequency, normal-pitch alerting bark to a high-frequency, less variant, more assertive and ritualistic vocalization. This pattern is characterized by two traits: the change in bark patterns occurs quickly and, once the dog has switched to the second class of vocalization, it is difficult to impossible to interrupt and does not respond to physical restraint. These changes are subtle, but if clients can intervene when the dog first reacts, the dog does not assume rigid postures and stereotypic vocalization. Unfortunately, with the exception of some work conducted on cues given to herding dogs (McConnell, 1990; McConnell & Baylis, 1985), there are few well-done ethological and sonographic studies that focus on canine vocalization. Dog barks are probably more variable that we believe.

Whether normal or abnormal, excessive or intensive canine vocalization causes problems for people because their neighbors complain, because there are laws enforcing silence in their area, or because the clients themselves are annoyed by the dog's barking. The key to controlling undesirable barking is to pursue the underlying diagnosis and to treat that. If the dog has separation anxiety, this must be treated. If the dog is being teased by children while in the yard, the dog should be removed from that circumstance. The next step is to teach the dog a more appropriate behavior with which to replace the barking.

Most dogs that bark continue to do so because they become more stimulated and, generally, more anxious. Dogs cannot learn another behavior to replace the barking unless the clients are present. If the clients are present, they can use a head collar with an indoor lead to correct the dog by closing its mouth and then encouraging the dog to sit and relax. The dog must sit until it is calm, and can be petted, rewarded, or told that it is "okay" only when calm and relaxed (see Appendix B: "Protocol for Deference: Basic Program" and "Protocol for Relaxation: Behavior Modification Tier I"). Clients must be able to respond to the dog within the first 30 to 60 seconds of the *onset* of the suite of behaviors that accompanies the barking. This means that clients have to pay attention. Clients should *not* pick dogs up and cuddle them, restrain them by pulling back on their collar, or tell them that it is "okay." All of these behaviors will make the barking worse and help to convince the dog that it is correct in pursuit of the vocalization. Clearly, starting to correct this behavior in young puppies correctly is important. The earlier that the clients intervene, the better.

Clients always want quick solutions. There are few. Remote or voice-activated shock collars cause pain. Although the pain does not appear to be excruciating, pain is only a useful stimulus for learning under certain conditions associated with avoidance of approach or manipulation. For most dogs, the barking is more rewarding than the shock is dissuading. Were this not true, the future frequency of the barking would drop precipitously, and this is not what is reported about shock collars. Dogs will often abort the particular barking bout for which they received the shock, but no data have been published that indicate that *frequency* of future bouts is affected. Furthermore, if barking is indicative of any underlying anxiety problems, shock will worsen the behavior in dogs with these anxieties. Even if the dog does become quiet, fear or another presentation of an anxiety is a common sequela. This is not the solution that clients want, and they should not be encouraged to pursue it.

There are some newer concepts in bark collars. Citronella collars (ABS System; ImmunoVet, Tampa, FL) spray the dog with a citrus oil mist when it begins to bark. Dogs tend to dislike this scent, but are not afraid of it or caused pain by it. The distasteful scent lasts long enough that the barking bout has passed, so that dogs can actually learn to decrease their barking behavior in the future. Clients know if dogs were barking in their absence because the house smells of lemon. Dogs learn to recognize if they are not wearing the collar, but as part of an integrated system emphasizing the teaching of a new behavioral pattern, these collars can help. Because they work without pain and in a way that helps the dog to quickly stop unsavory behavior, the clients will be more patient in working with the dog, which is a benefit.

Clients often think that it is cute that their dogs speak and talk to them. Dogs are great mimics and can learn to mimic "speaking" signals that the clients demonstrate. This is fine provided the dog "speaks" only when the client requests it and if the client can stop the speaking with a vocal command. Dogs that yap uncontrollably at clients and grumble when clients request that they stop barking and sit may have other problems, including dominance aggression. Some pushy dogs are very vocal and never show any signs of dominance aggression. This can be acceptable behavior if the client enjoys it *and* can control it by successfully telling the dog to stop.

Roaming

Dogs are social and curious. Most dogs would explore more space than that in which they live, given the option. Intact males roam more frequently than neutered males, and their tendency to roam can be decreased by almost 75% by castration (Hopkins et al., 1976). Intact male dogs seek out and congregate around sexually receptive females. Dogfights can occur under these conditions.

In urban environments normal exploration frequently results in dogs being killed or injured. Roaming dogs can pose serious public health risks from aggression and fecal contamination. Most urban areas have laws that restrict the extent to which dogs are allowed to roam. Controlling roaming is an important public health and community issue.

Dogs can be prevented from roaming by (1) leash walking them, (2) providing them with sufficient exercise, (3) giving them sufficient attention, (4) supervising them when fenced and not leaving them fenced for more than very short intervals, and (5) neutering them. These solutions all involve responsible pet ownership, and there is no substitution for it. Veterinarians should not feel obligated to negotiate with clients for suboptimal solutions that require less work on the client's part.

If clients wish to fence their dogs, they should know the following points.

1. Dogs that are fenced and have any territorial aggression will intensify that aggression if they can definitively identify their physical limits. That is what a fence does.
2. Just because the dog is fenced in a big yard, this does not mean that the dog is getting adequate exercise. Fenced dogs do not get much exercise and may get less than dogs that are leash walked, played with using Frisbees and balls, taken to agility training or obedience training, or involved in competitive jumping. These activities all should be alternative considerations for clients who report that their dog either destroys their yard, jumps the fence, or still seems "wired" when it comes inside.
3. Unless the dog is already housebroken, just confining it with a fence will not housebreak the dog.
4. Highly motivated dogs will break through an electric fence to get out, but generally not to get back in, can scale standard fences, and can dig under standard fences. Secure fences have corner posts placed in cement, underground extensions 1 m deep, and a roof and door that lock.

5. Dogs left unattended in fenced or walled situations are good and helpless victims for abuse.
6. Dogs left unattended in fenced or walled situations may be considered to be kept in an abusive context, in and of itself, under some of the more progressive, humane laws that focus on the well-being of pets.

Fence Running and Fence Fighting

Dogs that are left fenced will run the edges of the fence in response to the external stimulation of other dogs or people. If dogs are kenneled on opposite sides of a fence, vocal and physical displays can become exaggerated. In extreme cases dogs will charge the fence, sometimes grabbing and displaying in an aggressive manner to the inaccessible dog. Were these dogs able to mingle, the aggression would probably resolve. The noise and posturing is usually the result of the artificial restraint of the fence. Barriers truncate normal behavioral interactions and do not allow the dogs to resolve uncertainties or conflicts about their social relationships. Clients need to use common sense. Some dogs will fight when finally given access. This is more likely if their displays increase in intensity with exposure.

Some dogs run fences regardless of whether there is any external stimulation. These dogs have rules for how they travel along the fence, when they turn, and the direction in which they go. It is likely that this style of fence running is a manifestation of an OCD. It is a hallmark of the extreme nature of the problem that the clients are unable to intervene or to convince the dog to focus on them or another pet. Although not all dogs that are fenced exhibit this behavior, enclosing them in a fence might act as a facilitator for animals that have an underlying, unexpressed anxiety disorder.

Fence running in either of the above manifestations is *not* related to boredom. These dogs are stimulated, but thwarted.

Digging, Escaping, and Fence Jumping

Digging is a component of normal dog behavior. Domestic dogs dig for the following reasons: (1) to mark a scrape or elimination area, (2) to bury something, (3) to uncover something that they perceive is buried, (4) to thermoregulate, and (5) to play with something that plays back (e.g., soil, roots, stones).

Digging as part of normal elimination behavior has been discussed elsewhere. This type of digging usually involves the back feet and results in shallow scrapes and broadly dispersed soil cover. Digging as a marking behavior probably involves immediate (the behavior) and long-term (the mark) visual displays and long-term olfactory ones.

Digging to bury or uncover something (or to see if there is something to uncover) usually follows exploratory behaviors of sniffing, listening, and pawing and may be stimulated by visual, auditory, or olfactory cues. Some breeds, such as Jack Russell terriers, have been selected for tenacious sniffing and digging behaviors. Extensive digging of this nature is usually in response to some auditory or olfactory stimulus (e.g., to voles tunneling through leaves or snow). Clients should know that dogs vary greatly, both within and among breeds, in their desire to follow scent and buried creatures. Some dogs focus more on these stimuli and need to have an aerobic outlet for their activity and a more suitable outlet for their tracking needs. The latter can be met in competitive situations involving field trials, earth dog tests, lures, or retrieval in obedience (see Appendix C).

Soil has great thermal inertia, hence digging a hole into which they can crawl can help dogs in cold environments to conserve heat and dogs in hot environments to disperse heat. Dogs that are digging to conserve heat will also curl up, leaving the smallest possible surface area for passive radiant heat exchange, whereas dogs that dig to disperse heat will stretch out and pant. Panting provides for evaporative cooling, and increased contact with cool surfaces provides for heat exchange through conduction. Dogs that dig when it is cold should be provided with adequate shelter and clean bedding. Dogs that dig when it is hot can be accommodated with shelter or a small, shallow wading pool or an area that is walled off and filled with a slightly different soil type explicitly for their thermoregulation needs.

Dogs that dig as a form of self-play quickly learn that roots and soil play back. This is a formula for gardening disaster. The only remedy for this involves constant supervision so that the client can stop the dog as the digging begins, and active play should be increased. When dogs amuse themselves like this they are not communicating that they would like to be penned in a cement and chain-link fence kennel; rather, they are communicating that they can stimulate themselves but need aerobic play with people or objects that play back. Clients need to be helped to meet these pets' needs. More confinement will not suffice.

There is a learning component for any behavior, including digging. It is possible that the longer any digging in any of the above categories continues, the worse it will become. The dog learns, and the behavior becomes self-reinforcing. The occasional dog digs constantly in the absence of any of the above correlates. This digging is qualitatively and quantitatively different from the above descriptions. These dogs require few or no stimuli and dig in a focused, invariant pattern. As with most management-related behaviors, this form of digging may be a form of an anxiety or OCD. It usually does not respond to the above "quick" management solutions, although they should also be implemented, but can respond to behavioral and pharmacological treatment for anxiety or OCD.

Please ignore any advice about filling a hole that the dog has dug with water and then submerging the dog's head in the water (Koehler, 1962). Such advice is barbaric, inhumane, potentially injurious to both client and dog, and wrong.

Mouthing

Mouthing is a normal canine behavior. Dogs do not have hands with opposable thumbs and so use their mouths to grab and manipulate objects and individuals. Mouthing is a normal part of puppy play and adult caretaking (epimeletic) behaviors. Puppies mouth people as part of play because they are exhibiting attention-seeking behavior or they are teething. Mouthing can be cute (or at least is perceived to be cute) in some small puppies, but it should not be encouraged. Dogs of any age or size can injure someone, deliberately or not, when they mouth. If they are allowed to persist in this behavior they will hone their skills and mouth hard. Whether mouthing leads to nipping and biting does not matter: it can be injurious itself. Clients should *not* be encouraged to play with puppies or dogs of any age using their unprotected hands—this will only encourage more mouthing (see Appendix B: "Protocol for Teaching Kids (And Adults) to Play with Dogs and Cats"). Clients should not shove their hand to the back of the dog's throat, slap the dog under the chin, scruff the dog, or clap the mouth shut; all of these behavioral responses are potentially injurious to the dog, could make it feel threatened, and will, over time, increase the intensity, frequency, and stealth of the mouthing behaviors. Instead, clients should teach the dog more appropriate behaviors for getting attention (See Appendix B: "Protocol for Treating and Preventing Attention-Seeking Behavior"). These include sitting, being quiet, rolling on their back, bringing and dropping a toy, and so forth. It is particularly important that children learn how to deal with mouthing behaviors and that they do not mouth the dog back.

Coprophagia

Most dogs that are coprophagic (stool eating) are *not* fed a diet that is deficient in essential nutrients or vitamins, nor do they have a pancreatic enzyme disorder. For the coprophagia to be primarily of medical origin, poor diets and pancreatic enzyme deficits (and concomitant physical signs) would have to be overrepresented in the coprophagic group and underrepresented in the noncoprophagic group (Fig. 11-1). These criteria are seldom met. This does not mean that some dogs with digestive problems or poor or restricted diets will not eat their own or another dog's stool; they can and will. However, most of the dogs that are coprophagic do not have a physiological, gastrointestinal basis for this behavior.

No one has examined the role that scent and texture play in coprophagia, but there are numerous anecdotal reports of dogs actively seeking cat, rabbit, deer, and horse feces, and frozen canine feces. These substances are appealing to some extent to most dogs, suggesting that there might be evolutionary factors associated with coprophagia that are underappreciated.

	MEDICAL/ DIETARY CONDITION PRESENT	MEDICAL/ DIETARY CONDITION ABSENT
COPROPHAGIA PRESENT	A	B
COPROPHAGIA ABSENT	C	D

Fig. 11-1 Necessary and sufficient conditions for diet or physiological basis for coprophagia in dogs. For a medical or dietary condition to be responsible for coprophagia, A would have to be statistically overrepresented when compared with C in the population composed of A and C; A would have to be statistically overrepresented when compared with B in the population composed of A and B; and D would have to be statistically overrepresented when compared with C in the population composed of D and C. If the co-occurrence of A and D is not statistically greater than that of B and C, no associated functional relationship can be said to exist. As with most similar situations, few data are available to test any hypothesis of relationship.

Dogs, even extant wolves, have a well-documented history of scavenging for food, and coprophagia may be a behavior that is a remnant of that history. In the case of ingestion of herbivore feces, it has been suggested that the dogs may be supplementing their water-soluble (and, hence, replenishable) B-vitamin supply. At some level many coprophagic behaviors involve play, sampling, and learning. Coprophagia is probably modulated by a different neurochemical basis if it is directed toward another species' feces than if it is directed intraspecifically. Coprophagia is a normal behavior for a mother with young pups to exhibit, but no study has examined whether parous bitches are overrepresented in the coprophagic population when compared with nulliparous bitches. It has been postulated that coprophagia in puppies stimulates nervous system development through exposure to deoxycholic acid (Beaver, 1995).

The easiest way to avoid the development of coprophagia is to keep yards free of feces and supervise (and correct) dogs when they are in the yard or on leash walks. Parasite transmission is a risk for coprophagic animals, and they should be checked for parasite burdens frequently. Clients may have some limited success in stopping coprophagia by rendering the ingested feces distasteful. This means that the animal producing those feces should be provided with a food additive (e.g., monosodium glutamate) that will do this. If the client can treat the feces with an emetic agent just before ingestion, the aversive stimulus may be sufficient to abort subsequent coprophagic behaviors. These "treatments" appear to work best for animals that have just started the behaviors and who have not had extensive time to learn about coprophagia.

Some animals are so motivated by feces that they must be muzzled to prevent fecal ingestion. These animals may fit a different profile than that of the standard coprophagic patient. In an extreme case dogs may stimulate themselves to defecate and ingest their own feces directly from their rectum. These dogs defecate more frequently than normal and exhibit other anxiety-related behaviors. Dogs that behave like this are rare, but the extent to which their coprophagia is representative of an underlying anxiety disorder or OCD is unknown. Some of these dogs do respond to pharmacological intervention.

Rolling in Scents

Scent-rolling is a normal canine behavior (see Chapter 3). By rolling, dogs simultaneously disrupt the mark of another animal, deposit their own scent, and acquire some of the other animal's scent. They also groom by shedding some of their undercoat when they roll (see photo on p. 21). The extent to which the latter might be important in a masking situation useful in predation has not been fully explored. Dogs seem to find it pleasurable to roll in some scents that humans consider fairly offensive, which may mean that they are responding neurochemically to some pheromonal cue. Dogs do not have the same kind of vomeronasal organ as do ungulates or cats. It would be interesting to qualitatively and quantitatively compare rolling and Flehmen behaviors between these groups of animals.

Clients should learn to groom and to give their dogs baths, which will also help loosen and remove undercoat, and be reassured that rolling is a normal behavior. Once the dog has located the area that stimulates it to roll and has begun to drop, it is almost impossible to stop even the most obedient dog. If clients absolutely need to avoid this behavior, they will have to be vigilant, use a leash, and learn to read canine communication.

Mounting and Masturbation

Mounting and masturbation are normal canine behaviors.

Mounting occurs in both sexual and social contexts and is one of the first behaviors seen in play challenges in puppies. All mounting that is directed toward people is not about lust—it is usually about control, the solicitation of behavior, or both. If clients believe that they cannot slough off a dog that is mounting them, or they feel uncomfortable (even if they cannot articulate the reason) for shoving a dog down when the dog mounts them, they may be experiencing problems with dominance aggression. Mounting does not have to be a symptom of dominance aggression, but it can be a correlate of it. If the dog does not mount, it can still be dominantly aggressive. Collect the information first and make diagnos-

tic judgments later. Very pushy dogs can mount without ever becoming aggressive. Regardless, clients should not tolerate mounting by their dog, particularly if children are involved. If clients adhere to the "Protocol for Deference: Basic Program" and the "Protocol for Treating and Preventing Attention-Seeking Behavior" in Appendix B, the mounting behavior should resolve, and occasional incidents will be managed by telling the dog "no," "off," or "down."

Masturbation is a normal behavior that is exhibited by all social mammals. It can be pleasurable and may be a form of learning about sexual response in young puppies. Both males and females, neutered and intact animals can masturbate. Postures are varied and may involve animate (people or pets) or inanimate (chairs or stuffed animals) objects. Ejaculation may or may not accompany masturbation. Neutered animals can ejaculate. When a dog is castrated the bulbourethral glands, the source of the fluid for sperm transport, are left intact.

Masturbation can be accomplished because it is pleasurable or because it is a response to a stressful or anxious situation. Zoo animals masturbate disproportionately to their species-specific baseline. In extreme situations animals cannot stop masturbating, or masturbate so often or intensely that their ability to interact in other situations is profoundly and adversely affected. In such situations the masturbation can become ritualized. These dogs can respond to behavioral modification and drug treatment designed to address the underlying problem: the anxiety.

Maternal Neglect, Aggression, Infanticide, and Cannibalism

Common behavioral issues that arise during parturition include excessive nesting with concordant delays in labor or first-stage labor, restlessness, failure to attend to the first-born young, failure to eat the afterbirth, and awkward or inattentive nursing (Freak, 1968). All of these behaviors can be modulated by an attentive client. Maternal neglect, aggression to the puppies, and cannibalism of the mother's or another's pups are all rare circumstances. All of these behaviors increase in unstable resource and social environments, suggesting that there is a large underlying anxiety component to these behaviors.

There is some weak evidence that puppies that were neglected at an early age may not mother their puppies well. Few controlled experiments exist, but it makes sense that there is some learned component to maternal behavior. Puppies may be able to learn these behaviors from other animals, and it is not unusual to hear that a neutered male "mothered" the orphaned puppy. Dogs are communal caretakers of their young, so there is evolutionary precedent for this behavior. Neglect is more common if the mother is frequently disturbed after a history of abuse, fear, neglect, and malnourishment herself.

Some degree of protection of puppies from human

and animal intruders is normal, but all aggression must be appropriate and in context. Aggression should not be redirected to the puppies. In such situations it is best to remove the puppies—maternal aggression redirected to pups is *not* normal. Mothers that exhibit these behaviors should not be bred again; the recidivism rate for this form of aggression appears high, but there are few definitive data. It has been hypothesized that in extreme cases of fear or redirected aggression the mother will cannibalize the puppies. These situations are rare but have a reportedly high recidivistic rate. Furthermore, surviving pups may exhibit the same behavior toward their puppies and should not be bred. The more common scenario is for an intruder female to cannibalize another's pups. This is a response to the wild situation where only one female usually breeds. The breeding female actively and passively suppresses the breeding of other females in the group through hormonal and social means. In household situations with unstable social relationships, infanticide and cannibalism by another breeding female may be a risk. Such behaviors may have been evolutionarily conserved from the wild situation.

If the bitch appears unduly distressed about anyone's presence around the puppies, environmental disruptions should be minimized and the situation carefully monitored. Pups are most vulnerable for the first 2 to 3 weeks of life. If the clients can leave them, safely, with their mother for as long as possible, the mother will usually decide by 5 weeks that there is no risk. If any puppy is volitionally injured by the mother, particularly if this occurs within the first 2 weeks, the clients should remove and hand-raise the puppies and spay the bitch. Few drugs have been used to treat bitches who are poor mothers. Antianxiety agents, serotonin enhancers, and antidepressants have all been successfully used to treat humans, but most of these are transferred by the transplacental or transmammary route, which may necessitate bottle-feeding.

Pseudocyesis is more fully discussed in Chapter 6 but warrants brief mention here. Pseudocyesis, or false pregnancy, is most common 6 to 10 weeks after estrus in the absence of pregnancy. It is most common during the luteal phase of the cycle and may be a variant of normal behavior (Houpt, 1991a). Bitches experiencing pseudocyesis can have mammary enlargement (ranging from a slight increase to full lactation) and behavioral changes that include restlessness, nervousness, decreased activity and interaction, increased protectiveness of toys and nest material, increased nesting, and decreased appetite (Allen, 1986; Houpt, 1991a). These are the same signs that occur as pregnancy progresses.

The recidivism rate for pseudocyesis appears high, and dogs experiencing it may also be at increased risk for subsequent pyometra. Spaying is a definitive treatment but should be done after the signs associated with the luteal phase subside, or these will be prolonged. Making the dog more comfortable (bathing and gently massaging the glands) and leaving her unthreatened will also help the behaviors to diminish.

Excessive Water Consumption

Excessive water consumption should not be assumed to be an accurate representation of water intake, regardless of what the client says. Water consumption and urine specific gravity should be sequentially measured before intake is assumed to be "excessive." With this in mind, puppies are often polyuric and polydipsic and may use drinking as a chance to play. Water plays back and has a reflective surface that moves. These are characteristics that will stimulate more water consumption. If the puppy is healthy and growing normally and has variable periods when it does not spontaneously urinate, water can be provided in measured amounts on a scheduled basis. Urine output can be monitored. If most clients do this they will discover that the dogs are regulating input and outflow, and that the urine specific gravity does fluctuate during the day. These puppies can be safely restricted from playing in their water.

Older dogs may drink excessively because of numerous endocrine disorders; the potential for these should be fully evaluated. The minimum database required is a physical examination, urinalysis, complete blood cell count (CBC), and serum biochemistry profile. Additional tests, for example for alkaline phosphatase isoenzymes, may be required, depending on the dog's medical history.

Excessive is a relative term and must be evaluated in the context of input and outflow, the dog's activity level, and the dog's thermal environment. Only if there is *no* sign of organ, hypothalamic, or pituitary dependent disease, and if the dog is deemed to be truly polydipsic and hyposthenuric, should the water consumption be considered behavioral. "Psychogenic water drinking" (Fox, 1968a,c) is an undefined, catchall diagnosis that should be avoided as a diagnosis of first choice. It is very rare for a dog to drink water because it cannot help doing so. These dogs probably are exhibiting signs of anxiety disorders or OCD and may have an aberrant central CCK-B response to mouth opening. Treatment with behavioral modification is encouraged. Treatment with concomitant antianxiety medications may be recommended. Most of these agents also have secondary anticholinergic effects that could either help break or worsen the cycle, depending on the underlying mode of action of the problem. This is a condition that elegantly illustrates the importance of a hierarchical mechanistic approach as illustrated in Fig. 1-1.

Plant Chewing and Eating

Canids are more omnivorous than are felids. Ingestion of plants, including fruits and vegetables, can be normal behavior. Dogs will occasionally ingest plants, usually grasses, and then vomit. This has been interpreted as canine self-medication of GI distress, but the events of consumption and vomiting are confounded. Caution is urged for overinterpretation. Some plants are toxic for dogs, whereas others merely act as gastric irritants. Some anthelmintic agents are efficacious because of their irritant properties. Some plants contain natural larvacidal agents. The extent to which dogs that eat plants are treating themselves for parasitic conditions is unknown.

Ingestion of plants may indicate that the dog perceives a need for more fiber in its diet. Clients can meet these needs by choosing diets that are higher in fiber, by adding bran to the dog's food, or by adding cooked or raw vegetables to the dog's food. Sudden shifts in diet, particularly those that increase fiber, can cause diarrhea. All additions should be made gradually.

Plant chewing within the house can be a form of play behavior or attention-seeking behavior. These are best handled by instantaneous correction and encouragement of the replacement of the behavior with one that is more suitable. Puppies will explore all new situations and enjoy the feeling of chewing on plants. It is preferable to offer them frozen washcloths (watch for loose threads), ice, sterilized bones filled with peanut butter, Nylabones (Nylabone Toys, THF publications, Neptune NJ) or Kong toys (Kong Company, Lakewood, CO).

Pica and Stone Chewing

Pica is the ingestion of nonnutritive, nonfood items. Common foci for pica include fabric, plastics, sticks, and rocks. Some dogs exhibit an extreme form of this behavior toward stones, actively seeking and swallowing numerous rocks. The rocks chosen are usually large enough to require surgical removal. Gastroliths are not commonly used in carnivore digestion, and it is difficult to make a case for viewing stone ingestion in this context. Most pica, if exhibited by dogs that are past puppyhood, involves extreme focus on and selectivity of ingested objects. These behaviors are not normal and can become sufficiently intense that the dog disregards other activities. These behaviors are rare and poorly investigated. It is unclear if they are a manifestation of an OCD, if affected animals have central brain lesions, or if they are the result of aberrant CCK-B metabolism. Treatment is difficult and focuses on avoidance, early interruption and substitution of a more appropriate behavior, and the use of selective serotonin reuptake inhibitors (SSRIs).

Reintroduction After Hospitalization

Dogs appear to have fewer problems when one of the canine household returns from an enforced absence than do cats. Dog interactions are more direct than are those of cats, but dogs are not immune to fear of the unfamiliar. Dogs can avoid housemates if they smell strange, or if they are restrained by peculiar apparatuses (external fixation devices). Dogs that exhibit abnormal postsurgical behaviors, those that are chronically ill, or those who develop OCD may be avoided by their housemates. This can be normal. If there is no risk of aggression and neither party appears unduly stressed by the avoidance, there is no reason (from the dogs' standpoints) for the client to pursue treatment. Clients may have personal emotional needs that are left unmet if their pets are avoiding each other. Clients need to be counseled to put their pets' needs first, because, particularly in cases that involve a debilitating disease, the stress of forced interaction can make the patient worse.

If there is no chronic medical problem requiring management, the clients can begin to reintroduce their pets with the "Protocol for the Introduction of a New Pet to Other Household Pets" in Appendix B. In general, it is safest to keep pets separated until the clients are sure of their reliability, and introductions should be gradual and nonfearful. Any positive behaviors, including ignoring something that is potentially scary, should be rewarded (see the photos on p. 268).

Car Sickness

Dogs that become ill in the car do so because they have motion sickness or because they are afraid of some aspect of car travel. This could be leaving the house, traffic, noise, and so on. Assuming that the dog has no vestibular disease, car sickness is not complex to treat. As with most conditions it is best to prevent it, but if this is not possible, treating it early in the history of its development will minimize its complications.

Puppies should be taken for short car rides frequently. It is best to take puppies on short trips, at first, and to ensure that they have empty stomachs before doing so. Puppies vomit easily, and car travel will make most puppies that have just eaten vomit the first time they experience it. It is a mistake to stop the trip and return the puppy to home once it begins to salivate or vomit. It is far preferable to try to distract it or to relax it through massage (do not tell the dog it is "okay" or pet it if it is drooling or vomiting—this only reinforces the problematic behavior). Clients should keep washable towels in the car and be prepared to thrust them under the dog. If the puppy does not salivate, or if the salivation and emesis stop, a chew toy can be offered to the dog. It should learn to associate comfort behaviors and relaxation with car travel.

Profoundly fearful dogs will urinate and defecate either when put in the car or as soon as it begins to move. These dogs require a program of systematic desensitization. They should be taken to the car when it is not turned on and encouraged to enter and sit in the car as part of a game. If they do this without becoming

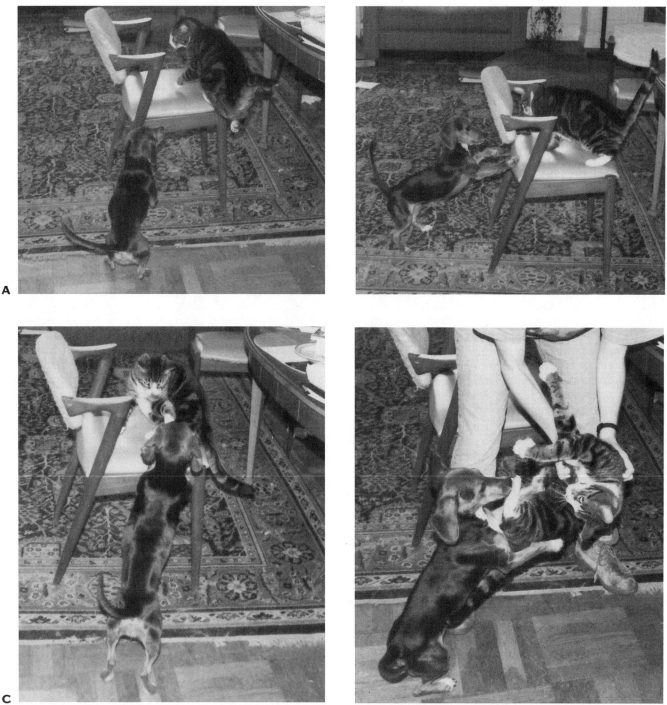

Appropriate introduction of new pets can help define future good relationships. The puppy is the new addition here. The cat can escape from him using three-dimensional space options that exclude him, but will play roughly with him as long as she retains control (A to C). The cat is less sanguine about their intimate interaction when she is forced to relinquish control. Note the defensive body posture, extended claws, and direct stare (D). (Photos by Emily Elliot and Nirit Rosenburg.)

distressed, they should get a treat. The client should practice this task multiple times a day for a few days. The clients should first practice with all of the car doors open, and then with them closed, but with the windows open. After the dog can do this it is safe to start feeding it part of its meals in the car. Once the dog willingly enters the car and eats, the clients can sit with the dog, providing treats and performing relaxation exercises (See "Protocol for Relaxation: Behavior Modification Tier I," in Appendix B) while the car engine is running but the car is not moving. After the dog has been able to successfully relax numerous times in these circumstances, the client should just move the car down the driveway or around the block and then take the dog out of the car, rewarding it with praise and treats for being good. As the dogs ceases to react adversely and continues to become more accustomed to and relaxed in the car, the client can very slowly begin to increase both distance and speed. If done correctly, the dog can be desensitized to car travel within days. Frequently refreshers are beneficial and dogs should learn to like going in the car.

Canine seat belts, gates, or crates are excellent ideas during car travel. These devices are something to which dogs should become accustomed early in their car travel career. They will make the dog more secure and protect it in an accident. Clients should *not* travel with pets roaming in the front seat or in their laps. The potential for client distraction and inattentiveness to road conditions is great.

Most dogs that have problems with car travel will respond to the above measures. For others dimenhydrinate (Dramamine) or small doses of beta-blockers or benzodiazepines can help.

This same type of early introduction/gradual exposure paradigm can be useful for other situations in which the dog is fearful or concerned, including bathing and nail clipping. The same caveats always apply: the circumstances should be made as pleasant as possible, good behaviors should be effusively rewarded, and no punishment or harsh discipline should be used.

Chasing Bicycles, Skateboards, In-Line Skaters, or Cars

Most dogs that chase things on wheels or joggers are not exhibiting predatory aggression, they are chasing the individual from their vicinity. Unfortunately, they are, de facto, successful at this and learn that they will be successful. Hence they begin to greet the quick-moving intruder with ever-increasing alacrity. Dogs tend to be most confident about any assertive behaviors the closer they are to home, and this pattern can be noted in the intensity with which they chase moving objects at the center of their range. As vehicles continue to move, the dog becomes less enthusiastic about pursuit. This is not because they are physically tired. Some dogs that behave in this manner are ex-

tremely territorially aggressive and can be a menace. The U.S. Postal Service has a policy of avoidance (and nondelivery) in these cases, but permits their employees to carry sprays designed to dissuade marauding dogs. Clients who have dogs that chase bicycles, trucks, skateboarders, in-line skaters, or joggers should confine their dogs. These are the quintessential self-reinforcing behaviors. Some of these dogs are actually playing, but they can be scary to those who are chased. Even if the dog does not have a problem aggression, people that it chases may not know this and could threaten the dog. Such threats could teach the dog to respond inappropriately.

Some of these dogs may be behaving in a predatory manner and will chase down and grab passing individuals. These dogs can be quite dangerous, not only because tearing wounds are likely, but because they do not truncate the stalk-and-grab sequence of the predation pattern. This manifestation of predatory behavior is qualitatively different from the silent stalk and pounce evinced by many dogs with predatory aggression. The extent to which such dogs might exhibit silent stalking and hiding before rushing from behind some blockade to exhibit the rest of the chase sequence is unknown. Once dogs engage in this sequence, they seem unlikely to inhibit their pursuit unless the person is able to escape. The responsible client action is to prohibit the dogs from being at large. In a litigious world, dogs that behave like this and are left unrestrained are invitations to lawsuits.

Hyperactivity

Hyperactivity is overdiagnosed in dogs. Most dogs that clients believe are hyperactive are either overactive or underexercised. Dogs that are truly hyperkinetic are unable to fully relax and have physiological signs that are concomitant with their hyperactive behavior (elevated baseline heart rate, respiratory rate, and temperature when at "rest" with lower than expected increases when exercised) (Voith, 1980d). Because many physiological conditions can produce these nonspecific changes, medical conditions that should be eliminated from a list of potential diagnoses include metabolic disease associated with liver dysfunction or aberrant glucose metabolism, endocrine (thyroid) disease, and neurological conditions such as encephalitis. It has been postulated that the rare, truly hyperactive dogs have a relative deficiency of central dopamine D_2 receptors (Burghardt, 1994). This hypothesis has not been fully evaluated, nor has the potential role for serotonin. Humans with attention deficit hyperactivity disorder (ADHD) may respond to treatment with selective serotonin reuptake inhibitors (SSRIs). The extent to which this more complex etiology and the potential treatment for hyperactivity are relevant for understanding the canine condition is unknown.

Dietary Problems

Obesity is a more common problem in dogs than in cats. It has been estimated that 20% to 30% of dogs are obese, whereas only 10% of cats are obese (Anderson, 1973; Darke, 1978; Mason, 1970). By definition, obesity and excessive intake are coupled. There appear to be breed differences in the extent to which obesity occurs, but genetic and management-related factors are confounded (Mugford, 1977). Labrador retrievers and Scottish terriers are overrepresented in the group of dogs that experience excessive intake (Houpt, 1982).

Spaying does increase appetite because estrogen (removed by spaying) suppresses appetite (Houpt et al., 1979). Treatment with benzodiazepines, progestins, and corticosteroids can also increase intake. Dogs will choose a diet that is 30% in protein (Romsos & Ferguson, 1983) and will increase intake if their diet is diluted (Janowitz & Grossman, 1949). Intake increases in winter with colder temperatures and decreases in the summer with warmer ones (Durres & Hannon, 1962). Dogs prefer palatable foods and will select novel ones (Beaver et al., 1992; Ferrell, 1984; Mugford, 1977). These factors all should be considered when evaluating "excessive" intake.

Excessive intake could also be associated with anxiety-related behaviors. Eating in humans can have an OCD manifestation, and a similar situation may occur in dogs (Fox, 1962).

Anorexia is rare in dogs and is usually associated with a primary illness. Fear associated with some aspect of feeding could also result in anorexia.

Postulated Breed-Specific Problems

It is arguable whether any problems are truly "breed specific"; however, humans have inadvertently selected for specific behaviors or suites of behaviors through the development of breeds and by specific training programs. For example, retired racing greyhounds may chase and pounce on small fuzzy things such as pet rabbits and kittens. Caution is urged. Many of these dogs have been specifically taught not to sit or to go down behind. In addition to having long forelimbs, which may make it more frightening to learn to lie down on tile floors, being specifically taught to stand erect can pose problems. Because some of the training methods are less than kind, overcoming fear may be an important aspect of teaching basic commands.

Another example can be found in herding dogs. Although individuals of herding breeds are taught specific moves, the tendency to "herd" has been specifically selected for. For some dogs the actual herding behaviors (blocking, nipping, and holding) may be default behaviors in the absence of any other command, become apparent in anxious and fearful situations, or become the behavioral focus of problems (e.g., problem aggressions like protective aggression). That such proclivities are very prominent in some lines should be no surprise. Anticipation and "shaping" can ameliorate these problems.

CASE 1

....

Signalment: "Bogie," 10-month-old, male, castrated, mixed breed pup

Initial problem: Tackling owner and stealing objects

History: This pup was adopted from a neighbor at 6 weeks of age. The neighbor had the mother, but she died after parturition and they have been hand-rearing the 8 pups. Bogie has always taken things out of the trash and chews tissues, dryer lint, cotton-tipped swabs, and so on. If anyone leaves their shoes unguarded, Bogey will chew on (and ingest) the laces. The toilet paper was always found draped all over the house; now it is kept on a very high shelf. The people have replaced the remote control for the television eight times. The children used to have plastic interlocking blocks. The house plants are history. The children do not have any socks without holes because the dog grabs them while they are dressing—tugging and chasing ensue. The pup steals pens, glasses, and other objects and does not relinquish these items even if people chase him. When anyone is watching television with his or her feet crossed, the pup watches the feet and grabs them, growling, when they move. Bogie tackles and grabs bathrobes when people are wearing them. The husband, who has primary care for the dog, kids, and house, has scratches and tooth marks all over his forearms and lower legs. The last visitors had to wrestle the dog to retrieve their jackets. And although the clients do not complain about it, when on a walk, Bogie takes all of them for a drag, coughing the entire time.

Physical Examination: This is a normal, healthy dog.

Previous Treatment: A trainer told the people to knee the dog in the chest every time he jumped. The clients were also told to step on Bogie's back toes if this persisted. The clients would call the dog up to their thigh by patting it and then step on its toes. The dog no longer comes for them when called, but barks at the clients instead. The dog also feints to the left when he jumps.

Diagnosis: This dog has attention-seeking behavior and inappropriate play behavior.

• •

Treatment: Treatment will involve behavior modification, primarily deference gestures (see Appendix B), the use of a head collar indoors and out, the use of a crate replete with acceptable chew toys when the dog is unsupervised, increasing aerobic exercise (Frisbee, lure-coursing), and provisioning with appropriate tug and chew toys. The clients are to bell Bogie and startle him with a water pistol when he starts to steal. With the use of a lunge line, he is taught to "come" (see Appendix B).

This case was mishandled from the beginning. The clients should never have permitted the dog to steal and play with their possessions. Chasing the puppy only encouraged him. The dog feints to the left when he jumps because he has learned to avoid being "kneed." No one should ever recommend this as a correction technique. It is abusive, can kill a dog, and does not work. The clients should be discouraged from baiting the dog to jump up on them so they can correct him. By doing so, the pup gets mixed messages. This dog can get better. All of his behavior problems could have been prevented if his people had received competent advice.

• •

Signalment: "Natasha," 8-month-old, 3.2 kg, spayed female Siamese cat. She is gorgeous, friendly, and outgoing and loved by the two adult daughters and their parents with whom she lives. She is an only cat.

Presenting complaint/problem: Biting and scratching

History: Natasha was obtained at a breeder at 9 weeks of age. The breeder had lavished love and attention on all the kittens with the hope of making them great pets. The two daughters brought the cat to the Behavior Clinic because she is becoming more aggressive. Everyone in the household has been scratched, and the cat is beginning to bite, although not severely. The clients made the appointment because they are worried about their father's health. He is elderly and diabetic and is losing his sight. The cat has always played roughly, but when he could see, the father was adept at avoiding or deflecting the cat's energies. Now, not only is the father unable to see and anticipate the aggressive behavior, but Natasha appears to be getting more aggressive. Because of his diabetic condition, it is important that he not be bitten or scratched by this cat.

Questioning revealed that the aggression is, and always has been, associated with play. This cat was well treated by the breeder between 3 and 7 weeks of age, the periods when cats are most sensitive to social stimuli. She was raised with exposure to people in varied situations and was left with her siblings until adopted. Because Natasha was so tiny the clients were afraid to correct the cat when she first started to attack their feet and ankles. The clients had also heard that most cat play is predatory behavior and assumed that the cat attacks were normal. And, they confessed, when she was small, her teeth and claws did not hurt very much. They all had thought that it was funny that this little fur ball would so confidently take on an adult human. Natasha would crouch behind doors and under furniture and spring at the clients when they passed. She would then continue to run. The clients enjoy this cat and learned that if they chased the cat, the cat would respond with rougher play. As she got bigger, the clients began to play back roughly with their hands and feet. Whenever anyone talked on the telephone the cat would attack their feet; the clients responded by bouncing their feet and wrestling with the cat, usually using their socks.

Physical examination: This is a healthy, normal cat.

Diagnosis: This cat has inappropriate play behavior that has become play aggression, and the clients largely facilitated it. Although it is true that cats complete their social play sensitive period by about 8 to 10 weeks of age and enter their social fighting sensitive period by 14 weeks of age, there was nothing remiss in this cat's upbringing that would induce either earlier and more fierce social fighting or predatory behavior. Many social fighting and predatory behaviors overlap in cats, and early weaning commonly precipitates earlier predatory behavior while suppressing normal play behavior. Natasha was not weaned early and had the benefit of experiencing extensive play with her siblings. One of the reasons early orphaned or weaned cats may play aggressively is that they are never corrected by other cats or kittens. The extensive role that intraspecific tactile, visual, and vocal signals may play in further shaping a more gentle, contextually appropriate play response has not been well investigated. Certainly, even if people can correct kittens by startling them as they start to exhibit undesirable behaviors, they are unable to give these other cues.

Natasha had no risk factors for play aggression, inappropriate play behavior, or predatory aggression before entering this household. Inappropriate responses from the clients taught the cat to intensify its play aggression. This, combined with her increased size, makes this cat potentially dangerous.

Treatment: The clients volunteered that they were afraid that they had been a significant factor in the development of this inappropriate behavior. They were very willing to stop playing with the cat using their body parts and were willing to play with toys that played back (stuffed mice on compressible springy cords, feathers, foil balls). They were also willing to carry compressed air canisters (commonly used to clean camera equipment) and blast Natasha at the first sign of any impending attack or rough play. Their concern was primarily for their father. Once the cat was fitted with a breakaway collar to which a loud bell had been attached, the father was able to also use the air canister technique. If the sound of the cat's bell intensified as it would with running and behaviors associated with pouncing, the father was to blast the cat. Even if he only shot the air into the vicinity of Natasha, the sound should startle her and act as a secondary reinforcer, or bridging stimulus, for the air blast. Finally, the clients were encouraged to increase Natasha's aerobic exercise, and to reward her when she was quiet and good. The latter was to include talking to her and slowly, softly petting and massaging her while she was sleeping, and rewarding her with tiny food treats when she sat quietly by them on the couch.

The clients wanted to know if they should use some medication to sedate Natasha. The answer is an emphatic no. Drugs should be a last resort in these cases, not a first. The clients were told that even if these measures did not fully ablate the play aggression, another nonpharmaceutical option was open to them: get another cat, preferably an older kitten that could take care of itself and would not be at risk from Natasha's rough play. The clients confessed that after the problem of Natasha's aggression surfaced, they doubted whether they would still be welcome in their parents' home if they brought in another cat.

Follow-up: A phone call 3 weeks later indicated that the play aggression had largely stopped. Natasha is still going after the clients' mother about three to four times a week while she cooks dinner. The mother had been less willing to correct the cat using startle because she was worried that it was a mean thing to do. The dangers of cat scratch and bite diseases were discussed (cat bites are a $25,000,000 per year human health industry in the U.S.) and the mother has more respect for the cat's teeth and claws. The father is delighted with the bell and the calm petting. He now spends hours petting and massaging Natasha and feeding her tiny treats when she stretches out fully for him. If he regains some sight, he has expressed an interest in teaching her some tricks.

Signalment: "Joey" 13-month-old, male castrated, 3.8 kg, domestic short-haired cat

Initial Problem: Nocturnal activity

History: The client obtained the cat at approximately 7½ weeks of age from a neighbor whose cat was the mother. The client and her husband are both professionals and work long days. They love this cat and have every known cat toy. The cat has two kitty condos and a bird video. They play with and chase the cat for about ½ hour when they come home at nights, and on weekends they take Joey outside, usually to the park, on his harness. On weekends Joey gets more exercise and attention than he does during the week. The clients are distressed about Joey's nocturnal activity. He has always been active at night and they went through a period where they chased him from the bedroom when he awakened them. Now, even if they close the door they hear noise all night long.

They are most disturbed by it at about 3 A.M. Books and magazines are found knocked on the floor in the morning, the throw pillows are off the sofa, plants are routinely uprooted, and Joey once shattered a group of cordial glasses after a party. The crowning blow came recently when they heard a loud tinkering of crystal and rushed downstairs to find Joey literally swinging from the chandelier. Some of their friends have children with attention deficit disorder and they wonder if this might be Joey's problem. They have also heard that cats can have problems with hyperthyroidism and are worried that this might be the reason for Joey's aberrant behavior. Their reason for coming to the clinic was to obtain medication to control Joey's behavior.

Physical examination: Joey is healthy, his thyroid gland was normal on palpation, and he shows no physiological signs of hyperactivity. In fact, he slept through part of the history.

• •

Diagnosis: Joey is a normal, young, active cat. He is not sufficiently stimulated during the day to overcome his otherwise perfectly normal feline predilection for nocturnal activity. The fact that he slept through part of the visit and that he is better on weekends both support this contention. It is the clients who must change what they are doing to get Joey to change.

Treatment: The clients need to increase Joey's aerobic play. Throwing balls, attaching toys that play back to belts on their waists (so that they move while the clients walk), and taking Joey with them whenever they get into the car so that he gets more stimulation will also help. Waking him up on weekends whenever they see him asleep during the daytime can be beneficial, as can feeding him his main meal just before bedtime. But nothing will take the place of stimulation and interaction that is the hallmark of normal young cat behavior. Accordingly, getting him another young cat could help (of course, they might both stay up at nights if the clients do not adhere to the other suggestions). Once the clients have cat-proofed the house so that Joey cannot break anything fragile and will not be injured by any of the household objects (toilets, dryers, electric cords), the clients can try earplugs so that they do not hear him tearing around. Finally, Joey might be happy as an indoor/outdoor cat if precautions are taken to keep him safe. These may include a kitty run, a kitty door, or an electronic cat fence. Outdoor cats are more prone to infections because of trauma and are not protected from wild or marauding animals.

If and only if they have done everything and still cannot sleep should medication be a consideration. A small amount of over-the-counter chlorpheniramine (2 to 4 mg orally) just before bedtime can be beneficial. The problem would have to be severe to warrant stronger drugs.

Discussion: Note that the clients wanted to use medication to suppress normal behavior. Veterinarians frequently call and ask my drug of choice for control of nocturnal activity. This is not the purpose of behavioral pharmacology. Behavioral pharmacology should be used as an adjuvant to treat abnormal behavior, not to suppress normal behavior. In really profound cases of nocturnal destruction a small amount of diazepam (0.5 mg) or alprazolam (0.25 mg) before bedtime may help. If the practitioner believes that the motor activity is not only undesirable but also abnormal (associated with fear or anxiety), other drugs can be beneficial. Regardless, before administering any benzodiazepine, tricyclic antidepressant, or nonspecific anxiolytic agent, premedication physical examinations, including auscultation and possibly a rhythm strip and serum biochemistry profiles and complete blood cell counts should be done. Cats can react idiosyncratically to psychotropic medications, particularly the benzodiazepines, with rare but tragic consequences. Furthermore, sole reliance on psychotropic medication to the exclusion of behavioral and environmental modification deprives the patient of the opportunity to explore behavioral adaptations, facilitated by the medication, that could make it happier. The welfare of the patient should be a concern, particularly for cats that are exhibiting normal behaviors that people find undesirable. An understanding of those behaviors, which are the result of a social system very different from ours, should be part of the covenant of cat guardianship.

12 ····· Treatment of Behavioral Problems

···

*I*n any situation there are three environments that potentially can be modified: the physical environment, the behavioral environment, and the pharmacological environment (Voith, 1979b, 1984c). These environments are not always independent and warrant some discussion.

The physical environment includes perceived and actual space considerations; any visual, olfactory, or auditory stimuli; other animals; relevant objects such as litter boxes; and any devices that might change an animal's perception, such as gauze curtains or the presence of background music. Although other animate objects may be part of the physical environment, they may potentially also interact within the behavioral environment. This is not requisite—the mere presence of a dog that can be seen through a window may be sufficient stimulus for an inappropriate behavior, even though that dog may never be an active participant in any behavioral interaction. Because perception is so critical in the evaluation of the physical environment, the time environment or the schedules of the clients must be considered. Some problems, such as separation anxiety in dogs, may develop when the only environmental change is one of time; day length shortens or the clients' schedules change. Part of the treatment must address this environmental change. The physical environment may be modified because it is a direct part of the problem (for example, insufficient space for exercise) or because changing the physical environment can help solve the problem, for example by providing dog houses to give each dog personal space in an unshared rain shelter.

The behavioral environment focuses on behavior modification, rather than alteration of the perceptual or tangible environment. The behavioral environment includes the individual and the social environment of anyone (human or animal) with whom the individual might interact. If there is another social group with whom the individual does not interact, but whose social interaction affects the individual (i.e., a group of cats whose play affects the resident dog, but who do not interact with it directly), this is also a component of the behavioral environment. In this example, if the dog barks every time the cats roughhouse, part of the treatment may be to teach the cats to play elsewhere or to not play in so rough a manner.

The third environment that the veterinarian can work to potentially modify, the pharmacologic environment, has two components: the endogenous environment and the exogenous environment. The former is influenced by hormones and physiological parameters. This is the environment that is influenced by neutering and disease. I mention the latter because there is a tendency to forget that an animal's behavior can change with physiological changes attendant with aging or illness. This type of endogenous change then affects the manner in which the animal interacts in the behavioral and physical environments. The exogenous pharmacological environment includes pharmacological intervention (drug therapy).

None of the three environments mentioned above is independent: they all interact—a perturbation in one can cause a shift in another.

It is critical to realize that behavior modification and the application of clinical comparative psychological treatment is not just fancy obedience training (*sensu* Mugford, 1984b). Although dogs are less reactive if lying down (because they must go through more movements to lunge or leave) when compared with sitting, and when sitting when compared with standing, the key is to change the dog's or cat's attitude about relaxation and assumption of deferential or anxiety-reducing behaviors. Animals may use obedience-type postures as part of a behavior modification program, but the context is different. That difference is the crux.

LEARNING AND MEMORY

Learning is complex and variable. The types of learning include (1) habituation, (2) associative (classical conditioning/operant conditioning), (3) perceptive/discriminative learning, (4) insight learning, (5) set learning (learning to learn), and (6) imprinting, a special type of early learning.

Much learning is not explained by classical or instrumental conditioning techniques—it occurs too quickly and appears irreversible. For such cases, the concept of imprinting has been developed (Hess, 1973; Lorenz, 1937, 1966). Imprinting is characterized by the following qualities: (1) it has a short sensitive period; (2) it is stable and irreversible; (3) it generalizes to like activities (i.e., it is supraindividualistic—the social orientation is to a group rather than an individual); (4) it tends to occur toward conspecifics, if available; (5) the strength of the imprinting bond depends on the effort (passive or active) spent to create it; and (6) the imprinted individual exhibits the appropriate behavior toward an object at adulthood (i.e. courtship and mating).

The neurophysiology of imprinting is interesting and suggests the relevance of similarities and differences to standard memory. Imprinting correlates with increased ribonucleic acid synthesis in the intermediate medial hyperstriatum ventrale (IMHV) in the dorsal forebrain. Electron microscopy has demonstrated increases in the synaptic area of the IMHV after imprinting, and the rate of neuronal firing in the IMHV is subsequently altered. Lesions of the IMHV quickly alter the ability to imprint, but leave associative learning unimpaired.

The neurotransmitters postulated to be involved in learning include acetylcholine; norepinephrine; dopamine; the pituitary peptides vasopressin, adrenocorticotropic hormone, and melanocyte-stimulating hormone; and serotonin (Rang et al., 1995). These effects should be considered when choosing behavioral medications. For example, anticholinergic drugs leave profound effects on both long-term and short-term memory. Pigs that are acetylcholinesterase impaired are slower to develop avoidance learning.

Short-term memory has been described biochemically as follows: (Rang et al., 1995) (1) receptors transduce proteins, (2) proteins activate amplifier enzymes (adenyl cyclase), (3) amplifier enzymes increase levels of the intracellular messenger cyclic adenosine monophosphate (cAMP), (4) the intracellular messenger activates protein kinases, and (5) the protein kinases modify the target proteins (via calcium and potassium channels), thereby modulating neuronal excitability and transmitter release. It is postulated that cAMP processes are also involved in the gene induction that occurs in long-term memory or long-term potentiation.

Behavior modification uses six main tactics that all involve learning: habituation, extinction, desensitization, counterconditioning, flooding, and avoidance/aversive conditioning. Before the specifics of this are discussed, some definitions of terms are required (Spreat & Spreat, 1982; Voith, 1986; Voith & Borchelt, 1982c).

PRINCIPLES OF BEHAVIOR MODIFICATION
Definitions Associated With Learning Paradigms

Habituation is an elementary form of learning. It involves no rewards. It is merely the cessation or decrease in a response to a stimulus that is the result of repeated or prolonged exposure to that stimulus. The stimulus can be positive, neutral, or negative. As would be expected, stimuli associated with potentially adverse consequences (negative stimuli) might be more difficult to extinguish with habituation than other stimuli. For example, for prey species, responses to sounds associated with predators should be difficult to habituate because they have been selected for and generally have an adaptive response (note that the predator does not have to be present very often for the

response to be rewarded). Furthermore, if such responses are even occasionally rewarded, the habituation response will be inhibited. In such circumstances, prolonged exposure to the stimulus might be expected to be associated with hypervigilance, exhaustion, and increased anxiety. In fact, this is one explanation for the feedback between anxiety and environmental events, even in situations where the anxiety is pathologic and potentially maladaptive.

When habituation is recommended for behavior modification, the goal is the *normal attenuation* of a response to something novel in the environment. The response to be habituated is attendant with an increase in intensity or frequency of exposure to the stimulus in circumstances where nothing horrendous happens. For example, a doorbell may startle a new puppy, but as the pup hears it more frequently in a benign context she may habituate to it (if inappropriately reinforced, she may not). People who move from the city to the country habituate to bird songs and insect calls.

Stimulus generalization is the quick habituation to a new stimulus that is only slightly different from the old.

Spontaneous recovery is a phenomenon that is associated with habituation. If there is an extended time between the time in which the animal last experienced a stimulus to which it had habituated and reexposure to the stimulus, the animal may again react. This is termed spontaneous recovery. Spontaneous recovery is usually easy to reverse if no overt fear is involved.

Dishabituation is the reinstatement of a habituated response as a result of exposure to a stimulus that provokes a response similar to the original. The classic examples of this involve mildly fearful responses: if habituation had just occurred to a certain hand gesture and another movement occurred that was also worrisome for the animal, the animal could dishabituate to the hand gesture. Rehabituation is the rule unless the event is compounded and made more fearful or the animal's reaction is extreme (suggesting something innate about the animal's response, not the event, itself).

Conditioning refers to associations between stimuli and responses. Classical conditioning does not involve a reward structure to make these associations. Operant or instrumental conditioning uses a reinforcement (reward or punishment) structure. Types of rewards or punishments commonly used are found in Box 12-1. In operant conditioning learning is fastest if the positive reinforcer occurs immediately (within 0.5 seconds). Delayed and intermittent reinforcements slow the acquisition of the response but work well to reinforce its maintenance (they enhance resistance to extinction). In addition to timing (quantity), value (quality) is also important. The more an animal values a reinforcer, the more quickly and reliably it will acquire the response. Hence, a food treat that dogs do

---

BOX 12-1
TYPES OF REINFORCERS

Rewards
- Food
- Touch
- Praise
- Play
- Attention
- Chewing or access to special chew toy
- Avoidance of discomfort

Punishment
- Physical pain
- Social or mental intimidation
- Fear
- Withdrawal of object, access to object, or attention ("time out")

Critical factors in punishment
- Timing—behavior as a process
- Consistency—vigilance *or* avoidance
- Appropriateness of intensity—watch behavioral response
- Conditioned punishment—secondary cues for distance situations

---

not usually get (cheese) will be better than their standard dog kibble in teaching them a new behavior. It is important to realize that not all dogs value food above all else; some value play with a ball or Frisbee, or love. Designing behavior modification programs that have a high probability of success requires understanding what the dog values and incorporating that into the program.

Reinforcement is the process that involves a stimulus or an event that increases the future probability that a certain behavior or class of behaviors will be performed. A positive reinforcer is a stimulus or an event that occurs after a response that leads to an increase in that response in the future. A negative reinforcer is an aversive event or stimulus that increases the frequency of a behavior, but does so through escape or avoidance.

Negative reinforcement is not to be confused with punishment. *Punishment* is the application of an aversive or negative stimulus, after or during a response, that leads to a decrease in the frequency of the response. Negative reinforcement is the withdrawal of a stimulus that then increases the probability of a behavior being repeated. In negative reinforcement, the animal responds more quickly to avoid a stimulus. The classic example of negative reinforcement is actually the correct use of choke collars: when the animal stops, the collar releases, and the animal is rewarded with release from choking for walking well. The sound the collar makes as it pulls and then slips acts

as a secondary reinforcer. One can see why this paradigm has been so abused for dogs that pull.

Both negative reinforcement and punishment differ from *omission training*, in which animals are taught that they are rewarded for *not* responding. For example, the dog that does not bark gets the treat. The signal (or secondary reinforcer) "Quiet" can indicate that the absence of sound will engender a reward. This technique is grossly misunderstood and underexploited in veterinary medicine.

A *schedule of reinforcements* is important for teaching or learning a behavior and for maintaining it. There are two main types of reinforcement schedules: continuous and intermittent. In a *continuous reinforcement schedule*, every occurrence is rewarded. This schedule type produces the fastest acquisition of a response. *Intermittent reinforcement schedules* can be of two types: ratio schedules and interval schedules. In ratio schedules, the animal is provided with a reward on either a fixed or variable basis. Fixed ratios mean that the reward comes, for example, every third time the animal successfully executes the behavior. Variable ratios are exactly that—sometimes the reward comes after two correct responses, sometimes after five. *Interval rewards* come after a set interval of time that can either be fixed or variable. Intermittent schedules are best for maintaining an acquired response. This dual strategy is the one used in the protocols in Appendix B.

Second-order reinforcers are signals that can be used at a distance that convey that the reward or the valuable stimulus is coming. Commonly used second-order reinforcers are words ("Good girl"), hand signals, and clickers or whistles. By carefully pairing these with the reward with which the response to the command has already been paired, second-order reinforcers can elicit the same response as the reward would (at least temporarily; one would not wish to suddenly switch from a first-order reward structure to only a second-order one without at least intermittent reinforcement about the coupling of the association—animals, including people, are smarter than that).

Stimulus and response generalization occurs when an operantly or classically conditioned response is provoked not only by the object or event that originally provoked it, but by objects or events that are similar to that original stimulus. The most common example of stimulus response generalization in dogs is to people in uniforms: if a delivery man or meter reader initially scared the dog or provoked a protective response, this response may then be generalized to others in uniform although the circumstances might not be the same. The more similar the original and subsequent stimuli, the more similar and intense the response. Stimulus and response generalization may be associated with the development of profoundly anxious or fearful and phobic responses, and understanding this may be tantamount to diminishing the worrisome behavior.

Extinction is the cessation of a response that occurs when reinforcement is stopped. The classical example of extinction of a response in dogs is the dog that jumps up on people for attention. If people pet the dog this continues; if they stop at once and continue to withhold attention, the dog will eventually extinguish its response because the reward is no longer there. The same example is classic for its illustration of the major pitfall for extinction: resistance to extinction. Any form of intermittent reinforcement—even occasional petting of the dog in response to her jumping—will enhance the continuation of the response. The more valuable the original reinforcer, the longer the reinforcement has been continuing. And the more uncertainty there is about whether the response has been truly removed (which is, after all, what occurs during intermittent reinforcement), the greater the resistance to extinction. Resistance to extinction can also occur even without reinforcement, if the reward was good enough and it is tightly coupled to the behavior. Because there is often an association between eliciting the reward and the intensity or rapidity of the performance of the behavior coupled with getting the reward, the intensity or frequency of the behavior one is attempting to extinguish usually increases at the beginning of an extinction process. It is critical at this juncture that clients not give in, although it may seem momentarily expeditious to do so, especially when they question whether they are losing their sanity. Giving in will only make extinction more difficult in the future because the animal has learned that although the client's threshold has increased, the animal can override it.

Extinction is the process by which normal or conditioned responses are decreased or attenuated by exposure to a stimulus that elicits the response in the *absence* of the reward. The new puppy that barks at the doorbell may get inappropriately reinforced by well-meaning owners who pick her up and reassure her. They are actually, and usually unintentionally, rewarding her for barking, so she continues to bark when the doorbell rings. This is now a conditioned response. If they consistently ignore her they will extinguish the response (if the sound of her own bark has not become self-reinforcing). Caution is urged since resistance to extinction is a very common phenomenon and occurs with very little reinforcement. The classic introductory psychology course story about this usually involves an elevator that is broken more often than not. Still, because it operates 1 in 10 or 1 in 20 times, most people still walk into the lobby and push the button on the off chance it works. They are exhibiting resistance to extinction as a result of an intermittent reinforcement schedule.

It is also important to realize that extinction does not work well for behaviors that are self-rewarding (chewing/scratching) or innate (urine marking).

Desensitization is a decrement in response that is produced by gradual exposure to a stimulus that elic-

its the response. If the puppy described above has become fearful of or stimulated by the doorbell, her bark, or the events occurring around the ringing of the doorbell, using a tape recording of the doorbell could help her stop the undesired response. If the tape is played very softly at first so that she does not react and is then only gradually increased in volume at increments designed to elicit no response, she may become desensitized to the doorbell.

In *counterconditioning*, negative or undesirable behavior is extinguished or controlled by teaching the animal to do another behavior (preferably favorable and fun) that competitively interferes with the execution of the undesirable behavior. This is best coupled with desensitization. When done correctly, it results in response substitution: the development of a positive behavior that is incompatible with the expression of the unwanted sequence (Mugford, 1984b; Thompson & Grabowski, 1977). Again, using the puppy example, she will learn faster if she is first taught to sit and stay and relax (the key here) in exchange for a treat. The dog must be absolutely quiet and calm, and convey by the look in her eyes, body posture, and facial expressions that she would do anything for the client. Once she can do this for exercises lasting a half hour or so, the desensitization component of the tape recording that gradually increases in volume is added. Performing the adoration act for a food salary is incompatible with or competitively exclusive of barking. If at any point she starts to act anxious or to not attend to the client, the tape recording should be lowered in volume until the dog can relax again. This is the key—the sitting and staying is merely a facilitator for the relaxation response. There is no sense to having the dog sit and stay if it is panting, salivating, its pupils are dilated, its ears are back, and it is clearly distressed. What is the dog learning? The gestalt of relaxation is the first step to changing the behavior. Counterconditioning coupled with desensitization is a very time-consuming technique. It means that one must constantly go back and repeat the exercises where there was a lesser response until there is none, and it means that one must attend to all the patient's communicatory signals. Bridging stimuli (recordings, signals) can be used to tell the animal to continue to relax because the reward is coming and can be useful as clients gradually withdraw from situations (Mugford, 1984b). It is hard work, but it works.

Clients who are least successful with this technique want both quicker fixes and less work. Inform them of the impossibility of either at the outset. Clients also want their dogs to be "quick," "fast learners," "A+ students," "achievers." These are all words that I have heard clients use as they whip through the counterconditioning and desensitization exercises so quickly as to provoke anxiety in the dog. This sabotages the program. Problem dogs have special needs. These needs do not reflect on the intelligence of the dog or on the abilities of the owners. These dogs may eventually be A+ students, but they will have to take a longer, harder path, and although the owners did not cause the dog's behavioral problems, they are constrained to accompany the dog on that path if the dog is to get better.

Flooding involves prolonged exposure at a level that provokes the response so that the animal eventually gives up. This is exactly the opposite of the approach taken in desensitization. It is far more stressful than any of the other therapy strategies and, used inappropriately, could damage the animal. If nothing else works for the puppy, flooding would involve enclosing the dog in a small space (a crate or small room) and constantly playing a tape of a doorbell louder than the actual bell until she ceases to bark or greatly decreases the frequency and intensity of her reaction (Levis, 1979; Young, 1982). The dog cannot be disturbed until this happens and that could take a while. One of the big risks is in creating a tremulous, fearful dog. In most cases flooding should be used as a last resort and should always be executed as humanely as possible. Animals cannot fear the clients and vice versa.

Overlearning is a phenomenon that is frequently used in training for specific events but may be underused in preventing fearful responses in dogs for whom one is concerned. Overlearning is the repeated evocation and expression of an already learned response. This accomplishes three things: (1) it delays forgetting, (2) it increases the resistance to extinction, and (3) it increases the probability that the response will become a "knee-jerk" one, or response of first choice, when the circumstances are similar. This last aspect can be useful in teaching any animal to overcome a fear or anxiety.

Overshadowing is the reduction in the influence of multiple stimuli by working on decreasing the response to one. Minimizing the effects of one stimulus decreases the effects of the others. This is a critical part of the paradigm for treating fears and anxieties, although it is seldom explicitly identified.

Shaping is a learning technique that works well for animals that do not know what a perfect response would be. It works through gradual approximations and allows the animal to be rewarded initially for any behavior that resembles the behavior that is desired as the final outcome. For instance, when teaching a puppy to sit, following a slight squat with a food reward will enhance the probability that squatting will be repeated. This squatting behavior is then rewarded only when it becomes more exaggerated, and finally, when it becomes a true sit. *Autoshaping* is classical conditioning that occurs simply because of repeated exposure (e.g., the cat comes when the can opener sounds).

Local enhancement is a form of trial-and-error learning that is combined with observation. Because of the latter, the former occurs faster. For example, a puppy learning to go through a dog door will eventu-ally figure it out, but the puppy will learn faster if it watches another dog go through the door.

Avoidance or *aversive conditioning* involves the presentation of an aversive stimulus in response to an inappropriate or undesirable behavior. The stimulus is intended to abort the behavior and to decrease the probability of its occurrence in the future. This is the correct definition of punishment. To be most successful the stimulus designed to abort the behavior must occur as early as possible but certainly within the first 30 to 60 seconds of the onset of the behavioral sequence and must be consistent and appropriate. The critical factors in punishment include (1) timing, (2) consistency, (3) appropriate intensity, and (4) the presence of a conditioned response. The latter means that when the undesirable behavior ceases, there must be some favorable stimulus or reward for the dog even if it is just praise or a pat. *This is the single most frequently ignored aspect of therapy for clients whose pets have behavioral problems; when the pets are not causing trouble, almost no one tells them how good they are. This is where the most ground is lost.* To reiterate, it is important to emphasize to clients that punishment must be as closely coupled with the inappropriate event as possible, must startle the animal to abort the behavior, must be appropriate in duration and intensity (it is never appropriate to beat a dog senseless, yet people tend to continue all forms of punishment long after the abortion of the event has occurred), and all of this must occur in a consistent manner that incorporates aborting the inappropriate behavior every time it occurs with rewarding the animal every time it is good. People resort to physical punishment as the correction method of choice. Notice that nowhere above does it say that punishment must be physical. The best punishment is nonphysical, noninteractive (e.g., "time out") (Nobbe et al., 1978). Furthermore, "good" punishment is just as hard work as is appropriately executed counterconditioning and desensitization. Punishment is never an "easy out" and has a high probability of backfiring unless the client understands that its focus is to decrease the probability of future inappropriate events. Local pain of the type caused by pinch collars, hitting, or electric (shock) collars *increases* aggression in dominantly aggressive dogs (Mugford, 1984b) and may induce other aggressions (Azrin & Holz, 1966). Species-specific responses are also important to consider. "Scruffing" a dog is likely to cause pain because flexor dominance does not persist in puppies, so we should not use it to correct puppies. Flexor dominance does, however, persist in kittens, and one sees adults of the same species use this response to correct kittens.

Aversive conditioning may be best used early in the development of the undesirable behavior. Early warning signs of most aggressions are recognizable if the client learns these early indicators. As emphasized above, for punishment to succeed it must occur, preferably within 1 second, but generally within the first 30 to 60 seconds, of the *onset* of the inappropriate behavior. The punishment should startle the animal sufficiently to interrupt the behavior and abort any attempt at immediate resumption (Blackshaw et al., 1990; Borchelt & Voith,1985). This value of surprise (startle device = unconditioned stimulus [UCS]) is based on the Rescorla-Wagner model of conditioning (Domjan & Burkhard, 1985). Learning does not automatically occur with any pairing of conditioned stimulus (CS)/unconditioned stimulus (UCS). It depends on the animal's previous experience, the presence of other stimuli, and the relevance to the animal of the pairing of the CS/UCS. This is a particularly important point when considering to what extent punishment should be used. Following a startle, the pup can be taught a more appropriate behavior, such as sitting and staying. This serves as a time out and teaches that the client is the leader in the situation and that the pup must take all cues as to the appropriateness of its behavior from the client. This is important, because at the crux of aggressive problems is the fact that these dogs are abnormal; they are incapable of making appropriate, in-context distinctions. These dogs exhibit inappropriate, out-of-context behavior. Early intervention must be aimed at getting the dog under excellent voice control and teaching it to make better context distinctions by taking cues from the client. The discriminative value of punishment should be used: the point is to change the behavior patterns, including those of the client. If they do not ignore good behavior, they will decrease the need for punishment.

Clients should be aware of the phenomenon of *learned helplessness*. This occurs when an animal is forced to be exposed to an uncontrollable situation, where no changes in its behavior effect a change in the environment. Random punishment or abuse leads to this. In such circumstances, further learning is disrupted.

INSTRUMENTAL LEARNING VERSUS CLASSICAL CONDITIONING

Instrumental learning and classical conditioning are different. *Instrumental learning* is usually used in behavior modification: the animal performs a voluntary response to get a reward or to avoid an aversive situation—the behavior is the instrument of the reward. *Classical conditioning* focuses on involuntary or reflex behaviors (salivating) and does not use rewards; instead, the animal learns to pair the reflexive or involuntary behavior with another neutral signal.

Classical conditioning is most often represented by the example of Pavlovian conditioning (Pavlov, 1927). In Pavlov's example a dog was shown meat. The dog then salivated. The next and subsequent times that the dog was shown meat, a bell was paired with the meat. Eventually the dog would salivate simply for the ringing of the bell, although meat was no longer involved. No rewards were used.

Note the following points:
1. In this example the meat was the unconditioned stimulus (UCS)—no "conditioning" was necessary to get the dog to learn what it was, and the salivation was the unconditioned response (UCR).
2. The dog did not learn to pair salivation with the meat; salivation is a response that is *unconditioned* or natural.
3. The bell is the neutral or CS (the stimulus starts out as neutral, having no innate association with meat, and becomes "conditioned" to be associated with it).
4. The bell is the stimulus with which the animal was going to be taught to make an association.
5. The salivary response that followed the bell was the conditioned response (CR)—a learned response that was *not* innate. Without this learning, coupling would not have occurred—dogs do not spontaneously salivate when a bell is rung.
6. Unlike in instrumental learning or operant conditioning (Skinner, 1938; Thorndike, 1911), no reward is used to reinforce the association.

In classical conditioning, the only reinforcement is the pairing in time of the neutral and unconditioned stimuli. The neutral stimulus should occur immediately before the unconditioned stimulus for conditioning to occur. If the neutral stimulus precedes the unconditioned stimulus by more than 0.5 seconds, learning does not occur as readily.

This observation about time periods has important ramifications for clients who wish to train their dogs to attend to them for a command and begin by using a whistle: a whistle will get the dog to attend to the client, but the word that the client now wishes the dog to associate with that attentive behavior must follow within 0.5 seconds of the dog alerting to the whistle if the dog is to learn as quickly as possible. Note that this is not the same as rewarding the dog to come. In this example, the whistle can act as a secondary reinforcer—a signal that the command to come will occur.

Another example in the use of a secondary reinforcer to enforce a behavior can be found in the housebreaking paradigm. Here, the response is not involuntary, but reflexive. When a bladder is full (UCS), emptying it becomes self-rewarding. Food treats are unlikely to compete with the reward of actual micturition. The conditioned stimulus is the *location* in which elimination occurs. For example, puppies will urinate wherever they are in the house when they have to urinate. If the client can anticipate this need and continually take the dog to the appropriate spot (CS), the act of micturition (UCR) in that area will become a CR. If the client wishes to reinforce a specific elimination posture, substrate preference, or elimination on command, instrumental conditioning involving a reward (praise or food) can be used. This will not reinforce the elimination behavior, but done correctly, could help with other choices.

In operant conditioning or instrumental learning, the paradigm always involves some sort of reward: cue = s = "sit"; response = R = "dog sits"; reinforcer = S = reward. Both forms of conditioning are used in behavior modification.

Rewards

Rewards must be appropriate for the particular dog's interest level. Most dogs will not work simply for the usual kibble, but will work for a little bit of cheese. Most of us will not work (or work as hard) for half our salary as we would for 150% of it. However, some dogs become so highly stimulated by the reward that they cannot focus on calmly learning the behavior that we are trying to teach them. The situation quickly spirals downhill. For counterconditioning to be successful, (1) the treat has to be something about which the dog cares, but which does not send it into a frenzy, and (2) the clients' timing must be sufficiently accurate that the dog is rewarded only when the dog is calm and attending to them, and they correct, ignore, or do not reward the dog if the dog's performance begins to slip. The optimum level of motivation/reactivity decreases as the complexity of the task increases — the dog has to pay more attention (Domjan &

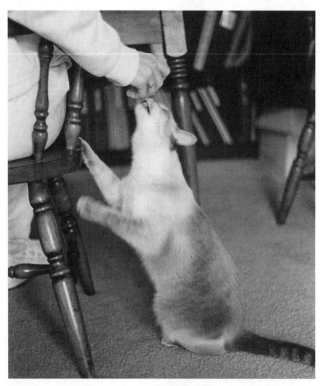

Cats, too, can learn to work with behavior modification programs that employ food treats. (Photo by Jesse F. Griffin.)

Burkhard, 1985; Miles, 1958 [Yerkes-Dodson Law]). Correcting a problem is not this simple. Calling a dog to come requires a basic and quickly executed response; it is easier to overcome intense reactivity in this time frame than it would be were one to ask the dog to sit for a long period of time while other dogs passed in the street. However, if the dog is too far away to readily respond to recall and the dog has learned that this command or request is difficult for the client to reinforce under these circumstances, no amount of reward will help. For every animal there is a window of desired attention/reactivity that can be reinforced with some form of reward (the form of reward may be different for different pets). The clinician's job is to help the client understand and use that window. A chart outlining the sentinel facets of instrumental conditioning is found in Box 12-2.

Clients should be cautious to not accidentally develop a reward-based operant conditioning paradigm. An example of this misstep is the development of attention-seeking behavior.

Finally, clients should be consistent with their reward structure. Unpredictability and instability increase frustration and hinder the development of adaptive behavioral responses (Post, 1989).

The Role of the Endogenous Pharmacological Environment: Hormones

Much attention has been focused on the role of hormones, primarily those that are sexually dimorphic, and their potential effects on undesirable behavior (Hart, 1974). Although 90% of all dominantly aggressive dogs may be male, testosterone *does not* cause dominance aggression. Instead, it would be more appropriate to view testosterone as a behavioral modulator that may facilitate the attainment and escalation of the aggressive state. If a dog is already aggressive, the difference between it in the neutered and unneutered form will be one of degree. The intact dog will react more easily, escalate the response more quickly, plateau in response at a higher level of aggressive intensity, become less reactive at a slower rate, and may return to a higher baseline state of vigilance after the event (see Fig. 6-2). Other dimorphic behaviors associated with the presence of testosterone include urine marking with lifted leg, roaming, and some types of mounting. Mounting is an unclear issue because it is a challenge and control behavior, as well as a sexual one; little work has been done to determine whether the nuances of the mounting behavior are identical in both situations. Castration results in an androgen drop within 6 hours of castration; the majority of the hormonal decrease is complete in 72 hours (Hopkins et al., 1976). Roaming in males decreases by roughly 90%, male-male aggression by roughly 75%, urine marking by approximately 60%, and mounting by 80%. Marking, mounting, and, to a lesser extent because of the modulator effect dis-

BOX 12-2
SCHEMATIC OF INSTRUMENTAL CONDITIONING TECHNIQUES

	Role for appetitive stimulus	Role for aversive stimulus
Positive reinforcement	Response produces appetitive stimulus not likely to occur otherwise	
Punishment		Response produces aversive stimulus not likely to occur otherwise
Negative reinforcement		Response eliminates or prevents (escape/avoidance) aversive stimulus that is more likely to occur otherwise
Omission training	Response eliminates or prevents occurrence of appetitive stimulus that is more likely otherwise	

cussed previously, fighting, are complex behaviors not wholly controlled by hormones. There is a significant learning component in these that many people neglect. If marking has been ongoing for some time, castration alone will *not* ablate it, but may decrease it. This is because of the learning component; the same logic holds for mounting.

Less attention has been paid to the role of female sex hormones and aggressive behavior, but recent work suggests a potential role for them (O'Farrell & Peachey, 1990). Female puppies that were already showing signs of dominance aggression became worse after spaying. For no other age and behavior group combinations did spaying have any effect. This observation agrees with some unpublished data from the Behavior Clinic at VHUP: although most dominantly aggressive dogs are male, when dominance aggression occurs in females it is a distinct syndrome. Females exhibiting dominance aggression are younger (usually less than 6 months of age) than the standard age cited for males (18 to 24 months of age) at onset, are more intensely aggressive in their early bouts, worsen quickly, and may have delayed or silent heat cycles if left intact. The issue of sex and aggression is more fully discussed in Chapter 6.

The discussion of any role for hormones in behavioral problems can be inflammatory. In some circles there is still resistance to performing ovariohysterectomy and castration of pets, despite voluminous data that indicate that the pets are safer (decreased roaming), healthier, and cannot contribute to pet overpopulation (Blackshaw & Day, 1994). Therefore it is not surprising that so much unwarranted emphasis is placed on the role of hormones in the development of behavioral problems. It is important to remember that sexual and social maturity occur at different times in all social mammals (sexual precedes social maturity). In a free-ranging situation, dogs or cats do not breed until they are 2 to 3 years of age. Hormonal factors related to sexual maturity are not to blame: breeding is controlled by factors related to social status. Hence it is inappropriate to insist that when dogs or cats begin to display behavioral problems at 2 to 3 years of age it is because of "hormonal changes." This simply cannot be logical and is not internally consistent. There surely is an interplay between most hormones (particularly those associated with the adrenal gland) and social status and stress. Hormones involved in social status and stress responses should interact at some level with sex hormones. There is further effect of behavior on brain chemistry and vice versa. Neurotransmitter levels also appear to be affected by adrenal hormones. However, to state that the behavioral changes that occur at social maturity are related to hormonal changes and either explicitly or implicitly, by treating with progestins and other hormones, to imply that the behavioral changes are related to sex hormones, is simplistic and wrong. If this were true, bitches that had gonadectomy at 6 to 8 weeks of age or at any time prepubertally would not experience the problems associated with social maturity.

As a final cautionary word about overemphasis of the endogenous pharmacological environment in the etiology and causality of behavioral problems, it is important to note that most aggression is a social, not a hormonal, condition. The behavioral effects of early spay and neuter programs have not been evaluated (Johnson, 1991; Kahler, 1993; Liberman, 1987). Hormones certainly can act as modulators. Accordingly, work continues on the effects of thyroid hormones and those associated with the hypothalamic-pituitary-adrenal axis. Expect elegant complexity.

SPECIAL CASES

Detailed protocols for the treatment and prevention of specific behavioral problems are found in Appendix B, so the specific treatment steps will not be repeated here. Certain topics, however, warrant slightly more extensive treatment.

Treating Canine Aggression

Factors Involved in Treatment

Diagnosis of aggression is relatively straightforward. The more difficult task is treatment. As stated previously, aggression, like diabetes, is not curable, but may be controllable in the majority of cases. In a retrospective analysis of prognosticators of aggressive cases seen at VHUP, client compliance and extent of effort was the single best determinant of success.

Until clients can seek qualified help for their pets, they should avoid circumstances known to precipitate the specific aggression. With therapy it may be possible to desensitize the dog to circumstances to which it reacts aggressively, but avoidance is key in minimizing danger. When this is explained to clients they tend to be concerned that avoidance means that the dog will now have control—that they are giving in to the dog. This is not what is happening; rather, the dog is not being given the chance to exert control in the manner to which it is accustomed—aggressively. Every time a dog experiences an aggressive event it learns from that event. It learns that it can react aggressively, thus reinforcing those tendencies. Even if the event is eventually aborted by an outside force, it learns the experience of exhibiting aggression. For this reason it is critical to stress avoidance of circumstances leading to aggressive events in the first phase of treatment.

Treatment of canine aggression is both rewarding and frustrating. Because of the potential danger and liability attendant with working with aggressive dogs, everyone involved in treating an aggressive animal must be realistic about what to expect and what they want to do and can handle. Requirements vary from one household to the next. A dog that could live safely and nonaggressively in a childless household may not be able to do so in one with children (Voith, 1981a). It would be unfair and perhaps dangerous to guarantee absolute reliability in *any* dog, even those with no prior history of aggression. Reisner et al. (1994) found that the less predictable the clients found their pets, the higher the euthanasia rate was. It is important to realize that "predictability" is complex but can be honestly evaluated if the clients are willing to learn about and monitor the dog.

There are both dog-driven and client-driven components to predictability of outcome. Dog-driven components largely influence assessment of predictability about aggression and include the dog's signaling intent (how clearly the dog signals) and the timing of the dog's signal with respect to the reaction (how much time occurs between them). The client-driven components include their ability to observe and read the signals and the ability to respond appropriately. Dog-driven and client-driven components are not independent. If the dog has a very short interval of time between the signal and the reaction, the clients will not be as able to respond appropriately. Dogs that give few overt signals and react quickly and clients who read signals poorly and cannot or will not react appropriately to them, are all poor prognosticators because of perceived danger, not necessarily because the dogs are unpredictable. Dogs that signal less clearly and react quickly may in fact be highly predicable, but they do not convey that predictability in as overt a fashion as dogs that give lots of signals and extensive amounts of time between signal and action.

Caution is urged for discrete use of terminology so that clients have an accurate assessment of the situation and their potential role in it. Only in such cases is the best chance for improvement present. By definition, a *first bite* means that the dog has not bitten previously; it may well have been previously aggressive. For those patients treated for aggression, the risks are far more apparent than for the majority of dogs for whom people rationalize less than pristine behavior. Knowing these risks may permit the clients to live safely with the dog and to improve its behavior.

Clients often want guarantees; there are no favorable ones, regardless of the issue discussed, and it would be inappropriate to give any, no matter how sympathetic the veterinarian wants to be. Most clients understand this and are gratified to be able to practice rational risk assessment and risk reduction. The Behavior Clinic at VHUP has a very high success rate with great improvement in more than 75% of all aggressive animals; 90% of aggressive patients improve to the extent that the clients are happy to keep them. Temporary relapses are not uncommon in households with clients who believe that their animals are cured and hence normal after behavior modification. Relapse can occur if clients cease to reinforce the dog's appropriate behaviors. In the case of dominantly aggressive dogs, such reinforcement may mean never letting the dog succeed with subtle, nonaggressive signs of control such as pushing. Euthanasia is a last resort but is preferable to "dumping" a dangerous animal on someone else. With early intervention and improved client education, euthanasia for behavioral problems may become the exception rather than the rule.

The principles of behavioral treatment are not complex but can be difficult to implement correctly. This difficulty lies in understanding exactly what is called for in the behavior modification technique and in the timing of the clients' response to the dog's behavior and communicatory gestures.

PREVENTION OF AGGRESSIVE DISORDERS

Traumatic experiences early in life appear to have a less defined role in the behavioral difficulties of dogs than they are postulated to have for humans (Eron, 1987; Simmel & Baker, 1980). Dogs experience developmental periods during which they are most plastic in terms of responses to certain stimuli. These periods are best defined as sensitive periods; if the animal is not exposed to the appropriate stimuli during these periods, it may never develop the appropriate or desired repertoire of behavioral responses. These periods have been well defined for dogs (see Chapter 3).

Pups that are hand-reared are at risk for developing inappropriate social behavior regarding other canids. If they live in isolation from other dogs during this period (rare) this is possible, but in very few cases of interdog aggression could this be suspected. This is not the norm, but regardless, it sometimes cannot be ruled out.

Pups that stay with breeders for extended periods of time (3 to 4 months of age) without exposure to novel circumstances and individuals may never respond appropriately to them. If these pups are exposed to many people, dogs, and new experiences, even if they stay with the breeder for an extended period, the benefit of exposure should generalize to strangers and changing environments. This is probably some of the logic for taking crated puppies to dog shows. The problematic situation associated with lack of exposure appears to be more common in kennelled pups. When adopted, these pups may exhibit fear of all new, nonkennel environments. This fear can be so crippling that these dogs are unable to go in and out of the house or walk on the street. With behavior modification and pharmacological intervention these dogs can improve, but they are probably never normal. Pfaffenberger and Scott (1959) maintain that pups kept in kennels beyond 14 weeks of age are never normal, exhibiting timidity and a lack of confidence. Pups that are brought home at 8 weeks of age and kept inside with one or a few clients may also find it difficult to make the transition to other environments.

It is clear that the best time to recommend that a client adopt a pup is between 7½ and 8½ weeks of age. At this time the pups are ready to be housebroken and are optimally poised to benefit from exposure to all socialization environments. There are two caveats to this rule of thumb. Later age is acceptable if the dog will be exposed to lots of different people, instead of just one person, at the breeder's. Furthermore, if housebreaking is important to the client, breeders should start this process if the pup remains with them. Remembering that pups learn from novel experiences at this time, the adoption process should not be scary, painful, or associated with horrific circumstances such as traumatic shipping, mutilation, tattooing, or severe punishment. Although observance and understanding of the appropriate periods is no guarantee that future problems will not develop, the client will be able to minimize the risk that future problems are the result of lack of exposure during these periods.

It is important to appreciate that some of the effects of developmental and sensitive periods may be mitigated by the personality of the individual puppy and by the intensity of attention that the animal receives. The extent to which mitigation of the effects of lack of exposure in early life is possible is unclear. Certainly, the one situation in which people have definitely caused the aggressive problem results not from lack of exposure, but from inappropriate exposure: abuse. Dogs that are abused may become fearful, fearfully aggressive, or outright aggressive. Which path is taken may be less influenced by the form of the abuse than by the underlying personality of the dog. Gene × environment interactions are well understood only for rigidly controlled, experimental situations. This does not describe dogs.

An ongoing study at the Behavior Clinic at VHUP to evaluate the effects of early intervention and client education on the development of behavioral problems in puppies has yielded some interesting early results. Regardless of the extent of work the different groups of clients are asked to do with their pups, equivalent proportions in each group are having problems. Each group has pups with severe problems, and each group contains picture-perfect pups. The difference appears to be that the groups that work most intensely with the dog require more from this dog and may provoke signs of resistance or problems earlier. We do not yet know if intervention and correction at an early age will make a difference, but the clients participating in the study are asking questions far earlier than does the average Behavior Clinic client and are working diligently to correct any undesirable puppy responses before the pups learn to incorporate them into their repertoire. Even without knowing outright whether aggression can be prevented, it appears that early intervention may be the next best option. Early intervention can be used only if problems are noted as they appear. Prospective use of the aggression screen (see Chapter 5) can allow clients and practitioners to chart changes in behavior through time and to determine whether any behavioral change is problematic. Such aggression screens can also be used as an objective measure for any improvement in the dog's behavior that occurs in the course of a treatment program.

An example of an aggressive situation that is relatively common and benefits greatly from early intervention is food-related aggression (Elliot & King, 1960). Food-related aggression is often a precursor of dominance aggression. Dogs that are aggressive around their food are also usually aggressive with table scraps, rawhide bones, and real bones. The latter two are excellent elicitors of this type of aggressive behavior. In general, food-related aggression is very difficult to treat; it is usually far simpler and safer to preclude treats, bones, and rawhides and to feed the dog in isolation. This removes possible triggers (O'Farrell, 1986). But what should the client do at the first signs of such aggression, before it has become an intractable problem?

All pups should be taught to sit and stay for verbal praise or food treats; no pup older than 7 weeks of age is too young to learn this. Clients should then routinely practice making the pup sit and wait to be fed and taking the dish away. The first signs of any aggression can be corrected with a sharp "no" and removal of the pup from the situation; the pup must then earn the food back by sitting and staying. The crux of this type of instruction is that the dog sees the client as the one from whom it must take the cues about the appropriateness of the behavior. Should the pup continue to threaten, it is already time to seek professional help. If the pup learns to relinquish its dish to the owner, the potential for dominance aggression later in life should still be discussed.

Dominance aggression commonly develops at social maturity, usually between 18 and 24 months of age (range, 12 to 36 months). Dogs that exhibit this behavioral syndrome challenge and threaten clients or other humans for control (by staring, barking, or growling when given commands, by leaning on people, growling or biting when disturbed while sleeping or when stepped over) will frequently have to have the last word when verbally corrected, and when physically punished, including hanging, will become more aggressive (see Appendix F for necessary and sufficient conditions for behavioral diagnoses). The condition is controllable with proper treatment, but it can be recognized before any biting has occurred if the clients are attuned to the previously mentioned signs. As soon as they recognize these early behaviors, clients need to start a program or schedule of behaviors that compels the dog to give in to the owner for everything it wants. This can be as simple as requiring the dog to sit and stay for all attention, food, play, egress or ingress, and grooming. The dog must learn to take all the cues about whether behavior is appropriate from the client. Absolutely no physical punishment should be used; to do so is to risk the dog intensifying its aggression to the client, thus putting the client in a risky situation. Early intervention can prevent this situation from becoming dangerous and injurious. It should be emphasized to clients that behavioral problems involving aggression are controlled, not cured, and that the dog will have to live with that level of discipline forever.

What about preventing aggression in dogs for whom all the right things were done in puppyhood? Can doing all the right things prevent aggression? There are few studies that have specifically addressed the following questions: (1) to what extent can any training or early intervention prevent the development of behavioral problems? and (2) are there specific circumstances that, if occurring sufficiently early in a dog's life, can either prevent or encourage the development of behavioral problems? These are difficult questions because at their root is the relative contribution of genetic and environmental components of behavior. The problem is as follows. If a puppy that would have had a tendency to be pushy and growl at the clients whenever requested to get off the bed or sit down is taught from 6 weeks of age to sit and be calm for anything it wants before exhibiting any signs of inappropriate behavior, it will not be possible to distinguish that dog from one that had no aggressive tendencies and was also taught the same behaviors. One might assume that both dogs came from the same population when they did not. This is the unascertainable type II error inherent in situations where no problems are apparent. We have no way of knowing if the problems do not exist because they would never have developed, regardless, or if teaching the dog a specific behavioral strategy before the expression of any problems shaped its behavior in a manner not compatible with the development of aggression. We know very little about the environmental and physiological conditions that allow the sequential development of any behavior, especially aggression. Even in cases for which a neuroanatomical modality has been proposed, prior exposure and experience appear to play a major role in the final expression of the aggressive behavior. The only groups we can define are the abuse group (discussed previously) and the group for whom early exposure to a specific behavioral strategy designed to encourage compliance does not prevent aggression. In the latter case we are further handicapped by our inability to know whether the dog would have exhibited even worse behavior had no early attempt been made. We are simply unable to tell whether the aggression was amenable to environmental shaping.

Inherent in this conundrum is the seldom addressed problem of defining aggression in a manner that allows ascertainment of risk for people involved in the interspecific interaction while defining some biologically meaningful parameters for predicting the dog's subsequent behavioral sequence (Frank, 1980). Certainly body posture and vocal communicatory displays can help in anticipating subsequent behaviors from which risk may be estimated, but these are not foolproof estimators of an underlying motivational state. Barking may indicate a lower level of aggression than do growling, snarling, snapping or biting, but some dogs bite without first having even barked. Dogs do tend to be more reactive when standing than when lying down with their head outstretched, and they do have to go through sitting/standing postures to spring when starting in a prone position, but they can do so sufficiently quickly as to render postural signals unusable. So where does this leave us? If any one of the three main sources of communicatory information we can easily glean from a dog (body posture, facial expression, or vocal displays) indicates any aggressive propensity, we should believe it, despite what the other sources may say. At worst, the dog may be experiencing conflict and indecision, and we have minimized the cost of error.

No work has been done on whether any of these sources is more indicative of potential aggression than any other, nor has anyone examined whether a dog exhibiting aggressive intentions using all communicatory sources is more aggressive than one not behaving thus. Much of the theory surrounding aggression supports the view that aggressive displays are associated with a willingness to avoid frank aggression. No studies have been done on dogs that exhibit lesser forms of aggression and the frequency of bites after those aggressive acts. We only tend to hear about dogs that exhibit specific precursor behaviors and bite or lunge. We are woefully ignorant of dogs that go no further than the precursor behaviors and of the factors that mediate this difference in outcome. These are questions that are amenable to empirical and experimental study; as the field of behavioral medicine progresses they will require addressing.

FACTORS AFFECTING THE SUCCESS OF TREATMENT

Five main factors contribute to the success of treatment. These are client compliance, age of onset, predictability of outbursts, duration of the condition, and the pattern of the behavioral changes in response to environmental, behavioral, and pharmacological intervention. Of these, client compliance may be the most critical. Veterinarians rely on clients to administer treatments as we have best learned to prescribe them and to report hopeful or worrisome changes. To do this they have to pay attention. This should be emphasized to the clients up front. If the behavioral therapy then fails, clients will not carry the burden of guilt for the failure if they truly complied. The remaining factors are related. The younger the animal was when the problem started, the less predictable the outbursts, the longer the condition has been present, and the more frequent and intense the rate and extent of the outbursts, the worse the prognosis. Part of the reason for this is because the degree to which the inappropriate behavior has been learned increases with the changes stated for these parameters. The ability of the client to recognize the potential for the aggressive event and to abort it before it happens cannot be overemphasized. Clients sincerely committed to treatment learn to do this wonderfully.

Effects of Clients' Behaviors

Any person can make any behavioral problem worse. With the exception of abusive or neglectful situations, most canine or feline behavioral problems are not created by people. Many feline behavioral problems, particularly those involving elimination, often reflect normal behaviors done in abnormal or undesirable contexts. People are usually truly not part of the problem (Neville, 1992). No text or article that has attempted to implicate people as causal in profound problems that are based in abnormal underlying behaviors has made the case (Serpell & Jagoe, 1995; O'Farrell, 1992). In a study designed to examine whether there is a causal relationship between clients' treatment of their pets and the pets' behavior problems, no correlational or causal relationship could be found (Clark & Boyer, 1993; Serpell & Jagoe, 1993; Voith et al., 1992). This does *not* mean that if clients do not change the way they respond to the pet that the pet will not continue with the problem. It *does* mean that, through ignorance or misinformation, the client can inadvertently worsen the problem. The client's emotional or psychological problems are the client's problems, not the dog's. Some clients who have benefited from psychological or psychiatric counseling may be more willing either to seek care for their pet or to be vocal about their experiences and how their experiences affected their willingness to seek care. This is not the same as attributing a causal role in the problem to clients. Although the clients' problems can affect the way they deal with their pets, the attitude of *any* clients will affect the way they deal with their pet. Clients without specific needs or problems could have a pet that is just as problematic as clients with what might be considered problems or unrealistic needs. There is a problem in attributing causality in the latter situation because it agrees with our own biases. Hypotheses regarding such associations can be tested and, if warranted, can be rejected (Voith et al., 1992). Accordingly, clients who have problems themselves and problem pets that may augment their own problems are a group that should be addressed by human psychologists or psychiatrists, but it is not appropriate to give the impression that unless the pets' problems are solved the clients' will not be, and that if the clients' problems are solved, the pets' problems will go away. This will lead to adaptationist story-telling and will interfere with understanding and treating pets' problems.

Correctly Using Deference Gestures as a Form of Counterconditioning

Ignoring dogs that frequently solicit attention and push clients around is a commonly recommended treatment (O'Farrell, 1992). Ignoring (or not rewarding the animal) certainly has a role, but attention seeking is a situation in which clients can co-opt the dog's behaviors to cause a favorable change that total removal of attention will not effect. When the dog solicits clients for attention, they should move away from the dog until the dog is attending to them (stand up and slough the dog off; become a log and then back away). If the dog leaves, fine. However, if the dog now looks at the clients, they can enforce this quiet, attentive behavior by teaching the dog that if it wants any attention, the dog must earn it, and the only way to do that is by sitting and being quiet. The client can request that the dog sit. If the dog does not do this after one or two tries, the client should ignore the dog. If the dog persists or yaps, the client can say "no." If the dog then still persists, the clients should abandon the dog. The dog will eventually seek out the clients. When this occurs, the clients can repeat the sequence until the dog sits. Eventually, the dog will sit and be quiet. If the client cannot do this, the option still exists of ignoring the dog unless engaged in carefully orchestrated and suitably rewarded interaction that is initiated by the client.

Once the dog does sit for attention and reward, the clients must be vigilant. Dogs that, when released, start pushing on the clients again have learned that the clients can be manipulated. These dogs can be quite sneaky and realize that if they do not paw at the clients, they can lean against them and the clients will not correct them. The clients must be ever vigilant for these subtle behaviors; all attention—even passive attention—must be earned. The dog earns attention through a deferential behavior—sitting and waiting quietly.

If the clients believe that they cannot be vigilant and their dog is very pushy, they can totally ignore the dog *except* when they are working with it. To give the dog ample opportunity to be reinforced and to ensure that it does not become pushier or more anxious as a result of the cataclysmic change in the clients' behavior, clients need to work with the dog frequently (six to eight times each day for 5 to 10 minutes at a time) emphasizing deference and counterconditioning. This is explained more fully to clients in the "Protocol for Deference: Basic Program (Appendix B-1), but the clinician should explain these two dichotomous choices clearly. Clients can segue from the latter into the former, but they still have to be consistent. For the dog's behavior to improve, clients must converge on a set of rules that both they and the dog can apply consistently. If clients switch rules (or apply none), the dog will manipulate the social environment and learn what behaviors are tolerated. The absence of rules is really another rule structure in which the participant in the interaction with the most structure (i.e., the dog) will persevere.

Treatment sessions should proceed for as long as progress can be made. Both clients and dog must be interested and not frustrated, *and* the dog should not be anxious. If the dog starts making mistakes and backslides and no amount of shaping and positive reinforcement can move the dog forward, find an exercise that the dog can successfully complete and stop. Studies have shown that intermittent reinforcement with longer interval schedules is among the most effective patterns to teach and enforce behavior. Longer sessions will allow clients to use this approach. Regardless, clients have to become good enough at watching the dog's cues that they can start increasing the interval between rewards and not teach the dog

that it requires a nonstop stream of reinforcement. An outline for implementing this approach is found in Boxes 12-3 to 12-8.

MISCELLANEOUS ISSUES
Signaling

Prevention involves reading signals. The ease with which this is done can be affected by the breed. Bradshaw and Nott (1995) found that there were qualitative and quantitative differences in signals involved in the maintenance of social relationships and hierarchy that were affected by attributes of breed (e.g., coat length, tail length).

Confinement

Confinement can either help dogs to relax if they find the area of confinement calming or reassuring, or the confinement can cause them to become claustrophobic and to panic. Evaluate the animal's responses to these two different circumstances first, and make an intelligent recommendation based on those observations.

BOX 12-3

TREATMENT PLAN: EMPHASIS ON AGGRESSION

1. Avoid provoking circumstances (learning and reinforcement component)
2. Teach signaling and anticipation
3. Logs?
4. Signs, warnings, cautions
5. Deferential behaviors (sit for all attention)
6. Behavior modification
   - Role of relaxation
   - Role of gradual change
   - Role of reward (salary)
   - Reinforce only appropriate behavior
7. Modification of physical environment
   - Crates
   - Banishment
   - Fences (caution with territorial dogs)
   - Incentives
   - Considerations of degree of reactivity (kennels?)
8. Gizmos
   - Head collars
   - Harnesses
   - Indoor leashes
   - Water pistols and air horns
   - Crates
   - Fences
   - Invisible fences
   - More appropriate toys (Boomer balls, Kong Toys, Kong Co., Lakewood, CO)
9. Role of neutering

BOX 12-4

STEPWISE APPROACH OUTLINE: EMPHASIS ON AGGRESSION

1. Accurately assess aggressive propensities (correct diagnosis critical; consider referral to a specialist)
2. Caution client
3. Design plan appropriate for patient and household
   - Role of neutering
   - Environmental modification
   - Behavioral modification
   - Gizmos
4. Premedication blood studies and examination
5. Recall client in 1 week
   - Assess progress
   - Answer questions
   - Question about specific responses
   - Use responses to confirm or reject your diagnosis
   - Modify plan
   - Schedule reexamination
6. Reexamination
   - Review modification procedures and responses
   - Start next phase of modification
   - Consider drug modifications

BOX 12-6

FACTORS AFFECTING THE SUCCESS OF TREATMENT

1. Age at onset
2. Duration of condition
3. Pattern of changes
4. Predictability of outbursts
5. Response to modification
6. Owner compliance affected by:
   - Understanding
   - Perception of danger
   - Fear
   - Ability to avoid
   - Known, reasonable goals and expectations

Gizmos

There are devices that can be extremely useful in the prevention and treatment of behavioral conditions, but many of these require knowledge of the learning principles discussed in this chapter. Others, if used inappropriately, can be inhumane or dangerous. A brief outline of the classes of devices available and their appropriate use will help.

The electronic age has discovered veterinary medicine, and there are a host of remote control motion de-

---

BOX 12-5

HELPFUL HINTS FOR MAKING THE BEHAVIORAL DIAGNOSIS

Diagnosis

1. Consider diagnosis as a hypothesis to be rejected or confirmed
2. Consider response to therapy as data to confirm or reject hypothesis
3. Realize that specific behaviors associated with the diagnosis are only correlations; therefore it is not necessary for the dog to exhibit every behavior associated with dominance aggression with everyone to be dominantly aggressive
4. Make a problem list
5. Make a frequency/circumstance/likelihood list
6. List diagnoses or problems
7. Cost of error minimization (diagnosis as a hypothesis)
8. Offer to call a specialist or refer to one

Cautions

1. *Any* dog that is aggressive for *any* reason can potentially be dangerous, even if you think that the aggression is *appropriate, in-context* behavior
2. Caution client about aggression, aggressive propensities, and availability of laws (different than dispensing legal advice)
3. Use a "Dog on Premises" sign
4. Warn friends, neighbors, and any relevant township people
   - Referral letters
   - Enlist help in treatment of dog
5. Catastrophic insurance policies
6. Define treatment objectives
   - Teamwork
   - Stop point
   - Disabuse of "cure" potential
7. Offer second (specialist) opinion
8. *Extreme caution* about recommending euthanasia, especially as a "treatment" of first choice
9. Maintain records!

BOX 12-7

POSTDIAGNOSIS OPTIONS

1. Treat in current home
2. Place in a home that will treat
3. Kill—caution for recommending euthanasia when treatment is available (e.g., from a specialist)

BOX 12-8

WHEN TO RECOMMEND PLACEMENT OR EUTHANASIA

1. Placement is an option if clients do not want to deal with the problem pet, or cannot, but the pet could get better in another home *and* that home knows about and is willing to deal with the problem (example: dog that is fearfully aggressive to children, but could go to a childless home; an older client recently lost a pet and will take dog, knowing about the problem with children and the poor leash manners; new owner is willing to work with the dog and will take all precautions).

2. After all therapies, including pharmacological intervention, have failed to produce a diminution in the behaviors and the clients are prisoners, ask them to consider euthanizing the dog; clients are unlikely to be able to place the dog, and this is far preferable to dumping it at a shelter; give the clients permission to not feel guilty, and offer to board the dog for a few days so they can see what it's like to live without the dog.

3. Consider euthanasia if, regardless of compliance on the clients' part and every therapy available, the aggression worsens; emphasize that the clients have not let the dog down.

4. If the dog is profoundly aggressive at the first visit, has all the poor prognosticators, and the clients are fearful of the dog, discuss the option of treatment, but tell clients that if at any point they decide to euthanize the dog, you will not disagree with them.

---

tectors, sound sensors, and containment devices available (Landsberg, 1984). These and their sources are listed in Appendix C.

Tones can alert dogs so that they attend to the client. The dog's alerting behavior must then be followed with instructions about what to do next and rewards for appropriate behaviors. Rewards can be coupled with another type of signal (a different tone or an ultrasonic technique) as a secondary reinforcer as a bridging stimulus that can signal the dog that the be-

havior has been good (e.g., Tattle Tale, KII Enterprises, Camillus, NY). Note that while helpful, the use of such devices requires that clients understand the principles of learning. These devices will not excuse clients from having to participate in the necessary work.

There are a variety of standard (air horn) and more exotic (high-frequency) audible devices that can startle the dog or cat with the intent to prohibit it from continuing in its activity. The client must understand that while useful, such devices do not automatically substitute a new and preferable behavior for the one that annoys them. Behavioral modification is still needed, but these gizmos provide the client with a range of options to use in startle techniques.

Electronic fences can be installed both indoors and out to confine the activities of both cats and dogs. A clever arrangement of these indoors can help protect children from pets and help orchestrate space sharing by pets. Clients should remember that highly motivated animals will sustain a shock to gain access to something that is highly desirable (e.g., attacking another cat). The same principle is used in key-coded electronic collars and pet doors. These can be installed in any door and will permit access to only the animal for whom the collar is coded. Clients also need to remember that animals that are kept segregated from parts of the household may require special arrangements to have their social needs met. Exclusion devices can be coupled with remote reward devices (Pavlov's Cat, Del West Enterprises, San Diego, CA) to encourage behaviors like scratching in a appropriate spot. When the animal performs the desired behavior it receives a treat or toy.

Some of the devices created to prevent human children from wandering from their parents (BeeperKid, Frontgate, Lebanon, OH) may be useful for aiding clients to monitor the location of their pets. These can be useful for housebreaking and teaching recall within boundaries using a two-piece electronic monitor that acts as a mobile perimeter sensor.

Devices that shock animals in the absence of the chance to substitute a more appropriate behavior will not encourage a paradigm shift in the animal's behavior. Electronic blankets that shock animals if they land on them may keep the pets from the sofa that is covered, but not from the bed that is not covered. Some of these devices will record the time that the animal jumped on the blanket, which may be useful for alerting clients to their pets' behaviors in their absence. If the client is covering every surface with such devices, there is more going on here than can be addressed with a gadget.

Electronic shock collars receive a lot of attention, but are probably overused (Polsky, 1994). The two basic types are those that act remotely in response to a stimulus (most bark collars) and those that are triggered by a hand-held unit. Shock can help any animal that can learn to avoid the object of focus. Timing is

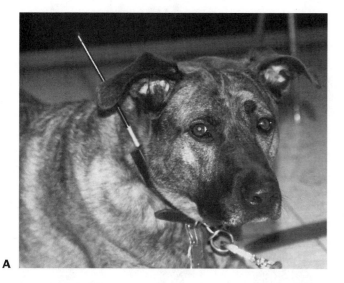

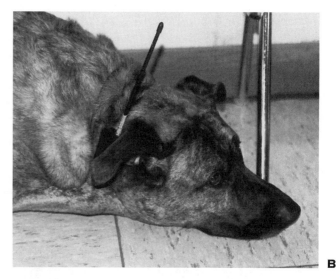

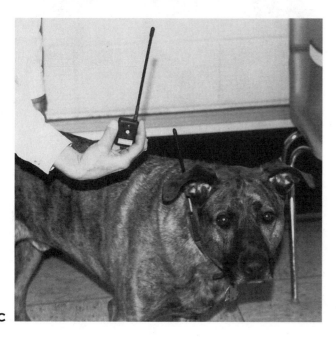

A and B, This dog is wearing a remotely activated shock collar. C, Hand-held control unit. The client actually uses this collar correctly and uses it in conjunction with active and passive behavior modification. The collar is used on this dog only in a particular circumstance: when he begins to lunge at another dog. This dog has been involved in some serious dog fights and weighs more than 60 kg. Once he reacts, no amount of physical intervention can stop a fight or prohibit damage. This dog is never allowed outside without a leash. The client has learned to recognize the behaviors associated with an anticipated lunge and seldom has to employ a shock. The collar has made the client more vigilant, not less. The dog has learned that if the antenna is by his ear (B) he cannot react to other dogs. If the collar is removed, his behavior pattern fully reverts, indicating that the collar hasn't changed his underlying behavior; it only controls his response. When he is wearing the collar he looks at the client when he sees another dog and sometimes whines as he stares at it. The collar also has not changed his underlying motivation. (Photos by K.L. Overall)

critical, and shocks should be instantaneous, and of just the right intensity to startle the animal so that it will abort the behavior and seek another replacement behavior. Inherent in this is teaching the dog a more appropriate behavior *and* rewarding spontaneously good behaviors. Remote-sensing bark/shock collars do not permit the latter two steps to occur. Those triggered by a hand-held unit should be used only in extreme circumstances, in the absence of other solutions, and only by clients who understand and are willing to comply with the amount of behavior modification involved. These clients will be rare, and this should never be a first-choice option. Shock collars are seldom used correctly, are more often overused or inappropriately used, can make any aggressive animal more aggressive, and may tell us more about the peo-

ple who feel that they have to rely on them than about the pet's problem, perceived or real. Dogs can learn to bark below any stimulus necessary to elicit the shock and will only become more anxious if shocked because they bark from anxiety. In a clinical study, nonelectronic citronella collars were found to be more efficacious, more humane, and better received by the clients than were remote electronic shock collars (Juarbe-Diaz, in press).

Options have never been better for controlling canine on-lead behavior. No-pull harnesses fit around the shoulders and apply pressure against the chest, encouraging the dog to slow when it bolts forward. Care must be taken to avoid under-arm rope burns and to not encourage the dog to learn to pull against the harness, but these can be great options for walks for dogs with cervical or tracheal problems or for use in a behavior modification program. Head collars provide more control and give signals that are similar to those that dogs use to communicate with each other. They are safe for dogs with tracheal and cervical problems, allow the client to gain leverage over any dog, especially the head, and in the case of the Promise System/Gentle Leader Canine Head Collar (Premier Pet Products, Richmond, VA), permit the clients to safely close the dog's mouth from a distance. Such collars can make it possible for clients to safely and efficaciously work with dogs that might otherwise pose too great a risk or of whom they are afraid. Both no-pull harnesses and head collars can also prophylactically encourage good behavior and are rapidly replacing choke collars in areas where they are widely available. "Protocol for Choosing Collars, Head Collars, and Harnesses" is found in Appendix B.

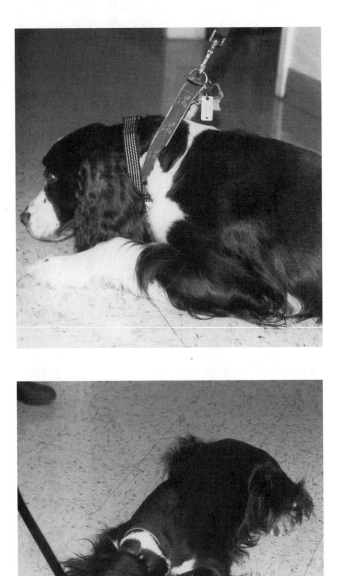

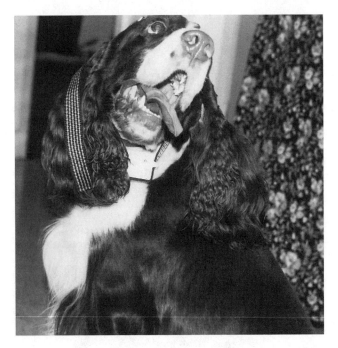

This dog is wearing a citronella bark collar. He lives in an urban apartment and barks at passersby. He has learned to bark just below the level that will trigger the collar, but this is not loud enough to cause the neighbors to complain. When the chamber empties (which is ascertainable by the weight change) he barks louder. He can wear this collar with a head collar (see third photo), which is used for all walks, and people comment on his angelic nature. (Photos by K.L. Overall)

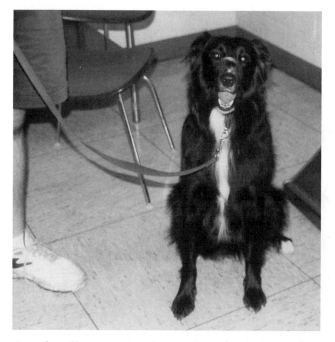

A profoundly aggressive dog can be calm and quiet and remain sitting with the help of a head collar. Notice that he is not snarling, that he can pant, and that the client can hold the leash loosely so that he can comfortably learn the behavior modification. (Photo by K.L. Overall)

Emotionality

"Increased emotionality" later in life has been purported to be associated with neonatal protein deficiency in laboratory mice (Hart & Hart, 1985a). It is not known if there is any association between this and decreased neonatal suckling behavior in dogs that later have problems (e.g., attention, hyperactivity, aggression). Studies on the effect of any aspect of diet on undesirable abnormal behaviors have not demonstrated a definitive link (Crowell-Davis, et al., 1994; Dodman et al., 1996).

Relaxation

Relaxation should not be underestimated as a technique to help in the treatment of fears and anxieties. In conditions such as trichotillomania in humans it has been as effective or more effective than competitive response training (de Luca & Holborn, 1984). It is important to realize that fear reduction and habituation may be related (Rachman & Levitt, 1988).

Age-Specific Ranks

There is no evidence that any "dominance" shown in puppies leads to dominance aggression in adults, nor is there evidence that rank hierarchies of puppies are maintained at social maturity, contrary to assertions made about this (O'Farrell, 1992).

Spaying

For dogs that require antianxiety medication, manipulation of ovarian cycles can be useful. This is usually best addressed by spaying. Removal of ovarian hormones may cause changes in response to medication, including behavioral drugs (e.g., tricyclic antidepressants). Spaying may encourage dogs to gain some weight; estrogen is catabolic. For weight loss or monitoring, starting with puppies, weigh the dog—numbers help.

Nontreatments

There are certain "treatments" that warrant discussion because they are foolish, dangerous, inhumane, or ill-conceived.

Tooth Removal. Animals whose teeth have been removed can still do damage. Occasionally they will stop biting (Houpt, 1991b) because the clients are more able to resist the dog's challenge if they are no longer fearful. Certainly, because the dog is now unable to enforce that challenge with its teeth, it may acquiesce to lower status; however, a very physically competent, confident animal will learn other ways to manipulate clients and could be just as dangerous in the new modality. Large dogs have powerful jaws. It would be a mistake to believe that because a dog is without teeth it has been rendered "safe" or that it can no longer cause injury.

Limb or Tail Removals. If animals are mutilating a body part, removal of the "offending" part, unless it is severely necrotic, is unlikely to help in the treatment of the problem. The problem is not local; it is global, and unless the neurochemical ramifications of the problem (e.g., the anxiety) are treated, the problem will not resolve. The animal will just chew more proximal parts.

Substitution of Activities. Although distraction and substitution can act as a mild form of punishment (O'Farrell, 1992), treatment of obnoxious behavior (stealing food, jumping) by the substitution of a nail clip, bath, ear cleaning and so on (Campbell, 1984) is *not* rational. All that will be encouraged is to teach the dog to dislike and avoid maintenance behaviors. The same logic is applicable to using a crate as punishment. "Time-outs" can occur in a variety of areas and should be short. The crate should be a good place that the animal can then go to reward the cessation of the obnoxious behavior and to give the client some mental and emotional space.

Remember, there is *never* any excuse to encourage inhumanity or abuse.

Mimicking Species-Typical Behaviors. People often impose pulling with a choker collar or scruff-shaking on a dog because they insist that this is what dogs do to dogs. Although intraspecific play and communication may involve bites and holds around the shoulders and neck, these behaviors are not analogous to those

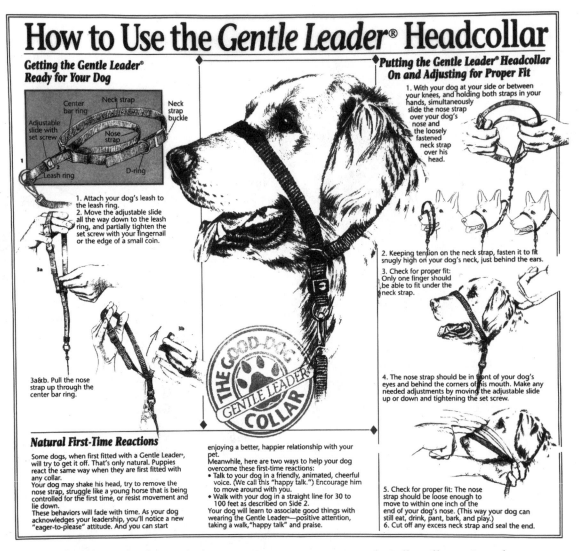

Fig. 12-1 Gentle Leader/Promise System Canine Head Collar illustration that demonstrates the use of innate responses encouraged by the collar. (From R.K. Anderson, 1995, Premier Pet Products, Richmond, Va.)

used by people. In a retrospective study on spinal pain, injury, or changes in dogs conducted in Sweden, Hallgren (1992) found that 91% of dogs with cervical anomalies experienced harsh jerks on lead or had a long history of pulling on the lead. Use of chokers was also overrepresented in this group. This strongly suggests that such corrections are potentially injurious. But are they species typical or mimics of such behaviors? In a study of mother-pup behaviors of litters from 190 breeders, 97.2% of breeders never witnessed scruff-shaking administered by the mother to pups (Hallgren, 1990). In thousands of cases of noted naturally occurring aggression of various forms between dogs, scruff-shaking was noted to be rare and unusual (Schulder & Netto, 1991). Head collars guide the head without injury, while concurrently co-opting the canine signals for control (e.g., manipulation of mouth and gentle pressure on rostral vertebrae [Fig. 12-1]). Corrections that work best are those that use the inherent communication repertoire. Violence seldom meets this criterion.

13 ····· Behavioral Pharmacology

···

*T*here is a potential and very real danger in including any discussion of behavioral pharmacology in a book of this nature. It would be unfortunate if this chapter's inclusion encouraged practitioners to reach for a drug as the first and only mode of treatment for behavioral problems. Facile drug use, particularly that executed in the absence of a diagnosis, is not a component of rational treatment and should be avoided. It is hoped that this will neither be the first, nor only, chapter in this book that is read. If I have encouraged the practitioner to try to treat any behavioral problem merely by reaching for a drug, I have done them, myself, and the field a disservice.

For the purposes of this chapter the terms *behavioral drugs/agents, psychoactive drugs/agents,* and *psychotherapeutic drugs/agents* are used interchangeably, unless otherwise noted. These agents comprise different classes of drugs and may have overlapping functions. A few words on the development of the terminology are warranted. The old term for antidepressant drugs is *thymoleptics.* Although no longer in common usage, this term is still occasionally used to link different classes of drugs. As is true for pets, one of the most common usages of behavioral drugs in human medicine was and is for the control of aggressive behavior. Most of the older behavioral drugs were either benzodiazepines or neuroleptics (antipsychotic/antischizophrenic drugs, or major tranquilizers). These have fallen into disfavor as a primary treatment for aggressive behavior because they lack a specific antiaggressive effect (*sic* mechanism) (Ratey & Gordon, 1993). Decreases in aggression associated with neuroleptics are usually the result of sedation and cognitive dulling, and thus neuroleptics can have adverse effects on the behaviors that they were intended to treat. In fact, it is underappreciated that the frequency of aggression can increase with frequency of treatment with neuroleptics and with increasing doses of these (Yesavage, 1984; Yudofsky et al., 1987). Furthermore, long-term treatment of aggression with neuroleptics (e.g., acepromazine) can include parkinsonian-like symptoms as a result of blockade of extrapyramidal dopaminergic inhibition in the corpus striatum (Ratey & Gordon, 1993).

Beta-blockers, serotonin agonists, and serenics (e.g., eltoprazine [DU 28853]) have fewer side effects, do not negatively affect cognition, and allow more rehabilitation. They positively influence the four axes of cognition, attention, arousal, and mood regulation (Sand & Ratey, 1986). Serenics leave defensive behaviors intact without the problems of sedation or muscle relaxation (Olivier & Mos, 1986). In a dose-dependent manner, serenics such as eltoprazine decrease aggression while concomitantly increasing social interest. In contrast, neuroleptic butyrophenones (e.g., haloperidol) decrease all forms of social interaction (Ratey & Gordon, 1993). These drugs are discussed in more depth later in the chapter. Appropriate usage of behavioral medication implies an appreciation of these advances and a willingness to integrate new information into treatment protocols.

Pharmacological intervention is often useful in facilitating behavior modification. In some cases, the use of psychotropic drugs is essential. However, whether the primary treatment of choice or used as an adjuvant to behavioral therapy, any pharmacological approach must be rational. As is true in human psychiatric medicine, it is almost always inappropriate to prescribe behavioral drugs in the absence of a treatment plan that included other therapies, such as behavior modification. This is true even for behavioral disorders with primarily an "organic" basis, because drug therapy does not ablate all signs of disorders in people in the absence of sustained behavioral therapy (Perse, 1988). Accordingly, clients should be dissuaded that drugs used to modify behavior are a "quick fix". Unfortunately, there is no substitute for hard work that will involve the entire family in a modification protocol; however, some medications may be able to make it easier to implement the modification. Clients and practitioners seeking quick-fix solutions undoubtedly will be disappointed. Inappropriate drug use only blunts or masks a resulting behavior without alteration of processes or environments that produced the behavior.

Before incorporating behavioral pharmacology into any treatment program, the practitioner should have (1) a reasonable diagnosis or list of diagnoses, (2) an appreciation for the putative mechanism of action of the available behavioral drugs, (3) a clear understanding of any potential side effects, and (4) some clear concept of how the drug being considered will specifically alter the behavior in question. This last point is critical because it not only helps clients to watch for side effects and improvements, but can help the practitioner in confirmation or rejection of the original diagnosis. Without these four guidelines, behavioral drugs may not be given long enough or at a sufficient dosage to attain the desired effect, the clients will be unable to participate in the evaluation process, there will be no objective behavioral criteria that will allow the veterinarian to assess improvement, and drug selection is liable to be similar to alchemy.

Client compliance is a crucial factor in the success of any behavioral case. It is critical that the veterinarian and the client communicate frequently and well about alterations in actual behaviors rather than relying solely on subjective client evaluations. This is particularly true when behavioral drugs are involved in the treatment plan. Pets cannot tell us when they begin to suffer from side effects of medication; therefore it important to teach clients to be observant and recognize specific signs of potential adverse reactions. Frequent practitioner-client communication is necessary for this to occur. Pharmacological treatment for behavioral problems does not have to be rare; rather, the client and veterinarian must have clear and reasonable expectations of exactly what behavioral changes can be expected with certain drugs, the time course over which these changes can be expected, and how the drug therapy fits into the overall treatment plan. As the field of behavioral medicine advances, most of the improvements in treatment probably will be based in behavioral pharmacology. Rational use will encourage this.

USING TREATMENT TO HELP TEST DIAGNOSTIC HYPOTHESES

The Newtonian medical model postulates that one biological abnormality has one cure. This assumes a direct linear causal relationship between the two. Most behavioral conditions are probably best represented by nonlinear models (i.e., those that represent multifactorial, heterogeneous disorders). Hence, there is no one drug to treat spraying. Feline spraying is caused by a variety of social circumstances and may be the result of the interactions of a variety of neural substrates. Likewise, not all aggression is neurochemically identical either in impetus or outcome. Diagnosis by pharmacological treatment is usually doomed to failure. *If* the clinician is using a drug that has very specific properties *and* is able to monitor very specific behavioral changes, pharmacological treatment can help the clinician reject an hypothesis about an underlying neurophysiological mechanism; however, response to drug treatment, alone, seldom confirms a causal link. Rational use of behavioral drugs can provide insight into factors affecting behavioral patterns, but only when modification of the pharmacological environment is part of an overall, integrative program that also considers the physical and behavioral, including social, environments can the therapy be considered appropriate and rational.

PREMEDICATION CONSIDERATIONS

Before the practitioner prescribes any drug, a complete behavioral and medical history should be taken. If the animal is older, has any metabolic or cardiac abnormalities, or is receiving any concurrent medical therapy, *caution is urged.* All animals should have a complete cell blood count (CBC) and serum biochemistry profile before treatment with any behavioral medication. Animals cannot tell us when they begin to feel ill. Because most behavioral drugs are metabolized through renal and hepatic pathways, knowledge of these baseline values is essential if needed to evaluate the extent to which mediation caused an alteration. Many of the more commonly (and oddly "safer") behavioral medications can have cardiac side effects. Baseline electrocardiograms (ECGs) are recommended for any patient with a history of any arrhythmia, heart disease, previous drug reactions with concurrent medications, and in the case of anesthesia or sedation. Cats with underlying cardiac disease (i.e., cardiomyopathy) are notoriously asymptomatic; baseline ECG may always be an option when treating cats with psychotropic medication. Liver dyscrasias and cardiac arrhythmias may not completely rule out the use of a drug, but knowing that they exist can serve as a guide to dosage and anticipated side effects. Once alerted to potential adverse reactions, clients are very willing to comply with all monitoring and with the extensive communication needs of behavioral cases. Clients should receive a complete list of all potential adverse responses and should be encouraged to communicate with the clinician at the first sign of any problem. A set of informed consent statements is found at the end of the chapter. These can be used as devices to help reduce liability, but really function to ensure that the practitioner and the client have discussed all options and concerns. Clients are often very distressed after a behavioral consultation and need a written reminder of situations for which they should be alert. A copy of an informed consent statement should be given to the client as part of the discharge instructions and one should be placed in the patient's file.

EXTRALABEL DRUG USE

Licensing and laws governing the use of prescription drugs vary between countries. This chapter reflects United States guidelines, and these may differ elsewhere. The Animal Medicinal Drug Use Clarification Act of 1994 (S-340) provides for the veterinary extralabel use of human drugs, including psychopharmacological agents, for pets if the following conditions are met: (1) there is a valid client/veterinarian/patient relationship, (2) the veterinarian is in compliance with the regulations promulgated by the secretary of Health and Human Services (HHS), (3) practitioners have established a diagnosis and need for treatment, (4) the drugs were prescribed under lawful written or oral order by a licensed veterinarian *and* records are kept, and (5) the extralabel drug used must have a specific rationale, and its use must be accepted under prevailing medical conditions (Brody, 1994). A valid client/veterinarian/patient relationship for situations involving behavioral problems means that a behavioral history was taken, a tentative diagnosis was formulated, and a treatment plan was developed. This precludes reaching for fluoxetine (Prozac) for Mr. Jones' cat simply because the cat is chewing at his tail and Mr. Jones believes that the drug may help. If veterinarians are uncomfortable with complying with these guidelines, they should refer their behavioral cases to a specialist in behavioral medicine.

CLIENT COMPLIANCE

Finally, the client household must be considered when the decision to use behavioral drugs is made. Substance abuse is rampant (in humans) and many drugs used for behavioral pharmacology have high abuse potential. The potential for abuse for each drug listed is discussed below. When considering whether to dispense a drug, both the client and the client's family must be considered. It is far safer to prescribe a smaller amount with only a few refills (and this may also be the law, depending on the agent and the state in which the veterinarian practices), after which time the client must consent to another consultation and evaluation of the pet before renewal of the medication. This strategy provides the veterinarian with the opportunity to objectively assess any questionable behaviors.

Veterinarians must consider the client's ability to administer the drugs as directed. For example, although diazepam can be effective in treating thunderstorm phobias, it has a relatively short half-life and must be administered before the storm begins. This makes its use impractical for many households. Clients should also be advised that many behavioral drugs must often be used for periods of 6 to 8 weeks before any change can be assessed, and for some conditions for which drugs are efficacious, therapy may ensue for the life of the patient. Should the latter be the case, CBC and serum biochemistry evaluations should be performed annually or as dictated by clinical signs. In turn, the results of these tests may indicate that the dosage of the medication be adjusted to meet the patient's behavioral and physiological needs.

PHARMACODYNAMIC CONSIDERATIONS

Before specifically discussing the classes of behavioral drugs and the individual agents, it would be useful to review and define some basic pharmacological terminology with an emphasis on behavioral pharmacology.

The following phenomena should be considered before choosing a behavioral drug. Most of the information in this section is adapted from Kaplan and Sadock (1993) and Rang et al. (1995). The characteristics of these phenomena are known for only a very few drugs when used to treat pets, but it may not be impossible to extrapolate from the human literature because many human drug studies used dogs, particularly for the evaluation of toxic effects.

1. *Receptor mechanism.* This refers to the cellular component that binds the drug and initiates its pharmacological effect (receptor agonist or antagonist). Most psychotherapeutic agents have a receptor that is also a receptor site for an endogenous neurotransmitter; hence, any response involving that neurotransmitter may be altered.

2. *Dose-response curve.* This curve plots the plasma drug concentration against the effects of the drug. The dose-response curve is related to potency, or the relative dose required to get a certain effect. For example, if 5 mg of drug A gives the same effect as 100 mg of drug B, drug A is more potent than drug B, although they are equivalent in their clinical efficacy.

3. *Therapeutic index.* This is the ratio of the median toxic dose (TD_{50}, or the dose at which 50% of the patients will become ill) against the median effective dose (ED_{50}, or the dose at which 50% of the patients will get better). Drugs with low therapeutic indices require more extensive monitoring than those with high therapeutic indices. Unfortunately, the data needed to evaluate these indices in pets are usually unavailable. Data from humans will help to formulate a target zone, particularly for dogs.

4. *Development of tolerance, dependence, or withdrawal phenomena.* Tolerance occurs when there is less response to a drug over time. It is usually associated with a physiological dependence because more drug is needed to achieve the same effect. True physiological dependence occurs when it is necessary to continue the drug to prevent withdrawal symptoms.

Pharmacokinetic interactions are defined by how the body handles the drug (i.e., the plasma concentration of the drug); *pharmacodynamic* interactions are defined by the effects of the drug on the body (i.e., receptor activities of the drug). These are different effects and can be factors in the extent to which therapeutic versus adverse effects are achieved. The *bioavailability* of a drug is the fraction of the ingested dose that gains access to the systemic circulation. This differs from *bioequivalence*, which is what we hope to attain with generic substitutes for trade name drugs. Bioequivalence means that all formulations of the drug will be clinically similar without untoward consequences on the basis of the drug's formulation.

Important properties to consider before dispensing any behavioral medication include absorption, distribution, metabolism, and excretion. Quantitative data on therapeutic dosages are seldom available for nonhuman species.

1. *Absorption.* Tablets dissolve slowly or quickly depending on (1) the drug's concentration and lipid solubility and (2) the local pH of the gastrointestinal (GI) tract, its motility, and its sur-

face area. Hence, if the animal has GI side effects from the drug, those effects have definitely changed the pharmacokinetic, and potentially changed the pharmacodynamic interactions of the medication. Absorption of most behavioral drugs is unknown for animals maintained as pets.

2. *Distribution.* A drug can be dissolved in the plasma, bound to dissolved plasma proteins (albumin) (interstitial or transcellular fluid), dissolved within blood cells (intracellular fluid), or bound to fat. Knowledge of how any behavioral drug responds to the compartments allows the clinician to understand the effects of the drug and to anticipate potential adverse effects.

If a drug is bound very tightly to plasma proteins, it will stay mainly in the plasma component and be metabolized and excreted before leaving the bloodstream; this greatly decreases the amount available to the brain. Drugs (e.g., lithium) that are water soluble and not bound to plasma proteins have a distribution in the brain that is controlled by the blood-brain barrier, the brain's regional blood flow, and that individual drug's affinity for receptors within the brain.

Lipid-*insoluble* drugs are confined mainly to the plasma and interstitial fluids and most do not enter the brain even after acute dosing. Conversely, lipid-*soluble* drugs (e.g., diazepam) reach all compartments and may accumulate in fat. This affects the long-term pharmacokinetics of the compound. This issue is discussed in depth below in the section on cats and diazepam.

The volume of the distribution (which differs for the cerebrospinal fluid [CSF] vs. entire body) varies with patient age, sex, and disease states in humans. One can only imagine the extent to which species and breed can also affect this.

Peak plasma level varies according to the route of administration and absorption. The half-life of a drug ($t_{1/2}$) is the amount of time it takes for half of the drug's peak plasma level to be metabolized and excreted. A first-pass effect can effect this because some drugs undergo extensive metabolism within the portal circulation, thereby decreasing the amount of drug that reaches the systemic circulation. Rapid first-pass effects greatly decrease the bioavailability of any compound. *Clearance* is a term that is used to indicate the amount of drug excreted in each unit of time. Generally, if a drug is administered repeatedly at intervals shorter than its half-life, the drug will reach 97% of its steady-state plasma concentrations in a time equal to 5 times its half-life.

Understanding drug metabolism may be particularly important because so many behavioral drugs have active intermediate metabolites. There are two broad classes of reactions seen in metabolic processes, and both of these subject the drugs to biotransformation. Phase I reactions involve hydrolysis, oxidation, and reduction. These processes generally produce more reactive products and may involve mixed

oxidase systems in which cytochrome P-450 plays a role (inducible, microsomal systems). The same psychoactive compound can undergo multiple routes of phase I reactions. For example, the tricyclic antidepressant (TCA) imipramine, a psychoactive agent commonly used in veterinary behavioral medicine to treat narcolepsy and anxiety-associated disorders, can undergo demethylation and produce an active intermediate metabolite, desmethylimipramine (40% metabolic products), can be hydroxylated (25% of metabolic products), or can be dealkylated (15% of metabolic products). Newly formed intermediate metabolites can repeat the cycle.

Phase II reactions involve conjugation (glucuronidation, glycine conjugation, sulfation, and so forth). These reactions usually form inactive metabolites that are more readily excreted than are parent products; however, *some* of the metabolites produced by these routes of biotransformation *can* be active. When contemplating metabolism it is also important to realize that induction of any enzyme system by other drugs could accelerate the hepatic metabolism of the behavioral drug. This also means that disease states can affect the extent to which renal and hepatic pathways are successful in metabolizing any psychoactive drug. Because of the involvement of renal and hepatic pathways, psychoactive (behavioral) drugs and their by-products are usually excreted in urine, feces, and bile, and may be found in sweat, milk, saliva, and tears. Hence, caution is urged in nursing animals.

Finally, total steady-state clearance ratios may not always reflect the ratio of metabolite-to-parent compound at the site of action. Predicting the latter is complex and one would need to know the extent to which the compound was bound to plasma proteins, the plasma/erythrocyte ratio, and the plasma/CSF ratio (Caccia & Garattini, 1990, 1992). This is one reason that changes in clinical signs are often used to gauge the efficacy of a particular behavioral drug, even in human psychiatric medicine.

Most drugs that are used for their antidepressant effects have at least one metabolite that is pharmacologically significant. Newer drugs such as fluvoxamine, paroxetine, and viloxazine are biotransformed but without active metabolites. This characteristic is one of the reasons that they are so receptor specific. Lithium is an exception to biotransformation; it is excreted unchanged in the urine. The discussion of its modality of action (see below) hints at why this may be true.

A short discussion of the neurotransmitters that are affected by psychoactive drugs follows (Box 13-1).

Biogenic Amines

Acetylcholine. Acetylcholine (ACh) receptors include the muscarinic ones (maChR) and the M_1-receptors, or "neural" receptors that are involved in slow excitation of ganglia and selectively blocked by pirenzepine (M_1-receptor antagonist). Cholinergic pathways include those in the caudal group leading from the

---

---

pons and medulla to the thalamus, those involving short interneurons in the corpus striatum and nucleus accumbens, those in the basal forebrain nuclei (magnocellular), septohippocampal pathways, and recurrent inhibitory pathways in the spinal motor neurons. The most common adverse effects of psychotherapeutic drugs are caused by a blockage of the mAChRs. These adverse effects are not common and may be dose dependent, but include blurred vision, constipation, decreased salivation, decreased sweating, delayed or retrograde ejaculation, delirium, decreased bronchial secretions leading to exacerbation of asthma, hyperthermia, changes in memory, narrow-angle glaucoma, photophobia, sinus tachycardia, and urinary retention. Muscarinic antagonists are associated with amnesia, whereas muscarinic agonists (e.g., arecoline), like centrally acting anticholinesterase drugs (e.g., physostigmine), improve performance of short-term memory. Agrin, a proteoglycan that is released by the nerve, is associated with Ach receptor clustering (Hall, 1995). This may be one key to postsynaptic neuronal differentiation, and may result in more attention paid to ACh in future investigations into the role of neurotransmitters in behavioral disorders.

Catecholamines. There are two main α-adrenoreceptor subtypes: α_1 and α_2. The α_1-receptors activate phospholipase C, which leads to the use of inositol (1,4,5)-triphosphate ($InsP_3$) and diacylglycerol (DAG) as second messengers. The α_2-receptors inhibit adenylate cyclase, which leads to formation of cyclic adenosine monophosphate (cAMP); hence, they are inhibitors of neurotransmitter release (primarily ACh) in central nervous system (CNS) neurons (for example, this is the postulated mode of action for clonidine). The three main β adrenoreceptor subtypes (β_1, β_2, β_3) all stimulate adenyl cyclase. All of these are similar in structure and all belong to the superfamily of G-protein–coupled receptors. Catecholamine responses vary according to receptor subtype. The order of agonist potency for α-receptors is norepineph-

rine (NE) > epinephrine (EPI) > isoproterenol (ISO), whereas for β-receptors the order is reversed (ISO > EPI > NE) (see Fig. 13-1 for biosynthetic and metabolic pathways).

Norepinephrine. Norepinephrine (NE) usually exerts an inhibitory effect through activation of β-adrenoreceptors (via increases in adenylate cyclase and concomitant increases in cAMP), although there are some excitatory effects on both α- and β- receptors. Norepinephrine has been postulated to affect (1) mood (NE decreases in depression and increases in mania), (2) functional reward systems, and (3) arousal. Norepinephrine agonists include norepinephrine, epinephrine, methylnorepinephrine, and clonidine. Norepinephrine antagonists include phenoxybenzamine, phentolamine, ergotamine, dihydroergamine, yohimbine, prazosin, and indoramin.

Interference with NE metabolism can occur presynaptically at calcium gates, synaptically at the vesicle, or in the synaptic cleft through effects on reuptake. The NE release from presynaptic neurons is calcium dependent. Anything that impedes the transport of Ca^{2+} into the presynaptic neuron decreases the amount of NE it releases. The NE is contained in the presynaptic vesicles that must fuse with the membrane to release the NE into the synaptic cleft. Reserpine blocks the transport and fusion of these presynaptic vesicles, depleting NE in the presynaptic neurons. Extracellular reuptake of NE at the level of the cleft is inhibited primarily by TCAs, cocaine, phenoxybenzamine, and amphetamines. Corticosteroids play a secondary role in inhibiting NE reuptake.

The primary NE pathways are in the dorsal and ventral adrenergic bundles; the most prominent cluster of NE neurons is in the locus ceruleus of the pons.

Serotonin or 5-hydroxytryptamine (5-HT). There are four main receptor subtypes for 5-HT. Types 1, 2, and 4 are G-protein–coupled receptors, whereas type 3 is a ligand-gated cation channel (see Fig. 13-2 for biosynthetic pathways).

1. The 5-HT$_1$ receptors are found predominantly in the brain. They are mainly neuronally inhibitory, both presynaptically and postsynaptically. 5-HT$_1$ receptors are G-protein–coupled receptors that linked to the inhibition of adenylate cyclase. This inhibition is linked to the inhibitory effects of 5-HT on NE release. The subclasses of these receptors vary in their effects. 5-HT$_{1A}$ receptors affect mood and behavior. 5-HT$_{1D}$ receptors affect cerebral blood vessels and appear to be involved in the development of migraine (hence the use of sumatriptan). These last two classes of receptor subtypes are the primary focus of many behavioral drugs. 5-HT$_{1C}$ receptors have more recently been recognized as 5-HT$_{2C}$ receptors are linked InsP$_3$ production, not to adenylate cyclase.

2. 5-HT$_2$ receptors are found mainly in the periphery and affect smooth muscles and platelets. The

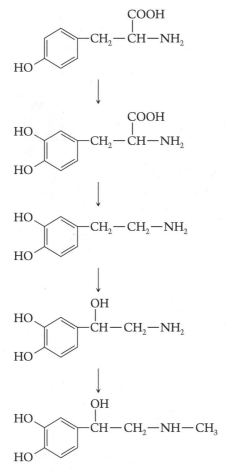

Fig. 13-1 Biosynthesis of catecholamines. (* Enzymes.)

most important of these appears to be the 5-HT$_{2A}$ receptor. This receptor may be responsible for the behavioral effects of lysergic acid diethylamide (LSD). These peripheral receptors are linked to phospholipase C, which acts as a catalyst for the formation of InsP$_3$ formation. They are primarily involved in cellular reactions in asthma and thrombosis.

3. 5-HT$_3$ receptors are found in the periphery of the nervous system, primarily in the nociceptive sensory neurons. They are linked directly to membrane ion channels and do not involve the use of any second messenger. They also occur centrally in the brain, and blocking agents appear to have diffuse anxiolytic effects, because the primary effect is an excitatory one. Ondansetron is a specific 5-HT$_3$ antagonist that is largely used as an antiemetic; however, antagonists of this receptor subtype class should also be anxiolytic.

4. 5-HT$_4$ receptors are found primarily in the GI tract where they increase cAMP production.

The specific agonists for these receptor subtypes are listed at right (Rang et al., 1995).

5-HT Receptor Subtype	Agonists
5-HT$_{1A}$	5-CT
	8-OH-DPAY
	Buspirone (partial)
5-HT$_{1B}$	5-CT
	Sumatriptan
5-HT$_{1D}$	5-CT
5-HT$_{2A}$	α-Me-5-HT
	LSD (CNS)
5-HT$_{2B}$	α-Me-5-HT
	LSD
5-HT$_{2C}$	α-Me-5-HT
5-HT$_3$	2-Me-5-HT
	Cl-Phenyl biguanide
5-HT$_4$	5-Methoxytryptamine
	Metoclopramide

5-CT, 5-carboxamidotryptamine; 8-OH-DPA, 8-hydroxy-2-(di *n*-propylamino)tetraline; α-Me-5-HT, α-methyl-5-HT; 2-Me-5-HT, 2-methyl-5-HT.

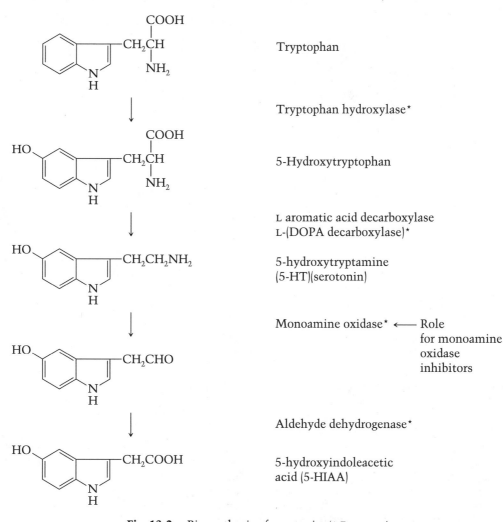

Fig. 13-2 Biosynthesis of serotonin. (* Enzymes.)

The synthesis, storage, release, reuptake, and degradation of 5-HT is similar in both the peripheral and central nervous system. The main factor in synthesis is the availability of tryptophan—hence, some of the more recent over-the-counter "remedies" for anxiety and insomnia. Urinary excretion of 5-hydroxyindoleacetic acid (5-HIAA) is a measure of 5-HT turnover, and this has been used to assess neurochemical abnormalities in human psychiatric patients. For example, during human migraine attacks urinary 5-HIAA increases sharply, whereas blood concentrations of 5-HT decrease, probably because of depletion of platelet 5-HT. Evaluation of urinary levels 5-HIAA technique has potential for veterinary medicine.

Centrally, 5-HT neurons are concentrated in the pons and the medulla, primarily in the caudate nuclei. They have diffuse projections to the cortex, the limbic system, the medial forebrain bundles, the hypothalamus, and the spinal cord. 5-HT stimulates peripheral nociceptive nerve endings and can cause either excitation or inhibition of CNS neurons, and thus have been implicated in control of appetite, sleep, mood, hallucinations, stereotypies, pain, and central emetic effects. Tryptamine has been termed both a neurotransmitter and neuromodulator (Mousseau, 1993).

Mechanisms of drugs affecting 5-HT include (1) increased production of 5-HT, (2) decreased uptake of 5-HT, (3) recruitment of more receptors, or (4) alteration of postsynaptic neuronal metabolism. The main class of 5-HT reuptake inhibitors are the TCAs (e.g., amitriptyline, imipramine, nortriptyline, clomipramine). Whereas TCAs also inhibit NE reuptake, the carrier affecting inhibition of 5-HT reuptake is different. Specific antagonists include spiperone,* methiothepine,* and ergotamine (partial antagonist). Agonists include 5-CT, 8-OH-DPAT, and, of clinical relevance, buspirone (partial agonist). Newer serenics like eltoprazine act primarily as specific $HT_{1\alpha}$ agonists.

*Not available in the United States.

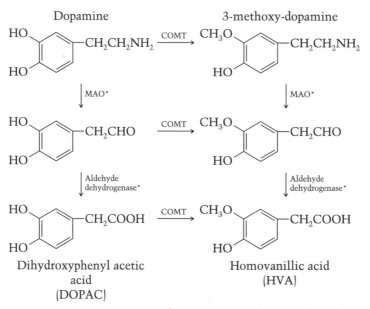

* Enzymes; *MAO*, Monoamine oxidase; *COMT*, caticol-O-methyl transferase.

Fig. 13-3   Primary dopamine metabolic pathways in the brain.

Dopamine. The distribution of dopamine in the brain is nonuniform but far more restrictive than that of NE. A large proportion of the brain's dopamine is found in the corpus striatum, the part of the extrapyramidal system concerned with coordinated movement. Dopamine has also been found to be high in some regions of the limbic system. Dopamine is metabolized by monoamine oxidase (MAO) and catechol-O-methyltransferase (COMT) into dihydroxyphenylacetic acid (DOPAC) and homovanillic acid (HVA) (Fig. 13-3). HVA is used as a peripheral index of central dopamine turnover. Presynaptic dopamine turnover appears increased in patients with early-onset schizophrenia; HVA is low in these patients, and this significant partial correlation between positive symptoms and serum HVA suggests a relative increase in the sensitivity of dopamine-associated responses in these patients (Steinberg et al., 1993). Dopamine has been implicated in an M_2-receptor–mediated increase in potassium (K^+) conductance in a slow inhibitory postsynaptic potential (IPSP).

Dopaminergic neurons form three major systems: (1) the nigrostriatal pathway, source of 75% of the brain dopamine (this is what is affected in Parkinson's disease); (2) the mesolimbic pathway; (3) the tuberoinfundibular system, source of prolactin release inhibition and growth hormone (GH) release stimulation.

All dopaminergic receptors are G-protein–coupled transmembrane receptors. There are two main classes of receptors: D_1 (includes D_1 and D_5), which are mainly postsynaptic inhibitory receptors; and D_2 (D_2, D_3, and D_4), which are presynaptic and postsynaptic inhibitory receptors. The D_1 receptors exhibit their postsynaptic inhibition in the limbic system, result-

ing in increases of cAMP as a second messenger, and are affected in mood disorders and stereotypies. D_2 receptors act through a decrease of cAMP as a second messenger. The D_2, D_3, and D_4 receptors are all affected in mood disorders and stereotypies. D_4 has specifically been implicated in schizophrenia and has been shown to be polymorphic in humans. Excess dopamine, as produced by dopamine-releasing agents (amphetamines and dopamine agonists, such as apomorphine) is correlated with the development of stereotypies.

Dopamine receptor antagonists compose most of the class of drugs referred to as antipsychotics (neuroleptics are the subset of antipsychotics known as major tranquilizers). These include (1) phenothiazines, (2) thioxanthenes, (3) dibenzoxazepines, (4) dihydroindoles, (5) butyrophenones, (6) diphenylbutylpiperidines, and (7) benzamides. Clozapine acts as a dopamine antagonist. Specific agonists include dopamine, apomorphine, and bromocriptine.

Gamma-aminobutyric acid. GABA is produced in large amounts only in the brain, and it has been estimated that GABA serves as a neurotransmitter in 30% of the synapses in the human CNS. It is the inhibitory neurotransmitter found in short interneurons. The only long GABA-ergic tracts run to the cerebellum and striatum. GABA is formed from glutamate via glutamic acid decarboxylase (GAD). It is destroyed by transamination, which is catalyzed by GABA-transaminase (GABA-T).

There are two main groupings of GABA receptors: $GABA_A$ and $GABA_B$. $GABA_A$ receptors, which belong to the class of ligand-gated ion channels, appear to mediate postsynaptic inhibition by increasing Cl^- influx. Barbiturates and benzodiazepines are a potentiators of GABA$_A$. GABA$_A$ receptors occur in a variety of peripheral neurons (autonomic ganglia cells) where GABA has no transmitter role; thus benzodiazepines appear to have no potent effects here. GABA$_B$ receptors are prevalent at presynaptic terminals and belong to the family of G-protein–coupled receptors. They increase K$^+$ conductance and decrease Ca^{2+} conductance. GABA$_B$ receptors are found at dopamine-releasing terminals of the striatum and peripheral sympathetic terminals.

GABA agonists include muscimol ($_A$) and baclofen ($_B$), whereas GABA antagonists include bicuculline ($_A$) and baclofen ($_B$).

Valproic acid (Depakene) increases GABA, by means of decreased catabolism. It has potent anticonvulsant effects and has been shown to be helpful in the treatment of some human bipolar disorders. Zolpidem (Ambien), an imidazopyridine is a newer hypnotic medication that binds GABA-benzodiazepine receptor complex but may not have the undesirable effects of benzodiazepines.

Nonbiogenic Amine Transmitters

Excitatory Amino Acids (EAAs). Excitatory amino acids are receiving much attention both for their role as central neurotransmitters and their abnormal levels in some aggressive, impulse, and schizophrenic disorders and in onset of childhood autism (Barthelemy et al., 1988; Hoehn-Saric et al., 1991; Rolf et al., 1993; Sahai, 1990). Increased binding of the glutamate antagonist MK-801 has been reported in Parkinson's disease and in dopaminergic nigrostriatal fiber degradation. It has been postulated that increased glutamine activity in the hippocampus and putamen may compensate for decreased dopaminergic activity. L-Glutamate and other acidic amino acids chemically excite spinal neurons. Glutamate and aspartate cause depolarization of neurons and may be involved in epileptogenesis. The main fast excitatory transmitters in the CNS are glutamate, aspartate, and, possibly, homocysteate. The Krebs cycle acts as the main source for glutamate and aspartate. Glutamate is formed from the Krebs cycle intermediate metabolite α-oxoglutarate by action of GABA-aminotransferase. The metabolic and neurotransmitter pools are linked by interconversion of glutamate and α-oxoglutarate. Glutamate is widely and fairly uniformly distributed in the CNS. It is involved in both carbohydrate and nitrogen metabolism. Glutamate is stored in synaptic vesicles and released by Ca^{2+}-dependent exocytosis. Hence, calcium channel blockers may play a role in the treatment of conditions that are associated with increased glutamate. Both barbiturates and progesterone suppress excitatory responses to glutamate (Sohn & Ferrendelli, 1976). Presynaptic barbiturates inhibit calcium uptake and decrease synaptosomal release of neurotransmitters, including GABA and glutamate (deBoer et al., 1982).

EEA substrates are either directly coupled to cation channel receptors (N-methyl-D-aspartate [NMDA], OC-amino-3-hydroxy-5-methyl-isoxazole [AMPA/Kainate]), or act through intracellular second messengers (metabotropic). NMDA channel receptors are highly permeable to Ca^{2+} and blocked by Mg^{2+}. These ions play a role in long-term potentiation. NMDA-operated ion channels are blocked by dizocilipine, ketamine, and phencyclidine. NMDA receptors require glycine as a co-agonist with glutamate and are more sensitive to endogenous glutamate than are AMPA channel receptors. Excessive Ca^{2+} production by NMDA receptor activity causes cell death through excitotoxicity. This may be one of the mechanisms through which aggression is affected. Tonic glutamate tone via NMDA receptor stimulation appears to modulate the firing rate and burst activity of some dopamine neurons (Christoffersen & Meltzer, 1995). Competitive NMDA-receptor antagonists include AP5 and CPP; unfortunately, these are not available in a form suitable for treatment.

Other Chemical Mediators. Nitric oxide (NO) and arachidonic acid metabolites (e.g., prostaglandins) can mediate neurotransmitter release. These are synthesized on demand and released by diffusion and therefore require no specialized vesicles or receptors. However, like encapsulated neurotransmitters (e.g., ACh) that are extruded through exocytosis after binding with the synaptic membrane, these chemical mediators are activated by an increase in calcium. Any change in NO may affect a change in glutamate, and excitotoxic and aggressive effects of glutamate may be partially modulated by NO (Snyder, 1995). Accordingly, calcium channel blockers may have profound behavioral effects. Their potential use to primarily treat behavioral problems is discussed below.

Classes of Drugs Useful in Behavior Modification

Classes of drugs that are useful in behavioral cases include, but may not be restricted to:
1. Antihistamines
2. Tranquilizers
3. Mood stabilizers/antipsychotics
4. Anticonvulsants
5. Progestins/estrogens
6. Sympathomimetics/stimulants
7. Monamine oxidase inhibitors
8. Nonspecific anxiolytics and tricyclic antidepressants
9. Narcotic agonists and antagonists
10. Miscellaneous drugs: β-adrenergic agents, calcium channel blockers, and so on

It is important to realize that many of the drugs in these classes have shared functions and mechanisms of action, and their effects may, in part, be dependent on the dosage schedule. For example, "anxiolytic drugs" can include benzodiazepines, 5-HT$_{1A}$ receptor agonists, barbiturates, and β-adrenoreceptor antagonists. Many drugs (e.g., benzodiazepines) act as hypnotics at high dosages, anxiolytics at moderate

TABLE 13-1 DRUG DOSAGES*

	Cats	Dogs
Acepromazine	1.1-2.2 mg/kg PO 0.11-0.22 mg/kg IM, SQ, IV	0.55-1.1 mg/kg PO 0.055-0.11 mg/kg IM, SQ, IV
Alprazolam	0.125-0.25 mg/kg PO q 12 h	0.125-1.0 mg/kg PO q 12 h (range can be so extreme as 0.01-0.1 mg/kg prn; should not exceed 4 mg/day); profound lethargy and incoordination will result)
Amitriptyline HCl	0.5-1.0 mg/kg PO q 12-24 h Start at 0.5 mg/kg PO q 12 h	1-2 mg/kg PO q 12 h to start
Atenolol*	6.25-12.5 mg/**cat** PO q 24 h	0.25-1.0 mg/kg PO q 12-24 h to 20-100 mg/**dog** PO q 8 h
Bethanecol Cl		2.5-10 mg/**dog** SQ q 8 h 5-25 mg/**dog** PO q 8-12 h
Buspirone	2.5-5 mg/**cat** PO q 8-12 h × 6-8 wk 0.5-1mg/kg PO q 8-12 h × 6-8 wk	1 mg/kg PO q 8-12 h (mild anxiety) 2.5-10 mg/**dog** q 8-12 h (mild anxiety) 10-15 mg/**dog** PO q 8-12 h (more severe anxiety) (use high dose for thunderstorm phobia)
Carbamazepine		4-10 mg/kg/day divided q 8 h 4-8 mg/kg PO q 12 h
Chlordiazepoxide		2.2-6.6 mg/kg PO prn (start low)
Chlorpheniramine	1-2 mg/**cat** PO q 12-24 h (low) 2-4 mg/**cat** PO q 12 h (high)	0.22 mg/kg PO q 8 h
Clemastine (time-released)	0.68 mg/**cat** PO q 12 h	0.05-0.10 mg/kg PO q 12 h
Clomipramine HCl	0.5 mg/kg PO q 24 h	1 mg/kg PO q 12 h × 2 wk, then 2 mg/kg PO q 12 h × 2 wk, then 3 mg/kg PO q 12 h × 4 wk or 2 mg/kg PO q 12 h × 12 wk
Clonazepam	1.5 mg/kg PO q 8 h	
Clorazepate	0.55-2.2 mg/kg PO prn 0.5-1.0 mg/kg PO q 12-24 h	0.55-2.2 mg/kg PO q 4 h 11.25-22.5 mg/dog PO q 24 h (~ 22.5 mg/**large dogs**; ~ 11.25 mg/**medium dogs**; ~ 5.6 mg/**small dogs**)
Dantrolene*	0.5-2.0 mg/kg PO q 12 h	0.5-2.0 mg/kg PO q 12 h
Dextroamphetamine		0.2-1.3 mg/kg PO prn 1.25 mg/**dog** PO prn (narcolepsy)
Diazepam	0.2-0.4 mg/kg PO q 12-24 h (start at 0.2 mg/kg PO q 12 h) As appetite stimulant, give q 8-24 h	0.55-2.2 mg/kg PO prn (1.0-2.2 mg/kg PO just before start)
Diethystilbestrol		0.1-1.0 mg/d for 3-5 days, then decrease to 1 mg/wk or 1 mg q 2-3 day
Diltiazem*†	0.5-1.0 mg/kg q 8 h (antiarrhythmic dose)	0.5-1.0 mg/kg PO q 8 h (antiarrhythmic dose)
Diphenhydramine		2.2 mg/kg PO q 8 h
Doxepin	0.5-1.0 mg/kg PO q 12-24 h	3-5 mg/kg PO q 8-12 h
Fluoxetine	0.5 mg/kg PO q 12-24 h (start at 0.5 mg/kg PO q 24 h) × 6-8 wk	1 mg/kg PO q 24 h × 6-8 wk
Flurazepam	0.1-0.2 mg/kg PO q 12-24 h (appetite stimulant)	0.1-0.5 mg/kg PO q 12-24 h (appetite stimulant)
Hydrocodone	0.25-1.0 mg/kg PO q 12-24 h 1.25-5.0 mg/**cat** PO q 12-24 h (start at 1.25 mg/cat PO q 12 h)	0.25 mg/kg PO q 8 h
Hydroxyzine		0.5-2.2 mg/kg PO q 8-12 h
Imipramine	0.5-1.0 mg/kg PO q 12-24 h (start at 0.5 mg/kg q 12 h)	1-2 or 2-4 mg/kg PO q 12-24 h (start at 1-2 mg/kg PO q 12 h) 0.5-1.0 mg/kg PO q 8 h (narcolepsy)
Levoamphetamine		1.0-4.0 mg/kg PO prn
Lithium		6-12 mg/kg q 12 h

*Includes those for drugs that may prove useful but that are not yet used for behavioral problems; caution is urged for indiscriminant use of agents that can induce bradycardia and possibly sudden death (indicated by †).

TABLE 13-1   Drug Dosages—cont'd

	Cats	Dogs
Medroxyprogesterone acetate (MPA)	10-20 mg/kg SQ, IM 50 (female)-100 (male) mg SQ, IM 3 times/year	5-10 mg/kg SQ, IM 11 mg/kg SQ, IM 3 times/year (caution; outdated; last resort only)
Megestrol acetate	2.5-5.0 mg/**cat** PO q 24 h 2.5-5.0 mg/**cat**/wk 5-10 mg/**cat** PO q 24 h × 1 wk then decrease q 2 wk to minimum effective dose	2.2-4.4 mg/kg PO q 24 × 7 days, decrease by half × 2 wk then continue to decrease by half every week 1.1-2.2 mg/kg PO q 24 h × 2 wk, decreasing by ½ q 2 wk
Methylphenidate HCI		5 + mg/**dog** (small) PO q 12 h; up to 20-40 mg/**dog** (large) 0.25 mg/kg PO q 24 h (narcolepsy)
Naloxone HCI		11-22 μ/kg SQ, IM, IV
Naltrexone	25-50 mg/**cat** PO	2.2 mg/kg PO q 12-24 h
Nortriptyline	0.5-1.0 mg/kg PO q 12-24 h	1.0-2.0 mg/kg PO q 12 h
Oxazepam	0.2-0.5 mg/kg PO 1 12-24 h 3 mg/kg PO (bolus) (appetite stimulant)	0.2-1.0 mg/kg PO q 12-24 h 0.2-1.0 mg/kg PO q 12-24 h
Pentazocine + naloxone		50 mg pentazocine + 0.5 mg naloxone/**dog** PO q 12 h
Phenobarbital*	2-3 mg/kg PO prn	2-6 mg/kg PO q 8-12 h
Phenoxybenzamine	1 mg/kg PO q 24 h	1 mg/kg PO q 12-24 h
Phenylpropanolamine		12.5-50 mg/**dog** PO q 8-12 h 1.0-4.0 mg/kg PO q 8-12 h
Promazine	2-4 mg/kg PO, IM prn	1.0-4.0 mg/kg PO, IM prn
Propranolol		Small: 5 + mg/**dog** PO q 8 h Large: 10-20 mg/**dog** PO q 8 h
Protriptyline		5-10 mg PO/**dog** q 12-24 h (narcolepsy)
Triazolam	2.5-5 mg/**cat** PO q 8 h	
Verapamil†	0.03 mg/**cat** PO q 12 h	0.5-1.0 mg/kg PO q 8 h

Range of doses indicated; see text for cautions and prohibitions.
NOTE: Some dosages extrapolated from those used in canine cardiac and gastrointestinal patients.
h, Hour(s); *IM,* intramuscularly; *IV,* intravenously; *PO,* orally; *prn,* as needed; *q,* every; *SQ,* subcutaneously; *wk,* weeks.
From Chapman & Voith, 1990a; Chrisman, 1995; Davenport, 1995; Dodman, cited in Marder, 1991; Fratta et al., 1976; Goldberger & Rapaport, 1991; Hart, 1980a, 1985c, 1991; Houpt, 1991b; Knecht et al., 1973; Lapras, 1977; Marder, 1991; Parker, 1983; Schwartz, 1993; Shell, 1995; Shouldberg, 1990, cited in Marder, 1991; Shull-Selcer & Stagg 1991; Voith, 1984c, Voith & Marder, 1988.

dosages, and mild sedatives at low dosages. Cellular mechanisms of action, despite the preceding discussion, are seldom fully understood. In general, behavior drugs are thought to act in one of four general ways: (1) they block receptors, preventing postsynaptic responses (antagonists), (2) they stimulate postsynaptic receptors (agonists), (3) they inhibit metabolic breakdown of the active compound in the synapse (e.g., selective serotonin reuptake inhibitors [SSRIs]), and (4) they metabolically stimulate the presynaptic neuron. One of these mechanisms can affect the others, as is the case for selegiline.

Dosages of the most common drugs used in behavioral medicine are found in Table 13-1.

Antihistamines. Antihistamines act by competitive inhibition of the H_1 receptor site. They are often used to treat drug-induced extrapyramidal signs and have mild hypnotic (more pronounced with diphenhydramine [Benadryl]) and sedative effects (more pronounced with hydroxyzine [Atarax]). The sedative effects usually appear within 30 to 60 minutes after administration and can last 4 to 6 hours. These drugs are well absorbed in the GI tract, can experience a 50% first-pass hepatic metabolic effect, and are largely excreted in the urine and feces.

Many of the classes of antihistamines have anticholinergic or atropine-like effects, or both, and so should be used cautiously in patients when such effects are undesirable or contraindicated (urinary retention, glaucoma, hyperthyroidism). Occasionally, for example, in dogs that may dribble urine, this anticholinergic effect is desirable; hence, for animals that may have inappropriate urination associated with mild situational anxiety, these side effects can be a boon.

The most common undesirable side effect, mild CNS depression, usually results in sleepiness. It is in the form of this side effect that these drugs may be useful in control of behavioral problems. Chlorpheniramine, an alkylamine, and diphenhydramine, an ethanolamine, may be useful as a mild sedative for animals that are either apprehensive of certain situations or overactive at inappropriate times. Indications include travel in the car, late-night activity patterns, and some unexplained pacing accompanied by vocalization when the client is home with the animal. Control of such problems may sufficiently modify the home environment that the client is more willing to make schedule adjustments or use behavioral modification that will ultimately lead to altered pet behavior, rather than pharmacologically controlled behavior.

The antipruritic effect of these compounds on dogs and cats is not impressive unless the drugs are used at relatively higher dosage (see Table 13-1); any benefit achieved may be related to the mild sedative effect (Griffin, 1991; Miller & Scott, 1994; Miller et al., 1992). One week trials of antihistamines including clemastine, chlorpheniramine, diphenhydramine, and hydroxyzine, have been recommended for the treatment of pruritus in dogs and cats, with the best effects being noted for clemastine and chlorpheniramine (Miller & Scott, 1994). For dogs that have pruritus and anxiety combined (and it is important to remember that the two are neurochemically linked), doxepin, when used as long-term therapy as part of an integrated treatment program, may help to maintain self-mutilatory conditions such as acral lick granuloma/dermatitis (ALD) at a tolerable level for both dog and client.

Although cyproheptadine is a potent antihistaminic and serotonin agonist (5-HT$_2$), antihistaminic drugs are not the drug of choice for chronic anxiolytic therapy. Nonspecific anxiolytics, TCAs, and some monoamine oxidase inhibitors (MAOIs) are much more preferred for this. Regardless, antihistamines should not be used within 2 weeks of MAOI treatment. Diphenhydramine should be used with caution in very small animals because the CNS depressant effects can be profound. Hydroxyzine falsely elevates urinary 17-hydroxycorticosteroids when assayed by Porter-Silber or Glenn-Nelson methods (Kaplan & Sadock, 1993).

Tranquilizers. Tranquilizers are used for their calming properties. They cause a decrease in spontaneous activity that generally results in a decreased response to external or social stimuli. This decreased responsiveness can profoundly interfere with any concomitant training or behavioral modification. In humans, tranquilizers are often successfully used to alleviate anxiety, although the accompanying sedative effects have rendered many of the newer anxiolytics, which have fewer sedative effects, more suitable. There are three main classes of tranquilizers that are commonly used in veterinary medicine: phenothiazines, benzodiazepines, and butyrophenones. Only the first two classes are discussed in depth below.

The *phenothiazines* include chlorpromazine (Thorazine), promazine (Sparine), acetylpromazine (acepromazine), perphenazine (Trilafon), trimeprazine tartrate (Temaril-P), propiopromazine (Tranvet), triflupromazine (Vesprin; Vetame), thioridazine, and piperacetazine (Psymod). The primary receptor site for chlor-

promazine (Thorazine) is a dopamine receptor, and phenothiazines act as dopamine antagonists. All phenothiazines have side effects from long-standing use that include cardiovascular disturbances, primarily hypertension, and extrapyramidal signs, including ataxia, muscle tremors, and incoordination. Interestingly, low-potency antipsycotics (e.g., phenothiazines) are more cardiotoxic than are high-potency drugs. Chlorpromazine prolongs QT and PR intervals, blunts T waves, and depresses the ST segment. Thioridazine has marked T wave effects. The tranquilizers are seldom used in continuous, long-term behavioral therapy in veterinary medicine (Jones, 1987).

Tranquilizers are largely inappropriate as a treatment for aggression because they blunt both normal and abnormal behavior, rather than treating the cause of the aggression. Acepromazine, in particular, should be used cautiously in restraint of aggressive dogs because they are more reactive to noises and startle when under its influence, and the level and duration of tranquilization varies, rendering the animal more unpredictable. This is an unacceptable and unwarranted effect for treatment of an aggressive animal. Sudden aggressiveness and periodic bouts of excitement have been reported in dogs treated with acepromazine (Waechter, 1982). Phenothiazines are well known for their potentiation of seizure activity; whether this characteristic is a factor related to the aggression effects is unknown. Use of acepromazine can also be problematic in the presence of pseudocyesis because prolactin is inhibited by dopamine and phenothiazines are dopamine antagonists.

Benzodiazepines include diazepam (Valium), chlordiazepoxide (Librium), clorazepate (Tranxene), lorazepam (Ativan), alprazolam (Xanax), triazolam (Halcion), and clonazepam (Klonopin). The exact mechanisms of action of the benzodiazepines are poorly understood, although the calming effects are postulated to be the result of their action on the limbic systems and reticular formation. Compared with cortical effects of treatment with barbiturates, the cortical function is relatively unimpaired by treatment with benzodiazepines. Wild animals have been reported to exhibit decreased aggressiveness and a "taming effect" when treated with diazepam.

The anxiolytic effects of benzodiazepines are distinct from their nonspecific consequences of CNS depression (e.g., sedation and motor impairment). At low dosages benzodiazepines act as sedatives and facilitate daytime activity by tempering excitement. At moderate dosages they act as antianxiety agents and may facilitate social interaction in a more proactive manner. At high dosages they act as hypnotics and facilitate sleep. Ataxia and profound sedation usually occur only at dosages beyond those needed for anxiolytic effects. Benzodiazepines decrease muscle tone by a central action that is independent of the sedative effect. Cats are very sensitive to this action. It is unclear whether some of the anxiolytic effects for which the benzodiazepines are so well known are attributable to

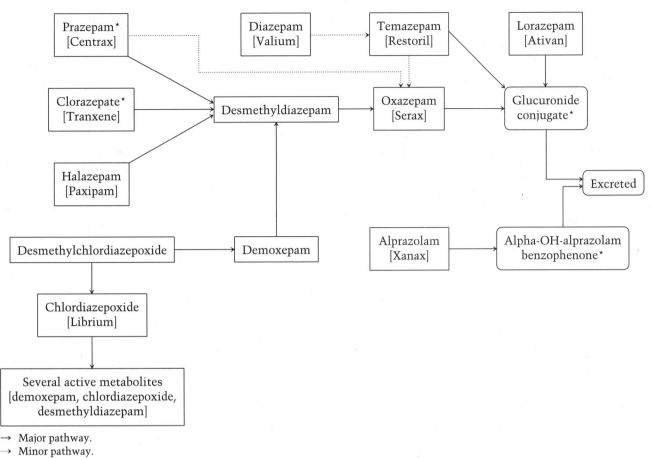

→   Major pathway.
⋯→   Minor pathway.
*   Pharmacologically inactive.

Fig. 13-4   Benzodiazepine metabolic pathways. (From Facts and comparisons: drug information, 1984; modified by A. E. Dunham.)

muscle relaxation because muscle tension is one of the nonspecific signs of anxiety. Some newer benzodiazepines (e.g., clonazepam) have muscle relaxation effects at smaller dosages than those needed for behavioral effects.

With the exception of clorazepate (Tranxene), all benzodiazepines are absorbed completely unchanged from the GI tract; clorazepate is converted to the active intermediate metabolite, desmethyldiazepam (nordiazepam) in the GI tract, and is then completely absorbed. The benzodiazepines vary widely in their half-lives, time required to attain peak levels, and so on, but absorption, attainment of peak levels, and onset of action are quickest for diazepam (Valium), lorazepam (Ativan), alprazolam (Xanax), triazolam (Halcion), and estazolam (ProSom). This rapid onset of activity is important for patients with medication prescribed to curb a single, situational burst of anxiety (e.g., thunderstorms). Alprazolam is particularly useful in blunting panic attacks associated with anticipation in separation anxiety and thunderstorm phobias (Shull, 1994).

All benzodiazepines have high lipid solubility, but the extent to which this is so varies fivefold with the individual compound. Benzodiazepines are widely dis-

tributed, and 80% to 99% is bound to plasma proteins. Estimates in cats suggest 94% plasma protein binding (Greenblatt et al., 1981, 1983). It should be noted that protein binding greatly decreases in patients with renal insufficiency. Any situation that causes hypoproteinemia or hypoalbuminea will increase the drug's volume of distribution. The average time to peak plasma levels is 1 to 3 hours (prazepam [Centrax] takes up to 6 hours), and there is a secondary peak plasma level 6 to 12 hours after enterohepatic circulation.

The primary route of metabolism of the benzodiazepines is through hepatic biotransformation. This is impaired in patients with chronic liver disease and could result in overdosing. Most of the drug product is excreted entirely in the urine as oxidized and glucuronide-conjugated metabolites.

The role of intermediate metabolites is critical in both the functioning and toxicity of the benzodiazepines (Figure 13-4). The common intermediate metabolite, *N*-desmethyldiazepam (nordiazepam), has a slow half-life: all 2-keto-benzodiazepines have plasma half-lives on the order of 30 to 100 hours in humans (Greenblatt et al., 1981). Hence attainment of steady-state plasma levels can take 2 weeks, and human patients can experience toxicity after 7 to 10 days. If a patient receives repeated doses of diazepam, the effects of *N*-desmethyldiazepam (nordiazepam) can be expected to be cumulative. This may be particularly important for cats when one considers that the plasma $t_{1/2}$ of diazepam in cats after IV injection is 210 minutes before the drug is metabolized to *N*-desmethyldiazepam (nordiazepam); only 3% of the intermediate metabolite is recovered in feline urine after 8 hours (Schwartz et al., 1965). This suggests that caution should be urged when any factors that can increase intermediate metabolite $t_{1/2}$ (obesity, repeated dosing, renal impairment) are involved.

Conversely, 3-OH-benzodiazepines (oxazepam, lorazepam, temazepam), on the other hand, have short half-lives (10 to 30 hours) because they are directly metabolized through glucuronidation and have no active intermediate metabolites. In humans, lorazepam (1 to 2 mg every 2 to 4 hours) has been more effective than carbamazepine for the control of acute agitation (Kaplan & Sadock, 1993).

The triazolodiazepines alprazolam and triazolam are hydroxylated before glucuronidation and have half-lives of 10 to 15 hours, and 2 to 3 hours, respectively, in humans. α-OH-Alprazolam, the active intermediate metabolite of alprazolam, is half as active as it, but has the same $t_{1/2}$.

The issues of intermediate metabolite activity and binding properties are important ones to consider before choosing a benzodiazepine for any patient, human or nonhuman. Although there have been recent reports of potential benzodiazepine toxicity in cats (Center et al., Hughes et al., 1996), the potential toxic effects of benzodiazepines have been recognized for years (Owen et al., 1970, 1971; Tedesco and Mills, 1982). *N*-desmethyldiazepam (nordiazepam), the intermediate metabolite of diazepam, has putatively been suggested to be responsible for most of the anxiolytic effects and side effects of diazepam in cats (Colter et al., 1984b; Overall, 1992b). The elimination half-lives of both diazepam and *N*-desmethyldiazepam (nordiazepam) are prolonged in obese patients because, although the total clearance does not change, the distribution of the drug does. Any drug that is lipophilic and has an active intermediate metabolite that also has a prolonged $t_{1/2}$ could be potentially toxic in individuals who are obese or those who may have compromised hepatic function. This effect should be particularly exaggerated in cats because they do not use glucuronic acid pathways as efficiently as do other species, and there is extensive binding or localization of diazepam and *N*-desmethyldiazepam in the cat (Placidi et al., 1976). Repeated elevation of alanine transaminase or gamma-glutamyl transferase activity (ALT/GGT) has been associated with acute hepatic necrosis after a challenge test with diazepam (Tedesco & Mills, 1982). This illustrates the importance of premedication blood studies, thorough behavioral and physical examinations, rational dosing, and monitoring of both favorable responses and potential side effects.

All benzodiazepines appear to potentiate the effects of GABA, an inhibitory CNS transmitter, through their affects on GABA binding sites and chloride channels. They are postulated to increase binding affinity of the GABA receptor for GABA, thereby increasing the flow of chloride ions into the neuron. $GABA_A$ receptors mainly occur postsynaptically and are directly coupled to chloride channels. When these chloride channels open, membrane excitability is decreased. $GABA_B$ receptors are primarily responsible for presynaptic inhibition and act by means of second messengers. There may also be at least two subtypes of CNS binding receptors: BZ_1 (Ω_1) and BZ_2 (Ω_2): BZ_1 receptors are thought to mediate sleep or hypnotic effects, whereas BZ_2 receptors are thought to mediate cognition, memory, and motor control. Benzodiazepines with fewer cognitive side effects (quazepam and halazepam) are more specific for the former. Binding of diazepam is highest in the cerebral cortex compared with the limbic system and midbrain, which are, in turn, higher than the brainstem and the spinal cord. This patterns appears to parallel that of $GABA_A$ receptors.

There are peripheral benzodiazepine receptors, which appear to be regulators of calcium channel function.

Two common, relevant usages of the concept of "tolerance" are used to discuss drug use. *Pharmacokinetic tolerance* is the product of lower blood concentrations with prolonged usage. This is a common sequela to use of drugs that induce hepatic microsomal enzymes. The second form of tolerance is *tissue tolerance*, which is often a result of changes in responsiveness of receptors. Benzodiazepines produce some degree of the latter, although the anxiolytic effects and dosages appear to be less prone to this than do the sedative effects and dosages. In studies of laboratory animals treated with diazepam, physiologic and behavioral dependency seems to be indicated by tremors, twitches, hyperactivity, and increased anxiety after withdrawal (File, 1990; Giorgi et al., 1988). Regardless, particularly for humans with opposable thumbs, appearance of withdrawal or discontinuation syndrome is a concern with the benzodiazepines (most of which are Drug Enforcement Agency (DEA) schedule IV drugs). These depend on the length of time the patient has taken the drug, the dosage, the rate at which the drug dosage is tapered, and the half-life of the compound. These are concerns for any veterinary patient, but because these drugs are controlled substances the practitioner also must evaluate the human household into which the medication might be sent. It is often an appropriate decision to not treat some animals with benzodiazepines because of the concerns for the clients. Regardless, because of the potential for these types of effects in animals the general recommendation should be as it is for humans—withdrawal of benzodiazepines should be through tapering by 25% per week. Benzodiazepines are primarily used to treat anxiety—both generalized and that associated with specific life events. They have also been used to treat human bipolar disorders (clonazepam [Klonopin]) and as an adjuvant to lithium therapy in acute mania. Panic disorder and social phobias in humans have been successfully treated with alprazolam and clonazepam. These drugs have not been frequently used in small animals, but they may have both more beneficial effects and fewer side effects than some of the traditional benzodiazepines.

Other adverse reactions to benzodiazepines include mild paradoxical reactions (most common in the first 2 weeks of use), hyperexcited states, anxiety, hallucination, increased muscle spasticity, insomia, and acute rage in human psychiatric patients and hyperactive children. The paradoxical excitement has been reported for cats treated with oral diazepam. If the excitement does not subside within 1 to 2 days of drug treatment or with a decrement in dosage, it is probably best to withdraw the drug.

Flumazenil is the competitive antagonist for benzodiazepines, but its use has not been explored in cats.

Long-term use of benzodiazepines in humans has been associated with isolated reports of neutropenia, jaundice, abnormal liver function, and decreased hematocrit. No long-term data evaluating effects on these parameters have been published for small animals.

Benzodiazepines have been successfully used in the inhibition of some forms of intercat aggression and for treatment of some manifestations of feline spraying. Diazepam appears to be effective in reducing substantially the incidence of feline spraying in about 75% of cases; the percentage is higher in castrated males, lower in spayed females, and higher in multicat households, and in 43% of all cases, spraying ceased totally (Marder, 1991). Cats that respond to diazepam stagger for the first 3 to 4 days of therapy; thereafter the staggering spontaneously resolves (Voith, personal communication, 1987; Overall, personal observation, 1987). This further suggests that intermediate metabolite is responsible for efficacy. If the spraying is related to aggressive or territorial behavior, the effect could be related to the tendency of benzodiazepines to increase friendly behavior. If the stimulus for spraying is marking that is related to anxiety about social status or territoriality, the effect could be mediated through anxiolytic actions. Little attention has been paid to these alternate modes of action. As a consequence, it is conceivable that many behavioral problems are actually syndromes that are multicausal. Such factors could contribute to the extent to which various treatments are effective to the exclusion of others in individual cases. Appreciation of multiple causality leading to singular signalment should lead to innovative and alternate therapies in "refractory" cases (see expanded discussion on this topic in Chapter 9).

Chlordiazepoxide (Librax) has also been reported to be efficacious in suppressing spraying behavior (Houpt, personal communication, 1989). It appears to have more a variable peak time and half-life than other benzodiazepines. Another benzodiazepine that has not been widely used but may be efficacious in such situations is alprazolam (Xanax) (Marder, 1991). The benzodiazepines vary in their kinetics; this may be the reason that some cats respond better to one type than another. The similar efficacy of each of the compounds is probably related to their common intermediate metabolite, desmethyldiazepam (nordiazepam).

Benzodiazepines have also been successfully used in the treatment of thunderstorm and other noise phobias (Shull-Selcer & Stagg, 1991; Voith & Borchelt, 1985b). They must be administered 3 to 4 hours before the onset of the fearful event so that there is an adequate level of the drug systemically to counteract the CNS and physiological effects of the anxiety at the onset of the stimulus. For thunderstorm phobias they need to be administered, minimally, at the first sign of a decrease in barometric pressure. Because benzodiazepines have short half-lives they need to be readministered as needed, generally every 3 to 6 hours during the phobic stimulus. Clorazepate dipotassium comes in a sustained-release form (Tranxene-SD) that may facilitate administration.

It should be noted that all benzodiazepines can interfere with the ability to learn and so may affect the progress of training programs.

No practitioner should just reach for any benzodiazepine to treat aggression; this approach could backfire. The disinhibiting effects of benzodiazepines, in fact, may lead to the precipitation of hostility or aggression. Cats treated with diazepam as an appetite stimulant have been reported to demonstrate increases in predatory aggression, possibly associated with changes in activity in the lateral hypothalamus (Pellis et al., 1988). Proaggressive responses have been noted in rats treated with low doses of benzodiazepines; aggression is decreased only at quite high doses (Mos & Olivier, 1989).

The butyrophenones (haloperidol and azaperone) have virtually no behavioral indications. Haloperidol has been shown to potentiate interpig aggression, but may have some use in treating obsessive-compulsive behaviors in animals. It has been used with mixed success to treat feather-picking in birds and some obsessive-compulsive disorder (OCD) in humans.

Mood Stabilizers/Antipsychotics. Mood stabilizers/antipsychotics such as lithium (available as a carbonate, Li_2CO_3 [Lithane], or citrate [Cibalith]) are useful in controlling the manic phase of manic-depression in humans and have been used in humans to treat schizoaffective disorder, cyclic major depressions, and impulse disorders that are not premeditated and seem untriggered. The lithium ion, monovalent and an alkali metal, is water soluble and therefore is not bound to plasma proteins; thus its distribution in the brain is determined by the blood-brain barrier, the brain's regional blood flow, and the drug's affinity with receptors in the brain. The receptor for lithium appears to be the intraneuronal enzyme inositol-1-phosphatase. This enzyme inhibition is postulated to lead to a decreased cellular response to neurotransmitters that are linked to the phosphatidylinositol second messenger system.

Because it is water soluble, lithium is completely absorbed and reaches peak serum levels within $1/2$ to 2 hours (4 to $4\frac{1}{2}$ hours when administered in the sustained release form) in humans. The half-life is about 20 hours, and steady-state levels are reached within 5 to 7 days of regular intake. Because lithium is water soluble, excretion is impaired if renal compromise is present. Toxic effects can be profound. Although no clinically significant effects on glomerular filtration may be apparent for many years of lithium treatment, clinically significant changes have been reported with long-term use (Gitlin, 1993). Furthermore, the range of toxicity and efficacy overlap. Most of the data for these dosage ranges in dogs are from animals treated with lithium or cyclic neutropenia. Lithium carbonate is usually administered to dogs at 6 to 12 mg/kg orally every 24 hours, which will generate a serum level of 0.8 to 1.2 mEq/L; the toxic level is 1.0 to 1.5 mEq/L. The use of lithium requires frequent blood monitoring (every 2 months) including creatine, triiodothyronine/thyroxine (T_3/T_4), and possibly a thyroid-stimulating hormone (TSH) assay, CBC, and ECG. At present drugs such as lithium are not widely used in companion animals. Should companion animals be found that are good models for human psychosis, this could change (see Reisner, 1994). Mood stabilizers have been shown to be effective in combination with TCAs in the management of human OCDs that do not respond to tricyclics alone (Insel, 1990). This effect has been postulated to be the result of the enhancement of function of presynaptic 5-HT receptors that have been sensitized by long-term TCA treatment (de Montigny, 1981). Combination therapy is underexploited in veterinary behavioral medicine.

Most of the typical "antipsychotics" are agents that have specific dopamine receptor effects. These can include clozapine and, to a lesser effect, bromocriptine. Clozapine (Clozaril; *do not confuse with clonazepam (Klonopin), entirely different drug*) may be an effective antiaggression agent (Volkava et al., 1993; Wilson, 1992). It functions through preferential blockage of the D_1- and D_2-mediated functions and appears to have a specific role in animal models of self-abuse (Meltzer, 1990; Ratey & Gordon, 1993). Bromocriptine (Parlodel), a derivative of ergot alkaloids, is a mixed dopamine agonist/antagonist. Its agonist effects are most profound at D_1 CNS receptors. Because it inhibits the anterior pituitary, its first use was for the treatment of galactorrhea and gynecomastia. Humans experience its anxiolytic properties at doses of 10 mg/day, and it has been effective in the treatment of OCD. It is long acting and has a plasma half-life of 6 to 8 hours. Bromocriptine has been used in depression *only* in experimental modes. Side effects include further depression if the patient experiences a decrease in dopamine and mania that has been associated with too much dopamine. Bromocriptine has shown some promise as a treatment for spraying cats when tested in a repository injectable form (Seksel, 1995), but has never been developed for market.

Anticonvulsants. Anticonvulsants include phenobarbital (a barbiturate), phenytoin (diphenylhydantoin; [Dilantin], a hydantoin), and primidone (Mysolene).

Barbiturates bind plasma proteins well. The extent to which these agents are lipid soluble depends on their side group. Barbiturates are metabolized by the liver and excreted by the kidneys and thus have half-lives that range from 1 to 120 hours. These compounds can induce hepatic enzymes and may actually decrease the functional level of circulating barbiturate and any concurrently administered drug. Barbiturates affect the GABA receptor–benzediazepine receptor–chloride ion channel complex. This latter effect has been the one desired for treating behavioral conditions; however, it is usually inappropriate, in the absence of a specific neurological diagnosis, to use barbiturates for treatment of behavioral problems. They have fallen into disuse for those purposes in human patients, largely being superseded by benzodiazepines and TCAs, but are still occasionally used if patients have profound side effects to the latter classes of drugs or for activation of a catatonic patient. This suggests that they are overused in veterinary behavioral medicine.

Phenobarbital has been successful in controlling excessive feline vocalization in cats when used in small doses. Long-term therapy with any of these agents requires blood monitoring because all agents are potentially hepatotoxic. With the exception of feline vocalization, there are currently few indications for these compounds in behavioral medicine that would not be better served by some other drug. Again, in dosages sufficient to inhibit aggression, administration of barbiturates results in a heavily tranquilized animal that exhibits altered normal and abnormal behaviors. Such effects produce pets that are unacceptable in their overall behavior to the client. Furthermore, the level of tranquilization is variable and unpredictable, making these drugs unacceptable for long-term control of aggression.

All barbiturates can affect the metabolism of anticoagulants, other anticonvulsants, corticosteroids, adrenocorticotropic hormone (ACTH), estrogen, and progesterone.

Although any of the above-mentioned anticonvulsants have been used to treat putative behavioral disorders, they all can have detrimental effects on cognition (Mayhew et al., 1992) and, largely because of this, *are no longer used to treat aggression in humans.*

This suggests that recommendations to use any of these anticonvulsants to treat overactive behaviors that may be incidences of psychomotor epilepsy (Dodman, 1992) or aggression (Houpt & Reisner, 1995) may be outdated. These drugs were originally tried in the treatment of aggression because some of them, particularly phenytoin (Dilantin), had appeared to be particularly effective in controlling hyperactivity and explosive aggression in humans.

The current anticonvulsant of choice for treating implosive aggression in humans (episodic dyscontrol) is carbamazepine (Tegretol), an iminodiabenzyl derivative of imipramine (Barratt, 1993). It is important to realize that this is only one form of human aggression (others include those that are medically related and premeditated with instrumental responses) and that there are relatively stringent diagnostic criteria associated with it. Carbamazepine has also been used in humans to treat temporal lobe epilepsy, trigeminal neuralgia, and acute mania. It has also been used, with some success, prophylactically in the treatment of bipolar disorder in humans. The efficacy of carbamazepine in such cases has been postulated to be the result of its effects on sodium ion channels and potential effects on peripheral benzodiazepine receptors in the brain. It also may potentiate α-adrenergic receptors. Carbamazepine is slowly and erratically absorbed from the GI tract and is better absorbed if ingested with food. In humans, it reaches peak plasma levels within 2 to 8 hours, has a half-life of 12 to 17 hours, and has an active intermediate metabolite that also has anticonvulsant properties. Carbamazepine has been used in dogs to treat motor activity that may be associated with seizurelike activity (Holland, 1988). Dosages overlap those in humans (400 to 1600 mg/day in divided doses) and, as with humans, the therapeutic concentration necessary to obtain antiepileptic effects (6 to 10 μg/ml) is lower than that necessary to obtain psychiatric or behavioral effects (8 to 12 μg/ml) (Parker, 1983); however, serum levels were not a useful guide for response. Carbamazepine can have profound side effects that include agranulocytosis, aplastic anemia (these occur in 1:20,000 human patients), and decreases in T3, T4, and the free T4 index, although the risk of hypothyroidism appears rare (based on references in Kaplan & Sadock, 1993).

Progestins/Estrogens. Progestins/estrogens include medroxyprogesterone acetate (Depo-Provera) and megestrol acetate (Ovaban, Megace), and diethylstilbestrol (DES). The former are frequently used in behavioral medicine because of their calming effects (possibly because of their ability to suppress the excitatory effects of glutamate [Sohn & Ferrendelli, 1976]) and their suppressant effects on male stereotypic behaviors. In rodents, progestins have been noted to decrease aggression without a decrease in general locomotor behavior (Fraile et al., 1988). In humans, cyclicity of epileptic seizures (decreases in seizure susceptibility) has been associated with increases in estrogen and progesterone. Progesterone has been reported to have anticonvulsant effects. Progesterone metabolites have been reported to be 10 to 50 times more potent than barbiturates in potentiating GABA-receptor–coupled Cl⁻ conductance in cultured embryonic rat hippocampal neurons (Taubøll & Gjerstad, 1993). Currently there are no direct applications for this. The most common use of progestins in veterinary behavioral medicine is as a nonspecific calming agent. There are generally better behavioral medications for this and ones that are more specific (hence safer).

Rational, competent use of these compounds includes physical examination and initial and repeated blood studies to monitor systemic side effects that may include diabetogenesis, gynecomastia, mammary gland hyperplasia, adenocarcinoma, endometrial hyperplasia/pyometra, adrenal cortical suppression, and bone marrow suppression (Peterson, 1987). DES has been used in the treatment of resting urinary incontinence, although there may be safer agents that are equally efficacious. Among these are bethanecol, which is particularly effective if the bladder is enlarged, and phenylpropanolamine (PPA), which is a sympathetic agonist. PPA is commonly used as a decongestant and diet aid; one of its side effects is increased bladder tone, necessitating contraindication in cases of urinary retention. Because of the profound range of potential side effects with progestins, some veterinarians insist that clients sign informed consent forms or releases before administration of these agents.

Progestins formerly had a role in some forms of aggression (Beaver, 1982c; Hart, 1974a, 1979c, 1980a; Knol & Egberink-Alink, 1989a,b) but should be used judiciously (if used) and may have been surpassed by newer antianxiety medication. The effect of progestins in aggression can be related either to the calming or feminization actions. Accordingly, they have also been used to successfully treat male stereotypic canine behaviors such as mounting and marking (Hart, 1979c). Spraying cats that do not respond to diazepam have been reported to respond to progestins (Hart & Cooper, 1984; Romatowski, 1989). Cats treated previously with progestins for spraying also responded to diazepam (Marder, 1991). Given the efficacy and relative safety of other classes of compounds, these may be best left as the *last drug tried*. Contraindications include breeding animals, animals with diabetes, and patients undergoing concurrent corticosteroid therapy. Enlargement of mammary glands has been reported in about 6% of cats treated with megestrol acetate. Although no tumors were reported in this study, metastatic breast disease has been reported in dogs after 3 years of progesterone treatment (Frank et al., 1979). Other studies have reported the development of adenocarcinomas in cats after prolonged treatment with repository progestins (Hernandez et al., 1975). Regardless, no animal should be treated with

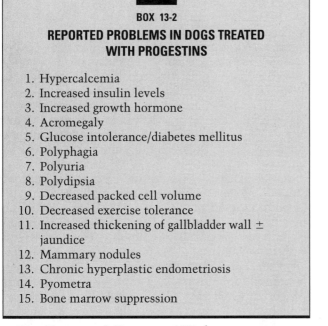

progestins without prior consent and disclosure, prior blood studies, and frequent follow-up blood tests, should treatment persist. A complete list of reported side effects of progestin use is found in Box 13-2. *Do not ever use these drugs as first-choice therapy.* I look forward to the day when they are never used.

Testosterone does not receive much attention when behavioral drugs are discussed, but this may change in the future. Recent evidence indicates that vasopressin disappears after castration. Testosterone binding sites in the medical amygdala interact with vasopressinergic neurons and sexual differentiation of vasopressinergic innervation of the lateral septum (peripheral testosterone) (references in Rang et al., 1995). This raises the question of whether antivasopressinergic drugs or medications (e.g., finasteride [Proscar]) would affect aggression. Finasteride is a specific inhibitor of steroid α-reductase, the enzyme that converts testosterone into the potent androgen dihydrotestosterone (DHT). Androgen antagonists (e.g., delmadinone (Tardak)) have been used in place of castration (O'Farrell, 1992). This appears to be largely for reasons of human vanity. Delmadinone has also been used to treat aggressive behavior in male dogs (Stabenfeldt, 1974). The following concerns should be addressed:

1. Male dogs can be involved in many kinds of aggression; treatment in the absence of a putative diagnosis is careless and could be a potential cause of litigation.
2. Dogs with a diagnosis of aggression should be neutered; most aggression appears to have some genetic basis.
3. There are far more specific drugs for the treatment of aggression; the best pharmacologic

treatment choices are the most specific and selective, while being the least restrictive.

Sympathomimetics/Stimulants. Stimulants such as dextroamphetamine (Dexedrine), methylphenidate (Ritalin), and pemoline (Cylert) have paradoxical effects in truly hyperactive animals: in these abnormal animals they have a calming function, whereas in normal individuals they produce excitement. Methylphenidate is commonly used in humans to decrease inattention and to increase self-control (Gadow et al., 1990). A case has been made primarily for short-term use, along with behavioral modification, to increase motivation (Arnold et al., 1973). The primary human usage is for the treatment of attention deficit–hyperactivity disorder (ADHD) and narcolepsy, although patients with the latter tend to become tolerant to the drugs over time. The half-life of dextroamphetamine is 8 to 12 hours and that of methylphenidate is 3 to 4 hours. Both of these are administered 2 to 3 times per day and reach peak levels in 1 to 2 hours. Pemoline has a very long half-life, allowing for dosing once every 24 hours. Because they are sympathomimetic amines with CNS stimulant activity, attendant effects include increased heart and respiratory rate, possible anorexia, and tremors with possible hyperthermia. Stimulants are contraindicated for patients with cardiovascular disease, glaucoma, concurrent MAO therapy, and hyperthyroidism. It is important that patients for whom these are prescribed for the treatment of hyperactivity be truly hyperactive, rather than overactive or energetic. Such patients should display physiological signs of hyperactivity (heart rate [HR], respiratory rate [RR] increases) in addition to the behavioral signs. If the condition worsens on administration of the drug, the condition is *not* a hyperactive one and may be better treated by behavioral therapy, changes in diet, and increases in exercise. Truly hyperactive states are rare in canine and feline patients (see review in Marder, 1991). Truly hyperactive dogs respond to treatment with 0.2 to 1.0 mg/kg methylphenidate with a $\geq$15% decrease in HR and RR 75 to 90 minutes after-treatment (Corson & Corson, 1976; Corson et al., 1971, 1980).

Monamine Oxidase Inhibitors and Tricyclic Antidepressants. Antidepressants that are commonly used in behavioral therapy are primarily MAOIs or TCAs. The former act by blocking oxidative deamination in brain amines (dopamine, norepinephrine, epinephrine, 5-OH-tryptamine). This results in an increase of these substances, stimulating mood elevation. They are seldom used in companion animal behavioral therapy and are best used in human therapy for nonresponsive, atypical depression. The exception to this is the MAO-B inhibitor, selegiline (Deprenyl), which is being used to treat what has been described as cognitive dysfunction in aged canines (Cummings et al., 1993; Head & Milgram, 1992; Milgram et al., 1990, 1993; Ruehl et al., 1994a,b). This is particularly interesting because in dogs, deamination of catecholamines is

TABLE 13-2 COMPARISON OF TRICYCLIC ANTIDEPRESSANTS

Drug	Anticholinergic Effect	Sedative Effect	NE Reuptake	5-HT Antagonism
Imipramine	++++	+++	++	+++
Doxepin	+++	++++	++	+++
Clomipramine	++++	+++	0	+++

After Koblenzer, 1993.
0 Effect absent or relatively small.
+ Some effect.
++ Pronounced effect.
+++ Large effect.
++++ Most notable effect.

TABLE 13-3 TCA SEDATIVE POTENTIAL

Potential	Agent
Greater	Amitriptyline
	Clomipramine
	Imipramine
	Nortriptyline
Lesser	Desipramine

controlled by MAO-A, not by MAO-B (Milgram et al., 1993). Selegiline is specific for dopamine and appears to decrease its deamination (Brandeis et al., 1991). This in turn slows destruction of the synaptic knobs of presynaptic neurons (Knoll et al., 1989; Milgram et al., 1990). Improved cognitive function is perceived at dosages of 0.5 to 1.0 mg/kg orally every 12 to 24 hours. Spontaneous behavior is unaffected at doses below 3 mg/kg orally every 24 hours, but above this level, the development of stereotypic behaviors has been reported.

MAOIs irreversibly inhibit MAO. With the exception of selegiline, most drugs in this class are MAO-A inhibitors (phenelzine [Nardil], isocarboxazid [Marplan], tranylcypromine [Parnate]). Maximum inhibition is experienced after 5 to 10 days, but it can take 3 to 6 weeks for the antidepressant effect to become apparent. A standard assay for efficacy is to measure platelet MAO activity. If it decreases by 80%, the patient is considered to have a therapeutic level of the drug. MAOIs (type A) are typically used in humans to treat agoraphobia, panic attacks, and depressions, whereas type B MAOIs have been successful in treating conditions associated with cognitive dysfunction (Parkinson's disease, Alzheimer's disease, Huntington's disease) (Kitani et al., 1992; Knoll et al., 1989; Milgram et al., 1990).

It is important to note that tyramine-containing foods should be avoided or decreased with MAO treatment. Finally, if MAOIs are administered concomitantly with TCAs, serotonin syndrome may result. The signs of this include autonomic instability, hyperthermia, rigidity, myoclonus, confusion, delirium, and coma.

TCAs are closely related in structure to the phenothiazine antipsychotics and hence have similar secondary side effects. They are commonly used to treat endogenous depression, panic attacks, phobic and obsessive states, neuropathic pain states, and enuresis in children. They may also be of use with attention deficits because they increase catecholamine action through norepinephrine reuptake inhibition; this may be particularly true for desipramine. These effects may be modulated through the postsynaptic receptor (Zametkin & Rapoport, 1987).

There are three major effects of TCAs that vary in degree depending on the individual drug: (1) sedation, (2) peripheral and central anticholinergic action, and (3) potentiation of CNS biogenic amines by blocking their reuptake presynaptically (Tables 13-2 to 13-6). The ability of TCAs to inhibit prejunctional reuptake of norepinephrine and serotonin is largely responsible for their antidepressant effect. Many TCAs also have potent muscarinic, α_1-adrenergic, and H_1 and H_2 blocking activity, which can account for their common side effects (dry mouth, sedation, hypotension). The H_1 and H_2 effects, however, may be useful in treating pruritic conditions (see Table 13-5).

The tertiary amines (amitriptyline [Elavil], imipramine [Tofranil] doxepin [Sinequan], trimipramine [Surmontil], and clomipramine [Anafranil]) are metabolized, in vivo, to secondary amines (desipramine [Norpramin], nortriptyline [Pamelor], and protriptyline [Vivactil]). These classes of antidepressants are among the most widely and safely used drugs (compared with benzodiazepines, phenothiazines, barbiturates, and sympathomimetic agents) in companion animal behavioral medicine. The tetracyclics (amoxapine [Asendin], loxapine [Loxitane], maprotiline [Ludiomil], and mianserin) have not been used in veterinary medicine.

TCAs are incompletely absorbed from the GI tract and have significant first-pass effects. They are over 50% protein bound and highly lipid soluble. TCAs reach peak plasma levels 8 to 12 hours after the last dose and reach steady-state levels after 5 to 7 days of the same dose. There is much variation in response in humans: a 30- to 50-fold difference in plasma levels of individuals given the same dose has been reported. No such data currently exist for domestic animals. Nortriptyline is slightly different from other TCAs in that it has a therapeutic window; plasma levels >150 μg/ml may reduce efficacy in humans. TCAs act primarily through a reuptake blockage of norepinephrine and serotonin. In the long term they may cause a decrease in number of β-adrenergic and 5-HT$_2$ receptors. Both of these systems are required for down-regulation to occur.

In general, TCA metabolites are more potent inhibitors of NE uptake, whereas parent compounds are more potent inhibitors of 5-HT uptake (Caccia & Garattini, 1992), and metabolites usually have similar or longer half-lives compared with the parent com-

TABLE 13-4 SIDE EFFECT PROFILE OF TRICYCLIC AND TETRACYCLIC ANTIDEPRESSANTS

	Anticholinergic Effects	Sedation	Seizures	Conduction Abnormalities
Tertiary Amines				
Amitriptyline	++++	++++	+++	++++
Clomipramine	++++	++++	+++	++++
Doxepin	+++	++++	+++	++
Imipramine	+++	+++	+++	++++
Trimipramine	++++	++++	+++	++++
Secondary Amines				
Desipramine	++	++	++	+++
Nortriptyline	+++	+++	++	+++
Protriptyline	+++	+	++	++++
Tetracyclic				
Amoxapine	+++	++	+++	++
Maprotiline	+++	+++	++++	+++

++++, High; +++, moderate; ++, low; +, very low.
From Kaplan and Sadock, 1993.

TABLE 13-5 NEUROTRANSMITTER EFFECTS OF TRICYCLIC AND TETRACYCLIC ANTIDEPRESSANTS

	Reuptake Blockade		Receptor Blockade		
	NE	5-HT	Muscarinic ACh	H$_1$	H$_2$
Imipramine	+	+	++	±	±
Desipramine	+++	±	±	−	−
Trimipramine	±	±	++	++	?
Amitriptyline	±	++	+++	++	++
Nortriptyline	++	±−	+	±	±
Protriptyline	+++	±	+	+++	−
Amoxapine	++	±	+	±	?
Doxepin	+	±	++	+++	+
Maprotiline	+++	−	++	±	?
Clomipramine	±	++	+	?	?

From Kaplan and Sadock, 1993.
− Little to no effect.
± Possible effect.
+ Some effect.
++ Large effect.
+++ Very large effect.
? Questionable effect or effect unknown.

pound. The metabolite/parent drug ratio for nortriptyline (active intermediate metabolite of amitriptyline) to amitriptyline is 0.2 to 3.4 (Caccia & Garattini, 1992; Mårtensson et al., 1984). The metabolite of nortriptyline—10-OH-nortriptyline—has a metabolite-to-parent compound ratio of 1.4 to 1.7 (Rudorfer & Potter, 1987). Imipramine's intermediate metabolite, norimipramine, is a more potent inhibitor of NE uptake than is imipramine (it is also an active intermediate metabolite of other antianxiety agents) and has its own active intermediate metabolite. The ratio of norimipramine/imipramine has been estimated to be 0.1 to 9.9 (Ereshefsky et al., 1988) and 0.2 to 0.3 (Mårtensson et al., 1984). Doxepin's intermediate metabolite, nordoxepin, fully retains the pharmacological properties of the parent compound, and its t$_{1/2}$ is 33 to 88 hours in humans compared with a t$_{1/2}$ of 8 to 25 hours with doxepin. The metabolite/parent compound ratio ranges from 0.1 to 3 (Ziegler et al., 1978). Norclomipramine is also a more potent inhibitor of NE than is clomipramine (Mårtensson et al., 1984), and the metabolite/parent compound ratio ranges from 0.4 to 5.9. Not only does this have profound implications for calculating the expected duration of effects, but it is interesting to note that the ability to formulate intermediate metabolites is subject to genetic polymorphism in the human population. This appears impaired in 5% to 10% of the white population because of a deficiency in an isoenzyme of cytochrome P-450 (Rudorfer & Potter, 1989).

Side effects may, but do not necessarily, include dry mouth, constipation, urinary retention, tachycardias and other arrhythmias, syncope associated with orthostatic hypotension and α-adrenergic blockade, ataxia, disorientation, and generalized depression and inappe-

tence. Symptoms usually abate on decrease or cessation of drug administration. Use is contraindicated in animals with a history of urinary retention and severe, uncontrolled cardiac arrhythmias. A cardiac consultation, including a rhythm strip, should be a part of standard, predispensation examination. The common side effects of TCAs as manifest on ECG include flattened T waves, prolonged QT intervals, depressed ST segments, ventricular tachycardia, and decreases in systolic arterial pressure (Nattel & Mittleman, 1984). At high doses TCAs have been implicated in sick euthyroid syndrome. In older or compromised animals, complete blood studies are urged because overdoses of TCAs are known to alter liver enzyme levels. Extremely high doses are associated with convulsions, cardiac abnormalities, and hepatotoxicity, but there are few data on hemotoxicity. TCAs can interfere with thyroid medication and should be used with caution in hypothyroid patients. There is a rare report of a respiratory depressant effect on ventilatory control in a patient with chronic obstructive pulmonary disease (COPD) who was treated with nortriptyline at therapeutic levels (Greenberg et al., 1993). Serotonin syndrome has been characterized by symptoms that may include confusion, restlessness, anxiety, double vision, myoclonus, ataxia, hyperreflexia, tremor, shivering, seizures, diarrhea, and diaphoresis (Sternbach, 1991).

TCAs are very successful in treating separation anxiety, generalized anxiety that may be a precursor to some elimination and aggressive behaviors, pruritic conditions that may be involved in acral lick dermatitis (ALD), compulsive grooming, and some narcoleptic

TABLE 13-6 COMPARISON OF CLOMIPRAMINE
WITH OTHER TCAs

Parent Compound	Metabolite	Norepinephrine/ Noradrenaline	5-HT
Desipramine	—	++	+
Imipramine	Desipramine	+++	++
Amitriptyline	Nortriptyline	++	++
Nortriptyline	—	+	+
Clomipramine	Desmethyl clomipramine	++	+++

+ Mild effect.
++ Moderate effect.
+++ Large effect.

disorders. Amitriptyline is very successful in treating separation anxiety and generalized anxiety (Snyder, 1982). Imipramine has been useful in treating mild attention deficit disorders in people and may be useful in dogs because it has been used to treat mild narcolepsy. Because of its norepinephrinergic effects, imipramine is not to exceed 5 mg/kg/day in humans. It is likely that similar recommendations are wise in treatment of dogs. Cats are more sensitive to all TCAs than are dogs, are more prone to the cardiac side effects, and should be monitored closely. It is wise to start at a lower dosage and one that is given less frequently. If cats have side effects when treated with a parent compound, they may respond well to one of its metabolites at the same dosage (i.e., 0.5 mg/kg orally every 12 hours of nortriptyline instead of amitriptyline). A TCA derivative, carbamazepine, has been successfully used to control aberrant activity in psychomotor seizures (Holland, 1988).

Clomipramine has been successful in the treatment of human OCD disorders (Ananth, 1986; McTavish & Benfield, 1990; Perse, 1988; Thoren et al., 1980) and in the treatment of panic attacks that have a component of repetitive behavior (McTavish & Benfield, 1990). It has also been successful in treating some cases of ALD in a small, noncontrolled study (Goldberger & Rapaport, 1991). It is possible that ALD is another multifactorial disorder with seemingly singular signalment, given that licking is the predominant sign (Shanley & Overall, 1992). Attempts are currently under way to identify which subset of patients with ALD will respond to clomipramine treatment (Overall, 1994n). More so than any of the other TCAs, clomipramine is thought to be selective as a serotonin reuptake inhibitor (Ananth, 1986; Flament et al., 1985). Favorable response to this drug, because of the class of serotonin receptors that is blocked (Miczak et al. 1989), has been considered diagnostic for OCDs; such protocols have been underexploited in veterinary medicine. Because clomipramine may have more side effects than some other TCAs, the strategy in humans has been to gradually increase the dose by 1 mg/kg

orally every 12 hours over a month (i.e., 1 mg/kg orally every 12 hours for 2 weeks, then 2 mg/kg orally every 12 hours for 2 weeks, then 3 mg/kg orally every 12 hours for 4 weeks; this will then be the maintenance dose; effects may not be apparent until weeks 4 to 6). This strategy has worked well in dogs (Overall, 1994n), although the dose is higher than recommended elsewhere, where only a constant dose is recommended (Houpt & Reisner, 1995).

Combination treatment has been used more frequently for humans than for veterinary patients. Concomitant administration of fluoxetine with amitriptyline at therapeutic levels potentiates both the amitriptyline and the intermediate metabolite nortriptyline (Aranow et al., 1989). There is probably also a reverse effect for fluoxetine and norfluoxetine, but their already long half-lives make this difficult to evaluate (El-Yazigi et al., 1995).

Nonspecific Anxiolytics. Nonspecific anxiolytics comprise some of the newer drugs developed for atypical depressions, nonspecific, generalized anxiety disorders, and some obsessive compulsive syndromes.

Buspirone, an azaspirone anxiolytic (along with experimental agents ipsapirone and gepirone), has been used or suggested for use in canine aggression of dominance or idiopathic origins, canine and feline ritualistic or stereotypic behaviors, self-mutilation and possible OCDs, thunderstorm phobias (Marder, 1991), and possibly feline spraying (Hart et al., 1993). Among its benefits are a low abuse potential, a probability of adverse withdrawal phenomena, and a low potential for cognitive impairment. It is well absorbed from the GI tract and attains peak plasma levels in 60 to 90 minutes. The half-life is short (2 to 11 hours); thus buspirone may require administration every 8 hours.

Buspirone shares no common features with the phenothiazines, benzodiazepines, or TCAs; it is anxiolytic and a partial serotonin agonist (Jenicke & Baer, 1988). Buspirone has no effect on 5-HT$_2$ receptors but has a high affinity for 5-HT$_1$ receptors. Buspirone acts as a 5-HT$_{1A/B}$ agonist at low dosages (Ratey & Gordon, 1993; Taylor, 1988; Taylor et al., 1985), and on this basis has been used to treat aggression associated with impaired social interaction in humans. Buspirone has also been postulated to have some dopaminergic effects, but if these are real, the extent to which they contribute to its efficacy is unknown. In a small trial for treatment of social phobia, buspirone was associated with a favorable response in half the patients; however, MAOIs seemed to produce a better response in this human population. Its use in treatment of human OCD has met with mixed results (Jenike & Baer, 1988; Pato et al., 1991; Robinson et al., 1989). Although used in human psychiatric medicine for over a decade, its use in veterinary medicine is new and shows promise, particularly in cases of anxiety associated with aggression or marking behaviors (Hart et al., 1993; Overall, 1994m).

Side effects of buspirone are relatively rare but may

include mild disorientation and GI symptoms. It has no anticonvulsant, cognitive, or withdrawal problems (Eison & Temple, 1986).

Newer derivatives of TCA are generally referred to as a group as serotonin specific reuptake inhibitors (SSRIs). These include fluoxetine (Prozac), paroxetine (Paxil), sertraline (Zoloft), and fluvoxamine.

Fluoxetine has at least one active intermediate metabolite, norfluoxetine. Both the parent and metabolite have R- and S-enantiomers. It has been postulated that the S-enantiomer is more potent than the right in inhibiting serotonin reuptake (Gram, 1994). The metabolite/parent drug ratio is 1 (Benfield et al., 1986). Fluoxetine reaches peak plasma levels in 4 to 8 hours and has a long half-life. Half-life for fluoxetine is 1 to 10 days and for norfluoxetine can be as long as 3 to 20 days. Both compounds are subject to extensive tissue binding and are cleared slowly. Accordingly, it can also take 2 to 3 weeks or longer to attain steady-state plasma levels, and it has been estimated that steady-state clearance takes more than a month (Benfield et al., 1986). Most of the effect of this compound seems to be by a highly selective blockade of the reuptake of 5-HT into presynaptic neurons. Fluoxetine appears to have no effects on NE or dopamine, no anticholinergic, no antihistaminic, and no anti-α_1-adrenergic activities; therefore most of the side effects associated with antidepressants are absent or minimized. Fluoxetine is commonly used in the treatment of depression, dysthymia, anxiety, and panic disorders in people. Concomitant use of TCAs or benzodiazepines increases the plasma levels of these agents and may prolong the excretion of fluoxetine. Coadministration of buspirone may decrease the efficacy of buspirone and potentiate extrapyramidal symptoms, but there have also been reports of synergistic effects. Fluoxetine should not be used with MAOIs or with L-tryptophan.

Fluoxetine is a specific serotonergic agent, far more potent than clomipramine (Fontaine & Chouinard, 1989; Pigott et al., 1991), that has been used with mixed results for the treatment of canine aggression (Marder, personal communication, 1994) and stereotypic behaviors in domestic animals (Houpt, McDonnell, personal communication, 1994). In humans, fluoxetine appears to be equally efficacious in the treatment of OCD, but has fewer side effects (Insel, 1990).

Serotonin agonists have been used to treat aggression in organically impaired patients and impulsive aggression in severe personality disorders in humans (Coccaro et al., 1990), although the need for studies far outstrips funding for them (Ratey & Gordon, 1993). There appears to be an inverse correlation between impulsive *externally* directed aggressive behavior and CSF-5-HIAA (5-hydroxyindoleacetic acid) (Linnoila & Virkkunen, 1992). Fluoxetine has been efficacious in the treatment and modulation of interdog aggression (Overall, 1995a). It has been useful in treating animal models of OCDs (wheel running, anorexia, weight loss) when imipramine has had no effect (Altemus et al., 1993). Fluoxetine also appears to be useful in treatment of companion animal panic and avoidance disorders, OCDs (spinning), and profound aggressions (Overall, 1995a), but contrary to reports in the popular press, it should not be used cavalierly to treat any condition that has a behavioral component and is certainly not a panacea for problem pets.

Paroxetine has not yet been used in companion animals, but has been efficacious in the treatment of depression, anxiety, and agitation associated with depression in humans. It is lipophilic and 95% protein bound and has a half-life of 24 hours. Hepatic metabolism produces only inactive metabolites. Paroxetine has been reported to be more potent than fluoxetine, fluvoxamine, and sertraline (Boyer & Feighner, 1992). It has little affinity for other receptor classes and thus has few CNS or autonomic side effects.

Sertraline may reach maximum plasma concentrations within 5 to 8 days, steady-state levels within about 7 days, and has a plasma elimination half-life of 26 hours when administered once a day. Its desmethyl metabolite is considerably less active than the parent compound. It is used in humans to treat depression but has not been used extensively in companion animals. Treatment effects in humans appear to require at least 3 to 5 weeks of constant dosing.

Fluvoxamine may be less specific in its effects on aggression than is fluoxetine. It more closely resembles amitriptyline in its sedative and anxiolytic effects, although it has fewer side effects. It reaches peak plasma levels within 1½ to 8 hours and has a mean plasma half-life of 15 hours after single dosing. The latter increases to 17 to 22 hours with repeated dosing in humans. Steady-state levels are reached within 10 to 14 days in humans treated for depression and OCD. Fluvoxamine undergoes extensive hepatic biotransformation, primarily through oxidative deamination, but its multiple metabolites appear to be of no treatment consequence. Its positive effects on the treatment of OCD are challenged by ritanserin (a specific 5-HT$_2$ receptor antagonist), indicating that the 5-HT$_2$ receptor may also be involved in this condition.

Narcotic Agonists/Antagonists. Narcotic agonists and antagonists have been useful in human OCDs (Herman et al., 1989; Pickar et al., 1982) and in domestic animal self-mutilation and ritualistic disorders (Dodman et al., 1987, 1988a,b). These include naloxone and naltrexone (pure antagonists) and nalorphine and pentazocine (mixed agonist-antagonists). Pure antagonists appear to block δ-, μ-, and κ-receptors equally. Naloxone reverses opioid-induced analgesia and may be a useful diagnostic tool for practitioners attempting to determine whether stereotypic behavior is associated with endogenous, self-stimulation of opioid receptors (Brown et al., 1987). Naloxone suppresses food intake in most domestic animals (Foster et al., 1981). Hydrocodone (Hycodan) can be useful in long-term treatment of canine acral lick granulomas and in self-mutilation by cats. The common human side effect of constipation does not appear to be a problem, but the drug is abusable by humans. Morphine opiates can be physiologically (and psychologically—if the dog is clever) addictive in dogs (Martin et al., 1974; Segall, 1964). Apomorphine, when given to early weaned pigs, prolongs nonnutritive suckling behavior (Sharman, 1978), an effect similar to that engendered by administration of dopamine.

Miscellaneous Agents

β-Adrenergic Receptor Antagonists (β-Blockers). β-Blockers are commonly used in humans to treat self-injurious behavior, intermittent explosive disorder, conduct disorders, dementia, brain disease/injury, autism, and schizophrenia. They have been primarily used in these conditions to decrease aggressive outbursts (Jenkins & Maruta, 1987; Ratey & Gordon, 1993). Older β-blockers (e.g., propranolol, a β_1 and β_2 blocker [Inderal]) that were originally used to treat aggression and somatic symptoms of anxiety have not been as successful as originally hoped in treating canine or feline aggression; propranolol has been used with mixed success in treating these aggressions and noise phobias (Shull-Selcer & Stagg, 1991). Although propranolol lowered HR and RR in cynomolgus monkeys *(Macaca fascicularis)*, there were no concomitant effects of β blockade on social dominance or aggressiveness, or on active aspects of affiliative behaviors such as grooming (Kaplan & Manuck, 1989). This lack of dramatic response may indicate that future treatment would do better to address physiological or behavioral causes of aggressive or phobic syndromes rather than to focus on the physiological correlates of the behaviors associated with these; newer β-blockers and more appropriate dosing may mean that this class of drugs will be more useful in the future.

β-Blockers are readily absorbed from the gastrointestinal tract and metabolized by the liver or excreted unchanged by the kidneys. They vary in the extent to which they are lipophilic: the more lipophilic the agent, the more likely it is to enter the brain and to have fewer peripheral side effects. β_1-Adrenergic receptors (those influencing chronotropic and inotropic function) are more numerous in the CNS than are β_2-adrenergic receptors (those influencing peripheral bronchodilation and vasodilation). Clinical responses of β blockade include, but are not restricted to, decreased cardiac output at rest and during exercise, possibly as a result of slowed sinus heart rate and decreased atrioventricular (AV) conduction and decreased systolic pressure on exercise. The exent to which any of these responses is manifest depends on the receptor specificity of the particular agent. For example, propranolol is lipophilic and nonselective in its receptor response; metoprolol is selective for β_1 receptors and is also lipophilic, whereas atenolol is not lipophilic, but also selective for β_1 receptors. Atenolol,

which is metabolized through renal rather than hepatic pathways, has a longer half-life than the other compounds and needs to be administered less frequently.

β-Blockers (antagonists) are contraindicated in asthma, COPD, diabetes, congestive heart failure (CHF), hyperthyroidism, peripheral vascular disease, and any situation in which atrial-ventricular (AV) conduction effects are a concern. β-Adrenergic receptors can increase plasma levels of chlorpromazine (Thorazine), thioridazine (Mellaril), and theophylline (Theo-Dur). If interaction of pharmacological agents is a concern, caution should be exercised if concomitant barbiturate or MAO therapy is ongoing. Barbiturates increase the elimination of β-adrenergic antagonists that are metabolized by the liver. Hypertensive crises and bradycardia have been reported in some humans treated concomitantly with MAOIs and β-adrenergic antagonists. Calcium channel blockers decrease myocardial contractility and AV nodal conductivity and could also adversely interact with these agents.

A related agent, clonidine (Catapres), an α_2-adrenergic receptor agonist, acts primarily as a hypotensive agent, but has been used to treat Tourette's syndrome, OCD, panic disorder, phobias, generalized anxiety, and mania in humans at a dose of 0.05 to 0.3 mg/day. It may have some use in animals for similar conditions.

Calcium Channel Blockers. The calcium ion acts as a major intracellular second messenger through its activation of calcium-dependent protein kinases. These kinases inhibit the influx of calcium into neurons through one type of voltage-dependent channel termed the L-type calcium channel. Specific calcium channel blockers or inhibitors include verapamil (Calan, Isoptin), diltiazem (Cardizem), and nifedipine (Adalat, Procardia). These have been successfully used to treat bipolar disorder, movement disorders, tardive dyskinesia, Tourette's disorder, and Huntington's disease in humans. Verapamil crosses the blood-brain barrier and reaches a CSF concentration that is 0.05% that of plasma (references in Kaplan & Sadock 1993). Calcium channel antagonists are underexplored in veterinary medicine, but may hold much hope for treatment of a variety of disorders including aggressions and anxieties.

Other Agents. Cholecystokinin (CCK) has been postulated to act as a mediator in panic attacks (Harro et al., 1993; Hughes et al., 1990) and has been implicated to have a role in situations involving self-medication with food. CCK has been postulated to be a physiological endogenous opioid antagonist (Wiesenfeld-Hallin & Xu, 1993). CCK-B receptors (central brain receptors) appear to be involved in the opening and closing of cat jaws (Singh et al., 1991) and may function in OCDs such as overgrooming and wool chewing or sucking. Unfortunately, the only specific CCK antagonists currently extant are very experimental. This is also true for excitatory amino acid (EEA) agonists and antagonists.

Combination therapy has been successful in humans but underexplored in veterinary behavioral medicine. In human patients with OCDs who do not respond to clomipramine alone, clomipramine-lithium and clomipramine-buspirone combinations have been successful (Insel, 1990); such protocols may have a role in veterinary medicine. There are also combination medications (chlordiazepoxide + amitriptyline [Limbitrol], chlordiazepoxide + clinidium bromide [Librax], dextroamphetamine + amphetamine [Biphetamine], meprobamate + benactyzine [Deprol], perphenazine + amitriptyline [Triavil]) that are commercially available. Some of these might be useful for treatment of anxieties in pets. In particular, Limbitrol might be useful in the treatment of some fears in dogs, (e.g., thunderstorm phobias).

Monitoring

Monitoring of side effects is critical for any practitioner dispensing behavioral medication. The first tier of monitoring involves the same tests mandated in the premedication studies, as discussed previously. Age-related changes in hepatic mass, function, blood flow, and plasma drug binding cause a decrease in clearance of some TCAs (Rudorfer & Potter, 1987). Accordingly, it is prudent to monitor hepatic and renal enzyme levels annually in younger animals, biannually in older, and always as warranted by clinical signs. Adjustment in drug dosages may be necessary with age. Furthermore, 3 of 82 patients treated for bipolar disorder bad creatinine concentrations that increased dramatically from baseline when treated with lithium; hence the recommendations are for creatinine activity to be evaluated routinely in humans if it is ≥1.6 mg/100 ml (Gitlin, 1993).

Ideally, measurement of blood concentrations of antidepressants should be the primary basis for establishing the course of action when the symptomatic response is not as expected. Unfortunately, because most behavioral conditions are not single entities and instead have complex symptoms and causes, and most behavioral drugs are not wholly receptor specific (Caccia & Garattini, 1992), this can be difficult. For TCAs, MAOIs, lithium, and second-generation antidepressants, adequate clinical response is not always achieved by various patients being given the same dose of the same drug. Accordingly, based on the symptoms, the best approach is a systematic one that optimizes benefits while decreasing the risks of therapy (Caccia & Garattini, 1992). This has been the approach taken, largely successfully, in behavioral medicine, although a study to attempt to determine correlations between serum levels of drug and patient response is under way (Overall & Beebe, unpublished, 1996).

Because of potential interactions, it is preferable to withdraw one class of drug before starting another. For SSRIs and MAOs the recommended drug-free time is 2 weeks (2+ half-lives, the general rule of thumb for withdrawal of any drug). It is preferable, when stopping a drug, to gradually reduce (wean) the dosage, rather than stopping abruptly. This not only minimizes any central withdrawal signs but allows the practitioner to determine the lowest dosage that is still effective. Long-term therapy may be the rule with many of these medications and conditions, but maintenance may be at a considerably lower level of drug than was prescribed at the outset. This is the only way the practitioner will discover this.

It is worth repeating that drugs commonly used in veterinary medicine (e.g., acepromazine) often have far more profound potential cardiotoxic effects than do drugs less commonly used (e.g., any of the TCAs). Regardless, rational treatment mandates cardiac monitoring at some level. If continuous cardiac monitoring (ECG, Doppler) is either not available throughout a surgical procedure or if the clinicians are concerned about the interactions of the behavioral drugs and their metabolites and the anesthetic agents, the behavioral drugs can be withdrawn, as above. Given that the time for weaning and the recommended period of cessation is equal to approximately twice the time needed to reach steady-state levels, this period can vary from 10 to 20 days for short-acting behavioral medications and can be 6 to 8 weeks for longer-acting ones such as clomipramine and fluoxetine. It is generally impractical to withdraw the latter. Regardless, the clinician should seriously consider the behavioral side effects associated with withdrawal (increased agitation and anxiety and increased catecholamine release associated with stress). This issue again illustrates how critical it is to *not* cavalierly dispense a drug. If an animal needs the medication as an adjuvant to behavioral therapy, to control some underlying neurochemical disorder, or to help it function normally and improve its welfare, careful monitoring before, during, and after surgery may be necessary. If the animal does not meet these requirements, the practitioner might question why the animal is being treated with behavioral drugs in the first place.

SPECIFIC BEHAVIORAL IMPLICATIONS FOR SPECIFIC DRUGS AND DRUG DOSAGES

A summary of the drugs useful in specific abnormal behaviors can be found in Box 13-3. Specific dosages for these drugs, listed alphabetically by compound, are found in Table 13-1.

Relevant DEA schedule information is listed below.
DEA Schedule II
High abuse potential
Severe physical dependency
Psychological dependency (humans)
No refills
No phone prescriptions
- Amphetamine
- Codeine
- Pentobarbital
- Methylphenidate

BOX 13-3
DRUGS USED FOR BEHAVIORAL DISORDERS

Cats

1. Urine marking/spraying
   - Alprazolam (Xanax)
   - Buspirone (BuSpar)
   - Clorazepate potassium (Tranxene and Tranxene-SD)
   - Chlordiazepoxide (Librium)
   - Clomipramine (Anafranil)
   - Diazepam (Valium)
   - Paroxetine (Paxil)
2. Intermale aggression related to sexual competition
   - Amitriptyline (Elavil)
   - Diazepam (Valium) (primarily for fear/noise-induced aggression)
   - Medroxyprogesterone acetate (MPA) (Depo-Provera) (outdated, last resort only)
   - Megestrol acetate (Ovaban, Megace) (outdated, last resort only)
3. Intercat aggression related to social hierarchy ± redirected aggression
   - Amitriptyline (Elavil)
   - Buspirone (BuSpar)
   - Clomipramine (Anafranil)
   - Diazepam (Diazepam)
   - Fluoxetine (Prozac)
   - Imipramine (Tofranil)
   - Nortriptyline (Pamelor)
   - Triazolam (Halcion)*
4. Compulsive grooming/wool sucking
   - Amitriptyline (Elavil)
   - Carbamazepine (Tegretol)
   - Chlorazepate potassium (Tranxene and Tranxene-SD)
   - Chlorphiniramine maleate (ChlorTrimeton)
   - Clomipramine (Anafranil)
   - Diazepam (Valium)
   - Diltiazem (Cardizem)*
   - Doxepin (Sinequan) (not wool sucking)
   - Hydrocodone (Tussigon, Hycodan)
   - Hydroxyzine (Atarax)
   - Naltrexone (Trexan)
5. Anxiety
   - Acetylpromazine maleate (Promace; acepromazine)
   - Amitriptyline (Elavil)
   - Atenolol (Tenormin)*
   - Buspirone (BuSpar)
   - Chlorazepate potassium (Tranxene and Tranxene-SD)
   - Diazepam (Valium)*
   - Diltiazem (Cardizem)
   - Oxazepam (Serax)
   - Phenobarbital (for travel in cars)
   - Promazine (Sparine)
   - Propranolol (Inderal)

Dogs

1. Dominance aggression—directed to people *only*
   - Amitriptyline HCl (Elavil), only in dogs that exhibit some indecision/anxiety
   - Atenolol (Tenormin)*
   - Diltiazem (Cardizem)*
   - Fluoxetine (Prozac)
   - Sertraline (Zoloft)
2. Male dimorphic behaviors: urine marking, mounting, roaming, intermale aggression
   - Amitriptyline (Elavil)
   - Clomipramine (Anafranil)
   - Fluoxetine (Prozac)
   - Medroxyprogesterone acetate (MPA) (Depo-Provera) (outdated, last resort only)
   - Megestrol acetate (Ovaban, Megace) (outdated, last resort only)
3. Fearful behavior/fear aggression
   - Amitriptyline (Elavil)
   - Buspirone (BuSpar)
   - Clomipramine (Anafranil)
   - Diltiazem (Cardizem)*
   - Fluoxetine (Prozac)
   - Propranolol (Inderal)
4. Noise phobias
   - Alprazolam (Xanax)
   - Atenolol (Tenormin)
   - Buspirone (BuSpar)
   - Chlordiazepoxide (Lithium)
   - Clomipramine (Anafranil)
   - Clorazepate dipotassium (Tranxene and Tranxene-SD)
   - Diazepam (Valium)—*do not use in dogs with any concurrent aggression, including fear aggression*
   - Verapamil (Isoptin)*
5. Hyperkinesis
   - Carbamazepine (Tegretol)
   - Dextroamphetamine
   - Levoamphetamine
   - Methylphenidate (Ritalin)

Drugs are listed in alphabetical order, not necessarily order of preference of use.

*May be useful but not yet routinely used.

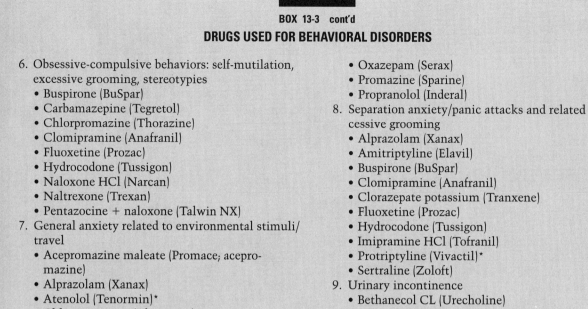

BOX 13-3 cont'd

DRUGS USED FOR BEHAVIORAL DISORDERS

6. Obsessive-compulsive behaviors: self-mutilation, excessive grooming, stereotypies
   - Buspirone (BuSpar)
   - Carbamazepine (Tegretol)
   - Chlorpromazine (Thorazine)
   - Clomipramine (Anafranil)
   - Fluoxetine (Prozac)
   - Hydrocodone (Tussigon)
   - Naloxone HCl (Narcan)
   - Naltrexone (Trexan)
   - Pentazocine + naloxone (Talwin NX)
7. General anxiety related to environmental stimuli/travel
   - Acepromazine maleate (Promace; acepromazine)
   - Alprazolam (Xanax)
   - Atenolol (Tenormin)*
   - Chlorpromazine (Thorazine)
   - Clonazepam (Klonopin)
   - Diazepam (Valium)
   - Diltiazem (Cardizem)*

   - Oxazepam (Serax)
   - Promazine (Sparine)
   - Propranolol (Inderal)
8. Separation anxiety/panic attacks and related excessive grooming
   - Alprazolam (Xanax)
   - Amitriptyline (Elavil)
   - Buspirone (BuSpar)
   - Clomipramine (Anafranil)
   - Clorazepate potassium (Tranxene)
   - Fluoxetine (Prozac)
   - Hydrocodone (Tussigon)
   - Imipramine HCl (Tofranil)
   - Protriptyline (Vivactil)*
   - Sertraline (Zoloft)
9. Urinary incontinence
   - Bethanecol CL (Urecholine)
   - Dantrolene (Dantrium)
   - Diethylstilbestrol (DES) **(Caution!)**
   - Phenoxybenzamine (Dibenzyline)
   - Phenylpropanolamine

Drugs are listed in alphabetical order, not necessarily order of preference of use.
*May be useful but not yet routinely used.

DEA Schedule III
Abuse potential less than schedule I and II
Moderate, low physical dependency
High psychological dependence (people)
New prescription after 6 months or 5 refills
- Compounds with codeine
- Hydrocodone
- Naltrexone
DEA Schedule IV
Low abuse potential
Limited physical dependence
Limited psychological dependence
Prescription after 6 months or five refills
- Benzodiazepines (treated as a schedule II drug in New York state)
- Phenobarbital
- Meprobate

• • •

Most of the future advances in therapy for behavioral medicine will probably be pharmacological. Newer developments in TCAs, specific and nonspecific anxiolytics, narcotic agonist-antagonists, and benzodiazepines will have great relevance for veterinary medicine. As the field of behavioral medicine expands, its paradigm hopefully will enlarge to include combination therapy and the implementation of neuropharmacological intervention as a diagnostic tool. At present, the veterinary practitioner can effec-

tively aid many common behavioral problems, with the glaring exception of most aggressions, with extant drugs. Pharmacological intervention is no replacement for competent history taking and behavioral modification; used rationally it is an adjuvant to these. Rational pharmacological therapy requires complete medical and behavioral histories, requisite laboratory tests, complete client understanding and compliance, and an honest and ongoing dialogue between the client and veterinarian that includes frequent followups and reexaminations. Executed thus, it is also possible to learn from cases that were not successful, as well as those that were.

Issues Yet to be Resolved

Behavioral pharmacology is a "hot" field; however, even in cases when treatment is successful, it should be remembered that the mechanism of change is seldom understood. Most agents are not sufficiently specific to allow testing of mechanistic hypotheses; however, responses may suggest neurochemical association. Most aggression is probably related to an underlying anxiety disorder and, as such, is the result of *many* neurochemical interactions. Particular attention should be paid to developments regarding glutamate, N-methyl-D-aspartate (NMDA) receptors, calcium channel blockers, and NO. It is likely that these factors interact at the level relevant for the treatment and prevention of most anxieties and aggressions.

INFORMED CONSENT STATEMENT

It has been recommended that your pet be treated with a medication that is not licensed for use in domestic pet animals. This means that use of it in your pet is considered "extra label." This does not mean that the drug is dangerous to pets, just that pets were not the subjects tested for approved use. We often know a lot about potential side effects of these medications because dogs and cats are the animals on which toxicity data have been collected by the drug company.

This medication has been chosen for your pet because it has been deemed to have the potential to be efficacious. This is not a guarantee that the medication will be efficacious in treating your pet's problem.

As with all medications, the medication that your pet will be taking may have potential side effects. Although side effects are rare and every effort has been made to minimize them, you should know what the potential side effects are since the occasional animal may not be able to tolerate the medication. The medication prescribed for your pet, **clomipramine (Anafranil)**, is a tricyclic antidepressant. It may cause a slight increase in thirst, but has not been associated with house-soiling accidents in pets. Potential side effects may include an increased heart rate, increased respiratory rate, vomiting, diarrhea, inappetence, lethargy, and fainting. Although these side effects are rare, and when experienced are usually transient, if your pet experiences any of them, please call us so that we can make informed decisions about your pet's care.

After you have read this statement, if you understand it and are willing to comply with it, please sign below. A copy will be provided for your information so that you can refer to it if needed.

Date:_____

Case #:_____

Client
Signature:_____

Clinician
Signature:_____

Telephone numbers to call if questions/
problems:_____

Fax number for questions/
problems:_____

INFORMED CONSENT STATEMENT

It has been recommended that your pet be treated with a medication that is not licensed for use in domestic pet animals. This means that use of it in your pet is considered "extra label." This does not mean that the drug is dangerous to pets, just that pets were not the subjects tested for approved use. We often know a lot about potential side effects of these medications because dogs and cats are the animals on which toxicity data have been collected by the drug company.

This medication has been chosen for your pet because it has been deemed to have the potential to be efficacious. This is not a guarantee that the medication will be efficacious in treating your pet's problem.

As with all medications, the medication that your pet will be taking may have potential side effects. While side effects are rare and every effort has been made to minimize them, you should know what the potential side effects are since the occasional animal may not be able to tolerate the medication. The medication prescribed for your pet, **amitriptyline (Elavil)**, is a tricyclic antidepressant. It may cause a slight increase in thirst, but it has not been associated with house-soiling accidents in pets. Potential side effects may include an increased heart rate, increased respiratory rate, vomiting, diarrhea, inappetence, lethargy, and fainting. Although these side effects are rare, and when experienced are usually transient, if your pet experiences any of them, please call us so that we can make informed decisions about your pet's care.

After you have read this statement, if you understand it and are willing to comply with it, please sign below. A copy will be provided for your information so that you can refer to it if needed.

Date:_____

Case #:_____

Client
Signature:_____

Clinician
Signature:_____

Telephone numbers to call if questions/
problems:_____

Fax number for questions/
problems:_____

INFORMED CONSENT STATEMENT

It has been recommended that your pet be treated with a medication that is not licensed for use in domestic pet animals. This means that use of it in your pet is considered "extra label." This does not mean that the drug is dangerous to pets, just that pets were not the subjects tested for approved use. We often know a lot about potential side effects of these medications because dogs and cats are the animals on which toxicity data have been collected by the drug company.

This medication has been chosen for your pet because it has been deemed to have the potential to be efficacious. This is not a guarantee that the medication will be efficacious in treating your pet's problem.

As with all medications, the medication that your pet will be taking may have potential side effects. While side effects are rare and every effort has been made to minimize them, you should know what the potential side effects are since the occasional animal may not be able to tolerate the medication. The medication prescribed for your pet, **nortriptyline (Pamelor)**, is a tricyclic antidepressant. It may cause a slight increase in thirst, but it has not been associated with house-soiling accidents in pets. Potential side effects may include an increased heart rate, increased respiratory rate, vomiting, diarrhea, inappetence, lethargy, and fainting. Although these side effects are rare, and when experienced are usually transient, if your pet experiences any of them, please call us so that we can make informed decisions about your pet's care.

After you have read this statement, if you understand it and are willing to comply with it, please sign below. A copy will be provided for your information so that you can refer to it if needed.

Date:_____

Case #:_____

Client
Signature:_____

Clinician
Signature:_____

Telephone numbers to call if questions/
problems:_____

Fax number for questions/
problems:_____

INFORMED CONSENT STATEMENT

It has been recommended that your pet be treated with a medication that is not licensed for use in domestic pet animals. This means that use of it in your pet is considered "extra label." This does not mean that the drug is dangerous to pets, just that pets were not the subjects tested for approved use. We often know a lot about potential side effects of these medications because dogs and cats are the animals on which toxicity data have been collected by the drug company.

This medication has been chosen for your pet because it has been deemed to have the potential to be efficacious. This is not a guarantee that the medication will be efficacious in treating your pet's problem.

As with all medications, the medication that your pet will be taking may have potential side effects. While side effects are rare and every effort has been made to minimize them, you should know what the potential side effects are since the occasional animal may not be able to tolerate the medication. The medication prescribed for your pet, **imipramine (Tofranil)**, is a tricyclic antidepressant. It may cause a slight increase in thirst, but has not been associated with house-soiling accidents in pets. Potential side effects may include an increased heart rate, increased respiratory rate, vomiting, diarrhea, inappetence, lethargy, and fainting. Although these side effects are rare, and when experienced are usually transient, if your pet experiences any of them, please call us so that we can make informed decisions about your pet's care.

After you have read this statement, if you understand it and are willing to comply with it, please sign below. A copy will be provided for your information so that you can refer to it if needed.

Date:_____

Case #:_____

Client
Signature:_____

Clinician
Signature:_____

Telephone numbers to call if questions/
problems:_____

Fax number for questions/
problems:_____

INFORMED CONSENT STATEMENT

It has been recommended that your pet be treated with a medication that is not licensed for use in domestic pet animals. This means that use of it in your pet is considered "extra label." This does not mean that the drug is dangerous to pets, just that pets were not the subjects tested for approved use. We often know a lot about potential side effects of these medications because dogs and cats are the animals on which toxicity data have been collected by the drug company.

This medication has been chosen for your pet because it has been deemed to have the potential to be efficacious. This is not a guarantee that the medication will be efficacious in treating your pet's problem.

As with all medications, the medication that your pet will be taking may have potential side effects. While side effects are rare and every effort has been made to minimize them, you should know what the potential side effects are since the occasional animal may not be able to tolerate the medication. The medication prescribed for your pet, **fluoxetine (Prozac)**, may cause a slight increase in thirst, but has not been associated with house-soiling accidents in pets. Potential side effects may include an increased heart rate, increased respiratory rate, vomiting, diarrhea, inappetence, lethargy, and fainting. In extremely high doses it has been associated with seizures. Although these side effects are rare, and when experienced are usually transient, if your pet experiences any of them, please call us so that we can make informed decisions about your pet's care.

After you have read this statement, if you understand it and are willing to comply with it, please sign below. A copy will be provided for your information so that you can refer to it if needed.

Date:_____

Case #:_____

Client
Signature:_____

Clinician
Signature:_____

Telephone numbers to call if questions/
problems:_____

Fax number for questions/
problems:_____

INFORMED CONSENT STATEMENT

It has been recommended that your pet be treated with a medication that is not licensed for use in domestic pet animals. This means that use of it in your pet is considered "extra label." This does not mean that the drug is dangerous to pets, just that pets were not the subjects tested for approved use. We often know a lot about potential side effects of these medications because dogs and cats are the animals on which toxicity data have been collected by the drug company.

This medication has been chosen for your pet because it has been deemed to have the potential to be efficacious. This is not a guarantee that the medication will be efficacious in treating your pet's problem.

As with all medications, the medication that your pet will be taking may have potential side effects. While side effects are rare and every effort has been made to minimize them, you should know what the potential side effects are since the occasional animal may not be able to tolerate the medication. The medication prescribed for your pet, **buspirone (BuSpar)**, may cause a slight increase in thirst, but has not been associated with house-soiling accidents in pets. Potential side effects may include an increased heart rate, increased respiratory rate, vomiting, diarrhea, inappetence, lethargy, and fainting. This drug may make some pets more assertive. Although these side effects are rare, and when experienced are usually transient, if your pet experiences any of them, please call us so that we can make informed decisions about your pet's care.

After you have read this statement, if you understand it and are willing to comply with it, please sign below. A copy will be provided for your information so that you can refer to it if needed.

Date:_____

Case #:_____

Client
Signature:_____

Clinician
Signature:_____

Telephone numbers to call if questions/
problems:_____

Fax number for questions/
problems:_____

INFORMED CONSENT STATEMENT

It has been recommended that your pet be treated with a medication that is not licensed for use in domestic pet animals. This means that use of it in your pet is considered "extra label." This does not mean that the drug is dangerous to pets, just that pets were not the subjects tested for approved use. We often know a lot about potential side effects of these medications because dogs and cats are the animals on which toxicity data have been collected by the drug company.

This medication has been chosen for your pet because it has been deemed to have the potential to be efficacious. This is not a guarantee that the medication will be efficacious in treating your pet's problem.

As with all medications, the medication that your pet will be taking may have potential side effects. While side effects are rare and every effort has been made to minimize them, you should know what the potential side effects are since the occasional animal may not be able to tolerate the medication. The medication prescribed for your pet, **diazepam (Valium)**, may cause your pet to be slightly ataxic for a few days. Potential side effects may include changes in heart and respiratory rates, vomiting, diarrhea, inappetence, lethargy, and fainting. Severe depression is not to be desired or expected. If your pet becomes depressed, stop the medication and call us immediately. This drug may make some pets more assertive. The rare cat may suffer toxic and potentially fatal side effects. Although these side effects are rare, and when experienced are usually transient, if your pet experiences any of them, please call us so that we can make informed decisions about your pet's care. Please be aware that this is a humanly abusable substance.

After you have read this statement, if you understand it and are willing to comply with it, please sign below. A copy will be provided for your information so that you can refer to it if needed.

Date:_____

Case #:_____

Client
Signature:_____

Clinician
Signature:_____

Telephone numbers to call if questions/
problems:_____

Fax number for questions/
problems:_____

INFORMED CONSENT STATEMENT

It has been recommended that your pet be treated with a medication that is not licensed for use in domestic pet animals. This means that use of it in your pet is considered "extra label." This does not mean that the drug is dangerous to pets, just that pets were not the subjects tested for approved use. We often know a lot about potential side effects of these medications because dogs and cats are the animals on which toxicity data have been collected by the drug company.

This medication has been chosen for your pet because it has been deemed to have the potential to be efficacious. This is not a guarantee that the medication will be efficacious in treating your pet's problem.

As with all medications, the medication that your pet will be taking may have potential side effects. While side effects are rare and every effort has been made to minimize them, you should know what the potential side effects are since the occasional animal may not be able to tolerate the medication. The medication prescribed for your pet, **selegiline (Deprenyl/Eldepryl)**, may have the potential side effects of changes in heart and respiratory rates, vomiting, diarrhea, inappetence, lethargy, and fainting. Although these side effects are rare, and when experienced are usually transient, if your pet experiences any of them, please call us so that we can make informed decisions about your pet's care.

After you have read this statement, if you understand it and are willing to comply with it, please sign below. A copy will be provided for your information so that you can refer to it if needed.

Date:_____

Case #:_____

Client
Signature:_____

Clinician
Signature:_____

Telephone numbers to call if questions/
problems:_____

Fax number for questions/
problems:_____

14 ····· Prevention of Behavior Problems

···

*E*veryone wants to prevent behavior problems. Behavioral problems and conditions are the single biggest killer of pets. Unfortunately, prevention of behavioral problems is not as simple as educating even a highly motivated client. Education and follow-through are only two of the factors that contribute to prevention of problems, but they are important factors (Campbell, 1992). Other factors include obtaining the type of pet and specific pet that best fits into the household and understanding the genetic basis of any problems. The latter is the responsibility of the breeder and will help breeders to eliminate dogs with problems from their breeding programs.

WHY GET A PET?

Not everyone needs a pet. One of the issues that should be discussed before clients get a pet is why they want one. Vanity purchases tend to become old fast, and dogs bought for guarding purposes can be a real handful later in life if the clients did not understand what they were getting. I have never heard this latter issue better discussed than when I was in Norfolk, Virginia, talking to the local veterinary association. All of the veterinarians present seemed to have large numbers of large, intact male dogs in their practices that either had problems with dominance aggression, protective aggression, or both. When I noted that they were all concerned about the same issue, and in such large numbers, one practitioner, a man, explained it in a paraphrase of the following sentiment (the words are not mine): "These big, macho guys want big, macho dogs to defend their wives and kids for the endless months they are at sea, but won't neuter them and don't do a lot of training. The wives and kids become reluctant victims." One practitioner in the area had been called by one of these wives who was barricaded in the bathroom with the cellular phone while the dog lunged against the door. This same phenomenon has been reported elsewhere: Joshua (1975) noted that when Alsatians (German shepherd dogs) were kept as symbols of power, their clients reveled in their aggressiveness. Male clients have been noted to choose male dogs more frequently than female dogs (Blackshaw & Day, 1994; Joshua, 1975), and concerns about misconceptions of age-specific, sexually dimorphic behaviors may be valid. The sailors above may have succeeded in getting exactly the type of dog that they mistakenly believed would provide their families with protection. Once this error

is made, it can be compounded by inadvertently reinforcing behaviors that clients mistakenly believe are associated with protection.

PICKING THE "RIGHT" PET: PREPET COUNSELING

Although prepet counseling is becoming more important, factors to consider in advising a client about a potential pet are seldom incorporated into the traditional veterinary curriculum. A service that advises clients about the attributes of different types of pets or breeds and in fact could serve to *discourage* pet ownership in some circumstances could be invaluable.

Formats in which this type of counseling can occur include Sunday afternoon open houses (these can rotate among practices in an area), community vaccination fairs, community health fairs, holiday parties, National Pet Week parties (the American Veterinary Medical Association [AVMA] will help provide materials for this), or free or low-cost individual appointments with one of the nurses. Slide shows or videotapes could be preloaded into tape players and prepared with or without an accompanying handout to be used as needed. Videotapes or posters illustrating the types of pets, and even the patients, in the practice can be displayed in the waiting room with breed- and age-specific information about characteristic behaviors, needs, or particular medical concerns. If money is a limiting issue (information that will generate a devoted clientele is among the cheapest investments in any practice), provide refreshments and ask for a minimum donation for them. This will pay for the nurse's time. If one of the foci of such meetings is to display advances in leashes and harnesses, the overhead generated from the purchase of Gentle Leader/Promise System Canine Head Collar (Premier Products, Richmond, Va), Haiti and Lupi (Safari Whitco, Bohemia, NY), Sporn/No-Pull Halter (Four Paws Products, Ltd., Hauppauge, NY) and other such products and will pay for the nurses' time, even if he or she spends most of it fitting harnesses.

The keys to any preventive program, whether medical or behavioral, are communication and motivation. Educating people is hard work. Support staff should be trained to always offer information. Posters can be placed next to displays that say "Ask us!" A fun fact of the week can be posted by the front desk (e.g., "Did you know that . . . until 4 weeks of age kittens cannot retract their claws?"). Support staff can be trained to encourage clients to ask questions by telling them something about their breed or their pet's behavior (e.g., "Oh, an Old English sheepdog puppy! How cute! Did you know that these dogs were developed for herding and driving conditions where the dogs had to move 35 miles per day?"). Obviously, this approach necessitates an educated staff, and education is not free. The extent to which such an investment in continuing education will pay off, particularly if the staff member is charismatic, enthusiastic, and interested in behavior, is vastly underestimated. Communicate the availability of prepet counseling through any means possible.

Factors to discuss with any client who is thinking of getting a pet are listed in Box 14-1, and they warrant some extensive discussion.

Type of Pet

The first decision should involve what type of pet the client wants. Box 14-1 focuses primarily on cats and dogs, but some clients with limited mobility might do better with something like a guinea pig. Guinea pigs are very social, big enough to cuddle, and do not live as long as some small dogs. Oddly, people sometimes resist getting a pet because they do not want to have to worry what will happen if they predecease the pet. Clients who love birds that talk must realize that the best talkers are also among the longest-lived of the birds. They require much work to teach them to talk, they only start to talk once out of babyhood, which can be protracted, and they tend to be the larger, more forceful psittacines and therefore can injure someone. Clients who want a Himalayan cat because of the way it looks need to check out the reality of the situation. These beautiful cats need a lot of grooming. Cats are wonderful, but people who want small, fuzzy dog-substitutes will be disappointed with the Himalayan no matter how fabulous the individual. Cats are *not* small dogs. On the other hand, people who never have had cats and acquire one through marriage are frequently shocked at how fabulous and loving they are. The debunking of myth is important: cats are *not* asocial, they *do* need attention. The time to deprive clients of the romance is *before* they get an inappropriate pet. Clients who seek information that is offered become realistic when allowed to make their own educated decisions.

Once the clients understand the basics of the social systems, extent of domestication (particularly important for comparisons between dogs and cats), any relevant health concerns (e.g., immunosuppressed individuals may not wish to have a pet with sharp claws, and they need to know how to control specific risks such as toxoplasmosis; people with allergies do best with animals that can be bathed frequently or do not shed as much, if a secretor), and general behavioral characteristics of the species in which they might be interested, they then need to focus on the range of sizes within that species.

BOX 14-1

ISSUES TO BE RAISED DURING PREPET COUNSELING

1. Role the pet is expected to play; reason for the pet
2. Specific expectations
   Size
   Activity level
   Specific needs (e.g., tracking, silent)
   Appearance, grooming needs
   Anticipated changes (puppy or aged dog)
3. Costs
   Adoption fee
   Neutering
   License
   Vaccines
   Fecal
   Food
   Cost of one major illness
4. Client's schedule and lifestyle
   Allergies
   Physical ability
   Work versus recreation time
   Age of client—provision in will
5. Breed-specific concerns
   Grooming
   Exercise
   Behavioral propensities (e.g., Abyssinians, hounds)
   Metabolic or genetic diseases
6. Common complaints with regard to breed, age, and sex
7. Average life expectancy
8. Myths about behavior
9. Return to the client's reason for getting the pet

Size of Pet

Size of pet can affect client mobility (many hotels will take small, but not large pets), amount and type of exercise required, grooming needs (regardless of coat length, bigger dogs take longer to groom than smaller), and the cost of maintaining a pet of that size. Larger animals are more expensive to feed and when they become ill the cost of medications scale with body mass: this means that the cost of treating a pet can scale geometrically, not arithmetically. People who have horses know this. Larger animals can be more difficult to exercise and have to be better behaved to make this painless; smaller animals can be horrendously behaved, yet still not pull an older lady into traffic. Finally, larger dogs produce larger amounts of feces. Cleaning up after this dog, regardless of weather conditions, is becoming a fairly standard regulatory practice. If this matters to the client, they should factor this consideration into their decision.

Activity Level

Activity levels can be associated with size (bigger, energetic animals need to cover more space than smaller, energetic animals), but it is more directly correlated with age and type of work for which the dog or cat was selected. Younger animals are more energetic. This pattern does not change until they reach social maturity (18 to 36 months of age for dogs; 24 to 48 months of age for cats). Specific breeds of dogs have been selected for endurance; this is true for many hound breeds and some herding/driving dogs such Old English sheep dogs. Not all large dogs need large amounts of exercise. Akitas were selected to play a relatively homebound protective role and need much less exercise than most people would predict. Of course, this does not mean that you can lock them in a box all day long and have a great puppy. Having a fenced yard is not a substitute for exercising a dog. Playing with the dog in the yard, letting all the dogs play together supervised while in the yard, taking the dog on long walks or to the park are all improvements on the concept of letting the dog raise himself or herself. There are self-made dogs, but they cannot expect to conform to the vagaries of human manners and social expectations.

Specific Needs

Clients need to identify whether they have specific needs they want the puppy to meet. People for whom silence is important might be ill served by the quintessentially cute Beagle puppy. People who want to raise search and rescue dogs may have more latitude in breed but need to look for dogs from lines with particular aptitudes. People who want hunting dogs not only need dogs with a natural aptitude, but also would like for those animals not to be overly reactive to noises. In a classic work by Stur (1987), it appears difficult, if not impossible, to spontaneously select for perfect hunting phenotypes that are perfectly noise resistant. Any competent evolutionary biologist would understand the difficulties in selecting for such performance criteria, and most breeders are not population geneticists. Given that limitation—and given human proclivities toward vanity—it is amazing that dog breeds are in as good shape as they are, regardless of the recent popular and highly critical approach to purebred dogs. Covarying traits are seldom appreciated when people decide that they want a breed of dog because it will serve a specific purpose. Dogs that are highly motivated to hunt have a different focus and may not meet the needs of a young child who needs to carry a pet around. Dogs that are highly motivated by scent can also be more difficult to housebreak if there are already household problems in that regard. There is no substitute for an honest self-assessment of client needs and expectations and common sense.

Appearance and Grooming Needs

The appearance of the dog or cat is often what attracts the client to the breed. It is fashionable to deride this approach, but there is actually much to be said about picking a pet at least partly because of its looks. The way a coat looks provides some idea of the amount of grooming the animal needs. If the client is sufficiently knowledgeable about coats, he or she can actually have much information about the pup's future behavioral proclivities (witness Chesapeake Bay retrievers). For a litigious world that is dealing with a plethora of dangerous dog laws, looks are important on another level: dogs that resemble the breeds about whom the laws are written (American pit bull terriers, rottweilers) do not get the benefit of the doubt. If the goal of getting the pet is to encourage social interaction, these breeds can, unfortunately, encourage avoidance. This should not be the death knell for someone who wants a dog of one of these breeds, but he or she must know the prevalent problems with perception. The same energetic behavior that may be encouraged in a fuzzy dog can be viewed as dangerous in one of these breeds. Although there is no basis in biological fact for many breed-specific perceptions, community problems can arise because of bias. Knowing about bias can help to ameliorate it.

Anticipated Changes

Finally, when addressing clients' specific expectations with their future pet, any developmental changes should be discussed. Puppies do not look as they will when adult. Data refute assertions that you can tell a puppy's future behavior and status based on how it behaves with its littermates. There are data that demonstrate that temperament tests *do not* reflect or predict later adult behavior (Young, 1988b). Some clients will be better served by adopting an older dog whose behaviors are known. Shelters, rescue organizations, and some breed groups can recommend these. Show dogs are often retired and available for placement in a "pet" home, often for free if the client will neuter the animal and meet the breeder's care conditions.

Breed-Specific Concerns

All behavior has environmental and genetic components. The variation in the genetic component is sufficient to produce a wide array of individual behavioral phenotypes in the absence of any specific breed. Hence, not all domestic long-haired cats or mixed-breed dogs look alike or demonstrate identical behaviors in response to like situations. This is true within and between litters. Evolutionary biologists since and including Darwin have recognized these differences. The extent to which behavioral plasticity is a function of genetics is a hotly debated issue in the fields of behavioral ecology and evolution. Some recent experimental evidence on desert toads living in highly variable environments indicates that selection may be operating to maintain developmental and concomitant behavioral plasticity, rather than one or a few modes, each of which would persevere under alternate conditions (Newman, 1989). These issues are important and relevant in discussing the issue of breeds.

One function of establishing and maintaining a breed is to canalize some of this overall genetic variation. Although domestic canine breeds have a relative body size that spans two orders of magnitude, such variation in size is absent in wild canids. The process of domestication alone relieved many of the pressures for which wild canid body size was a response, allowing the underlying genetic variation to respond to artificial selection. In the process of selecting for certain physical and behavioral traits within any breed, one has also selected for some variation in that trait. Accordingly, caution is urged in discussing what have been considered breed-specific behaviors. Selection, natural or artificial, cannot act if there is no underlying genetic variation. Some variation (termed additive genetic variance by quantitative geneticists) must be present for a trait to be developed. This is easy to visualize if one is considering a physical trait such as coat or feather color. It is less easy to realize that selecting for a behavioral trait, such as protectiveness, which is really a constellation of behaviors, will produce a *continuum* of protective behaviors, some of which will not be what the selector desired. In fact, some of these behaviors will be inappropriate, because they are not complete or forceful enough, and some will be unacceptable because they are too forceful and out of context. Under natural, instead of artificial, selection, these behaviors would have been selected against at their extremes; however, it would be an error to regard the wild environment as producing absolute phenotypes. The demographic and local climatic environments act in concert to determine what scope of the continuum of variation survives. In a very good year even the most inept hunter might live to reproduce and contribute genes to the next generation. This is the source of the additive genetic variance. That such genetic variance exists is demonstrated by the extent to which artificial selection has developed so many and such varied breeds in a few hundred years, while thousands of years of natural selection have not developed that degree of canine variability, although the initial stock should have been similar.

Hence, if a breed has been developed for certain specific behaviors (rather than overall survivability, as in the wild situation), one should expect some variation around that behavior and that some of this variation will result in inappropriate, out-of-context behavior. It is in this light that charges made about breed predilections should be viewed. This means that if one has selected a breed for protectiveness or guarding, some of the individuals in that breed may inappropriately protect or guard against objects that pose no threat. Some believe that herding behavior was developed from the first phases of predatory behavior (Bradshaw & Brown, 1990; Fox, 1978). It is conceivable that unless selection were extremely discrete, sufficient variation should exist so that the occasional herding animal exhibits inappropriate predatory behavior. This is commonly known by sheep ranchers (Green & Woodruff, 1988). Such concepts of genetic variability in the development of behaviors are difficult, but given the amount of misinformation regarding some breeds and prejudice toward others, the issue should be addressed.

Hart and Hart (1984b) and Hart and Miller (1985) have attempted to group breeds of dogs according to certain constellations of behavioral attributes. Although their classifications are based on subjective opinions (which can invoke prejudice and folklore) rather than objective classifications of individual behaviors, and their categories confound discrete behaviors and behavioral diagnoses, some overall patterns of behaviors correlated with breeds are apparent. Cluster analysis grouped animals according to reactivity, trainability, and aggression. It is no surprise that high trainability characterized most working and guard dogs; before selecting for any specific other behavior the ability to work with and be trained by people would have to be elaborated. Less reliable are the characterizations of aggression and reactivity, because these are both diagnoses and descriptions of amalgam behaviors. More recent studies have attempted to focus on specific behaviors (growling when disturbed while sleeping; stalking small animals, barking at approaching strangers). This is important because there is scant documentation of the frequency, duration, intensity, and pattern of occurrence of the actual behaviors that are involved in behavioral problems. It is only in this context that fair evaluations of breed-related behaviors should be made. Furthermore, because so little is known about normal behavior and behavioral precursors of serious problems, early signs are not recognized. A survey of the faculty and senior students at the Veterinary Hospital of the University of Pennsylvania (VHUP) and local practitioners revealed that virtually all individuals thought that there were more and less aggressive breeds and could rank these; the ranks of the three survey groups were different within and between groups, with no rank being statistically significant; and, with the exception of the majority of the students, few individuals in the other two survey groups could, when provided with a list of discrete behaviors, accurately identify those that were outright aggressive or precursory of future aggressive behavior (Overall, unpublished, 1990).

In summary, caution is urged regarding any generalizations about breed-based behaviors. It is best to view selection for specific behaviors as a risk assessment analysis. Breeds that have been selected for one or a few particular and specific behaviors may be more at risk for developing unsavory variation for those behaviors. This does not mean that dogs selected for protective behaviors are more aggressive than dogs for which this selective pressure was absent. It does mean that that breed may be more at risk for developing a disproportionate number of dogs that exhibit inappropriate, out-of-context protective aggression. Inherent in this concept is that any dog, regardless of breed, can also exhibit the inappropriate behavior. A further corollary is that dogs selected for tenacity and jaw strength in their in-context work (bull terriers, rottweilers, Rhodesian Ridgebacks), will, when they respond inappropriately or out of context in another behavioral setting, exhibit this same tenacity. Coupled with the physical traits attendant with such selection (large jaws, heavy musculature), they can and will do large amounts of damage on a first strike. These factors, rather than increased breed-specific aggression, are the cause of the severity of any inflicted wounds.

Some of the concerns associated with breed have already been mentioned with regard to specifically selected behaviors, but it is difficult to overemphasize the association between breed and exercise requirements, size, coat characteristics, lifespan, and medical and physical concerns (Clark & Stainer, 1983). Clients can seek worthwhile information about specific breeds from books, at dog shows, at obedience classes, from visits with breeders, and from visits to shelters. Pedigree/KalKan Foods have a computerized Select-a-Dog profile that suggests suitable breeds based on the client's needs or desires (Edney, 1987) (see Appendix C for addresses). Once the client is interested in a specific breed, the veterinarian or staff should thoroughly discuss grooming requirements (these can change with weather; not only do wet dogs smell like wet dogs, some breeds need special care after their coat gets wet), exercise needs, all behavioral propensities—including an explicit discussion of the behaviors for which the breed was developed (not all herding breeds do the same thing, for example)—and the metabolic and genetic diseases that have been recognized in that breed. The latter point is particularly important if clients will purchase a dog from a breeder. They need to ask if any of the recognized conditions (e.g., progressive renal atrophy [PRA] enzyme defects) have been found in that line. If screening tests are available, the dog, the dog's parents, or all these animals should be screened. Clients are entitled to this information but cannot get it if they do not know what to ask; even if they *do* know what to ask, they cannot get this information from a pet store. Although the American Kennel Club (AKC) has a *Breeder Referral Directory,* this directory serves mainly as a listing of breeders of particular breeds in specific geographic areas. Local clubs, such as the Mid-Atlantic States Australian Shepherd Club (an offshoot of the Australian Shepherd Club of America, not the AKC, which it predates) have set qualifying criteria for their breeders' directory. Any breeder wishing to be listed pays a nominal annual fee and the breeder must meet the following criteria: (1) be a member in good standing of the association, (2) be willing to warrant that all dogs used for breeding have been checked and found clear of any genetic faults (specifically, their eyes must be cleared annually by an American College of Veterinary Ophthalmologists [ACVO] board-certified canine ophthalmologist and the hips must be cleared and rated by the Orthopedic Foundation of America [OFA] [I imagine that they would accept the justification of a PENNHip or equally rigorous rating], (3) be willing to guarantee all the puppies, including those sold as pets, and (4) be willing to take a dog back at *any* time, should the client not be able to care for it. Listings are renewed annually. This is a very important step to setting a standard for respect for the breed and provides the client a benchmark by which puppy mill and pet store puppies are doomed to fall far short. Unless average clients understand these issues and the existence of such directories and screening services, they cannot use them. All dogs and cats (in most regions) in the United States, even where puppy mills are numerous and breed-specific problems are legion, need rabies vaccines; therefore at some point in theory they pass through the hands of a veterinarian. The best place for such information exchange to occur is from the professionals in the field.

A word about behavioral genetics is in order. Usually when people speak of behavioral genetics they are referring to the ability to select for dogs with good skills in a specific area (MacKenzie et al., 1985). There is more to behavioral genetics than selecting for specific aptitudes. As more is learned about problem behaviors, it is apparent that many of these are genetic, inherited, or organic. One of the reasons that the specific genetic basis of problem behaviors has received less attention than it should or could is that people still insist that if you do all the correct things with a puppy and "socialize" (a word I would like to eradicate from dog jargon behavior) the dog correctly, that dog will be problem-free at adulthood. Chapter 6 discusses the recent findings of the author and colleagues that dogs with dominance aggression may spill an excess amount of the neurotransmitter glutamate into their urine. This tendency appears to run in family lines. *Dogs and cats with recognized behavioral disorders should not be bred.* Clients should ask specifically about behavioral histories of the lines from which they are thinking of obtaining the kitten or puppy.

Clients should also consider whether they want a male or a female pet. The costs of neutering are different; unneutered animals can exhibit sexually dimorphic behaviors (unneutered males spray more, mark more, roam more, and fight more), and sizes and coat morphology of males and females can differ.

Age of Pet/Age of Client Mismatches

Many people have a specific breed of pet all of their lives. They have chosen that breed for particular reasons that others may not understand, but such clients are generally fairly knowledgeable about the breed. Breeds are subject to change. The very fact that certain "looks" in the show ring go into and out of fashion means that any breed of dog is constantly under selection for change. The clients who had a golden retriever 12 years ago may think that a lot of behavioral changes occurred in the breed between the time their old dog was a pup and when their new puppy was born. They would be right—breeds change behaviorally. Witness Doberman pinschers and German shepherds during the past 30 years. Clients also can have a very spectacular representative of a specific breed and think that their dog is representative of the breed standard. Both of these scenarios can be sources for disappointment about a new pet. Breeds are not static and changeless. Even clients who have had the breed before should fully update their knowledge.

Experienced dog and cat people can also fall into another trap when they go to "replace" a much beloved pet. Most clients understand that they cannot reincarnate their very special companion simply by getting another member of the breed, yet I have one client who ended up with almost 20 cats because she was looking for a cat that had the same temperament and personality as that of her cat that had died 4 years before. A gentle reminder about this potential pitfall can prevent heartbreak.

The more common pitfall for experienced dog and cat people is that, although they know how to raise a puppy or a kitten, they forget that they are perhaps 15 years older than the last time they assumed such responsibility. Two things have happened: the clients forgot that their soulmate also ate books as a puppy, and they, themselves, do not have the energy or priorities they had 15 years before. Acknowledgment of these issues may not deter, nor should it deter, someone from getting a puppy or kitten. However, in a frank discussion of these issues, particularly for people who have some mobility problems, I have seen people make the conscious choice to get a young adult, an older dog, or even an older puppy or kitten rather than a real youngster.

This approach is not without drawbacks. Older dogs may require more and costly medical care, and they may not live as long. Clients who do not wish to care for the teenager's pet when that child leaves for college might find a shorter-lived pet advantageous; however, older clients can be afraid to die and abandon another pet and so may be reluctant to replace a deceased companion. The potential problem of what to do with a pet that outlives the client should be addressed by people of any age who have pets. Pets need to be provided for in a will. If the client cannot find someone with whom they could share pet-care duties in the event of one or the other's death, arrangements can be made through charitable organizations. Organizations such as PhillyPAWS, a support group for pets of people with HIV/AIDS, has as one of its covenants the placement of pets left behind. This arrangement allows the pet to stay with the ill and dying individual when they may be most needed, thus removing a pressing concern for the client. My husband and I have a will that leaves the care of any pets that we may have when we die, along with sufficient funds to feed them and provide them with state-of-the-art veterinary care, to two close friends. These friends have a

reciprocal arrangement with us. One condition for obtaining a retired show champion Tibetan spaniel for my mother was that I take the dog if my mother predeceases her. These are logical and caring arrangements, but note the two important provisos: mutual agreement that is discussed beforehand (no one needs to inherit a "surprise" pet) and adequate financial arrangements to guarantee the pets' needs. Mary Lehman, a managing director of a major New York bank and the former head of its trusts and estates department, recommends both of these approaches and recommends outright bequeathing of funds, rather than the creation of a trust for the pets. The latter are expensive to create and administer and in most circumstances are not needed (*New York Times*, October 15, 1995).

One factor that may influence pet selection is the client's schedule. People who work (everyone) and who cannot take puppies with them so that they can go out frequently to eliminate will have a slower housebreaking process. People who work 18 hours a day, every day, may do better with a stuffed teddy bear than a young kitten. People who have several young children may have to reevaluate whether they want a pet at all, and, if so, how they are going to humanely meet that pet's needs for well-being. Sometimes an older pet can be saved from euthanasia and simultaneously meet everyone's needs. People with very young children must be able to supervise the children at all times when with the pet. This protects both the children and the pet. When clients cannot enforce direct supervision, the pet and children are separated. It is a myth that every child needs a pet. In already ravaged households, the addition of a financially burdensome, time-consuming pet can provide more stress than it can succor.

Finally, rough treatment of pets by children of any age should never be tolerated. Children should be taught to be gentle with pets and clear in their signals to them. Children need to respect that pets are a different species and may have problems of their own. Children should also be taught how to avoid dog bites (freeze; become small; and don't stare or scream) and how to approach strange dogs (be calm; ask permission to pet them). A coloring book that addresses these concerns is available from the Coalition for Safe Children and Dogs (Appendix C).

Financial Expectations

The American Humane Association (AHA) estimates that in the first year of a puppy's or kitten's life, the average client will spend between $900 (kitten) and $1500 (puppy). This *does not include* the purchase price of a breeding-quality purebred pet but does include the following: adoption fees or nonbreeder purchase, vaccinations, neutering, license fees, fecal examinations, preventive care, food, and the expense of one major illness. It is no secret that when financial times are tough, pets are brought to humane shelters in record numbers. There are two ways to prevent this

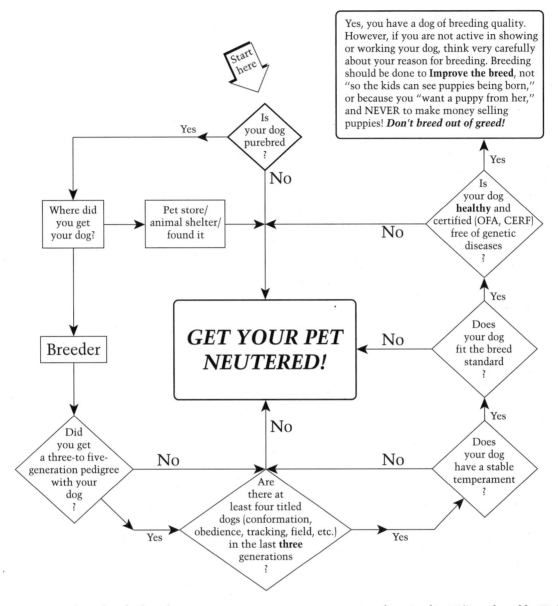

Start here

Is your dog purebred?

Yes, you have a dog of breeding quality. However, if you are not active in showing or working your dog, think very carefully about your reason for breeding. Breeding should be done to **Improve the breed**, not "so the kids can see puppies being born," or because you "want a puppy from her," and NEVER to make money selling puppies! ***Don't breed out of greed!***

Yes

No

Where did you get your dog?

Pet store/ animal shelter/ found it

Breeder

Is your dog **healthy** and certified (OFA, CERF) free of genetic diseases?

Yes

No

Does your dog fit the breed standard?

No

Yes

GET YOUR PET NEUTERED!

No

Did you get a three-to five-generation pedigree with your dog?

No

Yes

Are there at least four titled dogs (conformation, obedience, tracking, field, etc.) in the last **three** generations?

Yes

No

Does your dog have a stable temperament?

Yes

Fig. 14-1   Decision algorithm for breeding versus neutering: "Is Your Dog Breeding Quality?" (Developed by Esther Findling, Buffalo, NY, 1993; distributed by the American Kennel Club.)

problem—decrease the number of available pets through massive and continuous neutering, and control the market by enforcing realistic expectations. It is one of the brutal inequities in life that some of the people who most need the companionship and love of a pet are those least able to afford it. Community organizations and partnerships between private veterinarians and these organizations can address and remedy some of this unfairness, but such redress does not obviate the need for decreasing the pet population and shifting to a more responsible and responsive market.

The Issues of Neutering, Early Neutering, and Preventing Genetic-Based Problems

Early neutering and spaying (6 to 14 weeks of age) has been endorsed by the AVMA for shelter animals and is

safe and efficacious for any pet, provided the surgeon and anesthetist are skilled in neonatal techniques, (Fagella & Aronsohn, 1994; Kahler, 1993; Salmieri et al., 1991). Neutering and vaccination of even feral cats can be inexpensive. Zaunbrecker and Smith (1993) estimate that the average cost per cat is $6.95 ($5.15 for a female; $8.75 for a male), exclusive of time and capture. There is no evidence that early ovariohysterectomies/gonadectomies adversely affect growth or increase evidence of feline urological syndrome in cats (Stubbs & Bloomberg, 1995). In fact, long bones tend to grow in length rather than girth after castration (Armitage & Clutton-Brock, 1976).

When clients are unsure of whether to breed rather than neuter their pet, I often ask them to consider two things. I provide them with the flow chart on "Is Your

Dog Breeding Quality?" developed by Esther Findling of New York and distributed by the AKC (Fig. 14-1). The only change I would make in this flow chart is that I would move the behavior/temperament question to precede the one on breed standard. I also ask clients if they know that an emergency cesarean section can routinely cost more than $1000 without any guarantee of survival of the pups or the mother. In fact, 70% of all canine breedings result in the death of the mother and/or one or more of the pups. Breeding a dog is not currency in the bank, yet because clients pay so much for so many of their pets, they can see how multiplying that number by a litter of 10 or 12 puppies or 5 kittens looks like real money . . . and the children get to witness the "miracle of life." I once heard one of the directors of one of the major humane organizations in the country say that if that was what people wanted, children should get the full picture—they should witness the miracle of death of all the puppies and kittens that are unwanted, unloved, and not cared for. This sounds overly harsh, but is backed by pain most veterinarians feel. In a retrospective study conducted in Australia, Blackshaw and Day (1994) found that clients were often adverse to neutering their pets because they thought that the pet was too old, they did not want the pet to get fat, they did not have the money, they wanted to breed the pet, or they just did not agree with the idea. Further questioning revealed that clients believed that neutering removed more "maleness" in males than it did "femaleness" in females. Geriatric surgery does entail risks, but most pets should and could be neutered before their second heat cycle. Estrogen stimulates energy expenditure while decreasing appetite (Houpt et al., 1979), but overfeeding and underexercising of dogs contribute more to their age-related weight changes than does removal of the ovaries. Neutering is cheap compared with raising puppies or kittens; it should be factored into the a priori "costs" of having a pet. Issues of "maleness" and "femaleness" may reflect more on the client than they do on any biological reality.

PICKING THE SPECIFIC PUPPY: TEMPERAMENT TESTING

After clients have decided that want either a cat or dog and that they want a specific breed, they may be confronted with the choice of a specific individual from the litter. Clients frequently ask how they can pick the pup that is best for them. Less emphasis seems to be placed on picking the perfect kitten for a specific family, but this could be a function of people's often mistaken impressions about cat social systems. Clients should make a real effort to select kittens whose parents are friendly and outgoing and who have been raised in a household where they have been handled extensively by humans from weeks 2 to 7.

Puppy choice can be complex. If the puppy is coming from a humane shelter or is the last in the litter, the client may have no choice. It would be interesting to know whether clients who had a choice of a specific puppy were happier with the puppy and had fewer problems with it after a few years than clients who did not have a choice. These are two different issues and both raise complex questions, yet no studies have been done that address them. In an attempt to evaluate a puppy's propensities and either match it with an appropriate client or forewarn the client of these propensities, many breeders use temperament tests or puppy aptitude tests (PAT).

Given that behavioral problems are the most common problems that any pet dog or cat will face in its lifetime, and given that it is generally accepted that the genetic and physical environments interact to produce behavioral phenotypes, attempts have been made using early testing to predict the extent to which behaviors reflected by a puppy are manifest in later life. Temperament tests were originally developed for the purpose of evaluating and choosing service dog puppies that had temperaments that would be highly desirable for a service profession (Campbell, 1975). In the initial description, all breeds were evaluated according to the following traits: (1) excitability versus inhabitability, (2) active versus passive defense, (3) dominant versus submissive, (4) independence versus social attraction. Unfortunately, these are suites of behaviors, not individual events, individual behaviors, or behavior sequences, and the descriptions may confound the individual components. When this happens it means that one cannot identify independent patterns, one cannot suggest an underlying mechanism for those patterns, and one cannot then design a breeding program designed to enhance or minimize any underlying patterns. No breeding programs can be created in the absence of a hypothesis about the mechanism of the condition.

Regardless, temperament or aptitude testing is frequently used by breeders to assess obedience potential and to serve as a guide to the pup's future temperament so that he or she can be paired with the appropriate family (Campbell, 1975). The test has been adapted and refined for general use and includes two segments. The first deals with social attraction, following, restraint, social dominance, and elevation dominance; the second is concerned with responses associated with successful performance in obedience trials (retrieving, touch sensitivity, sound sensitivity, chase instinct, stability, and energy level) (Bartlett, 1979, 1987; Tamases-Fisher & Volhard, 1985). These tests usually use a scoring system of relative ranks from 1 to 5, 1 to 6, 0 to 5, or 0 to 6 (some organizations such as Canine Companions for Independence [CCI] have adapted the test and scoring to meet specific needs). In conservative interpretations, low scores are said to be correlated with assertive, reactive behaviors, whereas scores of 5 or 6 indicate more passive, withdrawn behaviors. Midrange scores are said to indicate dogs that are outgoing but responsive, deferential, and controllable. Other interpretations state that puppies with consistent scores of 1 are dominant and aggressive, and easily provoked to bite, whereas those with scores that are mostly 6s are independent, uninterested in people, and will not be demonstrably affectionate to people when older (The Monks of New Skete, 1991). There are no data to support either of these contentions, and they reflect the worst problems with interpretation of temperament test. The paradigm generally used is one of suitability versus unsuitability when defining temperament as the dog's suitability for a specific task or function (Tamases-Fisher & Volhard, 1985); however, assertions that dogs with low scores (primarily 1s) are suitable and best used for guard dogs are irresponsible. First, such statements do not separate social status (dominance) and agonistic behavior (appropriate or inappropriate aggression). Second, truly dominantly aggressive puppies should *not* be used for guard dog training because they will react regardless of whether the context is appropriate. With the exceptions of very few states, few police departments in the United States will take dogs with problem aggressions. This is because police officers *must* be able to rely on their dogs to react only under specified circumstances, whether they are trained to inhibit their bites or to proceed through an entire attack sequence.

Finally, it should be noted that some individuals who like to show their dogs in obedience prefer low- to low-medium–scoring dogs because they believe that these dogs have the drive to work. There are no published data regarding concordance of score on temperament test and success in obedience work.

Breeders who use the puppy aptitude test appear to be primarily pleased with the test for matching puppies to owners and to a lesser extent, for accurate predictions of temperament (Bartlett, 1987). However, available data, when they do exist, do not support any positive, significant trend. Fifty-nine percent of the breeders believed that the test was helpful in matching the puppies to the clients, but only 39.3% of 61 breeders surveyed agreed (but did not strongly agree) that puppy aptitude testing predicted "temperament." Seventy percent of the 61 breeders agreed strongly or agreed (two different category choices) that puppy aptitude testing was useful in anticipating training problems. The breeders themselves admitted in the same questionnaire that they often had trouble interpreting the results, and unfortunately, there have been no studies to determine whether the responses are repeatable. Without a repeatable response, any assertions about ability to predict future behavior or to match future clients with puppies must be viewed with utmost caution. The primary benefit of temperament testing, rather than accurately predicting adult temperament, appeared to be in anticipating training problems. However, it should be emphasized that most people who frequently use this evaluation protocol are interested in obedience trials. *These tests pose some serious problems for prospective clients who wish to predict the type of dog that their puppy will become.* It is worthwhile elaborating some of the more blatant problems.

First, it is important to remember that such tests are correlational. They provide no insight into factors that caused the pup to behave "appropriately" or "inappropriately," or with behaviors that rate a high versus a low numerical score. Second, because these tests are conducted when the pup is 7 weeks of age, there is an extended time for the later environment to play a role in the outcome of the dog's adult temperament. Also, if the gene × environment is of paramount importance in determining later behavior, it is unwise to place a large amount of faith in a test that may evaluate, however unreliably, only a small component of the former. Clients who use the test critically know this and use the trainability responses as foci for early intervention. Seven weeks was chosen as the best administration time in part because of the relative lack of environmental influences on preceding behavioral development. Third, the test evaluates the dog at one static period in its life; no measure of repeatability within the individual and no measure of progressive changes in behavior that might be useful for the prospective client exist.

Furthermore, no data exist on the predictability for specific behaviors associated with problems. Accordingly, it is inappropriate to view the restraint and dominance tests as accurate gauges of the dog's future regarding dominance and dominance-related problems. Dominance aggression generally develops between 18 and 24 months of age—at social maturity. Dominantly aggressive dogs generally have shown no signs of earlier aggression, although they may have shown some warning behaviors (staring at owner, pushing, leaning, resisting having feet or head handled, resisting/growling when being disturbed in sleep) that heralded the appearance of the full-blown behavioral syndrome.

Because most clients are unaware of the different impact of social (18 to 24 months of age) and sexual (6 to 12 months of age) maturity on behavior, they may believe that the dog "suddenly" became aggressive at 2 years of age. A good, thorough behavioral history usually reveals that the dog may never have bitten, but certainly showed many other behaviors concordant with incipient dominance aggression. These behaviors may have developed early or late and may have changed in frequency, duration, and intensity. Temperament testing invariably misses all such cases because they do not occur when the test is done.

This critique of temperament testing will be perceived by some as overly harsh. It is not. It is an attempt to superimpose the necessary and sufficient conditions for rigorous, objective evaluation on an area that is rife with personal opinion. No published data have ever supported the contentions in the popular literature regarding temperament tests.

It is more prudent to view such tests exactly as

cautious trainers do—as providing flags for behaviors that are inappropriate and must be addressed early. If, during such evaluations, the pup displays inappropriate or aggressive behavior, this is a warning sign, but not a condemnation. If the puppy is handled gently during one of these struggles and nips even after a few minutes and its aggression intensifies as the test continues and it exhibits these behaviors in a consistent and repeatable manner, that dog already has a problem that must be addressed. Such a puppy must be placed with a client who is both willing to address the problem and is competent to do so.

Failure to display inappropriate or aggressive behavior *does not* guarantee that behavioral problems will not develop. Scott and Beilfelt (1976) reported a very low correlation between age and social tendencies in the context of using aptitude tests to predict social behavior. Beaudet et al. (1994) tested 39 pups of 5 breeds (German shepherds, miniature poodles, beagles, Shiba Inu, and Shetland sheepdog) and found no predictability of future social tendencies on the basis of the test results obtained at 7 and 16 weeks of age. In a study of more than 400 dogs, Young (1988b) found absolutely no correlation between temperament testing at 7 weeks of age and subsequent behavior at 2 and 4 years of age. These data are far more reputable than are anecdotal reports from breeders for their particular breed. Given this perspective, the test can be valuable as an indicator of early problems and as a general guide to pairing pets and people with respect to whether the perspective clients are able to handle a dog that is a little rowdier than others, but it is not a predictor of future behavior. If breeders wish to claim that this is the successful function of the test, they should collect and publish data that would be generated by a scientific, longitudinal study. Otherwise caution is urged for overzealous interpretation.

If one is interested in refining aptitude tests, one can do what CCI is attempting. Their temperament tests have been adapted for a repeated-measures design—every month or bimonthly the same set of dogs are temperament tested under exactly the same conditions. This design was developed less to predict future temperament than it was to note changes in the behavior as they occur, and if the changes involve problem behaviors, correct them before they become unmanageable. If a client is interested in providing all the advantages for a future pet, this type of repeated-measures design can be a valuable tool once the initial database is established.

Finally, it should be emphasized that performance in the show or obedience ring is *not* correlated with perfect or even appropriate behavior in a home environment. Animals with behavioral problems from aggression to elimination win in show rings every day. Perfect behavior (especially when being handled by a professional) during a show does not mean that the animal has no behavior problems in everyday life. Hence, these animals *do not* need more obedience training to treat their behavioral problems; they re-quire the intervention of a specialist who can suggest a therapy that can be generalized to daily life and allow the pet to recognize and respond to contexts in which the behavior is inappropriate.

GENERAL GUIDELINES FOR SELECTING THE INDIVIDUAL PUPPY

As stated, if a purebred pup is desired, Fig 14-1 and its accompanying text should be followed. The best sources of purebred pets are *reputable* breeders who will follow strict breeding, health, and client screening guidelines; breed rescue organizations; and, for slightly older animals, humane shelters. An AKC certificate is not a guarantee of reputable breeding, and the majority of dogs produced by puppy mills have them. Puppy mills are cruel, inhumane, and are beginning to be subject—finally—to serious AKC, veterinary, and public censoring. Unless the local pet store specializes *only* in older pets from the neighborhood, it is best to avoid pet stores as sources of puppies simply because they feed the inhumane puppy mill industry. Pet store puppies also have been found to have a higher incidence than the general population of congenital defects (Hird et al., 1992; Ruble & Hird, 1993), and of infectious, gastrointestinal, and respiratory disease (Scarlet et al., 1994). Humane shelters also have a slightly higher incidence of infectious intestinal disease in their puppies than is true for the population derived from breeders. Interpreting these guidelines for use in cats is not difficult. Cats have behavioral and physical problems that run in family lines—these must be addressed. After this step, the choice of an individual animal can proceed in a similar manner for any purebred or mixed cat or dog litter. If possible, the client should see all of the kittens or puppies multiple times. There are no data about the future behavior or client satisfaction with first picks or last, but seeing the entire litter at various stages could give the client information about the range of personalities and relative changes as the puppy or kitten grows, as well as provide information about the parents. If the client picks a puppy or kitten at 3 weeks of age and then visits multiple times before taking the animal home, a bond will already have been formed. There are no data on whether clients will be more patient with the pet, but the anticipation and readiness can only be a positive aspect. If this opportunity is not available there are no negative connotations. One of my Aussies was "claimed" sight unseen the day she was born, another was hand-picked at 3 weeks of age, and the third was the last pick of the sex and color I desired. They have all been different and delights.

If possible, clients should see as many of the relatives of their prospective kitten or puppy as they can. They do not need to restrict themselves to one breeder to do this. This gives them the chance to see how related dogs behave at different ages. Previous breedings should not be ignored. Breeders can often put clients in touch with people who have a puppy from a previous breeding. Asking questions about a dog's behavior as it aged can be very valuable. For example, discovering that five of seven pups from a previous breeding were euthanized at 2 years of age because of aggression problems should set off loud warnings.

The individual puppy or kitten (or dog or cat) that catches the client's eye should have time to interact with the client both in a group and separately. Most humane shelters have now developed excellent facilities for clients to interact with the animals away from the commotion. If the pet is older, the shelter personnel or the person placing it for adoption can give the client their insights about the pet. These are not guarantees but are pieces of information that the client can critically consider. Clients should ask about specific contextual behaviors—for example, "When does the puppy play and for how long during each bout?" Knowledge of normal behavior or patterns can prevent misperceptions. If the puppy seems very quiet when the clients arrive, and they are delighted because they think that they are getting a calm pup, it might be beneficial to know that the dog is exhausted because it has played all morning—by tomorrow it will be a speed demon. Conversely, puppies that have been cooped up may seem frenetic at first, but if the clients spend 30 or so minutes with them, they might calm down. Clients should ask about daily patterns, any housebreaking progress, patterns of play with toys, mode of feeding, and the puppy's or kitten's response to food (do they fight with littermates, are they calm and so on.) No response to these queries can guarantee a future behavioral outcome, but the knowledge that clients gain may help them to have realistic expectations as they start. That can only help.

Clients should play with the puppy or kitten with toys, massage the animal, pick it up, crouch down and encourage the baby to come to them, and check the response to calm, verbal encouragement and to clapping. It is normal, especially for shelter animals, to sometimes be shy at first. Clients should be encouraged to let the animal come to them and not to rush them. If this takes a long time (30 minutes is extreme), the client is forewarned. Initial shyness is not an insurmountable problem, but if clients do not want to deal with this behavioral profile at first, they will not want to deal with it later.

Special commentary about recycled or rehomed pets is warranted. If a pet is obtained through a rescue organization or shelter, the kind of information that clients can obtain is restricted to what was reported to the shelter. Shelters are improving in elucidating information about behavioral problems that caused the pet to be placed and about correlating them with behaviors they have observed. Clients need to ask rigorous questions. The most common reasons that dogs and cats are placed in humane shelters involve aggression, overzealous (in the client's view) activity, and inappropriate or undesirable elimination. Many of these behaviors develop at social maturity; therefore it is no surprise that so many 2- to 3-year-old animals are in

humane shelters. Clients need to ask discrete and critical questions (e.g., "Does this dog have a history of growling, roughness, mouthing, or biting when children play with toys?" "Does this cat have any history of eliminating on carpets or spraying in the presence of other cats?"). These may not be reasons to not adopt a pet, but they are data that clients need. Full disclosure *may* turn away a prospective client, but when animal abuse and recycling is common, this may be the only chance that the animal has of finding a home where it can be helped. Placing an animal in a home from which it will later be ejected—or worse— is not placement. Many humane shelters now have staff members who are trained in behavior modification and offer classes or programs to help clients prevent or overcome some of their new pet's problems. These programs are models for the future and clients should ask about them.

Regardless of the age or source of the pet, dogs, in particular, should be encouraged to have superb public manners. Any client considering a pet should be willing to adhere to the established 10 principles of responsible pet ownership as recommended by the AKC:

1. Provide the pet with the basics of food, water, and shelter
2. Provide the pet with a safe living environment
3. Provide the pet with appropriate health care
4. Meet the social and emotional needs of the pet
5. Provide the pet with regular exercise and playtime
6. Provide the pet with training
7. Maintain the pet in a well-groomed manner
8. Spay or neuter the pet
9. Practice good neighbor and community citizenship—this means that the pet should be identified through use of tags, licenses, or permanent identification (microchipping is a good idea), and the clients should clean up after their pet (this includes not letting your cat dig up your neighbor's flowers)
10. Provide the pet with a lifetime commitment

STARTING ON THE RIGHT FOOT

After the clients have pursued prepet counseling, selected the type of pet they want, chosen the breed, and obtained the specific individual, the veterinarian and the veterinary staff *can* start to work on shaping the pet's behavior as he or she socially matures. Boxes 14-2 and 14-3 contain a summary of information to discuss at the first appointment. This information focuses on more global issues that are frequently involved in the placement or death of pets. If it is impossible to cover all of this information during the first examination, a series of short examinations, arranged as a package at one price, or a long first puppy or kitten visit (2 hours can be a realistic estimate), arranged as part of a package that includes all vaccinations, can be options. Videotapes, client handouts, and support staff participation are invaluable. If the puppy or kitten is to undergo a series of three vaccinations, the information can be outlined at the first visit and a schedule of topics to cover at that and subsequent visits developed. There are many variants on this approach and all are somewhat labor intensive; however, that labor pays off. Clients want information and will pay for it and later treatment if they received education first. Also, pets that are killed because of later behavioral problems do not generate income and do not contribute to an attitude and bond that encourages the generation of income. What veterinarians should *not* do on the first visit is rush the pup or kitten through in 5 minutes (because it is generally healthy) and quickly (and scarily—to the pet) vaccinate it.

First visits may not involve a vaccination, especially for fearful puppies or kittens; that activity may be better executed at the next visit, which may be the next day, when it could be done quickly after a temperature check if the first visit included a thorough physical examination. The first visit should involve acquaintance with the staff, play, fuss, treats, a physical examination, and possibly, a vaccination sneaked in at the end of play. Encourage clients to return between appointments to just visit—this is great for the puppy or kitten and them. Of course, they will ask your staff questions, but they can also be told up

---

BOX 14-2
WHAT TO DISCUSS AT THE FIRST DOG APPOINTMENT

1. Neutering and sexually dimorphic behaviors
   - Marking
   - Roaming
   - Mounting
   - Interdog aggression
2. Reproductive status and health
3. Nail trimming and injury
4. Housebreaking
5. Appropriate and inappropriate play behavior
6. Chewing and appropriate toys
   - Kongs
   - Nylabones
   - The problem with rawhide
7. Digging
8. Exercise needs
9. Breed-specific maintenance needs
10. Halters, leashes, harnesses, and collars
11. Development of pushy and aggressive behaviors
12. Crates
13. Canine good citizens and dog classes
14. Contagion and vaccines
15. Dog-dog interaction and parasites
16. Dental care and ability to handle
17. Most common reasons dogs are placed

BOX 14-3
WHAT TO DISCUSS AT THE FIRST CAT APPOINTMENT

1. Neutering and mating behavior
2. Spraying, sex, and reproductive status
3. Nail trimming and destruction
4. Litter aversions
5. Appropriate and inappropriate play behavior
6. Play aggression
7. Identification of status-related aggression
8. Harnesses, collars, and leashes
9. Diet and greenery
10. Predatory aggression and disease
11. Contagion and vaccinations
12. Normal behavior versus obsessive-compulsive behavior
13. Survivorship and indoor/outdoor cats
14. Dental care and ability to handle
15. Most common reasons cats are placed

---

front, when invited to drop in, that if the staff is too busy for the visit they will say so. During the first few visits clients should become familiar with the following procedures and be able to do them themselves:

1. Nail clipping—reticent clients can learn to use an emery board
2. Tooth brushing—with pediatric toothbrushes, gauze, or washcloths
3. Grooming
4. Temperature taking
5. Giving pills, particularly cats; practice with blanks and encourage the clients to give treats afterward
6. Ear cleaning
7. General lymph node palpation
8. Fitting, adjustment, and use of harnesses

These activities are outlined in the checklists in Boxes 14-4 and 14-5, and a list of demonstrations that should be provided for dogs is found in Box 14-6. Clients should practice these activities often, regardless of whether the pet "needs" them. Obviously, toenails should not be clipped or filed unless needed, but clients can manipulate the puppy's or kitten's toes and hold them in the way that they would when they clip them. This will make the actual activity easier. Repeated exposure of the new pet to these activities will help the client in two respects: (1) they will help render the pet more tractable and less fearful of manipulation, and (2) they will familiarize the client with "normal" so that they can report deviations.

Cats, in particular, benefit from the above measures. Cats should be harnessed and leashed and taken in the car frequently when they are young. Early exposure and desensitization will help save them from later trauma associated with visits to the vet. In par-

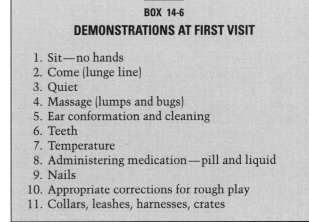

BOX 14-4

CHECKLIST FOR CLIENTS WITH NEW PUPPIES

To practice daily:
1. Brushing teeth
2. Taking temperature
3. Feeling lymph nodes
4. Swabbing ears
5. Sitting for *everything!*
6. Waiting at door
7. Entering and leaving vehicles
8. Relinquishment of toys
9. Grooming
10. Handling feet and nail manipulation
11. Belly rubs
12. Stop, come, and stay—gradual manner
13. Quiet times (crate?)
14. Undivided "quality time"
15. Gentle vocal communication—watch for signals in pup's response
16. Monitor food intake and urine and fecal output

BOX 14-5

CHECKLIST FOR CLIENTS WITH NEW KITTENS

1. Brushing teeth
2. Taking temperature
3. Feeling lymph nodes
4. Swabbing ears
5. Belly rub
6. Grooming
7. Quiet time
8. Undivided "quality time"
9. Handling feet and nail manipulation
10. Relinquishment of toys
11. Stop command
12. Aerobic play
13. Gentle vocal communication—watch for signals in kitten's response
14. Monitor food intake and urine and fecal output (emphasize special needs in cats)

BOX 14-6

DEMONSTRATIONS AT FIRST VISIT

1. Sit—no hands
2. Come (lunge line)
3. Quiet
4. Massage (lumps and bugs)
5. Ear conformation and cleaning
6. Teeth
7. Temperature
8. Administering medication—pill and liquid
9. Nails
10. Appropriate corrections for rough play
11. Collars, leashes, harnesses, crates

---

ticular, they should just come to the veterinarian's office for a "visit." Many later problems could be prevented if the first (and subsequent) exposure were not fear provoking.

Clients should be forewarned that all young animals experience periods of fear in their development. These are variable (but have been reported to be most common and apparent at 9 and 14 weeks, and 9 months) and normal. Animals also have "bad days" or can learn to be afraid if they are ill (their threshold might be lower) or if the stimulus is profound. Minor and transient fear and shyness are not problematic. If the response is not transient or if it is profound, clients should not wait to get help; the response will worsen. It is far better that the clients should seek your advice, only to be told that they do not have a problem, than to ignore the event, hoping that the response will "just go away."

All of the above advice is also applicable to older, rehomed dogs, although exposure may have to be more gradual until a reliable response is determined. Clients with adopted pets also should be encouraged to work through every item on the checklists in Boxes 14-4 and 14-5. Clients should be aware that pets with behavioral problems can live 3 to 4 months in their new home—the time it takes them to feel socially secure—before they manifest any of their prior problems. Accordingly, the clients should work as consistently with rehomed pets as they would with babies and be alert for any gradual changes. These changes need to be addressed as they arise.

EARLY INTERVENTION: THE ROLE OF TRAINING

Most dogs benefit from some form of training class, whether serious obedience training for show or obedience training for companion dogs. If a dog is participating in a current vaccination program, if it is well nourished and cared for, if no other animals present are overtly sick, and if good hygiene at the site is practiced, puppies can start in a kindergarten style class as early as 8 weeks of age. Early exposure and enrichment should be encouraged (Hubrecht, 1992). There is no reason to isolate or restrict them until they complete all vaccinations; in fact, there are data to indicate that pups that are exposed with the above restrictions have better immune responses when challenged (Jezyk, Personal communication, 1989). The earlier exposure to social and training situations occurs, the lower the probability of problems developing. At VHUP we start puppies as young as 8 weeks in a companion dog class designed for pups from 8 weeks to 6

BOX 14-7

CLIENT-PET HOMEWORK ASSIGNMENTS FOR COMPANION DOG CLASSES*

Puppy Class Homework for Week One

Practicing sit and stay

Day 1 SIT—LOOK—**Reward**—STAY 5×, then release OK! repeat 3×. Work at the above in five 10-minute sessions throughout the day until the dog will look at you when you say "look" without your holding cheese to your eye. When the dog has learned the word "look," *gradually* (2 seconds, 4 seconds, 6 seconds) increase the amount of time of eye contact 10 seconds before rewarding with food. *You should be smiling while the dog makes eye contact, so your expression must evoke trust not fear.*

Day 2 SIT—LOOK—STAY move your right foot back a step and return it in one fluid motion. In other words, don't hold your foot behind you. **Reward.** Repeat 5× release—OK! repeat 3× *Reminder: Your puppy should be making eye contact the whole time.*

SIT—LOOK—STAY move your right foot back and hold it there for 2 seconds. Return foot to normal standing position and **reward**. Repeat 5×, release—OK! repeat 3×.

SIT—LOOK—STAY move your right foot back, and return to original position without stopping one step away. **Reward**. Repeat 5×, release—OK! repeat 3×.

SIT—LOOK—STAY move your right foot back, then your left foot, stopping one step away for 2 seconds; return to original position. **Reward**. Repeat 5×, release—OK! repeat 3×. If your puppy seems good at this exercise, vary it by stepping at an angle by moving either right or left foot first.

Repeat this sequence with all repetitions three or four times during the day.

Day 3 Warm your puppy up by going through the Day 2 sequence without the repetitions. ***Reminder: Your puppy should be making eye contact the whole time.***

SIT—LOOK—STAY move your right foot back, then your left foot, stopping one step away for 5 seconds; return to original position. **Reward**. Repeat 5×, release—OK! repeat 3×. If your puppy seems good at

this exercise, vary it by stepping at an angle by moving either right or left foot first.

SIT—LOOK—STAY move two steps away from puppy and stop for 2 seconds; return. **Reward.** Repeat 5× release—OK! repeat 3×. If your puppy seems good at this exercise, vary it by stepping at an angle by moving either right or left foot first. *Reminder: Your puppy should be making eye contact the whole time.*

SIT—LOOK—STAY move two steps away from puppy and stop for 2 seconds; return. **Reward.** Repeat 5× release—OK! repeat 3×. If your puppy seems good at this exercise, vary it by stepping at an angle by moving either right or left foot first.

SIT—LOOK—STAY move two steps away from puppy and stop for 2 seconds; return. **Reward.** Repeat 5×, release—OK! repeat 3×. If your puppy seems good at this exercise, vary it by stepping at an angle by moving either right or left foot first.

Repeat this sequence with all repetitions three or four times during the day.

Day 4 Warm your puppy up by doing some of the *Day 1* (not Day 3) exercises.

SIT—LOOK—STAY move one step *forward* to the right of your puppy and return without stopping. **Reward.** Repeat 5×, release—OK! repeat 3×. It's good if the puppy turns its head in the direction you move, but it does not have to maintain eye contact. However, it must regain eye contact as soon as you return to your original position. You might have to help by saying *LOOK* before you reward the puppy.

SIT—LOOK—STAY move one step *forward* to the left of your puppy and return without stopping. **Reward.** Repeat 5×, release—OK! repeat 3×.

SIT—LOOK—STAY move one step *forward* to the left of your puppy and stop for 2 seconds; return. **Reward.** Repeat 5× release—OK! repeat 3×.

SIT—LOOK—STAY move one step *forward* to the right of your puppy and stop for 2 seconds; return. **Reward.** Repeat 5×, release—OK! repeat 3×.

*Instructions to puppy are in capital letters (SIT, LOOK, etc.) "OK" is used as a release signal to tell the puppy the exercise is finished.

---

months. We run a second class for dogs older than 6 months of age. The class is conducted as a series of four 2-hour weekly sessions. Each session starts with a play period that last about 10 minutes. We then ask the clients to restrain the pups (after week 1 this means *sit*) and have an informational section. During weeks 2 through 4 we use this first informational period to respond to questions from clients. The first informational period is then followed by a demonstra-

tion period, using one of the clients' dogs (these rotate). Clients then, in round-robin style, learn, practice, and demonstrate the exercise. The sequence is then repeated with play, information, and exercise, ending with 20 minutes for client questions. Client-pet teams are assigned homework for the following week. This is presented to them in the form of a handout (Boxes 14-7 through 14-9), and is part of a packet of handout information that they receive weekly. The

BOX 14-7—cont'd

CLIENT-PET HOMEWORK ASSIGNMENTS FOR COMPANION DOG CLASSES

SIT—LOOK—STAY move to the right in a circle around your puppy. **Reward.** *Reminder: Your puppy must make eye contact when you return.* Repeat 5×, release—OK! repeat 3×.

SIT—LOOK—STAY move to the left in a circle around your puppy. **Reward.** *Reminder: Your puppy must make eye contact when you return.* Repeat 5×, release—OK! repeat 3×. Repeat this sequence with all repetitions three or four times during the day. *If your puppy gets up when you move out of sight, note how far behind it you are when it breaks the stay, and back into starting position before you get to the breaking point. This should build the puppy's confidence after a few repetitions. Then, try going farther.*

Day 5 Warm your puppy up by doing the Day 4 exercises without the repetitions.

SIT—LOOK—STAY move two steps back from puppy and stop for 2 secs; return. **Reward.** Repeat 5×, release—OK! repeat 3×.

SIT—LOOK—STAY move two steps back from puppy and then move forward to the left in a now larger circle around your puppy. **Reward.** *Reminder: Your puppy must make eye contact when you return.* Repeat 5×, release—OK! repeat 3×.

SIT—LOOK—STAY move two steps back from puppy and then move forward to the right in a now larger circle around your puppy. **Reward.** *Reminder: Your puppy must make eye contact when you return.* Repeat 5×, release—OK! repeat 3×.

SIT—LOOK—STAY move two steps back from puppy and jog in place for 5 seconds; return. **Reward.** Repeat 5×, release—OK! repeat 3×. If your puppy seems good at this exercise, vary it by stepping at an angle by moving either right or left foot first.

SIT—LOOK—STAY move five steps back from puppy and jog in place for 5 seconds; return. **Reward.** Repeat 5×, release—OK! repeat 3×. If your puppy seems good at this exercise, vary it by stepping at an angle by moving either right or left foot first.

Repeat this sequence with all repetitions three or four times during the day.

Day 6 Warm your puppy up by doing the Day 5 exercises without repetitions.

SIT—LOOK—STAY move 10 steps back from puppy and return without stopping. **Reward.** Repeat 5× release—OK! repeat 3×. If your puppy seems good at this exercise, vary it by stepping at an angle by moving either right or left foot first.

SIT—LOOK—STAY move 10 steps back from puppy and stop for 5 seconds; return. **Reward.** Repeat 5×, release—OK! repeat 3×. If your puppy seems good at this exercise, vary it by stepping at an angle by moving either right or left foot first.

SIT—LOOK—STAY move 10 steps back from puppy and stop for 5 seconds and clap your hands; return. **Reward.** Repeat 5×, release—OK! repeat 3×. If your puppy seems good at this exercise, vary it by stepping at an angle by moving either right or left foot first.

SIT—LOOK—STAY move around the room for ten seconds and return. **Reward.** *Reminder: Your puppy must make eye contact when you return.* Repeat 5×, release—OK! repeat 3×.

Repeat this sequence with all repetitions three or four times during the day.

Puppy Class Homework for Week 1

Practicing Down

Two to three times per day, when your puppy is tired, sit on the floor and DOOOWWWN your puppy as you learned in class. Be sure your puppy is rolled over onto one hip, as we showed you in class. Give your puppy long, soothing strokes to encourage it to relax. Do *not* give a stay command yet (we're teaching stay with sit, and we'll add it to down later). If your puppy gets up, gently command DOOOWWWN again. Sit with your puppy for *a total of* 5 minutes. Release your puppy with OK! *before you stand up.* If your puppy falls asleep, gently wake it so you can release it from the down command. After a few days, when your puppy can lie quietly for 5 minutes, gradually increase the time, but do not exceed 10 minutes.

Developed by Emily Elliot, University of Pennsylvania School of Veterinary Medicine, 1996.

handout packets include information sheets on general canine behavior communication, hormones and reasons for neutering, housebreaking, and flea control. In addition, we include booklets prepared by various pet product companies on grooming, photographing dogs, playing with plastic disks, and problems. We spread the information over the series of four classes so that clients do not have "information overload"

and so that the information in the packets coordinates well with the information in that particular class. The room in which we hold the class has a chalkboard, and an outline of the schedule and topics for each class is posted at the start of the class. Class size is restricted to a maximum of six dogs. Because a veterinary teaching and research hospital has the advantage of student assistants, we always have lots of individ-

---

BOX 14-8

PUPPY CLASS HOMEWORK FOR WEEK TWO

Practicing Come (do *not* practice with sit—look—stay)

Day 1 If you need to, practice your footwork a few times without the dog. Do these exercises with the leash attached so that it tugs on the dog if it does not come when you back up.

PUPPYCOME (wait) take two steps backward SIT—LOOK—**reward.** Do *not* say stay, repeat 3× OK!

PUPPYCOME (wait) take two steps backward to the right, SIT—LOOK—**reward.**

PUPPYCOME (wait) take two steps backward to the right SIT—LOOK—**reward.**

PUPPYCOME (wait) take two steps backward to the right SIT—LOOK—**reward.**

PUPPYCOME (wait) take two steps backward to the right SIT—LOOK—**reward.**

OK! WHAT A GOOD PUPPY! *You just made a square.*

Now practice come by making a square to the left. Practice these exercises three or four times *in the house.* **Reminder:** You're setting your puppy up to succeed. Teaching these exercises outside where there are distractions is too much at first. Wait until Day 5.

Day 2 Warm up with any of the Day 1 exercises.

Now go through the Day 1 exercises without the leash. If your puppy doesn't come, put the leash back on.

Day 3 Warm up with any of the Day 1 exercises.

Get at least one other person to help you. Stand 10 feet apart with the dog with one person. The other person calls PUPPYCOME—SIT—LOOK—**reward**—OK! The first person calls PUPPYCOME—SIT—LOOK—reward—OK! *It is all right if the puppy wanders a bit after being released. After all, it is not being told to do anything. The next person should simply call the dog before it has moved very far.* Call back and forth three or four times. Not too much!

Try to practice at least twice during the day, at least 30 minutes apart.

Day 4 At odd times during the day when your puppy is wandering around the house *not particularly focused on anything,* call PUPPY-COME—SIT—LOOK—**reward**—OK! **Reminder:** Set your puppy up to succeed. Do not call if the puppy is sleeping or playing intently.

Day 5 Do the Day 1 exercises outside if it is not too cold or slippery. Otherwise do them in different rooms in the house.

Day 6 Do the Day 3 exercises outside *only* if you have a fenced area to use. Otherwise do them in the house again.

Practicing Sit and Stay

Every day, pick a different day's exercises from Week 1 and do them. Try them outside if you have a fenced yard.

Practicing Down

Every day, get on the floor and tell your puppy DOOWWN—**reward**—give long, relaxing strokes and gradually stop. Sit there with your puppy *without* stroking or rewarding with food. You can tell the pup it is good, but don't get it excited. Sit there with the puppy for 15 minutes. If it gets up tell it DOOWWN again but DO NOT reward with food, only verbal praise. Do not stroke the dog unless it seems tense. After 15 minutes release with OK! *before you stand up.*

Practice at least once a day; twice is better. Vary the length of time: sometimes 10 minutes, sometimes 20.

Reminder: Every day for 24 hours: Have your puppy sit for all food and attention. Practice encouraging deference.

---

ual one-on-one attention. However, we pay two student assistants to participate in each class so that there are always at least two or three "instructors" per session. This is beneficial when an unruly puppy needs to be babysat or worked with elsewhere while their clients need to listen and observe without a struggle. We do not make a profit with this arrangement, but neither do we lose money. Because we want students to be able to participate if they wish, we undercharge for the classes as a concession to their training. This type of reasonable class schedule can work in private practices, and some practices that have tried

it are letting their nurses conduct the classes, generating the salaries for this extra time from the class itself. Regardless, clients require high-quality, accurate information to make this type of class successful. Clients always want more than practitioners can give, and the ability to reach a reasonable compromise is important. These classes are not intended to be substitutes for obedience classes (note the title) but can prepare the dogs for later participation in such classes. Meanwhile, the dogs have learned to perform the basic behaviors that will allow their clients to not become frustrated with them: sit, stay, come, down, and walk nicely on a leash. These classes have been so successful that all the clients have asked that they be ongoing or extended. The clients usually arrive early to visit with each other and let the dogs play and practice. I once opened the inner door to the waiting room of VHUP at 8:30 on a Saturday morning to see a pug in one of the classes go flying past with a Lab in hot pursuit—and they came when called.

The pattern for the classes held at VHUP is found in Box 14-10. The homework assignments (see Boxes 14-7 through 14-9) were prepared by one of the veterinary students who helps conduct the classes (and who has dogs with obedience titles), Emily Elliot (University of Pennsylvania, School of Veterinary Medicine, 1996). The overall schedule (Box 14-10) sets an ambitious pace. If needed (and some groups will need it) the take it–drop it exercise can be deleted from the last class, and the other activities spread over 4, not 3 weeks.

WHAT ELSE?

Clients need one final piece of assistance to integrate their new pet into their household: how do they introduce this pet to the preexisting household members? These issues are outlined in Boxes 14-11 and 14-12 and addressed in the protocols in Appendix B.

Education is the best technique for problem prevention. Knowing common behavior problems and how and when they develop may not prevent them, but can help clients to recognize problems early when intervention is the easiest and most efficacious. There are special concerns for recycled pets that are outlined in Box 14-13. These are not generally insurmountable problems.

All clients with dogs should be familiar with the AKC's Canine Good Citizen Test. This evaluation tests a dog with regard to the following:

1. Overall appearance and response to grooming
2. Acceptance of a stranger
3. Walking on a loose lead
4. Walking through a crowd
5. Sitting for examination
6. Sit and down for examination
7. Stay in position
8. Reaction to another dog
9. Reaction to distractions
10. Reaction to being left alone

Dogs that can behave within some fairly wide ranges of tolerance with regard to the above will generally be very happy pets with people who love, value, and are pleased with them.

COMMON PROBLEMS: EARLY IDENTIFICATION AND SOLUTIONS

Given the above, there are a few problems that can be prevented outright and some that can be greatly diminished by early intervention.

Clearly, most management problems (see Chapter 11) can be prevented. Clients need to know the common management problems so that they can antici-

---

BOX 14-9
PUPPY CLASS HOMEWORK FOR WEEK THREE

Practicing Down—Stay

Instead of sitting on the floor, just lean over and DOOWWN your dog. Tell it to STAY and reward FREQUENTLY. When the dog can stay for 10 seconds with you standing in front of it, start moving your feet away as you did for the SIT—LOOK—STAY exercises. Progress only as much as your dog can succeed. Do not try for too much too fast. *Reminder*: Release your dog with OK! Do not inadvertently teach your dog to break the STAY by forgetting to release it or by asking it to do more than it can. *Reminder*: It is harder for the dog to look at you from its position lying on the floor; however, it should be paying attention: not sniffing or looking all around. Keep the dog's attention by talking to it, saying STAY and GOOD DOG.

Practicing Leash-Walking

Use the command LET'S GO instead of come on. Use THIS WAY to change direction. Take dog treats with you and practice SIT—LOOK—STAY every time you stop (e.g. at corners). *Reminder*: **Release your dog with OK!**

Practicing Sit—Look—Stay

Every day, pick a different day's exercises from Week 1 and do them. Try them outside if you have a fenced yard.

Practicing Puppy Come—Sit

Every day, pick a different day's exercises from Week 2 and do them. Add PUPPYCOME—SIT to your daily leash walks as I showed you in class.

Practicing Down for the Long Down

Every day, get on the floor and tell your puppy DOOWWN—reward—give long, relaxing strokes and gradually stop. Sit there with your puppy *without* stroking or rewarding it with food. You can tell the dog it is good, but don't get it excited. Sit with the dog for 15 minutes. If it gets up, command DOOWWN again but DO NOT reward with food, only verbal praise. Do not stroke the dog unless it seems tense. After 15 minutes release with OK! *before you stand up.* Practice at least once a day, twice is better. Vary the length of time: sometimes 10 minutes, sometimes 20.

Reminder: Every day for 24 hours: All attention is earned. Practice the deference protocol.

---

pate them. Clients should also learn to gradually expose the cat or dog to all maintenance behaviors it will require (see Box 14-4 and 14-5). Cats deserve par-

BOX 14-10

PATTERN FOR PUPPY AND ADULT DOG COMPANION CLASSES

Week 1

15 Minutes: Everyone introduces themselves and tells what kind of pet(s) they have and why they got this dog.

5 Minutes: Puppy play period—all pups let off lead to chase each other around. Clients can watch but not intervene. All dangerous objects have been removed before class, mops and disinfectant are available, and the staff is watching for problem or dangerous activities. (The clients will be afraid that their pups will be hurt; if the staff is vigilant this will not happen, and this is a good time to learn that pups play roughly—and can learn to inhibit their bites.) This is a good time to tell clients about nonverbal communication.

10 Minutes: Bathroom break for all concerned

5 Minutes: Discussion: leashes, collars, identification, halters, harnesses (some of the pups will be fitted with a head collar or no pull harness during the "stay" session)

25 Minutes: Teach sit with demonstrations using food treats and—*no hands.* Clients practice with their own dogs and staff help. Clients demonstrate.

5 Minutes: Play period

5 Minutes: Pass the puppy

10 Minutes: Information: diets, exercise, and gastric dilatation and volvulus; normal puppy behavior; normal elimination behavior and housebreaking

10 Minutes: Teach and demonstrate *stay* with treats. Clients practice with staff supervision. Clients demonstrate and integrate with *sit* command.

5 Minutes: Play period

5 Minutes: Pass the puppy

10 Minutes: Information about discussions for future classes and client questions. Do not be afraid to say that the information that they want is covered in the packet. (Escort the clients to the door unless you want to provide tea and coffee and another play period—if so, add a bathroom break.) Clients are really overloaded by this point and can only socialize, not absorb more information.

Week 2

15 Minutes: Questions from last week

5 Minutes: Puppy play period

10 Minutes: Bathroom break for all concerned

5 Minutes: Discussion: vaccinations, fecal examinations, and parasite infestations and treatment

25 Minutes: Review sit and stay from last week: demos! Start *come.*

5 Minutes: Play period

5 Minutes: Pass the puppy

10 Minutes: Information: brushing the dog's teeth and cleaning the ears—special grooming needs and brush/comb display

10 Minutes: Teach and demonstrate *down* with treats. Clients practice with staff supervision. Clients demonstrate and integrate with come.

5 Minutes: Play period

5 Minutes: Pass the puppy

10 Minutes: Information about discussions for future classes and client questions

Week 3

15 Minutes: Questions from last week

5 Minutes: Puppy play period

10 Minutes: Bathroom break for all concerned

5 Minutes: Discussion: nail trimming, basic emergency care, what to look for in a lymph node

25 Minutes: Review *sit, stay, come,* and *down.* Puppy-client team demos! Start *on* and *off lead* and *long down.*

5 Minutes: Play period

5 Minutes: Pass the puppy

10 Minutes: Information: giving a dog a pill and taking a temperature—the importance of knowing normal!

10 Minutes: Long down, continued. Clients practice with staff supervision. Clients demonstrate and integrate with *come* and *sit.*

5 Minutes: Play period

5 Minutes: Pass the puppy

10 Minutes: Information about discussions for future classes and client questions

Week 4

15 Minutes: Questions from last week

5 Minutes: Puppy play period

10 Minutes: Bathroom break for all concerned

5 Minutes: Discussion: breed-specific health concerns, growth, life expectancies, the death of a pet

25 Minutes: Review everything learned to date. Demonstrations by client-puppy teams. This is the time to institute corrections and suggestions.

5 Minutes: Play period

5 Minutes: Pass the puppy

10 Minutes: Information: classes available in the area, classification of agility training, obedience, conformation, high jumping, Canine Good Citizen (CGC) test (AKC), Pet Partners (Delta Society).

10 Minutes: Teach and demonstrate *take it–drop it* with rawhides and toys. Clients practice with staff supervision. Clients demonstrate and integrate with other tasks.

5 Minutes: Play period

5 Minutes: Pass the puppy

10 Minutes: Client questions and graduation certificate!

BOX 14-11

INTRODUCTION OF A NEW PUPPY OR KITTEN

1. Reminder—these are babies
2. Feeding and eating schedules
3. Avoid rough and inappropriate play
4. Crates or safe rooms when unsupervised
5. Close supervision—bells
6. Gradual introductions
7. Know about any predatory tendencies
8. Individual "quality" time
9. Age- and size-specific pet toys
10. Understand what it is that you want to reward

BOX 14-12

INTRODUCTION OF A NEW PET

1. Learn about any former problems
2. Do not do everything at once
3. Instruct children that fear can facilitate aggression
4. Separate from all other pets and children when not supervised
5. Gradually introduce under controlled circumstances (leash)
6. Use feeding opportunities
7. Individual quality time
8. Correct appropriately
9. No harsh physical punishment
10. Crates?
11. Be prepared for problems—do not get stuck in the middle
12. Do not expect all personalities to be the same
13. Consider age and personality matches and mismatches
14. Teach clients to read body language cues
15. Drugs?

---

ticular attention because they are most at risk (because of management styles) for intractable behaviors. Clients should learn to trim cat's nails, give them pills using treats and "fake" medications, and, if a long-haired cat, how to gently bathe and groom to prevent matting. Clients need to understand what is "normal." This also means that if their pet has been hospitalized, the return home could be met with anxiety-related behaviors from the other pets (vocalization, increased locomotion, changes in elimination behaviors) and changes in the patient's behavior that could include changes in elimination behavior.

Canine aggression is the most commonly seen suite of problems in the Behavior Clinic at VHUP, although general hospital clients most frequently complain about dogs jumping on people and pulling on the leash (Overall, unpublished, 1990; R.K. Anderson, personal communication, 1990). Aggressive syndromes have been well described. Early warning signs of most aggressions are recognizable if the clients learn what to look for early in their relationship with the dog. It is at this time that rational punishment will be the most successful. For punishment to succeed it must occur preferably in 1 second, but generally within the first 30 to 60 seconds, of the *onset* of the inappropriate behavior. The punishment should preferably startle the animal sufficiently to interrupt the behavior and abort any attempt at immediate resumption. The pup can then be taught a more appropriate behavior, such as sitting and staying. Sitting and staying serves as a time-out and teaches that the client is the leader in the situation and that the pup must take all cues as to the appropriateness of its behavior from the client. This is important, because at the crux of aggressive problems is the fact that these dogs are abnormal; they are incapable of making appropriate, in-context distinctions. Accordingly, a dog that is protectively aggressive will protect clients equally from a burglar and from a friend; fearfully aggressive dogs are afraid of both gentle and unfriendly approaches. These dogs exhibit inappropriate, out-of-context behavior. Early intervention must be aimed at getting the dog under ex-

cellent voice control and teaching it to make better context distinctions by taking cues from the client.

An example of an aggressive situation that is relatively common and benefits greatly from early intervention is food-related aggression. Food-related aggression is often a precursor of dominance aggression. Dogs that are aggressive around their food are also usually aggressive with table scraps, rawhide bones, and real bones. The latter two are excellent elicitors of this type of aggressive behavior. In general, food-related aggression is very difficult to treat; it is usually far simpler and safer to preclude treats, bones, and rawhides and to feed the dog in isolation. But what should the client do at the first signs of such aggression, before it has become an intractable problem?

All pups should be taught to sit and stay for verbal praise or food treats; no pup older than 7 weeks of age is too young to learn this (Voith, 1982a,b). Clients should then routinely practice making the pup sit and wait to be fed and taking the dish away. The first signs of any aggression can be corrected with a sharp, "no" and removal of the pup from the situation; it must then earn the food back by sitting and staying. The crux of this type of instruction is that the dog sees the client as the one from whom it must take the cues about the appropriateness of the behavior. Should the pup continue to threaten, it is already time to seek professional help. Should the pup learn to relinquish its dish to the client, the potential for dominance aggression later in life should be discussed.

Dominance aggression commonly develops at social maturity, usually between 18 and 24 months of age (range, 12 to 36 months) (Borchelt & Voith, 1986a). Dogs exhibiting this behavioral syndrome challenge and threaten clients or other humans for control by staring, barking, or growling when given commands, leaning on them, growling or biting when disturbed while sleeping or when stepped over, frequently having to have the last word when verbally corrected, and when physically punished, including hanging, becoming more aggressive. The condition is treatable and controllable with proper therapy, but it can be recognized before any biting has occurred if the clients are attuned to the signs above. As soon as they recognize these early behaviors, clients need to start a program or schedule of behaviors that compels the dog to give in to the client for everything it wants. This can be as simple as sitting and staying for all attention, food, play, egress or ingress, and grooming. The dog must learn to take all the cues about whether its behavior is appropriate from the client. Absolutely no physical punishment should be used; to do so is to risk the dog intensifying its aggression to the client, thus putting the client in a risky situation. Early intervention can prevent this situation from becoming dangerous and injurious. It should be emphasized to clients that behavioral problems involving aggression are controlled, not cured, and that the dog will have to live with that level of discipline forever.

The same principles of appropriate punishment and counterconditioning can be applied to most canine behavioral problems. Given what is known about developmental/sensitive periods, clients can be counseled about the best time to housebreak a pup (8½ weeks of age) and what to expect if they adopt an older pup. Such counseling should coincide with the first puppy visit to the veterinarian. In no case should the pup be physically punished after the fact for eliminating in the house; this only teaches the pup to be fearful of the approach of the client or of the area where it urinated or defecated, and in the latter case the dog will just find a new spot. Clients should be cautioned that puppies require frequent opportunities to urinate and defecate *and* to just smell the roses. Pups that are rigidly taken outside six times a day for 5 minutes with only one goal in mind will spend the 5 minutes smelling trees and watching butterflies; they will then eliminate in the house. Sniffing and movement are part of normal elimination behaviors. Pups should be taken outside 15 to 30 minutes after each meal for at least 20 minutes. This allows them sufficient time to both explore and eliminate. They should be praised and loved if they perform appropriately. If they do not urinate or defecate outside after this time, they should be carefully watched when brought back into the house. If the client spies on the pup and the pup starts to urinate or defecate, the client should startle the pup to stop the elimination and take it outside. Again, remember: the pup should be startled within the first 60 seconds of the onset of the behavior, the onset of the behavior includes the initial sniffing and circling, and the startle should be sufficient to abort the behavior, after which time the pup must be presented with an alternate substrate.

Behaviors such as jumping up, pawing, barking for attention, and pulling on the leash can be modified with the same counterconditioning techniques. Pups should be rewarded for appropriate behavior and ignored, in the case of jumping and pawing, for inappropriate behavior. Ignoring the dog must be a passive, rather than active process: the pup cannot be pushed down; instead, it must be sloughed off. To a pup that is desperate (whether with reason or not) for attention, pushing it away with a hand or foot can be seen as interacting. Even abuse, if that is the only attention a pup gets, can be viewed as interaction. Dogs with such behaviors also respond superbly to some of the newer training systems with dog halters (Gentle Leader/Promise System Canine Head Collar; Premier Products, Richmond; Va). These halters allow the clients to achieve and maintain excellent control over the dog's head and to lead the dog to positions that will earn the dog praise. The halters are wonderful devices for teaching new pups to walk on a leash and are godsends for people who have been dragged for years by their pets on leash-walks. Such devices should be used in conjunction with the principles of behavior modification already discussed.

Dogs that play too roughly and were early orphaned can be taught by the same methods to play more gently. Rambunctious play should never occur using hands and arms; toys are far more appropriate and help the pet to make contextual distinctions about what they can and cannot bite. Rough play is permissible if and only if the client can recognize the difference between play and nonplay growls, can interpret canine facial signals, can be trusted not to hurt the pup, and always, in a tug of war, is able to win, with the pet releasing the toy. Clients should *not* teach pups that they will be chased for toys or stolen objects unless they wish the pup to learn that such behavior will always elicit an interactive response from the client that the pup considers play.

Finally, pups should be exposed to a variety of stimuli early and frequently to take advantage of the developmental/socialization period when they most easily learn to accommodate novel situations (to 16 weeks). This is especially true if the dog will be expected to travel regularly in the car or on planes or be exposed to guns, bells, children, and so on. It is equally critical that during these exposures the pup not be horrified; therefore introductions to gunshots, for example, should be gradual and attenuated and associated with other good events. This approach does not guarantee that the pet will have no problems in later life, but will give the client the best chance and minimize the extent of future problems. Dogs are a lot like children; how they turn out is not all your fault.

THE ROLE OF TRAINING: WHAT IT WILL AND WILL NOT HELP

Obedience training, puppy kindergarten, and individual training all have their roles. They may function best to recognize early signs of possible behavioral problems rather than to prevent them. Certainly for some dogs with little other exposure to dogs, they can be very worthwhile. They are invaluable from the standpoint of getting the dog and the client to interact and in teaching the client, directly or indirectly, about variation in dog behavior and response to training. Once a problem develops, obedience training is an in-

appropriate substitute for intervention from a behavioral specialist. Such dogs are not just misbehaving, they are not normal, and to treat them as such, expecting normal responses to ever intensifying corrections, is dangerous to pet and client alike. The negative effect of inappropriate training, particularly regarding the use of physical punishment, is finally being addressed by those in the field (Myles, 1991). It is *never* appropriate to recommend to an client to hang a dog to subdue aggression. If the client cannot back the dog down, and this may take a fight to the death, the client is at risk of being injured. Furthermore, the dog is at risk of injured ocular vessels, tracheal and esophageal damage, and recurrent laryngeal nerve paralysis. This invariably leads to death.

Issues Yet to be Resolved

1. The big issue is still the one involving nature versus nurture. We know that how an animal is raised can and does affect its later behavior. We do not know to what extent later responses are influenced by genetics. It is interesting that, given the state of technology available to study genetics, we know so little in any quantitative sense of its effects on the development of normal, abnormal, or breed-related behavior.

2. The patterns of development of problem behaviors are largely unknown. Knowledge of such patterns is important if we are to understand what type of intervention is best applied at what point.

15 ····· Legal Issues in Behavioral Medicine

DEIDRE GANNON, Esq.

●●

*B*ecause of the geographic locale of the authors and the cases used in this book, most of the legal information in this chapter refers only to U.S. law. However, the issues raised (laws banning breeds, dangerous dogs) are issues that are relevant for all countries engaged in such debates, most notably Great Britain.

The legal system in the United States, with the exception of Louisiana, is based on the common law of England. Unlike the civil law countries, which are code based, the common law is constantly changing and evolving. This is especially true of the animal law areas.

During the past 10 to 15 years the spotlight of public opinion has focused on the animal world, in particular on dogs. The "pit bull" media blitz has resulted in a variety of vicious dog laws, some of which specifically ban certain breeds. Planned communities, such as condominiums, have expressly excluded animals by the language contained in the governing documents. The New Jersey Society for the Prevention of Cruelty to Animals filed charges against a man for killing a rat in his garden.

As a result, professional and semiprofessional organizations began to organize to positively affect legislation concerning animals and the people associated with them. Although more beneficial bills are being enacted, overall the animal world is becoming a highly regulated industry.

Veterinarians, by choice of profession, are part of this process. Thus the veterinarian needs to know not only how the law can potentially affect his or her practice, but how it could affect his or her client population and their animals.

The following text is an overview of a variety of basic legal concepts that affect animals and animal professionals together with more in-depth information on issues that may arise because of the American Veterinary Medical Association (AVMA) recognition of behavioral medicine as a specialty.

PROPERTY AND TITLE CONCEPTS

According to the law, animals are considered to be personal property, that is, a "thing" over which the client has the exclusive right to possess, use, and dispose of as he or she sees fit. Technically, the animal has no rights. The person, however, holds title to the animal and has various rights and responsibilities based on that ownership. Thus the statutes and case law that have been developed deal strictly with the actions of the client or other person in possession and control of the animal.

Although the concepts of property and title form the foundation of animal law, they are probably the most difficult to accept. It is hard to acknowledge that the living, breathing creature that showers us with unconditional love is no better than our refrigerator or any other appliance. Animals are an emotional subject, which makes the distancing required of the professional more difficult.

Despite rapid advances in other animal-related fields, the legal community has been slow to move away from historical concepts. Property law is especially well grounded in the past. Until recently there have been no pressing reasons to alter proven theory, especially where small animals are concerned.

Some progress has been seen in the large-animal fields because of the high value placed on particular species. For example, a person who contracts to sell a barren cow, who later discovers that the cow had conceived, can void the contract based on mutual mistake of fact. Obviously, a cow that can conceive is more valuable than one that cannot.

Progress also has been made in the valuation of horses. Courts regularly consider the racing or show career of the animal in addition to its potential stud or breeding potential.

However, this is not true in small-animal valuations. In most cases, the replacement value of a dog or cat is the price of a puppy or a kitten. Thus a top-winning show dog or obedience titlist has no more value than that of the mixed breed next door. Attempts to have show careers, stud and breeding potentials, training costs, and so forth taken into consideration have met with little success. Too few cases have been presented to the courts for review because of the high expense of the legal system as opposed to the expectations of recovery. Few, if any, attorneys will accept a small-animal case on a contingency basis. Although the attorney and the client may agree that the value of the animal is in the thousands of dollars, the attorney realizes that his percentage will most likely be based on a court valuation of a few hundred dollars. Only a few clients have the finances and strength of character to pursue these matters regardless of cost.

However, there has been some progress in the courts of equity where specific animals rather than money is involved. For example, a buyer contracts with the breeder to purchase the pick male puppy of a specific litter. The breeder decides to keep the pick male and tries to give the buyer a different puppy. The buyer wants only the specific puppy he has contracted for and brings suit against the breeder for specific performance. The courts have recognized that an animal is *unique property* that cannot be replaced by another animal or money damages. In other words, the buyer will not receive the benefit of the bargain unless he receives that specific puppy. Thus the court is likely to require that the breeder perform exactly as he has contracted to do with the buyer. The breeder will be ordered to turn over the pick male puppy to the buyer.

Although the courts of equity have their place, they are of limited use. The ideal is to move forward to the point where the legal system recognizes animals as "special property" and takes all possible factors into consideration during the valuation process. Should this occur, other areas of animal law will also benefit (e.g., service dog access, housing availability for animal owners) without the necessity for specific legislation. Meanwhile, it is important that animal professionals remember that their client is the person and that the animal is considered by law to be an object.

ANIMALS IN MODERN SOCIETY

Although all animals may be affected to some degree, dog owners have been the most affected in recent years by restrictions on ownership, liability for the actions of their animals, and insurance industry discrimination in providing coverage. Therefore the following sections will be presented and analyzed from the dog owner's perspective.

LEGISLATIVE ACTION

Although the federal government has involved itself in some animal legislation, the state and local governments have had the greatest impact. The tenth amendment to the Constitution, known as the reserve powers amendment, protects the sovereign powers of the individual states. Most important, for this discussion, is the inherent police power of state governments, which is often delegated to some degree to local governmental units.

The "police powers" give the governmental unit the right to enact public restrictions on private rights where they are reasonably related to the protection of the general health, safety, and welfare of the community. These are fairly broad based, discretionary powers. If challenged, the governmental unit need only show that the restriction is rationally related to the attainment of a legitimate governmental goal.

For example, few will disagree that "pooper scooper" laws requiring owners to clean up after their dogs are rationally related to the governmental goal of protecting the health of the community. Along the same lines, leash laws can be shown to be rationally related to the protection of the safety of the community. Although it is easy to make the connection between the law and the governmental goal in the above areas, the connection is not always as clear in local government's attempts to restrict the number of dogs owned, breeding bans, and breed-specific vicious dog ordinances. However, each of these has been attempted by governmental units throughout the United States and many have been upheld as a legitimate exercise of their police powers.

Local governmental units have enacted the most animal-related restrictions, but the state governments have the right of preemption. This is a judicial doctrine whereby a state can assert its supremacy over the multitude of local governments under its authority. This is usually done in areas of the law where uniformity is desired and the issue has attained sufficient importance that it has come to the attention of the higher governmental unit. The New Jersey Vicious Dog Act is a prime example of state preemption of a specific area from the jurisdiction of the local governmental units.

The federal government also has the power to preempt state action; however, this power is used only in those areas that have become so important that they require a national uniformity. The federal government does not lightly take sovereign powers away from the individual states. Thus national vicious dog laws are for the future. The attempt to enact a national lemon law failed. Classifying certain animal activities as protected as a result of the animal rights activists' actions *did* pass, and the extra-label drug use bill will be enacted into law on the national level in the United States.

This pyramid governmental structure is typical of a democratic society; however, it also allows for further subdivision. Approximately 20 years ago this occurred when the housing industry began building condominium developments. The documents creating these communities give certain powers over the development to a board of trustees that governs the association. Dogs already have become an issue because of the ownership structure of the condominium association. Ownership is divided into private ownership of the unit and common ownership of the grounds. When one person's dog causes destruction to the property of the whole community, the boards are often compelled to enact rules for the benefit of the whole community. Even if the municipality has enacted a two-dog limit, the condominium board may further restrict the owners to no dogs allowed.

Regardless of the level of legislation, those proposing the bills are usually well-meaning individuals who see a need for specific action. This does not necessarily mean that they are right or have the knowledge necessary to fairly and effectively impose further regulations on specific groups of people. The perfect examples of "legislative backfire" are the vicious dog and lemon laws. These two legislative areas affect veterinarians, their clients, and the relationship between the two.

Lemon Laws

Most "lemon laws" are structured to give the veterinarian sole decision-making power as to the fitness for sale of a particular animal. This is a broad power that must be exercised judiciously. In most cases the power is absolute and should not be used to accommodate the client's needs or desires. The greatest danger of abuse exists when the client has made an error either in the selection of a breed or a particular puppy. Rather than handling an error in judgment under the lemon law, the veterinarian should counsel the client to discuss the situation with the breeder. However, are all veterinarians capable of making judgments regarding the physical, mental, and emotional/behavioral fitness of all animals? If this were true, there would be no need for specialists within the profession. The average lawmaker is not fully aware of how specialized veterinary medicine has become over the years. The provision for a second opinion of the seller's choice does not necessarily make this any fairer to the animal, the buyer, the veterinarian, or the seller. If the lemon laws could be applied only to the problems that caused their enactment (e.g., puppy mills with atrocious conditions), this might create a different situation. However, too often such well-meaning legislation is applied to the private breeder, who takes great pains to do appropriate genetic testing, plans each breeding carefully, and raises each litter in the best conditions possible, because not every veterinarian can make judgments about all facets of the animal on presentation. Mistakes are made, and these can ruin the responsible breeder's reputation as well as bankrupting the small show kennel.

Furthermore, genetic testing is breed specific. Although a majority of breeds are routinely checked for hip dysplasia and eye problems, not all will be tested for hearing, blood disorders, or many of the rarer problems known to occur only in a handful of breeds.

Unlike Europe, which uses breed wardens to enforce stringent breeding practices, the United States exercises no control over the breeding of animals. It is the responsibility of each and every breeder to know their breed problems and to breed only those animals free of genetic defects. Some believe the lemon laws are, in effect, a way to legislate ethical breeding practices in the United States. Unfortunately, no individual veterinarian can be fully versed in each and every breed that might come into the office. In addition to the 150+ breeds recognized by the AKC, there are more than 300 other breeds recognized internationally.

Vicious Dog Laws

Vicious dog legislation,* although less veterinarian-intensive, can place unwanted obligations on members of the profession. Some breed-specific acts confer recognition of specific breeds on either an animal control officer, the local law enforcement personnel, or a veterinarian.

The more recent attempts at enacting breeding bans also puts pressure on the veterinarian community. Under some of these acts, a veterinarian who treats a litter and fails to inform the authorities that a litter was whelped in a restricted area (e.g., where only those licensed to breed animals would be allowed legally to do so) would be in violation of the law. However, on the other hand, clients may fail to seek veterinarian intervention because they have an illegal litter, resulting in harm to the animals involved.

Much more can be said about animals, specifically dogs, their place in modern society and legislation at all levels; however, that is beyond the scope of this chapter.

LIABILITY CONSIDERATIONS
Personal Injury

Every veterinarian should be cognizant of the potential areas of liability that his or her client may face merely by owning an animal. Veterinarian involvement is usually as an advisor or as an expert witness.

The most common situation involves a dog bite. The imposition of liability depends on the state in which the event occurs. Unless there is a unique statutory scheme, there will be either strict liability or known propensity.

Strict liability means liability without fault. Therefore if the dog bites, the owner is liable. Even if the owner was not in possession of the dog at the time, he or she will still be liable because *no showing of negligence* is required. The theory behind this is that the keeping of dogs is an ultrahazardous activity that has an inherent risk of injury. One New Jersey judge made the statement that ". . . all dogs have teeth. Therefore all dogs will bite . . ." while imposing the strict liability standard on the state (*Tanga v Tanga*, 94 N.J. Super 5, 222 A.2d 723 [1967]).

Until recently, the "known propensity" standard or the *"one-bite rule"* was in effect in most states. In order for liability to attach, there must be a showing of negligence on the part of the person in possession and control of the dog. A showing of negligence requires that the first person owe a duty of care to the second person. If the duty of care was present and the first person breached that duty and the injury to the second person was directly caused by that breach, then the first person would be liable to the second person.

---

*The reader is reminded that this is the description used in law, not in medicine; the word *vicious* is not an acceptable substitute for either a description or a diagnosis of aggression.

A definitive showing of a dog owner's duty of care to another person was that the dog had already bitten once. That first bite was presumed to put the owner on notice that the dog had a known propensity, or tendency, to bite. There is no requirement that this be a reported bite. Local authorities need not have been involved. This standard also includes the situation in which the owner should have known that the dog had the tendency to bite. Because the owner knew, or should have known, that a bite might happen, he or she owed a duty of care to others to properly contain and control the animal so that another bite did not occur. Actual knowledge is not required. Many landlords have been held liable for the actions of tenant-owned dogs under the known propensity standard. Case law presumes that the landlord would have knowledge of the animals on his or her property through routine inspections. Ignorance is no excuse.

This same duty of care can be extended to impose liability under the *doctrine of attractive nuisance.* In other words, a person who maintains animals on his or her property that are likely to attract children is under a duty to reasonably protect those children against dangers of that attraction. The theory is that the harm to the child is foreseeable. There is a social policy consideration in the protection of the young. That the child was a trespasser or the fact that all animals are likely to attract children is only a factor that might be considered. This is the same reasoning behind the obligation to enclose swimming pools with a fence.

In light of the above, the question remains as to what constitutes reasonable care/protection of another person/child. Although chain link and invisible fencing may be sufficient to keep the dogs in and the adult out, the adult being contributively negligent if trespassing on the premises, it is unlikely that it would be sufficient for a child. Given the worst-case scenario, securely fastened stockade fencing or chain link run with another secure chain link walkway surrounding it are the only outside enclosures that might be found to be reasonable precautions. The current social and political climate is far from animal friendly.

The most often asked question regarding the posting of signs fails under the same analysis. They are express notification that dogs are on the property. A child need only be able to read to have this constitute an attractive nuisance. In addition, designating the dogs on the premises as guard dogs is admitting that you know the dogs will bite, negating the one-bite rule even if it would be available.

There is a major difference between signs that say "Beware of Dog" and those that say "Be Aware of Dog." The former is an overt warning, whereas the latter is merely a notice that there are dogs on the property (i.e., keep gate closed). Equally acceptable are signs that say "Dogs on property" or "Large dogs on property." However, although signs that say "Forget the dogs, Beware of owner," may be cute, those that say "Trespassers will be eaten" or "Property protected by a pit bull" are not funny.

One final permutation of this analysis is "assumption of the risk," which is why veterinarians and their staff can rarely hold the owner of the animal liable if they are bitten in the course of professional treatment. Here the person injured has knowledge that the situation could be potentially dangerous and has voluntarily exposed himself to the risk of injury. There is implied consent regardless of the care or lack of care used. In some jurisdictions, the assumption of the risk doctrine has been abolished in favor of contributory negligence of the injured party in undertaking the risk. States with comparative negligence acts, whereby the responsibility for the damages between the parties is allocated to each according to his actions, have negated the need for the assumption of the risk doctrine.

Finally, note that biting is not the only action an animal can take that would impose liability on the owner. Under most modern statutes, any action that results in an injury would be sufficient reason. This would include scratching, jumping on, nipping, and so forth. Although these behaviors may constitute normal animal exuberance, they can create a liability situation. Remember, that, under the law, you take your victims as you find them. Whether your neighbor is an athletic 20-year-old or a 92-year-old lady with arthritis, your dog needs to be trained not to jump and leap in greeting. A little obedience training and control of the animal will go a long way and protect the owner and the animal.

Essentially, today's social and political environment is not animal friendly, and all owners need to be very, very careful in the maintenance of their animals.

Property Damage

Animals are often classified as nuisances. A nuisance, which can be either public or private, is an unreasonable interference with the free use and enjoyment of one's property. It originates from the unreasonable or unlawful use of property to the discomfort, annoyance, inconvenience, or damage to another. "Another" can include an individual, a family, a segment of the public, or even the public at large.

Various acts of animals and animal owners can constitute private or public nuisances. Some examples include continuously barking dogs, cats destroying gardens, the stench coming from a pig farm, and so forth.

The changing nature of communities makes this a potent weapon for unfriendly neighbors. Although some jurisdictions will hold that the new owner moved to the nuisance, others will consider the way the area has evolved in deciding whether a nuisance is present. You could have peacefully operated in the same location for 20 years and suddenly find that your business is considered a public nuisance. There is case law that supports the ability of local government to remove or abate the nuisance. Limiting the numbers of animals maintained in any one dwelling is an often used device. Although grandfather clauses can protect the existing use for a period of time, they really only maintain the status quo. Animal limits have proved to be highly effective in forcing people to move out of a restrictive community into less restrictive ones. In addition, this effect has encouraged other communities to adopt similar ordinances.

An unexpected result of limiting the number of animals one property may maintain is the partnering of those like situated. Two or more people may get together in different locations to mutually own a larger number of animals. This has already become apparent in dog fancy. However, there is potential for liability that few have yet to realize. For example, a coowned dog bites, the owner in possession claims bad temperament, the breeder-owner not in possession claims mishandling of the animal. The court declares joint and several liability for both parties. This situation may also become a future problem for veterinarians because of unknown ownership interests. Initial treatment agreements where the owner or other person presenting the animal for treatment agrees to indemnify the veterinarian against any claims by anyone else with an ownership interest in the animal may become necessary in the near future.

Property damage also includes instances when the animal itself is injured or killed or another animal is injured or killed. The analysis of liability imposition is the same as that regarding personal injury. However, some recent suits have given a new twist to the property damage issue: For example, "midnight raider" complaints, whereby a confined bitch in standing heat is bred by a dog that jumps the fence into the yard, breeds the bitch, and leaves. When seen and identified, the offending dog's owner could be cited for violation of the leash law. Because the dog is considered property of the owner, the dog cannot be held for trespass, but neither can the owner. If the bitch was scheduled for another stud dog, there may be damages available for the delay of the planned breeding. If the bitch conceives and requires veterinarian attention, the expenses may be chargeable to the raider's owners. This is an interesting area to watch over the next few years as animal owners are continuously being forced to be responsible owners.

The unfortunate side of greater governmental interference with animal ownership—greater willingness of individuals to bring suit for even the most minor infraction of their supposed rights, and the eternally irresponsible owner who ruins things for everyone—is that it is becoming more difficult for the responsible owner to maintain sufficient numbers of animals to remain active in the varied activities and events available. The size of one show kennel operation has been dramatically reduced because a breeder can exhibit only one or two dogs for a limited amount of time. Age alone requires that another dog be acquired to continue in the dog show sport.

Dog and cat fanciers especially do not want to give up their older show animal that is truly a member of the family just to get a younger one for show purposes. Although placement of the animal may not be in the best interests of the animal or the owner, governments and neighbors are putting a select group of people in that position almost daily. Would they be as agreeable if someone suggested the same should be done with their children after a certain number have been born?

BEHAVIORAL MEDICINE PRACTICE
General Practitioner

Every state has a statutory scheme to provide for the licensing of professionals. This is done because the states have an interest in ensuring a minimum level of competence/quality is being provided to the general public. Veterinarians are subject to professional licensing by the state. This licensing, which is considered a privilege and not a right, subjects the licensee to the requirements of the licensing board and any disciplinary procedures that may be in place should that person fall below the standard of conduct that has been set.

To avoid negligence in the practice of veterinary medicine, the law also requires that the licensed veterinarian meet certain minimum standards of care. Because of professional licensing requirements, this is an enhanced standard of care.

The law of negligence is based on the "ordinary man" standard of care. That is, requiring the person acting to conduct himself or herself as another "reasonable person of ordinary prudence" would do in the same circumstances. Should the person's conduct fall below the standard of the reasonable person, he or she may be liable for injuries or damages resulting from the substandard conduct.

Veterinarians, because of their special education and experience, are held to the "reasonable" veterinarian standard of care—in other words, the conduct of another veterinarian with similar training and experience with a similar type practice. In some states this requirement is further restricted to another similar veterinarian in the same locality, in others only to one similarly situated regardless of locality. Specialized training and board certifications as a specialist raise the standard of care even higher to that of another similarly situated specialist. Locality is irrelevant in the care of a specialist.

Negligence, which is an element of various tort or personal injury claims, is defined as the failure to exercise the degree of care that an ordinary person would exercise under the same circumstances. Although negligence is an element of malpractice, malpractice is defined as a professional's failure to exercise the degree of care that a professional similarly situated would have exercised in a professional relationship of like circumstances with his or her client.

This is where the veterinary-client relationship becomes problematic. Although most veterinary malpractice claims fail because fewer veterinarians than doctors will testify against each other, it is better to avoid the potential for a malpractice claim from the beginning of the relationship with each client.

The client is the person who legally owns the animal or who has the legal possession and control of the animal. The animal is only the property of the client on which you have been asked to exercise your professional expertise for the benefit of the client. To clarify further, if you are sued for malpractice, the client will be the one suing, not the animal. Therefore it is important that you communicate effectively with the client to prevent misunderstandings or false expectations. Be very careful how you phrase your prognosis. Make no promises, offer no guarantees, and qualify everything. Although I recommend an initial client treatment agreement for all clients, there should be a signed release for any surgical procedure or any other that may result in the injury or death of the animal. This is the minimum necessary to protect the practice.

Other members of a veterinary practice may also be subject to enhanced standards of care or may subject the supervising veterinarian to potential liability. Many states are now licensing various animal health professionals under a variety of titles including animal health technicians, registered veterinary technicians, and so forth. Those licensed as such will be subject to an enhanced standard of care of a person similarly licensed. However, technicians are only able to perform procedures on a client's animal under the supervision of the veterinarian, which makes the veterinarian liable for the action or inaction of the staff. This includes nontechnical staff members from receptionists to kennel help. Anyone who has direct contact with a client's animal is the responsibility of the supervising veterinarian. Great care must be used in hiring, training, and supervising all employees who have direct client/animal contact. Limits on discretionary activities within the practice must be clearly defined and enforced.

This is not true of third parties to whom a veterinarian may refer a client outside the veterinary practice. If a client should ask for a referral to a good obedience instructor and you know of one you think would be beneficial to the client and the animal, there is little, if any, potential liability in referring the client (See Box 16-1). However, I would recommend that you make a qualifying statement that you are not endorsing the school and would suggest that they call the trainer and discuss what they are looking for before enrolling. It should be made clear that the choice of a trainer is *the client's.* Your staff may also be put in the position of giving advice or recommending trainers. It would be a good idea to draft a series of handouts that address the most frequently asked questions and requested referrals so that no one inadvertently says or does the wrong thing.

Note the disclaimer at the end of the handout (Box 16-1). Disclaimers can save practitioners from many

---

SAMPLE HANDOUT: OBEDIENCE TRAINER REFERRAL

A number of our clients have expressed satisfaction with the following trainers:

ABC Dog Training School

Jane Doe Perfect Heelers

Northeast Obedience Club

Each organization has a number of trainers and you should contact them directly to discuss your particular needs and expectations before enrolling. Training is highly individualistic and not every trainer will be able to meet your needs. This Veterinary Clinic *does not* endorse or recommend any of the above organizations. These names are being provided at your request and for information purposes *only.* You are reminded that obedience school is not a substitute for behavioral treatment should your pet have a problem behavior.

---

problems. Although there are some obligations that cannot be waived and disclaimers will have no effect, a general disclaimer should be included just to be safe.

This precept is upheld by case law. In *Tramutols v Bartone* (63 NJ 9 [1973]), the court held that vicarious liability would not be imposed when a referral of a client or patient is made to an independent practitioner unless such a recommendation was made to one who is known to be incompetent and disreputable.

The question of *vicarious liability* for the actions of another really depends on the relationship of the parties together with the amount of control the veterinarian has over the management of the business. In referring to groomers or trainers located at their own facility, it would be doubtful that there would be any finding of an employer-employee relationship. The question becomes more difficult where the independent practitioner shares facilities with the veterinarian practice. Liability would most likely attach where the veterinarian exercised some degree of control over the other businesses in the same facility with his practice. The issue would be whether the veterinarian would have had the opportunity to alter the course of events.

Liability Considerations

The general practitioner is unlikely to become primarily involved in behavioral medicine; however, it is highly probable that one or more animals with mild to severe behavioral problems will be seen at the practice throughout the year. Most will be brought in for reasons other than behavior, and the veterinarian or technician will initially recognize the behavioral disorder.

The First Visit. There is minimal liability exposure

for the practice when the veterinarian sees the client's animal for the first time. Providing the appointment was made for a reason other than behavior problems, no one in the practice is likely to know or should have known that this particular client had an animal with a behavioral disorder. In addition, not all behavioral disorders have the potential, even if known, to create a situation where an incident will occur in which another client of the practice will be injured or harmed in a way that he or she would seek to impose liability on the owner, the practice, or both. Inappropriate urination is unlikely to cause harm to anything other than the floor. The difficult situation involves *inappropriate aggression*.

Even the first presentation of an aggressive animal is unlikely to cause any liability problems for the practice, but the front-office staff should be trained sufficiently to identify a potentially dangerous situation and have a plan in place to handle the problem. Much depends on the ability of the client to properly handle the animal. It is best to assume that the client is not completely competent. Putting such clients and the dog in an examining room away from the main traffic pattern or asking them to wait outside until called should avert the problem easily and quickly. The veterinarian who is scheduled to see this client should be apprised of the situation. Depending on the policy of the practice, the client's animal can be declined for future visits or a Halti (Safari Whitco, Bohemia, NY) or Gentle Leader/Promise System Canine Head Collar (Premier Products, Richmond Va) or muzzle can be required for all subsequent appointments. This should be noted in the chart and given in writing to the client. All notices intended to relieve the practice of potential liability should be in writing *and* sent by regular and certified mail. This is one situation when clients' feelings and reactions are of lesser consideration. If they do not agree or take offense, they are free to go elsewhere.

Depending on the severity and the cause of the disorder, the treating veterinarian needs to make some sort of recommendation. Whether the list includes an obedience trainer for minor management problems, a specialist at an animal behavioral clinic for further evaluation, or, in the worst-case scenario when the client refuses to seek further help, recommending euthanasia will be according to the policies and procedures of the practice and veterinarian. Caution is urged in recommending euthanasia as the sole option. It is far preferable to recommend assessment by a specialist who can give the client a more objective assessment of prognosis. Although the veterinarian does not have to continue to maintain a relationship with a client who condones dangerous behavior, pets are property, and it is the client who must make the decision about treating or not treating the pet. This is best done in an informed context, which also helps to maintain good interpersonal relations. Recommendations for the treatment to assist with the amelioration of aggressive behavior are not considered directly treating the animal and are unlikely to impose any liability on the person or practice making such recommendation. In fact, it is better to discuss the situation with the client and make recommendations than it would be to ignore the behavior and send the uninformed client and the animal back into the general public.

Additional Visits. Subsequent visits of the same animal pose a different situation. The veterinarian and the practice are now on notice that the dog is aggressive. As before, requiring the Halti or Gentle Leader/Promise System as a firm requirement for treatment should alleviate the potential for harm to other clients. The veterinarian, by agreeing to treat the aggressive animal even if for conditions other than behavior, assumes the risk and cannot hold the client liable should he or she or any the staff be injured. However, being on notice imposes a duty of care that is owed to other clients awaiting treatment when this animal is also present. Again, reasonable precautions can alleviate the potential problem. Have the client and animal enter through another door, have them wait outside until called, or sequester them in a treatment room off the main traffic pattern. Should an incident occur that results in injury to a person or other animal, and the veterinarian can establish that reasonable precautions were taken to protect the injured third party, and that no negligence or malpractice was shown, no liability attaches. The client in control and possession of the animal may be liable for the injury, but not the veterinarian or the practice.

Client reaction has an impact on whether the veterinarian continues treating the animal. Cooperative clients who accept that there is a problem and agree to follow all the requirements and recommendations from the veterinarian are probably good risks. A client who denies the problem or likes the animal's aggressive behavior are not a good risk. The client in denial may later agree and may eventually decide to work through the behavior and become an acceptable risk. The client who likes and may have trained or at least encouraged the aggression is a poor risk and should not be given a second appointment. The potential for an incident to occur and liability to attach is too great.

If the veterinarian has some specialized training and experience in behavioral medicine and wants to actively treat behavioral disorders, he or she must realize that *he or she will be held to an elevated standard of care even if not a board-certified specialist*. This is true of all behavior disorders, regardless of whether they have the potential for personal injury.

Specialists. The board-certified specialist is held to a much higher standard of care than the general practitioner, even if that veterinarian has specialized training and experience in that field. Board-certified specialists are held to the "reasonable board-certified specialist" standard. Because all areas of practice do not have large populations, this may cause a disparity of education, training, and experience when one person must be reviewed in light of another person. This will be true of the animal behavioral specialty for many years to come. Any newly recognized specialty must progress through a growth phase. Unfortunately, the legal community is under no obligation to verbally acknowledge the limits imposed by these developmental stages.

Several areas undoubtedly become potential "hot spots" in this area of practice, based on the experience of psychiatrists and psychologists in human medicine.

To date, the most frequent reason for a specialist in animal behavior to appear in court was as an expert witness for one of the two parties. Therefore the following is purely speculation on potential issues related to the AVMA recognition of a new specialty.

Often a client who takes an animal to a behavioral clinic does so as a last resort. The client is in a legal situation because of the animal's actions or at wits' end in trying to live with the animal and all else has already failed. The expectations and subsequent reliance on actual or perceived representations made by the practitioner will probably be low. The "last-ditch effort" frame of mind will engender cooperation. That behavioral medicine is a nonspecific area that often uses experimental or trial-and-error approaches will be readily accepted. Thus it is not surprising that veterinary training and rescue hospitals have highly motivated clients with high compliance and success rates as well as low euthanasia numbers.

Official recognition of a specialty automatically engenders changed attitudes in the client, as well as potentially increasing the client base. The term *specialist* immediately raises client expectations. It also legitimizes that area of practice, making it more acceptable to the general public. Historically, the same effect was seen in the psychiatric practices. Perhaps animal behavior specialists will be able to learn from their human medicine counterparts and protect themselves from the myriad pitfalls that have already been litigated under medical malpractice.

The first issue that arises is whether there should be client confidentiality between the client and veterinarian in the process of treating behavior disorders. Doctor-patient confidentiality is statutorily conferred and is not a common law creation. The purpose was to allow the patient to seek appropriate assistance from a physician without fear of betrayal or humiliation. The same has been applied to the psychotherapist-patient relationship because of the special therapeutic need to assure the patient that disclosures will not be made. The basis of the privilege is to encourage patients to seek needed therapy without fear. However, this privilege does not extend to a physician examining a patient for a purpose other than treatment; does not usually apply to a nurse, medical student, dentists, druggists, or chiropractors; and does not extend after the death of a patient. There is no statutory veterinarian-client privilege. Should there be?

It is doubtful that a legislature will be willing to grant a privilege to the veterinarian-client relationship. The basis of the doctor-patient privilege is to prevent betrayal or humiliation to the patient. The patient of the veterinarian is the animal. Can an animal be publicly embarrassed? The client is the person owning the animal. Would the seeking of treatment for the animal be encouraged because of a privilege or discouraged because of the lack of a privilege? Would the client be embarrassed by the diagnosis and treatment of the animal's disorder? Whereas a diagnosis of inappropriate aggression will put the owner on notice and could impose liability under the known propensity standard, public revelation of the disorder is unlikely to cause embarrassment or discourage the client from seeking treatment for the animal. Thus a privilege is unlikely to evolve in the veterinarian-client relationship, even when treatment is being supplied by a veterinarian behavior specialist.

However, the diagnosis of inappropriate aggression raises an entirely different issue. Does the veterinary behavior specialist, who has diagnosed an aggressive disorder and believes the animal is potentially dangerous to third parties, have a duty to warn?

Generally, one person does not owe a duty to control the conduct of a second person so as to prevent that person from harming a third person unless some special relationship exists between either the first and second person imposing such a duty, or between the first and third person, giving him or her a right to protection. Without a special relationship, the mere fact that a person knows or should have known that action on his or her part is necessary to protect another does not necessarily impose a duty to take such action.

The arguments against imposing a duty on the psychotherapist to warn a third party of potential danger from a second party who is the patient of the psychotherapist include (1) the inability to predict dangerousness with sufficient reliability, (2) potential for interference with treatment by negating confidentiality, (3) potential for deterring therapists from treating violent patients, and (4) increased commitments to mental or penal institutions.

Although not all of these objections apply to the veterinarian behavior specialist, some can be construed in the favor of not imposing a duty to warn. Interference with effective treatment is obvious. Few clients will take their animal to the clinic if the behavioral specialist is under a duty to warn the local authorities or even the community of the animal's potential dangerousness. This would be especially true in New Jersey, where the state has specific requirements for the licensing and containment of potentially dangerous dogs. Also, given the support that registration of sexual offenders has received, it would not be difficult to see a statutory scheme requiring the registration of animals that have been treated for a behavior disorder. Public policy would surely have an interest in protecting the public from animals with behavior disorders. There would not be the outcry of the ACLU or other organizations regarding further restrictions on animals and animal owners.

A duty to warn may discourage the treatment of aggressive animals since they are the most likely to evoke the duty. It may also result in increased recommendations to euthanize aggressive animals because of the fear of malpractice suits, as well as owners opting more often for that solution because they cannot, or will not, afford the licensing and confinement requirements necessary to keep such an animal.

Finally, animal behavior is a complex science like psychotherapy; however, the animal does not have the rights and intrinsic value of the human. Thus this would be a nonargument in animal situations.

The experiences of psychotherapists merit further mention. In *Tarasoff v. Regents of University of California* (551 P2d 334 [Super Ct 1976] [Tarasoff II]), a majority of the California Supreme Court imposed a duty to warn on the defendant therapists, holding, "When a therapist determines, or pursuant to the standards of his profession should determine, that his patient presents a serious danger of violence to another, he incurs an obligation to use reasonable care to protect the intended victim against such danger." The duty was based on the existing relationship between the patient and therapist.

In *McIntosh v Milano* (168 NJ Super 466 [Law Div 1979]), a psychotherapist's duty to warn was seen as analogous to a physician's duty to warn others of possible exposure to contagious or infectious diseases. The court stated, "A psychiatrist or therapist may have a duty to take whatever steps are reasonably necessary to protect an intended or potential victim of his patient when he determines, or should determine in the appropriate factual setting and in accordance with the standards of his profession . . . , that the patient is or may present a probability of danger to that person. The relationship giving rise to that duty may be found either in that existing between the therapist and the patient . . . or in the more broadly based obligation a practitioner may have to protect the welfare of the community . . . ."

However, in *Doyle v United States* (530 F Supp [CD Cal 1982]), a California court applying Louisiana law found that there was no duty to warn in this factual situation because the release of the patient was sufficiently distant from the time and location of the murder. They did state that California does recognize a duty to warn if the "victim is foreseeable and identifiable."

In *Bardoni v Kim* (390 NW2d 218 [Mich Ct App 1986]), the court held that "when a psychiatrist determines or, pursuant to the standard of care of his profession, should determine that his patient poses a serious danger of violence to a readily identifiable third person, the psychiatrist has a duty to use reasonable care to protect that individual against such danger."

Now consider the following fact situation: a large, mixed-breed mastiff-type dog is brought to a veterinary animal behavior clinic for treatment of perceived unprovoked aggression toward small children. The dog already has bitten the owner's 6-year-old son. On examination and evaluation it is apparent that the dog, at this time, is potentially dangerous to small children. The practitioner recommends a treatment protocol and cautions the owner about handling the dog pending resolution of the disorder. In conversation the owner tells the practitioner that there are several small children in the area including a 7-year-old next door who regularly comes onto her property. The owner takes the dog home and follows the treatment protocol precisely. She confines the dog to a chain link run when it is outside and supervises the dog at all times. A week after the clinic visit, the dog is outside the run, the owner runs in the house to answer the phone, and the child next door opens and enters the dog's run. The dog attacks and kills the child. Is the veterinarian behavior specialist liable in negligence for failure to warn the next-door neighbor? The neighborhood? The community? Local law enforcement personnel?

Under the reasoning applied to psychiatrists and therapists, the veterinary behavior specialist would probably be liable in negligence to the child's family for failure to warn the next-door neighbor of the potential danger presented by the dog because that child was readily identifiable and harm to the child was foreseeable. Will this be the case? Only time will tell.

Finally, will the recognition of a veterinary specialty in animal behavior affect nonveterinary trainers and behavioralists? The restrictions on practicing veterinary medicine apply only to the physical elements of treatment. Until the state legislatures find a need to regulate the practice of behavioral medicine to protect the public welfare, there will be little change. On the basis of concerns regarding the training and experience of trainers that have been expressed during recent years and attempts to informally license this group through various voluntary organizations, someone will raise the question and a statutory scheme will be developed. Most likely it will take the stance that behavior and training are separate entities. The behavioral specialist then will be required to be a licensed veterinarian considered equivalent to a psychiatrist. The nonveterinarian animal behavioralist will be equivalent to the psychologist with certain licensing requirements. Obedience trainers will, most likely, have their training protocols left intact with some restriction as to how much behavior modification can be effected in a training situation.

Now is the time for nonveterinarian animal behavioralists to take the initiative. As with many professions, there is a need for greater organization, more cohesiveness, and a set of minimum professional standards. The more internal controls that are in place when an outside authority decides to regulate, the less chance that the resulting regulation will be incorrect, intrusive, or both. Also, if a profession has a history of effective self-regulation, the outside authority will tend to work with the governing body rather than against it. There is no way to ward off future regulations, but there are ways to control and soften the impact.

Overall, veterinarian general practitioners will remain untouched by the process. Indeed, they will probably be left in the best position initially because they are unlikely to fall under the failure to warn issues because they are not specialists.

SUMMARY

Within the parameters of this book, this is merely an overview of a rapidly expanding area of the law. Changes will come quickly, and every veterinarian must be aware of the potential impact on the profession. These recommendations are minimal guidelines that should be seriously considered and implemented. As each practice eventually develops its own personality, the level of protection each chooses to implement will vary greatly. More, not less, will be the wave of the future. The denser the human population, the more high profile animals become, with a resultant spotlight being cast on animal care professionals.

GLOSSARY

Assumption of the risk: Where the injured party had knowledge that the situation was dangerous and voluntarily exposed himself or herself to the hazard created by the other person.

Attractive nuisance: In personal injury cases, this is a doctrine that imposes certain objections on a person who maintains something on his or her property that may attract a child onto the premises (e.g., obligation to fence a swimming pool).

Comparative negligence: The allocation of responsibility for damages between the two parties based on the relative negligence of each (eg., 50%-50%; 60%-40%).

Contributory negligence: The conduct of the injured party that falls below the level of care that he or she should exercise for his or her own protection.

Duty of care: The obligation to conduct oneself so as to avoid harmful matter.

Known propensity: Sometimes combined with the "one-bite rule" to imply knowledge of an animal's tendencies to the owner to impose a greater obligation of control. However, an actual bite may not be necessary if the animal's behavior should have alerted an owner to the potential of harm.

Negligence: A guideline to use the degree of care that a person of ordinary prudence (a reasonable person) would use under the same circumstances.

Nuisance: One person's unreasonable interference with another person's rights or interests in property.

One-bite rule: Where allowed, an animal is not considered vicious or potentially dangerous until it has bitten once. However, after the first bite, the animal is presumed to be vicious or potentially dangerous.

Police powers: The inherent power of state governments, which is often delegated in part to local government, to impose restrictions on the rights of individuals that are reasonably related to the promotion and maintenance of the general welfare of the public (e.g., leash laws).

Vicarious liability: The imposition of liability on one person for the actions of another (e.g., employer liable for actions of employees).

16 ····· Social Work and Behavioral Problems: Implications for Treating the Problem Pet and for the Family

ROBIN LEE SCHURR STAWASZ, MSW

···

THE IMPACT OF PETS WITH BEHAVIORAL PROBLEMS ON THE FAMILY

When treating a pet with a behavioral problem, it is crucial to consider the family. No behavioral treatment can be successful without the full involvement of the family. Understanding the pet's role within the family is essential for formulating treatment plans that are sufficient to remedy the problem and that can be executed within that family. For the purpose of this discussion, *family* is defined as the main social group that is the primary provider of the biological, social, and psychological needs of its members. This includes traditional and nontraditional families and close friends who regularly purchase pets together.

The role of pets in families has been informally understood but has just begun to be seen in a clinical light. It is known that pets offer benefits to individuals and families on biological, psychological, and social levels (Anderson, et al., 1984; Beck & Katcher, 1983; Cantazaro, 1988; Fogle, 1983; Friedman & Thomas, 1985; Podberscek, 1988; Ruckert, 1987; White & Watson, 1983). Veterinarians also recognize this:

> The health care given to companion animals may be as significant in terms of mental and emotional health of individuals in this society as the protection of the food supply is to their physical well-being (Anonymous, Association of American Veterinary Medical Colleges Council of Deans, 1979).

Most families with pets are families with young children, with the pets being obtained for companionship or pleasure. Of households with a youngest child who is younger than 6 years of age 67.4% have pets, and 78.7% of households in which the youngest child is greater than 6 years old have pets (Anonymous, AVMA, 1992). Most people consider their pets as part of the family and as "constant children" (Beck & Katcher, 1983; Voith, 1985).

Some researchers believe that the human-companion animal bond is stronger and closer than interper-

sonal relationships for some people. Forty-four percent of families state that the pet is the family member who receives the most attention or affection in the family (Cain, 1983). Barker and Barker (1988) found both dog enthusiasts and more typical clients perceive pets as being as close as one's spouse, child, or parent. This psychological attachment may be stronger with adults than with children. The length of ownership, the age of the adult client, family size, and the number of dogs or cats that the clients have had in the past reportedly have little effect on this particular relationship. Smith's (1983) work shows that when people compare their interaction with their pets with their interaction with other people, they become more strongly attached to their pets.

Different researchers have focused on various aspects of the role of pets within the family. Cain (1985) and Wessels (1984) built on work concerning triangles in the family system. In general, an emotional triangle forms as anxiety builds between a twosome and attention is then focused on a third object, which, for our purposes, is the pet. Pets are safe recipients of affection, anger, and emotional disturbance, and they can act as peacemakers, tension-breakers, and scapegoats. In this way, pets act much like a symptomatic child. Cain (1985) found 44% of families sometimes or always "triangled" their pets into their relationships.

Families often face a conflict when considering what to do about a pet that demonstrates a behavior problem, especially aggression, even though the pet can threaten the physical safety of the family. When the family is considering placing or euthanizing the pet, they face the possible loss of the triangular focus within the family system, as well as the loss of a strong emotional attachment (Wessels, 1984). If the animal has been triangled as described by Bowen (cited in Cain, 1985), a disruption in the relationship may result in an increase in interpersonal relationship difficulties. This increase in interpersonal relationship difficulties may be particularly pronounced if one person feels closer to the animal than other individuals in the household, yet, at the same time, other individuals in the household are the ones who may feel more threatened by the aggressive pet.

Human-companion animal interactions suffer when the animal's species-typical behavior is deemed unacceptable to the family or vice versa (Marder & Marder, 1985). A paradox arises because the family knows that the pet is an animal, but acts as if the pet is more like a child (Voith, 1985). Pet behavior is an important determinant of the success of the human–companion animal bond. When families assume the responsibilities of a pet, they also may take on the responsibility for the pet's behavior problems. They may feel guilt and a sense of failure when behavior problems develop. They may feel betrayed, as well as physically threatened, when an animal hurts them or hurts someone else. Their perception of the problem is often colored by their emotions. Often people deny that there is a problem, or they see themselves as the ones at fault or make excuses for the pet.

The pet with the behavior problem cannot be evaluated in a vacuum. The family must be an integral part of the evaluation, diagnosis, and treatment process. Although people seldom cause pets' behavioral problems—though through ignorance they may inadvertently reinforce or reward the problem—how the problem may be manifest depends greatly on both the household environment and how the family reacts to the problem. The extent to which treatment can be successful is largely dependent on the family system in which the pet lives. One critical point to emphasize to clients is that, although not everybody may have to do everything in all behavior modification programs, it is critical that *no one* in the family sabotages the process. When family members are unwilling to comply, the problems are far more complex than in cases just involving a pet with an inappropriate or undesirable behavior. Many times the pets become the scapegoats in a situation in which the people cannot resolve the conflicts between themselves. Given such cases, it would be inappropriate to view pets as entities separate from the family; each treatment program must be individualized for each separate family. More important, the emotional investment of the family in a pet must be respected when trying to understand why a family has kept a problem pet, particularly one that is aggressive.

THE ROLE OF THE FAMILY IN PREVENTION OF BEHAVIORAL PROBLEMS

Ideally, because very few pets with behavioral problems are fully cured but are excellent candidates for full control, it would be better if behavioral problems could be prevented. The extent to which most truly abnormal behaviors can be prevented is unknown. It is known that the earlier the intervention occurs, the lower the likelihood that the inappropriate behavior has been reinforced by learning paradigms. Many of the most common behaviors about which people complain, including jumping, cats scratching on furniture, animals eliminating in the house, and barking and digging, are management-related problems. All of these behaviors can be prevented. Because of the impact of any behavioral condition on a family, any time a client brings a new pet into any veterinary office, potential behavioral problems need to be discussed. This is particularly true concerning management-related problems or problems that early intervention or early management would greatly diminish. It is appropriate at the first veterinary visit of a new pet to discuss the family's roles with the pet and to discuss the implications of any behavioral problems for the family. It is also appropriate to discuss normal animal behavior, social structure, and anything that is known about breed predispositions. Ideally, it would be preferable to have a prepet consultation. In such consultations, the family members can be informed about the particular pet they are considering, and, in fact, they might reconsider their choice of either the pet or the breed. An example of a pet that may be inappropriate in a specific situation is a beagle in a small apartment in the city where all of the neighbors dislike noise. Beagles are hounds and have been selected to work in packs, but part of the way they do this is by baying. They can make excellent single-pet animals, although when they vocalize they do so with the voice characteristic of hounds. If the beagle is to be left alone for extended periods of time, the chances of a management-related problem developing derived from normal behavior are not small. The family's advance knowledge of this might allow them to make a different choice. Accordingly, both the veterinarian and the family must have a good sense of the role of the pet in the family, the interaction between family members and the pet, and how to develop and to reinforce acceptable behavior in the pet. Appendix C lists sources that help facilitate people choosing either a particular pet or a particular breed of dog and readings for people who decide to acquire a pet or those seeking to understand canine or feline social systems. It should be emphasized at the first visit that it is never too early to start working with any kitten or puppy. Proper obedience work in show situations often does not start until six to nine months of age. Regardless, dogs can be taught to "sit" and "stay" as early as six to eight weeks of age. Many of these animals benefit from puppy kindergartens, and many of them benefit from puppy socialization classes. Puppy socialization classes are nothing more than opportunities to teach good manners and to allow the puppies to play with other puppies. How to conduct these classes and instructions for clients on the first visit are discussed in Chapter 14. For young puppies and kittens, a good knowledge of reinforcing correct behavior and how to disabuse the animal of incorrect behavior greatly enhances prevention of behavior problems before they fully develop. Furthermore, the earlier that the family gets involved in working with the pet, the better the appreciation they will have for the development of the pet's behavior, the more they will be able to shape that behavior to their family's needs, and the more interested they will become in that pet as a member of their family.

Because of some potential genetic predispositions and some uncontrollable variables in pets' environments, no one can prevent all behavioral problems. Proper understanding of pet behavior can be very helpful in minimizing problems by attending to them in the earliest stages when treatment will be most effective and easiest to implement. Unfortunately, hindsight is often more effective than foresight in behavioral disorders. Families often feel guilty for either not recognizing the behavior problem in time or for contributing to it through their own mismanagement. The majority of clients at the behavior clinic articulate that they feel guilty that they have caused the problem, and this is particularly true for clients who have dogs who have been to obedience schools. Somewhere they have received the impression that dogs are a blank slate and whatever they do to them will create whatever the dog is. Accordingly, if the dog behaves wonderfully, they can take some credit for it, although often people state that they just have a great dog, but if the dog behaves inappropriately, obviously the clients are incapable of handling the dog. Nothing could be further from the truth. Most clients, with the glaring exception of clients who abuse dogs, should not be held responsible for the development of profound behavioral disorders. Management-related problems are not the issue here. In these profound behavioral disorder situations, as with most aggressions, the dog is clinically abnormal. The fact that the clients have been carrying the burden of the guilt that they caused this problem actually impedes them from getting proper care. They are embarrassed and confused because they often do not understand what they did that was so egregious—the answer is *nothing.* The unfortunate aspect of this situation is that the mentality that encourages clients to think that they are solely responsible for their pet's behavioral problems also prohibits them from getting help in a timely manner. Client education is obviously then critical.

Families may not realize that many factors contribute to the development of behavioral problems. Because families do not by themselves cause a problem and problems can develop in even the best and most prepared of families, emphasis must be placed on the family's understanding of the nature of the problem and the mitigated influences of these behaviors on family dynamics. It is important to relieve families of guilt feelings at the outset, because guilt is nonproductive and transfers the ownership of the problem from the pet to the family. In such situations, the family may be more reluctant to impose any needed restrictions on the pet. Such lack of objectivity potentially makes the pet more dangerous. If the animal is to be helped, the realization that it is the pet's problem and not the people's problem must occur. Only in such situations can the pet be treated in a safe manner. Families have to accept their lack of responsibility for another reason: if they do not, in the future they will repeat any management-related mistakes or mistakes that have inadvertently reinforced the animal's behavior.

THE ROLE OF THE CLINICIAN IN PREVENTION OF BEHAVIORAL PROBLEMS

The time for practitioners to start to develop a good relationship with the pet and the family so that any behavioral problems can be managed and treated is when they first see the pet. During subsequent examinations, practitioners should always ask about the pet's behavior and about any problems that may be attendant in age-specific groups. Sixty-eight percent of all clients coming to any practice at any point in time have a question about their pet's behavior, even if this question focuses on whether something is normal and at what point something should develop (Overall, unpublished data from VHUP and Philadelphia area surveys, 1990). Most clients do not ask their veterinarians these questions because they do not realize that veterinarians can provide behavioral information. To meet these needs veterinarians need to increase their awareness of behavioral issues and to inform their staff of their importance.

Weekly or monthly seminars for staff members to discuss behavioral cases that have occurred recently and the prevention of behavioral problems help everyone to become more aware of behavioral problems. These considerations are not important just in terms of creating better relationships with clients and their families (although that will serve to generate future income) or for meeting the needs of the pets, but they are also important in minimizing any damage to hospital staff. Nurses and technicians are often unaware of appropriate handling techniques, restraint techniques, and proclivities for aggressions in certain animals. The same misapprehensions that apply to behavioral medicine in general also can apply to the support staff. It is important both to minimize damage to people and to minimize horrible experiences for pets. Support staff must be aware of humane and kind restraint techniques and of problems that may arise with pets that already have behavioral disorders.

Practitioners can form close associations with local rescue groups and humane shelters and hold regular joint seminars on normal and abnormal animal behavior. It is important to educate the shelter staff about available treatment and management programs. The SPCA in Boulder, Colorado, is the first humane shelter to affiliate itself with a full-time animal behaviorist. Many shelters are doing excellent work in screening animals for potential behavior problems through both questionnaires and behavioral examinations. The point is not to euthanize more animals, but to ensure that animals that are surrendered to shelters receive the help they need.

The experience of dealing with a pet with a behavioral problem changes families' perspective of pet ownership. Their interaction with other pets they now have or will obtain in the future may become much more purposeful, and they may be able to carry out preventative measures more effectively in the future. They may have a better understanding of what to look for in a pet and what they are able to contribute to the relationship, as well as the dynamics of interaction of multiple pets in a home. Thus their decision of what type of pet to get in the future could be a good one, and intervention with a previous problem pet could prevent them from making similar management-related mistakes in the future. This results in more successful human-companion animal bonds and fewer dead pets.

THE NEED FOR COMMITMENT TO THE TREATMENT PROCESS BY THE FAMILY

A great deal of frustration can be felt by the family when they learn that the pet's behavior problem may not be easily or quickly remedied. Unfortunately, few people seek help as the behavior problem is developing; thus most behavior problems are long-standing and may be integrated into a pet's personality by the time that pet is seen by a specialist. Sometimes problems cannot be fully eradicated, and in the case of aggression, may not be *cured*; however, these problems might be fully *controlled* with appropriate measures. Management of the problem in an effort to immediately minimize the damage and danger potential of the pet must be done with any treatment of any problem. The intent is to minimize the impact of the pet's problems, as well as the problems themselves. The goal in cases where control is the best that can be hoped for must be to manage the problem through the behavior modification of the pet and through alteration of the home environment. If this will not be possible, and the clients are not willing to maintain the modifications that might be necessary, a breakdown in communication between them and the pet or within the family is likely. It is critical that all the people in the family be willing to work together at these initial stages even though it may require that they react to each other in ways to which they are unaccustomed. For example, a household that involves a teenage boy who has been in conflict with his parents about his desires and goals now might have to confine their conversations to soft tones rather than the yelling that previously was the major mode of communication. This is an actual case example—in this case the dog became aggressive whenever the teenage son was yelled at by the mother, but not when the son yelled at the mother. Unfortunately, in the triangularized manner, the son interpreted this to mean the dog was taking his side and that, obviously, his mother

was incorrect. It is easy to see how these rationalizations can spiral and how important it is to teach the dog not to have an inappropriate response. It is critical that everybody works toward the same goals. It is necessary to emphasize to the family that without proper management the pet might continue to pose a danger and inappropriate behavior will continually be self-reinforcing until it is changed.

Aggressive pets are special cases. Because any aggressive animal can pose a threat to the general public and the family, any clinician involved in such cases has a responsibility to discuss control of this potential for danger to others. Treatment often takes a prolonged period of time before the animal is nonreactive in specific situations, and management is going to be a lifelong course. If the clients are unwilling, either because of family problems or neighborhood problems, to work in their expanded social system of a neighborhood to minimize danger, it is unlikely that the pet's behavior will improve. It is also likely that the clients eventually will experience some legal problems. Unfortunately, the dog is usually at the crux of the legal problems (see Chapter 15). When the situation involves litigation, the simplest and most expedient choice is often euthanasia. It should be emphasized to clients that, regardless of how they feel about each other, if they care about the pet, they must realize that animals seldom get the benefit of the doubt in aggressive situations. Clients can be emotionally crippled by a euthanasia decision that was driven by liability concerns. This is particularly true if the clients had chosen to ignore what they knew was a problematic situation, or if they decided not to appropriately treat it. Clients need to be appraised of the importance of not setting a pet up to become a secondary victim in an aggressive situation.

Families often feel demoralized by behavioral problems, and it is critical to disabuse them at the outset of their role and causality of them. It would be untrue to say that they may not have affected the worsening of the problems. It is important to explain to people that knowledge of behavior medicine is incomplete and that most of these pets are clinically abnormal, rather than just misbehaving. Most pets that are simply misbehaving would respond to different family members with varying levels of obedience and would respond favorably to standard corrections. This does not apply to pets that are clinically abnormal.

Because of the extended period of therapy that is necessary for pets with behavioral problems, it is very easy for clients to become discouraged. Without being able to see rapid progress or return for their efforts, clients are very likely to diminish in their enthusiasm for treatment. If they do so, the animal invariably begins to exhibit more of the inappropriate behavior; the clients then assume treatment is not working and may give up on the treatment plan and on the animal. It is critical to emphasize to the clients that everybody goes through this phase of frustration and boredom. It can be likened to trying to lose 5 pounds on a diet; anybody who has ever tried to do this knows it is frustrating. Any time we change behavior patterns, whether they involve only the animal or they involve the entire family and their responses to the animal, it is a complex, tedious, difficult, frustrating endeavor. It needs to be emphasized to the clients that if they persist they will be rewarded with the appropriate changes. Often this can be a form of therapy for the clients themselves. We all need encouragement. If clients are able to succeed with a treatment schedule for an animal, we have seen instances where familiar relationships improve because of their commitment to working on something in a triangularized manner where they are not the direct focus of the work. Implicit in all of this is that every possible opportunity must be taken to minimize damage and danger. Without this, the clients will be unwilling to pursue therapy, and pursuit of therapy may not be the best option. Again, it is important to emphasize the role of at least benign cooperation if not active involvement of every member of the family. In any family in which any individual is going to sabotage the treatment, the problems are far more profound than just the pet's behavioral disorder, and therapy for the pet is unlikely to succeed in such a family.

Because the behavioral problem may be long-standing, and may be in part genetic, it is critical to emphasize to the clients that they will always have to monitor the animal, and perhaps even act in a stereotypic manner with it. For instance, a dominantly aggressive dog that has been well controlled with behavior modification programs designed to get it to "sit" and "wait" and "relax" for anything it wants and to defer to the client for anything the dog desires cannot suddenly be treated like a normal dog. If that dog has been operating under the impression that it must "sit" and "stay" for everything it wants for a year and a half, and suddenly the client decides that it would be perfectly acceptable for that dog to come up on the bed with him or her and have a biscuit, when in the past this has not been allowed, it may not be surprising when the dog exhibits aggression. The dog still is pushing the limits of the defined social system and the client has just made the rules blurry. It is helpful to start thinking about behavioral problems as being like diabetic conditions. We do not cure diabetes, but we do an excellent job of controlling it. Regardless, after diabetes is controlled, no one would dream of withdrawing the insulin. Analogies such as this one can help clients understand that it is critical that they continue to reinforce the choices they have outlined for the dog, and to reward the appropriate behaviors throughout the life of the dog. They should really be doing a little bit of work with the dog every day, the same way somebody who intends to stay in decent physical shape should be getting aerobic exercise daily. We would not expect our muscles to maintain tone without daily exercise; we should not expect our

pets' behavior to do that either. Accordingly, families must have an excellent understanding of what it means to manage versus treat the problem. There will be overlapping areas, and clients must have an appreciation of the difference between a control and a cure. With this understanding, families will have a better concept of the dynamics involved and a more valid expectation of prognosis.

Families must understand that because the pet's behavior problem may never be "cured," management becomes a lifetime issue. In families that demand a guarantee about a probability, life in general is going to problematic. It may help to point out that the probability of many events occurring is either higher or lower than people expect (for example, the probability of being hit by a car while crossing the street, or being struck by lightning is far greater than the probability of contracting acquired immunodeficiency syndrome from a blood transfusion; people are still fearful of blood transfusions). Clients must make their own choices. Any client who wants a guarantee about the outcome of any behavioral disorder has needs that cannot be met by the clinician, and the clinician should not feel guilty about that. Clinicians can give clients a ballpark figure and can cite the data known from the published literature, but it is wholly inappropriate to guarantee a client one outcome or another. Any client who will continually worry about whether the dog might have another aggressive event probably should never have dogs. It would be unfair to not be honest with them up front about this, because this will affect the way every individual in that family interacts with the dog. Often it is helpful to tell clients who are just mildly fearful that any aggressive dog can bite in certain situations, but dogs with aggressive propensities and defined aggressive disorders have a far greater potential for biting in those same situations. It can also be helpful to tell clients that dogs with diagnosed aggressive disorders are often far more manageable and may actually be safer than dogs that have no diagnosis because no one is in denial about those aggressive disorders. Clients whose dogs are not brought to veterinarians or behavioral specialists for treatment of aggression, but whose dogs continue to bite, very frequently make excuses for the dog. The dog for whom excuses are repeatedly made is far more potentially dangerous than a dog with a known aggression problem and clients who are willing to control it. Client education along these lines can create more responsible pet ownership and a far less anxious owner.

CHANGES THAT AFFECT THE PET AND THE FAMILY

The management of the immediate problem and treatment of any underlying cause often require changes in the family's and the pet's environment. As part of the process of behavior modification for the pet, often family members also have to modify many of their behaviors. Lifestyle changes within any family can be upsetting. For instance, in the treatment and management of an aggressive dog, much time is devoted to structuring interaction with the dog. Purposeful and restricted informal interaction with the pet must be closely supervised, and any interaction with people and animals both within and outside the household has to be controlled. These controlled changes may include things such as altering the dog's accessibility to areas of the house, changes in interactions with other pets in the home, and, potentially, a large financial commitment both to treatment and to any special needs that the animal may have (e.g., a crate). To change the pet's behavior, these changes will require major lifestyle changes on the part of the family. This may be particularly true if the family has children who have friends who come to visit. If the dog is territorially or protectively aggressive, or dominantly aggressive toward children, that dog cannot interact with those children until the dog's behavior starts to improve. This means that the dog must be locked up when the children come to visit or that no children are allowed to visit during the course of treatment. It is not sufficient that the 4-year-old runs to the door and announces that his friends are there and opens it and yells that the dog has to be put up. This is potentially a very dangerous situation, and the family must be willing to address the potential danger. For certain age groups, the parents must explain to their child's friends' parents that the dog has behavioral problems that are being treated. They must explain that no child will ever be put in danger, and that no child will be exposed to the animal until the animal's behavior is much improved. However, as a corollary, all visits must be announced so that the dog can be put in a crate before the visit.

Problems can develop when some members of the family are more committed to the pet and more willing to accept some changes than others. This not only leads to inconsistent treatment for the pet (given that so many of these pets already have anxiety disorders, this is the worst thing that could happen to them), but this also increases stress and conflict within the family. Because the behavior problem has already contributed to a high-stress environment within the family, such a conflict often makes the family situation much worse. If the pet has been incorporated into a triangled relationship, a preexisting conflict may be magnified by a conflict over the treatment. Conflicts over treatment can be minimized by involving as many of the family members as possible throughout the diagnostic and treatment process. Compromises and concessions can be built into the treatment program in the form of a verbal or a written contract so that all members of the family can have a similar view of the dynamics and importance of the process.

Just as behavior problems necessitate lifestyle changes, lifestyle changes can facilitate the development of behavioral problems. Changes in family structure or environment can dramatically alter a pet's otherwise stable environment, and the environment plays a role in determining the pet's behavior. Common situations when this occurs are births, deaths, remarriages, or a change of locale for some individual of the family, such as when children go off to college. A family's understanding of how a pet may be affected is critical; they may be able to take preventive measures to minimize problems. In such cases, it behooves the family to make any changes as gradually as possible while still giving attention to the pet. This is particularly true if a new spouse is on the scene or the family who has heretofore only had canine or feline children now adds a human baby. It is not unusual that the resident cat or dog becomes clinically depressed in such situations. They can develop marking behaviors or protective aggression regarding their original people. All of these changes in behavior weaken their original bond with their families. In such situations it is important that the animal understands that it is still a critical part of the household and is still important to the original people. In situations involving new babies, tips on how to do this are given in the "Protocol for Introducing a New Baby and a Pet" in Appendix B.

A little-addressed aspect of environmental change is the effect of moving or other changes on the older pet. Geriatric pets are finally beginning to receive the attention they deserve in the veterinary medical literature. Geriatric pets may be less able to physically accommodate some environmental changes, and it is important to realize that their sensory functions are not as sharp as before. There also appear to be old-age onset behavioral disorders including elimination disorders and separation anxiety disorders (Voith & Chapman, 1990). In many cases, cognitive changes occur. The special needs of the geriatric patient must be met. Some of these animals respond well to antianxiety medication and to special times set aside for them.

THE ROLE OF CHILDREN IN TREATMENT OF PETS WITH BEHAVIORAL PROBLEMS

Children are an essential aspect of a family who must be considered throughout any treatment process. First, the children's safety must be ensured and all threats to them eliminated. Children are often most vulnerable to an aggressive pet because of their physical inability to protect themselves and because of their lack of knowledge or inability to interact with pets appropriately. Children may not recognize potentially threatening nonvocal signals from pets. Children may not even recognize vocal signals that are threatening. Young children may have not yet developed many interpersonal communication skills, and thus it is often difficult for them to interpret the communicatory behaviors of another species. Similarly, if the dog or cat is more accustomed to interacting with human adults, the behaviors of a young child may seem garbled and contextually inappropriate to the pet. This represents a potentially toxic interaction; if children do not recognize the threat, they may unknowingly endanger themselves. The uncoordinated movements of an infant may actually make him or her appear as prey objects to some animals. Normal infant behaviors could inadvertently elicit predatory behavior. It is the responsibility of the adult family members and the clinician discussing the case with them to protect the children. This responsibility does not include only the children within the family, but any child who may come into the home or otherwise interact with the pet.

Children need to be kept safe. It is a myth that every child should have a dog or a cat. Children can be unpredictable, dogs can be unpredictable, and often the interaction is toxic. No child should be left alone, unsupervised, with a pet until the people are certain that that child will always act appropriately with that animal. This could mean that children will not be left alone with pets until they are between 7 and 10 years of age. Regardless, no pet should be left alone with an infant. This is not because cats are going to "suck the breath out" of babies, but rather because an infant not only looks like a prey item to an animal that may already have predatory tendencies, but also because infants are incapable of pushing off any animal that may be leaning next to them for warmth or love. Management efforts need to be aimed at minimizing dangers to children. If clients wish to have their pets present at all times during the infant and child development periods, they must realize that at certain times the animals may need to be on a harness in the home. If the clients are willing to do this, it would be best for both the children and the pets. It is important that children be positively reinforced for helpful interaction with the pet, and it is important that they are corrected instantly for inappropriate interaction. This can be done only if the pet is always with the adult when the adult is with the child, and if the child and pet are never alone together. Not only does this minimize danger to the child, but it also minimizes any further development of problems in the pet.

If children are involved, they must be considered in the discussion of the treatment plan. Because children often lack knowledge of or experience with interaction with animals, they may exhibit inappropriate behavior and elicit problem behaviors. Their immaturity may also create an environment that increases stresses on the pet. The presence of a child, especially the addition of a new baby, changes the social structure of the family; this can also affect the pet. When the pet loses its favored status to the new baby, it would not be unusual to see the appearance of attention-seeking behavior or other anxiety-related behaviors. For an animal whose previous behavior problem has been well controlled, any change in the family, but particularly the addition of a new child, could destabilize the treatment plan, and the behavioral problems may begin to reappear.

Any child older than 18 months of age is capable of working with a behavior modification program. Any child can be taught from infancy what age- and pet-specific appropriate behaviors are. One must not wait until 18 months of age to start to teach the child not to pull on the dog's tail. Two of the services that the Behavior Clinic at the Veterinary Hospital of the University of Pennsylvania now offers are short appointments to teach children how to interact appropriately with pets, and short prenatal appointments for expectant parents to teach them how the pets in their household may react to their baby and what they can do about that. Done correctly, pet-child interaction can be a wonderful experience for all concerned and may be important in creating a more humane child and adult. We can emphasize to people that this is just one more area from which they can derive great benefit from a pet.

A few comments on child abuse and pet abuse are warranted. Children who are abusive to animals often are later abusive to other people (DeViney et al., 1983; Felthous, 1980). A study of 53 families who met legal criteria for child abuse or neglect found that 32 (60%) of these families had pets that had been abused or neglected. In 47 (88%) of these families in which physical (contrasted with sexual) abuse occurred, the pet was also physically abused. These families did not differ from the overall population in their use of veterinary services, levels of basic pet care, or rates of pet sterilization (DeViney et al., 1983). This means that pet abusers and child abusers are found in all veterinary practices. A total of 2,694,000 children (34/100) are victims of abuse or neglect annually in the United States; the average age of these children is 7.23 years, more than half are girls, and 81% of the time the parent is the abuser (American Humane Association, 1992). Often the child learns violence from his or her parents and practices and hones violent skills on animals (pamphlet by P.A. Finch, "Breaking the Cycle of Abuse"; see Appendix C for source). It is critical that whenever any child is involved in the management of a pet's problem that the association between pet and child abuse be discussed. It can be discussed in a nonpejorative manner so that the family is not accused of encouraging any abusive activities or participating in them themselves. The data indicate that children who are allowed to act inappropriately with pets for whatever reason early in life transfer those rough and inappropriate social skills to their peers, to adults, and, later to their own children (Felthous, 1980; Talpia, 1971). In fact, although the AVMA emphasizes the need to preserve the clients' privacy, the one exception they specifically stipulate focuses on situations where the health and welfare of the individual, the animal, or others may be endangered (AVMA Directory, 1992). This is a view that has long been supported by the Latham Foundation and the Alpha Affiliates. Veterinarians will continue to play an expanded role in the overall health care system because of such factors (Arkow, 1994), especially with the importance placed on animal abuse by the human medical profession.

The American Psychiatric Association first included cruelty to animals in their diagnostic criteria for conduct disorder in 1987 (*American Psychological Association, Diagnostic and Statistical Manual of Mental Disorders* [third edition], 1987).

PLACING OR EUTHANIZING PETS WITH BEHAVIORAL PROBLEMS

Despite all of the therapies discussed in previous chapters and the interaction benefits discussed in previous paragraphs, alteration of the familiar environment and behavior modification for the pet are occasionally not options or do not create an acceptable change. If this is the case, the options that remain are placing or euthanizing the pet. If the clients have an interest in working with the pet, no matter how horrendous the problem, they should be encouraged to do so. Limits should be set on all behaviors to ensure that no one is injured, and a realistic schedule for behavioral, environmental, and pharmacological modification must be set. A reasonable schedule for reassessment and progress must also be set. If the clients decide to either relinquish or euthanize the pet after working as hard as possible on any modification programs designed, they will do so with far less guilt than if they had opted for euthanasia or placement of the pet initially.

For clients whose first reaction is to place the pet, the clinician should explore whether this is because they are fearful that they will not be able to accomplish the desired behavior change or because they do not wish to do the work. If they do not wish to do the work and that animal can be safely placed in another home, the best option for the animal is placement. Clients who are unwilling to work with their pets will invariably make the problems worse, and the pets will probably not get other things that they need, including adequate medical care.

It is not surprising that the primary reason that animals are surrendered to humane shelters are behavioral disorders (Marder & Marder, 1985; Sigler, 1991). Euthanizing a problem animal is preferable to shifting the problem to someone else. However, many animals with behavioral problems can improve in new environments simply because either the stimulus that prompts the problem behavior is not present (e.g., children may be absent for dogs that are fearful of children), or the person who adopts the pet is willing to work with the behavioral problems. Whenever a pet is placed in a new home because of a behavioral problem, absolutely full disclosure is necessary on the part of the client and the clinician. If that pet has been seen by a behavioral specialist or practitioner because of behavior problems, copies of all records must be sent to the new client. At the Behavior Clinic at the Veterinary Hospital at the University of Pennsylvania we never recommend placement unless the new family is willing to work with all of the protocols that we had originally outlined. If they are willing and they

understand the nature of the problem, there is certainly no reason that dog cannot be placed if the potential for improvement exists in the new environment. Preadoption interviews should occur and any questions should be answered at those times. Hiding information only dooms the pet to failure.

In many cases rescue services will take problem dogs provided the rescue service workers can talk to a specialist about the restrictions for such dogs. Rescue services are very interested in saving individuals of particular breeds and they have a vested interest in placing them in households where they will succeed. Many rescued animals become ideal pets, and placement in a new family can provide a quality environment that can help them get better.

If the client cannot work with the animal, or does not wish to do so, and that animal is too aggressive to be placed even in a specialized home, the only option is euthanasia. This should *not* be an option of first choice; however, one of the problems in seeking help is that clients are frequently told by others to euthanize their pet. This makes them reluctant to seek help from somebody willing to work with behavioral disorders or a specialist because they do not want to hear from somebody in authority that they should kill the animal. Because they have already been told by friends or family that euthanasia is the best thing to do, clients assume that this is what a specialist also will recommend. In fact, in 1993 at the Behavior Clinic at the Veterinary Hospital at the University of Pennsylvania, 100% of the clients were told by someone—a veterinarian, a friend, a trainer, or family members—to euthanize the animal and that they were "crazy for putting up with this behavior." In many cases, the clients are terrified of parting with the animal and are not willing to seek competent help because they are afraid they will be told that euthanasia is the only option. Clinicians must do everything possible to discourage this vicious cycle. In truth, most of these animals do not have to be euthanized. Even if the best option *is* euthanasia, it is still worth encouraging clients to work with the pet if they can do so carefully. Once the behavior modification programs are outlined and the restrictions to their environment and the animal's environment are proscribed, and appointments are made to assess progress, with written progress reports that indicate little or no success, most clients themselves make the very rational decision to euthanize the animal. There are benefits from this process that they would not have otherwise obtained. First, they made the decision themselves and know that they did all they could for their pet. This is invaluable in minimizing guilt. Second, they have learned about the social system of animals and about inappropriate behavior. Third, they have realized what is necessary to work with an animal with a problem and they have done it. If the animal did not succeed in those programs, the clients are able to accept that this outcome was not due to client failure. We always tell clients that euthanasia is not a decision that must be made hurriedly, that it is always an option later, but resurrections are difficult. However, we also tell clients that if at any time in the future they feel like prisoners, or they do not believe that they can live safely with this animal, or they do not want to continue living in the constrained manner that is dictated by the treatment, no one would think they were awful, evil, or horrible if they decide to euthanize the pet.

Whether the pet is placed in a new household or is euthanized, the loss of a pet can put a family into crisis and create true and intense grief. A clue that this grief is widespread is found in a discussion in an Ann Landers column (Jan 31, 1994). Clients discussed their grief, their other pets' grief at the death or loss of a pet, and the rituals (burial, presentation of the empty halter to the other horse) in which the clients participated. The stages of grief—anger, bargaining, guilt, depression, and acceptance (Kübler-Ross, 1969)—have been well identified and are exhibited for pets that are either placed or euthanized for behavioral problems. The length of time for clients to go through these stages can range from a few months to almost a year (Harris, 1984; Katcher & Rosenberg, 1979). Rarely this process goes on indefinitely. Pets also appear to grieve for animal companions, and their needs must be addressed in any situation involving euthanasia (Hetts & Estep, 1994).

We have been approached by veterinarians who have euthanized their own animals years ago because of behavioral problems and are still grieving for that animal. They are particularly grieving because they were unaware help was available. Imagine the burden a client faces when examining the option of placement or death for a pet that they love, but they know it may be too problematic to keep that pet in the absence of therapy. It is critical that behavioral medicine be integrated into all aspects of patient care.

Euthanasia is always an emotionally friable issue, but it may be a more complex decision for a pet with a behavioral problem than for a pet facing euthanasia because of a health problem. The family generally feels a greater level of responsibility for the pet's well-being and for the development of the problem, and the guilt that they may feel—rational or not—is compounded if they then assume responsibility of making the decision to end the pet's life. The feeling of failure for causing the problem originally, although irrational, and then not being able to solve it can be intense. Clients may know that euthanasia is rationally the best decision, but they are wracked with grief in their inability to fix or deal with the problem. These pets are often healthy and appear normal, and much of the time they are excellent pets. This makes the decision to euthanize these animals far harder than it is in an animal that is suffering from a terminal condition with decreasing quality of life. Furthermore, many pets with behavioral disorders are young and, if they were nor-

mal, could have many healthy years of life ahead of them. It is critical that the veterinary practitioner, the veterinary support staff, and the family support the clients after they have tried everything else and nothing has worked to treat these pets. Unfortunately, this is often problematic because most individuals do not understand why the clients kept the pet as long as they did and believe that they should have "gotten rid of it" sooner. People make snide remarks, congratulate clients, and exhibit an incredible lack of compassion and understanding about why the people would grieve over a pet that had such problems. In general, the same care and respect guidelines for euthanasia necessitated by medical constraints should be followed for the euthanasia of a problem pet. The practitioner and staff may not understand why the client is so emotionally bonded to the pet, but that bond should be respected. The euthanasia should be scheduled for a time of day when neither the veterinarian nor client is rushed (i.e., the beginning or the end of the day). Clients may request time with the pet alone before it dies. They should have this option. If the clients wish to be present, they should be allowed to remain with the pet as long as needed. This may necessitate the use of a separate room or entrance. This requires space and time, but can be critical in helping the client to later make the decision to get another pet. The pet should be adequately sedated before euthanasia. Because these are planned deaths, the clients can start this process by giving some tablets at home. Once the client makes the decision to euthanize the pet and the staff concurs, the staff should discuss with the client specifically what is involved in the euthanasia procedure (placement of catheters, reasons for sedation, type of drug), the physiological processes that occur during death (urination and defecation). Also, the clients should decide what they wish for the final deposition of the body. Choices should be described explicitly. For example, clients may not be aware that memorial markers at pet cemeteries are an option. Some clients prefer to bury their dog at home. If so, they may need instruction on how best to do this (Lee & Lee, 1992). After death, clean and arrange the pet's body so that the client can be with it comfortably, if desired. Finally, make sure the clients can drive safely before discharging them. Suggest that they bring someone to drive them. Offer them a cup of herbal tea. Even though they elected to kill this pet, send a sympathy card and call. You may not have shared their view and love of the pet, but that is irrelevant. This is a harder, more complex decision than the one to kill an animal that is clearly suffering. Consider working with a social worker for just this type of circumstance. A group of practitioners in an area can cooperate to retain the professional services of a social worker. If they do so, they will find that they needed that person as part of their team more than they knew.

If children are involved, they may not understand the need for the pet to be euthanized and are often angry at the adults in the family. Children may have skewed views of pet ownership and responsibility and do not understand some of the reasons the family is doing this. It is inappropriate in such cases to hide the decisions for the euthanasia from the child. It is inappropriate to tell the child that the pet has a terrible disease or a brain disorder. It is absolutely appropriate to discuss the reasons, although the child may not be able to intellectually accept them at that age. Honesty is critical.

It is also important to reassure a child that he or she will not be placed or euthanized if they misbehave. It is easier to do this if the client and family have seriously tried to overcome the problem. Distinctions must be made between how the family has responded to the pet's misbehaving and how they respond to the child's misbehavior, although this can be a wonderful lesson for the child on the importance of following rules and getting along with others in the family.

If a pet was lost because of placement or euthanasia, it is best for a family to complete their bereavement process and adapt to the loss before getting another pet. As mentioned before, this process takes anywhere from a few months to almost a year. Although the death of a pet does not stop the majority of people from replacement (Podberscek et at., 1988), this waiting period helps ensure that the new pet is not merely an attempted replicate for the lost pet. Otherwise, the new pets are often saddled with unrealistic expectations, and the clients become frustrated when the new pets do not behave as they desire. If children are a part of the family, a waiting period between pets will help them learn that pets are not replaceable and that loss and change are permanent. The entire family should be involved in any decision to get another pet. If there were problems with caretaking of the pet in the past, it can be expected that, unless these issues are resolved, they will become problematic for any future pets. The behavioral specialist, the practitioner, or a social worker or counselor working together should remain as a resource to the family throughout this decision-making process.

THE ROLE OF SOCIAL WORK IN ADDRESSING BEHAVIORAL PROBLEMS IN PETS

It is obvious from the preceding discussion that families play a crucial role in the identification and treatment of a pet's behavioral problem, particularly when abuse was involved in the development of the behavioral problem. Understanding family dynamics, including the family's communication patterns, role behavior, reinforcement strategies, and hierarchy, may be necessary for the successful treatment of a pet's behavior problem. Most behavioral specialists and practitioners have no special training in these areas. As with other situations in which clinicians find themselves dealing with problems for which they are not

trained, a specialist's advice should be sought. Specialists in family dynamics include psychologists, social workers, and trained counselors. Any of these individuals may be available to work with clinicians on a routine or consultation basis. It is most helpful if counselors are involved in the treatment process from the initial contact with the family if an interpersonal problem is expected. The social worker or counselor must have a good working knowledge of animal behavior to be able to integrate the pet's behavior within the family's behavior. Although the social worker or counselor is available to serve as a consultant for the behavioral clinician and for the practitioner, the counselor also plays an important role with the family. The many stressors encountered by families, including guilt associated with thoughts that they caused the behavior problem, the disruption of the family's status quo caused by the pet's problem, the grief associated with the placement or euthanasia of the problem pet, and the adaptation necessary with the lifestyle changes attendant with behavioral modification create a crisis for these families. If a pet is seen as a substitute child or is triangled into a dysfunctional relationship, a threat to this relationship compounds any preexisting problems within the family. The social worker or counselor is the professional who is especially prepared to deal with the developing crisis of the behavior problem, as well as with the preexisting family problems often present. Because differences often exist within the family concerning the understanding of the behavioral problem and the commitment to change, conflict can easily arise between family members, which further increases stress. Social workers or counselors are especially able to deal with such conflict and stress and are also available to aid the family with the difficult decisions associated with the loss of a pet through placement or euthanasia. They can also be available to provide follow-up grief counseling to help the family adjust to the change or loss. Social workers and counselors are better prepared to work with children in the family in an effort to better understand their interaction with the pet and to offer appropriate behavior modification for the children as part of the treatment plan. For a full and inclusive approach to the pet's behavioral problem and to offer all the services that a family might need, a social worker or counselor is a necessary part of a treatment team.

Social workers or counselors are not as commonly used in veterinary medicine as would be desired. Since 1980 the Veterinary Hospital at the University of Pennsylvania has had a social worker on staff. This individual is available routinely to all clients coming to the emergency service, the oncology service, and the behavior clinic. These are all services that require full attention to any emotional upheavals the family may be experiencing to assist them in understanding the disease, understanding the necessary treatment, and implementing the treatment if possible. The social worker is available on an as-needed basis to other services and is an integral part of the veterinary medical team. The social work/medical interaction has long been recognized in human medicine but is still new in veterinary medicine. Advocates who explain the procedures the patient is undergoing are also far more common in human medicine than in veterinary medicine. In the context of behavioral medicine, social workers or counselors can play the role of advocate and provide family support as well. Although most practices cannot financially sustain the services of a full-time social worker or counselor, many practices are able to work as a consortium and share the services of such an individual on a regular or on an as-needed basis. A small increase in general fees may greatly offset the provision of social worker counseling services as part of the overall care service. At the Veterinary Hospital at the University of Pennsylvania, we do not charge for these services but certainly accept donations for them. The same situation can be used in a practice consortium and could be made to pay for itself in terms of generated revenue by offering a resource that might be unavailable elsewhere.

Another method by which social workers and counselors can facilitate behavioral therapy is through group sessions for people with problem pets. These can be arranged in a similar manner to those arranged for people who are grieving for pets that have died.

A final example of how the staff, in conjunction with a social worker or counselor, can facilitate the treatment of a problem pet and how well a family can cope with that pet is the orchestration and formulation of a support network among clients whose pets have similar problems. This has been implemented quite successfully in a variety of practices for clients who are learning to deal with diabetic disease in their older animals or other high-maintenance medical conditions. The support network can be based on a "buddy system," in which a client who has experienced the situation in the past agrees to call new clients who have these problems, and new clients are provided with this buddy's name and telephone number. This network can also take the form of a book in which clients who have previously dealt with specific problems detail these experiences in a letter form, perhaps accompanied by pictures of their pet. The book can be made available to individuals either on an as-needed basis or in the waiting room. Certainly, the format of such a book detailing clients' experiences, accompanied by pictures of their pets and their family, can also be helpful when people are grieving for a pet that died, or for people who have had to make the painful decision of euthanizing or placing their pets. A variety of these types of books can be maintained and offered to the client either through the support staff at the veterinary hospital or in conjunction with the help of a social worker or counselor who can introduce clients to the multifaceted aspects of behavioral medicine.

Any of the above suggestions can be implemented either separately or alone, but attempts must be made to address the family's needs when dealing with any pet's problem. One of the primary problems faced by practitioners is that they do not have the time or tools to properly deal with the emotional constraints of clients who are severely troubled because of their pet's behavioral problems. In this instance, there is no substitute for competent, quality care that can be provided by a social worker or counselor.

References

Abbruzzese A, Swanson J: Jaundice after therapy with chlordiazepoxide hydrochloride. *N Engl J Med* 273:321-322, 1965.

Abel MS, McCandless DW: The kindling model of epilepsy. Animal models of neurological disease. II. Metabolic encephalopathies and the epilepsies. In: *Neuromethods*, eds. Boulton AA, Baker GB, Butterworth RF. Human Press Incorporated, Totowa, NY: 22:153-168, 1992.

Ablett P: Public reaction to control. In: *The Ecology and Control of Feral Cats.* Universities Federation for Animal Welfare, Potter's Bar: 60-62, 1981.

Abrantes R: The expression of emotions in man and the canid. *J Sm Anim Pract* 28:1030-1036, 1967.

Adamec RE, Stark-Adamec C, Livingston KE: The development of predatory aggression and defense in the domestic cat *(Felis catus):* III. Effects on development of hunger between 180 and 365 days of age. *Behav Neural Biol* 30:435-447, 1980a.

Adamec RE, Stark-Adamec C, Livingston KE: The development of predatory aggression and defense in the domestic cat *(Felis catus).* II. The development of aggression and defense in the first 164 days of life. *Behav Neural Biol* 30:410-434, 1980b.

Adamec RE: Behavioral and epileptic determinants of predatory behavior in the cat. *Can J Neurol Sci* 2:457-466, 1975a.

Adamec RE: Does kindling model anything clinically relevant? *Biol Psychiatry* 27:249-279, 1990a.

Adamec RE: Hypothalamic and extrahypothalamic substrates of predatory attack: suppresion and the influence of hunger. *Brain Res* 106:57-69, 1976a.

Adamec RE: The interaction of hunger and preying in the domestic cat *(Felis catus):* an adaptive hierarchy? *Behav Biol* 18(2):263-272, 1976b.

Adamec RE: The neural basis of prolonged suppression of predatory attack. I. Naturally occurring physiological differences in the limbic systems of killer and non-killer cats. *Aggr Behav* 1:315-330, 1975b.

Adamec RE: Role of the amygdala and medial hypothalamus in spontaneous feline aggression and defense. *Aggr Behav* 16:207-222, 1990b.

Adamec RE, Stark-Adamec C, Livingston KE: The development of predatory aggression and defense in the domestic cat *(Felis catus).* I. Effects of early experience on adult patterns of aggression and defense. *Behav Neural Biol* 30:389-409, 1980c.

Adamec RE, Stark-Adamec C, Livingston KE: The expression of an early developmentally emergent defensive bias in the adult domestic cat *(Felis catus)* in non-predatory situations. Appl Anim Ethol 10:89-108, 1983.

Ader R: Effects of early experience and differential housing on behavior and susceptibility to gastric erosions in rats. *J Compar Physiol Psychol* 60:233-238, 1965.

Adler L, Adler H: Ontogeny of observational learning in the dog *(Canis familiaris).* Devel Psychobiol 10: 267-272, 1977.

Agrawal HC, Fox MW, Himwich WA: Neurochemical and behavioral effects of isolation-rearing in the dog. *Life Sciences* 6:71-78, 1967.

Alexander C, Breslin N, Molnar C, Richter J, Mukherjee S: Counterclockwise scalp hair whorl in schizophrenia. *Biol Psychiatry* 32:842-845, 1992.

Allen WE: Pseudopregnancy in the bitch: the current view on etiology and treatment. J Sm Anim Pract 27:419-424, 1986.

Altemus M, Glowa JR, Murphy DL: Attenuation of food restriction–induced running by chronic fluoxetine treatment. *Psychopharmacol Bull* 29:397-400, 1993.

Altmann A: A field study of the sociobiology of rhesus monkeys, *Macaca mulatta. Annu NY Acad Sci* 102(2):338-435, 1962.

Aman MG: Efficacy of psychotropic drugs for reducing self-injurious behavior in the developmental disabilities. *Ann Clin Psychiatry* 5:171-188, 1993.

American Psychiatric Association: *Diagnositic and Statistical Manual of Mental Disorders,* 4th edition. Washington, DC, 1994.

Amlaner CJ Jr, Stout JF: Aggressive communication by *Larus glaucescens.* VI. Interactions of territory residents with a remotely controlled, locomotory model. Behaviour 66:223-251, 1978.

Anand BK, Brobeck JR: Hypothalamic control of food intake in rats and cats. *Yale J Biol Med* 24:123-140, 1951.

Ananth J: Clomipramine: an antiobsessive drug. *Can J Psychiatry* 31:253-258, 1986.

Andermann F, Andermann E: Startle disorders of man: hyperekplexia, jumping and startle epilepsy. *Brain Devel* 10:213-222, 1988.

Anderson RK, Foster RE: Promise: The Natural Behavior System. Morris Animal Foundation, Englewood, Co, 1995.

Anderson RK, Hart BL, Hart LA, eds.: *The Pet Connection: its Influence on Our Health and Quality of Life.* University of Minnesota Press, Minneapolis, 1984.

Anderson RS: Obesity in the dog and cat. In: *The Veterinary Annual 11,* eds. Grunsell CSG, Hill FWG. John Wright & Sons, Bristol: 182-186, 1973.

Angel C, DeLuca DC, Newton JAEO, Reese WG: Assessment of pointer dog behavior: drug effects and neurochemical correlates. *Pav J Biol Sci* 17:84-88, 1982.

Angel C, Murphree OD, DeLuca DC: The effects of chlordiazepoxide, amphetamine, and cocaine on bar-press behavior in normal and genetically nervous dogs. *Res Nerv Sys* 35:220-223, 1974.

Anonymous: Attitudes towards animals. *Pet Vet* March-April; 23-24, 1992a.

Anonymous: Cats across the world. *Anthrozöos* III:196, 1990.

Anonymous: Survey results, *Anim Behav Consultant Newslett* 4(2): 3-4, 1987.

Anonymous: Veterinary medical education—an issue for the '80s. Council of Deans, Association of American Veterinary Medical Colleges, Washington, DC: 11, 1979.

Appleby D: Socialization and habituation. In: *The Behaviour of Dogs and Cats,* ed. Fisher J. Stanley, Paul and Company, Ltd., Random House, London: 24-40, 1993.

Appleby MC: The probability of linearity in hierarchies. *Anim Behav* 31:600-608, 1983.

Apps PJ: Home ranges of feral cats on Dassen Island. *J Mammol* 67:199-200, 1986.

Aranow RB, Hudson JI, Pope HG, Grady TA, Laage, TA, Bell IR, Cole JO: Elevated anti-depressant plasma levels after addition of fluoxetine. *Am J Psychiatry* 146:911-913, 1989.

Archer J: *The behavioural biology of aggression.* Cambridge University Press, New York, 1988.

Archer J: Behavioural aspects of fear. In: *Fear in Animals and Man*, ed. Sluckin W. Van Nostrum, Wokingham, England: 56-85, 1979.

Arkow P, Dow S: The ties that do not bind. In: *The Pet Connection: its Influence on our Health and Quality of Life*, eds. Anderson RK, Hart BL, Hart LA. University of Minnesota Press, Minneapolis: 348-354, 1984.

Armitage PL, Clutton-Brock J: A system for classification and description of the horn cores of cattle from archeological sites. *J Archeol Sci* 3:329-348,1976.

Arnold LE, Kirilcuk V, Corson SA, Corson EO: Levoamphetamine and dextroamphetamine: differential effect on aggression in hyperkinesis in children and dogs. *Am J Psychiatry* 130:165-170, 1973.

Aronson LR, Cooper ML: Olfactory deprivation and mating behavior in sexually experienced male cats. *Behav Biol* 11:459-480, 1974.

Aronson LR, Cooper ML: Penile spines of the domestic cat: their endocrine-behavior relations. *Anat Rec* 157:71-78, 1967.

Arshavsky YUI, Gelfand IM, Orlovsky GN, Pavlova GA: Messages conveyed by descending tracks during scratching in the cat. I. Activity of the vestibulospinal neurons. *Brain Res* 159:99-110, 1978.

Arshavsky YUI, Orlovsky GN, Panchin YV: Responses of Deiter's neurons to tilt during scratching. *Neurophysiol Kiev* 10:229-231, 1979.

August JR: Dog and cat bites. *JAVMA* 193:1394-1398, 1988.

AVMA: *The Veterinary Services Market.* American Veterinary Medical Association, Center for Information Management, Schaumburg, Il, 1992.

Azrin NH, Holz WC: Punishment. In: *Operant Behavior: Areas of Research and Application*, ed. Honig WK. Appleton-Century-Crofts, New York: 380-447, 1966.

Azrin NH, Hutchinson RR, McLaughlin R: The opportunity for aggression as an operant reinforcer during aversive stimulation. *J Exp Anim Behav* 8:171-180, 1965.

Bacon WD, Stanley W: Avoidance learning in neonatal dogs. *J Compar Physiol Psychol* 71:448-452, 1970a.

Bacon WD, Stanley W: Effects of deprivation levels in puppies on performance maintained by a passive person reinforcer. *J Compar Physiol Psychol* 56:783-785, 1963.

Bacon WD, Stanley W: Reversal learning in neonatal dogs. *J Compar Physiol Psychol* 70:344-350, 1970b.

Bacon WD: Aversive conditioning in neonatal kittens. *J Compar Physiol Psychol* 83:306-313, 1973.

Baenninger R: Violence toward other species. In: *Targets of Violence and Aggression*, ed. Baenninger R. North Holland Press, New York: 5-43, 1991.

Baerends A, Stewart CN, Warren JM: Pattern of social interaction in cats *(Felis domesticus). Behavior* 11:56-66, 1957.

Baerends-van Roon JM, Baerends G: The morphogenesis of the behavior of the domestic cat: with a special emphasis on the development of prey-catching. North Holland Press, Amsterdam, 1979.

Baker TL, Mitler MM, Foutz AS, et al: Diagnosis and treatment of narcolepsy in animals. In: *Current Veterinary Therapy* VIII. *Small Animal Practice*, 8th edition, ed. Kirk RW. WB Saunders, Philadelphia: 755-759, 1983.

Bali VR, Hormeyer J: A surgical technique for urine spraying by castrated cats. *Kleintierpraxis* 31:313-364, 1986.

Balk J-H, Picetti R, Salardi A, Thiriet G, Dierich A, Depaulis A, le Meur M, Borrelli E: Parkinsonian-like locomotor impairment in mice lacking dopamine D$_2$ receptors. *Nature* 377:424-428, 1995.

Bandler RJ Jr, Flynn JP: Neural pathways from the thalamus associated with regulation of aggressive behavior. *Science* 183:96-99, 1974.

Bard P, Macht MB: The behaviour of chronically decerebrate cats. In: CIBA Foundation Symposium on the Neurological Basis of Behavior, eds., Wolstenholme GEW, O'Connor CM. J & A Churchill, London: 55-77, 1958.

Barker SB, Barker RT: The human-canine bond: closer than family ties. *J Mental Health Counsel* 10:45-56, 1988.

Barratt ES: The use of anti-convulsants in aggression and violence. *Psychopharmacol Bull* 29:75-81, 1993.

Barrett P, Bateson P: The Development of Play in Cats. *Behaviour* 66:106-120, 1978.

Barrette C: The "inheritance of dominance," or an aptitude to dominate. *Anim Behav* 46:591-591, 1993.

Barsanti JA, Downey R: Urinary incontinence in cats. *JAAHA* 20:979-985, 1984.

Barsanti JA, Finco DR: Feline urologic syndrome: medical therapy. In: *Current Veterinary Therapy.* VIII. *Small Animal Practice*, ed. Kirk RW. WB Saunders, Philadelphia: 1108-1111, 1983.

Barthelemy C, Bruneau N, Cottet-Eymard JM, Domenach-Jouve J, Garreau B, Lelord G, Muh JP, Peyrin L: Urinary free and conjugated catecholamines and metabolites in autistic children. *J Autism Devel Disord* 18:583-591, 1988.

Bartlett CR: Heritabilities in genetic correlations between hip dysplasia and temperament traits of seeing-eye dogs. Master's thesis, Rutgers University, New Brunswick, New Jersey, 1976.

Bartlett M: Follow-up: puppy aptitude testing. *Purebred Dog AKC Gazette* May: 64-71, 1987.

Bartlett M: A novice looks at puppy aptitude testing. *Purebred Dog AKC Gazette* March: 31-42, 1979.

Bastock M, Morris D, Moynihan M: Some comments on conflict and thwarting in animals. *Behaviour* 6:66-83, 1953.

Bateson P: The development of play in cats. *Appl Anim Ethol* 4:290, 1978.

Bateson P: How do sensitive periods arise and what are they for? *Anim Behav* 27:470-486, 1979.

Bateson P, Martin P, Young M: Effects of interrupting cat mothers' lactation with bromocriptine on the subsequent play of kittens. *Physiol Behav* 27:841-845, 1981.

Bateson P, Mendel M, Feaver J: Play in the domestic cat is enhanced by the rationing of the mother during lactation. *Anim Behav* 40:514-525, 1990.

Bateson P, Young M: Separation from the mother and the development of play in cats. *Anim Behav* 29:173-180, 1981.

Baxter LR: Brain imaging as a tool in establishing a theory of brain pathology in obsessive-compulsive disorder. *J Clin Psychiatry* 51(Suppl 2):22-25, 1990.

Baxter LR, Schwartz JM, Bergman KS, Szuba MP, Guze BH, Mazziotta JC, Alazaki A, Selin CE, Ferng H-K, Munford P, Phelps ME: Caudate glucose metabolic rate changes with both drug and behavior therapy for obsessive-compulsive disorder. *Arch Gen Psychiatry* 49:681-689, 1992.

Beach F: Coital behavior in dogs. VIII. Social affinity, dominance, and sexual preference in the bitch. *Behavior* 36:131-148, 1970.

Beach F: Effects of gonadal hormones on urinary behavior in dogs. *Physiol Behav* 12:1005-1013, 1974.

Beach F: Hormonal modification of sexual dimorphic behavior. *Psychoendocrinol* 1:3-23, 1975.

Beach F, Dunbar I, Buehler M: Competitive behavior in male, female, and pseudohermaphroditic female dogs. *J Compar Physiol Psychol* 96:855-874, 1982.

Beach FA: Coital behavior in dogs. III. Effects of early isolation on mating in males. *Behaviour* 30:218-238, 1968.

Beach FA, Dunbar IF, Buehler MG: Sexual characteristics of female dogs during successive phases of the ovarian cycle. *Hormon Behav* 16:414-442, 1982.

Beach FA, Gilmore RW: Responses of male dogs to urine from females in heat. *J Mammol* 30:391-392, 1949.

Beach FA, Le Boeuf BJ: Coital behaviour in dogs. I. Preferential mating in the bitch. *Anim Behav* 15:546-558, 1967.

Beaudet R, Chalifoux A, Dallaire A: Predictive value of activity level and behavioral evaluation on future dominance in puppies. *Appl Anim Behav Sci* 40:273-284, 1994.

Beaver BV: Animal behavior case of the month. *JAVMA* 203:651-652, 1993.

Beaver BV: Behavioral development and behavioral disorders. In: *Veterinary Pediatrics: Dogs and Cats from Birth to Six Months of Age*, ed. Hoskins J. WB Saunders, Philadelphia: 19-28, 1990.

Beaver BV: Characteristics of some dog breeds. *Vet Med Sm Anim Clin* 77:889-891, 1982a.

Beaver BV: Clinical classification of canine aggression. *Appl Anim Ethol* 10:35-43, 1983.

Beaver BV: Disorders of behavior. In: *The Cat: Diseases and Clinical Management*, ed. Sherding RG. Churchill Livingstone, New York: 163-184, 1989.

Beaver BV: Distance-increasing postures of dogs. *Vet Med Sm Anim Clin* 77:1023-1024, 1982b.

Beaver BV: Effectiveness of products in eliminating cat urine odors from carpet. *JAVMA* 194:1589-1591, 1989b.

Beaver BV: *Feline Behavior: A Guide for Veterinarians.* WB Saunders, Philadelphia, 1980, 1992.

Beaver BV: Feline behavioral problems other than house soiling. *JAAHA* 25:465-469, 1989c.

Beaver BV: Feline behavioral problems. *Vet Clin North Am: Sm Anim Pract* 6:333-340, 1976.

Beaver BV: Friendly communication by the dog. *Vet Med Sm Anim Clin* 76:647-649, 1981a.

Beaver BV: The genetics of canine behavior. *Vet Med Sm Anim Clin* 76:1423-1424, 1981b.

Beaver BV: Grass eating by carnivores. *Vet Med Sm Anim Clin* 76:968-969, 1981c.

Beaver BV: Hormone therapy for animals with behavioral problems. *Vet Med Sm Anim Clin* 77:337-338, 1982c.

Beaver BV: House soiling by cats: a retrospective study of 120 cases. *JAAHA* 25:631-637, 1989d.

Beaver BV: The marking behavior of cats. *Vet Med Sm Anim Clin* 76:792-793, 1981d.

Beaver BV: Mating behavior in the cat. *Vet Clin North Am: Sm Anim Pract* 7:729-733, 1977.

Beaver BV: Mental lapse aggression syndrome. *JAAHA* 16(6):937-993, 1980.

Beaver BV: Modifying a cat's behavior. *Vet Med Sm Anim Clin* 76:1281-1283, 1981e.

Beaver BV: Owner complaints about canine behavior. *JAVMA* 204:1953-1955, 1993a.

Beaver BV: Problems and values associated with dominance. *Vet Med Sm Anim Clin* 76:1129-1131, 1981f.

Beaver BV: Profiles of dogs presented for aggression. *JAAHA* 29:564-569, 1993b.

Beaver BV: *The Veterinarian's Encyclopedia of Animal Behavior.* Iowa State University Press, Ames, 1995.

Beaver BV, Fischer N, Atkinson CH: Determination of favorite components of garbage by dogs. *Appl Anim Behav Sci* 34:129-136, 1992.

Beaver BV, Terry ML, LaSagna LL: Effectiveness of products in eliminating cat urine odors from carpet. *JAVMA* 194:1589-1591, 1989.

Beck AM: *The Ecology of Stray Dogs: a Study of Free-Ranging Urban Animals.* Baltimore, York Press, 1973.

Beck AM: The epidemiology of animal bites. *Comp Contin Educ Pract Vet* 3:254-258, 1981.

Beck AM, Jones BA: Unreported dog bites in children. *Public Health Rep* 100:315-321, 1984.

Beck AM, Katcher AH: *Between Pets and People: the Importance of Animal Companionship.* GP Putnam's Sons, New York: 1983.

Beck AM, Loring H, Lockwood R: The ecology of dog-bite injury in St. Louis, Missouri. *Public Health Rep* 90:262-267, 1975.

Beebe AD, Overall KL: Feline behavioral disorders. In: *Handbook of Veterinary Internal Medicine*, ed. Morgan RV. Churchill Livingstone, New York: 1997.

Bekoff M: The development of social interaction, play, and meta-communication in mammals: an ethological perspective. *Q Rev Biol* 47:412-434, 1972.

Bekoff M: Development of agonistic behaviour: ethological and ecological aspects. In: *Multidisciplinary Approaches to Aggression Research*, eds. Brain PF, Benton D. Elsevier/North Holland, Amsterdam: 161-178, 1981.

Bekoff M: Ground scratching by male domestic dogs: a composite signal. *J Mammol* 60:847-848, 1979a.

Bekoff M: Scent-marking by free-ranging domestic dogs: olfactory and visual components. *Biol Behav* 4:123-139, 1979b.

Bekoff M: Social communication in canids: evidence for the evolution of a stereotyped mammalian display. *Science* 197:1097-1099, 1977.

Bekoff M: Social play and play-soliciting by infant canids. *Am Zool* 14:323-340, 1974.

Bekoff M, Daniels TJ, Gittleman JL: Life history patterns in the comparative social ecology of carnivores. *Annu Rev Ecol Systemat* 15:191-232, 1984.

Bekoff M, Mech LD: Simulation analyses of space use: home range estimates, variability, and sample size. *Behav Res Meth Instr Comp* 16:32-37, 1984.

Bekoff M, Tyrell M, Lipetz VE, Jamieson R: Fighting patterns in young coyotes: imitation, escalation and assessment. *Aggressive Behav* 7:225-244, 1981.

Belkin M, Yinon U, Rose L, Reisert I: Effect of visual environment on refractive error of cats. *Doc Ophthalmol* 42:433-437, 1977.

Benfield P, Heel RC, Lewis SP: Fluoxetine. A review of its pharmacodynamic and pharmacokinetic properties, and therapeutic efficacy in depressive illness. *Drugs* 32:481-508, 1986.

Bennett M, Houpt KA, Erb HN: Effects of declawing on feline behavior. *Companion Anim Pract* 2:7-12, 1988.

Berg IA: Development of behavior: the micturition pattern in the dog. *J Exper Psychol* 34:343-368, 1944.

Bergon D, DeHoff J: Medical costs and other aspects of dog bites in Baltimore. *Public Health Rep* 89:377-381, 1974.

Berman M, Dunbar I: The social behaviour of free-ranging suburban dogs. *Appl Anim Ethol* 10:5-17, 1983.

Bernstein, IS: Dominance: the baby and the bathwater. *Behav Brain Sci* 4:419-457, 1981.

Bernstein KS: A physiological reason for defecating outside the litterbox. *Vet Med Sm Anim Clin* 72:1549, 1977.

Bernstein P, Strack M: Home ranges, favored spots, time-sharing patterns and tail usage by fourteen cats in the home. *Anim Behav Consult Newsletter* 10(3):1-3, 1993.

Bernston GG, Hughes HC, Beattie MS: A comparison of hypothalamically induced biting attack with natural predatory behavior in the cat. *J Compar Physiol Psychol* 90:167-178, 1976a.

Bernston GG, Leibowitz SF: Biting attack in cats: evidence for central muscarinic medication. *Brain Res* 52:366-370, 1973.

Bernston GG, Beattie MS, Walker JM: Effects of nicotinic and muscarine compounds on biting attacks in cats. *Pharmacol Biochem Behav* 5:235-239, 1976b.

Bertram BCR: Social factors influencing reproduction in wild lions. *J Zool* 177:463-482, 1975.

Biben M: Predation and predatory play behavior of domestic cats. *Anim Behav* 27:81-94, 1979.

Bikash KS, Bikash CP: Factors associated with biting behavior of dogs. Environ Ecol 8(2):630-634, 1990.

Biller DS et al.: Polycystic kidney disease in a family of Persian cats. *JAVMA* 196:1288-1290, 1990.

Blackshaw JK: Abnormal behavior in cats. *Austral Vet J* 65:395-396, 1988.

Blackshaw JK: An overview of aggressive behaviour in dogs and methods of treatment. *Appl Anim Behav Sci* 30:351-361, 1991.

Blackshaw JK: Feline elimination problems. *Anthrozöos* 5:52-56, 1992.

Blackshaw JK: Human and animal interrelationships. Review series: 4. Behavioral problems of dogs: Part II. *Austral Vet Pract* 15:114-118, 1985a.

Blackshaw JK: Human and animal interrelationships. Review series: 3. Normal behaviour patterns of dogs. Part I. *Austral Vet Pract* 15:110-112, 1985b.

Blackshaw JK, Cook GE, Harding P, Day C, Bates W, Rose J, Bramham D: Aversive responses of dogs to ultrasonic, sonic, and flashing light units. *Appl Anim Behav Sci* 25(1-2):1-8, 1990.

Blackshaw JK, Day C: Attitudes of dog owners to neutering pets: demographic data and effects of owner attitudes. *Austral Vet J* 71:113-116, 1994.

Blackshaw JK, Sutton RH, Boyhan MA: Tail chasing or circling behavior in dogs. *Canine Pract* 19(3):7-11, 1994.

Blackwell NJ: Reflex dyssynergia in the dog (letter). *Vet Rec* 132:516, 1993.

Blanchard DC, Blanchard RJ: Affect and aggression: an animal model applied to human behavior. In: *Advances in the Study of Aggression*. Vol 1, eds. Blanchard RJ, Blanchard DC. Academic Press, New York: 1-62, 1984a.

Blanchard DC, Blanchard RJ: Inadequacy of pain-aggression hypothesis revealed in naturalistic settings. *Aggressive Behav* 10:33-46, 1984b.

Blanchard DC, Fukuga-Stinson C, Takahashi L, Flannelly KJ, Blanchard RJ: Dominance and aggression in social groups of male and female rats. *Behav Proc* 9:31-48, 1984a.

Blanchard RJ: Pain and aggression reconsidered. In: *Biological Perspectives on Aggression*, eds. Flannelly KJ, Blanchard RJ, Blanchard DC. Liss, New York: 1-26, 1984.

Blanchard RJ, Blanchard DC: Aggressive behavior in the rat. *Behav Biol* 21:197-224, 1977.

Blanchard RJ, Blanchard DC: The organization and modeling of animal aggression. In: *The Biology of Aggression*, eds. Brain PF, Benton D. Sijthoff & Noordhoff, Rockville, Md: 529-561, 1981.

Blanchard RJ, Flannelly KJ, Layng M, Blanchard DC: The effects of age and strain on aggression in male rats. *Physiol Behav* 33:857-861, 1984b.

Blanchard RJ, Kleinschmidt CK, Flannelly KJ, Blanchard DC: Fear and aggression in the rat. *Aggressive Behav* 10:309-316, 1984c.

Blecha F, Pollman DS, Nichols DA: Immunologic reactions of pigs regrouped at or near weaning. *Am J Vet Res* 46:1924-1937, 1985.

Borchelt PL: Aggressive behavior of dogs kept as companion animals: classification and influence of sex, reproductive status and breed. *Appl Anim Ethol* 10:45-61, 1983a.

Borchelt PL: Behavior development of the puppy in the home environment. In: *Nutrition and Behavior in Dogs and Cats*, ed. Anderson RS. Pergamon Press, New York: 165-174, 1984a.

Borchelt PL: Cat elimination behavior problems. *Vet Clin North Am: Sm Anim Pract* 21:257-264, 1991.

Borchelt PL: Development of behaviour in the dog during maturity. In: *Nutrition and Behavior of Dogs and Cats*, ed. Anderson RS. Pergamon Press, New York, 189-197, 1984b.

Borchelt PL: Separation-elicited behavior problems in dogs. In: *New Perspectives on Our Lives with Companion Animals*, eds. Katcher AH, Beck AM. University of Pennsylvania Press, Philadelphia: 187-196, 1983b.

Borchelt PL, Lockwood R, Beck AM, Voith VL: Attacks by packs of dogs involving predation on human beings. *Public Health Rep* 98:59-68, 1983a.

Borchelt PL, Lockwood R, Beck AM, Voith VL: Dog attack involving predation on humans. In: *New Perspectives on Our Lives with Companion Animals*, eds. Katcher AH, Beck AM. University of Pennsylvania Press, Philadelphia: 219-231, 1983b.

Borchelt PL, Voith VL: Aggressive behavior in cats. *Comp Contin Edu Pract Vet* 9:49-56, 1987.

Borchelt PL, Voith VL: Classification of animal behavior problems. *Vet Clin North Am: Sm Anim Pract* 12(4):571-585, 1982a.

Borchelt PL, Voith VL: Diagnosis and treatment of aggression problems in cats. *Vet Clin North Am: Sm Anim Pract* 12(4):665-671, 1982b.

Borchelt PL, Voith VL: Diagnosis and treatment of elimination behavior problems in cats. *Vet Clin North Am: Sm Anim Pract* 12(4):673-681, 1982c.

Borchelt PL, Voith VL: Diagnosis and treatment of separation-related behavior problems in dogs. *Vet Clin North Am: Sm Anim Pract* 12(4):625-635, 1982d.

Borchelt PL, Voith VL: Dominance aggression in dogs. *Comp Contin Edu Pract Vet* 8:36-44, 1986a.

Borchelt PL, Voith VL: Elimination behavior problems in cats. *Comp Contin Educ Pract Vet* 8:197-205, 1986b.

Borchelt PL, Voith VL: Punishment. *Comp Contin Educ Pract Vet* 7(9):780-788, 1985.

Bovée K, Rosin A, Hart BL: Urine spraying and marking in cats. In: *Textbook of Small Animal Surgery*, ed. Slatter D. WB Saunders, Philadelphia: II:1476-1754, 1985.

Boyd R, Silk JB: A method for assessing cardinal dominance ranks. *Anim Behav* 31:45-58, 1983.

Boyer WF, Feighner JP: An overview of paroxetine. *J Clin Psych* 53(Suppl.):3-6, 1992.

Bradshaw JWS: *The Behaviour of the Domestic Cat*. CAB International, Wallingford, England, 1992a.

Bradshaw JWS: Behavioural biology. In: *The Waltham Book of Dog and Cat Behaviour*, ed. Thorne C. Pergamon Press, Oxford: 31-53, 1992b.

Bradshaw JWS, Brown SL: Behavioral adaptations of dogs to domestication. In: *Pets, Benefits and Practice*, ed. Berger IH. British Veterinary Association Publications, London: 18-24, 1990.

Bradshaw JWS, Natynczuk S, Macdonald DW: Potential for applications of anal sac volatiles in domestic dogs. In: *Chemical Signals in Vertebrates.* V. eds. Macdonald DW, Natynczuk SE. Oxford University Press, Oxford: 640-644, 1990.

Bradshaw JWS, Nott HMR: Social and communication behavior of companion dogs. In: *The Domestic Dog: The Biology of Its Behavior,* ed. Serpell JA. Cambridge University Press, Cambridge: 115-130, 1992.

Brain PF: Differentiating types of attack and defense in rodents. In: *Multidisciplinary Approaches to Aggression Research,* eds. Brain PF, Benton D. Elsevier/North Holland, Amsterdam: 53-78, 1981.

Brain PF, Haug M: Hormonal and neurochemical correlates of various forms of animal aggression. *Psychoneuroendocrinol* 17(6):537-552, 1992.

Brandeis R, Sapir M, Kapon Y, Borelli G, Cadel S, Valsecchi B: Improvement of cognitive function by MAO-B inhibitor L-deprenyl in aged rats. *Pharm Biochem Behav* 39:297-304, 1991.

Braund KG: *Clinical Syndromes in Veterinary Neurology.* Williams & Wilkins, Baltimore: 1986.

Breazile JE: Physiologic basis and consequence of distress in animals. *JAVMA* 191:1212-1215, 1987.

Breitschwerdt EB, Breasile JE, Broadhurst JJ: Clinical and electroencephalographic findings associated with 10 cases of suspected limbic epilepsy in the dog. *JAAHA* 15:37-50, 1979.

Brisbon IL Jr, Austad SN: Testing the individual odour theory of canine olfaction. *Anim Behav* 42:63-69, 1991.

Brodbeck AJ: An exploratory study on the acquisition of dependency behavior in puppies. *Bull Ecol Soc Am* 35:73, 1954.

Brody MD: Congress entrusts veterinarians with discretionary extra-label use. *JAVMA* 205:1366-1370, 1994.

Brown KA, Buchwald JS, Johnson JR, Mikolich DJ: Vocalization in the cat and kitten. *Devel Psychobiol* 11:559-570, 1978.

Brown C, Murphree O, Newton J: The effect of in-breeding on human aversion in pointer dogs. *J Heredity* 69:362-365, 1978.

Brown KA, Buchwald JS, Johnson JR, Mikolich, DJ: Vocalization in the cat and kitten. Devel Psychobiol 11:559-570, 1978.

Brown PR: Flycatching in the Cavalier King Charles Spaniel (letter). *Vet Rec* 120(4):95, 1987.

Brown RF, Houpt KA, Schryver HF: Stimulation of food intake in horses by diazapam and promazine. *Pharm Biochem Behav* 5:495-497, 1976.

Brown SA, Crowell-Davis S, Malcomb T, Stuarts P: Naloxone-responsive compulsive tail chasing in a dog. *JAVMA* 190(7):884-886, 1987.

Brunner HG, Nelen M, Breakefield XO, Ropers HH, van Oost BA: Abnormal behavior associated with a point mutation in the structural gene for monoamine oxidase A. *Science* 262:578-580, 1993.

Buffington CA, Chew DJ, DiBartola SP:Lower urinary tract disease in cats: is diet still a cause? *JAVMA* 205:1524-1526, 1994.

Buffington, CAT, Blaisdell JL, Binns SP, Woodworth BE: Decreased urine glycosaminoglycan excretion in cats with inflammatory bladder syndrome (abstract). *J Urol* 149:509A, 1993.

Buitelaar JK: Self-injurious behaviour in retarded children: clinical phenomena and biological meachanisms. *Acta Paedopsychiatrica* 56:105-111, 1993.

Bullock JE: Acupuncture treatment of canine lick granuloma. *Calif Vet* April:14-15, 1978.

Burgess PR, Perl ER: Cutaneous mechanoreceptors and nociceptors. In: *Handbook of Sensory Physiology.* Vol. II: Somatosensory Systems, ed. Iggo A. Springer-Verlag, New York: 29-78, 1973.

Burghardt W Jr: Diagnosis and treatment of hyperactivity in dogs. Paper presented at 1994 AVMA Convention, San Francisco, Ca.

Burk T: Acoustic signals, arms races and the costs of honest signalling. *Florida Entomologist* 71:400-409, 1988.

Burke TJ: Feline reproduction. *Vet Clin North Am: Sm Anim Pract* 6:317-331, 1976.

Burns M, Fraser MN: *Genetics of the Dog: The Basis of Successful Breeding.* Oliver & Boyd, Edinburgh, 1966.

Burt WH: Territoriality and home range concepts as applied to mammals. *J Mammol* 24:346-352, 1943.

Caccia S, Garattini S: Formation of active metabolites of psychotropic drugs. An updated view of their significance. *Clin Pharmacokinet* 18:434-459, 1990.

Caccia S, Garattini S: Pharmacokinetic and pharmacodynamic significance of antidepressant drug metabolites. *Pharm Res* 26:317-329, 1992.

Cain AO: Pets as family members. In: *Pets and the Family,* ed. Sussman MB. Haworth Press, New York: 5-10, 1985.

Cain AO: A study of pets in the family system. In: *New Perspectives on Our Lives with Companion Animals,* eds. Beck AM, Katcher AH. University of Pennsylvania Press, Philadelphia: 72-81, 1983.

Cairns RB, Hood KE, Midlam J: On fighting in mice: is there a sensitive period for isolation effects? *Anim Behav* 33:166-180, 1985.

Campbell WE: *Behavior problems in dogs.* American Veterinary Publications, Santa Barbara, Calif: 1975, 1992.

Campbell WE: Correcting obnoxious behavior problems in dogs. *Modern Vet Pract* 62:933-934, 1984.

Campbell WE: The prevalence of behavioral problems in American dogs. *Modern Vet Pract* 67:28-31, 1986.

Cantanzaro TE: A survey on the question on how well veterinarians are prepared to predict their client's human-animal bond. *JAVMA* 192:1707-1711, 1988.

Carlson Kuhta P, Smith JL: Scratch response in normal cats: Hindlimb kinematics in muscle synergies. *J Neurophysiol* 64:1653-1667, 1990.

Caro TM: The effects of experience on the predatory patterns of cats. *Behav Neural Biol* 29:1-28, 1980a.

Caro TM: Effects of the mother, object play, and adult experience on predation in cats. *Behav Neural Biol* 29:29-51, 1980b.

Caro TM: Predatory behavior and social play in kittens. *Behav* 76:1-24, 1981a.

Caro TM: Predatory behavior in domestic cat mothers. *Behav* 74:128-148, 1980c.

Caro TM: Relations between kitten behavior and adult predation. *Zeitschrift für Tierpsychologie* 51:158-168, 1979.

Caro TM: Sex differences in the termination of social play in cats. *Anim Behav* 29:271-279, 1981b.

Carr GM: The behavioural ecology of feral domestic dogs *(Canis familiaris)* in central italy. XIXth Ecological Conference, Toulouse, Abstract 267, 1985.

Case DB: Survey of expectations among clients of three small animal clinics. *JAVMA* 192:498-502, 1988.

Cases O, Seif I, Grimsby J, Gaspar P, Chen K, Pournin S, Müller U, Aguet M, Babinet C, Shih J, de Maeyer E: Aggressive behavior and altered amounts of brain serotonin and norepinephrine in mice lacking MAOA. *Science* 268:1763-1766, 1995.

Cash WC, Blauch BS: Jaw snapping syndrome in eight dogs. *JAVMA* 175:709-710, 1979.

Castonguay TW: Dietary dilution and intake in the cat. *Physiol Behav* 27:547-549, 1981.

Center SA: Pathophysiology and laboratory diagnosis of hepatobiliary disorders. In: *Textbook of Veterinary Internal Medicine*, eds. Ettinger SJ, Feldman EC. WB Saunders, Philadelphia: 1261-1312, 1995.

Center SA, Elston TH, Rowland PH, Rosen D, Reitz BL, Brunt IE, Rodan I, House J, Banks S, Lynch L, Dring L, Levy J: Fulminant hepatic failure associated with oral administration of diazepam in 12 cats. *JAVMA* 209:618-625, 1996.

Centers for Disease Control: Encephalitis associated with cat scratch disease—Broward and Palm Beach counties, Florida, 1994. *MMWR*, 16 December 1994.

Chai CY, Wang SC: Cardiovascular actions of diazepam in the cat. *J Pharmacol Exp Ther* 154:271-280, 1966.

Chakraborty PK, Panko WB, Fetcher WS: Serum hormone concentrations and their relationships to sexual behavior at the first and second estrus cycles of the labrador bitch. *Biol Reproduct* 22:227-232, 1980.

Chance MRA: Attention structure as the basis of primate rank orders. *Man* 2:503-518,1967.

Chapin JL, Newton JEO: Parallel between antianxiety and cardiovascular effects of chlordiazepoxide in genetically nervous dogs. *Pav J Biol Sci* 14:1-9, 1979.

Chapman BL: Feline aggression: classification, diagnosis, and treatment. *Vet Clin North Am Sm Anim Pract* 21(2):315-327, 1991.

Chapman BL, Voith VL: Behavioral problems in old dogs. *JAVMA* 196:944-946, 1990a.

Chapman BL, Voith VL: Cat aggression redirected to people: 14 cases (1981-1987). *JAVMA* 196:947-950, 1990b.

Charney DS, Heninger GR: Abnormal regulation of noradrenergic function in panic disorders. *Arch Gen Psych* 43:1042-1058, 1986.

Charney DS, Woods SW, Nagy LM, Southwick SM, Krystal JH, Heninger GR: Noradrenergic function in panic disorder. *J Clin Psych* 51(12, Suppl. A):5-11, 1990.

Chase ID: Models of hierarchy formation in animal societies. *Behav Sci* 19:374-382, 1974.

Chastain CB, Graham CL, Nichols CE: Adrenocortical suppression in cats given megestrol acetate. *Am J Vet Res* 42(12):2029-2035, 1991.

Chesler P: Maternal influence in learning by observation in kittens. *Science* 166:901-902, 1969.

Chesney CJ: The response to progestagen treatment of some diseases in cats. *J Sm Anim Pract* 17:35-44, 1976.

Childs JE, Ross L: Urban cats: characteristics and estimation of mortality due to motor vehicles. *Am J Vet Res* 47:1643-1648, 1986.

Chrisman CL: Seizures. In: *Textbook of Veterinary Internal Medicine*, eds. Ettinger SJ, Feldman EC. WB Saunders, Philadelphia: 152-156, 1995.

Chrisman CL: *Problems in Small Animal Neurology*. Lea & Febiger, Philadelphia, 1982.

Christoffersen CL, Meltzer LT: Evidence for N-methyl-D-aspartate and AMPA subtypes of the glutamate receptor on substantia nigra dopamine neurons: possible preferential role for N-methyl-D-aspartate receptors. *Neuroscience* 67:373-381, 1995.

Chun Y, Berkelhamer J, Herold T: Dog bites in children less than four years old. *Pediatrics* 69:119-120, 1982.

Clark GI, Boyer WN: The effects of dog obedience training and behavioral counselling upon the human-canine relationship. *Appl Anim Behav Sci* 37:147-159, 1993.

Clark JM: The effects of selection and human preference on coat colour gene frequencies in urban cats. *Heredity* [Lond.] 35:195-210, 1975.

Clarke RS, Heron W, Feterstonhaugh ML, Forgays DG, Hebb DO: Individual differences in dogs: preliminary report on the effects of early experience. *Can J Psychol* 5(4):150-156, 1951.

Clifford DH, Boatfield MP, Daniels TJ: The social organization of free-ranging urban dogs. I. Non-estrus social behavior. *Appl Anim Ethol* 10:341-363, 1983a.

Clifford DH, Boatfield MP, Rubright J: Observations on fighting dogs. *JAVMA* 183:654-657, 1983b.

Clutton-Brock J: *A Natural History of Domesticated Animals*. British Museum (Natural History), Cambridge University Press, Cambridge, 1987.

Coccaro EF, Astill IL, Herbert JL, Shut AG: Fluoxetine treatment of impulsive aggression in DSM-III-R personality disorder patients. *J Clin Psychopharmacol* 10(5):373-375, 1990.

Coid J, Allilio B, Rees LH: Raised plasma metencephalin in patients who habitually mutilate themselves. *Lancet* 2:545-546, 1983.

Cole DD, Shafer JJ: A Study in Social Dominance in Cats. *Behav* 27:39-53, 1966.

Colgan P: *Animal Motivation*. Chapman & Hall, London, 1989.

Collard RR: Fear of strangers and play behavior in kittens with varied social experience. *Child Develop* 38:877-891, 1967.

Colter S, Gustafson JH, Colburn WA: Pharmacokinetics of diazepam and nordiazepam in the cat. *J Pharm Sci* 73:348-351, 1984.

Comfort A: Maximum ages reached by domestic cats. *J Mammol* 37:118-119, 1956.

Compaan JC, van Wattum G, de Ruiter AJH, van Oortmerssen GA, Koolhaas JM, Bohus B: Genetic differences in female house mice in aggressive response to sex steroid hormone treatment. *Physiol Behav* 54:899-902, 1993.

Coon H, Plaetke R, Holik J, Hoff M, Myles-Worsley M, Waldo M, Freedman R, Byerly W: Use of a neurophysiological trait in linkage analysis of schizophrenia. *Biol Psych* 34:277-289, 1993.

Coop CF, McNaughton N: Buspirone affects hippocampal rhythmical slow activity through serotonin I_A rather than dopamine D_2 receptors. *Neuroscience* 40:169-174, 1991.

Cooper L, Hart BL: Comparison of diazepam with progestin for effectiveness in suppression of urine spraying behavior in cats. *JAVMA* 200:797-801, 1992.

Coppinger R, Glendenning J, Torop E, Matthay C, Sutherland M, Smith C: Degree of behavioral neoteny differentiates canid polymorphs. *Ethology* 75:89-108, 1987.

Corbett LK: Feeding ecology and social organization of wild cats (*Felis silvestris*) and domestic cats (*Felis catus*) in Scotland. PhD Thesis, University of Aberdeen, Scotland,1979. Cited in: *The Domestic Cat: The Biology of its Behaviour*, eds. Turner DC, Bateson P. Cambridge University Press, Cambridge: 25, 1988.

Corson SA, Corson EO: Constitutional differences in physiological adaptation to stress and distress. In: *Psychopathology of Human Adaptation*, ed. Serban G. Plenum Press, New York: 77-94, 1976.

Corson SA, Corson EO, Decker RE, Ginsburg BE, Trattner A, Connor RL, Lucas LA, Panksepp J, Scott JP: Interaction of genetics and separation in canine hyperkinesis and in a differential response to amphetamines. *Pav J Biol Sci* 15:5-11, 1980.

Corson SA, Corson EO, Kirilcuk V: Tranquilizing effects of D-amphetamine on hyperkinetic untrainable dogs. *Federation Proceedings* 30:206, 1971.

Coyle JT, Puttfarcken P: Oxidative stress, glutamate, and neurodegenerative disorders. *Science* 262:689-695, 1993.

Craig W: Why do animals fight? *Internat J Ethics* 31:264-278, 1928.

Crawford MA, Kittleson MD, Fink JD: Hypernatremia and adipsia in a dog. *JAVMA* 184:818-821, 1984.

Crews WD Jr, Bonaventura S, Rowe FB, Bonsie D: Cessation of long-term naltrexone therapy and self-injury: a case study. *Res Devel Disabil* 14:331-340, 1993.

Cronin GM, Wiepkema PR, van Ree JM: Endogenous opioids are often involved in abnormal stereotyped behaviours of tethered sows. *Neuropeptides* 6:527-530, 1985.

Cronin GM, Wiepkema PR, van Ree JM: Endorphins implicated in stereotypies of tethered sows. *Experientia* 42:198-199, 1986.

Crowell-Davis SL, Barny K, Ballan J, LaFlamme DP: The effect of caloric restriction on the behavior of dogs (abstract). *Appl Anim Behav Sci* 39:184, 1994.

Crowell-Davis SL, Lappin M, Oliver JE: Stimulus-responsive psychomotor epilepsy in a Doberman Pinscher. *JAAHA* 25:57-60, 1989.

Cummings BJ, Su JH, Cotman CW, White R, Russell MJ: Beta-amyloid accumulation in aged canine brain: a model of early plaque formation in Alzheimer's disease. *Neurobiol Aging* 14(6):547-560, 1993.

Cummings JF, de Lahunta A, Braund KG, Mitchell WJ: Animal model of human disease: hereditary sensory neuropathy: nociceptive loss and acral mutilation in pointer dogs: canine hereditary sensory neuropathy. *Am J Pathol* 112:136-138, 1983.

Cummings JF, de Lahunta A, Simpson ST, McDonald JM: Reduced substance P-like immunoreactivity in hereditary sensory neuropathy of pointer dogs. *Acta Neuropathologica* (Berlin) 63:33-40, 1984.

Cummings JF, de Lahunta A, Winn SS: Acral mutilation and nociceptive loss in English Pointer dogs. A canine sensory neuropathy. *Acta Neuropathologica* (Berlin) 53:119-127, 1981.

Cunningham ML: Acute hepatic necrosis following treatment with amitriptyline and diazepam. *Brit J Psychiatry* 111:1107-1109, 1965.

Curzon G: Serotonergic mechanisms of depression. *Clin Neuropharmacol* 11(Suppl 2):S11-S20, 1988.

Czarkowska J: Changes of some postural reflexes during the first post-natal weeks in the dog. *Acta Neurobiologica* 43:27-35, 1983.

Daniels TJ: The social organization of free-ranging urban dogs. I. Non-estrous social behavior. *Appl Anim Ethol* 10:341-363, 1983.

Daniels TJ: The social organization of free-ranging urban dogs. II. Estrus groups in the mating system. *Appl Anim Ethol* 10:365-373, 1983b.

Daniels TJ, Bekoff N: Population and social biology of free-ranging dogs, *Canis familiaris*. *J Mammol* 70:754-762, 1989.

Danneman P, Chodrow R: History taking and interviewing techniques. *Vet Clin North Am Sm Anim Pract* 12:587-592, 1982.

Dantzer R: Behavioural, physiological and functional aspects of stereotyped behaviour: a review and a reinterpretation. *J Anim Sci* 62:1776-1786, 1986.

Dantzer R, Mormède P: Behavioural consequences of frustration and conflict in pigs. In: *Sisturned Behaviour in Farm Animals*, ed. Bessei W. Verlag Eugen Ulmer, Stuttgart: 87-100, 1982.

Dantzer R, Mormède P: Pituitary adrenal consequences of adjunctive behaviors in pigs. *Horm Behav* 15:386-395, 1981.

Dards, JL: The behaviour of dockyard cats: interactions of adult males. *Appl Anim Ethol* 10:133-153, 1983.

Daristotle L: Conference proposed to explore dog-bite issues. *JAVMA* 204:1853, 1994.

Darke PGG: Obesity in small animals. *Vet Rec* 102:545-546, 1978.

Darwin C: *The Origin of Species by Means of Natural Selection; or, the Preservation of Favored Races in the Struggle for Life*. D Appleton, New York, 1972 (orig. 1865).

Davenport DJ: Enteral and parenteral nutritional support. In: *Textbook of Veterinary Internal Medicine*, eds. Ettinger SJ, Feldman EC. WB Saunders, Philadelphia: 244-251, 1995.

Davis GC, Buchsbaum MS, Naber D, Pickar D, Post R, van Kammen D, Bunney WE Jr: Altered pain perception and cerebrospinal endorphins in psychiatric illness. *Ann NY Acad Sci* 398:366-373, 1982.

Davis JM: Socially induced flight reactions in pigeons. *Anim Behav* 23:597-601, 1975.

Davis RG: Olfactory psychophysical parameters in man, rat, dog, and pigeon. *J of Compar Physiol Psychol* 85:221-232, 1973.

Davis SJM, Valla FR: Evidence for domestication of the dog twelve thousand years ago in Natufian of Israel. *Nature* 276: 608-610, 1978.

Dawson TM, Dawson VL, Snyder SH: A novel neuronal messenger molecule in the brain: the free radical, nitric oxide. *Annu Neurol* 32:297-311, 1992.

Dawson VL, Dawson TD, London ED, Bredt DS, Snyder SH: Nitric oxide mediates glutamate neurotoxicity in primary cortical cultures. *Proc Natl Acad Sci USA* 88:6368-6371, 1991.

Dawson VL, Dawson TM, London ED, Bredt DS, Snyder SH: Nitric oxide mediates glutamate neurotoxicity in primary cortical cultures. *Proc Nat Acad Sci USA* 88:6368-6371, 1991.

Day C, Galef B: Pup cannibalism: One aspect of maternal behavior in golden hamsters. *J Comp Physiol Psychol* 91:1179-1189, 1977.

de Lahunta A: *Veterinary Neuroanatomy and Clinical Neurology*, 2nd edition. WB Saunders, Philadelphia: 1983.

de Luca RV, Holborn SW: A comparison of relaxation training and competing response training to eliminate hair pulling and nail biting. *J Behav Ther Exp Psych* 15:67-70, 1984.

Deag JM, Manning A, Lawrence CE: Factors influencing the mother-kitten relationship. In: *The Domestic Cat: The Biology of Its Behavior*, eds. Turner DC, Bateson P. Cambridge University Press, Cambridge: 23-39, 1988.

deBoer JN: The age of olfactory cues functioning in chemocommunication among male domestic cats. *Behav Proc* 2:209-225, 1977a.

deBoer JN: Dominance relations in pairs of domestic cats. *Behav Proc* 2:227-242. 1977b.

deBoer T, Stoof JC, van Duijn H: The effects of convulsant and anticonvulsant drugs on the release of radiolabeled GABA, glutamate, noradrenaline, serotonin, and acetylcholine from rat cortical slices. *Brain Res* 253:153-160, 1982.

Delius JD: Preening and associated comfort in birds. *Ann NY Acad Sci* 525:40-55, 1988.

de Luca RV, Holborn SW: A comparison of relaxation training and competing response training to eliminate hair pulling and nail biting. *J Behav Ther Exp Psych* 15:67-70, 1984.

Delville Y, Koh ET, Ferris CF: Sexual differences in magnocellular vasopressinergic system in golden hamsters. *Brain Res Bull* 33:535-540, 1994.

deMontigny C: Enhancement of the 5-HT neurotransmission by antidepressant treatments. *J Physiol* 77:455-461, 1981.

Denenberg VH: Developmental factors in aggression. In: *The Control of Aggression*, ed. Knutson JF. Aldine, Chicago: 41-57, 1973.

Dennenberg VH, Morton JRC: Effects of environmental complexity and social groupings upon modification of emotional behavior. *J Comp Physiol Psych* 55:242-246, 1962.

Derr M: The politics of dogs: how greed and AKC policies are endangering the health and quality of American dogs. *Atlantic Monthly* March: 49-72, 1990.

DeVries GJ, Best W, Slutter AA: The influence of androgens on the development of a sex difference in the vasopressinergic innervation to the lateral septum. *Develop Brain Res* 8:337-380, 1983.

Dewsbury DA: Fathers and sons. Genetic factors and social dominance in deer mice, *Peromyscus maniculatus. Anim Behav* 39:284-289, 1990.

Dewsbury DA, Hartung TG: Copulatory behavior and differential reproduction of laboratory rats in a two-male, one-female competitive situation. *Anim Behav* 28:95-102, 1980.

Dodman NH, Bronson R, Gliatto J: Tail chasing in a bull terrier. *JAVMA* 202:758-760, 1993.

Dodman NH, Miczek KA, Knowles K, Thalhammer JG, Shuster L: Phenobarbital-responsive episodic dyscontrol (rage) in dogs. *JAVMA* 201:1580-1583, 1992.

Dodman NH, Reisner I, Shuster L, Rand W, Luescher UA, Robinson I, Houpt KA: Effect of dietary protein content on behavior in dogs (Abstract). *JAVMA* 208:376-379, 1996.

Dodman NH, Shuster L, Court MH, White SD: Behavioral effects of narcotic antagonists. *J Assoc Vet Anesthetists* 15:56-64, 1988a.

Dodman NH, Shuster L, Court MH: Use of a narcotic antagonist in the treatment of a stereotypic behavior pattern (crib-biting) in the horse. *Am J Vet Res* 48:311-319, 1987.

Dodman NH, Shuster L, Court MH: Use of a narcotic antagonist (nalmefene) to suppress self-mutilative behavior in a stallion. *JAVMA* 192:1585-1586, 1988b.

Dodman NH, Shuster L, White SD, Court MH, Parker D, Dixon R: Use of narcotic antagonists to modify stereotypic self-licking, self-chewing, and scratching behavior in dogs. *JAVMA* 193:815-819, 1988c.

Domjan M, Burkhard B: *The Principles of Learning and Behavior.* Second Edition. Brooks/Cole Publishing Co, Pacific Grove, 1985.

Doty RL, Dunbar I: Attraction of beagles to conspecific urine, vaginal, and anal sac secretion odors. *Physiol Behav* 12:825-833, 1974.

Dumas C: Object permanence in cats *(Felis catus)*: An ecological approach to the study of invisible displacements. *J Comp Psych* 106:404-410, 1992.

Dunbar I: Behaviour of castrated animals. *Vet Rec* 96:92-93, 1975.

Dunbar I: How to Teach a New Dog Old Tricks: SIRIUS Puppy Training Manual. James and Kenneth Publishers, Oakland, 1991.

Dunbar I, Buehler M: A masking effect of urine from male dogs. *Appl Anim Ethol* 6:297-301, 1980.

Dunbar I, Buehler M, Beach F: Development and activational effects of sex hormones on the attractiveness of dog urine. *Physiol Behav* 24:201-204, 1980.

Dunbar I, Carmichael N: The response of male dogs to urine from other males. *Behav Neurobiol* 31:465-470, 1981.

Dunham AE: Population responses to global change: Physiologically structured models, operative environments, and population dynamics. In: Evolutionary, Population, and Community Responses to Global Change, ed. Kariva, P, Kingsolver J, Huey R. Sinauer Associates, Sunderland, MA, 95-119, 1993.

Dunham AE, Grant BW, Overall KL: Interfaces between biophysical ecology and population ecology of vertebrate ectotherms. Invited symposium paper at the December, 1987 American Society of Zoologists meeting. *Physiol Zool* 62(2):335-355, 1989.

Eckstein R: Use of electronic stimulation to treat acral lick dermatitis. Talk presented at AVMA Conference, San Francisco, Ca, 1995.

Edney ATB: Matching dogs to owners: 10 years of "Select-a-Dog." *J Sm Anim Prac* 28(11):1004-1008, 1987.

Egger MD, Flynn JP: Effects of electrical stimulation of the amygdala on hypothalamically elicited attack behavior in cats. *J Neurophysiol* 26:705-720, 1963.

Eichelmann B: Catecholamines and aggressive behavior. In: *Neuroregulators and Psychiatric Disorders*, ed. Usdin E. Oxford University Press, New York: 146-150, 1977b.

Eichelmann B: Neurochemical studies of aggression in animals. *Psychopharmacol Bull* 13:17-19, 1977a.

Eigenmann JE, Eigenmann RY: Influence of medroxyprogesterone acetate (provera) on plasma growth hormone levels and on carbohydrate metabolism, part II. *Acta Endocrinologica* 98:602-608, 1981a.

Eigenmann JE, Eigenmann RY: Influence of medroxyprogesterone acetate (provera) on plasma growth hormone levels and on carbohydrate metabolism, part I. *Acta Endocrinologica* 98:599-602, 1981b.

Eison AS, Temple DL: Buspirone: review of its pharmacology and current perspective on its mechanism of action. *Am J Med* 80(Suppl. 3B):1-8, 1986.

El-Yazigi A, Chaleky K, Gad A, Raines DA: Steady-state kinetics of fluoxetine and amitriptyline in patients treated with a combination of these drugs as compared with those treated with amitriptyline alone. *J Clin Pharmacol* 35:17-21, 1995.

Elkin I, Pilkonis PA, Docherty JP, Sotsky M: Conceptual and methodological issues in comparative studies of psychotherapy and pharmacotherapy. II: Nature and timing of treatment effects. *Am J Psych* 145:1070-1076, 1988a.

Elkin I, Pilkonis PA, Docherty JP, Sotsky M: Conceptual and methodological issues in comparative studies of psychotherapy and pharmacotherapy. I: Active ingredients and mechanisms of change. *Am J Psych* 145:909-917, 1988b.

Ellenbroek BA, Cools AR: Animal models with construct validity for schizophrenia. *Behav Pharmacol* 1:469-490, 1990.

Elliot O, King JA: Effect of early food deprivation upon later consummatory behavior in puppies. *Psychol Rep* 6:391-400, 1960.

Elliot O, Scott JP: The analysis of breed differences in maze performances in dogs. *Anim Behav* 13:5-18, 1965.

Elliot O, Scott JP: The development of emotional distress reactions to separation in puppies. *J Genetic Psychol* 99:3-22, 1961.

Elliott FA: Neurological factors in violent behavior (the dyscontrol syndrome). In: *Violence and Responsibility. The Individual, The Family and Society*, ed. RL Sadoff. SP Medical and Scientific Books, New York: 58-86, 1978.

Emlen ST, Oring LW: Ecology, sexual selection, and the evolution of mating systems. *Science* 197:215-223, 1977.

Ereshefsky L, Tran-Johnson T, Davis CM, LeRoy A: Pharmacokinetic factors affecting drug clearance and clinical effect: evaluation of doxepim and imipramine. New data and review. *Clin Chem* 3415:863-880, 1988.

Eron LD: The development of aggressive behavior from the perspective of a developing behaviorism. *American Psychologist* 10:435-442, 1987.

Eschalier A: Anti-depressants and pain mangement. In: *Serotonin and Pain*, ed. Besson J. Elsevier Science, New York: 305-325, 1990.

Everett GM: Observations on the behavior and neurophysiology of acute thiamine deficient cats. *Am J Physiol* 141:439-448, 1944.

Ewer RF: *The Carnivores.* Cornell University Press, Ithaca, NY, 1973.

Ewer RF: Further observations on suckling behaviour in kittens, together with some general considerations of the interrelations of innate and acquired responses. Behav 17:247-260, 1961.

Fagen R: *Animal Play Behaviour.* Oxford University Press, Oxford, 1981.

Fagen RM, Mankovich NJ: Two-act transitions, partitioned contingency tables, and the "significant cells" problem. *Anim Behav* 28:1017-1023, 1980.

Faggella AM, Aronsohn MG: Evaluation of anesthetic protocols for neutering 6- to 14-week-old pups. *JAVMA* 205:308-314, 1984.

Fält L: Inheritance of behavior in the dog. In: *Nutrition and Behavior in Dogs and Cats,* Anderson RS. Pergamon Press, New York: 183-187, 1984.

Feaver J, Mendl M, Bateson P: A method for rating the individual distinctiveness of domestic cats. *Anim Behav* 34:1016-1025, 1986.

Feder H, Shanley J, Barbera J: Review of 59 hospitalized patients with animal bites. *Pediatr Infect Dis J* 6:24-28, 1987.

Feldman HN: Domestic cats and passive submission. *Anim Behav* 47:457-459, 1994.

Feldman HN: Maternal care and differences in the use of nests in the domestic cat. *Anim Behav* 45:13-23, 1993.

Felthous AR: Aggression against cats, dogs, and people. *Child Psych in Hum Develop* 10:169-177, 1980.

Felthous AR, Kellert SR: Childhood cruelty to animals and later aggression against people: a review. *Am J Psych* 144:710-717, 1987.

Fenner WR: Diseases of the brain. In: *Textbook of Veterinary Internal Medicine,* eds. Ettinger SJ, Feldman EC. WB Saunders, Philadelphia: 578-628, 1995.

Ferrell F: Preference for sugars and non-nutritive sweetners in young beagles. *Neurosci Biobehav Rev* 8:199-203, 1984.

Ferris CF, Delville Y: Vasopressin and serotonin interactions in the control of agonistic behavior. *Psychoneuroendocrinol* 19:593-601, 1994.

Ferris CF, Delville Y, Irwin RW, Potegal M: Septohypothalamic organization of a stereotyped behavior controlled by vasopressin in golden hamsters. *Physiol Behav* 55:755-759, 1994.

Ferris CF, Foote KB, Meltser HM, Plenby MG, Smith KL, Insel TR: Oxytocin in the amygdala facilitates maternal aggression. *Ann NY Acad Sci* 652:456-457, 1992.

File SE: The history of benzodiazepine dependence: a review of animal studies. *Neuro Biobehav Rev* 14:135-146, 1990.

File SE: Interactions of anxiolytic and antidepressant drugs with the hormones of the hypothalamic-pituitary-adrenal axis. *Pharm Ther* 46:357-375, 1990.

File SE: New strategies in the search for anxiolytics. *Drug Design and Development* 5(3):195-201, 1990.

Finco DR, Adams DD, Crowel WA, et al.: Food and water intake and urine composition in cats: influence of continuous versus periodic feeding. *Am J Vet Res* 47:1638-1642, 1986.

Fisher GT: The danger of labelling aggression: understanding the types of aggressive behaviors, rather than labelling dogs, for more successful training. *Pure-Bred Dog/AKC Gazette* 107(7):52-56; 58-61, 1990.

Fisher J: *The Behavior of Dogs and Cats.* Stanley Paul, London: 1993.

Fitzgerald BM, Karl BJ: Home range of feral house cats *(Felis catus L.)* in a forest of the Orongorongo Valley, Wellington, New Zealand. *NZ J Ecol* 9:71-81, 1986.

Flament MF, Rappoport JL, Berg CJ: Clomipramine treatment of childhood obsessive-compulsive disorder. A double-blind controlled study. *Arch Gen Psych* 42:977-983, 1985.

Fleisher GR, Boenning DA: The treatment of animal bites in humans. *Comp Contin Edu Pract Vet* 3(4):366-370, 1981.

Floody OR: Hormones and aggression in female mammals. In: *Hormones and Aggressive Behavior,* ed. Svare BB. Plenum, New York: 39-90, 1983.

Fogle B: *The Dog's Mind: Understanding Your Dog's Behavior.* Howell Book House, New York: 1990.

Fogle B: *Pets and Their People.* Penguin Books, New York: 1983.

Folk GE Jr, Fox MW, Folk MA: Physiological differences between alpha and subordinate wolves in a captive sibling pack. *Am Zool* 10:487, 1970.

Fonberg E: Various relationships between predatory dominance and aggressive behavior in pairs of cats. *Aggressive Behav* 11:103-114, 1985.

Fonnum F: Glutamate: a neurotransmitter in mammalian brain. *J Neurochem* 42:1-11, 1984.

Fontaine R, Chouinard G: Fluoxetine in the long-term maintenance treatment of obsessive-compulsive disorders. *Psych Ann* 12:88-91, 1989.

Foster ES, Carrillo JM, Patnaik AK: Clinical signs of tumors affecting the rostral cerebrum in 43 dogs. *J Vet Intern Med* 2(2):71-74, 1988.

Foster JA, Morrison M, Dean SJ, Hill M, Frenk H: Naloxone suppresses food/water consumption in the deprived cat. *Pharmacol Biochem Behav* 14:419-421, 1981.

Foutz AS, Mitler MM, Dement WC: Narcolepsy. *Vet Clin North Am Sm Anim Pract* 10:65-80. 1980.

Fox MW: Abnormal Behavior in Animals. WB Saunders, Philadelphia: 1968a.

Fox MW: Aggression: its adaptive and maladaptive significance in animals. In: *Abnormal Behavior in Animals,* ed. Fox MW. WB Saunders, Philadelphia: 44-63, 1968b.

Fox MW: The anatomy of aggression and its ritualization in Canidae: a developmental and comparative study. *Behav* 35:242-258, 1969a.

Fox MW: Behavioral effects of rearing dogs with cat during the critical period of socialization. *Behav* 35:273-280, 1969b.

Fox MW: The behaviour of cats. In: *The Behaviour of Domestic Animals,* 3rd edition, ed. Hafez ESE. Williams & Wilkins Baltimore: 410-436, 1975.

Fox MW: A comparative study of the development of facial expressions in canids: wolf, coyote, and fox. *Behav* 37:49-73, 1970a.

Fox MW: *The Dog: Its Domestication and Behavior.* Garland STPM Press, New York: 1978.

Fox MW: The effects of short term social and sensory isolation upon behavior, EEG, and average evoked potential in puppies. *Physiol Behav* 2:145-151, 1967a.

Fox MW: Influence of domestication upon behavior of animals. *Vet Rec* 80:696-702, 1967b.

Fox MW: *Integrative Development of Brain and Behavior in the Dog.* University of Chicago Press, Chicago, 1971a.

Fox MW: Introduction: the concepts of normal and abnormal behavior. In: *Abnormal Behavior in Animals,* ed. Fox MW. WB Saunders, Philadelphia: 1-5, 1968c.

Fox MW: Neurobehavioral development and the genotype-environment interaction. *Q Rev Biol* 45:131-147, 1970b.

Fox MW: Neurobehavioral ontogeny: a synthesis of ethological and neurophysiological concepts. *Brain Res* 2:3-20, 1966a.

Fox MW: The ontogeny of behavior and neurologic responses in the dog. *Anim Behav* 12:301-310, 1964a.

Fox MW: Ontogeny of prey-killing in Canidae. *Behav* 35:259-272, 1969c.

Fox MW: Overview and critique of stages and periods in canine development. *Develop Psychobiol* 4:37-54, 1970c.

Fox MW: The postnatal growth of the canine brain and correlated anatomical and behavioral changes during ontogenesis. *Growth* 28:135-141, 1964b.

Fox MW: Psychogenic polyphagia (compulsive eating) in a dog. *Vet Rec* 74:1023-1024, 1962.

Fox MW: Psychopathology in man and lower animals. *JAVMA* 159:66-77, 1971b.

Fox MW: Psychosocial and clinical applications in the critical period hypothesis in the dog. *JAVMA* 146:1117-1119, 1965b.

Fox MW: Reflex development and behavioral organization. In: *Developmental Neurobiology*, ed. Himwich WA. Charles C. Thomas Publishers, Springfield, Ill: 553-580, 1970d.

Fox MW: The social significance of genital licking in the wolf (*Canis lupis*). *J Mammol* 53:637-640, 1972a.

Fox MW: Social behavior in three captive wolf packs. *Behav* 47:296-301, 1973a.

Fox MW: Socio-ecological implications of individual differences in wolf litters: a developmental and evolutionary perspective. *Behav* 41:298-313, 1972b.

Fox MW: Socio-infantile and socio-sexual signals in canids: a comparative and ontogenetic study. *Zeitschrift für Tierpsychologie* 28:185-210, 1971c.

Fox MW: *Understanding Your Dog*. Coward, McCann, and Geoghegan, New York, 1974.

Fox MW, Andrews RV: Physiological and biochemical correlates of individual differences in behavior in wolf cubs. *Behav* 46:129-140, 1973b.

Fox MW, Bekoff M: The behaviour of dogs. In: *The Behaviour of Domestic Animals*, 3rd edition, ed. Hafez ESE. Williams & Wilkins, Baltimore: 370-409, 1975.

Fox MW, Spencer J: Exploratory behavior in the dog: experiential or age dependent? *Develop Psychobiol* 2:68-74, 1969.

Fox MW, Stelzner D: Approach/withdrawal variables in the development of social behavior in the dog. *Anim Behav* 14:362-366, 1966a.

Fox MW, Stelzner D: Behavioral effects of differential early experience in the dog. *Anim Behav* 14:273-281, 1966b.

Fox MW, Stelzner D: The effects of early experience on the development of inter- and intra-species social relationships in the dog. *Anim Behav* 15:377-386, 1967.

Fox MW, Stelzner D: Spontaneous and experimentally induced abnormalities in the dog correlated with early experience and the critical period hypothesis. *Rec Advan Biol Psych* 8:39-49, 1966c.

Fraile IG, McEwen BS, Pfaff DW: Comparative effects of progesterone and alphaxalone on aggressive, reproductive and locomotor behaviors. *Pharm Biochem Behav* 30:729-735, 1988.

Frank DW, Kirton KT, Murchison TE, Quinlon WJ, Coleman ME, Gilbertson TJ, Feenstra ES, Kimball FA: Mammary tumors and serum hormones in the bitch treated with medroxyprogesterone acetate or progesterone for four years. *Fertil Steril* 31:340-346, 1979.

Frank H: Evolution of canine information processing under conditions of natural and artificial selection. *Zeitschrift für Tierpsychologie* 53:389-399, 1980.

Frank H, Frank M: On the effects of domestication on canine social development and behavior. *Appl Anim Ethol* 8:507-525, 1982.

Fraser AF, Broom DM: *Farm Animal Behaviour and Welfare*, 3rd Edition. Bailliére Tindall, London, 1990.

Fraser D: The effect of straw on the behaviour of sows in tether stalls. *Anim Prod* 21:59-68, 1975.

Fraser D: Observations of the behavioural development of suckling and early-weaned piglets during the first six weeks after birth. *Anim Behav* 26:22-30, 1978.

Fraser D, Rushen J: Aggressive behavior. *Vet Clin North Am Food Animal Pract* 3:285-305, 1987.

Fratta W, Mereu G, Chessa P, Paglietti E, Gessa G: Benzodiazepine-induced voraciousness in cats and inhibition of amphetamine-anorexia. *Life Sci* 18:1157-1165, 1976.

Frazer-Sisson DE, Rice DA, Peters G: How cats purr. *J Zool* 223:67-78, 1991.

Freak MJ: Abnormal behavior during pregnancy and parturition in the bitch. In: *Abnormal Behavior in Animals*, ed. Fox MW. WB Saunders, Philadelphia: 464-475, 1968.

Free NK, Winget CN, Whitman RM: Separation anxiety in panic disorder. *Am J Psychiatry* 150:595-599, 1993.

Freedman D: Constitutional and environmental interactions in rearing of four breeds of dogs. *Science* 127:585-586, 1958.

Freedman D: Some effects of early rearing on later obedience in dog. *Nordic Vet Med* 17:111-117, 1965.

Freedman DG, King JA, Elliot O: Critical periods in the social development of dogs. *Science* 133: 1016-1017, 1961.

Friedman E, Thomas SA: Health benefits of pets for families. In: *Pets and the Family*, ed. Sussman MB. Haworth Press, New York: 191-203, 1985.

Fromm GH, Nakata M, Kondo T: Differential action of amitriptyline on neurons in the trigeminal nucleus. *Neurol* 41:1932-1938, 1991.

Fuller J: Cross-sectional and longitudinal studies of adjustive behavior in dogs. *Ann NY Acad Sci* 56:214-224, 1953.

Fuller J: Photoperiodic control of estrus in the Basenji. *J Heredity* 47:179-180, 1956.

Fuller JL: Experiential deprivation and later behavior. *Science* 156:1645-1652, 1967.

Fuller JL: Hereditary differences in trainability of purebred dogs. *J Genetic Psychol* 87:229-238, 1955.

Fuller JL: Individual differences in the reactivity of dogs. *J Compar Physiol Psychol* 41:339-347, 1948.

Fuller JL, Clark LB: Effects of rearing with specific stimuli upon postulation behavior in dogs. *J Compar Physiol Psychol* 61: 258-263, 1966.

Fuller JL, Clark LB: Genotype and behavioral vulnerability to isolation in dogs. *J Compar Physiol Psychol* 66:151-156, 1968.

Gadow KD, Nolan EE, Sverd J, Sprafkin J, Paolicelli L: Methylphenidate in aggressive-hyperactive boys: I. Effects on peer aggression in public school settings. *J Am Acad Child Adolesc Psych* 29(5):710-718, 1990.

Gallo PV, Werboff J, Knox K: Development of home orientation in offspring of protein-restricted cats. *Develop Psychobiol* 17: 437-449, 1984.

Gallo PV, Werboff J, Knox K: Protein restriction during gestation and lactation: development of attachment behavior in cats. *Behav Neural Biol* 29:216, 1980.

Garney MJ, Tollefson GD: Association of affective disorder with migraine headaches and neurodermatitis. *Gen Hosp Psych* 10: 148-149, 1988.

Gartlan JS: Structure and function in primate society. *Folia Primatologica* 8:89-120, 1968.

Gedye A: Episodic rage and aggression attributed to frontal lobe seizures. *J Mental Defic Res* 33(part 5):369-379, 1989a.

Gedye A: Extreme self-injury attributed to frontal lobe seizures. *Am J Mental Retardation* 94:20-26, 1989b.

Geier S, Bancaud J, Talairach J, Bonis A, Szikla G, Enjelvin M: The seizures of frontal lobe epilepsy: a study of clinical manifestations. *Neurology* 27:951-958, 1977.

Genovese L, Summers B, deLahunta A: Behavioral cases with neurological complications. *AVSAB Newsletter* 16(2):2-3, 1994.

Gerber HA, Jochle W, Sulman: Control of reproduction and of

undesirable social and sexual behaviour in dogs and cats. *J Sm Anim Pract* 14:151-158, 1973.

Ghosh B, Choudhuri DK, Pal B: Some aspects of sexual behaviors of stray dogs, *Canis familiaris. Appl Anim Behav Sci* 13: 113-127, 1984.

Giger U, Jezyk PF: Diagnosis of inherited diseases in small animals. In: *Current Veterinary Therapy. XI. Small Animal Practice*, eds. Kirk RW, Bongura JS. WB Saunders, Philadelphia: 18-22, 1992.

Gilbert ME: Neurotoxicants and limbic kindling. In: *Vulnerable Brain and Environmental Risks.* Vol. 1. Malnutrition and Hazard Assessment, eds. Isaacson RL, Jensen KF. Plenum Press, New York: 173-192, 1992.

Ginsburg BE: Genetics as a tool in the study of behavior. *Perspect Biol Med* 1:397-424, 1958.

Giorgi O, Corda MG, Fernandez A, Biggio G: The abstinence syndrome in diazapine-dependant cats is precipitated by R015-1788 and R015-4513 but not by the benzodiazapine receptor antagonist ZK93426. *Neurosci Letters* 88:206-210, 1988.

Gitlin MJ: Lithium-induced renal insufficiency. *J Clin Psychopharm* 13:276-279, 1993.

Gittleman JL: Carnivore group living: comparative trends. In: *Carnivore Behavior, Ecology, and Evolution*, ed. Gittleman JL. Chapman & Hall, London: 183-207, 1989.

Goddard AW, Woods SW, Sholomskas DE, Goodman WK, Charney DS, Heninger GR: Effects of the serotonin reuptake inhibitor fluvoxamine on yohimbine-induced anxiety in panic disorder. *Psychiatry Res* 48:119-133, 1993.

Goddard M, Beilharz R: Early prediction of adult behavior in potential guide dogs. *Appl Anim Behav Sci* 15:247-260, 1986.

Goddard M, Beilharz R: A multivariate analysis of the genetics of fearfulness in potential guidedogs. *Behav Genet* 15:69-89, 1985b.

Goddard ME, Beilharz RG: A breeding program for guide dogs. First World Congress on Genetics Applied to Livestock Production, Madrid, Spain. Editorial Garsi, London and Madrid 3:371-376, 1974.

Goddard ME, Beilharz RG: Genetic and environmental factors effecting the suitability of dogs as guide-dogs for the blind. *Theoret Appl Genet* 62:97-102, 1982.

Goddard ME, Beilharz RG: Genetics of traits which determine the suitability of dogs as guide-dogs for the blind. *Appl Anim Ethol* 9:299-315, 1983.

Goddard ME, Beilharz RG: Individual variation in agonistic behaviour in dogs. *Anim Behav* 33:1338-1342, 1985a.

Golani I: Homeostatic motor processes in mammalian interaction: a choriography of display. In: *Perspectives in Ethology*, eds. Bateson PPG, Klopfer PH. Plenum Press, New York: 69-134, 1976.

Gold MS, Pottash ALC, Extein IL: "Symptomless" auntoimmune thyroiditis in depression. *Psychiatric Res* 6:261-269, 1988.

Goldberger E, Rapaport JL: Canine acral lick dermatitis: Response to anti-obsessional drug clomipramine. *JAAHA* 27:179-182, 1991.

Goldstein M, Kuga S, Kusano N, Meller E, Danxis J, Schwarz R: Dopamine agonist induced self-mutilative biting behaviors in monkeys with unilateral ventromedial tegmental lesions of brainstem, possible pharmacological model for Lesch-Nyhan syndrome. *Brain Res* 367:144120, 1986.

Goosen C: Some causal factors in autogrooming behavior of adult stump-tailed macaques *(Macaca arctoides). Behav* 49: 111-129, 1974.

Gordon F, Jukes MGM: Dual organization of the exteroceptive components of the cat's gracile nucleus. *J Physiol* 139:385-399, 1964.

Gorman JM, Gorman LK: Drug treatment of social phobia. Special issue: drug treatment of anxiety disorders. *J Affective Disorders* 13:183-192, 1987.

Gorman ML, Trowbridge BJ: The role of odor in the social lives of carnivores. In: *Carnivore Behavior, Ecology, and Evolution*, ed. Gittleman JL. Cornell University Press, Ithaca: 57-88, 1989.

Gosling LM: A reassessment of the function of scent-marking in territories. *Zeitschrift für Tierpsychologie* 60:89-199, 1982.

Grady TA, Piggott TA, L'Heureux F, Hill JL, Bernstein SE, Murphy DL: Double-blind study of adjuvant buspirone for fluoxetine-treated patients with obsessive-compulsive disorder. *Am J Psychiatry* 150:819-821, 1993.

Gram LF: Fluoxetine. *N Engl J Med* 331:1354-1361, 1994.

Grandin T, Deesing MJ, Struthers JJ, Swinker AM: Cattle with hair whorl patterns above the eyes are more behaviorally agitated during restraint. *Appl Anim Behav Sci* 46:117-123, 1995.

Gray J: *The Psychology of Fear and Stress.* McGraw-Hill, New York, 1971.

Green JS, Woodruff RA: Breed comparisons and characteristics of use of livestock guarding dogs. *J Range Manag* 41:249-251, 1988.

Green RW, Scott RC: Diseases of the bladder and urethra. In: *Textbook of Veterinary International Medicine: Diseases of the Dog and Cat*, ed. Etinger SJ. WB Saunders, Philadelphia: 1890-1936, 1983.

Green S, Marler P: The analysis of animal communication. In: *Handbook of Behavioral Neurobiology:* Vol. 3, Social Behavior in Communication, eds. Marler P, Vandenbergh JG. Plenum Press, New York: 73-158, 1979.

Greenberg D, Marks I: Behavioural Psychotherapy of uncommon referrals. *Br J Psych* 141:148-153, 1982.

Greenberg HE, Scharf SM, Green H: Nortriptyline-induced depression of ventilatory control in a patient with chronic obstructive pulmonary disease. *Am Rev Respir Dis* 147:1303-1305, 1993.

Greenblatt DJ, Shader RI, Abernethy DR: Drug therapy: current status of benzodiazepines. *N Engl J Med* 309:344-358, 1983.

Greenblatt DJ, Shader RI, Divoll M, Harmatz JS: Benzodiazepines: a summary of pharmacokinetic properties. *Brit J Pharmacol* 11(Suppl.):11S-16S, 1981.

Greene CE, Lockwood R, Goldstein EJC: Bite and scratch infections. In: *Infectious Diseases of the Dog and Cat*, ed. Greene CE. WB Saunders, Philadelphia: 614-620, 1990.

Griffen CE: A practical approach to pruritus. II. *Proc AAHA* 58: 93-99, 1991.

Griffin DR: *Animal Minds.* University of Chicago Press, Chicago, 1992.

Grunhaus L, Harel Y, Krugler T, Pande AC, Haskett RF: Major depressive disorder and panic disorder. *Clin Neuropharmacol* 11:454-461, 1988.

Gupta C, Bullock LP, Barden CW: Further studies on the androgenic, anti-androgenic, and syn-androgenic actions of progestins. *Endocrinol* 102:736-744, 1979.

Gupta MA, Gupta AK, Ellis CN: Anti-depressant drugs in dermatology. *Arch Dermatol* 123:647-655, 1987.

Gurski JC, Davis K, Scott JP: Interactions of separation discomfort with contact comfort and discomfort in the dog. *Develop Psychobiol* 13:463-467, 1980.

Gustavson CR, Garcia J, Hankins WG, Rusiniak KW: Coyote predation control by aversive conditioning. *Science* 184:581-583, 1974.

Guyot GW, Cross HA, Bennett TL: Early social isolation in the domestic cat: Responses during mechanical toy testing. *Appl Anim Ethol* 10:109-116, 1983.

Haefely W, Pieri L, Polc P: General pharmacodynamics neuropharmacology of benzodiazapine derivatives. In: *Psychotropic Agents.* Part II: Anxiolytics, Gerontopsychopharmacological Agents, and Psychomotor Stimulants, eds. Hoffmeister F, Stille G. Springer-Verlag, Berlin: 13-262, 1981.

Hailman JP: *Optical Signals: Animal Communication and Light.* Indiana University Press, Bloomington, 1977.

Halip J: Feline elimination problems. Presentation at AVMA, San Francisco, CA, 1994.

Hall ZW: Laminin β2 (S-Laminin): A new player at the synapse. *Science* 269:362-363, 1995.

Hallgren A: Mother and pups. *ABCN* 7(3)1-2, 1990.

Hallgren A: Spinal anomalies in dogs. *ABCN* 9(3):3-4, 1992.

Halterer JA, Herbert J, Hidaka C, Roose SP, Gorman JM: CSF transthyretin in patients with depression. *Am J Psych* 150:813-815, 1993.

Hamilton JB, Hamilton RS, Mestler GE: Duration of life and causes of death in domestic cats: influences of sex, godanectomy, and in-breeding. *J Gerontol* 24:427-437, 1969.

Hamner CE, Jennings LL, Sojka NJ: Cat *(Felis catus L.)* spermatozoa requires capacitation. *J Repro Fert* 23:477-480, 1970.

Hanno PM, Buehler J, Wein AJ: Use of amitriptyline in the treatment of interstitial cystitis. *J Urol* 141:846-848, 1989.

Hansen BD, Hardie EM: Prescription and use of analgesics in dogs and cats in a veterinary teaching hospital: 258 cases (1983-1989). *JAVMA* 202:1485-1494, 1993.

Harcourt AH: Activity periods and patterns of social interaction: a neglected problem. *Behav* 66:121-135, 1978.

Harding CF: Hormonal influences on avian aggressive behavior. In: *Hormones and Aggressive Behavior*, ed. Svare BB. Plenum Press, New York: 435-467, 1983.

Harless SJ, Turbes CC: Choline-loading: specific dietary supplementation for modifying neurologic and behavioral disorders in dogs and cats. *Vet Med Sm Anim Clinic* 77(8):1223-1230, 1982.

Harlow HF, Harlow MK: Psychopathology in monkeys. In: *Experimental Psychopathology*, ed. Kimmel HD. Academic Press, New York: 203-229, 1971.

Harrington FH, Mech LD: An analysis of howling response parameters useful for wolf packs censusing. *J Wildlife Manag* 46:686-693, 1982.

Harrington FH, Mech LD: Wolf howling and its role in territory maintenance. *Behav* 68:207-249, 1979.

Harris D, Imperato PJ, Oken B: Dog bites—an unrecognized epidemic. *Bull NY Acad Med* 50:981-1000, 1974.

Harro J, Vasar E, Bradwejn J: CCK in animal and human research on anxiety. *Trends Pharmacol Sci* 14:244-249, 1993.

Hart B, Murray S, Hahs M, Cruz B, Miller M: Breed-specific behavioral profiles of dogs: model for quantitative analysis. In: *New Perspectives on Our Lives with Companion Animals*, eds. Katcher A, Beck A. University of Pennsylvania Press, Philadelphia: 47-56, 1983.

Hart BL: Abolition of mating behavior in male cats with lesions in the medial preoptic-anterior hypothalamic region (abstract). *Am Zool* 10:296, 1970a.

Hart BL: Alteration of quantitative aspects of sexual reflexes in spinal male dogs by testosterone. *J Compar Physiol Psychol* 66:726-730, 1968.

Hart BL: The behavior of sick animals. *Vet Clin of North Am: Sm Anim Pract* 21:225-237, 1991.

Hart BL: *The Behavior of Domestic Animals.* W.H. Freeman Company, New York, 1985b.

Hart BL: Behavioral effects of long-acting progestins. *Feline Practice* 4:8-11, 1974a.

Hart BL: Behavioral indications for phenothiazine and benzodiazapine tranquilizers in dogs. *JAVMA* 186(11):1192-1194, 1985c.

Hart BL: Brain disorders and abnormal behavior. *Canine Practice* 4:10-12, 1977.

Hart BL: Breed-specific behavior. *Feline Practice* 9(6):10-13, 1979a.

Hart BL: Castration and urine marking in dogs. *JAVMA* 164:140, 1974b.

Hart BL: Effects of neutering and spaying on the behavior of dogs and cats: questions and answers about practical concerns. *JAVMA* 198:1204-1205, 1981a.

Hart BL: Environmental and hormonal influences on urine marking behavior in the adult male dog. *Behav Biol* 11(2):167-176, 1974c.

Hart BL: *Feline Behavior.* A Practitioner Monograph. Veterinary Practice Publishing, Santa Barbara, Calif, 1980.

Hart BL: Flehmen behaviour and vomeronasal organ function. In: *Chemical Signals in Vertebrates* 3, eds. Muller-Schwartze D, Silverstein RM. Plenum Press, New York: 87-103, 1983.

Hart BL: Gonadal androgen and sociosexual behavior of male mammals: a comparative analysis (review). *Psychol Bull* 81(7):383-400, 1974.

Hart BL: Inappropriate urination and defecation. *Feline Practice* 6:6-7, 1976.

Hart BL: Indications for progestin therapy for behavior problems in dogs. *Canine Practice* 6:10-14, 1979b.

Hart BL: Mating behavior in the female dog and the effects of estrogen on sexual reflexes. *Hormones and Behavior* 2:93-104, 1970b.

Hart BL: Medial preoptic-anterior hypothalamic area and socio-sexual behavior of male dogs: a comparative neuropsychological analysis. *J Compar Physiol Psychol* 86:328-349, 1974e.

Hart BL: Neurosurgery for behavioral problems: a curiosity or the new wave? *Vet Clin North Am: Sm Anim Pract* 12(4):707-714, 1982.

Hart BL: Normal behavior and behavioral problems associated with sexual function, urination, and defecation. *Vet Clin North Am: Sm Anim Prac* 4:589-606, 1974f.

Hart BL: Objectionable urine spraying and urine marking in the cat: evaluation of progestin treatment in godanectomized males and females. *JAVMA* 177:529-533, 1980a.

Hart BL: Olfactory tractotomy for control of objectionable urine spraying and urine marking in cats. *JAVMA* 179:231-234, 1981b.

Hart BL: Physiology of sexual function. *Vet Clin North Am: Sm Anim Pract* 4:557-571, 1974g.

Hart BL: Problems with objectionable sociosexual behavior of dogs and cats: therapeutic use of castration and progestins. *Comp Contin Edu Pract Vet* 1:461-465, 1979c.

Hart BL: Progestin therapy for aggressive behavior in male dogs. *JAVMA* 178(10):1070-1071, 1981c.

Hart BL: Role of prior experience in the effects of castration on sexual behavior of male dogs. *J Compar Physiol Psychol* 66:719-725, 1968.

Hart BL: Spraying behavior. *Feline Pract* 5:11-13, 1975.

Hart BL: Starting from scratch: a new perspective on cat scratching. *Feline Pract* 10(4):8-12, 1980b.

Hart BL: Successive approximation: the key to behavioral therapy. *Canine Pract* 5(5):8-14, 1978a.

Hart BL: Three disturbing behavioral disorders in dogs: idiopathic viciousness, hyperkinesis and flank sucking. *Canine Pract* 6:10-14, 1977.

Hart BL: Water sprayer therapy. *Feline Pract* 8:13-16, 1978b.

Hart BL, Barrett RE: Effects of castration on fighting, roaming and urine-spraying in adult male cats. *JAVMA* 163:290-292, 1973.

Hart BL, Cooper LC: Factors relating to urine-spraying and fighting in pre-pubertally gonadectomized cats. *JAVMA* 184:1255-1258, 1984.

Hart BL, Eckstein RA, Powell KL, Dodman NH: Effectiveness of buspirone on urine spraying and inappropriate urination in cats. *JAVMA* 203:254-258, 1993.

Hart BL, Hart LA: *Canine and Feline Behavioral Therapy.* Lea & Febiger, Philadelphia: 1985a.

Hart BL, Hart LA: Selecting pet dogs on the basis of cluster analysis of breed behavioral profiles and gender. *JAVMA* 186(11):1181-1185, 1985b.

Hart BL, Hart LA: Selecting the best companion animal: breed and gender specific behavioral profiles. In: *The Pet Connection: Its Influence on Our Health and Quality of Life*, eds. Anderson RK, Hart BL, Hart LA. University of Minnesota Press, Minneapolis: 180-193, 1984.

Hart BL, Haugen CM: Scent-marking and sexual behavior maintained in anosmic male dogs. *Communic Behav Biol* 6:131-135, 1971.

Hart BL, Haugen CM, Peterson DM: Effects of the medial preoptic-anterior hypothalamic lesions on mating behavior of male cats. *Brain Res* 54:177-191, 1973.

Hart BL, Leedy M: Identification of source of urine stains in multi-cat households. *JAVMA* 180:77-78, 1982.

Hart BL, Leedy MG: Analysis of the catnip reaction: mediation by olfactory system, not vomeronasal organ. *Behav Neurol Biol* 44:38-46, 1985.

Hart BL, Leedy MG: Female sexual response in male cats facilitated by olfactory bulbectomy and medial preoptic anterior hypothalamic lesion. *Behav Neurosci* 97:608-614, 1983.

Hart BL, Leedy MG: Stimulus and hormonal determinants of Flehmen behaviour in cats. *Hormones Behav* 21:44-52, 1987.

Hart BL, Melese-D'Hospital PY: Penile mechanisms and the role of the striated penile muscles in penile reflexes. *Physiol Behav* 31:807-813, 1983.

Hart BL, Miller MF: Behavioral profiles of dog breeds: a quantitative approach. *JAVMA* 186(11):1175-1180, 1985.

Hart BL, Voith VL: Changes in urine spraying, feeding and sleep behavior of cats following medial preoptic-anterior hypothalamic lesions. *Brain Res* 145:406-409, 1978.

Haskins R: A causal analysis of kitten vocalization: an observational and experimental study. *Anim Behav* 27:726-736, 1979.

Hatch RC: Effect on drugs on catnip-induced *(Nepeta cataria)* pleasure behavior in cats. *Am J Vet Res* 33:143-155, 1972.

Hauptman JG, Komtebedde J: Evaluation of surgical technique, ischiocavernosusmyectomy, for the treatment of chronic urine-spraying in the castrated male cat. *Vet Surg* 8(1):83-84, 1989.

Head E, Milgram NW: Changes in spontaneous behavior in the dog following oral administration of L-deprenyl. *Pharmacol Biochem Behav* 43:749-757, 1992.

Hellings JA, Warnock JK: Self-injurious behavior and serotonin in Praeder-Willi syndrome. *Psychopharmacol Bull* 30:245-250, 1994.

Hemmer H: Gestation period and postnatal development in felids. *Carnivore* 2:90-100, 1979.

Hendricks JC, Hughes C: Treatment of cataplexy in a dog with narcolepsy. *JAVMA* 194(6):791-792, 1989.

Hendricks JC, Lager A, O'Brien D, Morrison AR: Movement disorders during sleep in cats and dogs. *JAVMA* 194(5):686-689, 1989.

Hendricks JC, Morrison AR: Normal and abnormal sleep in mammals. *JAVMA* 178:121-126, 1981.

Hendricks JC, Morrison AR, Farnbach GL, Steinberg SA, Mann G: A disorder of rapid eye movement sleep in a cat. *JAVMA* 178:55-57, 1981.

Henik RA, Olsen PN, Rosychule RAW: Progestagen therapy in cats. *Compend Contin Edu Pract Vet* 7(2):132-142, 1985.

Henry JP: Biological basis of the stress response. *NIPS* 8:69-73, 1993.

Herman BH, Hammock MK, Egan K, Arthur-Smith A, Chatoor I, Werner A: Role for opioid peptide in self-injurious behavior dissociation from autonomic nervous system function. *Dev Pharmacol Ther* 12:81-89, 1989.

Hernandez FJ, Fernandez BB, Chertack M, Gage P: Feline mammary gland carcinoma and progestagens. *Feline Pract* 5(5):45-48, 1975.

Hess EH: *Imprinting: Early Experience and the Developmental Psychobiology of Attachment.* Von Nostrand Reinhold, New York, 1973.

Hinde RA: *Animal Behaviour.* 2nd Edition. McGraw-Hill, New York: 1970.

Hinde RA: The biological significance of territories in birds. *The Ibis* 98:340-369, 1956.

Hinde RA: The nature of aggression. *New Society* 9:302-304, 1967.

Hird DW, Ruble RP, Reager SG, Cronkhite PK, Johnson MW: Morbidity and mortality in pups from pet stores and private sources: 968 cases (1987-1988). *JAVMA* 201:471-474, 1992.

Hirsch B, Dubose C, Jacobs HL: Dietary control of food intake in cats. *Physiol Behav* 20:287-295, 1978.

Hoehn-Saric R, McLeod DR, Glowa JR: The effects of NMDA receptor blockade on the acquisition of a conditioned emotional response. *Biol Psych* 30:170-176, 1991.

Holland CT: Successful long term treatment of a dog with psychomotor seizures using carbamazepine. *Austral Vet J* 65:389-392, 1988.

Hölldobler B: Recruitment behavior in *Camponotus socius* (Hym: Formicidae). *Zeitschrift Verglichende Physiologie* 75:123-142, 1971.

Holliday TA: Clinical aspects of some encephalopathies of domestic cats. *Vet Clin of North Am: Sm Anim Pract* 1:367-368, 1971.

Holliday TA, Cunningham JG, Gutnick MJ: Comparative clinical and electroencephalographic studies of canine epilepsy. *Epilepsia* 11(3):281-292, 1970.

Holt PE, Gibbs C: Congenital urinary incontinence in cats: a review of 19 cases. *Vet Rec* 130(20):437-442, 1992.

Hopkins SG, Schubert TA, Hart BL: Castration of adult male dogs: effects on roaming, aggression, urine spraying, and mounting. *JAVMA* 168:1108-1110, 1976.

Hothersall D, Tuber DS: Fears in companion dogs: characteristics and treatment. In: *Psychopathology in Animals*, ed. Keehn JD. Academic Press, New York: 239-255, 1979.

Houpt KA: Abnormal behavior. *Vet Clin North Am: Lg Anim Pract* 3:357-367, 1987.

Houpt KA: Aggression in dogs. *Compend Contin Edu Sm Anim Pract* 3:123-128, 1979.

Houpt KA: Animal behavior and animal welfare. *JAVMA* 198:1355-1360, 1991a.

Houpt KA: Companion animal behavior: a review of dog and cat behavior in the field, the laboratory, and the clinic. *Cornell Vet* 75:248-261, 1985.

Houpt KA: *Domestic Animal Behavior for Veterinarians and Animal Scientists,* 2nd edition. Iowa State University Press, Ames, Iowa, 1991b.

Houpt KA: Ingestive behavior problems of dogs and cats. *Vet Clin North Am: Sm Anim Pract* 12(4):683-692, 1982.

Houpt KA, Coren B, Hintz HF, Hilderbrant JE: Effect of sex and reproductive status on sucrose preference, food intake, and body weight of dogs. *JAVMA* 174:1083-1085, 1979.

Houpt KA, Hintz HF, Shepherd P: The role of olfaction in canine food preferences. *Chemical Senses of Flavour* 3:281-290, 1978.

Houpt KA, Reisner IR: Behavioral disorders. In: *Textbook of Veterinary Internal Medicine,* 4th Ed, eds Ettinger SJ, Feldman EC. WB Saunders, Philadelphia: 179-187, 1995.

Houpt KA, Wolski TR: *Domestic animal behavior for veterinarians and small animal scientists.* Iowa State University Press, Ames: 1982.

Hubrecht RC: Enrichment in puppyhood and its effects on later behavior in dogs. *Lab Anim Sci* 45:70-75, 1995.

Hubrecht RC, Serpell JA, Poole TB: Correlates of pen size and housing conditions on the behaviour of kennelled dogs. *Appl Anim Behav Sci* 34:365-383, 1992.

Huey RB, Dunham AE: Repeatability of locomotor performance in a natural population of the lizard *Sceloporus merriami. Evolution* 41:1116-1120, 1987.

Hughes D, Moreau RE, Overall KL, van Winkle TJ: Acute hepatic necrosis and liver failure associated with benzodiazepine therapy in cats. *JVECC* 6(1):13-20, 1996.

Hughes H, Boden P, Costall B, Domeney A, Kelly E, Horwell DC, Hunter JC, Pinnock RD, Wooduff GN: Development of a class of selective cholecystokinin type B receptor antagonists having potent anxiolytic activity. *Proc Nat Acad Sci USA* 87:6728-6732, 1990.

Hughes KL, Faragher JT: Cat scratch disease (review). *Austral Vet J* 71(8):266, 1994.

Humphrey ES, Warner L: *Working Dogs: An Attempt to Produce a Strain of German Shepherds Which Combine Working Abilities with Beauty of Confirmation.* Johns Hopkins Press, Baltimore, 1934.

Hurni H, Rossbach W: The laboratory cat. In: *The U.F.A.W. Handbook on the Care and Management of Laboratory Animals,* 6th edition, ed. Pool TB. Longman Scientific and Technical, Harlow: 676-692, 1987.

Hutchinson R, Renfrew J: Stalking attack and eating behavior elicited from the same sites in the hypothalamus. *J Compar Psychol Physiol* 61:360-367,1966.

Iggo A: Cutaneous receptors with a high sensitivity to mechanical displacement. In: *Touch, Heat, and Pain,* eds. de Reuck AVS, Knight J. CIBA Foundation, London: 237-256, 1966.

Iggo A: Cutaneous sensory mechanisms. In: *The Senses,* eds. Barlow HB, Mollon JD. Cambridge University Press, Cambridge: 369-408, 1982.

Ihrke PJ: Diseases in dermatology. Proceedings of the 1995 Penn Annual Conference.

Immelmann K, Beer C: *A Dictionary of Ethology.* Harvard University Press, Cambridge, Massachusetts, 1989.

Impekoven M: Responses of laughing gull chicks *(Larus atricilla)* to parental attraction and alarm-calls, and effects of prenatal auditory experience on the responsiveness to such calls. *Behav* 56:250-278, 1976.

Insel TR: New pharmacologic approaches to obsessive-compulsive disorder. *J Clin Psych* 51(10)(Suppl)):47-51, 1990.

Insel TR: Toward a neuroanatomy of obsessive-compulsive disorder. *Arch Gen Psych* 49:739-744, 1992.

Insel TR, Donnelly EF, Lalakea ML, Alterman IS, Murphy DL: Neuroanatomical and neuropsychological studies of patients with obsessive-compulsive disorder. *Biol Psych* 19:741-751, 1983.

Inselman-Temkin BR, Flynn JP: Sex-dependent effects of gonadal and gonadotropic hormones on centrally elicited attack in cats. *Brain Res* 60:393-409, 1973.

Izawa M, Doi T, Ono Y: Grouping patterns of feral cats *(Felis catus)* living on a small island in Japan. *Japan J Ecol* 32:373-382, 1982.

Jackson LA, Perkins BA, Wenger JD: Cat-scratch disease in the United States. *Am J Public Health* 83(12):1707-1711, 1993.

Jacobs BL, Wilkinson LO, Fornal CA: The role of brain serotonin: a neurophysiologic perspective. *Neuropsychopharmacol* 3:473-479, 1988.

Jaeken J, Casaer P, Haegele KD, Schlechter PJ: Review: normal and abnormal central nervous system gaba metabolism in childhood. *J Inherited Metab Dis* 13:793-801, 1990.

Jaggy A, Oliver JE, Ferguson DC, Mahaffey EA, Glaus jin T: Neurological manifestations of hypothyroidism: a retrospective study of 29 dogs. *J Vet Intern Medicine* 8:328-336, 1994.

Jagoe A, Serpell J: Owner characteristics and interactions and the prevalence of canine behaviour problems. *Appl Anim Behav Sci,* in press, 1996.

James W: Dominant and submissive behavior in puppies as indicated by food intake. *J Genetic Psychol* 75:33-43, 1949.

James W: Observation of behavior of new-born puppies: method of measurement and types of behavior involved. *J Genetic Psychol* 80:65-73, 1952.

James WT: Social organization among dogs of different temperaments, terrier and beagles reared together. *J Compar Physiol Psychol* 44:71-77, 1951.

Jann M, Kurtz N: Treatment of panic and phobic disorders. *Clin Pharm* 6:947-962, 1987.

Janowitz HD, Grossman MI: Effect of variations in nutritive density on intake of food of dogs and rats. *Am J Physiol* 158:184-193, 1949.

Jenike MA, Baer L: Buspirone augmentation of fluoxetine in patients with obsessive-compulsive disorder. *J Clin Psych* 52(1):13-14, 1991.

Jenike MA, Baer L: An open trial of buspirone in obsessive-compulsive disorder. *Am J Psych* 145(10):1285-1286, 1988.

Jenkins SC, Maruta T: Therapeutic use of propranolol for intermittent explosive disorders (review). *Mayo Clin Proc* 62(3):204-214, 1987.

Jensen RA, Davis JL, Shnerson A: Early experience facilitates the development of temperature regulation in the cat. *Devel Psychobiol* 13:1-16, 1980.

John E, Chesler T, Barrett F, Victor I: Observational learning in cats. *Science* 159:1489-1491, 1968.

Johnston SD: Questions and answers on the effects of surgically neutering dogs and cats. *JAVMA,* 198(7):1206-1214, 1991.

Jones BA, Beck AM: Unreported dog bite and attitudes towards dogs. In: *The Pet Connection: Its Influence on Our Health and Quality of Life,* eds. Anderson RK, Hart BL, Hart LA. University of Minnesota Press, Minneapolis: 355-363, 1984.

Jones E, Coman BJ: Ecology of the feral cat *(Felis catus L.)* in South-Eastern Australia. III. Home ranges and population ecology in semi-arid North West Victoria. *Austral Wildlife Res* 9:409-420, 1982.

Jones RD: Use of thoridazine in the treatment of aberrant motor behavior in a dog. *JAVMA* 191:89-90, 1987.

Joshua JO: Responsible pet ownership. In: *Pet Animals and Society,* ed. Anderson RS. Balliére Tindall, London: 129-138, 1975.

Kahler S: Spaying/neutering comes of age. *JAVMA* 203:591-593, 1993.

Kahn RS, van Praag HM, Wetzler S, Asnis GM, Barr G: Serotonin and anxiety revisited (review). *Biol Psych* 23:189-198, 1988.

Kalin NH: The neurobiology of fear. *Sci Am* 268(5):94-101, 1993.

Kalmus H: The discrimination by the nose of the dog of the individual human odours and in particular the odours of twins. *Brit J Anim Behav* 3:25-31, 1955.

Kanarek RB: Availability and caloric density of the diet as determinants of meal pattern in cats. *Physiol Behav* 15:611-618, 1975.

Kanno Y: Experimental studies on body temperature rhythm in dogs. I. Application of cosinor method to body temperature rhythm in dogs. *Japan J Vet Sci* 39:69-76, 1977.

Kaplan HI, Sadock BJ: *Pocket Handbook of Psychiatric Drug Treatment.* Williams & Wilkins, Baltimore, 1993.

Kaplan JR, Manuck SB: The effect of propranolol on behavioral interactions among adult male cynomolgus monkeys *(Macaca fascicularis)* housed in disrupted social groupings. *Psychosom Med* 51:449-462, 1989.

Karsh EB: The effects of early handling on the development of social bonds between cats and people. In: *New Perspectives on our Lives with Companion Animals,* eds. Katcher AH, Beck AM. University of Pennsylvania Press, Philadelphia: 22-28, 1983.

Karsh EB: Factors influencing the socialization of cats to people. In: *The Pet Connection: its Influence on our Health and Quality of Life,* eds. Anderson RK, Hart BL, Hart LA. University of Minnesota Press, Minneapolis: 207-215, 1984.

Karsh EB, Turner DC: The human-cat relationship. In: *The Domestic Cat: The Biology of Its Behavior,* eds. Turner DC, Bateson P. Cambridge University Press, Cambridge: 159-177, 1988.

Katz RJ, Thomas E: Effects of para-chlorophenylalanine upon brain stimulated affective attack in the cat. *Pharmacol Biochem Behav* 5:391-394, 1976.

Kaufmann JH: Social relations of adult males in a free-ranging band of rhesus monkeys. In: *Social Communication Among Primates,* ed. Altman SA. University of Chicago Press, Chicago: 73-78, 1967.

Kerby G, Macdonald DW: Cats, society and the consequences of colony size. In: *The Domestic Cat: The Biology of Its Behaviour,* eds. Turner DC, Bateson P. Cambridge University Press, Cambridge: 67-81, 1988.

Kiley-Worthington M: Animal language? Vocal communication of some ungulates, canids, and felids. *Acta Zoologica Fennica* 171:83-88, 1984.

Kiley-Worthington M: *Behavioural problems of farm animals.* Oriel Press, Stockfield, England, 1977.

Kiley-Worthington M: The tail movements of ungulates, canids, and felids with particular reference to their causation and function as displays. *Behaviour* 56:69-115, 1976.

King JE, Becker RF, Markel JE: Studies on olfactory discrimination in dogs. III. Ability to detect human odour trace. *Anim Behav* 12:311-315, 1964.

Kiriike N, Izumiya Y, Nishiwaki S, Maeda Y, Nagata T, Kawakita Y: TRH test and DST in schizoaffective mania, mania, and schizophrenia. *Biol Psychiatry* 24:415-422, 1988.

Kitani K, Kanai S, Sato Y, Ohta M, Ivy GO, Carrillo MC: Chronic treatment of l-deprenyl prolongs the lifespan of male Fischer 344 rats. Further evidence. *Life Sci* 52:281-288, 1992.

Kizer KW: Epidemiologic and clinical aspects of animal bite injuries. *JACEP* 8(4):134-141, 1979.

Kleiman D: Scent marking in the canidae. *Symposium Zoological Society of London* 18:167-177, 1966.

Kleiman DG, Eisenberg JF: Comparisons of canid and felid social system from an evolutionary perspective. *Anim Behav* 21:637-659, 1973.

Klein E, Steinberg SA, Weiss SRB, Matthews DM, Uhde TW: The relationship between genetic deafness and fear-related behaviors in nervous pointer dogs. *Physiol Behav* 43:307-312, 1988.

Kling A, Kovach JK, Tucker TJ: The behavior of cats. In: *The Behaviour of Domestic Animals,* 2nd Edition, ed. Hafez ESE. William & Wilkins, Baltimore: 482-512, 1969.

Kling A, Orbach J, Schwartz NB, Towne JC: Injury to the limbic system and associated structures in cats. *Arch Gen Psychiatry* 3:391-420, 1960.

Klinghammer E, Goodman PA: Socialization and management of wolves in captivity. In: *Man and Wolf. Advances, Issues, and Problems in Captive Wolf Research,* ed. Frank H. DW Junk Publishers, Dordrecht: 31-59, 1987.

Knecht CD, Oliver JE, Redding K, Selcer R, Johnson G: Narcolepsy in a dog and a cat. *JAVMA* 162:1052-1053, 1973.

Knol BW, Egberink-Alink ST: Androgens, progestagens and agonistic behavior: A review. *Vet Q* 11:94-101, 1989a.

Knol W, Egberink-Alink ST: Treatment of problem behaviour in dogs and cats by castration and progestagen administration: A review. *Vet Q* 11(2):102-107, 1989b.

Knoll J, Dallo J, Yen TT: Striatal dopamine, sexual activity, and lifespan. Longevity of rats treated with l-deprenyl. *Life Sci* 45:525-531, 1989.

Ko GN, Elsworth JD, Roth RH, Rifkin BG, Leigh H, Redmond DE Jr: Panic-induced elevation of plasma MHPG levels in phobic anxious patients. *Arch Gen Psychiat* 40:425-430, 1983.

Koehler JE, Glaser CA, Tappero JW: *Rochalimaea henselae* infection. A new zoonosis with the domestic cat as reservoir. *JAMA* 271(7):531-535, 1994.

Koehler W: *The Koehler Method of Dog Training.* Hall Book House, New York, 1962.

Kolata RJ, Kraut NH, Johnson DE: Patterns of trauma in urban dogs and cats: a study of 1,000 cases. *JAVMA* 164:499-502, 1974.

Kolb B, Nonneman AJ: The development of social responsiveness in kittens. *Anim Behav* 23:368-374, 1975.

Komtebedde J, Hauptman J: Bilateral ischiocavernosus myectomy for chronic urine spraying in castrated male cats. *Vet Surg* 19:293-296, 1990.

Konrad KW, Bagshaw M: Effects of novel stimuli on cats reared in a restricted environment. *J Compar Physiol Psychol* 70:157-164, 1970.

Koolhaas JM, van der Brink THC, Roozendaal B, Boorsma F: Medial amygdala and aggressive behavior: interaction between testosterone and vasopressin. *Aggressive Behav* 16(3-4):223-229, 1990.

Koroffsky P: Identifying source of urine on rugs. *JAVMA* 191:917, 1987.

Kovach JK, Kling A: Mechanisms of neonate sucking behavior in the kitten. *Anim Behav* 15:91-101, 1967.

Krawiec D: Diagnosis and treatment of acquired canine urinary incontinence. *Companion Anim Pract* 19:12-20, 1989.

Krebs JR, Davies NB: *Behavioral Ecology: An Evolutionary Approach.* Third Edition. Blackwell Scientific, Cambridge, Ma, 1991.

Kremer HC: One-zero sampling in the study of primate behaviour. *Primates* 20:237-244, 1979.

Kretchmer KR, Fox MW: Effects of domestication on animal behaviour. *Vet Record* 96:102-108, 1975.

Kübler-Ross E: *On death and dying.* Macmillan, New York, 1969.

Kuhn G, Hardegg W: Effects of indoor and outdoor maintenance of dogs upon food intake, body weight and different blood parameters. *Zeitschrift für Tierpsychologie* 31:205-214, 1988.

Kuo ZY: The genesis of the cat's response to the rat. *J Comparative Psychol* 11:1-35, 1930.

Kuo ZY: Studies on the basic factors in animal fighting: VII. Inter-species co-existence in mammals. *J Genetic Psychol* 97:211-225, 1960.

Kuwabara N, Seki K, Aoki K: Circadian, sleep, and brain temperature rhythms in cats under sustained daily light-dark cycles and constant darkness. *Physiol Behavior* 38:283-289, 1986.

Kwochka KW, Short BG: Cutaneous xanthomatosis and diabetes mellitus following long-term therapy with megesterol acetate in a cat. *Compendium of Continuing Education for the Practicing Veterinarian* 6:185-192, 1984.

Landau HG: On dominance relations and the structure of animal societies: I. Effects of inherent characteristics. *Bull Math Biophys* 13:1-19, 1951.

Landsberg G: Products for preventing or controlling undesirable behavior. *Vet Med* October 970-983, 1994.

Landsberg GM: Cat owners' attitudes toward declawing. *Antrozoos* IV:192-197, 1990b.

Landsberg GM: The distribution of canine behavior cases at three behavior referral practices. *Vet Med* 86:1081-1089, 1991a.

Landsberg GM: Feline scratching and destruction and the effects of declawing. *Vet Clin North Am: Sm Anim Pract* 21:265-279, 1991b.

Lapras M: Proceedings of the Sixth World Congress, World Small Animal Veterinary Association. *Post Academisch Obderwijs Publikatie* 8(8):129-130, 1977.

Laundré J: The daytime behavior of domestic cats in a free-roaming population. *Anim Behav* 25:990-998, 1977.

Lawler DF, Sjolin DW, Collins JE: Incidence rates of feline lower urinary tract disease in the United States. *Feline Pract* 15(5):13-16, 1985.

Le Boeuf BJ: Copulatory and aggressive behavior in the prepubertally castrated dog. *Horm Behav* 1:127-136, 1970.

Le Boeuf BJ: Interindividual associations in dogs. *Behavior* 29:268-295, 1967.

Levine AS, Sievert CE, Morley JE, Gosnell BA, Silvis SE: Peptidergic regulation of feeding in the dog (*Canis familiaris*). *Peptides* 5:675-679, 1984.

Levinson P, Flynn J: The objects attacked by cats during stimulation of the hypothalamus. *Anim Behav* 13:217-220, 1965.

Levis DJ: Implementing the technique of implosive therapy. In: *Handbook of Behavior Intervention: A Clinical Guide*, eds. Foa EB, Goldstein AJ. John Wiley & Sons, New York: 92-151, 1980.

Leyhausen P: *Cat Behavior: the Predatory and Social Behavior of Domestic and Wild Cats.* Garland STPM Press, New York, 1979.

Leyhausen P: The communal organization of solitary mammals. *Symposium of the Zoological Society of London* 14:249-263, 1965.

Liberg O: Courtship behaviour and sexual selection in the domestic cat. *Appl Anim Ethol* 10:117-132, 1983.

Liberg O: Home, range, and territoriality in free-ranging house cats. *Acta Zoologica Fennica* 171:283-285, 1984a.

Liberg O: Social behaviour in free-ranging domestic and feral cats. In: *Nutrition and Behaviour in Dogs and Cats*, 2nd Edition, ed. Anderson RS. Pergamon Press, New York: 175-181, 1984b.

Liberg O: Spacing patterns in a population of rural free-roaming domestic cats. *Oikos* 35:336-349, 1980.

Liberg O, Sandell M: Spacial organisation and reproductive tactics in the domestic cat and other felids. In: *The Domestic Cat: The Biology of Its Behavior*, eds. Turner DC, Bateson P. Cambridge University Press, Cambridge: 83-98, 1988.

Liberman LL: A case for neutering pups and kittens at two months of age. *JAVMA* 191:518-521, 1987.

Line S, Voith VL: Dominance aggression of dogs towards people: behavior profile and response to treatment. *Appl Anim Behav Sci* 16(1):77-83, 1986.

Linnoila MI, Virkkunen M: Aggression, suicidality, and serotonin. *J Clin Psychiat* 53(10, Suppl.):46-51, 1992.

Linscheid TR, Pejeau C, Cohen S, Footo-Lenz M: Positive side effects in the treatment of SIB using the self-injurious behavior inhibiting system (SIBIS): Implications for operant and biochemical explanations of SIB. *Res Devel Disabil* 15(1):81-90, 1994.

Lockwood R: Dominance in wolves: useful construct or bad habit. In: *The Behavior and Ecology of Wolves*, ed. Klinghammer E. Garland STPM, New York: 225-244, 1979.

Lockwood R, Rindy K: Are "pit bulls" different? An analysis of the pit bull terrier controversy. *Anthrozoös* 1(1):2-8, 1987.

Loosen PT, Prange AJ Jr: Serum thyrotropin response to thyrotropin-releasing hormone in psychiatric patients: a review. *Am J Psychiatry* 139:405-416, 1982.

Lorenz K: The companion in the bird's world. *Auk* 54:245-273, 1937.

Lorenz K: *Man Meets Dog.* Translated by Wilson MK. Methuen, London, 1954.

Lorenz K: *On Aggression.* Harcourt, Brace & World, New York, 1966.

Love R, Eisenberg F: Avoidance reactions of domestic dogs to unfamiliar male and female humans in a kennel setting. *Appl Anim Behav Sci* 15:261-266, 1986.

Lucey JV, Butcher G, Clare AW, Dinan TG: Buspirone-induced prolactin responses in obsessive-compulsive disorder (OCD): Is OCD a 5-HT$_2$ receptor disorder? *Int Clin Psychopharmacol* 7:45-49, 1992.

Luescher UA, McKeown DB, Halip J: Stereotypic or obsessive-compulsive disorders in dogs and cats. *Vet Clin North Am: Sm Anim Pract.* Advances in Companion Animal Behavior 21(2):401-413, 1991.

Luiten PGM, Koolhaas JM, de Boer S, Koopmans SJ: The cortical-medial amygdala in the central nervous system organization of agonistic behavior. *Brain Res* 332:283-297, 1985.

Lulich JP, Osborne CA, Bartges JW, Polzin DJ: Canine lower urinary tract disorders. In: *Textbook of Veterinary Internal Medicine*, eds. Ettinger SJ, Feldman EC. WB Saunders, Philadelphia: 1833-1863, 1995.

Luxenberg JS, Swedo SE, Flament MF, Friedland R, Rapoport J, Rapoport S: Neuroanatomical abnormalities in obsessive-compulsive disorder detected with quantitative X-ray computed tomography. *Am J Psychiatry* 145:1089-1093, 1988.

Macdonald DW: The ecology of carnivore social behaviour. *Nature* 301:379-389, 1983.

Macdonald DW, Apps PJ: The social behavior of a group of semi-dependent farm cats, *Felis catus*: a progress report. *Carnivore Genetics Newsletter* 3:256-268, 1978.

Macdonald DW, Apps PJ, Carr GM, Kerby G: Social dynamics, nursing coalitions, and infanticide among farm cats, *Felis catus. Advances in Ethology* (Supplement to *Ethology*) 28:1-64, 1987.

MacDonald ML, Rogers QR, Morris JG: Aversion of the cat to dietary medium-chain triglycerides and caprylic acid. *Physiol Behav* 35:371-375, 1985.

MacDonald ML, Rogers QR, Morris JG: Nutrition of the domestic cat, a mammalian carnivore. *Ann Rev Nutr* 4:521-562, 1984.

MacKenzie SA, Oltenacu E, Houpt KA: Canine behavioral genetics—A review. *Appl Anim Behav Sci* 15:365-393, 1986.

MacKenzie SA, Oltenacu EAB, Leighton E: Heritability estimates for temperament scores in German shepherd dogs and its genetic correlate with hip dysplasia. *Behav Genetics* 15:475-482, 1985.

Maes J: Neuromechanisms of sexual behavior in the female cat. *Nature* 144:598-599, 1939.

Manning AM, Rowan AN: Companion animal demographics and sterilization status: results from a survey of four Massachusetts towns. *Anthrozöos* V(3):192-201, 1992.

Männistö PT, Peuranen E, Harro J, Vasar E: Possible role of cholecystokinin-A receptors in regulation of thyrotropin (TSH) secretion in male rats. *Neuropeptides* 23:251-258, 1992.

Manteca X: Animal behavior case of the month. *JAVMA* 206:317-318, 1995.

Marchlewski MT: Genetics studies on the domestic dog. *Bulletin of the International Academy of Political Science Letters, Clinical Science, Mathematics, Nat. Series* B:117-145, 1930.

Marder AR: Problems related to diet. *ABCN* 9(4):1-2, 1992.

Marder AR: Psychotropic drugs and behavior therapy. *Vet Clin North Am: Sm Anim Pract* 21:329-342, 1991.

Marder AR, Marder LR: Human-companion animal relationships and animal behavior problems. *Vet Clin North Am: Sm Anim Pract* 15:411-421, 1985.

Markl H: Manipulation, modulation, information, cognition: some of the riddles of communication. In: *Experimental Behavioral Ecology and Sociobiology*, eds. Hölldobler B, Lindaur M. Sinauer, Sunderlin, Massachusetts: 163-194, 1985.

Marks IM: The classification of phobic disorders. *Br J Psychiatry* 116:377-386, 1970.

Marks IM, Gelder MG: Different ages of onset in varieties of phobia. *Am J Psychiatry* 123:218-221, 1966.

Markwell PJ, Thorne CJ: Early behavioral development of dogs. *Can Pract* 12:32-34, 1985.

Marler P, Hamilton WJ III: *Mechanisms of Animal Behavior.* John Wiley & Sons, New York, 1966.

Mårtensson E, Axelsson R, Nyberg G, Svensson C: Pharmacokinetic properties of the antidepressant drugs amitriptyline, clomipramine, and imipramine: a clinical study. *Curr Ther Res* 36:228-238, 1984.

Martin P: The 4 whys and wherefores of play in cats: a review of functional, evolutionary, developmental, and causal issues. In: *Play in Animals and Humans*, ed. Smith PK. Basil Blackwell, Oxford: 71-94, 1984.

Martin P, Bateson P: Behavioral development in the cat. In: *The Domestic Cat: The Biology of its Behaviour*, eds. Turner DC, Bateson P. Cambridge University Press, Cambridge: 9-22, 1988.

Martin P, Bateson P: The ontogeny of locomotor play behaviour in the domestic kitten. *Anim Behav* 33:502-510, 1985.

Martin WR, Eades CG, Thompson WO, Thompson JA, Flanary HG: Morphine physical dependence in the dog. *J Pharmacol Exp Ther* 189:759-771, 1974.

Mason E: Obesity in pet dogs. *Vet Record* 86:612-616, 1970.

Mason GJ: Stereotypies: a critical review. *Anim Behav* 41:1015-1037, 1991.

Masserman JH, Siever DW: Dominance, neurosis, and aggression: an experimental study. *Psychosomatic Med* 6:7-16, 1944.

Masserman JH, Yum KS: An analysis of the influence of alcohol in experimental neuroses in cats. *Psychosomatic Med* 8:36-52, 1946.

Mavissakalian M: Differential effects of imipramine and behavior therapy on panic disorder with agoraphobia. *Psychopharmacol Bull* 25:27-29, 1989.

Mavissakalian M, Perel JM: Clinical experiments in maintenance and discontinuation of imipramine therapy in panic disorder with agoraphobia. *Arch Gen Psychiat* 49:318-323, 1992.

Mayes A: The physiology of fear and anxiety. In: *Fear in Animals and Man*, ed. Sluckin W. Van Nostrand Reinholt Company, New York: 24-55, 1979.

Mayr E: Teleological and teleonomic: A new analysis. In: *Learning, Development, and Culture*, ed. Plotkin HC. John Wiley & Sons, New York: 17-38, 1982.

Mayhew LA, Hanzel TE, Ferron FR, Kalachnik JE, Harder SR: Phenobarbital exacerbation of self-injurious behavior. *J Nervous Mental Dis* 180:732-733, 1992.

McCarty R, Southwick CH: Parental environment: effects on survival, growth, and aggressive behaviors of two rodent species. *Devel Psychobiol* 12:269-279, 1979.

McConnell PB: Lessons from animals trainers: the effect of acoustic structure on an animal response. In: *Perspectives in Ethology* 9th ed, eds. Bateson P, Klopfer P. Plenum Press, New York: 165-187, 1990a.

McConnell PB: Acoustic structure and receiver response in domestic dogs, *Canis familiaris*. *Anim Behav* 39:897-904, 1990b.

McConnell PB, Baylis JR: Interspecific communication in cooperative handling: acoustic and visual signals from human shepherds and herding dogs. *Zeitschrift für Tierpsychologie* 67:302-328, 1985.

McCrave EA: Diagnostic criteria for separation anxiety in the dog. *Vet Clin North Am: Sm Anim Pract* 21:247-256, 1991.

McCune S: The impact of paternity and early socialization on the development of cat's behaviour to people and novel objects. *Appl Anim Behav Sci* 45:109-124, 1995.

McDougle CJ, Goodman WK, Leckman JF, Holzer JC, Barr LC, McLance-Katz E, Heninger GR, Price L-H: Limited therapeutic effect of addition of buspirone in fluvoxamine-refractory obsessive-compulsive disorder. *Am J Psychiatry* 150:647-649, 1993.

McFarland DH: On the causal and functional significance of displacement activities. *Zeitschrift für Tierpsychologie* 23:217-235, 1966.

McGeer PL, McGeer EG, Wada JA: Glutamic acid decarboxylase in Parkinson's disease and epilepsy. *Neurology* 21:1000-1007, 1971.

McGrath JT: Jaw snapping dog (questions and answers). *Mod Vet Pract* 43:70, 1962.

McGregor PK: The singer and the song: on the receiving end of bird song. *Biol Rev* 66:57-81, 1991.

McKinley PE: Cluster analysis of the domestic cat's vocal repertoire. PhD dissertation, University of Maryland, College Park, 1982.

McQuay HJ: Opioids in chronic pain. *Brit J Anaesth* 63:213-226, 1989.

McTavish D, Benfield P: Clomipramine: an overview of its pharmacological properties and a review of its therapeutic use in obsessive-compulsive behavior and panic attack. *Drugs* 39:136-153, 1990.

Meier GW: Infantile handling and development in Siamese kittens. *J Compar Physiol Psychol* 54:284-286, 1961.

Meier GW, Stuart JL: Effects of handling on the physical and behavioral development of Siamese kittens. *Psychol Rep* 5:497-501, 1959.

Meir M, Turner DC: Reactions of housecats during encounters with a strange person: evidence for two personality types. *J Delta Society* 2:45-53, 1985.

Melese P: Detecting and neutralizing odor sources in dog and cat elimination problems (Abstract). *Appl Anim Behav Sci* 39:188-189, 1994a.

Melese P: New techniques in detection and neutralization of urine contamination. Handout for AVMA, San Francisco, Ca, July, 1994b.

Mellen JD: The effects of hand-raising on sexual behavior of captive small felids using domestic cats as a model. *Annual Proceedings of the American Association of Zoological Parks and Aquarium* 253-259, 1988.

Meltzer HY: The neuroendocrine profile of clozapine, an atypical antipsychotic agent. *J Clin Psychiat Monogr* 8:15-21, 1990.

Melzack R: The role of early experience in emotional arousal. *Ann NY Acad Sci* 159:720-730, 1968.

Melzack R, Scott TH: The effects of early experience on the response to pain. *J Comp Physiol Pyschol* 50:155-161, 1957.

Mendl M: The effects of litter-size variation on the development of play behaviour in the domestic cat: litters of one and two. *Anim Behav* 36:20-34, 1988.

Meric SM: Polyuria and polydipsia. In: *Textbook of Veterinary Internal Medicine*, eds. Ettinger SJ, Feldman EC. WB Saunders, Philadelphia: 159-163, 1995.

Mertens C: Human-cat interactions in the home setting. *Anthrozöos* 4(4):214-231, 1991.

Mertens C, Schär R: Practical aspects of research on cats. In: *The Domestic Cat: the Biology of Its Behaviour*, eds. Turner DC, Bateson P. Cambridge University Press, Cambridge: 179-190, 1988.

Mertens C, Turner DC: Experimental analysis of human-cat interactions during first encounters. *Anthrozöos* 2:83-97, 1988.

Messent PR, Serpell JA: An historical and biological view of the pet-owner bond. In: *Inter-Relations Between People and Pets*, Fogle B. Charles C. Thomas Publishers, Springfield, Illinois: 5-22, 1981.

Michael RP: Observations upon the sexual behavior of the domestic cat *(Felis catus L.)* under laboratory conditions. *Behaviour* 18:1-24, 1961.

Miczek KA, Mos J, Olivier B: Serotonin, aggression and self-destructive behavior. *Psychopharmacol Bull* 25:399-403, 1989.

Miles RC: Learning in kittens with manipulatory, exploratory, and food incentives. *J Comp Physiol Psychol* 51:39-42, 1958.

Milgram NW, Ivy GO, Head E, Murphy MP, Wu PH, Ruehl WW, Yu PH, Durden DA, Davis BA, Paterson IA, Boulton AA: The effect of L-deprenyl on behavior, cognitive function, and biogenic amines in the dog (review). *Neurochem Res* 18(12):1211-1219, 1993.

Milgram NW, Racine RJ, Nellis P, Mendonca A, Ivy GO: Maintenance on L-deprenyl prolongs life in aged male rats. *Life Sci* 47:415-420, 1990.

Miller WH Jr, Scott DW, Wellington JR: Non-steroidal management of canine pruritus with amitriptyline. *Cornell Vet* 82:53-57, 1992.

Miller WH, Scott DW: Medical management of chronic pruritus. *Comp Contin Edu Pract Vet* 16:449-462, 1994.

Moelk M: The development of friendly approach behavior in the cat: a study of kitten-mother relations and the cognitive development of the kitten from birth to eight weeks. In: *Advances in the Study of Behavior* 10th, ed. Rosenblatt J. Academic Press, New York: 164-224, 1979.

Moelk M: Vocalizing in the house cat: a phoenetic and functional study. *Am J Psychol* 57:184-205, 1944.

The Monks of New Skete: *The Art of Raising a Puppy*. Little, Brown, Boston, 1991.

Montgomery SA, Bullock T, Fineberg N: Serotonin selectivity for obsessive-compulsive and panic disorders. *J Psychiatry Neurosci* 16:30-35, 1991.

Moreau PM, Lees GE: Incontinence, enuresis, nocturia, and dysuria. In: *Textbook of Veterinary Internal Medicine*, eds. Ettinger SJ, Feldman EC. WB Saunders, Philadelphia: 164-168, 1995.

Morgan M, Houpt KA: Feline behavior problems: the influence of declawing. *Anthrozöos* III:50-53, 1990.

Morton ES: On the occurrence and significance of motivation-structure rules in some bird and mammal sounds. *American Naturalist* 111:855-869, 1977.

Mos J, Olivier B: Quantitative and comparative analyses of pro-aggressive actions of benzodiazepines in maternal aggression of rats. *Psychopharmacol* 97:152-153, 1989.

Mos J, Olivier B, van Oorschot R: Behavioural and neuropharmacological aspects of maternal aggression in rodents. *Aggressive Behavior* 16:145-163, 1990.

Mosh SL, Ludvig N: Kindling. In: Recent Advances in Epilepsy, number 4, eds. Pedley TA, Meldrum BS. Churchill Livingstone, New York: 21-44, 1988.

Moss SP, Wright JC: The effects of dog ownership on judgements of dogbite likelihood. *Anthrozöos* 1:95-99, 1987.

Moulton DG, Ashton EH, Eayers JT: Studies in olfactory acuity. 4. Relative detectability of n-aliphatic acids by the dog. *Anim Behav* 8:117-128, 1960.

Mousseau DD: Tryptamine: a metabolite of tryptophan implicated in various neuropsychiatric disorders. *Metab Brain Dis* 8:1-44, 1993.

Moyer KE: Kinds of aggression and their physiological basis. *Communications Behav Biol* 2(A):65-87, 1968.

Moynihan M: Control, suppression, decay, disappearance and replacement of displays. *J Theoretical Biol* 29:85-112, 1970.

Moynihan N: Why is lying about intentions rare during some kinds of contests? *J Theoretical Biol* 97:9-12, 1982.

Mrosobsky N, Sherry DF: Animal anorexics. *Science* 207(4433): 837-842, 1980.

Mugford RA: Aggressive behavior in the English cocker spaniel. *Vet Annual* 24:310-314, 1984a.

Mugford RA: Behaviour problems in the dog: In: *Nutrition and Behaviour in Dogs and Cats*, ed. Anderson RS. Oxford, Pergamon Press: 207-215, 1984b.

Mugford RA: External influences on the feeding of carnivores. In: *The Chemical Senses and Nutrition*, eds. Kare MR, Maller O. Academic Press, New York: 25-50, 1977.

Murphree OD: Inheritance of human aversion and inactivity in two strains of pointer dogs. *Biol Psychiatry* 7:23-29, 1973.

Murphree OD, Angel C, DeLuca DC, Newton JEO: Longitudinal studies of genetically nervous dogs. *Biol Psychiatry* 12:573-576, 1977.

Murphree OD, DeLuca DC, Angel C: Psychopharmcologic faciliation of operant conditioning of genetically nervous catahoula and pointer dogs. *Pav J Biol Sci* 9:17-24, 1974.

Murphree OD, Dykman RA: Litter patterns in the offspring of nervous and stable dogs. I: behavioral tests. *J Nerv Mental Dis* 141:321-332, 1965.

Murphree OD, Dykman RA, Peters JE: Genetically determined abnormal behavior in dogs: results of behavioral tests. *Conditional Reflex* 1:199-205, 1967.

Murphree OD, Newton JEO: Cross-breeding and special handling of genetically nervous dogs. *Conditional Reflex* 6:129-136, 1971a.

Murphree OD, Newton JEO: Schizokinesis: fragmentation of performance in two strains of pointer dogs. *Conditional Reflex* 6:91-100, 1971b.

Murphree OD, Peters JE, Dykman RA: Behavioral comparisons

of nervous, stable, and crossbred pointers at ages 2, 3, 6, 9, and 12 months. *Conditional Reflex* 4:20-23, 1969.

Musi B, DeAcetis L, Alleva E: Influence of litter gender composition on subsequent maternal behavior and maternal aggression in female house mice. *Ethology* 95:43-53, 1993.

Myles S: Trainers and chokers. How dog trainers affect behavior problems in the dog. *Vet Clin North Am: Sm Anim Pract* 21:239-246, 1991.

Namikas J, Wehmer F: Gender composition of litter affects behavior of male mice. *Behav Biol* 23:219-224, 1978.

Natoli E: Behavioral responses of urban feral cats to different types of urine marks. *Behaviour* 94:234-243, 1985.

Natoli E: Mating strategies of cats: a comparison of the role and importance of infanticide in domestic cats *(Felis catus L.)* and lions *(Panthera leo L.). Anim Behav* 40:183-186, 1990.

Natoli E: Spacing pattern in a colony of urban stray cats *(Felis catus)* in the historic center of Rome. *Appl Anim Behav Sci* 14:289-304, 1985.

Natoli E, de Vito E: Agonistic behaviour, dominance rank, and copulatory success at a large, multi-male feral cat, *Felis catus L.,* colony in central Rome. *Anim Behav* 42:227-241, 1991.

Natoli E, de Vito E: The mating system of feral cats living in a group. In: *The Domestic Cat: The Biology of Its Behaviour,* eds. Turner DC, Bateson P. Cambridge University Press, Cambridge: 99-108, 1988.

Nattel S, Mittleman M: Treatment of ventricular tachyarrhthmias resulting from amitriptyline toxicity in dogs. *J Pharm Exp Therapeut* 231:430-435, 1984.

Natynczuk S, Bradshaw JW, Macdonald DW: Chemical constituents of the anal sacs of domestic dogs. *Biochemical Systematics and Ecology* 17:83-87, 1989.

Neamand J, Sweeny WT, Creamer AA, Conti PA: Cage activity in the laboratory beagle: a preliminary study to evaluate a method of comparing cage size to physical activity. *Lab Anim Sci* 25:180-183, 1975.

Neff WD, Diamond IP: The neural basis of auditory discrimination. In: *Biological and Biochemical Basis of Behavior,* eds. Harlow HF, Woolsey CN. University of Wisconsin Press, Madison, Wi: 101-126, 1958.

Neitz J, Geist T, Jacobs JH: Color vision in the dog. *Visual Neuroscience* 3:119-125, 1989.

Nelson RJ, Demas GG, Huang PL, Fishman MC, Dawson VL, Dawson TM, Snyder SH: Behavioral abnormalities in male mice lacking neuronal nitric oxide synthase. *Nature* 378:383-386, 1995.

Nelson RW, Meric SM, Hawkins EC, Turrel JM: Diseases of the thyroid gland. In: *Handbook of Small Animal Practice,* ed. Morgan RV. Churchill Livingstone, New York: 507-520, 1988.

Nemeroff CB, Simon JS, Haggerty JJ Jr, Evans DL: Antithyroid antibodies in depressed patients. *Am J Psychiat* 142:840-843, 1985.

Nesbitt GH, Kedan GS: Differential diagnosis of feline pruritus. *Compend Contin Educ Pract Vet* 7:163-172, 1985.

Netto WJ, Van der Borg FA, Siegers JF: The establishment of dominance relationships in a dog pack and its relevance for the man-dog relationships. *Tidjschrift voor Diergenesskunde* 117(Suppl. 1):51-52S, 1992.

Neville PF: Behaviour patterns that conflict with domestication. In: *The Behaviour of the Domestic Cat,* ed. Bradshaw JWS. CAB International, Oxon: 187-204, 1992.

Neville PF: Treatment of behaviour problems in cats. *Practice* 13:143-150, 1991.

Neville PF, Bradshaw JWS: Unusual appetites. *Bull Feline Advisory Bureau* 28:5-6, 32, 1991.

Neville PF, Remfry J: Effects of neutering on two groups of feral cats. *Behaviour* 94:234-243, 1984.

Newman RA: Developmental plasticity of *Scaphiopus couchii* tadpoles in an unpredictable environment. *Ecology* 70:1775-1787, 1989.

Newton JEO, Dykman RA, Schapin JL: The prediction of abnormal behavior from autonomic indices in dogs. *J Nervous Mental Dis* 166:635-664, 1978.

Nobbe OE, Niebuhr BR, Levinson M, Tiller JE: Use of time-out as punishment for aggressive behavior. *Canine Pract* 5:12-18, 1978.

Noyes R Jr: Beta-adrenergic blocking drugs in anxiety and stress. *Psych Clin North Am* 8(1):119-132, 1985.

O'Farrell V: Behavior problems in dogs: aggression towards people. *Vet Ann* 30:196-199, 1990.

O'Farrell V: *Manual of Canine Behaviour.* BSAVA Publications, Cheltenham, England, 1992.

O'Farrell V, Peachey E: Behavioural effects of ovariohysterectomy on bitches. *J Sm Anim Pract* 31:595-598, 1990.

Oliver JE Jr, Lorenz MD: *Handbook of Veterinary Neurologic Diagnosis.* W.B. Saunders, Philadelphia, 1983.

Olivier B, Mos J: Serenics and aggression. *Stress Med* 2:197-209, 1986.

Olm DD, Houpt KA: Feline house-soiling problems. *Appl Anim Behav Sci* 20:335-345, 1988.

Olney JW: Excitatory amino acids and neuropsychiatric disorders. *Biol Psychiatry* 26:505-525, 1989.

Olney JW: Neurotoxicity of NMDA receptor antagonists: An overview. *Psychopharm Bull* 30:533-540, 1994.

Olsen SJ: *Origins of the domestic dog: The Fossil Record,* University of Arizona Press, Tucson, Arizona, 1985.

Ortize de Zarate JC, Ortize de Zarate CO: Hair whorl and handedness. *Brain Cognition* 16:288-230, 1991.

Osborne CA, Johnson GR, Kruger JM, O'Brien TD, Lulich JP: Etiopathogenesis and biological behavior of feline vesicourachal diverticula. *Vet Clin North Am: Sm Anim Pract* 17:697-733, 1987.

Osborne CA et al: Feline lower urinary tract disorders. In: *Textbook of Veterinary Internal Medicine,* 3rd edition, ed. Ettinger SJ. WB Saunders, Philadelphia: 2057-2082, 1989.

Osborne CA, Kruger JM, Lulich JP, Polzin DJ: Feline lower urinary tract diseases. In: *Textbook of Veterinary Internal Medicine,* eds. Ettinger SJ, Feldman EC. WB Saunders, Philadelphia: 1805-1832, 1995.

Ounsted C: Aggression and epilepsy rage in children with temporal lobe epilepsy. *J Psychosomatic Res* 13:237-242, 1967.

Overall KL: Animal behavior case of the month. Intrasexual interdog aggression in two pugs. *JAVMA* 207:305-307, 1995b.

Overall KL: Animal behavior case of the month. Use of buspirone (BuSpar) to treat spraying associated with intercat aggression. *JAVMA* 205:694-696, 1994m.

Overall KL: Animal behavior case of the month. Use of fluoxetine (Prozac) to treat complicated interdog aggression. *JAVMA* 206:629-632, 1995a.

Overall KL: Canine aggression: Part I. *Canine Pract* 18(2):40-41, 1993b.

Overall KL: Canine aggression: Part II. *Canine Pract* 18(3):29-31, 1993c.

Overall KL: Canine aggression: Part III. *Canine Pract* 18(4):32-34, 1993d.

Overall KL: Choosing drugs for spraying cats. *Feline Pract,* in press, 1996.

Overall KL: Commentary on "Buspirone for use in treating cats . . ." *Advances Sm Anim Med Surg* 7(14):4-5, 1994h.

Overall KL: Diagnosing and treating undesirable feline elimination behavior. *Feline Pract* 21(2):11-15, 1993a.

Overall KL: Diagnosis and treatment of management related feline behavioral disorders. *Feline Pract* 22(1):13-15, 1994i.

Overall KL: Feline aggression. Part I. The role of early socialization. *Feline Pract* 22(4):25-26, 1994j.

Overall KL: Feline aggression. Part II. Common aggressions. *Feline Pract* 22(5):16-17, 1994k.

Overall KL: Feline aggression. Part III. The role of social status in hierarchical systems. *Feline Pract* 22(6):16-17, 1994n.

Overall KL: Practical pharmacological approaches to behavioral problems. In: Purina Specialty Review: Behavioral Problems in Small Animals. 36-51, 1992b.

Overall KL: Preventing behavior problems: Early prevention and recognition in puppies and kittens. In: Purina Specialty Review: Behavioral Problems in Small Animals. 13-29, 1992a.

Overall KL: Recognition, diagnosis, and management of obsessive-compulsive disorders. Part I. *Canine Pract* 17(2):40-44, 1992c.

Overall KL: Recognition, diagnosis, and management of obsessive-compulsive disorders. Part II. *Canine Pract* 17(3):25-27, 1992d.

Overall KL: Recognition, diagnosis, and management of obsessive-compulsive disorders. Part III. *Canine Pract* 17(4):39-43, 1992e.

Overall KL: Sex and aggression. *Canine Pract* 20(3):16-18, 1995c.

Overall KL: State of the art: Advances in pharmacological therapy for behavioral disorders. *Proceedings NAVC* 8:43-48, 1994a.

Overall KL: A stepwise approach to treating the aggressive canine. *Proceedings NAVC* 8:52-54, 1994c.

Overall KL: Stereotypic and ritualistic behaviors. *Proceedings NAVC* 8:55-57, 1994d.

Overall KL: Treating canine behavioral disorders. I. Understanding and implementing behavior modification. *Canine Pract* 18(6):24-28, 1993e.

Overall KL: Treating canine behavioral disorders. II. Prevention and early intervention for aggression. *Canine Pract* 19(1):19-22, 1993f.

Overall KL: Treating canine behavioral disorders. III. Is there a role for temperament testing and obedience training? *Canine Pract* 19(4):19-21, 1994g.

Overall KL: Understanding the interaction between feline aggression and elimination disorders. *Proceedings NAVC* 8:58-60, 1994e.

Overall KL: Use of clomipramine to treat ritualistic motor behavior in dogs. *JAVMA* 205:1733-1741, 1994n.

Overall KL: Uses for newer anxiolytic and antipsychotic drugs. *Proceedings NAVC* 8:49-51, 1994b.

Owen G, Hatfield GK, Pollock JJ, Steinberg AJ, Tucker WE, Agersborg HPK: Toxicity studies of lorazepam, a new benzodiazepine, in animals. *Arzneim Forsch* 21:1065-1073, 1971.

Owen G, Smith THF, Agersborg HPK: Toxicity of some benzodiazepine compounds with CNS activity. *Toxicol Appl Pharmacol* 16:556-570, 1970.

Owens D, Owens M: Social dominance and reproductive patterns in brown hyaenas *(Hyaena brunnea)* of the central Kalahari desert. *Anim Behav* 51:535-551, 1996.

Paape SR, Shille VM, Seto H, Stabenfeldt GH: Luteal activity in the pseudopregnant cat. *Biol Repro* 13:470-474, 1975.

Packer C: The ecology of sociality in felids. In: *Ecological Aspects of Social Evolution*, eds. Rubenstein DI, Wranghan RW. Princeton University Press, Princeton: 429-451, 1986.

Packer C, Gilbert DA, Pusey AE, O'Brien SJ: A molecular genetic analysis of kinship and cooperation in african lions. *Nature* 351:562-565, 1991.

Packer C, Pusey AE: Cooperation and competition in lions. *Nature* 302:356, 1983.

Packwood J, Gordon B: Stereopsis in normal domestic cat, Siamese cat and cat raised with alternating monocular occlusion. *J Neurophysiol* 38:1485-1499, 1975.

Palazzolo BL, Quadri SK: The effects of aging on the circadian rhythm of serum cortisol on the dog. *Experimental Gerontology* 22:379-387, 1987.

Palen GF, Goddard GV: Catnip and oestrus behavior in the cat. *Anim Behav* 14:372-377, 1966.

Panaman R: Behavior and ecology of free-ranging female farm cats *(Felis catus L.) Zeitschrift für Tierpsycologie* 56:59-73, 1981.

Panciera DL: Hypothyroidism in dogs: 66 cases (1987-1992). *JAVMA* 204:761-767, 1994.

Parker AJ: Behavioral signs of organic disease. In: *Textbook of Veterinary Internal Medicine*, 3rd edition, ed. Ettinger SJ. WB Saunders, Philadelphia: 70-74, 1989.

Parker AJ, O'Brien DP, Sawchuk SA: The nervous system. In: *Feline Medicine*, ed. Pratt PW. American Veterinary Publications, Santa Barbara, Calif, 421-510, 1983.

Passanisi WC, Macdonald DW: Group discrimination on the basis of urine in a farm cat colony. In: *Chemical Signals in Vertebrates*, vol 5, eds. Macdonald DW, Muller-Schwarze D, Natynczuk SE. Oxford University Press, Oxford: 336-345, 1990.

Pato MT, Pigott TA, Hill JL, Grover GN, Bernstein S, Murphy DL: Controlled comparison of buspirone and clomipramine in obsessive-compulsive disease. *Am J Psychiat* 148:127-129, 1991.

Paton D: Communication by agonistic displays: II. Perceived information and the definition of agonistic displays. *Behaviour* 99:157-175, 1986.

Patronek GJ, Glickman LT, Moyer MR: Population dynamics and the risk of euthanasia for dogs in an animal shelter. *Anthrozoös* VIII:31-43, 1995.

Patronek GJ, Rowan AN: Determining dog and cat numbers and population dynamics. *Anthrozoös* VIII:199-205, 1995.

Paul SM, Skolnick P: Comparative neuropharmacology of antianxiety drugs. *Pharmacol Biochem Behav* 17(Suppl. 1):37-41, 1982.

Pavlov IP: *Conditioned Reflexes. An Investigation of the Physiological Activity of the Cerebral Cortex.* Oxford University Press, London, 1927.

Pawlowski AA, Scott JP: Hereditary differences in the development of dominance in litters of puppies. *J Compar Physiol Psychol* 49:353-358, 1956.

Pellis SM, O'Brien DP, Pellis VC, Teitelbaum P: Escalation of feline predation along a gradient from avoidance through "play" to killing. *Behav Neurosci* 102:760-777, 1988.

Perse T: Obsessive-compulsive disorder: A treatment review. *J Clin Psychiatry* 49:48-55, 1988.

Perse TL, Greist JH, Jeffereson JW, Rosenfeld R, Dar R: Fluvoxamine treatment of obessive-compulsive disorder. *Am J Psychiatry* 144:1543-1548, 1987.

Peters RP, Mech LD: Scent-marking in wolves. *American Scientist* 63:628-637, 1975.

Peterson ME: The effects of megestrol acetate on glucose tolerance in growth hormone secretion in the cat. *Res Vet Sci* 42:354-357, 1987.

Pettijohn T, Wong T, Elert P, Scott JP: Alleviation of separation distress in three breeds of young dogs. *Developmental Psychobiology* 10:373-381, 1977.

Pfaffenberger CJ, Scott JP: The relationship between delayed socialization and trainability of guide dogs. *J Genet Psychol* 95:145-155, 1959.

Pickar D, Vartanian F, Bunney WE, et al.: Short-term naloxone administration in schizophrenic and manic patients. *Arch Gen Psychiatry* 39:313-319, 1982.

Pigott TA, Altemus M, Rubenstein CS, Hill JL, Bihari K, L'Heureux F, Bernstein S, Murphy DL: Symptoms of eating disorders in patients with obsessive-compulsive disorders. *Am J Psychiat* 148:1552-1557, 1991.

Pinckney LE, Kennedy LA: Traumatic deaths from dog attacks in the United States. *Pediatrics* 69(2):193-196, 1982.

Pitman RK: Animal models of compulsive behavior. *Biol Psychiatry* 26:1898-198, 1989.

Placidi GF, Tognoni G, Pacifici GM, Cassano GB, Morselli PL: Regional distribution of diazepam and its metabolites in the brain of cat after chronic treatment. *Psychopharmacol* 48:133-137, 1976.

Plutchik R: Individual and breed differences in approach and withdrawal behavior in dogs. *Behaviour* 40:302-311, 1972.

Podberscek AL, Blackshaw JK: Dog attacks on children: report from two major city hospitals. *Austral Vet J* 68:248-249, 1991.

Podberscek AL, Blackshaw JK, Beattie AW: The behavior of laboratory colony cats and their reactions to a familiar and unfamiliar person. *Appl Anim Behav Sci* 31:119-130, 1991.

Podberscek AL, Blackshaw JK, Bodero DAV: An evaluation of human-cat associations. *Austral Vet Pract* 18:16-20, 1988.

Pollack MH, Otto MW, Tesar GE, Cohen LS, Meltzer-Brody S, Rosenbaum JF: Long-term outcome after acute treatment with alprazolam or clonazepam for panic disorder. *J Clin Psychopharmacol* 13(4):257-263, 1993.

Pollard JS, Baldock MD, Lewis RFV: Learning rates and use of visual information in five animal species. *Austral J Psychol* 23:29-34, 1971.

Polsky RH: Developmental factors in mammalian predation. *Behav Biol* 15:353-382, 1975a.

Polsky RH: Electronic shock collars: Are they worth the risks? *JAAHA* 30:463-468, 1994.

Polsky RH: Hunger, prey-feeding, and predatory aggression. *Behav Biol* 13:81-93, 1975b.

Post RM: Introduction: emerging perspectives on valproate in affective disorders. *J Clin Psychiat* 50(3):3-10, 1989.

Potegal M: The reinforcing value of several types of aggressive behavior: a review. *Aggressive Behavior* 5:353-373, 1979.

Prendergast D: *The Wolf Hybrid*, second ed. Rudehaus Enterprises Gallup, NM, 1989.

Prescott CW: Reproduction patterns in the domestic cat. *Austral Vet J* 49:126-129, 1973.

Pyke T, Greenberg H: Norepinephrine challenge in panic patients. *J Clin Psychol* 6:279-285, 1986.

Raab, A, Dantzer R, Michaud B, et al: Behavioral physiological and immunological consequences of social status and aggression in chronically coexisting resident and intruder dyads of male rats. *Physiol Behav* 36:223-228, 1986.

Rabb GB, Woolpy JH, Ginsburg BE: Social relationships in a group of captive wolves. *Am Zool* 7:305-311, 1967.

Rachman S: *The Meanings of Fear.* Penguin Educational, Baltimore, 1974.

Rachman S, Levitt K: Panic, fear reduction and habituation. *Behav Res Ther* 26:199-206, 1988.

Radinsky L: Evolution of the felid brain. *Brain, Behavior, and Evolution* 11:214-254, 1975.

Raemaekers JJ, Raemaekers PM: Field playback of loud calls to gibbons *(Hylobates lar):* territorial, sex-specific and species-specific responses. *Anim Behav* 33:481-493, 1985.

Ralls K: Mammalian scent marking. *Science* 171:443-449, 1971.

Randall W, Lasko V: Body weight and food intake rhythms and their relationships to the behavior of cats with brainstem lesions. *Psychosomatic Science* 11:33-34, 1968.

Randall W, Swenson RW, Parsons V, Elbin J, Trulson M: The influence of seasonal changes in light on hormones in normal cats and in cats with lesions of the superior colliculi and pretectum. *J Interdisciplin Cycle Res* 6:253-266, 1975.

Randolph JF, Center SA, Reimers TJ, Scarlett JM, Corbett JR: Adrenocortical function in neonatal and weanling Beagle pups. *Am J Vet Res* 56:511-517, 1995.

Rang HP, Dale MM, Ritter JM, Gardner P: *Pharmacology.* Churchill Livingstone, New York, 1995.

Ratey JJ, Gordon A: The psychopharmacology of aggression: toward a new day. *Psychopharmacol Bull* 29:65-73, 1993.

Rauschecker J, Marler P, editors. *Imprinting and Cortical Plasticity.* John Wiley & Sons, New York, 1987.

Redbo I: Changes in duration and frequency of stereotypies and their adjoining behaviours in heifers, before, during and after the grazing period. *Appl Anim Behav Sci* 26:57-67, 1990.

Redbo I: Stereotypies and cortisol secretion in heifers subjected to tethering. *Appl Anim Behav Sci* 38:213-225, 1993.

Reed CA: A review of the archeological evidence of animal domestication in the prehistoric east. In: *Prehistoric Investigations in Iraqi Kurdestan*, eds. Braidwood RJ, Howe B. The Oriental Institute of Chicago, Chicago: 119-145, 1964.

Rees P: The ecological distribution of feral cats and the effects of neutering on a hospital colony. In: *The Ecology and Control of Feral Cats*, ed. The Universities Federation for Animal Welfare. UFAW, Potter's Bar, 1981.

Reiman EM, Fusselman MJ, Fox PT, Raichle ME: Neuroanatomical correlates of anticipatory anxiety. *Science* 243:1071-1074, 1989.

Reinhard DW: Aggressive behavior associated with hypothyroidism. *Can Pract* 5(6):69-70, 1978.

Reis BJ: The chemical coding of aggression in the brain. *Advances Behav Biol* 10:125-150, 1974.

Reis D: Brain monamines in aggression and sleep. *Clin Neurosurg* 18:471-502, 1971.

Reisner I: The pathophysiologic basis of behavior problems. *Vet Clin North Am: Sm Anim Pract* 21:207-224, 1991.

Reisner I: Use of lithium for treatment of canine dominance-related aggression: a case study (abstract). *Appl Anim Behav Sci* 39:193, 1994.

Reisner IR, Hollis NE, Houpt KA: Risk-factors for behavior-related euthanasia among dominant-aggressive dogs: 110 cases, (1989-1992). *JAVMA* 205(6):855-863, 1994.

Reisner IR, Houpt KA, Erb HN, Quimby FW: Friendliness to humans and defensive aggression in cats: The influence of handling and paternity. *Physiol Behav* 55:1119-1124, 1994.

Remmers JE, Gautier H: Neural and mechanical mechanisms of feline purring. *Respir Physiol* 16:351-361, 1972.

Rheingold HL, Eckerman CO: Familiar social and nonsocial stimuli and the kitten's response to a strange environment. *Dev Psychobiol* 4:71-89, 1971.

Rice RG, Starbuck GW, Reed G: Accidental injuries to children. *N Engl J Med* 255:1212-1219, 1956.

Richards SM: The concept of dominance and methods of assessment. *Anim Behav* 44(4):914-930, 1974.

Richardson JS, Zaleskey WA: Naloxone and self-mutilation. *Biol Psychiatry* 18:99-101, 1983.

Rickels K, Schweizer E: Clinical overview of serotonin reuptake inhibitors. *J Clin Psychiat* 51(Suppl. B):9-12, 1990.

Ricketts RW, Goza AB, Ellis CR, Singh YH, Singh NN, Cooke

JC: Fluoxetine treatment of severe self-injury in young adults with mental retardation. *J Am Acad Child Adolesc Psychiatry* 32:865-869, 1993.

Rieger I: Scent rubbing in carnivores. *Carnivore* 2(1):17-25, 1979.

Rigdon JD, Tapia F: Children who are cruel to animals—a follow-up study. *J Operational Psychology* 8:27-36, 1977.

Robins LN, Helzer JE, Weissman MM: Lifetime prevalence of specific psychiatric disorders in three sites. *Arch Gen Psychiatry* 41:949-958, 1984.

Robinson DS, Shrotriya RS, Alms DR, Messina M, Andany J: Treatment of panic disorder: Non-benzodiazepine anxiolytics, including buspirone. *Psychopharmacol* 25:21-26, 1989.

Robinson I: Behavioural development of the cat. In: *The Waltham Book of Dog and Cat Behaviour*, ed. Thorne C. Pergamon Press, Oxford: 53-64, 1992a.

Robinson I: Social behaviour of the cat. In: *The Waltham Book of Dog and Cat Behaviour*, ed. Thorne C. Pergamon Press, Oxford: 79-95, 1992b.

Robinson R: *Genetics for Cat Breeders*, 2nd edition. London, Pergamon Press, 1977.

Robinson R, Cox HW: Reproductive performance in a cat colony over a 10-year period. *Laboratory Animals* 4:99-112, 1970.

Rolf LH, Haarmann FY, Grotenmeyer K-H, Kehrer H: Serotonin and amino acid content in platelets of autistic children. *Acta Psychiatr Scand* 87:312-316, 1993.

Rolls ET: A theory of emotion and its application to understanding the neural basis of emotions. In: *Psychobiological Aspects of Relationships Between Emotion and Cognition*, ed. Gray JA. Lawrence Erlbaum Associates, Hove, Hillsdale: 161-199, 1990.

Romand R, Ehret G: Development of sound production in normal, isolated, and deafened kittens during the first postnatal months. *Developmental Psychobiology* 17:629-649, 1984.

Romatowski J: Problems in interpretation of clinical laboratory test results. *JAVMA* 205:1186-1188, 1994.

Romatowski J: Use of megestrol acetate in cats. *JAVMA* 194:700-702, 1989.

Romsos DR, Ferguson D: Regulation of protein intake in adult dogs. *JAVMA* 182:41-43, 1983.

Roselli CE, Handa RJ, Resko JA: Quantitative distribution of nuclear androgen receptors in microdissected areas of the rat brain. *Neuroendocrinol* 49:449-453, 1989.

Rosenblatt JS: Stages in the early behavioural development of altricial young of non-primate animals. In: *Growing Points in Ethology*, eds. Bateson PPG, Hind RA. Cambridge University Press, Cambridge: 345-383, 1976.

Rosenblatt JS, Turkewitz G, Schneirla TC: Early socialization in the domestic cat as based on feeding and other relationships between female and young. In: *Determinants of Infant Behavior*, ed. Foss BM. Methuen, London: 51-74, 1961.

Ross LA: Urinary system: Introduction. In: *Handbook of Small Animal Practice*, 2nd edition, Morgan RV. Churchill Livingstone, New York: 555-557, 1992.

Ross S: Suckling behavior in neonate dogs. *J Abnormal Sociol Psychol* 46:142-149, 1951.

Ross S, Ross J: Social facilitation of feeding behavior in dogs: I. Group and solitary feeding. *J Genetic Psychol* 74:97-108, 1949a.

Ross S, Ross J: Social facilitation of feeding behavior in dogs: II. Feeding after satiation. *J Genetic Psychol* 74:293-304, 1949b.

Rosser EJ: Diagnosis of food allergy in dogs. *JAVMA* 203:259-262, 1993.

Rossier J, French ED, Rivier C, Ling N, Guilemin R, Bloom FE: Foot-shock induced stress increases β-endorphin levels in blood but not brain. *Nature* 270:618-620, 1977.

Rothschild AJ, Benes F, Hebben N, Woods B, Luciania M, Bakanas E, Samson JA, Schatzberg AF: Relationships beteen brain CT scan findings and cortisol in psychotic and nonpsychotic depressed patients. *Biol Psychiatry* 26:565-575, 1989.

Rowan AN, Williams J: The success of companion animal management programs: a review. *Anthrozöos* 1:110-122, 1987.

Rowell TE: The concept of social dominance. *Behav Biol* 11:131-154, 1974.

Rowell TE: *The Social Behavior of Monkeys*. Penguin, Harmondsworth, 1972.

Roy A, Linnoilia M: Suicidal behavior, impulsiveness and serotonin. *Acta Psychiatr Scand* 78:529-535, 1988.

Rozkowska E, Fonberg E: Salivary reactions after ventromedial hypothalamic lesions in dogs. *Acta Neurobiologica Experimentia* 33:553-562, 1973.

Rubin HD, Beck AM: Ecological behavior of free-ranging urban pet dogs. *Appl Anim Ethol* 8:161-168, 1982.

Ruble RP, Hird DW: Congenital abnormalities in immature dogs from a pet store: 253 cases (1987-1988). *JAVMA* 202:633-636, 1993.

Rudorfer MV, Potter WZ: Antidepressants. A comparative review of the clinical pharmacology and therapeutic use of the "newer" versus the "older" drugs. *Drugs* 37:713-738, 1989.

Rudorfer MV, Potter WZ: Pharmacokinetics of antidepressants. In: *Psychopharmacology: The Third Generation of Progress*, ed. Meltzer HY. Raven Press, New York: 1353-1363, 1987.

Ruehl WW, DePaoli A, Bruyette D: L-deprenyl for treatment of behavioral and cognitive problems in dogs: preliminary report of an open label trial (abstract). *Appl Anim Behav Sci* 39:191, 1994a.

Ruehl WW, DePaoli A, Bruyette D: Pretreatment characterization of behavioral and cognitive problems in elderly dogs. *J Vet Int Med* 8(2):178, 1994b.

Russell PA: Fear-evoking stimuli. In: *Fear in Animals and Man*, ed. Schluken W. Van Nostrand Reinhold, New York: 86-124, 1979.

Sacks JJ, Sattin RW, Bonzo ME: Dog-bite related fatalities from 1979 through 1988. *JAMA* 262:1489-1492, 1989.

Sahai S: Glutamate in the mammalian CNS. *Eur Arch Psychiatry Clin Neurosci* 240:121-133, 1990.

Salmieri KR, Bloomberg MS, Scruggs SL, Shille V: Gonadectomy in immature dogs: effects on skeletal, physical, and behavioral development. *JAVMA* 198:1193-1203, 1991.

Salzen EA: Fear in animals and man. In: *Fear in Animals and Man*, ed. Sluckin W. Van Nostrand Reinhold Company, New York: 125-163, 1979.

Sampson D, Willner P, Muscat R: Reversal of antidepressant action by dopamine antagonists in an animal model of depression. *Psychopharmacol* 104:491-495, 1991.

Sand S, Ratey J: The concept of noise. *Psychiatry* 49:290-297, 1986.

Sarter M, Markowitsch HJ: Involvement of the amygdala in learning and memory: a critical review, with emphasis on anatomical relations. *Behavioral Neurosci* 2:342-380, 1985.

Sayetta RB: Pica: an overview. *AFP* 33:181-185, 1986.

Scarlett JM, Saidea JE, Pollock RVH: Source of acquisition as a risk factor for disease and death in pups. *JAVMA* 204:1906-1913, 1994.

Schaffer CB, Phillips J: The Tuskegee behavior test for selecting pet therapy dogs (abstract). *Appl Anim Behav Sci* 39:192, 1994.

Schaller GB: *The Serengeti Lion: A Study of Predator-Prey Relations*. University of Chicago Press, Chicago, 1972.

Scheel D, Packer C: Group hunting behaviour of lions: a search for cooperation. *Anim Behav* 41:697-709, 1991.

Schenck CH, Hurwitz TD, Mahowald MW: REM sleep behavior disorder: an update on a series of 96 patients and a review of the world literature. *J Sleep Res* 2:224-231, 1993.

Schenck CH, Mahowald MW: Motor dyscontrol in narcolepsy: rapid eye movement (REM) sleep without atonia and REM sleep behavior disorders. *Ann Neurol* 32:3-10, 1992.

Schenkel R: Submission: its features and functions in the wolf and dog. *Am Zool* 7:319-330, 1967.

Schilder MGH, Netto WJ: On punishment and aggression. *Anim Behav Consultant Newsletter* 8(3):2-3, 1991.

Schmidt PM, Chakraborty PK, Wildt DE: Ovarian activity, circulating hormones, and sexual behavior in the cat. II. Relationships during pregnancy, parturition, lactation, and postpartum estrus. *Biological Reproduction* 28:657-671, 1983.

Schneier FR, Saoud JB, Campeas R, Fallon BA, Hollander E, Copran J, Liebowitz MR: Buspirone in social phobia. *J Clin Psychopharm* 13:251-256, 1993.

Schneirla TC, Rosenblatt JS, Tobach E: Maternal behavior in the cat. In: *Maternal Behavior in Mammals*, ed. Rheingold HR. John Wiley & Sons, New York: 122-168, 1963.

Schwartz MA, Koechlin BA, Postma E, Palmer S, Krol G: Metabolism of diazepam in rat, dog, and man. *J Pharmacol Exp Ther* 149:423-435, 1965.

Schwartz S: Naltrexone-induced pruritus in a dog with tail-chasing behavior. *JAVMA* 202(2):278-280, 1993.

Scott J: Social genetics. *Behavior Genetics* 7:327-346, 1977.

Scott J, Shepherd J, Werboff J: Inhibitory training of dogs: effects of age at training in Basenjis and Shetland Sheepdogs. *J Psychol* 66:217-252, 1967.

Scott JP: The analysis of social organization in animals. *Ecology* 37:213-221, 1956.

Scott JP: Critical periods in the development of social behavior in puppies. *Psychosomatic Med* 20:42-54, 1958.

Scott JP: Critical periods in behavioural development. *Science* 138:949-958, 1962.

Scott JP: The evolution of social behaviour of dogs and wolves. *Am Zool* 7:373-381, 1967a.

Scott JP: Evolution and domestication of the dog. In: *Evolutionary Biology*, vol 2., eds. Dobzhansky T, Hecht M, Steere W. Appleton-Century-Crofts, New York: 243-275, 1968.

Scott JP: The process of primary socialization in canine and human infants. Monographs of the Society for Research in Child Development 28:1-49, 1963.

Scott JP, Beilfelt S: Analysis of the puppy testing program. In: *Guide Dogs for the Blind: Their Selection, Development, and Training*, eds. Pfaffenberger CJ, Scott JP, Fuller JL, Ginsburg BE, Bielfelt SW. Elsevier, New York: 39-75, 1976.

Scott JP, Bronson F, Trattner A: Differential human handling in the development of agonistic behavior in Basenji and Shetland Sheepdogs. *Devel Psychobiol* 1:133-140, 1968.

Scott JP, Charles N: Genetic differences in the behavior of dogs: a case of magnification by thresholds and habit formation. *J Genetic Psychol* 84:175-188, 1954.

Scott JP, Fuller JL: *Genetics and the Social Behavior of the Dog*. University of Chicago Press, Chicago, 1965.

Scott JP, Marston MV: Critical periods affecting normal and maladjustive social behavior in puppies. *J Genetic Psychol* 77:25-60, 1950.

Scott JP, Stewart JM, DeGhett UJ: Critical periods in the organization of systems. *Devel Psychobiol* 7:489-513, 1974.

Scott PP: Cats. In: *Reproduction and Breeding Techniques for Laboratory Animals*, ed. Hafez ESE. Lea & Febiger, Philadelphia: 192-208, 1970.

Searle AG: Gene frequencies in London's cats. *J Genet* 49: 214-220, 1949.

Sechzer JA, Brown JL: Color discrimination in the cat. *Science* 144:427-429, 1964.

Segall S: Opium addiction in the dog. *JAVMA* 144:603-604, 1964.

Segrest M, Clifford D: Are Pit Bulls different? Part 1. *Community Animal Control* 5:14-17, 1986a.

Segrest M, Clifford D: Are Pit Bulls different? Part 2. *Community Animal Control* 5:16-17, 1986b.

Seitz PFD: Infantile experience and adult behavior in animal subjects. II. Age of separation from the mother and adult behavior in the cat. *Psychosomatic Medicine* 21:353-378, 1959.

Seksel K: Use of bromocriptine in spraying. *Appl Anim Behav Sci* 46:132, 1995.

Seligman ME: Phobias and preparedness. *Behav Ther* 2:307-320, 1971.

Seligman ME, Mineka S: Conditioned drinking produced by procaine, NaCl, and angiotensin. *J Comp Physiol Psych* 77(1):110-121, 1971.

Selye H: The Story of Adaptation Syndrome, Montreal, ACTA.

Serpell J: The domestication and history of the cat. In: *The Domestic Cat: The Biology of Its Behavior*, eds. Turner D, Bateson P. Cambridge University Press, Cambridge: 151-158, 1988.

Serpell J, Jagoe JA: Early experience and the development of behaviour. In: *The Domestic Dog: Its Evolution, Behaviour, and Interactions with People*, ed. Serpell J. Cambridge University Press, Cambridge: 80-102, 1995.

Serpell JA: The influence of inheritance and environment on canine behaviour—myth and fact. In: Canine Development Throughout Life. Waltham Symposium, #8, ed. Edney ATB. *J Sm Anim Pract* 28:949-956, 1987.

Shaikh MB, Dalsass M, Siegel A: Opioidergic mechanisms mediating aggressive behavior in the cat. *Aggr Behav* 16:191-206, 1990.

Shalter MD, Fentress JC, Young GW: Determinants of response of wolf pups to auditory signals. *Behaviour* 60:98-114, 1977.

Shanley KS, Overall KL: Psychogenic dermatoses. In: *Current Veterinary Therapy. XI. Small Animal Practice*, eds., Kirk RW, Bongura JD. WB Saunders, Philadelphia: 552-558, 1992.

Shanley KS, Overall KL: Rational use of antidepressants for behavioral conditions. *Veterinary Forum* 11:30-34, 1995.

Sharman DF: Brain dopamine metabolism and behavioural problems of farm animals. *Advances Biochem Psychopharmacol* 19:249-254, 1978.

Sharman DF, Mann SP, Fry JP, Banns H, Stephens DB: Cerebral dopamine metabolism and stereotyped behaviour in early-weaned piglets. *Neuroscience* 7:1937-1944, 1982.

Sheard MH: Lithium in the treatment of aggression. *J Nervous Mental Dis* 160:108-118, 1975.

Sheldon JW: Wild Dogs: *The Natural History of the Nondomestic Canidae*. Academic Press, San Diego, 1992.

Shell LG: Feline hyperesthesia syndrome. *Feline Pract* 22(6):10, 1994.

Shell LG: Sleep disorders. In: *Textbook of Veterinary Internal Medicine*, eds. Ettinger SJ, Feldman EC. WB Saunders, Philadelphia: 157-158, 1995.

Shouldberg N: The efficacy of fluoxetine (Prozac) in the treatment of lick and inhalant allergic dermatitis in canines. *Proc Am Acad Vet Derm Am Coll Vet Derm* 1990:31-32, 1990.

Shull EA: Analysis and treatment of noise phobias. Paper presented at AVMA, San Francisco, July 1993.

Shull-Selcer EA, Stagg W: Advances in understanding and treatment of noise phobias. *Vet Clin North Am: Sm Anim Pract* 22:353-367, 1991.

Sibly RM, Smith RH: Behavioral Ecology: *Ecological Consequences of Adaptive Behaviour*. Blackwell Scientific Publications, Oxford, 1985.

Siegal A, Edinger H, Koo A: Suppression of attack behavior in the cat by the prefrontal cortex: role of the mediodorsal thalamic nucleus. *Brain Res* 127:185-190, 1977.

Siegal A, Pott CB: Neural substrates of aggression in flight in the cat. *Prog Neurobiol* 31:261-283, 1988.

Siegel A, Edinger H, Dotto M: Effects of electrical stimulation of the lateral aspect of the prefrontal cortex upon attack behavior in cats. *Brain Res* 93:473-484, 1975.

Sigler L: Pet behavioral problems present opportunities for practitioners. *AAHA Trends* 4:44-45, 1991.

Signoret J-P: Influence of the sexual receptivity of a teaser ewe on the mating preference in the ram. *Appl Anim Ethol* 1:229-232, 1975.

Simmel EC, Baker E: The effects of early experieinces on later behavior: a critical discussion. In: *Early Experiences and Early Behavior: Implications for Social Development,* ed. Simmell EC. Academic Press, New York: 3-13, 1980.

Simonson M: Effects of maternal malnourishment, development and behavior in successive generations in the rat and cat. In: Malnutrition, Environment and Behavior, ed. Levitsky DA. Cornell University Press, Ithaca, 1979.

Singh L, Lewis AS, Field MJ, Hughes J, Woodruff GN: Evidence for involvement of the brain cholecystokinin B receptor in anxiety. *Proc Natl Acad Sci USA* 88:1130-1133, 1991.

Skinner BF: *The Behavior of Organisms.* Appleton-Century-Crofts, New York, 1938.

Slabbert JM, Rasa OAE: The effect of early separation from the mother on pups in bonding to humans and pup health. *J South Afr Vet Assoc* 64:4-8, 1993.

Sloan M: Of wolves, wolf hybrids and children. *Latham Letter* 12(3):11-13, 1991.

Slobodchikoff CN: *The Ecology of Social Behavior.* Academic Press, San Diego, 1988.

Smiley LE, Schotte CS, Ginsburg BE: Analysis of the vocalizations of coyote-dog hybrids: a preliminary report. Paper presented at the Animal Behavior Society Meeting, University Park, Penn, 1977. Cited in MacKenzie et al, 1986.

Smirnova T, Laroche S, Errington ML, Hicks AA, Bliss TVP, Mallet J: Transsynaptic expression of a presynaptic glutamate receptor during hippocampal long-term potentiation. *Science* 262:433-436, 1993.

Smirnova T, Stinnakre J, Mallet J: Characterization of a presynaptic glutamate receptor. *Science* 262:430-433, 1993.

Smith BA, Jansen GR: Behavior and brain composition of offspring of underfed cats. *Fed Proc* 36:1108, 1977a.

Smith BA, Jansen GR: Maternal undernutrition in the feline: brain composition of offspring. *Nutrition Reports International* 16:497-512, 1977b.

Smith BA, Jansen GR: Maternal undernutrition in the feline: behavioral sequelae. *Nutrition Reports International* 16:513-526, 1977c.

Smith DW, Gong BT: Scalp and hair patterning: Its origins and significance relative to early brain and upper facial development. *Teratology* 9:17-34, 1974.

Smith SL: Interactions between pet dog and family members: an ethological study. In: *New Perspectives on Our Lives With Companion Animals,* eds. Beck AM, Katcher AH. University of Pennsylvania Press, Philadelphia: 29-36, 1983.

Smith WJ: *The Behavior of Communicating: An Ethological Approach.* Harvard University Press, Cambridge, Massachusetts, 1977.

Smith WJ: Consistency in change in communication. In: *The Development of Expressive Behavior: Biology-Environment Interactions,* ed. Zivin G. Academic Press,San Diego, California: 51-76, 1985.

Smith WJ: Message, meaning and context in ethology. *American Naturalist* 99:405-409, 1965.

Smith WJ: Referents of animal communication. *Anim Behav* 29:1273-1275, 1981.

Snyder SH: Neurotransmitters and CNS disease: schizophrenia. *Lancet* 30 October 1982:970-973, 1982.

Snyder SH: No endothelial NO. *Nature* 377:196-197, 1995.

Soares CJ: The companion animal in the context of the family system. In: *Pets and the Family,* ed. Sussman MB. Haworth Press, New York: 49-62, 1985.

Sohn RS, Ferrendelli JA: Anticonvulsant drug mechanisms. Phenytoin, phenobarbital, and ethoxsuximide and calcium flux in isolated presynaptic endings. *Arch Neurol* 33:626-629, 1976.

Sojka NJ, Jennings LL, Hamner CF: Artificial insemination in the cat *(Felis catus L.). Lab Anim Care* 20:198-204, 1970.

Soubrie P: Reconciling the role of central serotonin neurons in human and animal behavior. *Behav Brain Sci* 9:319-335, 1986.

Southwick CH: Effect of maternal environment on aggressive behavior of inbred mice (abstract). *Am Zool* 7:794, 1967.

Southwick CH: Effect of maternal environment on aggressive behavior of inbred mice. *Communications in Behavioral Biology* A 1:129-132, 1968.

Sprague RH, Anisko JJ: Elimination patterns in the laboratory Beagle. *Behaviour* 47:257-267, 1973.

Spreat S, Spreat SR: Learning principles. *Vet Clin North Am: Sm Anim Pract* 12:593-606, 1982.

Stabenfeldt GH: Physiologic, pathologic, and therapeutic roles of progestins in domestic animals. *JAVMA* 164:311-317, 1974.

Stanley W, Bacon W, Fehr C: Discriminated instrumental learning in neonatal dogs. *J Compar Psychol Physiol* 70:335-343, 1970.

Stanley WC, Elliot O: Differential human handling as reinforcing events and as treatments influencing later social behavior in Basenji puppies. *Psychological Reports* 10:775-788, 1962.

Stead AC: Euthanasia in the dog and cat. *J Sm Anim Pract* 23:37-43, 1982.

Stein DJ, Hollander E, Chan S, DeCaria CM, Hilal S, Liebowitz MR, Klein DF: Computed tomography and neurological soft signs in obsesssive-compulsive disorder: detection with magnetic resonance imaging. *Psychiatr Res Neuroimaging* 50:143-150, 1993.

Steinberg JL, Garver DL, Moeller FG, Raese JD, Orsulak PJ: Serum homoranillic acid levels in schizophrenic patients and normal control subjects. *Psychiat Res* 48:93-106, 1993.

Sterman MB, Wyrwicka W, Roth S: Electrophysiological correlates and neural substrates of alimentary behavior in the cat. *Ann NY Acad Sci* 157:723-739, 1969.

Sternbach H: The serotonin syndrome. *Am J Psychiatry* 148:705-713, 1991.

Stogdale L, Delack JB: Feline purring. *Comp Cont Educat Pract Vet* 7:551-553, 1985.

Strack M, Bernstein P: A game of cat and house: home ranges, favored spots, and time-sharing patterns of 14 house-bound domestic cats. Abstract presented at the ABS, UC-Davis, July 1993.

Stubbs W, Bloomberg MS: Implication of early neutering in the dog and cat. *Semin Vet Med Surg (Sm Anim)* 10:8-12, 1995.

Stur I: Genetic aspects of temperament and behavior in dogs. *J Sm Anim Pract* 28(11):957-964, 1987.

Stur I, Kreiner M, Mayrhofer G: Investigation into judging temperament parameters in dogs. *Wiener Tieraerztliche Monatsschrift* 76:290-294, 1989.

Suomi SJ, Kraemer CW, Baysinger CM, Delizio RD: Inherited

and experimental factors associated with individual difference in anxious behavior displayed by rhesus monkeys. In: *Anxiety: New Research and Changing Concepts*, eds. Klein DF, Rabkin J. Raven Press, New York: 179-199, 1981.

Sutin J, Michael RP: Changes in brain electrical activity following vaginal stimulation in estrous and anestrous cats. *Physiol Behav* 5:1043-1051, 1970.

Sutin J, Rose J, Van Atta L, Thalmann R: Electrophysiological studies in an animal model of aggressive behavior. *Res Publ Assoc Res Nerv Ment Dis* 52:93-118, 1974.

Swedo SE, Pietrini P, Leonard HL, Schapiro MB, Rettew DC, Goldberger EL, Rapoport SI, Rapoport JL, Grady CL: Cerebral glucose metabolism in childhood-onset obsessive-compulsive disorder: revisualization during pharmacotherapy. *Arch Gen Psychiatry* 49:690-694, 1992.

Syme GJ: Competitive orders as measures of social dominance. *Anim Behav* 22:931-940, 1974.

Symons M, Bell K: Canine blood groups: description of 20 specificities. *Anim Gen* 23:509-515, 1992.

Tamases-Fisher G, Volhard W: Puppy personality profile. *AKC Gazette*, March: 36-42, 1985.

Tan P, Counsilman J: The influence of weaning on prey-catching behavior in kittens. *Zeitschrift für Tierpsychologie* 70:148-164, 1985.

Tancer ME, Stein MB, Bessetle BB, Uhde TW: Behavioral effects of chronic imipramine treatment in genetically nervous pointer dogs. *Physiological Behavior* 48(1):179-181, 1990.

Tapia F: Children who are cruel to animals. *Child Psychiatry and Human Development* 2:70-77, 1971.

Taubøll E, Gjerstad L: Comparison of 5α-pregnan-3α-01-20-one and phenobarbital on cortical synaptic activation and inhibition studied *in vitro*. *Epilepsia* 34(2):228-235, 1993.

Taylor DB: Buspirone: a new approach to the treatment of anxiety. *FASEB J* 2:2445-2452, 1988.

Taylor DP, Elson MS, Riblet LA, Vandermaelen CP: Pharmacological and clinical effects of buspirone. *Pharmacology, Biochemistry and Behavior* 23:687-694, 1985.

Tedesco FJ, Mills LR: Diazepam (Valium) hepatitis. *Dig Dis Sci* 27:470-472, 1982.

Teicher M: Biology of anxiety. *Med Clin North Am* 72:791-813, 1988.

Terenius L, Wahlstrom A, Lindstrom L et al.: Increased CSF levels of endorphines in chronic psychosis. *Neuroscience Letters* 3:157-162, 1976.

Terlouw WM, Lawrence AB: Long-term effects of food allowance and housing on development of stereotypies in pigs. *Appl Anim Behav Sci* 38:103-126, 1993.

Thompson RT, Heron W: The effects of early restriction on activity in dogs. *J Compar Physiol Psychol* 47:77-82, 1954.

Thompson T: Aggressive behaviour of Siamese fighting fish. In: *Aggressive Behaviour*, eds. Garattini S, Sigg EB. Excerpta Medica Foundation, Amsterdam: 15-31, 1969.

Thompson T, Grabowski J: *Behavior Modification of the Mentally Retarded*. Oxford University Press, New York, 1977.

Thompson WR, Heron W: The effects of early restriction on activity in dogs. *J Compar Physiol Psychol* 47:77-82, 1954.

Thompson WR, Melzack R, Scott TH: "Whirling behavior" in dogs as related to early experience. *Science* 123:939, 1956.

Thoren P, Asberg M, Cronholm B: Clomipramine treatment of obsessive-compulsive disorder. *Arch Gen Psychiatry* 37:1281-1285, 1980.

Thorndike EL: *Animal Intelligence*. MacMillan, New York, 1911.

Thorne CJ: Feeding behaviour in the cat—recent advances. *J Sm Anim Pract* 23:555-562, 1982.

Thorne FC: The inheritance of shyness in dogs. *J Genetic Psychology* 66:275-279, 1944.

Thyer BA, Parrish RT, Curtis GC et al.: Ages of onset of DSM-III anxiety disorders. *Comp Psychiatry* 26:113-122, 1985.

Tinbergen N: The functions of territory. *Bird Study* 4:14-27, 1957.

Todd MB: Inheritance of the catnip response in domestic cats. *J Heredity* 53:54-56, 1962.

Tompkins DC, Steigbigel RT: Rochalimea's role in cat scratch disease and bacillary angiomatosis. *Ann Intern Med* (5 & 6) 118:288-290, 1993.

Toner BS, Miller DI Jr: Olfactory discrimination of individual human odors using experienced tracking police and work dogs. *Anim Behav Consult Newsletter* 10(4):2-4, 1993.

Troutman CM: Cat owners and their use of veterinary services. *JAVMA* 193:1217-1219, 1988.

Tsirka SE, Guanlandris A, Amaral DG, Strickland S: Excito-toxin-induced neuronal degeneration and seizure are mediated by tissue plasminogen activator. *Nature* 377:340-344, 1995.

Tuber DS, Hothersall D, Peters MF: Treatment of fears and phobias in dogs. *Vet Clin North Am: Sm Anim Pract* 12(4):607-623, 1982.

Tucker AO, Tucker SS: Catnip and the catnip response. *Economic Botany* 42:214, 231, 1988.

Turnbull PF, Reed CA: The fauna from the terminal Pleistocene of Palegawra Cave, a Zorzian occupation site in northeastern Iraq. *Fieldiana Anthropology* 63:81-146, 1974.

Turner DC: The ethology of the human-cat relationship. *Animalis Familiaris* 3:16-21, 1988.

Turner DC: The ethology of the human-cat relationship. *Swiss Arch Vet Med* 133:63-70, 1991.

Turner DC, Bateson P: *The Domestic Cat: The Biology of Its Behavior*. Cambridge University Press, Cambridge, 1988.

Turner DC, Feaver J, Mendl M, Bateson P: Variations in domestic cat behaviour towards humans: a paternal effect. *Anim Behav* 34:1890-1892, 1986.

Turner DC, Meister O: Hunting behaviour of the domestic cat. In: *The Domestic Cat: The Biology of Its Behaviour*, eds. Turner DC, Bateson P. Cambridge University Press, Cambridge: 111-122, 1988.

Turner DC, Mertens C: Home-range size, overlap, and exploration in domestic farm cats *(Felis catus)*. *Behaviour* 99:22-45, 1986.

Turner DC, Stammach-Geering MK: Owner assessment and the ethology of human-cat relationships. In: *Pets, Benefits, and Practice*, ed. Berger IH. British Veterinary Association Publications, London, 1990.

Turner P, editor: *Pliny's Natural History* in Phileman Holland's Translation. Centaur Press, London, England, 1962.

Uhde TW, Boulenger J-P, Roy-Byrne PP, Geraci MF, Vittone BJ, Post RM: Longitudinal course of panic disorder. *Prog Neuropsychopharmacol Biol Psychiatry* 9:39-51, 1985.

Ulrich R: Pain as a cause of aggression. *Am Zool* 6:643-662, 1966.

Underman A: Bite wounds inflicted by dogs and cats. *Vet Clin North Am: Sm Anim Pract* 17:195-207, 1987.

Van Winkle T, Summers B, deLahunta A: Behavioral cases with neurological complications. *AVSAB Newsletter* 16(2):3-4, 1994.

Van der Velden NA, De Weerdt CJ, Brooymans-Schallenberg JHC, Tielen AM: An abnormal behavioural trait in Bernese Mountain Dogs (Berner Sennenhund): a preliminary report. *Tijdschrift Diergeneesk* 101:403-407, 1976.

Van Hooff JARAM, Wensing JAB: Dominance and its behavioral measures in a captive wolf pack. In: *Man and Wolf*, ed. Frank

H. Dr. W Junk Publishers, Dordrecht, The Netherlands: 219-252, 1987.

Van Ness JJ: Electrophysiological evidence of sensory nerve dysfunction in 10 dogs with acral lick dermatitis. *JAAHA* 22:157-160, 1986.

Van Putten G, Dammers J: A comparative study of the well-being of piglets reared conventionally and in cages. *Appl Anim Ethol* 2:339-356, 1976.

Van Putten G, Elsof WJ: Inharmonious behaviour of veal-calves. In: *Disturbed Behaviour in Farm Animals*, ed. Bessei W. Verlag Eugen Ulmer, Stuttgart: 61-71, 1982.

Vandenberg JG: The effect of gonadal hormones on the aggressive behavior of adult golden hamsters. *Anim Behav* 19:589-594, 1971.

Verberne G, de Boer J: Chemocommunication among domestic cats, mediated by the olfactory and vomeronasal senses. *Zeitschrift für Tierpsychologie* 42:86-109, 1976.

Villablanca JR, Olmstead CE: Neurological development in kittens. *Devel Psychobiol* 12:101-127, 1979.

Villars TA: Hormones and aggressive behavior in teleost fish. In: *Hormones and Aggressive Behavior*, ed. Svare BB. Plenum, New York: 407-433, 1983.

Vochteloo JD, Koolhaas JM: Medial amygdala lesions in male rats reduce aggressive behavior: interference with experience. *Physiol Behav* 41:99-102, 1987.

Voith VL: Animal behavior problems: an overview. In: *New Perspectives on Our Lives with Companion Animals*, eds. Katcher A, Beck A. University of Pennsylvania Press, Philadelphia: 181-186, 1983a.

Voith VL: Applied animal behavior and the veterinary profession: A historical account. *Vet Clin North Am: Small Anim Pract* 22:203-206, 1991.

Voith VL: Attachment of people to companion animals. *Vet Clin North Am: Sm Anim Pract* 15:289-295, 1985.

Voith VL: Behavior disorders. In: *Textbook of Veterinary Internal Medicine*, ed. Ettinger S. Saunders, Philadelphia: 208-227, 1983b.

Voith VL: Behavioural problems. In: *Canine Medicine and Therapeutics*, eds. Chandler EA, Sutton JB, Thompson DJ. Blackwell Scientific Publications, Oxford: 499-537, 1984a.

Voith VL: Diagnosing dominance aggression. *Mod Vet Pract* 62(9):717-718, 1981b.

Voith VL: Fear-induced aggression in dogs. Part I. *Canine Pract* 3(5):14-18, 20, 1976a.

Voith VL: Fear-induced aggressive behavior. In: *Canine Behavior*, ed. Hart BL. Veterinary Practice Publishing Company, Santa Barbara, Ca: 59-62, 1980a.

Voith VL: Fear-induced aggressive behavior. Part II. *Modern Vet Pract* 3(6):14-16, 1976b.

Voith VL: Female reproductive behavior. In: *Current Therapy in Theriogenology* ed. Morrow D. WB Saunders, Philadelphia: 839-843, 1980b.

Voith VL: Functional significance of pseudocyesis. *Modern Vet Pract* 61(1):75-77, 1980c.

Voith VL: Hyperactivity and hyperkinesis. *Modern Vet Pract* 61(9):787-789, 1980d.

Voith VL: Intermale aggression in dog. *Modern Vet Pract* 61(3):256-258, 1980e.

Voith VL: Learning principles in behavioral problems. *Modern Vet Pract* 60(7):553-555, 1979a.

Voith VL: Looking at the attachment between people and their pets: Behavior problems of pets that arise from the relationship between pets and people. In: *Interrelations Between People and Pets*, ed. Fogel B. CC Thomas Publisher, Springfield, Il: 271-294, 1981c.

Voith VL: Multiple approaches to treating behavior problems. *Modern Vet Pract* 60(8):651-654, 1979b.

Voith VL: Owner/pet attachment despite behavior problems. In: *Pet Loss and Human Bereavement*, eds. Kay WJ et al. Iowa State University Press, Ames: 135-142, 1984b.

Voith VL: Play: a form of hyperactivity and aggression. *Modern Vet Pract* July:63-64, 1980f.

Voith VL: Play behavior interpreted as aggression or hyperactivity: case histories. *Modern Vet Pract* 61:707-709, 1980g.

Voith VL: Possible pharmacological approaches to treating behavior problems in animals. In: *Nutrition and Behavior in Dogs and Cats*, ed. Andersen RS. Pergamon Press, Inc., Oxford: 227-234, 1984c.

Voith VL: Principles of learning. *Vet Clin North Am: Equine Pract* 2:485-506, 1986.

Voith VL: Profile of 100 animal behavior cases. *Modern Vet Pract* 62(6):483-484, 1981d.

Voith VL: Prognosis of treatment for aggressive behavior of dogs towards children. *Modern Vet Pract* 61(11):939-942, 1980h.

Voith VL: Teaching sit-stay. *Modern Vet Pract* 63(5):317-320, 1982a.

Voith VL: Teaching the down-stay. *Modern Vet Pract* 63(5):425, 1982b.

Voith VL: Therapeutic approaches to feline urinary behavior problems. *Modern Vet Pract* 61(6):539-542, 1980.

Voith VL: Treatment of dominance aggression of dogs towards people. *Modern Vet Pract* 63:149-152, 1982c.

Voith VL, Borchelt PL: Diagnosis and treatment of dominance aggression in dogs. *Vet Clin North Am: Sm Anim Pract* 12(4):655-663, 1982a.

Voith VL, Borchelt PL: Diagnosis and treatment of elimination behavior problems in dogs. *Vet Clin North Am: Sm Anim Pract* 12(4):637-644, 1982b.

Voith VL, Borchelt PL: Elimination behavior and related problems in dogs. Compendium of Continuing Education for the Practicing Veterinarian 7:537-546, 1985a.

Voith VL, Borchelt PL: Introduction to animal behavior therapy. *Vet Clin North Am: Sm Anim Pract* 12(4):565-570, 1982c.

Voith VL, Borchelt PL: Separation anxiety in dogs. Compendium of Continuing Education for the Practicing Veterinarian 7(4):42-53, 1985b.

Voith VL, Borchelt PL: Social behavior of domestic cats. Compendium of Continuing Education for the Practicing Veterinarian 8(9):637-646, 1986.

Voith VL, Marder AR: Canine behavior disorders. In: *Handbook of Small Animal Practice*, ed. Morgan RV. Churchill Livingstone, New York: 1033-143, 1988.

Voith VL, Wright JC, Danneman PJ: Is there a relationship between canine behavior problems and spoiling activity, anthropomorphism, and obedience training? *Appl Anim Behav Sci* 34:263-272, 1992.

Volkava J, Magno-Zito J, Vitrai J, Czobor P: Clozapine effects on hostility and aggression in schizophrenia (letter). *J Clin Psychopharmacol* 13:287-289, 1993.

Vom Saal FS: The intrauterine position phenomenon: effects on physiology, aggressive behavior, and population dynamics in house mice. In: *Biological Perspectives on Aggression*, eds. Flannelly KJ, Blanchard RJ, Blanchard DC. Liss, New York: 135-179, 1984.

vom Saal FS: Sexual differentiation in litter-bearing mammals: influence of sex of adjacent fetuses in utero. *J Anim Sci* 67:1824-1840, 1989.

vom Saal FS: Variation in phenotype due to random interuterine positioning of male and female fetuses in rodents. *J of Reprod Fertil* 62:633-650, 1981.

Waechter RA: Unusual reaction to acepromazine maleate in the dog. *JAVMA* 180:733-74, 1982.

Waddington CH: *The Strategy of Genes.* Allen & Unwin, London, 1957.

Walker R: Understanding aggression. In: *The Behaviour of Dogs and Cats,* ed. Fisher J. Stanley, Paul & Company, Ltd., Random House, London: 41-51, 1993.

Waller GR, Price GH, Mitchell ED: Feline attractant, Cis, trans-nepetalactone: metabolism in the domestic cat. *Science* 164:1281-1282, 1969.

Walls R, Murphree O, Angel C, Newton J: A multi-variate discriminate analysis of behavioral measures in genetically nervous dogs. *Pavlov J Biol Sci* 11:175-197, 1976.

Walther FR: Artiodactyla. In: *How Animals Communicate,* ed. Sebeok TA. Indiana University Press, Bloomington: 655-714, 1977.

Waring GH: *Horse Behavior.* Noyes Publishers, Parkridge, New Jersey, 1983.

Warren J, Levy S: Fearfulness in male and female cats. *Animal Learning and Behavior* 7:521-524, 1979.

Waterman K, Purves SJ, Kosaka B, Strauss E, Wada JA: An epileptic syndrome caused by medial frontal lobe seizure foci. *Neurol* 37(4):577-582, 1987.

Wayne RK: Molecular evolution of the dog family. *Trends Genetics* 9(6):218-224, 1993.

Wayne RK, Benveniste RE, Janczewski DN, O'Brien SJ: Molecular and biochemical evolution of the carnivora. In: *Carnivore Behavior, Ecology, and Evolution,* ed. Gittleman JL. Cornell Unviersity Press, Ithaca, New York: 465-494, 1989.

Wemmer C, Scow K: Communication in the felidae with emphasis on scent marking and contact patterns. In: *How Animals Communicate,* ed. Sebeok TA. Indiana University Press, Bloomington: 749-766, 1977.

Wenzel B: Tactile stimulation as reinforcement for cats and its relation to early feeding experience. *Psychological Reports* 5:297-300, 1959.

Werner BE, Taboda J: Use of analgesics in feline medicine. *Comp Cont Educ Pract Vet* 16:493-499, 1994.

Wessels DT: Family psychotherapy methodology: a model for veterinarians and clinicians. In: *Pet Loss and Human Bereavement,* eds. Kay WJ et al. Iowa State University Press, Ames: 175-184, 1984.

West MJ: Play in domestic kittens. In: *The Analysis of Social Interaction,* ed. Cairns RB. Lawrence Erlbaum, Hillside, New Jersey: 179-193, 1979.

West MJ: Social play in the domestic cat. *Am Zool* 14:427-436, 1974.

Whalen RE: Sexual behavior of cats. *Behaviour* 20:321-330, 1963.

White B, Watson TJ: *Betty White's Pet Love: How Pets Take Care of Us.* William Morrow and Company, New York, 1983.

White SD: Naltrexone for treatment of acral lick dermatitis in dogs. *JAVMA* 196:1073-1076, 1990.

White SD, Sequoia D: Food hypersensitivity in cats: 14 cases (1982-1987). *JAVMA* 194:692-695, 1989.

Wiepkema PR: On the identity and significance of disturbed behaviour in vertebrates. In: *Disturbed Behaviour in Farm Animals,* ed. Bessei W. Verlag Eugen Ulmer, Stuttgart: 8-17, 1982.

Wiepkema PR, Koolhaas JM, Oliver-Aardema R: Adapative aspects of neuronal elements in agonistic behaviour. *Progr Brain Res* 53:369-384, 1980.

Wiesenfeld-Hallin Z, Xu XJ: Role of cholecystokinin Type B re-

ceptor in nociception studied with peptide agonists and antagonists. *Meth Neurosci* 11:148-169, 1993.

Wilbur RH: Pets, pet ownership and animal control: social and psychological attitudes, 1975. In: Proceedings of the National Conference on Dog and Cat Control. American Humane Association, Denver: 21-34, 1976.

Wildt DE: Effect of transportation on sexual behavior of cats. *Lab Anim Sci* 30:910-912, 1980.

Willeberg P: Epidemiology of naturally occurring feline urologic syndrome. *Vet Clin North Am: Sm Anim Pract* 14:455-469, 1984.

Willis MB: Breeding of dogs for desirable traits. *J of Sm Anim Pract* 28(11):965-983, 1987.

Willis MB: *Genetics of the Dog.* Howell Book House, New York, NY, 1989.

Wilson M, Warren JM, Abbott L: Infantile stimulation, activity, and learning by cats. *Child Development* 36:843-853, 1965.

Wilson WH: Clinical review of clozapine treatment in a state hospital. *Hosp Commun Psychiatry* 43:700-703, 1992.

Winkler WG: Human deaths induced by dog bites, United States, 1974-1975. *Public Health Reports* 92:425-429, 1977.

Winslow CN: Observations of dominance-subordination in cats. *J Genetic Psychol* 52:425-428, 1938.

Winslow CN: Social behavior of cats. II. Competitive, aggressive and food-sharing behavior when both competitors have access to the goal. *J Compar Psychol* 37:315-326, 1944.

Wise JK, Yang J-J: Dog and cat ownership 1991-1998. *JAVMA* 204:1166-1167, 1994.

Wise JK, Yang J-J: Veterinary service market for companion animals, 1992, part I: companion animal ownership and demographics. *JAVMA* 201:990-992, 1992.

Wise RA, Dawson V: Diazepam-induced eating and lever pressing for food in sated rats. *J Compar Physiol Psychol* 86:930-941, 1974.

Wolfle TL: Control of stress using non-drug approaches. *JAVMA* 191:1219-1221, 1987.

Wolfle TL: Policy, program and people: the three P's to well-being. In: *Canine Research Environment,* eds. Mench JA, Krulisch L. Scientists' Center for Animal Welfare, Bethesda: 41-47, 1990.

Wolpe J: Parallels between animal and human neuroses. *Proc Ann Psychopathol Assoc* 55:305-313, 1967.

Wolski TR: Social behavior of the cat. *Vet Clin North Am: Sm Anim Pract* 12(4):693-706, 1982.

Wright J: The development of social structure during the primary socialization period in German Shepherds. *Developmental Psychobiol* 13:17-24, 1980.

Wright J: The effects of differential rearing on exploratory behavior in puppies. *Appl Anim Ethol* 10:27-34, 1983.

Wright J: Severe attacks by dogs: characteristics of the dogs, the victims, and the attack settings. *Public Health Rep* 100:55-61, 1985.

Wright JC: Canine aggression toward people: bite scenarios and prevention. *Vet Clin North Am: Sm Anim Pract* 21(2):299-314, 1991.

Wright JC: Reported dog bites: are owned and stray dogs different? *Anthrozöos* 4:113-119, 1990b.

Wright JC, Nesselrote MS: Classification of behavioral problems in dogs: distributions of age, breed, sex and reproductive status. *Appl Anim Beh Sci* 19:169-178, 1987.

Wuensch KL, Cooper AJ: Preweaning paternal presence and later aggressiveness in in male *Mus musculus. Behavioral Biol* 32:510-515, 1981.

Wyrwicka W: Imitation of mother's inappropriate food preference in weanling kittens. Pavlov J Biol Sci 13:55-72, 1978.

392 Clinical Behavioral Medicine for Small Animals

Yesavage JA: Correlates of dangerous behavior by schizophrenics in hospital. *Psychiatr Res* 18:225-231, 1984.

Young MS: Aggressive behavior. In: *Clinical Signs and Diagnosis in Small Animal Practice*, ed. Ford RB. Churchill Livingstone, New York: 135-150, 1988a.

Young MS: The evolution of domestic pets and companion animals. *Vet Clin North Am: Sm Anim Pract* 15(2):297-309, 1985.

Young MS: Puppy selection and evaluation. In: *Dogs: Companions or Nuisances?* Public Seminar Werrebee Veterinary Clinic Center 22:8-15, 1988b.

Young MS: What do "puppy tests" test? Paper presented at annual meeting of Animal Behavior Society, Raleigh, NC, 1985.

Young MS: Treatment of fear-induced aggression in dogs. *Vet Clin North Am: Sm Anim Pract* 12(4):645-653, 1982.

Yudofsky S, Silver J, Schneider S: Pharmacologic treatment of aggression. *Psychiatr Ann* 17:397-407, 1987.

Yudofsky SC, Silver JM, Jackson W Endicott J, Williams D: The overt aggression scale for the objective rating of verbal and physical aggression. *Am J Psychiatry* 143:35-39, 1986.

Zagrodzka J, Fonberg E: Amygdalar area involved in predatory behavior in cats. *Acta Neurobiologica Experimentia* 37:131-136, 1977.

Zametkin AJ, Rapoport JL: Neurobiology of attention deficit disorder with hyperactivity: where have we come in 50 years? *J Am Acad Child Adolesc Psychiat* 5:676-686, 1987.

Zangwill KM, Hamilton DH, Perkins BA, Regnery RL, Plikaytis BD, Hadler JL, Cartter ML, Wenger JD: Cat scratch disease in Connecticut—epidemiology, risk-factors, and evaluation of a new diagnostic test. *N Engl J Med* 329:8-13, 1993.

Zaumbrecker KI, Smith RE: Neutering of feral cats as an alternative to eradication programs. *JAVMA* 203:449-452, 1993.

Zeuner FE: *A History of Domesticated Animals*. Harper & Row, Publishers, Inc., New York, 1963.

Ziegler VE, Biggs JT, Wylie LT, Rosen SH, Hawf DJ, Coryell WH: Doxepin kinetics. *Clin Pharmacol Ther* 23:573-579, 1978.

Zuckerman M: Serotonin, impulsivity, and emotionality. *Behav Brain Sci* 9:348-349,1986.

Appendix A

CLIENT QUESTIONNAIRES

••

A-1 PRELIMINARY CLIENT QUESTIONNAIRE

Please complete these questions and return the questionnaire before the appointment if possible. Otherwise please bring it with you at the time of the appointment. All of your answers are confidential. PLEASE REMEMBER THAT YOU ARE REQUESTED TO BRING PROOF OF RABIES VACCINATION TO YOUR APPOINTMENT.

1. Pet's Name _____

   Your Name _____

2. Breed of Dog or Cat _____ Color _____

3. Age of Pet _____

4. Date of Birth of Pet (if known) _____

5. Sex _____

6. Is your pet spayed or castrated?   ☐ Yes   ☐ No

   If yes, at what age? _____

   Date neutered _____

   Reason for neutering _____

   Any behavioral changes after neutering? _____

7. If your pet is not neutered, do you plan to breed this dog or cat?

   ☐ Yes   ☐ No

8. Has this dog or cat ever been bred?

   ☐ Yes   ☐ No

   If female, did she experience heat cycles before neutering?

   ☐ Yes   ☐ No

   Age of first heat, if applicable _____

   Date(s) of heat cycle(s) _____

9. How old was your pet when you first acquired it? _____

10. Has this pet had other owners?

    ☐ Yes   ☐ No

    If so, how many? ☐ 1 ☐ 2 ☐ 3 ☐ 4 ☐ Unknown

    Why was this pet given up? _____

11. How long have you had this pet? _____

12. Where did you get this pet? _____

    ☐ Stray/Found

    ☐ Breeder

    ☐ SPCA/Humane shelter

    ☐ Breed Rescue Service

    ☐ Newspaper adoption advertisement (not breeder)

    ☐ Pet store

    ☐ Friend

    ☐ Other (Please explain) _____

13. Why did you get this pet? _____

14. When was your pet last vaccinated for:

    Distemper/Feline rhinotracheitis, etc. (date, if you know it) _____

    Rabies (date, if you know it) _____

15. Is this pet (please check all that apply):

    ☐ Allowed to run free, unsupervised

    ☐ Fenced/kenneled/run

    ☐ Leash-walked, only

    ☐ Outside, unleashed but supervised

    ☐ Indoors only

    ☐ Outdoors only (primarily cats)

16. What percentage of the day does your pet spend inside?

    _____

    What percentage of the day does your pet spend outside?

    _____

    What kind of a living situation do you have?

    ☐ Apartment

    ☐ Townhouse/condominium

    ☐ House with small yard

    ☐ House with large yard

    ☐ Farm

17. How many times is your dog or cat walked or let out per day?

    ☐ 0 ☐ 1 ☐ 2 ☐ 3 ☐ 4 ☐ 5 ☐ 6 ☐ 7 ☐ 8

    If your pet is walked, what is the average length of time for each walk (in minutes)? _____

18. How often is your pet fed meals each day?

    ☐ 1 ☐ 2 ☐ 3 ☐ 4

    How often is your pet fed treats (cat treats, dog biscuits, chewies) each day?

    ☐ 0 ☐ 1 ☐ 2 ☐ 3 ☐ 4

How often is your pet fed snacks from the table (i.e., human food) each day?

☐ 0 ☐ 1 ☐ 2 ☐ 3 ☐ 4

19. What exactly is your pet fed (include brand names)?

_____

20. Does your pet have any allergies? ☐ Yes ☐ No

Please specify _____

21. Does your pet have any preexisting or current medical problems?

☐ Yes ☐ No

If so, what are they? _____

22. Is your pet currently taking any medication to prevent heartworm?

☐ Yes ☐ No Brand _____

Is your pet currently taking any other medications?

☐ Yes ☐ No Types _____

23. Do you have any other pets besides this one?

☐ Yes ☐ No

If so, are any of these other pets ill?

☐ Yes ☐ No

24. Has your household changed since acquiring this pet?

☐ Yes ☐ No

If so, how?

☐ Death of human in family

☐ Death of pet in family

☐ Divorce

☐ Marriage

☐ Baby born

☐ Child moved

☐ Pet added

☐ Family moved

☐ Family schedule changed (lost or gained jobs)

☐ Other

25. Please list the people, *including yourself*, currently living in the household.

Name	Sex	Age	Relationship (Self, husband, wife, mother-in-law, etc.)	Occupation

Please mark with an asterisk (*) any of the above who are coming to the clinic with the pet. If anyone *Not listed* is coming with the pet, who are they (i.e., friend, neighbor)?

26. Please list all the animals in the household.

Name	Breed	Sex	Age Obtained	Age Now

Refer to the chart above and, using numbers, label which pet was obtained first, second, etc.

27. Do you know how many animals were in this pet's litter?

☐ Yes

Number = _____ (_____ females _____ males)

☐ No

28. Why did you choose this specific animal from the litter?

_____

29. Why did you choose this specific breed?

_____

30. Have you had this particular breed before?

☐ Yes ☐ No

31. Have you had pets before?

☐ Yes ☐ No

32. Have you had dogs before?

☐ Yes ☐ No

33. Have you had cats before?

☐ Yes ☐ No

34. Have you had birds before?

☐ Yes ☐ No

35. Where does your pet sleep (check all that apply; we know pets move at night)?

☐ In or on your bed

☐ On its own bed in your bedroom

☐ In its crate in your bedroom

☐ On its own bed in another room

☐ In a crate in another room

☐ On the floor next to your bed

☐ In another room, voluntarily, anywhere it wants

☐ In another room because it is locked from your bedroom, anywhere it wants

36. How often do you play with toys or play games with the pet inside the house daily (on average)?

    □ 0   □ 1   □ 2   □ 3   □ 4   □ 5   □ >5

    How long does each play bout last, on average (in minutes)? _____

37. How often do you play with toys or play games with the pet outside the house daily (on average)?

    □ 0   □ 1   □ 2   □ 3   □ 4   □ 5   □ >5

    How long does each play bout last, on average (in minutes)? _____

38. Describe, in detail, how you prepare to leave the house when the pet will be left alone. Do you ignore your pet, do you seek it out and say goodbye, do you make a fuss over it, etc.?

39. What does your pet do as you prepare to leave?

For Dogs Only

40. What is your dog's obedience school history?

    □ No school—trained yourself

    □ Puppy kindergarten

    □ Group lessons—basic

    □ Group lessons—advanced

    □ Private trainer at house

    □ Private trainer—sent to trainer

41. Age when dog started lessons/training _____

42. Who took the dog to obedience school? _____

43. How did the dog do in obedience school? _____

    Does the dog have any obedience titles? _____

44. What commands does the dog know and how well?

    □ Sit   Perfect   Usually OK   Needs work

    □ Stay   Perfect   Usually OK   Needs work

    □ Lie down   Perfect   Usually OK   Needs work

    □ Come   Perfect   Usually OK   Needs work

    □ Wait   Perfect   Usually OK   Needs work

    □ Heel   Perfect   Usually OK   Needs work

    □ Fetch   Perfect   Usually OK   Needs work

    □ Drop it   Perfect   Usually OK   Needs work

    □ Other _____

45. Is there anything else you would like to tell us about your dog's training?

For Cats Only

40. How many litter boxes do you have?

    □ 0   □ 1   □ 2   □ 3   □ 4   □ 5   □ 6   □ >6

41. Describe the litter boxes (check all that apply and put in parentheses the number of boxes for which the description is true).

Description	Number
□ Open	( )
□ Covered	( )
□ Square	( )
□ Rectangular	( )
□ Large	( )
□ Small	( )
□ Deep	( )
□ Shallow	( )
□ Liner	( )
□ No liner	( )

    □ Other—please specify: _____

42. What kind of litter material do you put in the box(es) (check all that apply)?

    □ Clumpable, recyclable

    □ Plain clay

    □ Deodorized

    □ Playground sand

    □ Anything you can get with a coupon

    □ Ashes

    □ Potting soil

    □ None (empty box)

    □ Gravel/rock

    □ Sawdust/wood chips

    □ Wheat husks

    □ Recycled, pelleted newspaper

    □ Shredded paper or paper toweling

    □ Other—please specify: _____

43. Where are the litter boxes (check all that apply)?

    □ Closet

    □ Kitchen

    □ Bathroom

    □ Bedroom

    □ Attic

    □ Entryway

    □ Pantry

    □ Basement

    □ Stairwell

    □ Other—please specify: _____

Feel free to include a diagram of your cat's litter box locations if you think that it would help us understand the situation.

44. Describe, in detail, how your cat uses the litter box. For example, does it scratch in the litter before eliminating? Cover up feces? Scratch outside box?

45. Are the front feet declawed?

    ☐ Yes

    ☐ No

Age declawed _____

Are the back feet declawed?

    ☐ Yes

    ☐ No

Age declawed _____

Is there anything else you would like to tell us about your cat's behavior?

46. What is (are) the behavioral problem(s) that you wish to address, and how much of a problem do you consider the behavior to be? Please use the chart below.

47. Why have you kept the pet despite its behavior problem?

48. Are you concerned that you may have caused the problem?

    ☐ Yes   ☐ No

Why? _____

49. Do you feel guilty about this problem?

    ☐ Yes   ☐ No

Why? _____

50. Have you considered finding another home for this pet?

    ☐ Yes   ☐ No

51. Have you considered euthanasia (putting your pet to sleep)?

    ☐ Yes   ☐ No

52. Did someone recommend euthanasia before your visit here?

    ☐ Yes   ☐ No

53. If you think that it would help us understand your pet's problem, attach a map of your house or the relevant areas of your house (i.e., locations of litter boxes or dog beds, locations of fences, etc.).

Problems	Very Serious	Serious	Not Serious

A-2 BEHAVIORAL HISTORY AT CLIENT/PATIENT VISIT*

Patient _____

Client _____

Date of Appointment _____

1. Chief complaints

    a.

    b.

    c.

    d.

2. Precipitating reason for visit

3. Number of total bites

    ☐ 0   ☐ 1   ☐ 2   ☐ 3   ☐ 4   ☐ 5   ☐ >5

4. Number of bites that broke skin

    ☐ 0   ☐ 1   ☐ 2   ☐ 3   ☐ 4   ☐ 5   ☐ >5

5. Number of bites reported and to whom (i.e., local authorities, hospital, humane society).

    Number reported

    ☐ 0   ☐ 1   ☐ 2   ☐ 3   ☐ 4   ☐ 5   ☐ >5

    Reported to: _____

6. Was there legal action taken against the owner as a result of the bite(s)?

    ☐ Yes

    ☐ No

7. Frequency of occurrence of the undesirable behavior(s):
    Complaint 1 _____

    ☐ Daily

    ☐ Weekly

    ☐ Monthly

    Percent of time that animal is in situation and during which undesirable behavior occurs:

    ☐ Less than 25%

    ☐ 25% to 50%

    ☐ 51% to 75%

    ☐ 76% to 100%

    Complaint 2 _____

    ☐ Daily

    ☐ Weekly

    ☐ Monthly

Percent of time that animal is in situation and during which undesirable behavior occurs:

☐ Less than 25%

☐ 25% to 50%

☐ 51% to 75%

☐ 76% to 100%

Complaint 3 _____

☐ Daily

☐ Weekly

☐ Monthly

Percent of time that animal is in situation and during which undesirable behavior occurs:

☐ Less than 25%

☐ 25% to 50%

☐ 51% to 75%

☐ 76% to 100%

Complaint 4 _____

☐ Daily

☐ Weekly

☐ Monthly

Percent of time that animal is in situation and during which undesirable behavior occurs:

☐ Less than 25%

☐ 25% to 50%

☐ 51% to 75%

☐ 76% to 100%

8. Has the frequency or the intensity of the occurrence of the behavior changed since the problem started?

    ☐ Yes

    ☐ No

    If so, how and when?

9. Record a detailed description of events and how long ago each event occurred.

    Most recent incident: Date _____

    Second most recent incident: Date _____

    Third most recent incident: Date _____

10. Chronological development of the problem; other significant incidents:

---

*If time is severely limited, questions 1 through 21 can be completed at home by the client, with questionaire A2 returned before the visit.

11. Duration of problem ____ Days ____ Months ____ Years

12. Corrections and/or medical therapy to date and outcome

13. Age of animal when it first began showing signs of the problem _____

    Client's impression:

    Practitioner's impression:

14. Do you know if the parents engage in similar behaviors as the presented animal?

    ☐ Yes, they do

    ☐ No, they do not

    ☐ Do not know

    If so, what behaviors are exhibited and by whom?

15. Does the client know if any littermates are engaging in same behaviors?

    ☐ Yes, they do

    ☐ No, they do not

    ☐ Do not know

    If so, what behaviors are exhibited and by whom?

16. Describe interactions between pets in the household.

17. How does the pet react to strangers?

18. How does the pet behave in veterinary offices and while being examined?

19. Has the pet ever been in a boarding kennel?

    ☐ Yes

    ☐ No

    If yes, how did the pet behave at the boarding kennel?

20. Has the pet ever been to a groomer?

    ☐ Yes

    ☐ No

    If so, how did the pet behave at the groomer?

21. Describe, in detail, 24 hours of a typical day in the pet's life starting with where the pet is when it wakes up in the morning.

Do not ask the following, but if, at any time during the interview, either of the following occurs, check yes and record the comment. If none of these topics are mentioned, check no at the end of the session. Record who makes the comments as well as what the comments are.

22. Describe the general activity level of the pet and interesting behaviors the pet engaged in over time as the interview progresses.

23. How did the animal interact with the client?

24. How did the animal interact with the practitioner during the physical examination and interview?

25. How did the animal react to strangers entering the room, noises in the room, being left alone in the room, other pets in the room, etc.

26. Describe the general activity level and behaviors that the people engaged in over time as the interview progresses.

27. How did the clients interact with the pet?

28. How did the clients interact with each other?

29. How did the clients interact with the practitioner?

30. Did the client express guilt that he or she caused the problem (regardless of what was stated on the entry questionnaire)?

    ☐ Yes

    ☐ No

31. Diagnosis and summary of problems

    a.

    b.

    c.

    d.

    e.

32. Does the pet need reexamination?

    ☐ Yes

    ☐ No

    How many?

    ☐ 1   ☐ 2   ☐ 3   ☐ >3

33. Describe plan for reexamination, including procedures to be practiced

34. Was any placement recommended or discussed?

    ☐ Yes

    ☐ No

    If so, when?

35. Was euthanasia recommended or discussed?

    ☐ Yes

    ☐ No

    Under what circumstances?

36. Was any laboratory work submitted?

    ☐ Yes

    ☐ No

    If so, which tests?

    Were there any abnormal results?

37. Was a head collar or a no-pull harness given (circle and specify)?

    ☐ Yes

    ☐ No

38. Were any behavioral medications or drugs prescribed?

    ☐ Yes

    ☐ No

    If so, which medications and at what dosage?

39. Which handouts were given (check all that are relevant)?

    ☐ Protocol for Deference: Basic Program

    ☐ Protocol for Relaxation: Behavior Modification Tier 1

    ☐ Behavior Modification Tier 2: Protocol for Desensitizing Dominantly Aggressive Dogs

    ☐ Behavior Modification Tier 2: Protocol for Desensitization and Counterconditioning Using Gradual Departures

    ☐ Protocol for Teaching Your Dog to Uncouple Departures and Departure Cues

    ☐ Tier 2: Protocol for Desensitizing and Counterconditioning a Dog (or Cat) From Approaches From Strangers

    ☐ Tier 2: Protocol for Desensitizing and Counterconditioning Dogs to Relinquish Objects

    ☐ Tier 2: Protocol for Desensitization and Counterconditioning to Noises and Activities That Occur by the Door

    ☐ Protocol for Dogs With Protective and/or Territorial Aggression

    ☐ Protocol for Dogs With Interdog Aggression

    ☐ Protocol for Dogs With Dominance Aggression

    ☐ Protocol for Treating and Preventing Attention-Seeking Behavior

    ☐ Protocol for Basic Manners Training and Housebreaking for New Dogs and Puppies

    ☐ Protocol for the Introduction of a New Pet to Other Household Pets

    ☐ Protocol for Cats With Elimination Disorders

    ☐ Protocol for Introducing a New Baby and a Pet

    ☐ Protocol for Dogs With Separation Anxiety

☐ Protocol for Dogs With Fearful Aggression

☐ Protocol for Cats With Intercat Aggression

☐ Protocol for Cats With Play Aggression

☐ Protocol for Redirected Aggression in Cats (and Dogs)

☐ Protocol for Status-Related Aggression in Cats

☐ Protocol for Treating Fearful Behavior in Cats and Dogs

☐ Protocol for Dogs and Interactions With Food, Rawhide, Biscuits, and Bones

☐ Protocol for Handling and Surviving Aggressive Events

☐ Protocol for Teaching Children (and Adults) to Play With Dogs and Cats

☐ Protocol for Choosing Collars, Head Collars, and Harnesses

☐ Protocol for Cats With Pica or Inappropriate Ingestion Conditions Including Wood Sucking

☐ Protocol for Cats With Barbering (Self-Mutilation)

40. What is the prognosis?

☐ Excellent

☐ Good

☐ Fair

☐ Guarded

☐ Poor

A-3   QUESTIONNAIRE FOR CATS WITH ELIMINATION DISORDERS

Questions 1 to 14 are summarized in a tabular form below for easy compilation of information.

1. How many litter boxes are available for the cat(s)?

2. How many of the litter boxes are covered?

3. What are the sizes of the boxes?

4. Where are the boxes?

5. How deep is the litter in each of the boxes?

6. Are liners ever used?

7. If liners are used, are they scented?

8. List all the types of litter used for each box.

9. Are any of the litters scented?

10. Does the cat respond differently to any of the above styles of boxes or litters, sizes of box, or depths of litters?

11. How frequently is the litter changed?

12. How frequently is the litter box washed and replaced?

13. Are deodorants used in the cleaning process?

14. How many cats actually share a litter box?

TABULAR ANSWERS FOR QUESTIONS 1-14

	Box 1	Box 2	Box 3	Box 4
1. Number of boxes				
2. Is the box covered?				
3. Size of box				
4. Location of box				
5. Depth of box				
6. Liner?				
7. Liner scented?				
8. Type of litter				
9. Litter scented?				
10. Response?				
11. Frequency of changing litter				
12. Frequency of washing box				
13. Deodorants used in cleaning?				
14. Number of cats sharing box				

15. What does the cat do in the litter box: does it get in, does it stand outside, does it dig in or out?

16. Is the cat ever allowed outside?

17. Does the animal eliminate in the presence of other animals or people, or is the elimination behavior secret?

18. Will the cat immediately use a freshly cleaned litter box?

19. Has the cat ever had any variation in whether it covers its feces or urine, and is any of that variation associated with the presence or absence of any other situation or cat?

20. Does the cat ever vocalize while it eliminates?

21. Will the cat spray against the back of a covered litter box?

22. Does the animal ever use a shower or a bath tub for elimination? If so, how frequently?

23. What other areas (get a complete list with locations and frequency of use) are ever used for elimination?

A-4 CANINE AGGRESSION SCREEN

KEY: NR = no reaction; SL = snarl/lift lip; BG = bark, growl (aggressive, *not* alerting bark); SB = snap/bite; NA = not applicable

This screen can be used in three ways: (1) to note the presence or absence, at any time, of any of the behaviors; (2) to log the baseline behavior, noting how many times the behavior occurs, given the number of times it is attempted, per unit time (i.e., per week); and (3) to log frequencies of the occurring behaviors, given the number of times the circumstance has been encountered, during treatment so that these numbers can be compared with (2). Note if the reaction is consistent in style or is directed toward only one person or is present in only one restricted circumstance. If this screen is being used as a client log, the circumstances must be evaluated for all people to whom the dog reacts. For any use, it is worth noting whether the dog is subjectively becoming more or less intense (or harder or easier to interrupt) in its behavior (>I [intensity], <I, relatively). If this screen is being used only for the initial consultation, note whether the dog has been worsening in intensity or frequency in any category. Interpretation of this screen is found in Chapter 6.

	NR	SL	BG	SB	NA
1. Take dog's food dish with food					
2. Take dog's empty food dish					
3. Take dog's water dish					
4. Take food (human) that falls on floor					
5. Take rawhide					
6. Take real bone					
7. Take biscuit					
8. Take toy					
9. Human approaches dog while eating					
10. Dog approaches dog while eating					
11. Human approaches dog while playing with toys					
12. Dog approaches dog while playing with toys					
13. Human approaches/disturbs dog while sleeping					
14. Dog approaches/disturbs dog while sleeping					
15. Step over dog					
16. Push dog off bed/couch					
17. Reach toward dog					
18. Reach over head					
19. Put on leash					
20. Human pushes on shoulders					
21. Dog mounts, pushes on shoulders					
22. Human pushes on rump					
23. Dog mounts, pushes on rump					
24. Towel feet when wet					
25. Bathe dog					

	NR	SL	BG	SB	NA
26. Groom dog's head					
27. Groom dog's body					
28. Human stares at dog					
29. Dog stares at dog					
30. Take muzzle in hands and shake					
31. Push dog over onto back					
32. Stranger knocks on door					
33. Stranger enters room					
34. Dog in car at toll booth					
35. Dog in car at gas station					
36. Dog on leash approached by dog on street					
37. Dog on leash approached by person on street					
38. Dog in yard—person passes					
39. Dog in yard—dog passes					
40. Dog in veterinarian's office					
41. Dog in boarding kennel					
42. Dog at groomer					
43. Dog yelled at					
44. Dog corrected with leash					
45. Dog physically punished—hit					
46. Someone raises voice to client in presence of dog					
47. Someone hugs/touches client in presence of dog					
48. Squirrels, cats, small animals approach dog					
49. Bicycles, skateboards nearby					
50. Crying infant					
51. Playing with 2-year-old children					
52. Playing with 5- to 7-year-old children					
53. Playing with 8- to 11-year-old children					
54. Playing with 12- to 16-year-old children					

KEY: NR = no reaction; SL = snarl/lift lip; BG = bark, growl (aggressive, *not* alerting bark); SB = snap/bite; NA = not applicable.

A-5 HISTORY SHEETS FOR ANIMALS WITH STEREOTYPIC AND RITUALISTIC BEHAVIORS

1. Into which of the following categories does the behavior fit?
   - ☐ Grooming (chewing/biting/licking self)
   - ☐ Hallucinatory (staring/tracking/attacking invisible prey)
   - ☐ Consumptive (consuming rocks, dirt, other objects/sucking wool)
   - ☐ Locomotory (circling/chasing tail/freezing/scratching)
   - ☐ Vocalization (rhythmic barking/barking/howling/growling)

2. Was there a change in the household or an event that was associated with the development of the behavior?

3. Is there any time of day when the behavior seems more or less intense? If so, what is usually going on at that time of day?

4. Is there a person/other pet in the presence of whom the behavior seems more intense? If so, who is this and what is their association to the pet?

5. What is the attitude of the pet while performing the behavior (i.e., distressed, self-absorbed, fearful)?

6. Does the animal respond to its name or seem aware of its surroundings during the behavior? Is it aware that you are calling it? How can you tell?

7. Can you convince the pet to stop the behavior by either (1) calling it or (2) using physical restraint?

8. What kinds of things, if any, will interrupt the behavior once it has started (i.e., noises, treats, toys)?

9. What does the client do when the behavior begins?

10. Is there a location in which the animal prefers to perform the behavior?

11. For ingestion, what types of objects are consumed? Be as specific as possible (e.g., type of rug, fabric, or sweater).

12. Is there a pattern to the behavior? What are the duration, frequency, and characteristics of the events themselves?
    Duration: days, weeks, months
    Frequency: hourly, daily, weekly, monthly, sporadic
    Pattern: after meals, in the morning (specify)

13. Does any event or behavior routinely occur immediately before the behavior begins?

14. Does any event or behavior routinely occur immediately after the behavior ceases?

15. Has the pet's general behavior changed in any way since the onset of the atypical behavior (e.g., the dog is more aloof, more aggressive)?

16. Has the pet's diet recently been changed?

17. Is there any other relevant information?

A-6 QUESTIONNAIRE FOR REEXAMINATION

Reexamination

☐ 1   ☐ 2   ☐ 3   ☐ 4+

Current Problems

1.

2.

3.

4.

5.

Problems Still to be Worked on After Reexamination

1.

2.

3.

4.

5.

Medications and Dosages

1.

2.

3.

Response to Medication (Changes in pet's behavior, problems, improvements, appearance of undesirable behaviors) (Be specific and check all that apply.)

☐ Profound side effects (specify)

☐ Minor side effects (specify)

☐ No side effects

☐ Wholly improved (100%)

☐ Decrease in frequency or extent of behaviors by 75% to 90%+

☐ Decrease in frequency or extent of behaviors by 50% to 74%

☐ Decrease in frequency or extent of behaviors by 25% to 49%

☐ Decrease in frequency or extent of behaviors by less than 25%

☐ No change at all

☐ Pet worse

Behavioral Questions

1. Have there been any incidents of the problems for which the client sought help since the client and the pet were last seen for an examination/consultation? If so, what happened, what were the circumstances, and how did the pet react? (Be specific.)

2. How is the client handling the situations that specifically gave him or her trouble (e.g., confining the pet when visitors come, getting a pet sitter when they go to work)? How are these efforts working, and what does the animal do when the client uses them?

3. Have there been any *new* behaviors (desirable or undesirable) that have developed since the first appointment or since beginning the behavior modification programs? If so, what specific behaviors have developed and in what circumstances do they occur?

4. Have there been any changes in the household (pet and human) since the patient was last seen?

5. Is this animal using a canine head collar or a no-pull harness?

   ☐ Yes

   ☐ No

   If so, has this helped with any of the problem behaviors? If so, which ones? Does the client have any questions about the appropriate use of head collars or harnesses?

6. How far has the client progressed in Tier 1 of the behavior modification programs? Is the client successfully and consistently exercising the behaviors discussed in the deference program?

7. Are there any parts of the programs with which the pet or client is having more difficulty than others?

8. Is there any family member who is having more trouble with the programs than others?

9. To whom does the pet currently best listen? Is this a change? Why does the client perceive that this difference exists (one person works with the pet more, one person still hits the pet)?

10. Does the client perceive any problems with the behavior modification techniques that you have asked to be used with the pets? Does the client dislike them, think they are too easy, think that the pet is too smart for them, not understand that they are not "obedience" programs? Is this interfering with the client's ability to shape a more appropriate behavior for the pet?

11. How does the client feel that the pet is progressing with regard to the intensity of the problems? Do he or she think that the pet is:

    ☐ Worse (behavior occurs more intensely than it did in the past)

    ☐ No change

    ☐ 25% improved (behavior is about three fourths of the intensity it would have been in the past; easier to interrupt)

    ☐ 50% improved (behavior is about half of the intensity it would have been in the past; easy to interrupt, can prevent)

    ☐ 75% improved (behavior is about one fourth of the intensity it would have been in the past; very easy to interrupt and prevent)

    ☐ 90%+ improved (behavior is easily prevented; it seldom occurs and, when it does, it is easy to interrupt).

12. How does the client feel that the pet is progressing with regard to the frequency of the problems? Does he or she think that the pet is:

    ☐ Worse (behavior occurs more frequently than it did in the past)

    ☐ No change

    ☐ 25% improved (behavior is about three fourths of the number of times it would have been in the past; easier to interrupt)

☐ 50% improved (behavior is about half of the number of times it would have been in the past; easy to interrupt, can prevent)

☐ 75% improved (behavior is about one fourth of the number of times it would have been in the past; very easy to interrupt and prevent)

☐ 90%+ improved (behavior is easily prevented, it seldom occurs and, when it does, it is easy to interrupt).

13. Has the program helped the clients in dealing with the pet (i.e., they are more relaxed, understanding, less tense, more confident, more informed)?

14. What have the reactions of others (neighbors, veterinarians, relatives) been to the pet-client participation in behavioral therapy?

15. Have the clients found that, in their discussions with others about the pet, other people have made helpful suggestions? If so, what, specifically, were these suggestions?

Questions Specifically for Clients With Cats With Elimination Problems

1. Have the clients changed the number of litter boxes? If so, how many do they have?

2. Have the clients tried other litters? If so, what types?

3. Which litter and litter box arrangement has worked best?

4. Have there been any incidents of inappropriate or undesirable elimination since the last appointment? If so, where and when?

5. Have the clients tried confining the cat or startling it with a water pistol or fog horn? If so, what was the response?

Summary Observations

1. How did the pet interact with the practitioner, client, nurses? (Be specific.) Is this a change from the last visit? If so, how is it different?

2. What is the pet's activity level? Is this a change?

3. Is there any difference in opinion about the progress of the pet either between the clients or between the client and the practitioner? If so, what is the discrepancy?

4. Is there any other information that the client or the practitioner believes is relevant for the reexamination (changes in diet, other illnesses)?

Appendix B

CLIENT HANDOUTS

••

CONTENTS

INTRODUCTION TO THE BEHAVIOR MODIFICATION PROTOCOLS

The following protocols are the ones used with clients and problem pets at the Behavior Clinic at the Veterinary Hospital of the University of Pennsylvania (VHUP). They have been developed and refined to meet the pets' needs and to minimize the client's confusion about how to work with a problem dog. These protocols were developed with much help, input, and initiative from the students who have worked in the Clinic. Some of these were modeled after and share commonalities with suggestions and programs (published and unpublished) of Drs. Ian Dunbar (Dunbar, 1991), Bruce Fogle (Fogle, 1990), Roger Mugford (Mugford, 1992), and Victoria Voith (Voith, 1982a,b; unpublished), and trainers Carol Lea Benjamin (Benjamin, 1985), and David Weston (Weston, 1990), and Ruth Ross (Weston and Ross, 1992). After I began to develop client handouts for treatment of specific problems, many practitioners asked for and received copies of early editions of the protocols for their use. Their comments and suggestions have been invaluable. Alterations were made by my student assistants, generations of students, and me to address the peculiar needs of problem pets and their people. Accordingly, as more is learned about behavioral problems and their treatment, these protocols will evolve.

These protocols are written for the average client. Practitioners should ensure that they themselves can understand and execute these protocols before recommending them to clients. In all cases the initial round of behavior modification should occur under the practitioner's supervision with his or her guidance. Videotaping the clients can help illustrate where they have not best responded with the dog or where the dog was signaling some intention or anxiety that the client missed or did not understand. Only after clients understand the program, have had it demonstrated to them, and can execute some part of it flawlessly with their pet should they begin to practice in earnest by themselves. The reasons for this are as follows:

1. These are *not* obedience exercises. At the outset clients should be disabused of the notion that this is fancy obedience. First, although sitting is part of obedience training, the goal of these programs is not just to have the dog sit, but also to relax and be receptive to changing its behavior while doing so. It is critical that clients understand and appreciate this difference. Dogs that are stressed or anxious cannot successfully learn a more appropriate behavior, and they certainly cannot associate that behavior with having fun or with good things. Second, if clients perceive that all we are doing is trying to teach the dog what it has already learned in training class, they will not see the need to comply. If we offer nothing different, what

is the point of behavior modification? It is the practitioner's job to teach clients that behavior modification and obedience training, although sharing many similarities, differ in the premise, interactive reward structure, goal, and outcome. Most dogs that undergo behavior modification have had some form of training and know how to sit. For a dog to do this successfully in a class (or even a show) situation, the dog does not have to be relaxed. That is not true for behavior modification.

2. The biggest problem is appropriate timing of rewards and corrections. Dogs read nonvocal communication or body language far better than most humans do. It is easy for them to subvert the exercise and to shape the behavior of the client. Problem dogs have been doing this already. Someone from outside the relationship needs to be able to comment on timing problems and instruct clients as to when to change their posture, their tone, or their quickness of praise or reward. Most clients are quite good at learning to do this, but they need help. After the initial demonstration the clients should show the practitioner what they are doing to find out if it is correct or if the practitioner can make recommendations. This can be done in a quick 10- to 15-minute appointment (and support staff can be responsible for this), or clients can send a videotape and make an appointment for a critique in person or by telephone. If the clients do not see any improvement or are having serious difficulties, the following problems may exist: (a) they are pushing the dog too hard, too fast (common in today's faster-is-better world), (b) they are giving confusing signals, or (c) their timing is wrong. This is hard work—it is not magic. The practitioner needs to provide help along the way.

3. The practitioner must work *with* the client. In the case of a very fearful or very aggressive dog, the practitioner may not be able to demonstrate the exercises or fit a halter during the first visit. In such cases, after fully cautioning clients about possible risks, the practitioner can ask whether the clients feel comfortable attempting the first round of the behavior modification protocols while the practitioner talks them through it. For reasons of liability it is important to explain that this is *not* the desired technique; however, if clients cannot eventually work with the dog or if the clients are perpetually afraid of the dog, the situation will be hopeless.

   If the practitioner can work with the dog, he or she should do so both to teach the dog the appropriate behaviors and to demonstrate to the clients what is desired. Viewing a videotape that can be played back and critiqued after the session can help. When the dog works well with the practitioner, it is the clients' turn. It is of no benefit if the dog is perfect for the practitioner, but a horror for clients. It is not sufficient to demonstrate the protocols successfully without then giving the clients the chance for emulation. It is irrelevant that the dog is perfect for the practitioner—the practitioner does not go home and live with the dog. The clients must be able to accomplish the protocols; hence, it is inappropriate simply to send them home with sheets of paper.

4. Finally, if there is potential for a dangerous behavior that will need to be corrected or avoided, it would be optimal if clients do not discover this when there is no one to help them. A run-through of the program will minimize, but not ablate, this chance.

These programs use praise and food treats as rewards. They do not use hand signals. A brief commentary on these facets is warranted.

Many humans have a tremendous resistance to using food rewards for dogs. The charitable explanation for this is that they do not understand that a food reward is *not* a bribe, but rather a salary. A bribe comes *a priori* (before the desired behavior) as a lure to distract or compete with the dog's current focus so that it does not commit a behavior that the clients are otherwise impotent to control. This is a sad, but common situation in which clients find themselves. A reward or salary comes *a posteriori* (after the desired behavior) in exchange for a behavior perfectly executed in response to a request from the clients. This means that the dog is attending to the clients' desires, awaiting their intentions, deferring to their needs, and responding appropriately, for which it has learned it can *earn* a reward.

Clients are generally receptive to these differences and quickly realize that not only have they been bribing their dogs, but also that they have not felt good about themselves for doing so. A reward structure sets the standard for compassionate but disciplined control.

The less charitable reason that many humans dislike food rewards, preferring to use only praise, is that they feel the need to control, dominate, and subjugate. Dogs are good targets for these needs.

When clients tell me that they want the dog to work only for praise, I always ask them why they feel that way. I seldom hear a logical, internally consistent reason, but I often hear that they want the dog to be willing to respond to their vocal commands or that the dog should obey them. This is about *them*, not about the dog. It is valuable and important for dogs to respond to vocal commands, but these can be coupled with salaries or rewards for a more consistent, reliable, attentive, and collaborative response. Psychologists have demonstrated that intermittent, unpredictable, but not *rare*, reward structures improve performance on any task. Clients are usually receptive to this logic, especially after a demonstration. They have to make the decision to comply; when asked if they would work at their job without a salary, most clients readily admit that they would not perform or work without some tangible reward. If the clients execute this reward schedule appropriately, their dog will often be willing to work largely for vocal commands and praise.

Some dogs work better for play (the receipt of a ball) than they do for food rewards. This is perfectly acceptable, although a little more difficult for clients to execute. *All* dogs should have praise coupled with the salary. As the dog progresses, the praise continues while the treats become intermittent to maintain the dog's interest and attention.

Hand signals are commonly used in obedience and can be useful for dogs and clients. These protocols are for use with problem dogs or young pups. They need every bit of help available. Hand signals are a needless distraction in such cases. Once the dogs master the programs, they will have no problems coupling the learned vocal cues to visual ones. Until then, these dogs should work in calm, quiet circumstances without distraction for vocal cues and a consistent reward structure. Dogs can learn all the words for the commands that they will need for these programs. Hand signals at this stage only distract their attention from the behavior modification process; for very aggressive dogs, such signals put the person using them at risk. Without exception, dangling body parts in front of an aggressive dog is not recommended and will make the animal more anxious. If clients wish to add hand signals later, they can easily do so by using the same principles enforced here: kindness, clarity, and consistency.

B-1 PROTOCOL FOR DEFERENCE: BASIC PROGRAM

Dogs' social systems are very similar to those of humans. They live in extended family groups; they have extensive and extended parental care; they work as a group or a family to help care for the offspring; they nurse their young before feeding them semisolid, then solid, food; they use play as one form of developing social skills; they communicate extensively vocally and nonvocally; and, most important, they have a social system that is based on deference to others. Fights for status or control are notoriously rare among wild canids such as wolves. Except in what humans perceive to be abnormal social conditions, most human social relations are structured by negotiation and deference to others rather than by violence. Deference-structured hierarchies mean that the individual to whom others defer may differ depending on the social circumstances. Status and circumstances are not absolute. In the human situation, a child may defer to his parents' requests but then be the leader on the playground to whom other children defer. Dogs are similar.

Much has been written about dogs viewing their human families as their packs. Although the pack comparison is not exact, dogs are social and generally look to their people for guidance. Dogs often become problems when they cease to do this or if they never do this. This program is the first step in both *preventing* such problems and in *treating* all forms of behavioral problems. All social animals create some form of rule structure. This structure allows them to communicate with each other. Because dogs are so similar to humans in so many ways and so frequently appear to be attentive to every word, it is assumed that they are complying with human rule structure. Puppies actually need guidance in how to do this, and problem dogs need to have a consistent, benign, kind rule structure explicitly spelled out for them. This is a kind of benign doggie boot camp: if the dog knows a consistent rule or behavior that will get the attention of its people, the dog will then be receptive to guidance. This is a form of discipline. People often confuse discipline with violence or abuse. The following program should be executed without violence or physical abuse. In fact, for most dogs, withdrawal of attention is a far more profound correction than is physical abuse. Abused dogs or those consistently mismanaged with physical punishment either learn to override the punishment or learn to seek it because it may be their most common contact.

The intent of this program is to set a baseline of good behavioral interaction between the client and pet and to teach the dog that it must consistently defer to people to receive attention. This is done in a safe, kind, passive manner and is more difficult than clients frequently acknowledge. The reason is as follows: if the clients are talking, reading, or watching television and the dog comes up to them and rubs, paws, or leans against them, the clients usually passively reach out and touch or pet the dog. The *dog* controlled that entire interaction. Score: dog, 1; human, 0—and the people do not even know that they were conveying any signals other than affection to the dog.

Under no circumstances can the clients touch, love, or otherwise interact with the dog unless the dog defers and awaits their attention. This is done by having the dog sit. Sitting need not be prolonged (5 to 15 seconds), and very young puppies may not do it perfectly because they are wiggle worms. Regardless, pups as young as 5 weeks of age can learn to sit and attend to the client (look at them for cues, make eye contact, look happy and attentive while being

quiet) in exchange for a food treat. As soon as the puppy sits, the person should say "Good girl (boy)!" and give a tiny treat of something special. Also praise and pet the pup (see "Teaching Sit," below).

For a dog that already knows how to sit, the only problem is going to be to reinforce this for everything that the dog wants. The rule is: *the dog must sit and be quiet to earn anything and everything it wants for the rest of its life.* This includes sitting for the following:

- Food and feeding
- Treats
- Love
- Grooming
- Being able to go out—and come in
- Having the leash, halter, or harness put on
- Having feet toweled
- Being *invited* onto the bed or sofa (if desired)
- Playing games
- Playing with toys
- Having a tick removed
- Having a wound checked
- Being petted or loved
- Attention
- *Anything the dog wants!*

All the dog must do is put its bottom on the floor or ground, be quiet, look at the client, and await the client's cue. This takes only seconds, but its value is inestimable. *All* dogs should learn this, and *no* dog is too old to learn this. If the dog is older or arthritic, it might be more comfortable lying down. All puppies should be raised with this simple but powerful deference behavior. This *will not* take away a dog's spunk, fire, or individuality. It *will* allow the client to have a far better relationship with the dog and to control the dog. The latter can be critical if the dog puts itself in a potentially injurious position.

If the client has a very pushy or very energetic dog, the client may find that constantly monitoring and correcting the dog's behavior is exhausting. If this happens, the client will become angry with the dog and will not practice the behavior modification correctly, *and* the client will eventually be worn down by the dog. If the latter happens, the dog will have learned to hone its obnoxious behaviors. For such clients, a better option may be to banish and ignore the pet, unless they are actively working with them. This is *not* the same as the withdrawal of affection recommended by many training manuals. Withdrawal of affection will make anxious dogs more anxious and will make clients feel sad, angry, or guilty. Such circumstances will worsen, not improve, the situation. However, by giving themselves permission *not* to have to monitor the dog's every breath, clients can then better comply with this protocol and the protocol for relaxation: behavior modification Tier 1 when they are with the pet. In fact, unless clients are absolutely willing to exhibit the extensive degree of vigilance recommended here, it is preferable to banish the dog to a place where it can be ignored but not neglected. Such places should be dry and comfortable, protected from the elements, safe, and somewhat amusing for the dog. Amusement or stimulation can be provided by toys, balls, marrow bones, or Kong toys filled with peanut butter. Caution is urged in using food with *any* dog with *any* food-associated aggressions. Clients must be able to retrieve the dog and then induce it to practice these protocols. If clients choose to actively banish or ignore the dog as a part of the method for enforcing the protocol for deference, they must be willing to establish and maintain regularly scheduled periods of interaction in which the deference protocol is *always* enforced and in which Tier 1 and Tier 2 of the behavior modification protocols can be practiced. This will take a minimum of 20 minutes twice a day. Several (8 to 12) 10- to 15-minute sessions per day are preferred when banishment is used. Remember, *any time* the dog is with the client, the protocol for deference *must* be enforced. This means no attention for the dog unless the dog is quietly sitting.

What does such a protocol do to treat or prevent problem behaviors?

1. Sitting and deferring for everything the dog wants, forever, reinforces the innate social structure of the dog and teaches it to look to its people for cues about the appropriateness of its behavior.
2. Deference behaviors can act as a form of "time out": they give the dog respite from a situation so that it does not worsen. The dog can learn that if it responds to a person's request to sit, the person will help it decide what the next best behavior is. This is a great relief to dogs that are anxious about appropriate responses (i.e., many dogs with behavioral problems).
3. Deference behaviors allow the dog to calm down. A sitting dog is less reactive than one that is running around; thus these behaviors allow the dog to couple a verbal cue, a behavior, and the physiological response to that behavior. This has a calming effect.
4. Deference behaviors, consistently reinforced, allow the dog to anticipate what is expected and to be able to *earn* attention.

Points to Remember

1. Starting immediately, the dog must earn everything that it wants for the rest of its life. The dog does this by quietly sitting and staying for a few moments (deferring to you).
2. The dog is requested to sit by using its name and then saying "Sit." This can be repeated every 3 to 5 seconds as needed (this is *not* an obedience class exercise).
3. If the dog resists or refuses to comply—*walk away from the dog*. The dog will eventually follow. When the dog appears or demands attention, ask it to sit as prescribed above. If the dog resists, walk away from the dog. Sooner or later this dog will capitulate. Outlast it.
4. As soon as the dog sits, reward it with praise. A food reward will hasten the process for a dog that does not know how to sit. The next step is to teach the dog "stay" (see "Teaching Stay"). Remember that the dog must stay until released. Because the point of this protocol is to enforce deference that is generalizable, quick releases are desired. Later you can practice long stays and downs as part of an overall relaxation and behavior modification program (see "Protocol for Relaxation: Behavior Modification Tier 1").
5. Watch for subtle, pushy, defiant behaviors that the dog may exhibit. Expect to occasionally make mistakes—do not fight with the rest of the family about it. This will not help the dog. Expect to be a little frustrated. Remember that dogs read body language far better than you do and that they are watching for their opportunity. Use that watchful behavior and shape it into deference behaviors.
6. Remember that everyone in the household must be consistent and work with the dog. Children need to be monitored to ensure their safety and to help them not teach the dog the wrong behavior. Children must understand

the difference between a food salary and a bribe and must be taught not to tease the dog. Dangling food in front of a dog at a distance is an invitation to get up and lunge. Everyone must return to the dog to reward it, tell it to stay, and quickly couple verbal praise with the food treat that should magically appear on an unfolded, flat hand.

7. Reward the dog. This should be fun—for everyone.

Teaching Sit

Consider using a food reward or salary, particularly if the dog must reshape undesirable behaviors. Many humans have a tremendous resistance to food rewards for dogs. The charitable explanation for this is that they do not understand that a food reward is not a bribe, but rather a salary. It is important to understand the difference and to avoid bribes.

A bribe comes a priori (before the desired behavior) as a lure to distract or compete with the dog so that it does not commit a behavior that the clients are otherwise impotent to control. This is a sad but common situation in which clients find themselves. A reward or salary comes a posteriori (after the fact) in exchange for a behavior perfectly executed in response to a request from the clients. This means that the dog is attending to the clients' desires, awaiting their intentions, deferring to their needs, and responding appropriately, for which it has learned it can *earn* a reward.

Clients are generally receptive to these differences and quickly realize not only that have they been bribing their dogs, but also that they have not felt too good about themselves for doing so. A reward structure sets the standard for compassionate but disciplined control.

Food rewards may not be necessary to teach and enforce deference behaviors to dogs that already know how to sit; they can be very useful in teaching puppies that do not know how to sit how to do so. Puppies are babies and have short attention spans. Food helps them focus.

If the food treat is held in one of the client's hands between two fingers and that hand is first placed in front of the pup's nose and then raised up and back, the pup's head will begin to move to follow it. Gradually the pup will sit because it is easier and more comfortable to do so. If the client is saying "Sit (2 to 3-second pause), sit (2 to 3-second pause)," and so on while doing this and as soon as the puppy accidentally sits says, "Good dog!" and *instantly* gives the treat, the pup will be reinforced in the appropriate time. This must be repeated until the puppy does it flawlessly and without hesitation. This generally takes less than 30 minutes for a pup that has not yet developed bad or inattentive behaviors.

Is it necessary to push on the puppy's bottom to make it sit? No, and given how big people are and how small puppies can be, it might be unwise to do this. This is especially true for dogs that might be predisposed to later hip problems. There are three other choices:

1. Clients can gently put a hand behind the puppy's bottom so that as the dog backs up, it bumps into the hand. The client can then gently shape the puppy to sit and reward as mentioned previously.
2. Clients can have another person stand behind the pup with his or her feet near the pup's haunches; as the pup backs up the person's feet and legs will shape the puppy's body in the sit position.
3. A Gentle Leader/Promise System Canine Head Collar or Halti can be used to help the client quickly teach the pup to sit. See "Protocol for Choosing Collars, Head Collars, and Harnesses" for more information.

Teaching Stay

"Stay" can be more difficult to teach than "sit" because the tendency is to rush the dog and proceed at a pace more suitable for the person than for the dog. This response is rooted partly in the client's feelings that if the dog does not comply instantly, the dog is stupid and the client is in error. This is not true, so everyone can stop feeling guilty. There is much variation in dogs' abilities to relax and stay, and clients often unwittingly give inconsistent signals with their body language. Among the most common of the inconsistent signals is talking to the dog over one's shoulder and telling it to stay while going away from the dog. Dogs that do not know "stay" will not learn it by this approach and will be distressed.

Before the dog can learn to stay, it first must know how to sit. If the dog is physically more comfortable lying down, that is fine. This is not an obedience class, no points will be awarded, and no trophies will be given. The point is to start the animal in a posture of deferential behavior. Sitting is a less reactive posture than is standing, and lying down is less reactive than sitting. Some dogs are calmer lying down, so it is preferable for them.

Next, tell the dog to sit, verbally praise it, say *"stay,"* and take a microscopic step backward. Repeat "stay," go back to the dog, repeat "stay," and reward. A sample sequence proceeds as follows:

"Bonnie—sit—good girl! (treat)—stay—good girl—stay (take a step backward while saying stay—then stop) stay Bonnie—good girl—stay (return while saying stay—then stop)—Bonnie—good girl (treat)—okay!" (the releaser and Bonnie can get up).

Note the Following

1. Use the dog's name—this will get it to attend to you. You can use it frequently, unlike in obedience, provided it attends to you. In fact, the name should be the cue to orient toward you. If the dog does not look at you immediately, put the treat near your eye. The dog needs to focus. (You can couple the treat next to your eye with the vocal signal "look.")
2. Repeat the commands. This is *not* obedience—the dog needs your reassurance. As the dog improves or learns more, repeat the commands less frequently and at greater intervals. This is what psychologists call "shaping" a behavior.
3. Reward the dog appropriately. Eventually the food treats will appear less predictably. At the outset the dog needs everything possible to help it.
4. Remember to use one or two words consistently as a *releaser*—and remember that if you use those words while talking to the dog, the dog will get up. If the dog gets up before released, make it stay and stay again, and wait 3 to 5 seconds before you release the dog. This prevents jack-in-the-box behavior.

As the dog becomes more experienced and masters staying at a short distance, *gradually* increase the distance between you and the dog. *Do not* go from getting the dog to stay within 1 meter of you to walking across the room. The temptation will be great and you will have only provoked conflict and anxiety in the dog, which defeats your goal. A more detailed approach to reinforce stay is found in the "Protocol for Relaxation: Behavior Modification Tier 1."

This protocol can be done with the dog on lead with a head collar. Head collars, when coupled with long-distance leads, allow you to reinforce sitting and to correct the dog if it gets up.

B-2 PROTOCOL FOR RELAXATION: BEHAVIOR MODIFICATION TIER 1

Introduction

This program is the foundation for all other behavior modification programs. Its purpose is to teach the dog to sit and stay *while relaxing* in a variety of circumstances. The circumstances change from very reassuring ones with you present to potentially more stressful ones when you are absent. The purpose of the program is not to teach the dog to sit; sitting (or lying down, if the dog is more comfortable) is only a tool. The goals of the program are to teach the dog to relax, to defer to you, to enjoy earning a salary for an appropriate, desirable behavior, and to develop, as a foundation, a pattern of behaviors that allow the dog to cooperate with future behavior modification (generally desensitization and counterconditioning). This protocol acts as a foundation for teaching the dog context-specific appropriate behavior. The focus is to teach the dog to rely on you for all the cues as to the appropriateness of its behavior so that it can then learn not to react inappropriately.

About Food Treats

This program uses food treats. Please read the logic behind this approach in the "Protocol for Deference: Basic Program." Remember, the treats are used as a salary or reward—not as a bribe. If you bribe a problem dog, you are defeated before you start. It is often difficult to work with a problem dog that has learned to manipulate bribes, but there are creative ways—often involving the use of head collars—to correct this situation. First, find a food that the dog likes and that it does not usually experience. Suggestions include boiled, slivered chicken or tiny pieces of cheese. Boiled, shredded chicken can be frozen in small portions and defrosted as needed. Individually wrapped slices of cheese can be divided into tiny pieces suitable for behavior modification while still wrapped in plastic, minimizing waste and mess. Consider the following guidelines in choosing a food reward:

1. Foods that are high in protein may help induce changes in brain chemistry that help the dog relax
2. Dogs should not have chocolate because it can be toxic to them
3. Some dogs do not do well with treats that contain artificial colors or preservatives
4. Dogs with food allergies or those taking monoamine oxidase inhibitor (MAOI) drugs may have food restrictions (cheese, for dogs taking MAOIs [deprenyl])
5. Dog biscuits generally are not sufficient motivation, but some foods are so desirable that the dog is too stimulated by them to relax—something between these two extremes is preferred
6. Treats should be tiny (less than half the size of a thumbnail) so that the dog does not get full, fat, or bored
7. If the dog stops responding for one kind of treat, try another
8. Do not let treats make up the bulk of the dog's diet; the dog needs its normal, well-balanced ration

The Reward Process

Rewarding dogs with food treats is an art. Learning to do so correctly helps the dog focus on the exercises and keeps everyone safe. To prevent the dog from lunging for the food, keep the already prepared treats in a little cup or plastic bag behind your back and keep one treat in the hand used to reward the dog. That hand can then either be kept behind your back so that the dog does not stare at the food or can be moved to your eye so that you can teach the dog to look happy and make eye contact with you. The food treat must be small so that the focus of the dog's attention is not a slab of food but rather your cues. A treat of the correct size can be closed in the palm of the hand by folding the fingers and will not be apparent when held between the thumb and forefingers. When presenting the dog with the treat, bring the hand, with a lightly closed fist, up quickly to the dog (do not startle the dog) and turn your wrist to open your hand.

When starting the program, let the dog smell and taste the reward so that it knows the anticipated reward for the work. If the dog is too terrified to approach, you can place a small amount of the treat on the floor. Then ask the dog to "sit"; if the dog sits instantly, say "Good girl (boy)!" and instantly open your hand to give the dog the treat instantly while saying "stay."

Getting the Dog's Attention

If the dog does not sit instantly, call its name again. As soon as the dog looks at or attends to you, say "Sit." If the dog will not look at you and pay attention, do not continue to say "Sit." If you continue to give a command that you cannot reinforce, the dog learns to ignore that command. If necessary, use a whistle or make an unusual sound with your lips to get the dog's attention. As soon as the dog looks at you, say "Sit." Use a cheerful voice. Some people may have to soften or lower their voice almost to a whisper to get the dog to pay attention to them. Often this is because they have given all their previous commands to the dog by yelling. The dog has very successfully learned to ignore this.

If the dog is looking at you but not sitting, approach the dog to close the distance, raise the treat gently to your eyes, and request "sit." Often just moving toward a dog helps the dog sit. Not only have you decreased the distance, but you appear taller and to be over the dog; such behaviors are used in canine communication to get the lower (in relative elevation) dog to obey the desires of the higher one. You can use these innate dog behaviors as long as you are careful. Never back up a dog that is growling. Never corner a fearful dog. Never continue to approach a dog that acts more aggressively the closer you come. Remember, the point of the program is to teach the dog to relax and look to you for the cues about the appropriateness of its behavior. The dog cannot do this if upset.

If the dog still will not sit, consider using a head collar. By using a long-distance lead you can request that the dog "sit" and gently enforce this from a distance by pulling on the lead. Reward with a treat as soon as the dog sits.

Cautionary Note:

If your dog is aggressive or if you are concerned about approaching it, do not do any of these exercises off-lead until the dog is perfect on-lead. Fit the dog with a head collar and work with the dog only on a lead at the outset. The halter allows you to close the dog's mouth if the dog begins to be aggressive. This is an ideal correction because it meets the rule that psychologists have established for ideal "punishment": you have interrupted the dog's inappropriate behavior within the first few seconds of the beginning of the behavior so that the dog can learn from the experience. Be gentle but consistent. Taking your anger or fear out on the dog will only worsen the behavior. As soon as the dog responds to the halter and calmly sits, reward the dog and continue. *Never reward a dog that is growling, lunging, barking, shaking, or urinating.*

After the dog sits for the first time you are ready to begin the program. Remember the following guidelines:

1. Use the dog's name to get the dog to orient toward you and to pay attention. If this does not work, use a whistle or a sound to which the dog is not accustomed.
2. Once the dog is attending to you (paying attention) say "sit" and give the dog 3 to 5 seconds to respond. If the dog *does* sit, reward it instantly; if not, repeat the "sit" command in the same calm, cheerful voice. You may want to experiment with voices to see the tonal qualities to which your dog best responds.
3. Do not worry about using the dog's name frequently or about repeating the commands if the dog responds. This is not obedience class, but if you later wish to take the dog to obedience class, the dog will do well *if* it did well on these programs. Making the adjustment will not be a problem.
4. Do not chase the dog around the room to try to get it to comply with you. If necessary, choose a small room with minimal distractions and use a leash. A head collar provides even more instantaneous response. *Use head halters and other collars kindly.*

A sample sequence could look like this:
"Bonnie—sit—(3-second pause)—sit—(3-second pause)—Bonnie, sit—(move closer to the dog and move the treat to your eye)—sit—(Bonnie sits)—good girl! (treat)—stay—good girl—stay (take a step backward while saying "stay"—then stop) stay Bonnie—good girl—stay (return while saying "stay"—then stop)—stay Bonnie—good girl! (treat)—okay (the releaser and Bonnie can get up)!"—(Bonnie happily gets up and watches calmly for your next signal.)

Note that you talk nonstop to the dog during these programs. This type of talking is not allowed in obedience classes but is desperately needed with inexperienced puppies and problem dogs. These dogs need all the cues that they can get. They need the constant guidance and reassurance of hearing your voice with clear instructions. These instructions and reassurances should occur in the context of shaping or gradually guiding their behavior toward more appropriate behaviors. You will have to learn to read subtle cues that your dog is giving and use these to your advantage. You will find it easier than you believe. The one thing that you absolutely *cannot* do is to talk a continuous stream to the dog without receiving the context-appropriate responses to your requests. If you rush through everything, you will only stress the dog and teach it to ignore everything you say. This is not good. A corollary of this admonition is that it is necessary to use consistent terminology and brief phrases and to do so in an environment when no one else is carrying on long, loud, distracting conversations.

Avoiding Problems

Do not push or pull on your dog or tug on its collar to get the dog to sit. These types of behaviors can be viewed as challenges by some dogs and may make them potentially dangerous. Use the methods discussed previously. If you really believe that the dog needs some physical help in sitting, use a head collar.

Do not wave your hands or the treat around in front of the dog. This acts as a distraction and confuses the dog. Part of the point of this program is to make the dog calmer and less confused. Excitable behavior on your part or unclear signals can make your dog more anxious. This does not help.

It is important to be calm. Your dog will make mistakes. This does not reflect on you. Problem dogs and new puppies require a lot of patience. The people who have had the most success with these protocols have been those who work the hardest and most consistently.

Do not let your dog be a jack-in-the-box. You must control the situation, and you must achieve that control by convincing the dog to defer to you. If the dog gets up to get the treat every time it is offered, the *dog* just controlled the situation. If the dog does this, consider whether you were too far away from the dog when you offered the treat. If so, move closer. Ideally, the dog should be able to get the treat just by stretching its neck. The dog should not need to get up. If you have a small dog, this may mean that you need to squat down to offer the reward. Be careful if the dog is aggressive because your face is now close to the dog. If you are close enough for the dog to do the exercise properly and the dog still gets up, close your hand over the treat and say "No." One advantage of holding the treat in this manner is that you can safely deny the dog the treat as the last second if the dog acts inappropriately. Then ask the dog to sit again. After the dog sits, say "Stay," wait 3 to 5 seconds, say "Stay" again, and *then* give the treat. The two "stays" with the period between them will reinforce the dog that it cannot get up when it wants to—the dog must be released. By asking the dog to stay twice, you are telling it that whenever it makes a mistake, it must do *two* things to recover from it. A sample sequence follows:

"Susie—sit—(3 to 5-second pause)—sit—(Susie sits)—good girl!—stay (start to give treat and dog gets up)—no!—(close hand over treat)—sit—(Susie sits)—stay—(3 to 5-second pause)—stay—good girl!—stay—(give treat)—okay!" (Dog is now allowed to get up and does so.)

Do *not* tell the dog that it is good if it is not. *Do not* reward shaking, growling, whining, or any other behavior that may be a component of the behavior you are trying to correct. If the dog gets impatient and barks for attention, say "No! Quiet!—stay—good girl—stay—good girl—(treat)—stay. . . ." If a vocal command is not sufficient to quiet the dog, remember that a head collar (especially the Gentle Leader/Promise) can be pulled forward to close the mouth and abort the bark before it starts, so that your correction is the most appropriate possible.

Finally, if you accidentally drop a food treat and the dog gets up to get it, do not correct the dog (the dog did not make the mistake and you did not deliberately drop the treat). Just start at the last point.

The Protocol

The Protocol is a program that was designed so that your dog could learn from it without becoming stressed and without learning to ignore the tasks because they were too predictable. The protocol intersperses long activities with short ones. You may have to adjust some activities to your particular needs. The pattern is actually spelled out in the program. It is preferable to reward the dog *only* for performing each task perfectly. If this is not possible for your dog, you can use a "shaping" procedure in which you first reward the dog for a behavior that approaches that indicated in the task. The next time you do the task, the behavior *must* be closer to perfect to be rewarded. If the program is done correctly, your dog will perform the task perfectly within a short time.

The Protocol is a foundation for desensitizing and counterconditioning your dog to situations in which it reacts inappropriately. The pages can be used as one day's tasks, or you may proceed at the dog's pace (which may be faster or slower). Some exercises are weird (asking you to run in circles or talk to people who do not exist), but these can be very helpful in getting dogs to learn to relax in a variety of circumstances. Before you start the actual exercises, you must practice with the dog so that it can sit perfectly for 15 seconds without moving. Do this with food treats as described previously. Once your dog can sit this way and look happy and as if it worshipped the ground you walk on, you are ready for the more challenging stuff.

Theoretically the tasks are grouped in 15- to 20-minute units. Your dog may have to go more slowly or may be able to go quickly. *This is not a race, and people who push their dogs too quickly create additional anxiety problems!* Watch your dog's cues. Once the animal can sit for 15 seconds perfectly, reward it only when it approaches perfect *behavior* or perfection on the other exercises. Use the shaping behaviors discussed previously if needed. If the dog really cannot perform an exercise or task, return to one that the dog knows flawlessly, reward the perfect performance, and stop. Every member of the family is to work 15 to 20 minutes per day with the dog, but it may be less anxiety provoking and more stimulating for the dog if this is done in three or four 5-minute segments.

If everyone in the family cannot or will not work with the dog, the people who are not participating *must not* sabotage the program. They minimally must comply with "The Protocol for Deference." If they cannot or will not do this, they should not be interacting with the dog at all. If there is a problem with noncooperation in the household, the dog will not behave as well as it can.

Remember that the keys to success are consistency and appropriate rewards. This means that, although we want you to work 15 to 20 minutes once or twice per day, you should work only for as long as both you and the dog are enjoying and benefitting from the program. If this means that you use six 5-minute intervals to accomplish three or four of the tasks, that is fine. Please do not end on a bad note. If the dog's behavior is deteriorating or its attention is dissipating, do one final, fun, easy exercise and stop. By pushing the dog past its limits, you induce anxiety, and the dog backslides.

When the dog is able to perform all of the tasks and exercises both on- and off-lead in one location (the living room), repeat them all in other rooms and circumstances (the backyard or the park—use a lead here). When the dog performs all the tasks perfectly in all places with all household members, you are ready for Tier 2 of the protocols, which focuses on your dog's specific problems.

If at any point you cannot get past one task, try breaking that task into two or three component parts. If this still does not help, call the veterinarian who recommended the program and who is working with the dog's behavior problems. He or she will be able to help you determine the root of the problem. Please do not just continue accepting suboptimal responses. The goal is to improve your dog's behavior. Videotaping while you work with the dog can help. Not only can you show the veterinarian what you are doing, but also you can be a more objective critic of your approach if you are not also an active participant.

Finally, remember that the dog will give you lots of cues about how it feels. We are rewarding the physical changes associated with relaxation and happiness and so will also reward the underlying physiological states associated with this (parasympathetic part of the autonomic nervous system). This means that if the dog is relaxed, its body is not stiff, the jaws hang relaxed and are not tense, the ears are alert or cocked but not rigid, its head is held gently at an angle, and the eyes are calm and adoring, you will be rewarding the nervous system responses that help your dog learn. If you mistakenly reward fear, tension, aggression, or avoidance, you will not make as much progress. If it is easier for you and the dog to be relaxed if the dog is lying down, do that.

Good luck, and do not get discouraged. Many dogs go through a period of 3 to 7 days when their behavior gets worse before it improves. For the first time in their life the dogs have a rule structure they must follow, and they get frustrated while learning it. As they discover they are rewarded for being relaxed and happy, their behavior will improve. These programs are more difficult for the people, in many ways, than they are for the dogs. Stick with it!

A sample map/floor plan is provided that illustrates a physical layout that works well for these types of protocols.

PROTOCOL TASK SHEETS

The task is listed on the left. To the right is a space for your comments about the degree of difficulty of the task for the dog, how many times it had to be repeated, or other questionable behaviors that appeared during the task. You should discuss these with your veterinarian at the reexamination appointment.

Remember after each task to verbally praise the dog and reward it with a treat for perfect performance before going on to the next task. Each set of exercises is designed for a day or a block of time. Warm-up and cool-down periods are provided.

At the first sign of any anxiety (lips retracted, pupils dilated, head lowered, ears pulled down and back, trembling, scanning), return to an exercise with which the dog is more comfortable or break down the exercise that produced these behaviors into smaller steps.

Day 1: Dog's Task	**Comments about response or difficulty**
Sit for 5 seconds	
Sit for 10 seconds	
Sit while you take 1 step back and return	
Sit while you take 2 steps back and return	
Sit for 10 seconds	
Sit while you take 1 step to the right and return	
Sit while you take 1 step to the left and return	
Sit for 10 seconds	
Sit while you take 2 steps back and return	
Sit while you take 2 steps to the right and return	
Sit for 15 seconds	
Sit while you take 2 steps to the left and return	

Sit while you clap your hands softly once
Sit while you take 3 steps back and return
Sit while you count out loud to 10
Sit while you clap your hands softly once
Sit while you count out loud to 20
Sit while you take 3 steps to the right and return
Sit while you clap your hands softly twice
Sit for 3 seconds
Sit for 5 seconds
Sit while you take 1 step back and return
Sit for 3 seconds
Sit for 10 seconds
Sit for 5 seconds
Sit for 3 seconds

Day 2: Dog's Task

Sit for 10 seconds
Sit while you take 1 step back and return
Sit while you take 3 steps back and return
Sit for 10 seconds
Sit while you take 3 steps to the right and return
Sit while you take 3 steps to the left and return
Sit for 10 seconds
Sit while you take 3 steps to the right and clap your hands
Sit while you take 3 steps to the left and clap your hands
Sit for 5 seconds
Sit for 10 seconds
Sit while you walk one fourth of the way around the dog to the right
Sit while you take 4 steps back
Sit while you walk one fourth of the way around the dog to the left
Sit for 10 seconds
Sit while you take 5 steps back from the dog, clapping your hands, and return
Sit while you walk halfway around the dog to the right and return
Sit while you walk halfway around the dog to the left and return
Sit for 10 seconds
Sit while you jog quietly in place for 3 seconds
Sit while you jog quietly in place for 5 seconds
Sit while you jog quietly in place for 10 seconds
Sit for 10 seconds
Sit while you jog one fourth of the way around the dog to the right and return
Sit while you jog one fourth of the way around the dog to the left and return
Sit for 5 seconds
Sit for 10 seconds

Day 3: Dog's Task

Sit for 10 seconds
Sit for 15 seconds
Sit while you take 2 steps backward and return
Sit while you jog 5 steps backward from the dog and return
Sit while you walk halfway around the dog to the right and return
Sit while you walk halfway around the dog to the left and return
Sit while you take 10 steps backward and return
Sit for 15 seconds
Sit while you take 10 steps to the left and return
Sit while you take 10 steps to the right and return
Sit for 20 seconds
Sit while you walk halfway around the dog to the right, clapping your hands, and return
Sit for 20 seconds
Sit while you walk halfway around the dog to the left, clapping your hands, and return
Sit for 10 seconds

Comments about response or difficulty

Comments about response or difficulty

Sit while you jog 10 steps to the right and return
Sit while you jog 10 steps to the left and return
Sit while you jog in place for 10 seconds
Sit for 15 seconds
Sit while you jog in place for 20 seconds
Sit for 10 seconds
Sit while you jog backward 5 steps and return
Sit while you jog to the right 5 steps and return
Sit while you jog to the left 5 steps and return
Sit for 5 seconds while you clap your hands
Sit for 10 seconds while you clap your hands
Sit for 10 seconds
Sit for 5 seconds

Day 4: Dog's Task

Sit for 10 seconds
Sit while you jog backward 5 steps and return
Sit for 20 seconds
Sit while you jog halfway around the dog to the right and return
Sit while you jog halfway around the dog to the left and return
Sit while you move three fourths of the way around the dog to the right and return
Sit while you move three fourths of the way around the dog to the left and return
Sit while you jog backward 5 steps, clapping your hands, and return
Sit for 10 seconds
Sit while you clap your hands for 20 seconds
Sit while you move quickly backward 10 steps and return
Sit while you move quickly 15 steps backward and return
Sit for 20 seconds
Sit while you jog halfway around the dog to the right and return
Sit while you jog halfway around the dog to the left and return
Sit while you walk quickly 15 steps to the left and return
Sit while you walk quickly 15 steps to the right and return
Sit for 20 seconds
Sit while you move three fourths of the way around the dog to the right and return
Sit while you move three fourths of the way around the dog to the left and return
Sit while you walk all the way around the dog
Sit while you walk approximately 20 steps to an entrance and return
Sit while you walk approximately 20 steps to an entrance, clapping your hands, and return
Sit while you walk around the dog, quietly clapping your hands, and then return
Sit for 20 seconds
Sit while you jog quickly around the dog
Sit for 20 seconds
Sit for 10 seconds while you clap your hands

Day 5: Dog's Task

Sit for 5 seconds
Sit for 15 seconds
Sit while you walk quickly 15 steps to the right and return
Sit while you walk quickly 15 steps to the left and return
Sit while you walk approximately 20 steps to an entrance and return
Sit while you walk approximately 20 steps to an entrance, clapping your hands, and return
Sit for 20 seconds
Sit while you walk around the dog, clapping your hands
Sit for 20 seconds
Sit for 10 seconds
Sit while you walk quickly backward, clapping your hands, and return
Sit while you walk approximately 20 steps to an entrance and return
Sit while you walk approximately 20 steps to an entrance, clapping your hands, and return

Sit while you go to an entrance and just touch the doorknob or wall and return

Sit for 10 seconds

Sit while you walk quickly backward, clapping your hands, and return

Sit while you walk approximately 20 steps to an entrance and return

Sit while you walk approximately 20 steps to an entrance, clapping your hands, and return

Sit while you go to an entrance and just touch the doorknob or wall and return

Sit for 20 seconds

Sit while you walk approximately 20 steps to an entrance, clapping your hands, and return

Sit while you go to an entrance and just touch the doorknob or wall and return

Sit for 10 seconds

Sit while the doorknob is touched or you move into entryway and return

Sit for 10 seconds

Sit for 15 seconds while you clap your hands

Sit for 10 seconds while you jog in place

Sit for 5 seconds

Day 6: Dog's Task

Sit for 10 seconds

Sit for 20 seconds while you jog back and forth in front of the dog

Sit for 15 seconds

Sit while you walk approximately 20 steps to an entrance and return

Sit while you walk quickly backward, clapping your hands, and return

Sit while you go to an entrance and just touch the doorknob or wall and return

Sit for 20 seconds while jogging

Sit while you walk around the dog

Sit while you walk around the dog, clapping your hands

Sit for 15 seconds

Sit for 20 seconds

Sit for 30 seconds

Sit while you walk quickly backward, clapping your hands, and return

Sit while you go to an entrance and just touch the doorknob or wall and return

Sit while you open the door or go into the entranceway for 5 seconds and return

Sit while you open the door or go into the entranceway for 10 seconds and return

Sit for 30 seconds

Sit while you walk quickly backward, clapping your hands, and return

Sit while you go to an entrance and just touch the doorknob or wall and return

Sit for 10 seconds

Sit while you go through the door or the entranceway and return

Sit while you go through the door or the entranceway, clapping your hands, and return

Sit while you open the door or go though the entranceway for 10 seconds and return

Sit for 30 seconds

Sit while you disappear from view for 5 seconds and return

Sit for 20 seconds

Sit for 10 seconds while you clap your hands

Sit for 5 seconds

Day 7: Dog's Task

Sit for 10 seconds

Sit for 20 seconds while you clap your hands

Sit while you take 10 steps backward and return

Sit while you walk around the dog

Sit while you go through the door or the entranceway and then return

Sit while you go through the door or the entranceway, clapping your hands, and return

Sit while you open the door or go through the entranceway for 10 seconds and return
Sit for 30 seconds
Sit while you disappear from view for 5 seconds and return
Sit while you go through the door or the entranceway and return
Sit while you go through the door or the entranceway, clapping your hands, and return
Sit while you open the door or go through the entranceway for 10 seconds and return
Sit for 30 seconds
Sit while you disappear from view for 10 seconds and return
Sit while you disappear from view for 15 seconds and return
Sit for 10 seconds
Sit for 15 seconds
Sit for 5 seconds while you clap your hands
Sit while you jog in place for 10 seconds
Sit while you jog three fourths of the way to the right and return
Sit while you jog three fourths of the way to the left and return
Sit while you go through the door or the entranceway, clapping your hands, and return
Sit while you open the door or go through the entranceway for 10 seconds and return
Sit for 30 seconds
Sit while you disappear from view for 15 seconds and return
Sit for 10 seconds
Sit for 5 seconds

Day 8: Dog's Task

Comments about response or difficulty

Sit for 10 seconds
Sit for 15 seconds while you jog and clap your hands
Sit while you back up 15 steps and return
Sit while you circle the dog and return
Sit while you disappear from view for 20 seconds and return
Sit while you disappear from view for 25 seconds and return
Sit for 5 seconds
Sit for 5 seconds while you sit in a chair (placed 5 feet from the dog)
Sit for 5 seconds
Sit for 15 seconds while you jog and clap your hands
Sit while you back up 15 steps and return
Sit while you circle the dog and return
Sit while you disappear from view for 20 seconds and return
Sit while you disappear from view for 30 seconds and return
Sit for 5 seconds
Sit while you circle the dog and return
Sit while you disappear from view for 20 seconds and return
Sit while you disappear from view for 25 seconds and return
Sit for 5 seconds while you sit in a chair near the dog
Sit while you disappear from view for 10 seconds, sit in a chair for 5 seconds, and return
Sit for 10 seconds
Sit for 20 seconds while you jog and clap your hands
Sit for 15 seconds while you run around the dog
Sit for 10 seconds
Sit for 5 seconds while you turn around
Sit for 5 seconds while you sit in a chair near the dog
Sit while you disappear from view for 10 seconds, sit in a chair for 5 seconds, and return
Sit for 10 seconds

Day 9: Dog's Task

Comments about response or difficulty

Sit for 5 seconds
Sit for 10 seconds while you turn around
Sit for 5 seconds while you jog
Sit while you walk around the dog
Sit while you jog around the dog
Sit while you jog around the dog, clapping your hands

Sit while you jog twice around the dog
Sit for 10 seconds
Sit for 15 seconds while you clap your hands
Sit for 20 seconds
Sit while you move three fourths of the way around the dog to the right and return
Sit while you move three fourths of the way around the dog to the left and return
Sit while you disappear from view for 10 seconds and return
Sit while you circle the dog and return
Sit while you disappear from view for 20 seconds and return
Sit while you disappear from view for 25 seconds and return
Sit for 5 seconds while you sit in a chair near the dog
Sit while you disappear from view for 10 seconds, sit in a chair for 5 seconds, and return
Sit for 10 seconds
Sit while you bend down and touch your toes
Sit while you stretch your arms
Sit while you stretch your arms and jump once
Sit while you touch your toes 5 times
Sit while you stretch your arms and jump 3 times
Sit for 15 seconds
Sit for 10 seconds
Sit for 5 seconds

Day 10: Dog's Task

Comments about response or difficulty

Sit for 5 seconds while you clap
Sit for 10 seconds while you touch your toes
Sit for 15 seconds while you sit in a chair
Sit while you walk quickly 15 steps to the right and return
Sit while you walk quickly 15 steps to the left and return
Sit while you walk approximately 20 steps to an entrance and return
Sit while you disappear from view for 5 seconds and return
Sit while you disappear from view for 10 seconds and return
Sit while you disappear from view for 15 seconds and return
Sit for 10 seconds
Sit for 5 seconds
Sit while you walk quickly 15 steps to the right and return
Sit while you walk quickly 15 steps to the left and return
Sit while you approximately 20 steps to an entrance and return
Sit while you disappear from view for 5 seconds and return
Sit while you disappear from view for 10 seconds and return
Sit while you disappear from view for 15 seconds and return
Sit while you disappear from view for 5 seconds, knock softly on the wall, and return
Sit for 5 seconds
Sit while you disappear from view for 5 seconds and return
Sit while you disappear from view for 10 seconds and return
Sit while you disappear from view for 15 seconds and return
Sit while you disappear from view for 5 seconds, knock softly on the wall, and return
Sit while you disappear from view, knock quickly but softly on the wall, and return
Sit for 5 seconds
Sit while you disappear from view for 10 seconds, knock softly on the wall, and return
Sit for 10 seconds
Sit for 5 seconds

Day 11: Dog's Task

Comments about response or difficulty

Sit for 5 seconds
Sit for 10 seconds
Sit while you disappear from view, knock quickly but softly on the wall, and return
Sit for 5 seconds

Sit while you disappear from view for 10 seconds, knock softly on the wall, and return
Sit for 30 seconds
Sit while you disappear from view, ring the doorbell, and immediately return
Sit while you disappear from view, ring the doorbell, wait 2 seconds, and return
Sit for 30 seconds
Sit while you disappear from view, ring the doorbell, and immediately return
Sit while you disappear from view, ring the doorbell, wait 5 seconds, and return
Sit for 30 seconds
Sit while you disappear from view, ring the doorbell, and immediately return
Sit while you disappear from view, ring the doorbell, wait 10 seconds, and return
Sit for 5 seconds while you jog around the dog
Sit while you walk around the dog
Sit while you jog around the dog
Sit while you jog around the dog, clapping your hands
Sit while you jog twice around the dog
Sit for 10 seconds
Sit for 15 seconds while you clap your hands
Sit for 20 seconds
Sit while you move three fourths of the way around the dog to the right and return
Sit while you move three fourths of the way around the dog to the left and return
Sit while you disappear from view for 10 seconds and return
Sit while you circle the dog and return
Sit for 10 seconds
Sit for 5 seconds

Day 12: Dog's Task

Sit for 10 seconds
Sit for 5 seconds while you clap your hands
Sit for 15 seconds
Sit for 20 seconds while you hum
Sit while you disappear from view for 20 seconds and return
Sit while you disappear from view for 25 seconds and return
Sit for 5 seconds while you sit in a chair near the dog
Sit while you disappear from view for 10 seconds, sit in a chair for 5 seconds, and return
Sit for 15 seconds
Sit for 20 seconds while you hum
Sit while you disappear from view for 20 seconds and return
Sit while you disappear from view for 25 seconds and return
Sit while you move three fourths of the way around the dog to the right and return
Sit while you move three fourths of the way around the dog to the left and return
Sit while you disappear from view for 10 seconds and return
Sit while you circle the dog and return
Sit for 10 seconds
Sit while you disappear from view, knock quickly but softly on the wall, and return
Sit for 5 seconds
Sit while you disappear from view for 10 seconds, knock softly on the wall, and return
Sit for 30 seconds
Sit while you disappear from view, ring the doorbell, and immediately return
Sit while you disappear from view, ring the doorbell, wait 2 seconds, and return

Comments about response or difficulty

Sit for 30 seconds
Sit while you disappear from view, say "hello," and return
Sit while you disappear from view, say "hello," wait 3 seconds, and return
Sit for 10 seconds
Sit for 5 seconds

Day 13: Dog's Task

Sit for 5 seconds
Sit for 15 seconds while you hum
Sit for 15 seconds while you clap your hands and hum
Sit while you disappear from view for 20 seconds and return
Sit while you disappear from view for 25 seconds and return
Sit for 5 seconds while you sit in a chair near the dog
Sit while you disappear from view for 10 seconds, sit in a chair for 5 seconds, and return
Sit for 5 seconds
Sit for 10 seconds
Sit while you disappear from view, knock quickly but softly on the wall, and return
Sit for 5 seconds
Sit while you disappear from view for 10 seconds, knock softly on the wall, and return
Sit for 30 seconds
Sit while you disappear from view, ring the doorbell, and immediately return
Sit while you disappear from view, ring the doorbell, wait 2 seconds, and return
Sit for 30 seconds
Sit while you disappear from view, say "hello," wait 5 seconds, and return
Sit while you disappear from view, knock or ring the doorbell, say "hello," wait 5 seconds, and return
Sit for 30 seconds
Sit while you disappear from view, say "hello," wait 5 seconds, and return
Sit while you disappear from view, knock or ring the doorbell, say "hello," wait 5 seconds, and return
Sit for 20 seconds while you hum
Sit for 15 seconds while you clap your hands
Sit for 5 seconds
Sit while you jog around the dog
Sit for 10 seconds while you clap your hands and hum
Sit for 5 seconds while you jog in place
Sit while you jog around the dog, humming

Day 14: Dog's Task

Sit for 10 seconds
Sit for 10 seconds
Sit for 5 seconds while you clap your hands and hum
Sit while you run around the dog
Sit while you walk back and forth to the door
Sit while you leave the room, quickly knock or ring the doorbell, and return
Sit for 5 seconds
Sit for 10 seconds
Sit for 10 seconds
Sit for 5 seconds while you clap your hands and hum
Sit while you run around the dog
Sit while you walk back and forth to the door
Sit while you leave the room, quickly knock or ring the doorbell, and return
Sit for 5 seconds
Sit for 10 seconds

Sit while you disappear from view for 10 seconds, knock softly on the wall, and return

Sit for 30 seconds

Sit while you disappear from view, ring the doorbell, and immediately return

Sit while you disappear from view, ring the doorbell, wait 2 seconds, and return

Sit for 30 seconds

Sit while you disappear from view, say "hello," wait 5 seconds, and return

Sit while you disappear from view, knock or ring the doorbell, say "hello," wait 10 seconds, and return

Sit for 30 seconds

Sit while you disappear from view, say "hello," wait 10 seconds, and return

Sit while you disappear from view, knock or ring the doorbell, say "hello," wait 10 seconds, and return

Sit for 20 seconds while you hum

Sit for 20 seconds

Sit for 5 seconds

Day 15: Dog's Task

Sit for 10 seconds

Sit for 5 seconds

Sit for 15 seconds while you clap your hands and hum

Sit while you disappear from view, knock or ring the doorbell, say "hello," talk for 10 seconds, and return

Sit for 20 seconds while you hum

Sit while you disappear from view, say "hello," invite the imaginary person in, wait 5 seconds, and return

Sit for 10 seconds

Sit for 5 seconds

Sit while you disappear from view, say "hello," invite the imaginary person in, wait 10 seconds, and return

Sit while you disappear from view, say "hello," talk (as if to someone) for 5 seconds, and return

Sit for 5 seconds while you clap your hands and hum

Sit while you run around the dog

Sit while you walk back and forth to the door

Sit while you leave the room, quickly knock or ring the doorbell, and return

Sit for 5 seconds

Sit while you leave the room, knock or ring the doorbell for 3 seconds, and return

Sit while you leave the room and knock or ring the doorbell for 5 seconds

Sit while you leave the room and talk for 3 seconds to people who are not there

Sit while you leave the room and talk for 5 seconds to people who are not there

Sit while you leave the room and talk for 10 seconds to people who are not there

Sit while you run around the dog

Sit for 10 seconds while you sit in a chair

Sit for 30 seconds while you sit in a chair

Sit for 15 seconds while you clap your hands and jog

Sit for 5 seconds

For Future Repetitions

- Repeat all tasks in different locations.
- Repeat all tasks with all family members.
- Repeat all tasks with only every second or third task being rewarded with a treat. (Remember praise!)
- Repeat with only intermittent treat reinforcement. (Remember praise!)

You and your pet are now ready for Tier 2.

Comments about response or difficulty

B-3 BEHAVIOR MODIFICATION TIER 2: PROTOCOL FOR DESENSITIZING DOMINANTLY AGGRESSIVE DOGS

Before desensitizing your dog to gestures or actions that may inadvertently encourage the dog to exhibit dominance aggression, you should have been working with the first two behavior modification protocols: "Protocol for Deference: Basic Program" and "Protocol for Relaxation: Behavior Modification Tier 1." In addition, you should have been complying with the "Protocol for Dogs With Dominance Aggression." The purpose of this program is to begin to shape the dog's undesirable behaviors into behaviors that are more desirable. You need to continue to observe the recommendations in "Protocol for Dogs With Dominance Aggression."

At the outset of these tasks, one person should be able to request that the dog sits and stays, both on- and off-lead, in the same format as recommended in Tier 1. The person giving the dog cues or commands (the rewarder or handler) is the one responsible for rewarding appropriate behaviors with food treats. Because the dog has already completed Tier 1 of the program with this person, the dog should not view this situation as confrontational. The goal of this protocol is to desensitize and countercondition the dog to gestures that it may or has considered challenging. This protocol requires the cooperation of a second person, the helper. The helper is to stand (or sit, if necessary) approximately 3 meters from the dog, off to the side of the animal. This means that the dog knows that the person is there and can see the person in its peripheral vision but that the dog can still attend to and focus directly on the person giving the cues. With one arm bent at the elbow and held at waist height and with the palm of that hand facing the floor, the second person should start to make small circles in the air. As the dog learns to ignore this distraction and relax while receiving treats as a reward for the relaxation, the helper will gradually make larger circles, move them from waist to shoulder height, approach the dog, make the gestures quicker, form the movements closer to the dog, and, eventually, reach down, press on the dog, and roll the dog over. This is a kinder, less threatening, more beneficial outcome than an "alpha roll," a "dominance down," or other forceful "dominance" exercises.

The program starts with the helper forming small circles close to his or her own body. While the dog sits quietly and attentively and looks as happy as possible (remember—unhappy or anxious dogs do not learn well to change their behavior), the size of the circles can be increased. If the dog remains relaxed, the helper can step closer to the dog, again decreasing the circle size. After the dog relaxes, the circle size is increased. Remember, larger gestures, closer to or over the dog, are potentially big threats to dominantly aggressive dogs. Repeating the pattern of small circles—larger circles—relaxation—approach—small circles—relaxation—larger circles—relaxation, and so on, the helper should continue to approach the dog.

The team should work to the point at which the dog is able to sit quietly and remain inattentive to the handler with the rewards when large circles are made over the dog's head. Gradually the helper will approach the dog and attempt to touch and then push on the dog.

The program will take you through all the necessary steps. Remember, the following rules apply for this tier of the protocols as well as for the others:

1. You are only to reward the dog when it reacts appropriately. Never bribe the dog.

2. If the dog becomes distressed or anxious and cannot successfully complete some part of the program, back up and slowly work on the exercises with which the dog has problems. If the dog just cannot get past one suite of tasks, contact the veterinarian with whom you are working. Regardless, make sure that each session ends on a positive note.

3. Keep sessions short—15 to 20 minutes once or twice a day. If either you or your dog have trouble with that time block, use shorter but more frequent sessions (5-minute sessions eight times per day). Shorter sessions may work better for some dogs that appear to be unable to complete a suite of exercises.

4. If at any time you feel that the dog is becoming aggressive or if you or your helper feel threatened, stop for a few minutes and then resume.

5. If the dog appears to lose interest after a few days, make sure that you are rewarding it at the appropriate times in the response sequence. You may also need to change rewards at some point and use the dog's propensity to be interested in novel items.

6. If you or your helper feel safer or more comfortable with the dog on-lead, practice for the first few times with the dog on-lead. It may be best to work with a head collar. This can be an excellent idea because some dogs view all hand signals as threats and the Gentle Leader Promise System allows you to close the animal's mouth, thereby both preventing an injury and issuing a correction at the most appropriate time. If you use a halter, hold the leash in one hand and reward with the other. If you choose to just use a leash, put it under your foot with a small amount of slack. This leaves both your hands free, but requires that you can quickly slip your other foot across the leash so that the dog's head is held closer to the floor.

During these tasks the dog should remain attentive to the person giving the cues and rewards while the helper performs the potentially distracting activities. A brief glance at the helper is acceptable *if and only if* the dog is immediately responsive to a quick request to look at the handler (use the dog's name as you see the dog turning toward the helper: "Sparky, here!") *or* if the dog spontaneously returns its attention to the handler.

The helper forms small circles close to his or her body. When the dog sits quietly and attentively, the circles are increased in size and speed. If the dog remains relaxed, the helper can step toward the dog, again returning to the smaller circle size that is less threatening. As the dog relaxes the circle size should again be increased. It is sometimes helpful if the rewarder anticipates the next phase of the helper's actions and gets the dog's attention before the animal has time to be concerned. For example, as the helper steps forward, the rewarder could say "Sparky!" (use an upbeat tone) and reward the dog (if it behaves appropriately) *as* the helper makes his or her move. Go slowly. Large or quick gestures can be threats to dominantly aggressive dogs. By proceeding slowly, the helper can continue to approach the dog with progressively more complicated desensitization gestures.

Clients are often frustrated by this slow approach. Remember that regardless of your stage in the program, there are earlier tasks that you would not have been able to execute without the commitment to the desensitization and counterconditioning.

The helper eventually works to the point at which the dog is able to sit quietly and remain attentive while the helper makes large circles over the dog's head. The circling hand should gradually be lowered until it just touches the dog's fur. If the dog permits this, the helper can gradually begin to apply more pressure to the dog with each pass of his hand. *Watch the dog carefully as the touching begins.* Many dominantly aggressive dogs will tolerate gestures that do not involve physical contact but will become aggressive at the least intimate contact. The rewarder is responsible for monitoring the dog's facial and eye gestures for the *least* sign of displeasure. At the first sign of this, the helper should back off. It is far wiser to not take any chances. You can always return to working at a less reactive level and gradually build to a more intimate level. A dog that may be unable to tolerate contact while off-lead may be able to learn to do it—and enjoy it—while on-lead wearing a head halter. Use every available option.

The objective of this program is to gradually work up to the point at which the helper can push the dog to the ground without any resistance. Once this is possible, the entire program should be repeated in different rooms, indoors and outside, and from different positions relative to the dog (behind the dog and, the more threatening position, in front of the dog). Everyone in the household should practice as both the rewarder and the helper. The ultimate hope is that people will be able to rush up and hug the dog. *Not all dogs will attain this level of behavioral change.* Caution is urged, and some dogs may *never* be able to be hugged and surrounded by strangers. One of the benefits of these programs is that you will become aware of gestures that signal the dog's limits and can decide whether you wish to attempt to modify these.

A sample map/floor plan is provided that illustrates a physical layout that works well for these types of protocols.

Comments about response or difficulty

Dog's Task

Make small circles at 3 meters
Make large circles at 3 meters
Make small circles at 2.5 meters
Make large circles at 2.5 meters
Make small circles at 2 meters
Make large circles at 2 meters
Make small circles at 1.5 meters
Make large circles at 1.5 meters
Make small circles at 1 meter
Make large circles at 1 meter
Make small circles at 0.5 meters
Make large circles at 0.5 meters
Make small circles at 0.25 meters
Make large circles at 0.25 meters
Bend at the waist at 0.25 meters and make small circles above the dog's head
Bend at the waist at 0.25 meters and make large circles above the dog's head
Make small circles immediately above the dog's head
Make large circles immediately above the dog's head*
Quickly and lightly brush the dog's fur while circling above the dog's back*
Repeat the above and brush for a slightly longer time*
Repeat, increasing pressure slightly*
Repeat, with petting pressure*
Press gently on the dog's shoulders*
Press moderately on the dog's shoulders*
Press firmly on the dog's shoulders*
Press firmly on the dog's back*
Keep increasing pressure on the dog until the dog is pushed to the ground*
Massage the neck, shoulders, and hips*
Roll on to back so that the dog's belly is exposed*
Massage the belly, groin, and chest gently*

*CAUTION: These gestures can be viewed as threats by the dog; observe the dog's signaling carefully and do not take risks. Not all dogs will succeed at the highest levels, but frequent repetitions often allow them to do so.

For Future Repetitions

- Repeat all tasks in different locations.
- Repeat all tasks with all family members.
- Repeat all tasks with only every second or third task being rewarded with a treat. (Remember praise!)
- Repeat with only intermittent treat reinforcement. (Remember praise!)

B-4 BEHAVIOR MODIFICATION TIER 2: PROTOCOL FOR DESENSITIZATION AND COUNTERCONDITIONING USING GRADUAL DEPARTURES

Dogs with separation anxiety often begin to experience anxiety at the first cue that you will be leaving the dog's sight. The first set of protocols concentrated on uncoupling cues for departure from the actual event and on reinforcing general relaxation and responsiveness to your vocal cues (see "Protocol for Deference: Basic Program" and "Protocol for Relaxation: Behavior Modification Tier 1"). This program concentrates on desensitizing and counterconditioning the dog to being left alone for gradually longer periods.

It is not sufficient that the dog does not bark or destroy something when left alone. The goal of this program is to reinforce relaxation and behaviors associated with actually feeling calm when left alone (i.e., happy looks, lowered heart rates, and slowed respiration). Once again, *go slowly*. It is particularly important that dogs with separation anxiety do not become stressed or made more anxious during this protocol. Speed is *not* a measure of success—behavior is. Remember to shape the dog's behavior by rewarding even the smallest, incremental hint that the dog is more relaxed than previously. If at any time you notice outward physical and physiological signs that the dog is becoming anxious while working, break the suite of tasks on which you were working into smaller components. Outward physical and physiological signs of stress or anxiety can include panting, increased heart rate, lowered head with ears retracted, lips pulled back horizontally, dilated pupils, "redder" eyes with or without movement, shaking or shivering, whimpering or whining, and blowing in and out of "cheeks." If you see any of these signs, the dog is too distressed to effectively learn to change its behavior. Backtrack and return to a level at which the dog does not react inappropriately and can respond happily. Break the tasks with which the dog had difficulty into smaller components. All of the following tasks can be broken into smaller components. Everyone in the family who is involved with the dog must be able to successfully complete the program.

When the program is completed in one calm area, it must be expanded to other areas: other rooms, indoors or outside, inside a fence or outside, and so on.

Remember to use the dog's behavior to help you decide how to adapt the protocol for the dog's specific needs. If the dog is perfectly calm when left in a car but is distressed when someone leaves, start by practicing the tasks in the car. If the dog is calm when all but one person leaves the house but panics when that person leaves, start by practicing with departures involving people for whom the dog does not panic. If the dog appears to keep a good calendar and does not become distressed when people leave on weekends, start by practicing the tasks in the protocol repeatedly on weekends.

Remember to shape the dog's behavior by rewarding even the smallest signal that it is more relaxed with each succeeding task. Be patient. Do not become angry. Do not punish the dog. Stop and return later if you are feeling stressed.

A sample map/floor plan is provided that illustrates a physical layout that works well for these types of protocols.

NOTE: As usual, for the following tasks always remember to return to the dog and reward it after completing the task.

Day 1: Dog's Task

Sit for 5 seconds
Sit for 10 seconds
Sit for 20 seconds
Sit while you take one step back
Sit while you take two steps back
Sit while you take one step to the side
Sit while you take two steps to the side
Sit while you take three steps back
Sit while you take three steps to the side
Sit while you walk around the dog
Sit while you take 10 steps backward and return
Sit while you go through the door or the entranceway and return
Sit while you open the door or go into the entrance for 10 seconds and return
Sit while you take one step to the side
Sit while you take two steps to the side
Sit while you take three steps back
Sit while you take three steps to the side
Sit while you walk around the dog

Comments about response or difficulty

Day 2: Dog's Task

Sit for 20 seconds
Sit while you take 10 steps backward and return
Sit while you go through the door or the entranceway and return
Sit while you open the door or go into the entrance for 10 seconds and return
Sit for 30 seconds
Sit while you disappear from view for 5 seconds and return
Sit while you go through the door or the entranceway and return
Sit while you touch a doorknob
Sit while you rattle a doorknob
Sit while you turn the doorknob, but do not open the door

Comments about response or difficulty

Sit while you touch a doorknob
Sit while you rattle a doorknob
Sit while you turn the doorknob, but do not open the door
Sit while you open the door a few centimeters and quickly close it
Sit while you open the door 0.25 meters and the close it
Sit while you open the door 0.5 meters and the close it
Sit while you walk back 10 steps
Sit while you rattle the doorknob
Sit while you open the door 0.5 meters and then close it
Sit while you open the door 1 meter and then close it
Sit while you step into the door but remain in view

Day 3: Dog's Task

Sit while you turn the doorknob, but do not open the door
Sit while you open the door a few centimeters and quickly close it
Sit while you open the door 0.5 meters and then close it
Sit while you open the door 1 meter and then close it
Sit while you step into the door but remain in view
Sit while you step into the doorway
Sit while you step through the doorway
Sit while you step through the doorway, close the door just slightly, and
   immediately return
Sit while you step through the doorway, close the door, wait 5 seconds,
   and return
Sit while you disappear from view for 10 seconds and return
Sit while you disappear from view for 15 seconds and return
Sit for 10 seconds
Sit for 15 seconds
Sit while you disappear from view for 15 seconds and return
Sit while you step through the doorway, close the door, wait 10 seconds,
   and return
Sit while you step through the doorway, close the door, wait 20 seconds,
   and return
Sit while you go out of the door and firmly close it
Sit for 20 seconds
Sit for 10 seconds
Sit for 5 seconds

Day 4: Dog's Task

Sit for 10 seconds
Sit while you go out of the door and close it:
   and wait 5 seconds
   and wait 30 seconds
   and wait 45 seconds
   and wait 90 seconds
   and wait 2 minutes
Sit while you go out of the door and close it:
   and wait 3 minutes
   and wait 4 minutes
   and wait 5 minutes
   and wait 7 minutes
   and wait 10 minutes

Comments about response or difficulty

Comments about response or difficulty

Continue as above until the dog can sit quietly and relax while left alone for 30 minutes. Generally, if the dog can be relaxed while left alone for 30 minutes, the dog will be able to relax when left alone for normal durations, prohibiting any startling or disastrous consequences. This means that if your dog is afraid of thunderstorms and one occurs while it is left alone, relapse is possible. Treat all of the problems.

For Future Repetitions

- Repeat all tasks in different locations.
- Repeat all tasks with all family members.
- Repeat all tasks with only every second or third task being rewarded with a treat. (Remember praise!)
- Repeat with only intermittent treat reinforcement. (Remember praise!)

Antianxiety medications may help some dogs that otherwise are unable to succeed in this program. Remember, if it is decided that medication could benefit your dog, you need to use it *in addition* to the behavior modification, not instead of it.

B-5 PROTOCOL FOR TEACHING YOUR DOG TO UNCOUPLE DEPARTURES AND DEPARTURE CUES

There are two components to beginning to teach dogs to *not* react anxiously when you leave them. The first involves resisting the normal tendency to reassure an unhappy dog, and the second involves teaching the dog not to respond to cues that tell it you might leave. Tier 2 of the program actually teaches the dog the third component, gradually learning to be left alone.

Dogs that become distressed after you have left probably became distressed before you left. You need to be alert for such cues as panting, pacing, whining, digging, trembling, not eating, and so on and ensure that you do not inadvertently reward such cues by telling the dog that it is "okay." The dog does not think it is okay, and you are rewarding and reinforcing the dog for being anxious. Rather, before the dog becomes distressed, even if it has just awakened, make every effort to reward the calm behavior. Talk happily to the dog, groom slowly, or massage and rub the dog's belly and chest. If the dog becomes upset when you leave, do not fuss over the dog. Try some of the initial Tier 1 exercises to determine whether these will calm the dog. If they do, reward the dog profusely. If they do not, proceed to leave, placing the dog in a crate or pen, if that is normal, and do not fuss over the dog. See "Protocol for Dogs with Separation Anxiety" for further details.

It is important to start to teach the dog that it can divorce the signals you give when you are about to leave from its anxiety at your departure. Remember, dogs read body language better than humans. The cues that you need to work on include all of those that induce anxiety as described previously.

When you are not leaving, start to go through the same routine that you pursue when departing. For example, if you always take your briefcase to work, pick it up and then watch television or read a book. If you always go to the health club with a gym bag, pick up your gym bag and make dinner. If you only wear high heels and makeup when you go to work, wear them instead on a Sunday and spend the day by the fire reading the newspaper. You get the idea.

Remember, you are responsible for identifying the cues that start to upset your dog. All dogs are different. Some dogs only react when the keys are picked up, others only when the car is started, some because of the hour at which their people awake when going to work, and still others because of the presence or absence of a meal or a type of food. These are typical examples; your dog may respond to something different.

Any specific event that triggers anxiety in your dog should be uncoupled from your actual departure.

In addition to using cues that signal to the dog that you are leaving, and then staying home, you can use cues that tell the dog you are staying home and then leave. For example, if you only eat breakfast on weekends when you stay home, start eating breakfast on weekdays. If you only wear jogging clothes on weekends, wear them to work and change there.

On days when you are not leaving the dog, you can start to develop some specific cues that tell the dog that you are not leaving. For example, you could play a specific, easily recognizable piece of music. You can then use this piece of music to help teach the dog to relax when you are leaving (or, by remote control, when you are not there). This is called a bridging stimulus and can be very useful in cases of milder anxieties or as animals begin to recover.

The anxiety induced by the specific event that your dog associates with your departure is often a self-fulfilling prophecy. If the dog can be taught to not become anxious in the first place at the time when the cues are given, this will help the dog learn to not be anxious when you are gone. Remember that what we know about anxiety indicates that it is a *cascade type of phenomenon:* once you get upset, it is easier to become more upset more quickly.

Antianxiety medications may help some dogs that otherwise are unable to succeed in this program. Remember, if it is decided that medication could benefit your dog, you need to use it *in addition* to the behavior modification, not instead of it.

B-6 TIER 2: PROTOCOL FOR DESENSITIZING AND COUNTERCONDITIONING A DOG (OR CAT) FROM APPROACHES FROM STRANGERS

The "Protocol for Desensitizing and Counterconditioning a Dog (or Cat) From Approaches From Strangers" is written primarily for dogs, but the clever client can adapt it for cats. It is intended to be started after "Protocol for Deference: Basic Program" and "Protocol for Relaxation: Behavior Modification Tier 1" have been successfully completed. This protocol will work for animals that respond inappropriately (fearfully, aggressively, or fearfully aggressively) to either strange animals (primarily dogs) or people. The execution of this protocol requires the cooperation of several people and sometimes another dog or cat. If the dog's problem involves other dogs, a second dog will be required. If the dog is very aggressive toward or fearful of other dogs, the first dog that works with this one should preferably be one to which this dog is accustomed and to which it does not respond. Later another dog, generally one not in the household, will be required.

It is best to set these tasks up in a T-shaped hallway. If you do not have a T-shaped hallway, the dog can be placed in a room off a hall. The point of this physical restriction is to allow the dog, even when using its peripheral vision, to see a stranger for only a brief moment at the outset of the protocol. A momentary glimpse lessens the dog's anxiety and allows the desensitization techniques emphasized in Tier 1 to be used.

Ask the dog to sit and stay, or to lie down and stay if this is more relaxing for the dog, in the doorway or hall. Have the dog facing the hallway where the person or dog will approach. The further the dog is from the door or hall, the less the dog will be able to see of the approaching stranger, and the more momentary any glimpse of the person or dog will be. Use this. If your dog is very anxious, move the dog far away from the approacher. Only when your dog has become relaxed at this long distance should you gradually move it closer to the approacher and repeat the tasks described in this protocol. As soon as your dog sits, stays, and relaxes, reward it with a small treat. Make sure that what you are rewarding is that the dog remained relaxed and was attentive to you. As the stranger passes, the dog is permitted to quickly glance at the stranger but should not react inappropriately or anxiously by putting his hair up, whining, growling, barking, trembling, salivating, or looking distressed. At all times the dog should look happy and look at you adoringly. If the dog looks at the approacher for more than a moment, as soon as you say the dog's name (in a happy, upbeat voice), the dog should look at you and be relaxed. Remember that a tone of voice that conveys that you are worried for the dog or angry that the dog is not instantaneously responding only increases the dog's anxiety. If you approach this task gradually, the dog will eventually respond instantaneously; it just may be unable to do so right at the outset.

The dog must look at your face and eyes—not at the food rewards. Once the dog does not react at all, you can make the rewards intermittent, but at the outset you need to reward the dog for its constant attention. Be very quick with the food rewards: as soon as the dog responds to your call or voice command, give the reward. The potentially anxiety-provoking event—the movement of the approacher—should be timed to coincide with and take place during the reward phase of the exercise. The following tasks can be varied by having the stranger approach the dog from the front

and from the back, but you should start with the dog facing you and sitting sideways to the approach of the stranger.

If cooperative strangers are not available or for further practice, these exercises can be performed in shopping centers, parks, or other busy places using fortuitous strangers *if* and only if you have good control over the dog's head and can be confident that it does not pose any risk to the strangers (dog or human). For dogs that need reassurance or a little more restraint, practice these exercises using a head collar. This not only prevents the dog from bolting but also allows you to safely turn the dog's head away from someone else and toward you within the time frame (the first few seconds of the behavioral process) that will allow the dog to learn from and be rewarded for the correction.

These same tasks can be used for dogs that have problems with interdog aggression. Instead of having a stranger walk by, have someone (preferably a person with whom the dog is comfortable) walk by with another dog. Begin the exercises with the strange dog walking next to the wall in the hall. This places the approaching dog as far away as possible from the one with the problem *and* uses the person as a buffer and signal to relax for the dog with the problem. After all tasks have been successfully and calmly completed the first time, repeat the same exercises with the strange dog walking on the *opposite* side of the person who is walking down the hallway.

If a strange dog is not available, you can first use another dog of your own or use dogs that are behind fences or in the park, leashed. Remember, other dogs may have problems, too, and you not only need to protect other dogs from your dog (use a head halter), but you also want to protect your dog from them. This is often not easy to do if any of the other dogs run free. Use sound judgment and err on the side of caution.

If your dog has problems only with a particular dog or a particular class of dogs, start with a dog or class of dogs with which there is no problem and then gradually begin to use the problem dog. You may need to do so intermittently at first.

You will need the cooperation of other people and dogs to succeed in this protocol. You can get this cooperation by being cautious and ensuring that your dog can injure no one else. Head halters can speed the rate at which the dogs can learn these exercises because they correct the dog before it can become fully upset and experience a cascade phenomenon of inappropriate behavior. Head halters also can provide an extra degree of protection for the approacher dog and should be used for both dogs in all circumstances when the problems exist between the dogs. If you cannot find appropriate strangers (dogs or people) with which to practice the approaches, ask if your veterinarian can set these up in his or her practice. If at first you practice under extremely controlled circumstances (the veterinarian's office), you eventually need to practice under less controlled circumstances.

Again, for each step you are rewarding the dog; not just for not reacting, but also for relaxing and being happy and confident while it does not react. If you have difficulty with any of the following tasks, break them down into simpler, smaller, more manageable tasks. Your dog's behavior will tell you what is manageable. Do not make the dog more fearful. It is better to work for three 5-minute periods that the dog enjoys than for one 15-minute period when the dog becomes distressed.

The intent of this program is to teach the dog that someone can walk quickly up to it, touch it while making noise, and keep going. If the problem is with another dog, the intent is to teach the dog that another dog can pause in front of it, sniff, and then pass without ensuing problems.

Dog's Task	**Comments about response or difficulty**

The dog sits, stays, and relaxes while:

A stranger passes quietly and quickly down the opposite end of the hall

A stranger passes quietly and at a moderate pace down the opposite side of the hall

A stranger passes at a slow pace down the opposite side of the hall, making a slight noise (i.e., scuffing of feet)

A stranger passes at a slow pace down the opposite side of the hall, making slightly more noise (i.e., the jangling of keys)

A stranger passes quietly and quickly down the center of the hall

A stranger passes quietly and at a moderate pace down the center of the hall

A stranger passes slowly down the center of the hall, making a slight noise

A stranger passes slowly down the center of a hall, making more noise

A stranger passes quietly and quickly down the near side of the hall

A stranger passes quietly and at a moderate pace down the near side of the hall

A stranger passes quietly and at a slow pace down the near side of the hall

A stranger passes at a slow pace down the near side of the hall, making a slight noise

A stranger passes quietly down the near side of the hall, pausing momentarily in the doorway

A stranger passes quietly down the hall, taking one tiny step into the doorway and momentarily pausing

A stranger passes quietly down the hall, taking one brief step into the doorway, pausing briefly, and glancing at the dog

A stranger takes two steps into the doorway

A stranger takes two steps into the doorway and briefly pauses

A stranger takes two steps into the doorway, briefly pauses, and glances at the dog

A stranger takes three steps into the doorway

A stranger takes three steps into the doorway and briefly pauses

A stranger takes three steps into the doorway, briefly pauses, and glances at the dog

A stranger walks quietly and quickly through the doorway and passes the dog

A stranger walks quietly and quickly past the dog, and reaches slightly toward the dog

A stranger walks quietly and quickly past the dog and briefly reaches close to the dog

A stranger walks quietly and quickly past the dog, briefly reaching slightly toward the dog

A stranger walks moderately quickly past the dog, briefly reaching slightly more toward the dog

A stranger walks at a slow pace past the dog

A stranger walks at a slow pace, briefly reaching toward the dog

A stranger walks at a slow pace, briefly reaching slightly closer toward the dog

A stranger walks at a slow pace, briefly pausing next to the dog

A stranger walks at a slow pace, briefly pausing next to the dog and glancing at it

A stranger briefly pauses next to the dog, glances at it, and reaches slightly toward it

A stranger briefly pauses, glances, and reaches slightly more toward the dog

A stranger pauses and looks at the dog (*do not stare*) for 5 seconds

A stranger pauses and looks at the dog (*do not stare*) for 10 seconds
A stranger pauses and looks at the dog (*do not stare*) for 20 seconds
A stranger pauses and looks at the dog (*do not stare*) for 30 seconds
A stranger pauses and looks at the dog (*do not stare*) for 45 seconds
A stranger pauses and looks at the dog (*do not stare*) for 1 minute
A stranger pauses next to the dog for 1 minute then reaches slightly toward the dog
A stranger pauses for 1 minute and reaches closer to the dog, almost touching it
A stranger pauses for 1 minute, reaches closer to the dog, and touches it
A stranger pauses for 1 minute, reaches down, and pets the dog

For Future Repetitions
- Repeat all tasks in different locations.
- Repeat all tasks with all family members.
- Repeat all tasks with only every second or third task being rewarded with a treat. (Remember praise!)
- Repeat with only intermittent treat reinforcement. (Remember praise!)

Antianxiety medications may help some dogs that otherwise are unable to succeed in this program. Remember, if it is decided that medication could benefit your dog, you need to use it *in addition* to the behavior modification, not instead of it.

B-7 TIER 2: PROTOCOL FOR DESENSITIZING AND COUNTERCONDITIONING DOGS TO RELINQUISH OBJECTS

Some dogs have difficulty relinquishing objects about which they care. These can range from objects such as bones, whose value people can generally appreciate, to illogical objects such as seeds harvested outside and brought into the house. All dogs should be able to relinquish possessions of any kind to their people on request. Not only is this a sign that they are willing to be deferential to their people, but also it is a behavior that could save their life some day if the object that they are so fiercely protecting can hurt them.

The point of this protocol is to teach the dog to relinquish any object to its person *on request.* If you cannot teach the dog to willingly relinquish one class of objects—and this may happen if those objects are bones—it would be far preferable to omit these from the dog's repertoire forever. Remember, the goals of this program are twofold: by decreasing the dog's anxiety if it is inappropriately protecting an object, it is hoped that the dog will learn to relax and be less anxious when presented with the object, and, finally, minimization of any danger to any person who may come in contact with the dog when it is protecting the object, regardless of whether the person thinks that such protection is rational. When dogs learn to behave appropriately, they become safer.

Before starting this tier of the behavior modification programs, all dogs should have successfully completed "Protocol for Deference: Basic Program" and "Protocol for Relaxation: Behavior Modification Tier 1." To begin the tasks in this protocol, select an object in which the dog has no interest—a paperweight or a rock from outdoors. The object should have *no value to the dog* and certainly should not frighten the dog. Ask the dog to sit and stay or to lie down and stay, and relax, and then place the object about 2 to 3 meters from the dog so that the dog can see the object. Reward the dog for relaxing. Instruct the dog to stay; then pick up and quickly return the object. Return to the dog and reward the dog if it relaxed and did not move. Continue to pick up and replace the object, moving it progressively closer to the dog in a gradual manner. Each time you pick up and replace the object, remember to return to the dog and reward the dog if it ignored the movement of the object and relaxed (see the following task sheets). If at any point the dog picks up the object, ask the dog to drop it. This is a command that all puppies should learn, and you can use this protocol to teach it. If the dog drops the object, tell the dog that it was good, but do not reward it with a food treat. After this, ask the dog to wait or stay for 5 to 10 seconds; if it does so, reward the dog with a food treat. If the dog does not drop the object after a second request, you can either isolate the dog or leave the room.

If you leave the room you have denied the dog both your attention and control of the situation. The dog will ultimately seek you out. When it does, ask the dog to sit, request that it wait, and pursue some exercises from Tier 1. Then start with the tasks in this protocol again.

Isolating the dog may be difficult if the dog also has any aggressions toward you. Aggressions involving possession often coexist with other aggressions that may involve people. Alternatively, you can use a Gentle Leader/Promise System Canine Head Collar when you work with the dog. If the dog does grab the object, you can safely interrupt the theft in the act and reinforce the dog's relaxation. If you are concerned about your ability to take an object directly from the dog, you should use a head collar for the first round of these exercises.

After the dog is able to sit quietly and relax, even if the object is removed from directly in front of it, select a different item with which to work with the dog. The next object should be one about which the dog cares slightly more. Repeat the entire protocol as listed in the following task pages. Continue to repeat all of the tasks, sequentially selecting an item that is progressively more interesting to the dog.

Finally, if your dog is able to complete the entire protocol and appear relaxed and happy when you pick up even the most valued of its items, you may wish to start "take it—drop it." This is another exercise that all puppies should learn. Start with objects in which the dogs have a mild interest (a broken squeak toy) and proceed to objects in which the dog has a keen interest (a rope toy or plush dog toy). Consider using rawhides or real bones *if and only if* your dog is not aggressive around food. It is ideal to start puppies by teaching them to relinquish rawhides, but if you begin to have problems with aggression, talk to your veterinarian. It is always safer to deny rawhides and real bones to dogs that have the potential for problem behaviors. The dogs will not be deprived if you do so.

Finally, remember all of the work that you emphasized in Tier 1 of the protocols. Use body language cues to tell whether the dog is relaxed or distressed. Distressed dogs cannot learn or focus and may shake, tremble, whine, salivate, move their eyes from side to side, pull the corners of their lips horizontally backward, and so on. Remember, for these protocols to work best, it is not sufficient that the dog is just sitting and staying. The dog must be relaxed while doing this. Dogs that can learn to enjoy the exercises will progress at the fastest rate. As for the other protocols, if at any point the dog continues to have difficulty with the tasks, divide them into smaller units and continue. If the dog works best for three 5-minute periods instead of one 15-minute period, do the former first and then work up to the latter.

Dog's Task	Comments about response or difficulty

The dog should sit, stay, and relax when:

The object is placed on the floor 3 meters away from the dog; briefly retrieve and replace the object

The object is placed on the floor 2.5 meters away from the dog; briefly retrieve and replace the object

The object is placed on the floor 2 meters away from the dog; briefly retrieve and replace the object

The object is placed on the floor 1.5 meters away from the dog; briefly retrieve and replace the object

The object is placed on the floor 1 meter away from the dog; briefly retrieve and replace the object

The object is placed on the floor 0.5 meters away from the dog; briefly retrieve and replace the object

The object is placed on the floor 0.25 meters away from the dog; briefly retrieve and replace the object

The object is placed on the floor 10 centimeters away from the dog; briefly retrieve and replace the object

The object is placed on the floor 5 centimeters away from the dog; briefly retrieve and replace the object

The object is placed on the floor 2 centimeters away from the dog; briefly retrieve and replace the object

The object is placed on the floor, touching the dog's feet; briefly retrieve and replace the object

For Future Repetitions

- Repeat all tasks in different locations.
- Repeat all tasks with all family members.
- Repeat all tasks with only every second or third task being rewarded with a treat. (Remember praise!)
- Repeat with only intermittent treat reinforcement. (Remember praise!)

Advanced Section (And For Puppies)

Have the dog sit and relax while you hold out an object in which the dog is interested and do the following:

Dog's Task

Put the object in the dog's mouth or, if the dog will take the object itself, offer it with the request to take it and let the dog hold it for 1 second, then repeat above

Put the object in the dog's mouth or, if the dog will take the object itself, offer it with the request to take it and let the dog hold it for 1 second, then repeat above

Put the object in the dog's mouth or, if the dog will take the object itself, offer it with the request to take it and let the dog hold it for 2 seconds, then repeat above

Put the object in the dog's mouth or, if the dog will take the object itself, offer it with the request to take it and let the dog hold it for 3 seconds, then repeat above

Put the object in the dog's mouth or, if the dog will take the object itself, offer it with the request to take it and let the dog hold it for 4 seconds, then repeat above

Put the object in the dog's mouth or, if the dog will take the object itself, offer it with the request to take it and let the dog hold it for 5 seconds, then repeat above

Put the object directly under the dog's nose or gently in its mouth and say, "Take it"; before the object can be fully grasped say, "Good boy (girl)!" and then say, "Drop it"; reward the dog for allowing you to take the object, although the dog never truly held it. Gradually advance to letting the dog hold the object for, at first, a very short time. Reward the dog with praise or a tiny treat when it responds to "drop it." Slowly increase the amount of time that the dog can have the object before you request that the dog drop it.

Comments about response or difficulty

Repeat the previous exercises with progressively more fascinating (for the dog) objects.

Ultimately, you should be able to request that the dog take and drop virtually anything.

Antianxiety medications may help some dogs that otherwise are unable to succeed in this program. Remember, if it is decided that medication could benefit your dog, you need to use it *in addition* to the behavior modification, not instead of it.

B-8 TIER 2: PROTOCOL FOR DESENSITIZATION AND COUNTERCONDITIONING TO NOISES AND ACTIVITIES THAT OCCUR BY THE DOOR

Some dogs that cannot be left alone become anxious whenever any activity occurs by doors. Some dogs that are fearfully aggressive or those that are protectively or territorially aggressive react whenever anyone comes to a door and rings the doorbell or knocks. Because the reaction level at the door is a key in the dog's increasing anxieties, clients often need to work separately on desensitizing and counterconditioning the dogs to noises and activities around the door. This protocol is designed to help you teach your dog to relax and to be calm in such circumstances. As with the other protocols, it is expected that you have completed "Protocol for Deference: Basic Program" and "Protocol for Relaxation: Behavior Modification Tier 1." You may use this program to help with the last part of Tier 1.

Place the dog in the middle of the room (see suggested layout drawing) with its side facing the door. This allows the dog to use peripheral vision but will not draw all attention to the door. It is best to have two people to practice this protocol: one person acts as the rewarder, and one person acts as the stranger. It is best at first if the stranger is a person with whom the dog is comfortable.

The goal of the protocol is to get the dog to relax when given a cue to do so, despite the fact that someone is at the door. Some people prefer that the dog be permitted to bark once or twice as a warning before being quiet. This may be possible, but for some dogs, even reacting to that limited extent may send them into a cascade of behavior that is undesirable and inappropriate. It is not sufficient that the dog is sitting or lying quietly—it must not be showing any of the physical signs of underlying physiological stress (shaking, trembling, panting, salivating, increased heart rate, averted gaze, frequent eye movements, and so on). Relaxed animals can learn, and animals that enjoy the tasks learn faster.

When the dog is sitting or lying down and is relaxed, give instructions to the stranger to begin to knock softly and briefly (see the following task list). You should review the plan with the stranger before you practice with the dog so that you two can communicate without confusion. This helps prevent anxiety in the dog. As soon as you hear or anticipate that you will hear the knock, call the dog to look at you. As soon as it looks at you, say, "Good boy (girl)!" and reward with a treat. If the dog glances quickly at the door but otherwise does not appear to be upset and either spontaneously returns its gaze to you or responds to a soft signal from you (pursing of your lips, clearing your throat, saying the dog's name, and so on), you can reward the dog. If the dog reacts or stares at the door, call the dog to you; farther away from the door, repeat, with the stranger knocking more softly. If this does not work and the dog continues to react, take the dog out of the room, practice some tasks from Tier 1 when the dog is calm enough to successfully do so, and start again at a softer level of knock with more distance between the dog and the door.

A Gentle Leader/Promise System Canine Head Collar can help correct the dog at the door at the point in the behavioral sequence of reacting to the door when the dog is best able to learn from the experience (when it first starts). You can also prevent the full-blown inappropriate behavior and help the dog relax while using a head collar.

Finally, if you must remove the dog from the room, you will be best served by being able to do so with a verbal command. If your dog will not respond to a verbal command to come when it is upset, you will need a head collar to kindly and gently lead the dog toward a more appropriate behavior. If you have any doubts that you can easily correct the dog with a verbal command, or if you or the stranger are concerned about personal safety, please use a head collar. If you work with the dog, it will learn to couple the verbal command with the collar direction, and you will gradually be able to work off-leash. If this never happens, it is not a disaster. Provided you are with the dog, you can use a head collar and a long-distance lead to correct inappropriate door behavior. Do not leave leads or head collars on an unsupervised dog; the dog could injure itself.

If you do not have someone to help you practice the tasks, you can still participate in this protocol. Make a tape recording of the tasks as listed with appropriate pauses between them, and start with the volume very low. As your dog's behavior improves, increase the volume. This also works well for dogs that react more to the people on the other side of the door than they do to the sounds.

The following tasks will help you teach your dog to react more appropriately at the door. Remember that you can use a baby gate to keep the dog in a room away from the door so that you do not get into a contest of wills at an entryway. If the dog is less upset under gated circumstances, you can progress more quickly with the program because the dog will not continue to learn from and reinforce its inappropriate behavior.

Dog's Task

Dog sits and relaxes while:
Person knocks briefly and softly
Person knocks softly for 5 seconds
Person knocks softly for 10 seconds
Person knocks moderately and briefly
Person knocks moderately for 5 seconds
Person knocks moderately for 10 seconds
Person knocks normally, briefly
Person knocks normally for 5 seconds
Person knocks normally for 10 seconds
Person knocks loudly for 5 seconds
Person knocks loudly for 10 seconds
Person bangs on the door briefly
Person bangs on the door for 5 seconds
Person bangs on the door for 10 seconds

Comments about response or difficulty

Person rings the doorbell briefly
Person rings the doorbell for a normal length of time
Person rings the doorbell for 5 seconds
Person knocks on the door normally and turns the knob
Person opens the door 2 centimeters
Person opens the door 5 centimeters
Person opens the door 10 centimeters
Person opens the door, steps into the doorway, and then closes the door
 (do not enter)
Person opens the door, steps through the doorway into the room, then
 exits
Person opens the door, enters the room, and closes the door behind him
 or her

Once the dog can sit and stay while a familiar person can come to and through the doorway, repeat the task list with someone who is less familiar to the dog.

For Future Repetitions
* Repeat all tasks in different locations.
* Repeat all tasks with all family members.
* Repeat all tasks with only every second or third task being rewarded with a treat. (Remember praise!)
* Repeat with only intermittent treat reinforcement. (Remember praise!)

Antianxiety medications may help some dogs that otherwise are unable to succeed in this program. Remember, if it is decided that medication could benefit your dog, you need to use it *in addition* to the behavior modification, not instead of it.

B-9 PROTOCOL FOR DOGS WITH PROTECTIVE AND/OR TERRITORIAL AGGRESSION

Dogs with protective or territorial aggression protect people or places regardless of whether there is actually a threat. This is an inappropriate, out-of-context response and one that is potentially dangerous to the person or other animal that the dog perceives is trespassing. A dog that was behaving appropriately would either take its cues as to the appropriateness of its behavior from its people or from the context. Dogs that make good contextual distinctions generally give some low-level threat (a bark or a growl) and then make their decision about whether the threat is real on the basis of response that they receive. This is one reason that it is foolish to bark back at or growl at a barking or growling dog: the dog correctly perceives your response as a threatening answer and then becomes more aggressive. Children are particularly tempted to behave in this in appropriate manner and should be explicitly taught not to do so.

Clients often find protective and territorial behaviors desirable in their dogs and want the dogs to protect them and their property. If there truly is a threat (an attack or a break-in), it appears that dogs treated for problem protective or territorial aggression will still react to repel the intruder. It is almost impossible to teach dogs to act in an appropriately protective manner unless they show signs of interest. Once the dog appears to be willing to protect, those traits can be enhanced through training. The problem is that appropriate protection and inappropriate protective aggression are two very different circumstances. Clients are often concerned that if they control their dog's inappropriate, out-of-context protective or territorial aggression that their dog will no longer protect them or their property if there is a threat. This is not true, and it is kinder and safer for everyone to take action to ensure that the dog learns not to react inappropriately.

Dogs can protect people or animals in their household from other people and other animals (protective aggression), or they can protect a space (crate, car, yard, room, house) from other animals or people (territorial aggression). These become problematic behaviors because the dog responds as if there is a threat when none exists. For example, when someone hugs the client in the presence of the dog, the dog threatens or bites the person hugging the client. In this example the dog exhibits the same behavior that it uses to repel an intruder who physically threatened the client.

Some dogs react inappropriately even if no one touches their person—if the client stops to talk to someone on the street the dog may start to growl. Clients often report that these dogs do not react if the client does not acknowledge the presence of the passerby, whereas other clients complain that their dog begins to react even if the dog sees another person on the street. Both behaviors are a part of a continuum of problematic behavior. In either case the person that the dog threatens can be a total stranger (e.g., a delivery person) or someone known to them, but not well (e.g., the client's cousin). Only in rare cases will the dog inappropriately protect one household member from another. This situation sometimes arises when children are involved. Dogs that are not sure whether the threat is real may protect the child against being yelled at or hit by the parent. If no physical abuse of the pet or child is, or has been, involved, this is an undesirable, exaggerated, and inappropriate response. One of the requirements that will then be factored into the treatment of the dog will be to find ways to correct the child that do not put the dog in the position of threatening the individual who is correcting the child. On the other hand, if abuse has been involved, an aggressive response can be a learned survival tactic.

It is a common belief that dogs are territorial animals and that they will protect their turf (bed, crate, house, yard). Animals often protect such areas but usually do so by marking and posturing, rather than by threats and violence. The dog that responds to another dog that walks past its crate by growling, snarling, and lunging without first posturing, staring, or waiting to see if the other dog takes the bed is acting out of context—the dog perceived a threat where there was none. The dog that guards the front of its crate from children by pacing and scanning is acting inappropriately—there is no threat. The dog that is loose in the yard and snarls frantically at anyone who comes into the yard has a problem. The dog that will not let anyone enter the house, instead positioning itself by the door and then lunging and snapping at anyone who attempts to enter, is not exhibiting appropriate behavior. Some dogs will be fine with strangers off-lead but vigorously protect their people when on-lead. Some dogs are fine in the yard but become very aggressive when they are put behind a fence, which leaves no doubt as to the extent of their turf. Usually dogs that exhibit protective or territorial aggression do so because they are unsure whether there is a problem. This causes them to be anxious in any similar circumstance. Accordingly, this protocol, as for Tier 1 of the behavior modification protocols, emphasizes removing sources of the dog's anxiety.

Dogs with protective and territorial aggression can be perfectly appropriately behaved in other circumstances. If no one approaches them on the street, they can be well behaved with the family. If no one enters the yard or if they are in the house when someone enters the yard, they can be well behaved. Some dogs that defend their yards or beds are perfectly fine and nonreactive when not near those locations. Both of these aggressions can have extremely variable patterns associated with them; however, both share in common demonstration by the dog of the out-of-context, inappropriate, exaggerated, preemptive defense behaviors in the absence of a true threat.

The best improvement is seen for dogs whose people can very **discretely** identify the situations in which the dog will respond inappropriately. At first, these situations are to be totally avoided. After the dog has successfully completed Tier 1 of the behavior modification protocols, Tier 2, which focuses on teaching the dog not to react to the cues that are associated with the inappropriate aggression, can be begun. The following checklist is designed to help you control or avoid basic and common situations in which most dogs with these problems will react.

Checklist

☐ 1. Avoid any and all situations that may elicit the aggressive behavior. If you cannot instantly stop the inappropriate behavior by use of a verbal command, the dog should be removed from the situation. For example, if you cannot answer the door without the dog barking and growling and without having to cling to the dog's collar while it snarls and snaps, the dog cannot go to the door with you. Simply tell the person to wait a minute and place the dog in another room behind a closed door or in its crate until the person has left or is well settled into the house.

2. Some people want to be able to take their dog to the door expressly for protective purposes. Regardless, as your dog's behavior improves, this will be a task that it will be expected to negotiate without inappropriate reaction. If you cannot instantly abort the aggressive behavior with a verbal command, consider a head collar for all situations in which your dog might react. A Gentle Leader Promise System Canine Head Collar can allow you to interrupt the dog as it begins to react inappropriately, can close the dog's mouth, humanely, rendering the dog safer, and can help you remove the dog from the situation without an intensification of the behavior. All of these are critical for the dog's learning process. The head collar can be worn indoors so that the dog can be corrected at doors or as people within the household pass by. Do not leave head collars, or any other device on which any animal can become hung, on the dog when the dog is not being directly supervised.

3. Warn your neighbors that head collars are not muzzles. This means that the dog can still bite, although now you have the option of closing the dog's mouth to prevent this. Obviously, no one should tease the dog, but for clients who need for the dog to be able to protect them, this behavioral flexibility is important. Use of head collars still permits *appropriate* protective aggression. Do not make excuses for inappropriate aggression. For problem dogs, inappropriate aggression is far more common than appropriate aggression; do not let your dog manipulate you.

4. If the dog growls or lunges, say "*No*" sharply and disrupt the situation by leaving or by bringing the dog into another room. The use of a head collar can facilitate this. For the dog to learn from the correction, it must occur within the first 30 to 60 seconds of the onset of the suite of behaviors in which the aggression occurred (i.e., within the first few seconds of the aggression). If you cannot use a verbal command that reliably achieves this result alone, you need to use a lead and preferably a head collar. For dogs that may also have dominance aggression, which can cooccur with protective and territorial aggression, grabbing the dog when it reacts can put the client at risk. These dogs should be wearing head collars so that the risk can be minimized.

5. Dogs can be let out of a room in which they have been placed *only* under the following circumstances:

   • The dog is quiet and calm
   • The dog, when released, willing and perfectly performs a few exercises from Tier 1 of the protocols, thus demonstrating willingness to defer to the clients and to take cues as to the appropriateness of its behavior from them
   • If the visitor is still present, the dog is introduced to him or her on a head collar; the visitor does *not* solicit the dog, instead letting the dog come to him or her; when the dog comes, the visitor requests that the dog sit; the dog complies, and the visitor verbally praises the dog but otherwise ignores it.

If these are not possible, the dog stays banished.

6. Warn your neighbors and friends that *any* dog that is aggressive, for whatever reason, can be dangerous and that it is important that they comply with your instructions to minimize danger to the dog and to themselves. Emphasize that such compliance will help the dog improve. This is also true for dogs that are protective or territorially aggressive with other dogs. In such circumstances the other dog must also be able to respond appropriately.

7. Sudden arm gestures or motions can be perceived as a threat to dogs with protective aggression. Caution people to avoid them and be alert for potential problems so that you can avoid them.

8. If your dog continues to bark, growl, or ignore you in any circumstance and working through a series of Tier 1 tasks that the dog knows well does not help the dog relax, sequester or banish the dog to another room. Taking attention, and control for attention, from these dogs is one of the most effective and safest disciplinary actions. As soon as the dog is quiet or subdued, it can be released, but you must do this as for number 5, above.

9. If your dog exhibits territorial aggression only when you are in the house, make sure that the dog is placed behind a secure door when any repair person comes. This should also hold true for a friend's visit if you cannot enforce numbers 5 through 7, above.

10. If your dog exhibits territorial aggression only when you are not present, never leave this dog in a situation where it can have or obtain access to delivery people, repair persons, and so on.

11. No dog with territorial aggression should ever be left alone, loose outside. The dog knows what it considers its turf; humans do not.

12. If your dog has protective aggression, it should not be put in the situation where it is with you in a fenced yard; someone that they may perceive as a threat can enter.

13. Never leave a dog with territorial aggression behind a fence, electric or otherwise. The fence defines their boundaries absolutely and will render the dog more confident and dangerous. Remember, visitors cannot see an electric fence and so are deprived of any warning. Problem dogs forfeit their freedom in these contexts. There is no room for negotiation.

14. If you decide to build a pen or run for your dog, make sure that it is not near any sidewalks, driveways, service areas (propane tanks), doorways, or any other areas to which strangers might need or have access. Not only does the logic in number 13 above hold here, but the dog's behavior will worsen by exposure to what the dog perceives to be threatening circumstances. Furthermore, the dog could pose a risk to others.

15. If your dog protects its crate, bed, or eating area, do not facilitate this. Selectively exclude the dog from areas by using baby gates, or make the exact location of the protected area (e.g., the dining location) unpredictable. If your dog decides to protect these areas from another animal in the house, do not leave them alone unsupervised. Always make sure that they are separated behind secured doors when not supervised, *and* place the dog that is being territorial in a place that is a less desirable area that is not as defendable or worthy of defense (e.g., a spare room, rather than your bedroom). The animal that is behaving appropriately should always have free reign and be able to move, unimpeded, throughout the rest of the house. You may have to move the area in which you keep

the aggressive animal frequently so that the animal does not begin to feel that it is *its* area.

□ 16. Get a "Dog on Premises" sign. This is not an admission of a dangerous dog; it is a civically responsible reminder that a dog is on the property. Anyone who has a dog should have such a sign.

□ 17. If you have a dog that you know is protective, territorially aggressive, or both and small children come to visit, banish the dog, regardless. Children can be unpredictable and may inadvertently provoke an aggressive dog. Do not talk yourself into taking the chance.

□ 18. Do not use any form of physical punishment.

□ 19. Remember that by correcting your dog's problem aggressions you will not remove any appropriate protective behaviors.

□ 20. Consistently practice and enforce "Protocol for Deference: Basic Program" and "Protocol for Relaxation: Behavior Modification Program Tier 1." When you and your dog have successfully completed Tier 1, you will be ready to move on to the relevant components of "Tier 2: Protocol for Desensitizing and Counterconditioning a Dog (or Cat) From Approaches From Strangers" and "Protocol for Desensitizing and Counterconditioning to Noises and Activities that Occur by the Door."

Antianxiety medications may help some dogs that otherwise are unable to succeed in this program. Remember, if it is decided that medication could benefit your dog, you need to use it *in addition* to the behavior modification, not instead of it.

B-10 PROTOCOL FOR DOGS WITH INTERDOG AGGRESSION

Interdog aggression can be highly variable, but it generally appears between 1 and 3 years of age and is more common between dogs of the same sex. This makes sense because interdog aggression generally focuses on issues of social status and control, which become apparent at social maturity (approximately 18 to 36 months of age in dogs). Interdog aggression can occur between dogs that are either unknown or known to each other. In the latter case it can be initiated by a young dog that is becoming socially mature or by the older dog that perceives the changing status of the younger dog.

Very few dogs are aggressive to other dogs because they never learned how to interact with them when they were young. Dogs focus primarily on the parent(s) and litter mates until they are 5 to 8 weeks of age, when they become very receptive to interaction with people. Puppies form hierarchies within the litter, and these social orders are maintained both by some agonistic behavior (posturing, vocalizing, and snapping) and by active and passive deference by the other pups (rolling on the back and urinating or looking away). The few studies of this issue indicate that these puppyhood hierarchies appear to have no association with the relative status of the animals when they reach social maturity. Hence they should not be associated with any interdog aggressions that are related to social status. It *is* conceivable (but probably rare) that some dogs that never see other dogs when they are puppies might have some problems relating to other dogs; however, these problems are often related to fear (see "Protocol for Treating Fearful Behavior in Cats and Dogs" and "Protocol for Dogs With Fearful Aggression"). The majority of dogs that have problems with interdog aggression have a problem with relative social status and have had no untoward experiences as puppies.

Interdog aggression is not associated with sexual maturity (approximately 6 to 9 months of age), although there is a role for testosterone in interdog aggression. Testosterone, the male hormone that is greatly decreased by castration (the removal of the testicles), stimulates dogs to roam and mark with urine. These two behaviors take dogs into the path of other dogs, increasing the chances for a conflict about status or rank between two dogs that do not live in the same household. Testosterone also facilitates fighting: intact (noncastrated) male dogs react quickly, react to a higher level overall, and take longer to calm down. Castration greatly decreases roaming, urine marking, and fighting between dogs and appears effective in diminishing all of these behaviors in about 60% of all dogs with such problems. It is important to remember that all behaviors have learned components. The fact that a hormone facilitates the development of a form of aggression does not mean that diminishing that hormone will simply "fix" the problem. If a dog has exhibited a series of behaviors for a long time (e.g., years), that dog has learned about the behavioral patterns and his response. Accordingly, simply removing the hormones that help that response does nothing about the learned component. That is a role for behavioral modification.

The situation with intact (nonspayed) female dogs is not so simple. Hormonal cycling does not appear to facilitate aggression between female dogs in the same sense that testosterone facilitates aggression between male dogs; however, clients often report that many intact bitches experience "mood" changes before and during estrus (heat). Many bitches also experience changes in appetite and activity levels during or preceding their heat cycles. If there were some mild status-related problems between the female dogs in the household, they might be exaggerated at such times. If there is an intact male dog in the house, he might become highly motivated to pursue one of the female dogs and further disrupt the social order. There are few in-depth studies of any association between female hormones and aggression, but available studies indicate that female hormones do not play a large role in interdog aggression.

Both male and female dogs are healthier if they are neutered. Not only do fewer infectious and cancerous problems related to the reproductive tract develop, but females, if spayed early, have a lower risk of mammary cancer. Furthermore, roaming can be fatal to a dog. No dog is a match for a car, and, in many areas, dogs are driven off private property by guns. Most communities and townships have "dog at large" ordinances that prohibit free-ranging, wandering dogs. This is safer for the dog and for people.

Dogs that react to unknown dogs generally do so for two reasons: they are either afraid or they perceive, with or without cause, that the other dog represents a social or hierarchical threat. Dogs that fear other dogs can be spontaneously afraid of them or be afraid because they have been attacked. These problems are addressed in the "Protocol for Treating Fearful Behavior in Cats and Dogs" and "Protocol for Dogs With Fearful Aggression."

Dogs that react as if there is a challenge about social status when there is none are reacting inappropriately and out of context. If there is a challenge (staring, hackling up, placing a paw on shoulders, growling, snarling, snapping) of any kind, a reaction might be appropriate, but it is important to remember that, as for people, rules apply to many normal social behaviors in dogs. If the approaching dog just stares at your dog and your dog lunges for the other dog's throat, refusing to let go even when the other dog is whimpering and has rolled over, your dog is not behaving appropriately.

Most interdog aggression occurs between housemates, and it occurs more commonly between same-sex housemates. It is not unusual for two dogs to have lived together harmoniously for 2 years before problems occur. These problems are not related to "inappropriate or incomplete early socialization" or because someone did something to the dogs. The development of these problems reflects the intrinsic change that all social animals experience when they become socially mature. The more common scenario for interdog aggression within a household involves the younger dog that was fine as a puppy but, now that it is becoming socially mature, challenges the older dog. Challenges to the other dog can include blocking access to a bed or crate; lying on the other dog on a couch; stealing the other dog's biscuits, rawhides, or toys; blocking the other dog's access to food, shoving past the other to get out or in a door or car first, and posturing in a ritualized display where the challenger approaches the other dog's shoulders in a perpendicular manner.

Challenges can involve staring, vocalizing, or outright aggression. Challenges may start with staring and escalate to aggression. Regardless, it is important to treat the problem as soon as it becomes apparent. The longer that it is allowed to persist, the worse the dogs' behavior will become.

A similar scenario can occur even if the younger dog is not challenging the older animal. In such cases the older dog begins to sense the change in the younger dog and spontaneously starts to react. Alternatively, the younger dog may try out some of the behaviors that develop with age (pushing on another dog) and not be the least bit aggressive, but the older dog perceives the younger dog as a serious problem and becomes aggressive.

In general, the dog that is challenged responds in one of three ways: (1) it acts absolutely deferential and shows the other dog that it is not interested in holding a higher rank (rolling on its back and urinating, looking away, waiting for the other dog to be first at everything), (2) the dog fights back and wins or loses and that outcome is accepted by both dogs, or (3) both dogs jockey for status and each is unwilling to concede status to the other. In the last situation the aggression continues and may be prolonged, confusing, and dangerous. In the second situation the situation resolves, but the process of resolution is still potentially dangerous. Most behavior modification recommended for dogs with interdog aggression is derived from the first situation.

Much has been written about ranking dogs numerically and determining the "alpha" dog. Such paradigms usually fail in profound cases of interdog aggression because the situation is not that simple. Interdog aggression is associated with status relationships between dogs. These relationships are not absolute. They change with age and health status. The manifestations of the relationships can be affected by the people who are present and by how those people interact with the animals. Some relationships apply only to feeding and sleeping orders. Because dog hierarchies, like those of people, are not linear, the amount of aggression exhibited may depend on which dogs were where and when they were there. A dog that challenges one dog may not care about another dog in the household that, to all outward appearances, seems to act the same and be the same age and sex. Chances are they are not acting identically, and it is in the subtleties that the problems with the relationship occur.

Treatment of interdog aggression focuses on setting and maintaining a new social order. In general, reinforcement is given to the dog that is best able to maintain social status when this is contested in a fight. (Generally, but not always, the younger, the larger, and the more physically fit the dog is the more confident it is). Preferential treatment or attention reinforces that dog as the higher ranking dog. In some households in which the problem dog (C) attacks one dog (A) but mildly pushes around another dog (B), the dogs might respond to all being reinforced in a linear manner (A over B and C, B over C). How this is best done warrants some discussion, but two important cautions must be issued.

First, never physically punish these dogs. Doing so only raises their level of distress, and they may feel that they have to fight you. This reaction could manifest itself as fear, pain, or redirected aggression. None of these choices is good, and you could make a bad situation worse.

Second, if possible, never reach between two fighting dogs. Most people have good intentions and want to separate fighting dogs to prevent injury to them. If you place your body parts between the dogs, the dogs might accidentally mistake you for the other dog and injure you. When this happens, the dogs usually withdraw, but the damage is already done. Instead, if you know your dogs have a problem, watch them closely whenever they are together and keep cardboard, a broom, a bucket of water, a hose, or a blanket handy. These are all "remote-control" items that can be used to separate the dogs safely. In general, once the dogs are apart, they start to calm down and you can remove the aggressor. Removing the victim if the aggressor is unrestrained may enhance the helplessness of the victim to the aggressor. If no small children, high-strung people, or nervous animals are in the house, a loud noise such as that generated by a foghorn can also help separate the animals. Remember that any animal that is injured is in pain and is frightened. These animals can bite without being malicious. Avoid this by transporting them by means of blankets and loose muzzles.

Checklist

☐ 1. First, separate all dogs involved in the interdog aggression at all times when unsupervised. This will not be difficult for interdog aggression involving dogs on the street but can be difficult within a household. If the aggressor can be identified, that dog should be confined to the less desirable room (a spare bedroom, rather than your bedroom; a pen in the heated, well-lit basement, rather than the kitchen where the dogs are fed). All other dogs should have free range. If more than one dog is actively problematic, the problem dogs should be confined and the nonproblem dogs can be left loose. If every dog is a problem, they should all be kept in crates where they cannot see each other or threaten each other.

If your dog reacts only to other dogs on the street, avoid them until you have completed "Protocol for Deference: Basic Program" and "Protocol for Relaxation: Behavior Modification Program Tier 1" and can begin "Tier 2: Protocol for Desensitizing and Counterconditioning a Dog (or Cat) From Approaches From Strangers." Always walk your dog on a head collar. At the first sign of any inappropriate behavior, ask the dog to sit and relax. Close the dog's mouth with the head collar. If the dog still reacts, turn it around immediately and ask it to sit and relax. If the dog still reacts, remove the dog from the situation as quickly as possible. Use the head collar to close the dog's mouth and lead it to a place where it can sit and relax.

☐ 2. Bell the dogs with different sounding bells. If they are loose you must be willing to supervise them. The bell will signal you when the aggressor is approaching and when the problem dogs are close together. The dogs can approach each other if and only if you are confident that you can control them from a long distance. If not, you have three choices:
   a. Crate one or both dogs.
   b. Keep one dog behind a baby gate.
   c. Use harnesses or head collars on each dog and restrain them so that they cannot interact with each other.

☐ 3. Choose an order in which to reinforce the dogs. Hints about what will be most successful can be derived from the dogs' behaviors, as follows:
   a. For example, you have two dogs and the younger one has begun to passively challenge the older dog; the older dog is snarling and most of the time the younger dog backs off. The older dog is larger and stronger than the younger dog, just as healthy, and not much older. Reinforce the older dog over the younger dog.
   b. The older dog perceives a threat from the younger dog, but the younger dog is not actively challenging the older one. The older dog is weaker than the younger dog, and, although the younger dog is sweet, it is huge. Reinforce the younger dog.
   c. The younger dog is actively challenging the older dog and is getting very aggressive. The older dog is fighting back and the younger one is meeting the

challenge. The older animal is arthritic and weaker, but the dogs are fairly evenly matched in size. It will break your heart, but reinforce the younger dog.

d. One of the dogs perceives a challenge, and the other one does not seem to be bothered. The challenger is becoming more violent, but the recipient continues to actively and passively defer. The last time the challenged dog rolled over on its back and the other moved in for the kill. *Caution:* this is the problem scenario. Reinforce the challenged (deferential) dog. This may be very difficult to execute successfully, but if you cannot give this dog some status (regardless of whether it's the younger or older dog), it will be a terrific victim. Remember, these aggressions are inappropriate and out of context. *Do not assume that the dogs will not injure each other.* They can seriously disable or kill each other in such circumstances. If the dog that is deferential cannot hold its status, you must either keep the dogs continuously separated or find another home for one of the dogs. If you decide to place the challenger, that dog can go only to a home where it will be the only dog.

Reinforcing the chosen dog has active and passive components. First, separate them as discussed previously. Second, enforce higher status by feeding one dog first, letting it outside before the other dog, giving it a treat or toy first, walking it first, playing with it first, grooming it first, and so on. You can also have the dog sleep in a crate or on a bed in your room or on your bed (if you like this and the dog never growls at you while you are sleeping), whereas the other dog is banished to a room or crate outside your room. Each dog needs daily individual attention. The dog that is being reinforced should always get the attention first in the presence of the other dog if this can be done quietly. If necessary, restrain the other dog with a harness. If you are walking the dogs as a group, make sure that the dog that is "out in front" is the dog that you are trying to reinforce.

☐ 4. Fit all dogs with Gentle Leader/Promise System Canine Head Collars or a harness, and gradually reintroduce them to each other when there is no attention being given. For example, watch television while they both sit quietly, secured at a distance where they can see each other but cannot lunge and connect. If the problem dog stares at the dog you are trying to reinforce, squirt it with a water pistol or a compressed air canister. If the dog that you are reinforcing stares at the other, ignore it if the other dog does not growl. If the other dog growls, use the air canister or water pistol. If the aggression intensifies, remove that dog and banish it. If the dog that you are reinforcing stares at the other dog and the other dog looks away, reward them both with food treats—that is exactly the behavior you are trying to reinforce.

☐ 5. Make sure that you have followed "Protocol for Deference: Basic Program" and "Protocol for Relaxation: Behavior Modification Program Tier 1." The next phase focuses on desensitizing the dogs to each other. This is true whether your dog reacts to dogs within the household or to strange dogs on the street (see "Tier 2: Protocol for Desensitizing and Counterconditioning a Dog (or Cat) From Approaches From Strangers" and "Protocol for Introducing a New Baby and a Pet" [the principles are the same].

Antianxiety medications may help some dogs that otherwise are unable to succeed in this program. Remember, if it is decided that medication could benefit your dog, you need to use it *in addition* to the behavior modification, not instead of it.

B-11 PROTOCOL FOR DOGS WITH DOMINANCE AGGRESSION

The most common behavioral problem with dogs that are aggressive is dominance aggression. Any dog that is aggressive for any reason can be potentially dangerous to humans and to other dogs, but dogs with dominance aggression can be particularly dangerous because their problem is rooted in a struggle with people over control.

Much has been written about dogs' perception of people as part of their pack. This simplifies the situation. It is more likely that dogs and humans are able to live successfully together in all the situations that they do because dog and human social systems are so similar. Dogs live in extended family groups, have extended parental care, and use extensive vocal and nonvocal communication. More important, dogs have social systems that are based on deference, not on physical violence and control.

Many people envision dogs as constantly fighting for control and status. In fact, every study of wolf and wild dog behavior has indicated just the opposite: *aggression and violence are the exceptions.* The key to the domestication of pet dogs and to humans' working and service relationships with them is based in this social similarity: both social systems are maintained by deference structures and extensive signaling systems that communicate deferential and other behaviors. This means that there is a hierarchy and that some animals in both systems are higher ranking and others are lower ranking, but this hierarchy is relative, not absolute. Status can be affected by the relative age and sex composition of the social group and by performance or skills. Because dogs share so much in common with people regarding social structure, they also share many signals that we can recognize. Most people are able to recognize the message conveyed by dog signals, but many people have trouble with cat signals. Cats are not derived from animals that share our social systems, and we have not selected them to act in the same capacities as we have selected dogs. Canine signals are recognized because of convergent social systems. Unfortunately, this also presents a problem.

The same type of signal can be given in a context in which we, as humans, would recognize the signal to mean one thing and the dogs would recognize it to mean another. For example, most people state that they think that their dogs are giving them a "hug" when the dog places its paws on the person's shoulders. More often than not, this is not a hug, but rather a challenge. In communication between dogs, pressing on another using the front feet is an unambiguous challenge. Dogs do not "hug" in the same context as do humans. In fact, many humans have been squeezed by others under the guise of a hug and correctly recognized the gesture as a threat. This is the importance of *context*.

The issue of mimicry further complicates the interpretation of situations involving "hugs" or "smiling." People can teach their dogs to hug on command or unintentionally teach them to do this by rewarding with attention what the people perceive as loving behavior. Another example of mimicry occurs when clients say that the dog "smiles" at them when they play. First, dogs do not have the same facial musculature as people (that is why they do not have as many facial expressions) and do not technically "smile" in the same sense as humans. We all know what we mean when we see a very happy dog with mouth open and mouth pulled back, but it would not be correct to attribute to that gesture all of the interpretations humans use when they talk about "smiling." In some human cultures smiling is a threat. Second, in interactions between dogs the "smile" is not seen. However, dogs are great mimics and can learn to be rewarded with love and praise for a facial expression that the human finds pleasing.

The preceding discussion is very important in treating dominantly aggressive dogs because most people do not recognize the majority of behaviors that are correlated with dominance aggression as problematic. *These dogs are focused on control;* to help them it is imperative for the client to recognize and abort even subtle behaviors associated with dominance aggression. Dominantly aggressive dogs routinely dislike being pushed from a sofa or a bed, will act aggressively when a human stares at them, dislike having their shoulders or back pushed on, may react aggressively when someone reaches over their head (even if this is only to put on a leash), may become aggressive when corrected verbally or with a leash, and intensify their aggression if physically punished.

Many such dogs are quite subtle and cause clients to redirect their activities. These dogs will lie in front of doors or furniture so that the person has to avoid those areas and may lean against or have a paw resting on the client at every opportunity. Clients often ask how they can distinguish these behaviors from those that are merely pushy or attention seeking. Clients can learn to carefully test and determine whether the response is appropriate in the specific context. If the dog leans against you simply to get attention, you should be able to physically move the dog without the dog becoming aggressive. This may be too risky a test for some dogs that are thought to be dominantly aggressive. Clients can learn to look for more subtle cues. Dogs that lean on you to be close or for attention do not stiffen, open their eyes, and then move so that they are again touching or pressing on you—most dominantly aggressive dogs do. Dogs that are seeking closeness usually respond to verbal cues to get off or down and then use solicitous behavior (turning their head on their side, rolling over, whining, wagging their tail, putting their ears loosely back, and so on). Dogs with dominance aggression may "talk back," become stiffer, or become aggressive. Caution is urged.

Not all household members may be equally victimized by dominantly aggressive dogs. Young children are often perceived as a threat by some dogs because the children are at the same eye level as the dog and their staring is perceived by the dog as a threat. The more compliant person in the household may be victimized more frequently than the person who is firm with the dog because the dog is sure of its position relative to the person who sets rules but is only sufficiently confident to push around someone who is not confident. Conversely, some dominantly aggressive dogs know that they can push compliant people and thus do not challenge them. Instead they challenge the person who is more forceful. Dominance aggression is a highly variable condition. Any dog that is aggressive for any reason can be potentially dangerous. Every year dogs kill people. The first rule in treating aggressive dogs must be to take all precautions to ensure people's safety. These same precautions will also keep the dog safe.

Before discussing specific instructions pertaining to dominantly aggressive dogs, it is necessary to address one final area of confusion. Many people confuse dominance with dominance aggression. A dog can be dominant without being dominantly aggressive. Dominant dogs can be pushy, can talk back, can snort at people, but are never aggressive in the listed contexts. They are pushy. There is no evidence that pushy puppies will become the dominant dogs in a household grouping of dogs, and there is no evidence that pushy dogs become dominantly aggressive. By definition, dominance aggression is a manifestation of inappropriate, out-of-context responses to specific situations related to control. Pushiness or dominance is a personality style. In fact, many people prefer pushy or dominant dogs because they work well in obedience situations and because some people believe that these dogs are "personality plus." Regardless, they should never be inappropriately aggressive.

Finally, dominance aggression usually develops at social maturity. This generally occurs between 18 and 36 months of age in dogs, although it can occur later or earlier and still be normal. This explains why your dog may be perfectly normal as a puppy and then at about 2 years of age seem to suddenly change. Although the majority of dominantly aggressive dogs are male, this condition is not controlled by hormones, although the presence of testosterone may exacerbate the aggression. The fact that dominance aggression occurs at social maturity is another hint that clients did not "cause" the problem. Some female puppies that exhibit true dominance aggression are very young (8 to 24 weeks); these dogs may have been exposed to androgen in utero. Although they represent an exception to the social maturity rule, these dogs still respond to behavior modification.

Finally, recent evidence indicates that many dogs exhibit dominance aggression because they are unsure of their role in the social hierarchy. Aggression in such situations may have its roots in anxiety. It is critical that the treatment of the aggression focuses on decreasing anxiety. A fair, enforceable rule structure will accomplish this without resorting to physical violence or attempting to be solicitous and will reassure the dog.

The key to treating all aggressive dogs, especially dominantly aggressive dogs, is to avoid all the circumstances in which the dog might be provoked to react inappropriately. This means that you must be a good observer of your dog. If your dog growls whenever you stare at it, do not stare. This instruction is in conflict with instructions commonly found in training manuals, but consider the following logic. You are asking the dog to respond to your challenge (the stare) with a challenge. An anxious dog will only become more anxious if you pursue the threat. The behavior here is truly abnormal: the dog *cannot* back down from a threat. If you do so, you put yourself at risk for intensification of your dog's aggression. You are not giving in to the dog; you are avoiding a circumstance in which the dog might manipulate you and in which its anxiety can only intensify. As you progress through the protocols and Tiers 1 and 2 of the behavior modification programs, you will gradually teach the dog that it must defer to you to get any attention. These rules also lessen the dog's anxiety. Later you will desensitize the dog to situations in which it responds inappropriately. You cannot do all of this simultaneously. Remember, every time a dog has an inappropriate response, three things happen:

1. The dog learns from it and learns your weaknesses and fears (dogs read nonverbal communication well, probably better than you do).
2. You reinforce the inappropriate behavior simply because it continues to happen.
3. The dog backslides because it is upset and made more anxious by an aggressive event. Most dogs act as if they find the circumstance of their exhibition of aggression traumatic; they realize that something untoward hap-

pened but cannot escape it. Remember, these dogs do not disobey simply to disobey you; they are behaving this way because they are abnormal and need help.

The safest strategy in dealing with any aggressive dog, particularly one that is dominantly aggressive, is to give the dog attention only when it defers to you (see "Protocol for Deference: Basic Program"). This simple rule is generalizable to every situation in which the dog can ever find itself and will help enforce the types of behavior that not only help the dog, but also that you desire.

Checklist

☐ 1. Do not reach for the dog or the dog's collar or pull its legs. First, have the dog sit and stay, then you can push a leash or preferably a Gentle Leader/Promise System Canine Head Collar on the dog. All head collars allow you to control the direction of the dog's body and more safely control the dog. The Gentle Leader/Promise System Canine Head Collar allows you to close the dog's mouth if it becomes aggressive. This keeps you safe and stops the dog from intensifying the aggression when the dog can best learn from it. If you cannot reach over the dog without eliciting an aggressive event, use a lasso-type leash to walk the dog.

☐ 2. Do not disturb the dog while it is resting, sleeping, or lying in front of a door or on the sofa or bed. Do not walk over the dog. Always ask the dog to come to you and then to sit and stay. Make sure that you do not shove the dog from a sofa or bed or push it away if it paws at you or pushes on you. Always give the dog warning of your intentions and then ask the dog to come and sit and stay for any attention.

☐ 3. If the dog scratches at or jumps on you or others, do not push or shove the dog down. Instead, turn away, fold your arms, and slough the dog off.

☐ 4. If necessary, walk the dog only on a head collar. Warn your neighbors that it is not a muzzle but that the dog is undergoing some behavior modification. Ask them to help you help the dog.

☐ 5. Do not play aggressively with the dog (slapping at it or wrestling). Play *only* with toys. You can greet the dog with a soft sock toy and play tug *only if* you start the game with the dog sitting, you ask the dog to take the toy, the dog takes the toy only on command, the dog relinquishes the toy when requested, and . . . you always win the game. If you cannot do all of these facets exactly, do not play tug with the dog— you are setting it up to fail.

☐ 6. Do not let the dog sleep on your bed. You may not even be able to let the dog sleep in your bedroom. This minimizes the potential for an inadvertent threat when you are sleepy and least able to anticipate problem behavior. The key is to set the dog up to succeed not to fail.

☐ 7. Feeding time may be a reactive situation. Many dogs with food-related aggression also have dominance aggression. If necessary, feed the animal in a separate room with the door closed to avoid any aggressive incidents. If you have small children you should be able to lock the door. If you give the dog table scraps, all scraps should be placed in the dog's dish. The dog should not be allowed to beg at the table and must sit and wait at all times before approaching its dish. Do not feed the dog from the table if it becomes aggressive around food because this creates a potentially explosive and difficult-to-control situation.

☐ 8. *Do not physically punish the dog. No exceptions.* You will always lose because the dog will become more anxious or aggressive. If the dog growls or lunges, tell the dog "no" and disrupt the situation. You can do this by asking the dog to come into another room and sit or by leaving the dog. If the dog is wearing a head collar, pull the collar shut and say, "no," then quickly lead the dog away from the inciting event. If it is necessary to remove the dog from the room or from a situation, wait for the dog to become calm, then practice a few of the sitting and staying exercises so that it realizes it must act appropriately to get "good" attention. Remember, try to avoid any aggressive events.

☐ 9. Warn your friends and neighbors that any aggressive dog can be potentially dangerous and that they must comply with your instructions to minimize danger to the dog and to themselves. If needed, when people visit have the dog in another room and introduce it only on the Gentle Leader/Promise System Canine Head Collar and only when everything has become quiet. If you cannot do this, the dog may not mingle.

☐ 10. If the dog continues to bark, growl, or ignore you in any circumstances and returning to an exercise or task that the dog knows well still does not work, abandon the dog or sequester it in another room. Banishment is the most potent form of correction that you can use because it removes the dog's ability to control any part of the situation. These dogs are usually anxious and rely on the constant interaction and manipulation to reassure themselves. Removing that option and replacing it with a consistent rule structure that helps the animal relax can be the first step to teaching a more appropriate behavior.

☐ 11. Once the dog is controlled with the two tiers of the behavior modification protocols and the techniques discussed previously, it is important to continue to reinforce the appropriate behavior in the dog for the rest of its life. Lapses invariably result in regression. This is because these dogs need reassurance. Aggression is not cured, but it can be controlled. Dominantly aggressive dogs are not normal, but they can learn to behave normally.

Antianxiety medications may help some dogs that otherwise are unable to succeed in this program. Remember, if it is decided that medication could benefit your dog, you need to use it *in addition* to the behavior modification, not instead of it.

B-12 PROTOCOL FOR TREATING AND PREVENTING ATTENTION-SEEKING BEHAVIOR

Many dogs and cats are very attached to their people and often solicit attention from them. The manner in which they do so can affect the manner in which the people interact with them. Pets that receive little attention from clients, those that are particularly needy for attention, or those that may never have had any guidelines set about acceptable behavior may resort to extremes to get attention.

Dogs may jump on their people, constantly nudge them, pull at their clothing, nip at them, or bark at them. Cats may scratch people, paw at them, pull their clothing, howl, pounce, or stroll up and down their person's body when that person is asleep. Sometimes pets become destructive or eliminate in inappropriate places. Both cats and dogs can learn to steal objects or knock them from forbidden surfaces if this gets them attention. Many cats scratch furniture because they know that it will result in someone chasing them.

It is important to remember that if an animal is severely needy of attention, for whatever reason, it will get that attention by any means possible. For an animal that craves attention, even negative attention is better than none. There is a parallel with children: if a kick is the only attention a young child receives, he or she will return for that kick. It is important that pets do not learn that misbehavior is the best way to satisfy their need for attention. This is particularly true for the pets that are overly anxious. These animals are not just misbehaving—they are abnormal, and negative attention can worsen their behavior. Many aggressive dogs are anxious.

The biggest obstacle in treating this mild but annoying behavioral problem is not the pet—it is our own tendency to automatically reach out and touch any animal that brushes against us. We are more likely to do this especially if our defenses are down—when we are reading a newspaper, napping, or watching television. Cats and dogs know this and take advantage of it. If the problem is bad enough to be annoying, people must be vigilant if they are to correct it.

The mode for the treatment of attention-seeking behavior is the same as for prevention. Although most attention-seeking behaviors are not dangerous, like aggression, they are annoying, and annoying behaviors prompt complaints. Annoying behaviors cause people to take their pets to shelters. It is critical to control such behaviors. Fortunately, this is not difficult.

First, people should establish a regular schedule of interaction. *Some degree of predictability is particularly important for anxious animals.* The person should focus on the pet at a regular time for at least 15 minutes twice a day. Scheduling this interaction makes it easier to do and allows both the person and the pet to look forward to it. During this time the pet could be taught obedience exercises (cats learn to fetch quite well for a food treat) or tricks (the American Humane Society has a videotape on this subject) or could be walked or encouraged to participate in aerobic exercise. The latter could be good for both the client and the pet. Some people who have treadmills can teach their larger dogs to use them. For people and pets with more sedentary style, the attention can involve grooming, massage, or petting and talking. Behavior modification exercises designed to teach a pet to sit, stay, and relax can help. It is important to tailor the type of interaction to both the person's and the pet's needs. Very young puppies and kittens have a huge requirement for aerobic, interactive play. A walk will not meet this need, but throwing a ball or frisbee might. The exuberance of youth will turn into obnoxious attention-seeking behavior if the dog's or cat's needs are not met. Structured time for play and attention provides an outlet for the pet but also ensures that the person does not feel guilty when he or she wants some quiet, non-pet time. Play provides an opportunity to strengthen the pet-person bond. That strengthened bond, coupled with an improved understanding of the pet's needs and behaviors, will make the person more patient with the pet and more receptive to its needs. All of these should decrease the pet's need to solicit attention through inappropriate or undesirable behaviors.

Whenever the person and pet are not interacting during the scheduled times, some mechanism must be used to reinforce the pet's good behavior and discourage its undesirable behavior. If the cat or dog demands attention by using one of the behaviors described previously, the person should ignore the pet. If the pet backs off or sits down and awaits the person's attentions, the pet should be commended and petted or caressed. If the person wants to then interact extensively with the pet, that's fine; but the point is that the person should be allowed to say no without being mauled or bothered.

Regardless, do not push the pet down. If the pet does not automatically back off, slough the animal off (stand up or back up and let them fall off) and say, "No! Down." As soon as the dog backs off, have the dog sit (cats can be taught this, too, but people generally do not seem to be as interested in training cats) and say, "Good dog (cat)!" If the dog acts like a jack-in-the-box and comes back jumping, move further away and refuse to interact until the dog sits. Then repeat the reward. If the person is consistent, the pet will eventually learn. It is important that the person *not* push the pet down or shove it away using his or her feet. Dogs, especially, will interpret this as play and, rather than being corrected, will interpret the correction as fun.

Cats are very adept at getting people to play with them using their feet; every time the person moves his or her foot, the cat plays back by grabbing him or her again. It is important to stand still to dissuade the cat. If the cat persists, startle it. Use the minimum amount of startle necessary to get the animal to stop the behavior. Remember, the object is not to cause a fear or anxiety disorder. Once the cat stops the undesirable behavior, redirect its activity to a toy. Cats often nibble on their people for attention either when they are sitting in the person's lap or when the person is asleep. Any cat that does this should be unceremoniously dumped from the lap or bounced from the bed by moving the bedcovers. It is important that the cat not be able to misinterpret the person's response as play.

If these measures do not correct the behavior, it is time to intensify your response. Get an air canister (the pressurized air used to clean computers and cameras), a foghorn, or a battery-operated water pistol. Use a holster and keep the behavior modification device of choice handy. If more than one person is being victimized, everyone needs to be so equipped. As soon as the cat or dog even looks like it might push on you or swat at you, startle the animal with the air canister or the water pistol. The earlier in the sequence of the attention-seeking behaviors that interruption occurs, the better the response.

If you need to be reminded to pay close attention to the pet, sew a bell to its collar. The point of any of these devices is to startle the animal sufficiently so that it aborts the behavior and leaves. As soon as you see the animal again, ask it to do a more appropriate behavior and reward it.

If the pet becomes aggressive when you ask it to perform a deferential behavior (e.g., sitting), more severe problems than attention-seeking behavior exist and you should get help in dealing with them.

If the pet still persists and is not aggressive, consider banishing the animal to another, neutral room. You can effectively banish aggressive pets by removing yourself to a place they cannot go. Remember, these pets are desperate for attention, and the worst punishment that they can receive is to be deprived of the potential to get attention. Do not cuddle them or verbally reassure them that you are not a bad person while you are doing this; this only either reinforces the undesirable behavior or sends mixed signals. Do not leave them in isolation. Give them the chance to demonstrate that they have corrected the behavior. When they are good, let them out and ask them to do a more appropriate behavior (sitting or waiting for grooming) and then reward them. Remember not to let the animal out until it has stopped any inappropriate attention-seeking behaviors, including meowing and barking.

The final step is the easiest and most frequently ignored: reward the pet when it is calm. People tend to ignore these pets when they are sleeping or being good because they are so used to them being pests and do not want to disturb them. This is unfortunate because this is the perfect time to talk calmly to the pet and, if the animal is stretched out, to rub its belly or gently massage it. The pet is now doing exactly what you wish it would do more often—encourage it! Tell the animal it is terrific and give it a food treat.

Finally, for dogs, this type of appropriate behavior can be reinforced daily by requiring that the dog briefly defer to you by sitting and staying for anything it may want. This includes love, grooming, eating, going out, playing, having a leash put on, being petted, or even having a wound examined. This is an excellent start to getting a dog to take all the cues as to the appropriateness of its behavior from you. All dogs should learn this, and any dog older than 6 weeks of age can learn it quickly. Make sure that as soon as the dog's bottom does hit the ground, you tell it that it is wonderful.

CHECKLIST

☐ 1. Regular interaction schedule:
15 minutes in the morning
15 minutes in the evening

☐ 2. Correct with saying "no" and sloughing off. Redirect activity to more appropriate objects (toys).

☐ 3. Do not push down.

☐ 4. If the behavior persists, use a battery-operated water pistol, a foghorn, or an air canister. Use these judiciously and do not use a foghorn if any animal in the house is afraid of noises, if there is a young baby, or if your neighbors would be disturbed.

☐ 5. If the behavior still persists—banish the dog. Release and reinforce the good behavior with a command and reward the dog when it is quiet.

☐ 6. Reward the dog whenever it is quiet and calm.

☐ 7. For dogs, reinforce at all times that the dog must sit and stay for anything it wants.

B-13 PROTOCOL FOR BASIC MANNERS TRAINING AND HOUSEBREAKING FOR NEW DOGS AND PUPPIES

The following steps are designed to help you begin training and housebreaking any dog. They are divided into two sections: puppies and older dogs.

Puppies

Puppies become adept at interacting with other dogs between the ages of 4 and 8+ weeks and with people between the ages of 5 and 10 weeks. They learn to explore new surroundings between 5 and 16 weeks, and if they are not exposed to these by about 10 weeks of age they can become neophobic (fearful of the unfamiliar). This means that dogs that miss these "socialization" or sensitive interaction periods do not necessarily develop problems associated with that lack of experience, but they may be more at risk for such problems. The following recommendations are designed to minimize risk. Accordingly, in the first 2 months that you have the puppy, you should make sure that the pup interacts with other dogs and people of all ages and sexes, experiences cars and traffic noises, meets other animals it lives with such as farm animals, and gets accustomed to environments in which the adult dog is expected, by you, to function. If you intend to show the dog, take the pup to shows early, even before it is old enough to be entered.

The best time to start training a dog to eliminate in a desired location is when the puppy is between $7\frac{1}{2}$ and $8\frac{1}{2}$ weeks of age. This is when the puppy is best able to start to choose a preferred substrate and to act on that choice. This does not mean that the puppy will not have accidents after that time: it will, but the foundations for easier housebreaking are best laid at that age.

Some puppies are not as developmentally advanced as others at the same age and may do well forming a preference for an area for urination and defecation but may not have the physical muscle and nervous control necessary for extended periods without accidents. There is much variation in the rates at which puppies develop, just as with human children. This control comes with age if the puppy is appropriately reinforced and if there is no physical problem.

If you have truly done everything "right" and the 6- to 9-month-old-puppy is still not completely housebroken, it is important to look for an underlying medical problem, such as an infection, that may be contributing to or causing the problem. Sometimes a slight amount of dribbling, particularly if the dog is excited, can be normal. For example, although not true for every dog, it is not uncommon for female puppies to dribble urine because of some of the hormonal and anatomical differences that distinguish them from male dogs. This usually improves with age, but in some cases when it does not, the puppy may respond to the hormones that become abundant during an estrous or heat cycle. This usually starts at about 9 months of age and continues about every 6 months if the puppy is not spayed or neutered (ovariohysterectomized).

A word on spaying and castration is in order. Spayed pets are healthier pets. They are less likely to roam, are not at risk of dying of uterine infections or unintended pregnancies, and have a greatly decreased risk of mammary cancer if spayed no later than $1\frac{1}{2}$ years of age. If the decision is made to allow the puppy to have a heat cycle, the owner is absolutely responsible for always keeping the puppy on a leash, in sight, and away from male dogs for the extended period before, during, and after the actual discharge phase of the cycle. Otherwise the puppy *will* become pregnant. Fifteen to 20 million unwanted pets are killed annually in humane shelters in the United States. No one needs any unwanted and unplanned puppies, and it is an unkindness to allow a *puppy* to bear puppies. Even if the dog is a superior quality breeding dog, no responsible breeder would encourage or allow a *puppy* to be bred and have babies.

Castration is also an excellent idea for male puppies that are not to be bred. They fight less with other dogs, they urine-mark less frequently, they roam less, and they are healthier. If your dog is not an absolutely top-quality breeding animal (i.e., all parents and grandparents are free of any genetic disease or problem, its temperament and those of its parents and grandparents are flawless, and its pedigree is liberally sprinkled with champions), *do not breed the animal; neuter it*. This is a kindness. Most of the dogs brought to humane shelters are purebred dogs, and 60% of all breedings result in the death of either the mother or one or more of the puppies.

With the considerations in mind, barring any physical problems, housebreaking a puppy is time consuming because it requires attention to the puppy's signals and consistent action, but it is much easier than trying to correct inappropriate elimination behaviors that could have been avoided by the right approach at the start.

Crates

Decide whether you will crate-train the puppy. This is generally an excellent idea for most puppies and can be an essential step in the housetraining process. Small, enclosed areas encourage the pup to develop conscious muscle control to inhibit elimination at inconvenient times.

Crates are available from pet stores, mail order houses, and some kennel clubs that may rent them. If you are planning to travel with the pet, buy a crate. Airlines require it, and you can even check in to some of the finest hotels if you are willing to crate the dog.

Some pups immediately feel more secure when left alone in a crate with blankets, toys, food, water, and, if the crate is large enough, an area for paper for urination and defecation. Get a bigger crate if the pup will spend all day in it. Young (8-week-old) puppies need to eliminate every hour (more if eating, playing, or just awakening) and will need an area they can start to use for this. If the crate is small, an older puppy will be unlikely to soil it; however, no puppy can be expected to last 8 to 10 hours without urinating or defecating.

Crates should always be placed in family areas, not in the damp, dark basement or the garage. You want the puppy to learn to love going into the crate. Feed the puppy in the crate with the door open: ask the puppy to sit and wait (see "Protocol for Deference: Basic Program" and "Protocol for Relaxation: Behavior Modification Tier 1"), put the food inside, and release the puppy. Teach the puppy to wait to go into the crate by using biscuits to reward the dog for restraint. Correctly *reward* with treats or toys; *do not bribe*. Remember, a bribe is an action taken to lure an animal away from an undesirable behavior that rewards the animal a priori; a reward is an action taken a posteriori when the animal has willingly complied with a request. A reward is a salary; a bribe is blackmail.

Each day give the puppy a toy, a blanket, and something to chew (a biscuit, a big sterilized bone that has been stuffed with peanut butter, a Nylabone [TFH Publications, Neptune, NJ] [these are available for purchase from good pet suppliers], or a KONG toy [Kong Co., Lakewood, CO] stuffed with peanut butter), and put the puppy into the crate for some quiet time. This is quiet time for all of you and will provide you with the ability to give the dog a safe place to relax and calm down ("time out") whenever the puppy is driving you crazy and you do not have the patience to work with the pup. Puppies are babies and need their own quiet time, too. During these short (5 to 10 minutes to start) sessions, stay quietly in the room with the pup, but do not respond to attempts to get your attention. The puppy is capable of amusing itself. As the pup becomes more accustomed to the crate, extend the period of time that the dog is in it and go to other areas of the house. Before you release the pup from the crate, ask the pup to sit. When the pup does sit, praise it. When the puppy is let out of the crate, do not fuss over the pup for a few minutes or it could learn to associate release from the crate with lots of attention. Do this later after the pup has performed a few "sits" and "downs" for you.

The crate should be kept clean. If it is soiled, use hot water and nonirritating soap or baking soda and vinegar and rinse well and dry. Use an odor neutralizer. Crates should be placed in well-lit areas but not where they will get the heat of the afternoon sun—the puppy could easily overheat and die. Timers can be used on lights so that the pup is not left alone in the dark. Radios and televisions can be turned on for auditory company and to mask scary street sounds ("white noise").

Never leave anything around the pup's neck (a loose or choker collar) that can tangle and hang on any part of the cage or anything in it. The puppy could strangle and die a painful death.

The crate has three main purposes:

1. To encourage the dog to start inhibiting the urge to eliminate
2. To keep the puppy safe from all the disasters from electric cords to toxic substances that lurk in the average home
3. To keep you sane when the puppy is too rambunctious

Puppies *are* rambunctious. They need an *aerobic* outlet for their energy. The crate is *not* meant to keep them incarcerated or to substitute for that need for aerobic exercise. Do not think that you can keep the puppy in the crate for 8 to 10 hours per day and then not have to play energetic games at night. If you need an animal you can keep caged for most of its young life, consider a gerbil.

Alternatives to Crates

If you are not going to crate your puppy, confine it to one area (kitchen, den, sunporch) at first. This gives the dog a greater sense of security when you are not home and minimizes damage. Leave a radio and a light on for the pup. Expand the areas to which the pup has access gradually, only when the puppy has not eliminated or destroyed anything in the area to which it was previously confined. Baby gates are useful. If you will be gone for more than 2 to 3 hours, the puppy will have to urinate or defecate and you must provide the pup with an area to do this (litter box or newspaper, see following discussion). Make sure that the room is puppyproof: no cupboards with chemicals or toxic substances that the dog can enter; no strings, ropes, slippers, magazines, or mail the dog can shred or ingest and possibly cause an intestinal obstruction. As with a crate, the dog should have a blanket, water, toys, and a few biscuits. Caution is urged in confining puppies to bathrooms, where they have been known to drown in toilets, or in kitchens, if they can reach and turn on the stove accidentally.

Elimination Paradigm

Puppies develop substrate preferences for urination and defecation. This means that if you teach a dog to urinate on newspaper, the pup will learn to seek out that substrate. This can be a problem if you have not finished reading the newspaper and place the unread section on the floor. Although it is more difficult to teach a puppy to go outside to urinate and defecate after it has learned to use newspaper, it is not impossible. It is preferable to teach the dog to go outside at the outset, but this may not fit your schedule. The following are options:

1. Take the puppy outside every 1 to 2 hours. Puppies have high metabolisms and small bladders. Let the puppy sniff a bit; do not just pull the pup and keep walking. Sniffing is an important part of the elimination sequence in dogs. If the dog is just rampantly plowing ahead sniffing, instead, stop and walk quickly back and forth. *Do not jerk the dog.* Sensibly walk the puppy with a head collar or harness (see "Protocol for Choosing Collars, Head Collars, and Harnesses"). Use a short rather than extendable lead so that you can quickly correct the dog and respond to its cues. This movement simulates normal dog elimination precursor behavior. The pup will eventually squat—pay attention and praise it. When the dog is finished, tell the pup that it is brilliant. You can give the pup a little piece of biscuit as it squats on a desired substrate (grass); this may help encourage the association between squatting on that substrate and good experiences.

2. Regardless of the frequency of your other walks, take the pup out 15 to 45 minutes after each time it eats. These are the range of times that it takes after food is eaten for the intestine to be stimulated. "Food" includes biscuits and rawhides, both of which stimulate elimination. Watch for behaviors that tell you the dog may be ready (pacing, whining, circling, a sudden stopping of another behavior) and intercept the animal. If you pick the pup up and it starts to leak or the act of picking up the pup starts the leak, get a cloth and clamp it to the pup's genitals. This will stimulate the pup to associate inhibition of elimination with those muscle groups. It also keeps the floor cleaner. Again praise the dog as it is squatting and *immediately* after it has finished.

3. Take the puppy out immediately after any play *and* naps or after it has awakened at night. If this is the first walk of the day, put your clothes on and have your cloth ready before you even approach the crate.

4. If you must train the pup to paper or a litter box, put the box or paper in one place, preferably close to a door. Take the puppy to the paper frequently and praise the pup if it squats. You may want to put heavy-gauge plastic under the newspaper to protect the underlying substrate in case the pup misses or the urine soaks through the paper. Getting the puppy outdoors still requires you to be home for a while. While the dog is being trained to paper, you still must take it out at least three or four times a day (after meals, awakening and play). Praise the puppy immediately during and after the squat. To wean the puppy from the paper, gradually start to move the paper 1 to 2 inches per day closer to the door. Spy on the puppy during weekends and, as it begins to squat on the paper, rush outside and wait for the dog to urinate or defecate. This also helps stop the dog from being fearful outside. Praise the pup in excess. Paper training may slow the process of getting the puppy to develop an outdoor substrate preference but may be your only option. Some people with small

dogs elect to have the dog permanently trained to paper or a litter box. That is easier for small dogs and fine if it works for you, but if you do not want the dog to rely on these devices, you must go through the amount of work described here.

5. If you have an older dog that is housebroken, take it with you when you take the pup out. Dogs learn very well by observing, and this may speed up the process.

6. Dogs are generally faster to housebreak for defecation than urination. This may be related in part to the fact that puppies urinate more frequently than they defecate. For some very "clueless" dogs, it can help to take either a urine-soaked sponge or a piece of feces to the area you would prefer the pup to use. This may help the animal learn to associate its scent pattern with the area, but it cannot be used in the absence of the other steps previously mentioned.

7. For puppies that are older (7 to 9 months) and still seem to have no awareness of appropriate elimination behavior, diapers can help. This is *not* a substitute for the process previously described, but an addition. Dog diapers or britches are available at pet care outlets and are sold primarily for females in season (heat). The uncomfortable sensation of a damp diaper next to the skin helps teach some dogs to inhibit themselves. You must be willing to bathe and powder any dogs that might soil themselves to prevent urine burns or fecal contamination. A thin layer of petroleum jelly can help provide a protective coating.

In addition to all these steps it is important to note that even if you have 120 acres and the dog will have free range, you need to be standing next to the dog, rewarding it for eliminating on an appropriate substrate, or the association will *not* be made. It is not acceptable to do this through a window or when the pup comes back in. Free-range dogs learn to eliminate anywhere. This is not what you want.

Reward the puppy with a longer walk and more play outside after it eliminates. Do not play with the puppy or allow it to play with other dogs before it eliminates. If the only time that the pup has to watch the air, chase leaves, and hear birds is when it is outside to eliminate, you may be worsening your housebreaking problems. If the pup is brought back in right after eliminating, the dog can learn both to avoid or postpone elimination outside and to save walks for exploration. After all, the pup can always eliminate indoors.

Finally, if you want your dog to start to learn to eliminate on command, give the command, and no other interaction, until the pup does it. Say "empty" or "go pee," and make sure that your last command coincides with a squatting event. Then tell the dog it is brilliant. Use this with play after elimination and your pup will be more than willing to do your bidding.

Punishment

You will notice that no mention of punishment for housebreaking has been made because punishment has virtually no role in housebreaking a dog. Animals and people make associations between acts and consequences; this is how we learn. Finding a puddle of urine in the rug and the dog cringing *does not* mean that the dog knows it has erred. This action probably means that this has happened before: you have come home, grabbed the dog, dragged the dog to the urine, and hit the dog. The dog *has* made an association: you come home and the dog gets hit, but it is the wrong association (or at least one you did not intend for the dog to learn). In fact, if you have punished the pup, the pup probably cringes when you come home even if it has not urinated on the rug, but you do not notice.

You *must* couple the correction exactly with the action that needs correcting. If you see the puppy start to squat (preferably) or in the act of urinating or defecating on the rug, *startle it:* a sharp "no," coupled with a loud noise (clapping of hands, banging of a pot, blasting a foghorn) will startle the pup. Use the lowest level of stimulus necessary to achieve the startle. For some very meek pups this might just be saying "Shame. . . . " The concept of shame probably does not exist for dogs, but your tone of voice will be very potent. The startle merely interrupts the behavior and gives you a chance to reinforce a better behavior. After the pup is startled, grab the pup and take it outside, praising the pup when it urinates or defecates on an appropriate substrate. Psychologists have shown that we learn best and most quickly when surprised, thus startling the dog with an unpleasant stimulus when you catch it in the act is the best way to teach association of unpleasant actions with eliminating in the wrong place.

There is *never* any excuse to hit or beat a dog.

Early Training

No puppy is too young to learn to earn what it wants by sitting and staying. All pups should be taught to sit and stay for walks, food dishes, water, play attention—anything. The fastest way to teach this is with food treats—tiny pieces of biscuits, treats, jerky, or even cheese. This technique allows you to use only voice commands so that your moving hands do not distract the pup. Later you can add hand signals and other cues. The puppy will accidentally sit the first time: hold the treat in one hand in front of the dog's nose; gradually move it close to the ground and repeat "sit" until its bottom is on the ground. *Instantly* open your hand for the treat and say "good pup." As the puppy matures you can begin to expect it to distinguish between "sit" and "down" by using those words to mean only what they say; at first, the pup only has to get its bottom on the ground (see "Protocol for Relaxation: Behavior Modification Tier 1"). At first, use the words "sit" and "down" to mean exactly that, but reward the pup if it does either; reinforce the dog to distinguish between the commands by being particularly enthusiastic if it does so. You will gradually shape the behavior. Later, as the pup is more mature, you only reward it for "down" when it lies down and "sit" when it sits instead of lying down. The earlier you start to teach a dog to look to you for cues and to defer to you for anything it desires, the better. All dogs should be taught discipline, manners, and to respond to clients' requests. This is particularly true for large-breed dogs that can be unpleasant, at best, and dangerous, at worst, when out of control. No dog needs to be hit or otherwise physically or verbally abused to learn to do this.

Older Dogs

The same basic training and housebreaking rules apply for older dogs, but older dogs can be more difficult to housebreak because they may have to unlearn some less favorable behaviors. Older puppies or dogs who have been in kennels for extensive periods may have developed a preference for the substrate on which they were kept.

While doing all of the previously mentioned exercises, you must be very vigilant whenever the dog is around substrates it had used in the past. Expect to do a lot of monitoring and correcting. Spying on the dog can be made easier by putting a bell on the dog's collar. Incarcerate the dog any time you cannot monitor it. *Be patient.* If you have ever tried to lose 5 pounds, you know how hard it is to break a habit.

Put a cow bell, sleigh bells, or jingle bells on a string by the door and teach the dog that when it bats the bell, you open the door and let it out. Demonstrate this the first few times by taking the dog's paw and saying "knock," and whacking the bells. Then tell the dog "good dog" and let it out. This process will give you an auditory cue for when the dog has to go outside so that you can further reinforce the good behavior. You must be willing to take the dog out every time that the bell rings when you are home. Dogs can learn not to ring when you are not there. You can hasten this learning by placing the bells on the door only when you are home and removing them when you are not home. This is also a useful technique for older puppies.

On the positive side, these older dogs are usually so grateful that they were rescued and can now be loved they will work wonderfully for praise and interaction. Use this.

Checklist for Housebreaking a Puppy

- ☐ 1. Put bells on the puppy so you know where it is at all times; this way you can interrupt and correct it
- ☐ 2. Crate the puppy
- ☐ 3. Take the puppy to a desired area
  - Immediately on awakening
  - Immediately after playing (especially if the puppy voluntarily slows play)
  - 15 to 30 minutes after any food

- Minimum of 6 to 8 times per day
- Every 1 to 2 hours optimal
- ☐ 4. Restrict the puppy's access
- ☐ 5. Maintain regular feeding times and no free access and take up food after 30 minutes
- ☐ 6. Walk the puppy on a leash!
- ☐ 7. Do not allow play until the puppy has eliminated
- ☐ 8. Take 15- to 20-minute walks
- ☐ 9. Permit sniffing
- ☐ 10. Concentrate in one area—take small steps
- ☐ 11. Allow play and interaction after elimination
- ☐ 12. Reward the puppy after elimination
- ☐ 13. Appropriate corrections—startle
- ☐ 14. Reinforce scent (older dog, feces in correct area)
- ☐ 15. Use a variety of substrates (show or traveling dogs)
- ☐ 16. Use vocal commands (empty, potty, go pee)
- ☐ 17. Be patient
- ☐ 18. Use odor eliminators and appropriate cleaning
- ☐ 19. Provide nonelimination-associated aerobic play

Checklist for Housebreaking an Older Dog

- ☐ 1. See puppy checklist
- ☐ 2. Identify preferred substrate
- ☐ 3. Gradually switch preferred substrate
- ☐ 4. Concentrate on rewarding appropriate behavior
- ☐ 5. Startle when caught in the act
- ☐ 6. Crate—use natural inhibition
- ☐ 7. Short lead for leash corrections
- ☐ 8. Walk and reinforce the dog frequently; teach dog how to "knock" at door using a bell, for example

B-14 PROTOCOL FOR THE INTRODUCTION OF A NEW PET TO OTHER HOUSEHOLD PETS

When you first bring home a new pet, expect a period of transition and adjustment for the other pets in the household. You may find that some pets hide from the new addition, whereas others might try to push it around. Sometimes the original pets will start behaviors designed to get your attention including barking, pawing, stealing items, or pushing the new addition out of the way and jumping on you. All of these can be normal and are not worrisome if they change within a week or two. If the animals in the household do not revert to normal behavior within a short time or if they become aggressive, a problem exists that will not go away on its own. The sooner you seek help from a qualified specialist, the better.

Before introducing *any* new pet, make sure it is healthy, has up-to-date vaccinations, and that test results for fecal parasites are negative. It is particularly important that all new cats are checked for their viral titer (feline immunodeficiency virus [FIV], feline leukemia virus [FeLV]) status. Cats with positive results should not be brought into a negative household.

You can make the transition easier for new pets by using gradual introductions. The new pet should be kept separate from the other pets whenever they are not closely supervised. This advice may be extreme, but it is designed to ensure that no injuries occur and that the social system of the original pets is not suddenly fragmented. The original pet(s) should have access to the same areas of the house as previously. If the dog was crated, the crate can still be used. If access was restricted to the first floor, this pattern should continue. The new pet should be placed in a neutral area (den, finished basement, brightly lit bathroom) with toys, a blanket, water, a litter box if the new pet is a cat, and anything else that it might need. It is important that the new pet *not* be placed in an area that is considered highly desirable by the other pets. Areas of high value usually include places where the people spend a lot of time with the pets (bedrooms) or where the pets choose to stay when they are alone (around food dishes or on window sills that are good perch sites). If your dog is always crated, you can accustom the dog quickly to a new dog by crating the new dog across the room where it can be seen by the original one. As the dogs become more accustomed to each other, their crates can be moved gradually closer together until they are side by side.

Be sure that the area in which you are confining the new pet is "pet-proof." This means that toilet seats should be down, electric cords should be tied up and put away, sockets should be protected with child guards, and any valuable or fragile items should be moved. New pets will explore, and that exploration should not endanger them. If the new pet is a very young puppy or kitten, you may wish to crate it for its own protection (see handout on "Protocol for Basic Manners: Training and Housebreaking for New Dogs and Puppies"). Crates do not afford total protection from willful and determined claws and teeth of an uncrated animal, but they do greatly minimize the risk of damage.

Whenever any animal is isolated for any reason it is critical that the animal receive a lot of social attention whenever possible. This is especially true for new pets. When you come home greet the original pets (make all the dogs sit first) and let them out, if this is your normal routine. Do not rush—when people are stressed and rush they may either facilitate undesirable interactions between the pets or not be as attentive to cues about impending problems as they otherwise would. Introduce the new pet gradually. First, spend some time alone with the new pet. Then bring the new pet outside on a leash or harness and let the other pets explore him or her. If you anticipate problems, the other animals also can be on leashes or harnesses. If you have too many animals to adequately monitor under these circumstances, the new pet can be placed in a crate or cage in the center of a room and the other pets can explore the caged pet.

The best time to perform gradual introductions is when the animals are calm. Start by petting the original pets and telling them that it is "okay" only if it is truly okay; do not reward hissing, growling, or biting. When you tell a pet it is "okay" when it is upset, you are not calming the animal—you are rewarding the inappropriate behavior. If the animals in the household are calm and either ignore each other or act friendly despite the new addition, you can feed them within sight of the new pet. This distance should be close enough that they can easily see and watch each other, but not so close that they become upset. Once you find this distance you can move their food dishes closer together by an inch a day until they are side by side. If you ever have an aggressive encounter, back off from that distance and return to the last distance where neither pet reacted. Leave the dishes there for a few days and then gradually start to move them again. Feeding and petting the animals in each other's presence teaches them that good things happen when they are together and calm. For this to be successful, neither side can react violently. If a pet does react this way, banish that animal to a neutral zone *immediately* and try again when it is calm. If it again reacts violently, banish the pet for the rest of the day or evening and try later in the day or during the next morning.

Some aggressive and undesirable interactions are not violent but are still not conducive to the development of a good relationship between the pets. You can learn to watch for subtle behaviors that can signal potential problems, should the recipient of those behaviors not be able to change the course of the interaction. In dogs these behaviors include piloerection (hair lifting on scruff, neck, or back), staring, snarling, stalking, side-by-side posturing with growling or lip lifting, and pinning the other animal by grabbing its neck. Cats are masters of subtle threats, and their biggest nonvocal threats include a direct stare and an elevation of the rump and the base of the tail with or without piloerection. Hissing, snarling, and pouncing are also threats but are less intimidating to many animals than the display just described. If you *believe* that the new pet either is losing the contest or is terrified, or is becoming so aggressive that it might injure the original pet, separate the animals. *Do not put your hands or other body parts between the animals.* This is the single most common way in which people are injured by pets. Use cardboard, brooms, loud noises (whistles, foghorns), or water pistols to separate the animals. If you can identify the aggressor, banish *that animal* to neutral turf. If you cannot identify one aggressor, banish every animal to different pieces of neutral turf.

If the new pet is sitting in close proximity to the other pets and everything seems to be going well, tell all the animals that they are good and give them all small food treats and petting, if they like to be petted. This works best if you have two people so one can hold the new pet while the other deals with the other animals. If you are working with two people, switch roles so that the new pet does not associate its rewards with only one person. This can still be accomplished with one person by using leashes, harnesses, and crates. Leashes can be tied to furniture or doorknobs that are at a distance that will allow the pets to sniff each other and react, but not so close as to permit them to lunge at and injure one another. Never leave a tied pet unsupervised even for a minute; it could strangle and die.

The entire time that you are doing this exercise—and it could take hours or weeks—make sure that each pet has 5 to 10 minutes alone with you each day when all you do is pay attention to that pet. This attention could be grooming, playing with a toy, or just petting and massage. Make sure that the pet is happy and relaxed at these times. If you know in advance that you are getting a new pet, you may want to establish these periods of individual attention in advance of the new arrival. If these periods follow a regular schedule, the pets will learn to anticipate them. It may decrease their anxiety about the new addition because they can rely on them.

Once you are able to get the pets to react to each other in a positive manner or not to react at all when restrained, remove the restraints. Be vigilant and keep a water pistol, foghorn, air canister, or whistle with you to interrupt any dangerous situations. If the animals are all behaving well, remember to reward them with praise and treats.

Once you have done the above, you are ready to let the animals out of your sight. Put a bell on the new animal by sewing a bell to its collar so that you always know where it is. This will allow you to spy on any potentially problematic interactions and to interrupt them before they create problems. During this period when you are beginning to provide the pets with free access, remember to provide additional water dishes, litter boxes, beds, and toys so that you minimize competition and the potential for aggressive interaction.

The keys to success are patience and observation. It is critical that the animals are not inadvertently encouraged to become hostile or nervous in each other's presence by well-meant but misplaced reassurance for inappropriate behaviors. Expect that the social system may shift. The dog that you always thought of as the "boss dog" may not only be relegated to a lower position, but may also prefer that. Let the animals set their own pace. In many cases the pets never become close companions but are reasonably content leading separate lives under the same roof. This is far more preferable to frank aggression. Do not push the animals too hard or push for relationships they clearly do not want; this could backfire and you could undo most of the good behavior that you had achieved.

If your pets have lived in the same household but have begun to have some problems with interaction, the previously mentioned protocol can also help them (for more detailed information for dogs, see "Protocol for Dogs with Interdog Aggression"). The pet that is the victim of the aggressive behavior should be fed, walked, and given attention before the aggressor. This reinforces its right to some valued status. If confinement of one pet becomes necessary, confine the aggressor in a neutral or lower quality room. Do not confine the aggressor where it would rather spend time; this only convinces the animal that the contest is meritorious. When you reintroduce the pets, do so gradually as described previously. Move from introductions under controlled circumstances to ones in which the animals are being monitored from a distance. Let their behaviors tell you when you are ready to progress. Put a bell on the collar of the aggressor. At the first sign of any aggressive behavior, and defi-

nitely within 30 to 60 seconds of the onset of the behavioral *progression*, startle the aggressor with a foghorn, air canister, or water pistol. This means that you should not wait to startle the cat until it has pounced on the kitten, but that you startle it as soon as it stares at the kitten. Timing is everything. The startle must be sufficient that the behavior is aborted but not so profound that the animal becomes terrified. At that time reassure the victim, and after *all animals have been* calmed, engage them both in behaviors that are incompatible with aggression (i.e., feeding and petting). If the aggression persists, banish the aggressor until it is calm, then try again. If the aggression continues, banish the aggressor until later in the day or the next morning.

If the aggression—either between new pets or pets already in the household—continues, you can try a behavioral modification technique called "flooding." Done incorrectly this can be very traumatic and damaging. Consider consulting a behavioral specialist to see if this is necessary. It can be a wonderful last resort. In flooding, one animal is kept confined or otherwise restrained while it is reacting inappropriately in the presence of the other animal. It is kept in that restrained or confined situation until the level of the inappropriate reaction diminishes by at least 50%. Obviously you could not keep an animal on a leash for days without respite, but an aggressive animal can be crated for an extended period with food, water, toys, and litter box, if necessary, and a blanket while the other animal is either locked in a room with it or placed in a similar cage facing the aggressor. If one animal is loose, you should realize that it could injure the caged animal or be injured by sticking its paws through the crate. If the animals become more aggressive and upset, flooding does not work and is counterproductive and should be stopped. Usually the effect is a positive one, and the crated aggressor realizes that the other animal also has a right to share the house. This technique is a last resort and should not be attempted without qualified advice.

Finally, pharmacological intervention may succeed where other therapies have failed. There are many newer anxiolytics available which, when used correctly and prescribed by qualified individuals, may be useful adjuvants to behavioral and environmental modification. In very extreme cases of interanimal aggression in which all other therapies, including pharmacological, have failed, the best, kindest, and safest solution may be to place one of the animals in a new home.

Checklist for Introducing a New Pet to Other Household Pets

☐ 1. Separate the pets when they are unsupervised.
☐ 2. Crate one or more of the pets.
☐ 3. Pet-proof the home.
☐ 4. Gradually introduce the pets using food and rewards.
☐ 5. Introduce the pets during quiet times by using leashes and harnesses.
☐ 6. Use water pistols, air canisters, foghorns, or whistles to interrupt any aggression.
☐ 7. Be familiar with the physical signs of impending aggression and know how to safely interrupt such behavior.
☐ 8. Put a bell on the new animal when you are ready to introduce it to the household unsupervised.
☐ 9. Flooding?
☐ 10. New home?

B-15 PROTOCOL FOR CATS WITH ELIMINATION DISORDERS

The steps below are designed to help resolve substrate and location preferences and substrate and location aversions that are commonly experienced by cats. These steps are intended to help reinforce a cat's appropriate litter box use. Remember that the feline social system may also affect the behavior of a cat that is not using the litter box. Note any interactions that might be compounding the problem.

1. All affected areas must be cleaned with an odor eliminator.
2. After cleaning, cover affected areas with heavy-gauge plastic both to change the tactile sensation for the cat and to prevent further penetration in the event of elimination.
3. Encourage the client to use multiple litter boxes, generally one more than there are cats, unless there are more than five cats; large numbers of cats may render the stimulus too strong. These litter boxes should be placed in a variety of locations and be of a variety of styles (open, covered, deep, shallow, big, small).
4. Litter should be scooped daily, and most litters should be dumped totally every other day. The exceptions to this are the newer, clumpable litters; these do not have to be discarded as frequently but do need to be "topped up." Many cats differ in their preference for litter depth. Boxes should be washed weekly. Some old boxes may be so permeated with scent that they should be discarded.
5. A variety of litters should be offered to the cat in a variety of boxes. If the cat is using soft substances, consider softer litters: No. 3 blasting sand, playground sand, shredded newspaper or toweling, sawdust, or wood chips (not cedar). Many clients at the Behavior Clinic at the Veterinary Hospital of the University of Pennsylvania (VHUP) are now using recyclable, clumping litters with almost universally excellent results. Be creative and persistent. Consider trying one of the new trays where urine passes through rocks onto a pad below. Watch the cat and find out what works. Use this information to plot your strategy. Some cats prefer very little or no litter.
6. Cats are not trained to litter boxes; this is a behavior that develops in the absence of human intervention as kittens. Accordingly, a cat with an elimination problem cannot be trained to use a litter box; however, it can be encouraged to use a specific substrate by taking the cat to the litter box frequently, waiting with it, and praising it whenever it uses the box.
7. If the cat is observed squatting outside the box, punishment works if the cat is startled within the first 30 to 60 seconds of the onset of the behavior (that includes circling, facial expressions, and digging) *and* the startle is sufficient to make the cat abort the behavior and leave. Foghorns, water pistols, whistles, and tins of pennies all work with some cats. Foghorns are usually inappropriate in apartments, although clients derive much satisfaction from their use. Regardless, physical punishment, including rubbing the cat's nose in the soiled area, is useless after the fact and is potentially dangerous to the client and injurious to the cat during the act.
8. Some cats may need to be confined to a restricted area at first. If you do this, make sure that the cat has the same choice of litters and boxes mentioned previously and that you give much attention to the cat during its confinement. If the cat was very social beforehand, confinement must be arranged to meet the cat's social needs. If the behavior of the other cats in the household changes when one is isolated, this hints at a social problem that may need to be addressed as part of the treatment for the elimination disorder. Access to the rest of the house can be expanded once the cats are using litter appropriately in the confined area. It is important that the expanded access be closely supervised both because of the potential relapses and because of potential social problems that may not have been previously recognized. A bell sewn to the cat's collar can act as a reminder that supervision is necessary. Access should be gradually expanded—do not give the cat free access to the entire house all at once after 6 weeks of confinement. If the cat has truly learned and demonstrated a preference for a litter or box style, this will be generalized to the rest of the house if the reintroductions are gradual. Remember that the number of boxes still must be maintained at the increased number and all cleanliness rules still apply.

Antianxiety medications may help some cats that otherwise are unable to succeed in this program. Remember, if it is decided that medication could benefit your cat, you need to use it *in addition* to the behavior modification, not instead of it.

Checklist

1. General
   - Scoop litter boxes daily
   - Dump litter at least every other day
   - Wash the litter box in hot, soapy water once a week; use no ammonia products, and make sure that the box is well rinsed and dried
   - Clean soiled areas with an odor eliminator; repeat and cover with plastic to prevent resoiling
   - Take the cat to the box often and praise for scratching and/or use of substrate (If this scares the cat, do not do it.)
   - Provide one more box than the number of cats
   - Change litter types, depths, and box styles
2. Location
   - Follow general instructions
   - Place a scent deterrent in the area (mint or deodorant-scented soap or something you know the cat dislikes)
   - Place food and/or water dishes on the spot(s)
   - Place a litter box on the spot
3. Substrate
   - Follow general instructions
   - Try different litters
     Types tried:

     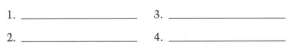

   - Try with and without litter box liners
   - Try covered versus open boxes
   - Try different depths of litter, including *no* litter

B-16 PROTOCOL FOR INTRODUCING A NEW BABY AND A PET

The addition of a new baby to a household can upset the social environment of that household and can upset the pets in the household. Steps can be taken to greatly reduce the probability of this happening by following the instructions below. These instructions are primarily designed for two-parent families. However, it is possible to implement most of the instructions if only one parent is available; notations about this have been made throughout. Please remember that *no animal should be left alone unsupervised with an infant for any reason.* This is not because most animals are innately aggressive toward infants, but rather because no infant would be capable of pushing an animal away if that animal cuddles up to them either for love or for heat. Until the child is old enough to behave absolutely appropriately with the pet (and that could be as old as 10 years of age), do not let children interact alone with the pets until you know how they will respond in those circumstances. This protects both the child and the pet.

Step 1

Before the baby comes, get the pet used to a regular schedule that you believe is realistic and that will be kept when the infant is present. Start the feeding and walking schedule that the animal will experience once the infant comes. This schedule will probably be radically different than the current schedule, and it is best that they do not experience all the changes at once when the baby arrives. Include in the schedule a 5- to 10-minute period daily when you will attend only to the pet's needs. This period will represent its quality time and can occur either in one bout or in two. During this time, pet the animal, groom it, scratch it, play with toys, talk to it, massage it, and so on. Maintain the schedule no matter what, and make it one that can be implemented in the presence of the infant. This may necessitate setting an alarm clock 5 minutes earlier or agreeing that even if a baby cries at some point, you will not interrupt the interaction with the pet during those periods if the baby is not overly distressed and if the pet is not distressed by the child's cries. You might also find that this is a time you can set aside for you to relax; the grooming, massage, and conversation with the pet will help you relax. Be realistic and do not feel guilty. Five or 10 minutes of concentrated attention is probably more time than you give the animal as a block now. Although everybody will have to adjust to an infant's schedule, this is one way that you can tell the animal that it is still important to you and it counts. Realize that if you have multiple pets, each will need at least 5 minutes of undivided attention each day. If you have pets that get along particularly well with each other, you can certainly team them up to play with or to talk to them, but remember that the more animals you have, the more difficult it will be to give them all of the things that they need.

Step 2

Start the dog on a leash-walking schedule that you anticipate can be maintained with a baby. Make your schedule realistic and implement it before the arrival of the child. It would be preferable if the schedule changes could be made as early as possible before the arrival of the child. This is a good time to consider changing the mechanism you use to walk your dog. If you are using a choke collar or a regular buckle collar and the dog does not behave properly instantaneously, now is the

time to teach the dog to walk in a head halter (either a Halti or, preferably, a Gentle Leader Promise System Canine Head Collar) or to teach it to walk on a no-pull harness (Lupi or Sporn harness). This is the time to get the pet under control so that you are able to take the dog with you everywhere you go with the baby where dogs are welcome, *and* you want the dog to behave well. In addition, you do not want to struggle with a baby in a backpack or in a stroller and a dog that is pulling. That is a potentially dangerous scenario that is potentially injurious for all three of you. You may want the protection of the dog, the company of the dog, and the necessary exercise for the dog when you are with the baby. A well-controlled dog will give you this. In addition, if you are unable to take the dog everywhere you take the baby, the dog will learn that the baby has displaced it in that role in the family. Although it is inappropriate to use terms such as *jealousy* when discussing the manner in which the pet treats the baby, any dog or cat will realize that it is not getting the same amount of attention. Pets will also realize that this attention has been transferred to another individual. This phenomenon could then promote attention-seeking behaviors that are designed to be competitive with the attention the infant is now getting. The more often you can exercise the dog (or cat, if the cat enjoys the exercise) with the child, the better everybody's relationship will be. As soon as you learn that an infant will be arriving, obtain and learn to use a device such as the Gentle Leader Promise System Canine Head Collar, a Halti, or a no-pull harness.

Step 3

Again, *before* the baby arrives, allow the pet to explore the baby's sleeping and diaper changing area. For the same reasons discussed previously, you do not wish to wholly exclude the dog from every place the baby will be. These areas will provide smells that are interesting to the dog or cat. Let the dog or cat become familiar with them. You will be using baby powder, lotions, diapers, and baby objects before you have the baby. Let the dog or cat become accustomed to these by sniffing and even pawing or nosing at them.

If the dog or cat tries to drag any baby items off, correct it by telling it "No" and asking the animal to relinquish the object. If you are unable to get the dog to relinquish the object, now is the time to start teaching the dog more appropriate manners, such as "sit," "stay," "drop," "down," "take it," and "drop it." If your dog cannot do these before the arrival of the baby, you will have serious management problems. Now is the time, when you have some time, to address them. It is insufficient to say that your dog has been to an obedience class if the dog still does not respond to you instantaneously for a vocal command. Mechanisms for teaching dogs these types of behaviors are discussed in the "Protocol for Deference: Basic Program" and "Protocol for Relaxation: Behavior Modification Tier 1."

Do not let the pet make a habit of sleeping in or on any of the baby's furniture. It will only seem like a further correction when you do not allow the pet to do so once the baby arrives. Do let the animal become familiar with the area.

If your pet has had toys that are stuffed animals that may look just like infant or baby toys, expect that the pet will think that it can play with the baby's toys. If you are willing to wash these, there is nothing wrong from a health standpoint; however, the big problem will be that the dog may round up and take all of the infant's toys. As the baby ages, the dog may drag the toys from the baby's hand. Babies can be unintentionally, but tragically, injured under such circumstances. It may be preferable to shift the dog to toys that do not closely resemble the toys the baby may have. Such toys can have different scents or different sounds associated with them. If your dog can "sit" and "stay" and take an object and "drop it" at your request now, you can use that behavior to teach both the baby and the dog how to interact appropriately with each other later in life.

Step 4

When the baby is born, have your spouse (or whomever is caring for the pet at that time) take home some articles of clothing that the baby has used. This will teach the animal not only that these new clothing smells are part of its new repertoire, but also that there is an infant involved. Allow the pet to smell these items. Leave them around the house.

It is also best to make arrangements for the pet to be cared for in your home in advance of the arrival of the infant. Advance notice is good because the animal will be rushed around in a surprising manner, left with strangers, and shifted quickly from one place to another, only to return home to discover the infant. It is preferable to have the dog watched for in your home because this decreases the dog's stress level. A dog, especially if it does not like being in a kennel or has never been kenneled, may become more anxious and fearful when removed to the kennel. The pet can learn to associate the advent of this fear and anxiety with the advent of a new arrival.

Step 5

When the baby comes home, you will need help. Someone, whether or not he or she is your spouse, should hold the baby while you go in to greet the animals. You have been missing from the household while either having or going to meet the baby, and the pets will have missed you. You should be able to greet and pay attention to the animals without having to tell them to go away and without having to risk them inadvertently knocking you over or scratching the baby. If you have a dog that jumps, the dog should be put in another room until everything is calm and you can get inside to greet it. You may want to introduce any jumping dogs or dogs that are difficult to control or exuberant to the rest of the family on a leash if it provides more control, but first you should greet the dog or cat exuberantly. Remember, you have been gone and that is potentially scary for pets. After the greeting process, the baby should be held by someone else and kept out of the way. When you are ready to start to introduce the pets to the new baby, harnesses and leashes can be very helpful. Introductions should only be begun once all pets are already quiet and calm and everything is back to a more normal situation. This could take 15 to 30 minutes. During this time the pets might be curious about the baby, but they must first calm down from the earlier rambunctious mode.

Step 6

Once the initial pandemonium has ceased, you are ready to start formally introducing the pets to the new baby. Your spouse, or a friend who is helping you, should sit comfortably on the couch with the baby. You can then be responsible for controlling and monitoring the pet. The pet should be able to smell the baby and explore. Pets should be leashed or otherwise restrained in case they make any sudden aggressive (or even nonaggressive) movements toward the baby. If the pet is fearful of the baby, talk to the pet gently, rub it, massage it, and encourage it to smell the infant. *Do not hold or dangle the child in front of the pet.* This could cause the pet to lunge. It is a wholly inappropriate and potentially dangerous behavior. The animals and the baby will get used to each other on their own terms; certainly, any infant that is dangling over a pet is in an abnormal social circumstance. If you are alone, you can put a harness on the pet and tie the harness to solid, stationary pieces of furniture with a leash. If you do this, you can then sit down at a distance where the pet can sniff the infant but not lunge. You can still verbally reward the pet while enforcing this safe distance.

Remember to be calm at all times. Although one lick might be acceptable, you should be able to tell the animal to stop *instantly*. If the animal is unable to respond to a verbal correction, licking is not acceptable. If the animal hisses or growls at the infant, you must be able to verbally correct those behaviors. If not, take the animal and put it in another room until it is calm. As soon as it is calm, you can try this again in the same circumstances. Do not reassure the pets that it is "okay" and that "Mommy" and "Daddy" still love the pet; an aggressive behavior toward an infant is *not* okay. The animal must learn that if it wants favorable attention from you, it must behave in a favorable manner toward the newest addition to the family.

If you have trouble getting the animal to calm down or getting it to respond to a verbal correction (this might be particularly true with cats), you can try using a water pistol. Squirt the animal as it begins to hiss or look aggressive. Remember that cats that take showers will not respond quickly to water, and you may have to use a higher power water pistol or one that has a small amount of lemon juice or vinegar added to the water in it. Remember that the point of any correction is to *startle* the animal so that it aborts the behavior, *and* you can then reinforce a more appropriate behavior. The point of these corrections is not to terrify the animal. In fact, terrifying the animal or brutally punishing the pet will grossly misfire and will teach the animal that any time the infant is present horrible things happen. Corrections are best done in the first 30 seconds of the beginning of the behavioral sequence, and that behavioral sequence usually starts with a look. Cats' eyes usually become huge, the ears are moved back, the hair is up, and the cat might arch its back, duck its neck and retract its lips or sound nasty. Please do not wait for a pounce or a swat to correct any animal.

Step 7

When there is only one spouse at home with the infant during the first few weeks, pets should be restrained or confined in the presence of the infant. It is impossible for you to be sitting on the couch, ministering to a baby, and prevent a pet attack if the situation arises. The key is to avoid any aggression or any circumstances in which the pet might be unsure of what the appropriate behavior would be. If the pet is a dog, it can be leashed at a distance with either a head halter or a harness or, if the dog does not pull, a neck collar. The animal can still be close to the baby and the client can pet it, but the dog cannot lunge and reach the baby. Baby gates also work well for some dogs. If the dog is prone to run through baby gates, a new baby is a potent stimulus. If you are tying the animal, make sure that the full extent of the animal's reach, including the extent of the neck and head, is at least one dog length away from the child. This is because you will invariably be nursing the baby, typing on a computer, and the fax machine and the doorbell will ring at the same time. Any dog that is problematic may wait for a moment when your guard is lowered to lunge at the baby. Cats are more difficult, but many cats adjust well to leashes and harnesses; otherwise, many cats do not object to being banished from the room for short periods of time.

Step 8

If, after 3 weeks or so, the pet accepts the baby with no untoward behavior, it can be unleashed. Regardless, the pet still needs to be closely supervised and observed. It is best if one spouse tends to the pet while the other tends to the baby. It is important that if two people are to share caretaking duties and the responsibility for reinforcing appropriate behavior, that one person does not always reinforce the dog. Sharing and trading off the attention for the dog and the baby is critical for both people so that the dog learns to associate the warm, loving environment with everybody. For dogs that do not respond well to voice commands and for whom the baby is a strong stimulus, the dog should never be alone with the child, even in passing, until the child can fend for himself or herself. In many cases that dog should not be alone with the child if only one adult is available until the dog can be taught to react more appropriately to the child. Please do not believe that a muzzle could protect an infant or a young child from damage from a dog. Muzzles may prevent bites, but they do not dissuade the dog from lunging and pushing on the child. Infants and young children are particularly susceptible to crush injuries and, in many cases, skulls have been fractured by a dog that lands on a child in play without the intention to do damage.

Step 9

If the pets do not pose a hazard (tripping, falling, jumping, grabbing) and they are truly just being social, there is no reason, once they are accustomed to the new baby, that they cannot accompany the parent around the house and be with the baby while he or she is being changed, bathed, and so on. In fact, this helps facilitate the future interaction between the child and the pet and may help the child become a kinder, more humane individual by learning age-appropriate pet behavior. Regardless, any dog so treated should be very responsive to voice commands so that no struggle should ever ensue in getting the dog to comply with a desired behavior.

Step 10

Under no circumstances should any pet be allowed to sleep in a room with an unattended infant or young child. Use a baby monitor, an intercom, or a room monitor, and close the door. Predatory tendencies are far less of a concern than is the fact that a dog or cat could inadvertently smother a child. The amount of guilt associated with a tragedy would be unbearable for both the new parent and for the pet.

Step 11

If the pet is aggressive or frightened around the child, you should start exposing the pet to children very gradually. Go back to Steps 5 and 6. Such pets must be supervised in all interactions with children. Remember that even muzzled animals can harm infants. Predatory aggression is the most common form of aggression shown by dogs to very young infants, whereas aggression caused by pain or fear is frequently associated with older children (18 to 36 months of age). These children are often uncoordinated and may inadvertently hurt a pet by their play or their ambulatory capabilities. Older pets that may be arthritic or that have painful hips or shoulders are particularly at risk, as are those with chronic ear conditions. These are areas that children frequently grab. Young children should be taught to treat pets gently: no pulling, no tugging, and no pounding on them. Again, this is especially important if the pet is old, ill, or arthritic because any dog that is in pain may use a bite as its only defense against a rambunctious child.

Finally, there has been a well-documented link between animal abuse and child abuse. Children who abuse animals will progress to abuse of other individuals and will abuse their own children in the future. In turn, many children who are abused will abuse pets. If your child has a problem complying with age-specific, appropriate, humane, and gentle handling conditions of pets, it could be that the child has a problem or has observed this behavior from friends. If so, this potential problem should be explored. On the very positive side, appropriate pet-child behavior can be a wonderful experience and can help make the children more humane and socially well-adjusted.

B-17 PROTOCOL FOR DOGS WITH SEPARATION ANXIETY

Dogs with separation anxiety traditionally destroy objects in the house, destroy sections of the house, or urinate, defecate, vomit, or salivate when they are left alone. The amount of time that they can be left alone without these problems can be very variable. In profound cases of separation anxiety, dogs can be left alone for no more than 10 or 15 minutes before they panic and exhibit these behaviors associated with anxiety.

In many cases of separation anxiety the inappropriate behavior is only apparent after a schedule change. For instance, the dog may be fine until 5:30 or 6:00 P.M. when the client is accustomed to coming home. If the client's schedule changes and now he or she is not home until 7:30 P.M., the dog may start to panic at 6:00.

There are idiopathic changes that occur in some older dogs and, for no apparent reason, a dog that has been able to be left alone all its life can no longer be left alone.

In some cases the fear of being left alone can be associated with horrific events. These events include being caught in a fire, being in the house when a burglary was attempted, or being in the house when an alarm system sounded. In these situations dogs may have a worse experience than dogs for whom separation anxiety develops more gradually and may benefit at the outset from stronger medications.

Dogs that are at risk for separation anxiety include those rescued from humane shelters, those rescued from laboratory situations, those rescued from the street, and those that have spent extended periods in kennels or with one older housebound person.

The following steps are designed to teach these dogs that they do not have to be fearful and that they do not have to have panic attacks when they are left alone. Remember, the dog's separation anxiety can be extremely variable; although most dogs respond by having a smaller space where they can feel secure, some dogs panic at being put in a crate. If the dog panics when put in an enclosed space, no matter how airy the crate or what type of room, do *not* force the dog to be crated. This will only make the situation worse.

Step 1

The first step of this program—designed to teach dogs to not be anxious when left alone—involves teaching the dog the first tier of the behavior modification program. This program is designed to teach the dogs to "sit," "stay," and "relax" while the client does a variety of behaviors, some of which may be upsetting to the dog, in a benign and protected circumstance. When the dog can perform all of these behaviors perfectly for everyone in the household in each room in the house without reacting and perform them outside without reacting, the dog is then ready to start the second tier of the behavior modification programs. For the dog with separation anxiety, the second tier of behavior modification programs involves teaching the dog to be left alone for gradually increasing increments of time. Until the dog is absolutely ready for that program, it would be best if the dog were not left alone. Because some dogs react inappropriately only when one person leaves the house, it would be optimal if that individual could take the dog to work. If that is not possible, having a dog sitter in the house or putting the dog in a kennel during the day are other suggestions. If the dog must be left at home, it is best to put the dog in either a crate if it is comfortable there or in a small isolated area. This is discussed in the following step. In addition, it is critical that

the animal respond to programs designed to support and encourage deferential behavior throughout the day. The "Protocol for Deference: Basic Program" is designed to teach the dog that it must "sit" and "stay," look happy and relaxed, and earn all of its attention 24 hours a day. Remember that dogs with separation anxiety are anxious. They are not anxious only when they are left alone—they are probably anxious in a variety of contexts, and it is important to teach them to relax at any opportunity you get. The more you can make their relaxation behaviors generalize to everyday life, the better. It is critical that both programs to teach deferential behavior and the programs to teach the dogs to take all cues as to the appropriateness of their behavior are practiced minimally twice each day for 15 to 20 minutes by every member in the household. If there are several household members, each person can practice once a day, but each person must practice at least once a day. If everybody practices twice a day, the dog's behavior will improve more quickly. The harder you work and the more intensely you work, the better.

Step 2

Crate the dog or isolate it in a small room when you are not at home. Ensure that the crate and the room are puppy-proof (i.e., no dangling cords, no uncovered electrical outlets, no open areas of water, such as a toilet, in which a pet can drown). Make sure that the dog has a blanket or bedding, water, toys, and a biscuit. Never leave a loose collar, a Gentle Leader/Promise System Canine Head Collar, or any other head collar on a dog while it is in a crate. In fact, it is probably best to remove buckle collars while crating dogs because any dog can catch any collar on a crate and potentially strangle to death. This may be particularly true for an anxious dog that constantly moves around. Anything that can be destroyed should be removed from the room and, if necessary, acrylic plastic sheets can be placed against the walls so that if the animal becomes upset, it does not do any further damage. Once the dog starts to do damage, it is possible that this will become a self-perpetuating cycle. *Never use the crate as punishment.* Crates and safe rooms must be areas where the dog is content and feels secure.

Step 3

Make sure that the crate or safe room is in a brightly lit, temperature-controlled area. No dog will enjoy being thrown in a dank, dark garage just because that is the easiest place to clean up. Leave a television or radio and lights on for the dog while you are gone, and make sure that there is a signal that will tell the dog 15 to 20 minutes before you are going to return that you will be returning. You can place an additional light and a radio on a timer. If the dog can learn to respond to this through short departures over the weekend, you can use it in the behavior modification program. You can try this by setting a light and timer and coming into a room where the dog is sitting and relaxing for short periods. Every time you come in, the light should come on. Every time you leave, reset it. If you can work up to 15 or 30 minutes, you may be able to use this as a signal throughout the day that you will be coming home.

Step 4

If you are unable to get a pet sitter, you can have somebody come into the house to visit the dog during the day. This works well particularly for dogs who can go 3 hours but not 4 hours without attention. In some cases dogs are fine when left alone in cars, but they are not fine in houses. Do not leave the dog alone in the car unless you are positive the dog will not destroy it. For some people, being able to take the dog and leaving it in the car is an option. It may not work for everybody and, until you know how the dog is going to behave, it would be inappropriate to subject the dog to an entire day in a vehicle. It is also inappropriate to subject dogs to this if you live in climates that are either too hot or too cold. Remember that when it is 80° F, the inside temperature in a car often reaches 140° F to 160° F. Dogs can die within minutes at such temperatures.

Step 5

Regardless of how the dog behaves to timer desensitizations, set a light on a timer so that it will come on 30 minutes before you come home. This acts as a first cue for the dog.

Step 6

Some dogs behave best if they can observe the outside world. If your crate can be *placed* by sliding glass doors or if you have an outdoor run that is sturdily enclosed, including a roof, and no one can steal or abuse the dog, some dogs do much better if they are outside. This is an option worth investigating. It is not a substitute for behavioral therapy but can be an adjuvant to it.

Step 7

Identify cues that make your dog realize that you are about to leave (see "Protocol for Teaching Your Dog to Uncouple Departures and Departure Cues"). These are usually cues such as putting on makeup, grabbing your briefcase, dressing in a suit, getting up at 6:00 A.M. and putting on work clothes immediately, and picking up your keys. Desensitize the dog to any of these cues. For example, pick up your keys but do not go anywhere, put on makeup and high heels on the weekend, leave for your legal practice wearing a jogging suit, use a different door than you usually do, change your pattern of things that you do before leaving. Start to water the plants before you leave instead of rushing out the door. Anything to decouple the cues the dog uses as a signal for your departure from the dog's actual initiation of anxiety-based behaviors (these include pacing, panting, whining, pupil dilation, movements of ears, frequent solicitation of attention, hiding, and jumping up and down in solicitation of behavior) will help. If you work intently on these for several weekends, you can uncouple the cues in a relatively short time.

Step 8

Finally, most of these dogs require some form of antianxiety medication to improve. Most antianxiety medications have rather limited side effects and have tremendous benefits. After you finish the first tier of the behavior modification program, your dog will begin the second tier designed to get the animal to not react to gradual departures. At that point the need for medication can be reassessed, but starting a regimen of antianxiety medication provides real benefits at that time.

B-18 PROTOCOL FOR DOGS WITH FEARFUL AGGRESSION

Fearful aggression is the second most common canine aggression. Dogs that are fearfully aggressive frequently are called *fear biters*. Many fearfully aggressive dogs do not bite; instead they growl or bark aggressively in situations that upset them. Such situations can include approaches from other dogs, approaches from all people, approaches from children, approaches from people or dogs in specific places, interactions involving a certain kind of noise, and so on. In some rare cases dogs become fearfully aggressive because they have been excessively punished or abused. Puppies that are physically punished for housebreaking accidents can become fearfully aggressive. Some dogs that are fearfully aggressive have not had any bad experiences—they are naturally anxious and fearful. These dogs are not normal but can respond well to treatment.

Fearfully aggressive dogs generally react inappropriately when they sense an intrusion and worsen if they feel cornered. They do not actually have to be cornered to feel this way. Approaching a dog that is fearfully aggressive can be sufficient to intensify its aggressive response. Many dogs continually threaten by barking, growling, or snarling but they do not bite. These behaviors can be accompanied by postures that include slinking, lowering or tucking of the tail, ears pulled horizontally back, piloerection (hair standing on end) over the regions of their neck and shoulders, hips, and tail. Some dogs urinate or salivate while exhibiting the aggressive behaviors. Just because a dog has not ever bitten before does not mean that it will never do so. Fearfully aggressive dogs often bite from behind when the interaction is ending. These dogs often back up immediately after they have been aggressive. This does not mean that the dogs will not bite from the front; biting from the front is their only recourse if they are cornered. Such dogs feel cornered if they have no other means of escape. Situations that can make them feel cornered include when the dog is crated, when it is under a table, when it is in a corner, or when it is under a blanket.

A special class of fearful aggression can develop in households with small children. This type of fearful aggression is usually directed toward children that are 2 to 5 years of age. Because these children are very active, they may fall over the dog when playing and unintentionally hurt the dog. This may be especially true for older dogs that have physical ailments such as arthritis or for dogs that have chronic or periodic ear infections. If the dog begins to associate pain or discomfort with the presence of the child and the child continues to pursue interaction, the dog may act aggressively because it fears being hurt again. In the case of a dog with periodic ear infections, the clients think that the dog has always acted appropriately in the past and do not understand the sudden snap at the child until they realize that the dog's ears are severely infected again.

Children of all ages should be taught age-specific appropriate behaviors for interacting with pets. No child should be allowed to tug on an animal's ears or tail. Children should learn to play with animals using toys, not their body parts. Children should learn to respect that pets are another species and that because of that they may not always understand that the child did not mean to hurt them. Children should learn to respect that animals have teeth and claws and can use those to defend themselves. Until the parent is positive that both the dog and the child are safe together, they should not be left alone unsupervised—no exceptions.

The treatment of fearful aggression involves treating both the fear and the aggression. Because these animals are already fearful, it is important that nothing in the course of treatment worsen this fear. These animals are not the same as those that are fearful without being aggressive. Dogs that are fearfully aggressive are potentially dangerous to the animals or people in whose presence they exhibit this response and must be treated with appropriate respect and caution.

Checklist

☐ 1. Do not reach toward the dog, especially if the dog is cornered or if there is no way that the animal can escape from or avoid you (e.g., when the dog is under a table or in a crate). Instead, call the dog to you and ask it to sit and relax. When the dog relaxes, give it a treat.

☐ 2. Do not disturb the dog when it is resting. This could startle and frighten the dog. Instead, call the dog to you and ask it to sit and relax. When the dog relaxes, give it a treat.

☐ 3. *Never* physically correct or punish the dog. Physical correction scares these dogs and will worsen their behavior. Furthermore, it teaches them that their aggressive response is the correct one because it was met with aggression. Consider using a Gentle Leader/Promise System Canine Head Collar. Once the dog is fitted with this collar, the halter can be used indoors when the dog is supervised. You then have the option of correcting the dog by closing its mouth and then taking it safely out of the room, away from the inciting event. Remember to reward the dog when the dog is calm. If the dog is not calm, ignore it.

☐ 4. Try to avoid any and all situations in which the dog may react aggressively.

☐ 5. Do not tell the dog it is "okay" when the dog becomes aggressive—it is not okay. You may be trying to reassure the dog, which is understandable, but you are reinforcing inappropriate behavior.

☐ 6. Warn your friends and neighbors that any dog that is aggressive can be potentially dangerous. Ask them to cooperate with you and avoid situations that may distress the dog. These may be as simple as not reaching toward the dog to pet it. When your friends come to visit, place the dog in another room if needed. When everyone has settled down, the dog can be introduced to the people if and only if:

   • The dog has been quiet in the area in which it was placed
   • The dog appears to have an interest in coming out of that area
   • The dog can he introduced on a head collar
   • The dog successfully sits and waits on command (see "Protocol for Deference: Basic Program")
   • Your friends agree to let the dog approach them and then to request that the dog sit and relax for a verbal request

If the dog and the visitors can do all of these things, the visitors can reward the dog with small treats. This also helps the dog learn not to react in such situations.

☐ 7. Minimize or avoid sudden movements or loud noises.

☐ 8. If the dog approaches any visitor (canine or human), the dog should be asked to sit and relax. People should be requested not to stare at the dog.

☐ 9. If small children are involved, interaction with the dog should be allowed only when supervised. A head collar should always be used, and the children should practice asking the dog to sit before giving it attention. If the visitors are small children, the dog should be placed in another room before their arrival. This will protect the children, save the dog from being placed in the situation of potentially making a mistake, and save the dog much anxiety. The dog should always have a "safe" room or area that is away from the situations (i.e., children) that are associated with the fearful aggression. This area should be comfortable and should not be used as punishment.

☐ 10. If the problem involves individuals or situations that occur in the house, put a bell around the dog's neck so that you know where it is. This allows you to monitor the dog's movements and to either avoid or correct any inappropriate behaviors.

☐ 11. After you have completed "Protocol for Deference: Basic Program" and "Protocol for Relaxation: Behavior Modification Program Tier 1," you may begin Tier 2, which focuses on desensitizing the dog to the situations in which it reacts.

As with other conditions, many dogs with fear aggression can benefit from antianxiety medication. Antianxiety medication is not a substitute for behavioral therapy but can augment it.

B-19 PROTOCOL FOR CATS WITH INTERCAT AGGRESSION

Cats, like dogs, can be aggressive to other cats for a variety of reasons. This protocol focuses on cats that are aggressive to other cats because of concerns about status or rank. Some of these cats may have other problems; therefore it may be necessary to refer to the appropriate protocol for help with those problems.

Cat social systems have been less intensely investigated than have those of dogs. When given the choice and sufficient food resources, cats tend to live in family groups of related females. One or a few males usually control all the mating. Cats are seasonally polyestrous (meaning that they come into heat more than once a year, but there is a seasonal effect) and they are induced ovulators (meaning that mating causes them to ovulate and ends their heat cycle, usually with a pregnancy). The social system of cats means that not all males will have mates. This is the primary reason that intercat, in this case intermale, aggression is seen—males fight with each other over access to family groups and to females in heat. Most cats in urban areas in the United States are both indoor cats and neutered; thus intermale intercat aggression is not a common problem for most people with pet cats. It can still be a common problem for people who live in areas where there are feral or free-ranging cats.

For the previously mentioned situation to occur, it is not sufficient that male cats are sexually mature—that happens at about 6 months of age. They must also be socially mature. Social maturity occurs in cats sometime between 2 and 4 to 5 years of age. There has not been much research in this area, but studies of free-ranging domestic cats indicate that cats in this age group start to take some control of the social groups and their activities. Social maturity is an event independent of sex or reproductive status (i.e., it also happens for neutered animals). When cats become socially mature, some of them fight over status within a household. These fights can be between males, between females, or between males and females. Fights may be less common between females than in the other pairings, because females live within family groups, but there are no data to indicate that this is so. Regardless, the cats will contest resources or access to resources. The resources may be food, water, perch sites, sunny windows, areas where the cats can survey the environment (French doors or picture windows), attention from people, and so on. There may be no true or actual threat to access to these resources. The change can be in one cat's perceptions of how much control it wants over the environment, over access in the environment, and over its housemates' behaviors.

Typically, intercat aggression occurs either between cats that have only recently been introduced or between those that have known each other since kittenhood. Regardless, it usually occurs when one of the cats becomes socially mature or when that cat perceives that another cat in the household is becoming socially mature. Clients often comment that the cats lived together perfectly well for the first 3 years of their lives and they find the new aggression particularly puzzling.

Cats can exhibit both active and passive aggression. Studies have shown that cats that are more familiar with each other or those that are less evenly matched often exhibit passive aggression. Cats that are less familiar with each other and those that are evenly matched often exhibit active aggression. Very confident cats are superb at exhibiting passive aggression. Unfortunately, clients often fail to recognize one cat's behaviors in this context as aggressive and may not realize that an aggressive situation is developing until the other cat either begins to hide, fight back, or hiss when it sees the aggressor.

Behaviors involved in active aggression include hissing, swatting, piloerection, stalking, wrestling, and biting. Passive aggression can be subtle but is usually unmistakable once clients know what signs to look for. Cats that are very confident do not back down from other cats; they may even set up the social situation so that the cat that they are challenging is denied access to an area, must avoid an area, or must take a tortuous path to get to something that it wants. Passive aggression involves stares and a lowering of the head and neck while elevating the rump and piloerecting the tail and tail base and may be accompanied by a low growl.

Cats that are controlling, confident, and successful at this usually only have to use passively aggressive strategies. These cats will stare at another cat and the second cat will leave the room. If the second cat reenters the room and sees the aggressor, its presence alone may cause the second cat to flee. The victims of passive aggression are often found to spend increasingly large amounts of time away from the family, in areas of the house that others do not use (the basement), or spend time only with the clients when the aggressor is absent. This form of aggression can be very difficult to recognize because of its subtlety.

Clients often notice that the controlling, passively aggressive cat may also exhibit marking in the presence of the other cats or in their absence. The most common form of marking involves rubbing of the cheeks ("bunting"), head, chin, and tail on people, doorways, and furniture at cat height. Unfortunately, marking can also involve urine.

Urine marking generally acts as a flag for some form of aggression. Marking can involve squatting and urinating or defecating (nonspraying marking) or, the behavior with which people are more familiar, spraying, in which the cat treads and kneads, raises its tail, and flicks the tip of it while spraying urine on a vertical surface. Spraying is a sexually dimorphic behavior. This means that males more frequently exhibit it. Regardless, both males and females spray, and neutering animals of either sex reduces the frequency of marking but does not completely eliminate it. Spraying or nonspraying marking can be exhibited in either active or passive aggression by either the aggressor or the victim. It is not necessary for marking to be present for intercat aggression to occur.

Active aggression is far more physically risky than is passive aggression. In some but not all circumstances, if one cat is willing to defer to the other (let it eat first, let it have the best perch sites, groom it), the aggression will resolve. This is the theory behind tolerating some aggression when cats are initially introduced (see "Protocol for the Introduction of a New Pet to Other Household Pets"). However, if one cat refuses to tolerate the other or neither cat will acquiesce to being the lower-ranking cat, the aggression will intensify. Cat bites are very injurious because of the depth of the puncture. All cat bites—to people and cats—should be treated by competent medical help as soon as possible.

Treatment for intercat aggression focuses on establishing a social order that is tolerable for all cats involved and that minimizes danger. These cats may never be best friends, but perhaps they can live together nonstressfully. As is the case for interdog aggression, if one cat is acting deferentially to another and the cat to which it is acting deferentially is still aggressive, great pains must be taken to give status to the cat that is being victimized. Because the aggression between the cats often has been ongoing for a long time before the clients recognized it—particularly if it involved passive aggression—the treatment of intercat aggression may be difficult. In some cases the best solution may be to place or find a new home for one of the cats. Unfortunately, the cat that is most easily placed is the cat that is being victimized. Because this is a condition involving social status, the introduction of more cats into any household with aggressive cats may put the new cats at risk for entering into the aggressive cycle. The more cats in the household, the greater the potential for aggressive problems.

Checklist

☐ 1. Neuter all cats.

☐ 2. Trim all nails as short as possible.

☐ 3. Whenever the cats are not directly supervised, separate the cats involved in the aggression. This may mean that two of three cats in the household can stay together, but that the third one must be isolated. The cat that is the aggressor should be banished to the less valuable or less desirable area. Do not lock the aggressor in a dark closet, a dank basement, or a cold garage—this only teaches the cat to avoid you. Instead, if the aggression occurs in the bedroom or in front of the picture window, let the cat that is being victimized have the valued area and put the aggressor into a neutral area (a spare room). Remember to provide water and litter boxes for all cats.

☐ 4. Determine whether you can find a distance at which the cats can see each other but at which they do not react aggressively while they eat. If you can, you have a reasonable chance of being able to convince the cats to tolerate each other. Place a food dish for each cat at this distance. Make sure the food is something they crave. You may have to forgo ad libitum (free choice) feeding with aggressive cats. Give the cats small amounts of food and use frequent feeding opportunities. If you can find a distance where the cats eat happily and show no signs of aggression or fear, let them eat at that distance for a few days, then gradually start to move the dishes closer together 2 cm at a time. The goal is to have the cats eat side by side. If you can achieve this goal the cats usually will tolerate each other. If you reach a distance where the cats exhibit aggression, anxiety, or fear, move the dishes back to the last place where the cats seemed happy. Gradually try moving the dishes closer together again. If you cannot succeed in moving the dishes closer after repeated tries, let the cats eat at a distance at which they are happy. Remember, it is important to reduce anxiety, especially for the victim. Be vigilant for subtle signs of aggression such as staring. Monitor feeding time and intake. If you notice that the victimized cat is no longer finishing food that it likes or is eating quickly and leaving, threats are probably involved.

☐ 5. If marking is involved, refer to the "Protocol for Cats With Elimination Disorders."

☐ 6. When you are able to supervise the cats, they can mingle under the following conditions:

- When they each have a bell on their collars that allows you to distinguish between individuals
- If you hear the problem cats approach, you are willing to visually monitor the situation
- If you carry a water pistol, a compressed air canister, a whistle, or a foghorn with you at all times, and at the first sign of any aggression you interrupt the cat by directing the device toward the aggressor (use some common sense in your choice of a device to interrupt and correct the cats; if your cat loves to play in water, water pistols will not deter it unless they have a small amount of vinegar or lemon juice in them; if you have a fearful animal or a baby in the house, or if you live in an apartment, a foghorn may not be the best choice)
- If the threats escalate to frank aggression, do not reach between the fighting animals—instead make sure that a blanket is available that can be thrown over the animals or a broom or a piece of cardboard is available that can be shoved between the cats.

☐ 7. Use harnesses and leashes for all involved cats. If there are two or more people in your household, each should take turns monitoring each of the cats. If you are alone, attach the leash of the aggressive cat to a piece of furniture and hold the leash of the other cat. The cats should be restrained at a distance at which they cannot connect with each other even if they lunge. Find a food treat that the cats crave (small pieces of cooked shrimp, chicken livers, tinned sardines or anchovies, or tiny pieces of shredded chicken). Any time the cats ignore each other, tell them that they are terrific and give them a treat. If the aggressor voluntarily looks away from the other cat, reward that. If the victimized cat stares at the aggressive cat, reward that. Do not give a treat to any cat that shows any signs of aggression, fear, or anxiety. These signs include shaking and hiding.

☐ 8. Use a harness to correct the cat verbally or with a startle at the first sign of any aggression. If the aggression continues, banish the aggressive cat.

☐ 9. Use the harnesses to arrange the cats so that they cannot reach each other. Then alternate between the involved cats and groom and massage each cat. Start with the cat that is being victimized by the aggression. The goal is to get them to not react and to ignore each other. Any cat that reacts aggressively is banished. You can couple a favorable response to food treats. If the cats ignore each other, gradually begin to move them closer together. They should not become distressed or aggressive by the moves; if they do, separate them and try again at a greater distance.

☐ 10. If the cats are able to lie side by side without becoming distressed or aggressive and if they can eat together, you can leave them alone for gradually increasingly longer amounts of time. If you notice, at any time, that any cat is injured or is avoiding the other cat, repeat the previously mentioned steps. Some cats will never tolerate being close together but can live perfectly happy, separate lives in the same house.

☐ 11. Cats generally require and use more space than the average house or apartment affords them. The addition of three-dimensional space can help. Consider the addition of kitty condos, cardboard boxes, beds, and crates to all rooms once you have started to reintroduce your cats.

Some problematic cats benefit from antianxiety medication. This may be an option for your cat. The role of medication should be to augment behavior modification, not replace it.

B-20 PROTOCOL FOR CATS WITH PLAY AGGRESSION

Cats experience early kittenhood stages of both social play (3 to 12 weeks of age) and social fighting (14+ weeks of age). Much of kitten play is associated with skills useful for later hunting behavior. In fact, play becomes particularly well developed at about 6 to 8 weeks of age when cats develop good eye-paw coordination and are able to sense and respond to olfactory threats. Cats are superb solitary hunters and can begin to show independent predatory behavior by 5 weeks of age. Their mothers begin to teach predatory behavior as early as 3 weeks of age, and in large cat groups family members will continue to guide hunting skills for months. Studies have shown that cats that are weaned early (orphaned kittens that are hand-raised by humans or those born to mothers that are ill or do not have enough milk) exhibit very early predatory behavior and that predatory behavior replaces some play behaviors.

These normal cat behaviors are seen in an intensified form with play aggression. Play aggression is usually directed toward people but certainly can be directed toward other, generally older, animals in the household.

Play aggression is usually associated with early weaning and a shift to more predatory behaviors or with rough play from clients. In the former case the kitten plays roughly because its brothers and sisters or mother does not correct it when it hurts them. There is also probably some component of the actual way cats play with each other, when compared with the way they play with people, that is important but unexplored. In the latter case the kittens are taught to play aggressively by the people.

Treatment of play aggression focuses on three major strategies:

1. Avoiding the circumstances that encourage the cat to play in this manner
2. Being attentive to the behaviors that are associated with the play aggression and interrupting (correcting those)
3. Giving the cat a more appropriate outlet for its play and energy

Cat bites and scratches cause disease. They can be seriously dangerous to someone who is already ill, is immunocompromised, or has poor circulation. You are not being mean by controlling your cat's aggression. If anything, your relationship with your cat will improve.

Checklist

☐ 1. Learn to recognize the early signs of play aggression in your cat. Play aggressive cats will hide behind doors or around banisters, crouching and waiting for any movement. They then will spring, using both teeth and claws, before quickly fleeing. Expect the cats to hide in these locations and beware; correct the cat at the first sign of any of these behaviors. Some cats will startle at the sound of a loud noise like a clap; some need a stronger stimulus such as a water pistol, foghorn, or compressed air canister. Cats that like to play in water may not respond to water. The point is not to bathe or mist the cat; the point is to *startle* the cat so that it aborts the aggressive attack. Startle, which is a form of punishment, works best if it interrupts the cat in the act of committing the inappropriate behavior. The earlier in the sequence of events that this happens, the better.

☐ 2. Do not physically punish the cat. This only teaches the cat that you will play back roughly, and the cat will respond with intensified violence. Furthermore, if the cat is small or a young kitten, you could seriously injure the cat. People observe that mothers carry kittens around by the neck with their teeth and reason that kittens will not be hurt by pinches and so on. This is not true; cats have extremely sensitive pressure receptors around their face and at the base of their teeth and can correct kittens in ways humans cannot. Furthermore, cats are often communicating other information to the kitten at that time that we are not capable of evaluating.

☐ 3. Put a bell on the cat's collar (use a breakaway collar). This is particularly important for cats that play with your moving body parts or clothing or those that are adept at hiding and waiting for you to pass by. Many of these cats hide under furniture and then attack toes when you sit down and move your feet. The bell will let you know exactly where the cat is and will allow you to do steps 1 and 2 above.

☐ 4. *Do not* play roughly with your hands. Do not wrestle with the cat, grab the cat by the head and shake it, move your hands back and forth so that the cat chases them, or pull the cat's tail. Whenever you are playing with the cat you must use a toy. If you do not use a toy, the cat will not learn to distinguish your body parts from items of play. If the cat misses the toy and grabs or scratches your hand or arm, stop the play and act mortally wounded. If you cannot make a sound that will startle the cat or if this is not your style, you can quickly blow in the cat's face. The point is to startle the cat so that it stops the aggressive event and learns from that experience. If it is done correctly, this action will decrease the probability of the cat exhibiting the inappropriate behavior in the future. There are many stuffed kitty toys on the market or you can make some from stuffed socks. Make sure that the toys you choose for your cat do not have loose threads or parts that can be chewed off; these can easily become lodged in the cat's intestines. Check your cat's toys for wear frequently and replace them if they are damaged or if you are in doubt.

☐ 5. Increase the amount of your cat's aerobic exercise. You can throw rolled-up tin foil or paper for the cat to bat around the room. You can rig a scratching post so that the cat gets a treat if it scratches energetically at the top of the post. If your cat likes catnip, you can use a toy system with catnip "mice" and springs that are attached to kitty condos. You can attach a toy to an extendible, flexible, elastic roping that you tie to your waist; that way, wherever you walk the cat will be able to chase a moving toy.

☐ 6. If all else fails or if you are not averse to it and your cat is young or is a kitten, consider getting another cat. You should try to select one that is also outgoing; you do not want a very young kitten that could be injured by your cat's rough play. Another cat often provides the perfect foil for your cats' aggressive play. Cats are more social than is commonly appreciated. It is not much more difficult to care for a second cat, and the company will provide your cat with an additional outlet for play. Furthermore, if the second cat plays appropriately, it will be able to correct your aggressive cat in a way that makes sense within a feline social system.

☐ 7. Make sure that your cat has its claws trimmed and kept short. If your cat uses a scratching post covered with sandpaper, this is very easy. Regardless, provide your cat with something besides you to scratch. Logs, scratching posts, and tree branches can be useful.

☐ 8. If your cat persists in its aggressive play, banish it to another room. When the cat is calm, let the cat out and repeat the above instructions. Most play is about attention—eventually this will work.

☐ 9. If anyone is injured by the cat, seek immediate competent medical help.

B-21 PROTOCOL OR REDIRECTED AGGRESSION IN CATS (AND DOGS)

Redirected aggression is more common in cats than it is in dogs. This protocol is written primarily with cats in mind, but it can be easily adapted to dogs by applying the same principles and guidelines.

Redirected aggression can be difficult to diagnose because the circumstances that precipitate it are not often witnessed. Accordingly, the people who are watching the redirected event, unless it is directed toward them, think that the primary problem is interanimal (interdog or intercat) aggression. Redirected aggression is potentially a very dangerous problem; the recipient of the aggression seldom anticipates it and is usually traumatized by the aggression because it appears so out of context to them.

The classic example of redirected aggression involves two cats that are sitting in a window. Unknown to one of the cats, the other sees another cat outside. Because that cat cannot have access to the one that is outside and is agitated by that, the cat redirects its aggression toward its housemate. This behavior involves both an aggressive response that is related to the social system *and*—this is very important—frustration at not being able to resolve the perceived social conflict. Another example of redirected aggression involves the dog that is chasing the cat. A person stops the dog from chasing the cat and the dog redirects its aggression to the person. In such cases, when there are no physical barriers that thwart the continuation of the aggression, it is very important to distinguish true redirected aggression from an accidental bite. An accidental bite is one that occurs to persons or animals simply because they found themselves between fighting animals. In these cases the animal generally releases the person as soon as it realizes that it made a mistake. In redirected aggression the animal acts as if it is angry at the person or animal who interrupted it and pursues the new victim of its aggression.

Unfortunately, redirected aggression can be so contextually inappropriate, so unexpected, and so traumatic that the recipient of the aggression becomes instantly and intensely fearful of the aggressor. This aggression can change the entire social hierarchy in the household and cause the victim to hide and become withdrawn. If the aggressor has had a problem with the victim in the past, this provides a good opportunity to further victimize that cat. Full-blown interact aggression can then develop. If the recipient of the redirected aggression fights back, fighting back can either start or exaggerate an already existent cycle of intercat aggression.

It is not necessary that the aggressor continue to be aggressive for the victim to be fearful. The context is so inappropriate that a recipient can learn to be fearful on the basis of *one* exposure. Similarly, after only one experience the aggressor may learn to associate its inability to pursue an individual or circumstance in which it was initially thwarted with the presence of the housemate. For example, every time the aggressor sees the housemate, regardless of whether the outdoor cat is present, it experiences the same full-blown set of behaviors as when the initial event occurred. No wonder the feline housemate now hides from the aggressor.

Treatment of redirected aggression is very difficult. In addition to the checklist below, you need to use all of the relevant procedures in "Protocol for Cats With Intercat Aggression" or "Protocol for Dogs With Interdog Aggression." Caution is critically important. These animals are not acting normally and can injure another individual.

Checklist

☐ 1. Identify the primary source of the animal's initial upset. If the cats sit in the window, look outside for signs of an intruder cat (e.g., smells of urine, buried feces, paw prints, spraying against the window, or nose prints on the glass). Do anything you can to prevent the circumstances in which the initial aggression occurred from reoccurring (put a lace curtain in the window or ask your neighbors to keep their cat indoors). If you know that the aggression has happened when the dog was corrected for chasing the cat, separate them so that the chase cannot happen. Try to ensure that the precipitating stimulus is eliminated from the behavioral environment.

☐ 2. Separate the individuals involved in the redirected aggression when not supervised. Make sure that the victim or recipient of the aggression has the most freedom to roam or to select a preferred resting spot.

☐ 3. Reward the aggressor for ignoring the victim by praising it or using food treats.

☐ 4. Make sure that the victim has all the attention first and that each cat or dog gets 5 to 10 minutes of individual, calming attention (grooming or massage) alone each day.

☐ 5. Adhere to instructions in the "Protocol for the Introduction of a New Pet to Other Household Pets." Start as if these two pets have never known each other.

☐ 6. Put a bell on the aggressor and observe it closely. Startle the aggressor at the first signs of any aggression, including staring. If the aggressor's mere presence seems to frighten the victim or recipient of the aggression, banish the aggressor. Try to ensure that the recipient sees you do this.

☐ 7. Particularly for cats, redirected aggression is so horrific that each of the cats requires antianxiety medication. The medications chosen for each cat are usually different because the desired effects are different (rendering one cat less fearful while rendering the other less reactive and aggressive). Remember, these medications are adjuvants to, not substitutions for, behavioral and environmental modification.

☐ 8. If nothing works after months of effort and compliance, consider placing one of the animals in another home. This is a difficult condition to treat, it may have a high relapse rate, and it may be safer to place one of the animals. Because the problem involves a specific complex circumstance, finding new homes is a good option because it totally alters the circumstance.

☐ 9. If the patient involved in the redirected aggression is a dog, remember that canine redirected aggression can be associated with dominance aggression. Ensure that this is not also a problem, and if it is, treat it.

B-22 PROTOCOL FOR STATUS-RELATED AGGRESSION IN CATS

Cats do not have social systems that are identical to those of dogs or humans, but they still have a system wherein some individuals have higher rank or lower rank than others. Usually any conflicts about controlling status occur only with other cats. Occasionally some cats manipulate people in a manner similar to that of dominantly aggressive dogs. This has been termed *assertion*, or *status-related aggression*.

Some cats have been described as disliking attention or as rejecting petting ("the leave-me-alone bite"). This certainly can be a component of status-related aggression, but for many cats, rejection by biting is only an indicator of an underlying problem. If clients watch these cats closely, they often note that the cat stares at them and that, for reasons they cannot explain, they will avoid the cat's stare. Some cats constantly block clients' access to furniture or to pathways by standing in the way. Some cats rub everywhere a particular person has been or rub (or even spray) the people that they are trying to control. As long as the cat is not aggressive in these situations, there should be few concerns, but many of these cats actively solicit attention by jumping into a client's lap and then biting the client if they are petted or shifted. Cats with very exaggerated status-related aggression may lie on their people, batting at them to make them settle in positions that the cat controls and then biting the people if they do not do this or if they move. Some cats block accessways and stare at or hiss at the person who tries to go around them. Clients find themselves not doing things that they would otherwise do because they feel uncomfortable about it. These cats are very successful at passively controlling their people. This can be true to such an extent that many people do not realize it is happening.

Clients complain that, at times, these cats like to be petted, but at other times they are savage if they try to cuddle the cats. This occurs because the cat has to control the situation. When the cat initiates the petting, it might tolerate petting if the client does not get very manipulative (which may be how cats perceive effusive petting and cuddling); when the client initiates the petting, the cat often resists by using aggression. A hallmark of these cats, unlike many of those exhibiting other forms of aggression, is that they seldom swat with their claws first. Instead they become stiff, may twitch their tail, erect the hair down their back and tail, put their ears back, dilate their pupils, unsheathe their claws, growl, and bite.

A final similarity between these cats and dogs with dominance aggression is that both occur at social maturity. Social maturity begins later (probably between 2 and 4 years of age) in cats than in dogs. Clients are often unable to understand why the cat "changed." The client did not necessarily "do" anything to cause the change; the change is related to the manner in which the cats now perceive the world. The same thing happens to humans in their teens and early 20s.

The key to controlling status-related aggression is the same as that for controlling dominance aggression—do not let the cat have control. This is more difficult than it sounds because most of the cat's behaviors have been so passive that the client has not even recognized them as aggressive. Do not give up. These cats may never be cuddly (and you would be well advised to never expect them to be so), but they can learn to live harmoniously in the household and will usually do well with a cat that is cuddly. Finally, it is critical to remember that these cats are potentially very dangerous. Cats with profound status-related aggression look for openings when the person is unsuspecting (e.g., when they are talking on the telephone) and will bite without preamble and then leave.

Checklist

☐ 1. Avoid all situations in which you know that the cat might react inappropriately.

☐ 2. Be suspicious of these cats when they jump into your lap. Watch them carefully. At the first sign of any unsheathed claws, tensing of muscles, twitching of tail, movement of ears, or rippling of back, stand up and let the cat fall from your lap. Do not pick them up or shove them. These are challenges, and you will be bitten. This all happens quickly.

☐ 3. If you feel that you cannot react quickly enough in the previously mentioned situation, or the cat does not give a lot of warning *(which is not unusual)*, keep a foghorn, air canister, or water pistol with you at all times. At the first sign of aggression or if any of the above appear, blast the cat. Later, when the cat is calm, talk to it sweetly and give it a treat. Do not pet the cat or dangle body parts in front of the cat.

☐ 4. If the cat appears calm in your lap, you can pet the cat once or twice. You, not the cat, always must terminate the attention and regulate the amount of it. Do not get involved in a love fest—you are putting yourself at risk. Always keep the cat a little hungry for attention. Stand up and let the cat fall from your lap before it is ready to stop the attention.

☐ 5. If you are too fearful of the cat to work on Steps 2 to 4 above, do not interact with the cat. Do not feel guilty—the cat does not feel guilty.

☐ 6. Put a bell on the cat's collar (use a breakaway collar) so that you know where the cat is at all times. Monitor its movements. Do not let the cat surprise you with a manipulative attack. Carry a water pistol, foghorn, or air canister with you at all times and use it.

☐ 7. Do not let the cat control your access to something. Ask the cat to move. Try throwing a toy that the cat will chase. If the cat will not move, use something like a broom to gently move the cat. Do not use your hand—the cat will perceive this as a challenge (the broom may also be a challenge), and you will not be able to fight back.

☐ 8. You can teach the cat to do tricks that require the cat to defer to you in exchange for small food rewards (tiny pieces of tinned shrimp or sardines, boiled chicken livers, or shredded boiled chicken). Decide what you want the cat to do (lie down or reach up and touch your hand with his or her paw). Using the food treat, guide the cat into that position using a command (e.g., "down" or "shake") and as soon as the cat accidentally or initially does the behavior say "Good Simba (or whatever)" and give the cat the treat. Keep the cat a little hungry by offering smaller meals so that you can practice these deference exercises frequently. Keep a water pistol or other deterrents handy. If at any time the cat's pupils dilate, its ears go back, or it shows any of the other signs discussed previously, blast the cat. Wait until the cat comes to you for attention before interacting again, and watch to make sure that it is not setting you up for a challenge.

□ 9. If the cat rubs against you and marks you, remove yourself from the situation after one or two rubs. *Then* the cat *cannot* control the situation or passively believe or demonstrate that it has manipulated you.

□ 10. Remember, dogs and cats do not have identical social systems. Not all the same behaviors will be exhibited by dogs and cats, nor will the signals "mean" the same thing in the same context. If you are more familiar with dogs than cats, watch your cat's specific behaviors. Bruce Fogle's book *Know Your Cat* can help.

□ 11. Some cats are so persistent that they would benefit from antianxiety medication. Remember that this is to be used in addition to, not instead of, behavioral and environmental modification.

□ 12. If you do not wish to monitor the cat, isolate it when you cannot or will not be able to work with it. This can be as simple as closing a door.

□ 13. Finally, some cats are too dangerous to keep in some households. If that is the case, very few of them can go to another very special home. Please do not turn these cats loose on the streets.

□ 14. If anyone is scratched or bitten by your cat, seek competent medical help immediately. Cat bites and scratches become infected easily and can be dangerous.

B-23 PROTOCOL FOR TREATING FEARFUL BEHAVIOR IN CATS AND DOGS

Fearful behavior can be either idiopathic (meaning that it developed endogenously and, although it is not understood what triggers it, that nothing happened externally to cause it) or associated with some causal event (teasing by a child or being bitten by another animal). Fear is poorly understood in both human medicine and in veterinary behavioral medicine, but it can be crippling for anyone experiencing it.

In the first 2 months of life both cats and dogs go through periods that have often been called *socialization periods* but might best be called *sensitive periods*. During these periods kittens and puppies begin to explore the world around them. If deprived of age-appropriate experiences at such times, animals may be at risk for behaving inappropriately in those situations later in life. For example, cats that are not handled by people until 14 weeks of age never become friendly or outgoing toward people. Dogs that do not see people until after 5 to 8 weeks of age (when they are first aware that humans exist) may become fearful of *any* approaches—friendly and not—to people. In general, a very small amount of exposure to a stimulus is required during puppyhood or kittenhood to ensure that the animal does not become afraid. A good rule of thumb is that the more nontraumatic exposure that the animal can have, the better. For kittens, being exposed to people from 3 to 7 weeks of age is much more important than people anticipated. Puppies should also be exposed to people early, although they tend to focus more on their littermates than they do on people until they are about $1\frac{1}{2}$ months old.

It is important to give young animals a good start. The "Protocol for Basic Manners Training and Housebreaking for New Dogs and Puppies," "Protocol for the Introduction of a New Pet to Other Household Pets," and the "Protocol for Treating and Preventing Attention-Seeking Behavior" are helpful.

A small amount of fear in unfamiliar situations is good and adaptive. This is what stops us from doing foolish and potentially fatal things. Fear becomes an *abnormal* response when it actively interferes with normal social interaction. It has been postulated that many animals and humans with fear-related problems have an underlying abnormality with their brain chemistry. This should not be surprising and may be why so many of these animals respond so well to antianxiety medication. Some very profound fearful and panic behaviors in dogs appear to begin to be displayed at social maturity (18 to 36 months of age). This also happens during the analogous developmental stage in humans but is currently poorly understood in both cases.

The keys to treating fear include the following:

1. Early recognition of the fearful response because permitting the animal to continually or repeatedly become fearful only reinforces the fearful behavior
2. Avoidance of situations that induce the fear
3. Gradual desensitization and counterconditioning of the animal to the stimuli that have made it fearful
4. Rewarding the animal any time that it does not act fearful

Checklist

☐ 1. For a dog, practice "Protocol for Deference: Basic Program" and "Protocol for Relaxation: Behavior Modification Tier 1." Only after you have completed these can you begin to work with the specific Tier 2 protocols that are designed to desensitize and countercondition the pet to the problematic situations. The concepts behind these programs can easily be adapted for cats—and cats can be trained to respond to food rewards.

☐ 2. Until you reach the second phase of the behavior modification programs, make sure that you avoid all the circumstances in which the pet could become distressed.

☐ 3. If you must expose the pet to something that distresses it, consider using a mild sedative or tranquilizer. Discuss with your veterinarian whether this is appropriate. These medications are not appropriate for every pet but may prevent the animal from learning to become even more fearful. Tranquilizers and sedatives are *not intended* for daily use. They are for occasional situations (e.g., going to the veterinarian) when animals must be exposed to problem situations.

☐ 4. Whenever the pet is calm, tell the pet that it is brilliant and give it love and food treats.

☐ 5. Do not tell the pet that it is okay when it is not okay. No abnormally fearful response is okay. Although your intentions are good, you are giving the pet conflicting signals. If the pet will permit it, you can lay a hand or arm firmly on the pet and press, but do not pet the animal or tell it that it is okay.

☐ 6. Do not try to bribe the animal into not being fearful—it will not work. What will work is to teach the dog or cat to sit for a food treat and then gradually introduce the fearful situation so that the pet learns to associate it with good things. That is the principle behind Step 1.

☐ 7. Do not force the animal to be in a situation in which it becomes progressively more panicked. Many people think that if the puppy is upset, you should drag it to the thing that upsets it and the pet will "get over it." This concept is wrong—you are making the problem worse. Observe the pet's behavior; if it tries to escape in a more active manner, looks away, pants, shakes, drools, or widens its pupils, the dog is stressed and scared. Remove the animal from the situation as soon as possible, or ignore the pet until it is calm.

☐ 8. Do not use physical punishment. It is guaranteed to worsen the problem and may make the dog aggressive.

☐ 9. Warn friends who might interact with the animal how you would like them to interact with the pet. Emphasize that it is important for them to help the pet. If your friends do not comply, separate them and the pet.

☐ 10. Do not forcibly extract a fearful animal from an area where it is hiding. You may be bitten and this will be an even worse event for the pet. Instead, speak calmly and try to coax the animal from its hiding place. If this is not effective, try leaving a dish of food a slight distance away from the hiding place and just sit there. When the pet comes out, do not reach for it—just talk softly. The animal will eventually come to you. Let the pet set the pace of the interaction. Be calm.

☐ 11. Head collars can help dogs relax because they do not permit the dog to intensify the fearful behavior. Consider this option.

☐ 12. Antianxiety medications are not tranquilizers. They do not alter an animal's perceptions by drugging the animal; they act to increase levels of specific neurotransmitters. If your pet is profoundly fearful, these drugs may help you implement the behavior modification. Some dogs and cats need antianxiety medication on a daily basis and may need medication for life. This is further evidence that these problems are rooted in brain chemistry.

B-24 PROTOCOL FOR DOGS AND INTERACTIONS WITH FOOD, RAWHIDE, BISCUITS, AND BONES

Myths about feeding dogs are almost as numerous as myths about dog behavior. Dogs are omnivorous but have strong carnivorous tendencies. This means that they may prefer meat, given a choice, but will also opportunistically supplement their diet with fruits, berries, and herbs. Dogs will scavenge if given the chance. Although this tendency is a serious public health problem in cities, it is interesting to note that scavenging garbage is a major mode of support for wolves in some areas of Italy. Because of the perception of dogs as obligate carnivores, many people think that their dogs must have bones or rawhides, pigs' ears, pizzle sticks, cows' hooves, and so on. It is not necessary for dogs to have any of these for good nourishment, but most dogs value these treats. The problem arises when dogs protect these items and become aggressive around them. This protocol is designed to help you understand how some of these problems develop and how to avoid incidents of aggression.

New Puppies

Puppies should learn early in life that they do not have to compete for food. This means that when the pups first experience semisolid food they should be fed from multiple dishes, or ones with central wells that disperse the pups. Frequent feedings are best because puppies learn that there will be enough food when they are hungry. If puppies are given treats or bones, *all* puppies must be included; they may need to be separated so that they do not fight. No one puppy should be permitted to control access to all the treats or all food or to threaten its littermates' access to those. Experimental work has shown that if puppies are given a bone, they will structure a hierarchy around that bone. The hierarchy can change, but both its maintenance and its shifts are affected by threats and challenges. This is exactly what we do not want to encourage with our pets.

No puppy that is old enough to be adopted is too young to learn to sit (See "Protocol for Deference: Basic Program"). For reasons involving social stability, ease of housebreaking, immunological health, and the pup's ability to handle social change, the earliest a puppy should be adopted into a new home is between $7\frac{1}{2}$ and $8\frac{1}{2}$ weeks of age. However, puppies as young as 5 weeks of age can learn to sit for a few seconds for a food treat, and excellent breeders take advantage of this. Breeders should start to request that pups sit for treats and for feedings at this age. Doing so will accomplish several goals: (1) the dogs will start to learn to be calm before eating and when they want anything: the food dish will not be placed on the floor until the dog is quiet and sitting; (2) the dogs will learn that physically contesting each other for food does not work, and, in fact, is associated with not getting the food; and (3) clients will be able to shift hierarchies either by preferentially feeding in a certain order or feeding in a random and changing order. If there are no problem aggressions within the litter, the latter is preferable because, to some extent, it removes the client's influence over food from the social system. If this pattern of activity is enforced by the breeder, the clients' task will be easier when they encourage their dogs to sit and wait when they are ready to put the food dish on the floor.

Once it is in its new home, the puppy should be taught to sit for *all* food treats (rewards for behavioral protocols, biscuits, and bones). The puppy should also be taught "wait" if the food is in a dish. Puppies have short attention spans and should not be forced to sit or wait long. As they mature, they can be asked to wait for increasingly longer periods, but starting with a few seconds is reasonable. The easiest way to accomplish this is as follows.

The dog should be asked to sit. As the dish is picked up (and it is best to do this so that the area where the dish is placed is right next to where the dog will sit, which prevents the client from inadvertently encouraging the puppy to get up and make a mistake), the client should say "sit" and gently place a hand in front of the dog's chest, under the chin and say "wait." The pup only has to wait a few seconds. The client can then say "okay" and either put the dish down and allow the dog to eat or hold the dish while the dog eats. The latter is easier if the dog either growls at any movement once the dish is down or if the dog wolfs down its food once the dish is down. Holding the dish allows the client to feed the dog small amounts at first and then add food gradually so that the dog is helped to eat more slowly. If the puppy becomes excited every time the dish is slightly withdrawn, only small amounts of food should be placed in the dish at any one time. Refilling the dish will give the client the opportunity to repeat the "sit, wait, okay" sequence frequently and will help the puppy reinforce its own appropriate behavior to these commands. Such repetition is tedious for the client but invaluable for the pup.

After the dog learns "wait," the client should start teaching the dog to sit while the client is permitted to take the dish, regardless of whether the dog has finished eating. This is important because at some point the client may need to retrieve the dog's dish back with food still in it. The easiest way is to hand-feed the dog the small amounts discussed previously and say "wait" with a slightly restraining hand placed on the chest. Move the dish away for a short while, get the dog to look quickly up at you ("Magda, look!"), and then quickly say "good girl" or "good boy" *and reward the dog with the food.* If the dog has problems with this sequence, (anything from wiggling and not looking at you to growling), teach the dog to sit and wait for an empty dish. Practice taking the dish away and giving it back frequently with times that vary from a few seconds to 30 seconds. Once the dog's behavior is perfect, start to add food to the dish. At first let the dog lick a small amount of food from your hand while your hand is in the dish, then add the food directly to the dish, always practicing "wait" and taking the food away, finally reaching the point where you can take the dish from the dog using the commands "sit" and "wait" when the dish contains food and is on the ground or floor. Remember, new food items are naturally desirable, and a puppy that has been wonderful for presentation and removal of puppy chow might not be so wonderful for the presentation and removal of boiled chicken. Anticipate such problems and only offer tiny amounts of new food in the manner recommended previously.

Older Dogs

Food-related aggression is a problem with some dogs. When a dog has food-related aggression, it will guard its food, treats, rawhides, or real bones from other dogs or from people. This type of aggression can be associated with other problem aggressions but is a valid diagnostic category on its own. If your dog is only aggressive around food but does not challenge you in other contexts, do not assume that you do not have a serious problem. Any inappropriate or undesirable canine aggression can cause a person to be maimed or killed. The presence of food is ubiquitous in our life and may be a particular problem for small children who either carry food with them or who constantly smell like food. Even if you decide not to actively treat any food-related aggression in your dog, understanding it can help you avoid it and can render your pet safe and loving.

Food-related aggression can be quite variable. Some dogs begin to growl softly from a great distance and increase the intensity of their growling as people approach. Some dogs growl while shaking and gulping their food, and some dogs stare at anyone within their view while they are eating and snarling. The logic supporting the safe resolution of all of these behaviors is similar—if possible, feed the animal where it is undisturbed. Food-related aggression may be tightly coupled to survival skills that have been honed over years of evolutionary time and treating it safely may require more effort than the average person is willing to expend. Not treating the aggression is not the same as ignoring it—a conscious decision to not treat food-related aggression means (1) that the people involved understand that the behavior is abnormal, undesirable, and dangerous, (2) that they do not wish to work with the dog to change the behavior, and (3) that they will avoid eliciting the behavior at all costs so that they are safe and so that they do not help the dog reinforce the undesirable response. These are active, conscious choices. They are not the same as living with a dog that growls when it is fed and tolerating that behavior. In the latter situation the client is actually passively reinforcing or encouraging the inappropriate behavior. Dogs, like people, hone their skills every time they are allowed to exhibit a certain behavior, even if this behavior is inappropriate. Clients who do not wish to actively teach the dog a more suitable behavior than aggression in the presence of food or those who cannot or are too afraid to work with the animal *must avoid all circumstances* in which the aggression will be apparent.

Avoidance includes the following steps:

1. The dog is fed at discrete times from a dish and is either kept sequestered until the dish is placed on the floor, at which point the dog is given access to the food and the people leave the area, or the dog is asked to sit, stay, and wait until the dish is put down. The dog does not approach the dish until released ("Okay!") and the humans leave. Some dogs are fine when people are present but react aggressively when other dogs or cats are present. They, too, must follow this first step.
2. The dog is never fed from the table or fed food scraps when food is being prepared.
3. The dog is always behind a barrier (a gate, a door, or in a crate) when people are eating or preparing food (or when other dogs are eating, if the problem is aggression toward other dogs in the presence of food). This means that the dog is banished from family barbecues; however, this is safer than permitting the dog to be present. Also, the anxiety level of the people decreases dramatically if they are not worried that there might be a dog bite. If people are stressed or distressed because of concern about the potential for a dangerous event, they will have little patience for the pet and will be less understanding of the pet's special needs, which can be modified with work. Put the dog in another space and do not feel guilty.
4. Any treats (dog biscuits or table scraps) must be placed in the dog's bowl in a room where the dog is undisturbed and must be of a nature that the dog can finish them in

one session. The latter requirement is particularly important for dogs that guard food. If the client knows that the dog hoards and protects biscuits, even biscuits may need to be deleted from the dog's diet unless they are sufficiently small to be finished within minutes of presentation. This is particularly important advice in the case of dogs that hide their biscuits in sofas or other places because the client will not know where the dog has stashed its treats and could then inadvertently be victimized by the dog when they approach the cached biscuit.

5. Some dogs respond inappropriately only to very high-quality treats such as bones, rawhides, pig ears, pizzle sticks, cow hooves, or chew sticks. If these treats cannot be finished in one setting (and most cannot), the most simple, easiest solution is to remove them from the dog's diet forever. This is not cruel, injurious, or deprivational for the dog—it is good common sense. The dog is forbidden to experience something that other dogs have and would find enjoyable; however, this cost is small compared with the guilt any client would feel if a child's skull were crushed because the child came between the dog and a bone. If dogs inappropriately protect food items, people must be responsible for ensuring that they do not help the dog orchestrate a disaster by setting them up to fail. This is a particular risk when small children are involved. Even if the dog is behind a closed door with a rawhide treat, the child could open the door and pay profoundly for that innocent gesture.

Clearly, it is easy to avoid situations that provoke food-related aggression, and in most circumstances, this is a far preferable choice to treating the problem. This aggression should only be treated if the clients can guarantee that they can always control the dog's access to food. If they cannot do this (and *no* household with children can do this), they should not even entertain the notion of treating the aggression. Instead, it is preferable to believe that the aggression will occur when the opportunity is provided and that all provocational opportunities must be avoided.

Treatment involves the same approaches as mentioned previously: gradual exposure to small amounts of a food that is not highly valued. The amounts and quality of the food are increased only if the dog relaxes and does not respond. The client can start by hand-feeding the dog small amounts of dog food. All food will come only from the client's hand and will be relinquished only when the dog is lying down, is quiet, and is calm. If the client is too fearful to do this, the aggression should not be treated, and instead the client should practice avoidance.

When the dog can accept all food from the client's hand without reacting adversely, the client should start stroking the dog during feeding. This should continue until the client can massage the dog while providing food, and the dog's response is calm and friendly. This process could require several months.

After the dog relaxes to the touch when fed, the client should introduce a dish in the manner recommended previously. After giving the dog ever-increasing amounts of massage while holding the dish *and* having the dog respond favorably, the client is ready to start introducing food in a dish.

At first a small amount of food should be offered. The dog should be taught "sit," "wait," and "okay" and can only get the food when the client says "okay." After the dog has finished the small amount of food, the dog must be taught to sit and stay (or lie down and stay) while the client reaches for the dish, refills it, and replaces it. If the dog growls or lunges at any point in the sequence, the client should abandon the dog and return to try again when the dog is calm. If the dog gets up, the client must move the food to where the dog cannot see it and repeat the sequence of sit, stay, and wait. The client may have to do this many times before the dog responds appropriately, but repetition is far better than allowing the dog to become aggressive and control the situation. If the client does not have the patience to pursue such a repetitious course, it is better to not treat the aggression and use avoidance to control the problem.

Finally, once the client can fill and offer, reach for, get, and refill the food dish, the client can start practicing leaving the dog and returning while the dog is eating. At first the client should only move a few centimeters from the dog and then return. The dog should never react inappropriately. If the dog does react, the client must repeat that sequence until the dog is calm. Ultimately the client should be able to put the dish down, leave the room, return, request that the dog sit (with food still in the dish), take the dish, and have the dog relax throughout. This can take months to accomplish and may never be wholly successful. If not wholly successful, the client will have at least learned the dog's limits

and then must take great pains to control any potential danger attendant with that limit (i.e., avoid the situation).

The client can repeat the previously listed steps for any food-related substance to which the dog reacts: dog food, rawhides, real bones, or scraps. Clients should note that real bones and rawhides often elicit a much more exaggerated response than any food in a dish. If there is any doubt about the client's ability or desire to work successfully with the dog, the client should avoid all potentially provocative situations, even if this means that the dog is forever deprived of rawhide. The dog will not suffer from the absence of rawhide.

Anyone who works with a dog with food-related aggression may feel more secure if the dog is fitted with a head collar. The Gentle Leader collar is the ideal choice in this situation because the client can quickly, humanely, and safely close the dog's mouth, thus avoiding any untoward events.

It is perfectly all right and sensible for anyone to decide to not work with a dog with food-related aggression, instead choosing avoidance. No one should feel guilty for this decision.

B-25 PROTOCOL FOR HANDLING AND SURVIVING AGGRESSIVE EVENTS

No one wishes to be victimized by an aggressive cat or dog, but it is a sad commentary on the frequency of this event that more than 50% of all children in the United States 11 years of age and younger have been bitten by a cat or dog. Understanding which canine and feline behaviors indicate a potentially aggressive response and knowing how not to provoke an aggressive response can help people avoid attacks by animals. If the person behaves cautiously and appropriately, even if the attack cannot be avoided, damage from the attack can be minimized. Most serious bites to people that occur in the United States and Europe involve dogs; therefore this protocol focuses primarily on avoiding dog bites, but the information can also be adapted to avoiding injury by cats.

The Unknown or Unfamiliar Dog

Dogs that are unknown to individuals pose a different set of problems when considering the potential to be bitten than do familiar dogs. Most dogs that bite people in public places or in their communities are not strays—they are owned by someone and may be a good pet for them, but they are loose and free ranging. Some general information about the behavior of free-ranging dogs can help people avoid being bitten.

1. Dogs in groups may be more confident and more reactive than are single dogs.
2. Single dogs may be more wary but may still bite if cornered.
3. Dogs become bolder and more confident if close to their home turf. Unfortunately, if the dog is unknown to the person, knowing where the dog's home turf is can be difficult.
4. Dogs can view stares as threats.
5. Dogs will chase individuals who are running away from them in one of two ways: as they would chase an intruder or as they would chase prey. In both cases four-footed animals with large shearing teeth have all the advantages.
6. Children who shriek are far more liable to elicit active pursuit than those who are quiet.
7. Throwing stones, sticks, or any item or aggressively waving your arms at a dog that is aggressively pursuing you is far more likely to intensify the dog's aggression than it is to mollify the dog.
8. Young children and older people are more at risk for serious injury than are young adults. Individuals in both of these age groups are less likely to be able to successfully retreat from and fend off an attack because they may not be able to move in a coordinated manner or because they cannot anticipate the event. In fact, the mortality rate for people in these groups is much higher than for adults.
9. Although it is inappropriate and incorrect to say that certain breeds are more aggressive than others, larger breeds do more damage when they attack. The greater the size or person mismatch, the more damage that will be done. If the person attacked is a child, the chance of serious and often fatal injury increases dramatically.

With these points in mind, children should be encouraged to *not* play with unfamiliar dogs. Under no circumstances should children play with dogs that are not theirs unless they are supervised by a sentient adult. This advice is as much for the dog's protection as it is for the child's. Both children and dogs can be unpredictable, and the interaction can occasionally be toxic. Many dogs only respond aggressively to a child after an extended period of abuse, but the dog will never get the benefit of the doubt. People should protect their dogs and their children.

If an unfamiliar or at-large dog approaches a child in a public place, the child should tell an adult immediately and the adult should tell someone responsible for the maintenance of the open space. If the dog is clearly friendly and solicitous, the adult may make the decision to take the dog home, but any dog that is exhibiting any wariness or threat should be avoided at all costs. Threat postures in dogs include wide-legged stances with lowered heads, growling and baring of teeth, pupil dilation and staring, and piloerection. Dogs that wag their tails are only indicating their willingness to interact: they are *not* communicating that they are friendly. People should remember that interactions can be good or bad.

If a person is approached by a worrisome dog, he or she should take the following actions: (1) avoid staring at the dog; instead look at the dog obliquely out of the corner of the eye; (2) back up slowly, ensuring not to trip over anything; (3) keep arms and legs to the side—do not flail arms or make sudden bolting movements; (4) talk calmly and soothingly to the dog in a low voice if this seems to calm the dog; if the dog intensifies its growl, clearly this is not a good idea; (5) hold oneself as tall as possible; (6) move as directly as possible to a safe area—inside a building or car, behind a truck, or so on. This is the same advice that is given in wilderness situations for handling the approach of mountain lions, bears, or wolves. It is good advice.

Do not assume that because the dog stands still that you can start to run. You can only run if you can get inside a building in a few steps. Running triggers a chase response in a dog, and you have to turn your back to run—do not do it.

Once you are away from the dog, call for help and wait until it comes.

Practice the previously mentioned techniques with children. Furthermore, teach children that if the dog is jumping at them, they should fall directly and silently to the ground, curl up in a ball, and cover their head with their hands and arms. Kids should be taught to look like armadillos when threatened by advancing, threatening dogs. This is also good advice for anyone who accidently trips during the process of getting away from a dog.

Finally, if the dog makes contact with you, stay calm, stay silent, and do not get into a tug of war over any of your body parts. This last piece of advice is difficult to enact, but it is important. In situations involving actual bites from dogs, the majority of the damage is done when a person tries to pull an arm or afflicted area from the dog's mouth. The dog's innate response is to tighten its hold with its jaws and to shake the victim. These last two behaviors are the prime culprits in profound attacks that result in debility and death. Be calm; once the dog releases its grip, follow the previously mentioned steps and try to get away.

If children are grabbed by dogs, *do not struggle* with the dog for the child—the child will be further injured. Instead, look for something to throw over (a blanket) or at (a bucket of water) the dog to stop the behavior. Be calm and quiet. Encourage the child to be quiet and to go limp. Try to distract the dog. If you are successful with this advice the outcome may still be awful, but it will always be much worse if you get into a physical contest with the dog.

Known Dogs

Known dogs, in this context, are defined as dogs that are known to have a problem aggression and may pose a risk to the people who live with them. The first step in the treatment of any canine or feline aggression is for the clients to avoid *any* circumstances that are known to be associated with aggression. This means that clients are responsible for protecting children and unsuspecting friends from their dog. If safety requires that the dog be banished when people come to visit, the dog is banished. Clients will feel more guilty if their dog mauls a child than if the dog spends the day in the bedroom. If the visiting children are going to run free, the bedroom in which the dog is ensconced must be locked. Remember, kids can be unpredictable. In the absence of any other information, clients should assume that if their dog has a problem aggression that they cannot take a chance with that aggression and with people whom the dog does not know. Dogs become more reactive when people are excited, and problem dogs, in particular, become more reactive in unfamiliar, noisy circumstances. A little common sense and discipline can save a lot of heartbreak.

Clients must protect themselves from their pet's aggression by learning to give the pet cues that encourage appropriate behavior and separate cues that tell the pet that it will be ignored by the client rather than being rewarded with interaction. This means that clients must change their own behavior to change the pet's behavior. Although it is true that the clients invariably did not cause the pet's problem, they have the responsibility for fixing it. If clients know that the dog is more aggressive when it is allowed to sleep on their bed, the dog is no longer allowed to sleep on their bed unless the clients can ask the dog to get off the bed and lie down, *and* the dog complies willingly. If not, the dog cannot be in the bedroom with them because they will always be at risk. If clients know that the dog growls every time clients groom or pet the dog, clients must avoid grooming or petting until the dog can lie down and relax for this. Use of a Gentle Leader head collar can hasten this response and render the dog safe. Under no circumstances must clients ever believe that they have to put their own safety at risk to make progress in changing their pet's behavior. This is absolutely wrong.

Clients should remember that dogs read body language much better than people and will pick up on any uncertainty. Whether they can smell "fear" is unimportant; they will take advantage of any pause or uncertainty in the clients' behavior to take control of the situation and exhibit aggression. If clients cannot be calm, confident, and patient when working with the dog, they have a low probability of changing the dog's behavior. Clients also need to remember that *every* time that a dog or cat with a problem behavior is allowed to exhibit that behavior, it is reinforced. The pet learns how to do the behavior better with exposure, experience, and repetition. Avoidance is the key.

If clients take all precautions and the dog still threatens them, the clients should back away in the manner described previously for unknown dogs. Clients whose dogs have known aggression problems have an advantage over the situation above—they are able to keep devices like blankets, water pistols, air horns, and spray canisters on their person or in the room where they interact with the dog so that they can distract the dog or protect themselves should the dog intensify its aggression. If clients give the dog a command to sit, whether part of a behavior modification program or not, and the dog begins to growl or otherwise become aggressive, they should gently try to get the dog to relax using a verbal command. If this does not work, the clients should release the dog (not reward it) and slowly back away. It is far better to ignore the dog than to struggle to "win" or "dominate" the dog. Clients invariably succeed at doing neither but instead teach the dog more about the clients' fears and the extent to which the dog can manipulate them. Even if the clients must repeatedly avoid the dog, this is preferable to physically contesting the dog. If clients are consistent, the dog will ultimately approach and be willing to exhibit deferential behaviors in exchange for the clients' requests. In extreme cases this can take days. It sounds hard-hearted, but the dog will not starve to death. However, in these extreme cases, if clients are overly sympathetic for the dog, the dog will manipulate them and the behavior modification process will backslide. If the dog continues to threaten the clients and avoidance does not elicit deference, the clients should orchestrate the situation so that the dog is behind a closed door or in a safely fenced area. Sometimes just letting the dog into the backyard can interrupt the aggression and the clients can begin the modification process again. Keep the dog behind a barrier for as long as is necessary for the dog to calm down. Clients feel guilty and sympathetic to the dog and try to interact with it before the animal can rationally learn anything from the interaction. Such responses usually intensify the aggression. The longer it takes the dog to calm down, the worse the prognosis (i.e., if the dog was snarling yesterday and 20 hours later still cannot be approached for feeding, clients may wish to question their success in reliably changing this behavior into a safe and loving one).

If the dog bites the client, the client should freeze and not struggle with the dog. Do not get into a struggle over body parts. Go limp, look away, become small and quiet, and slowly retreat at the first opportunity.

Client anger and a sense of disappointment and betrayal are normal, but dogs with problem aggressions cannot respond rationally to those feelings. Clients should remove themselves from the situation as quickly as possible. Leave the dog alone to be quiet. Clients should not punish the dog physically, no matter how angry or hurt they are—this will only make matters worse. The client should seek any required medical care and then calmly approach the dog using the deference and relaxation measures that the dog has been taught. If the client is either too fearful or too physically or emotionally injured to do this or no longer wants to work with the dog after such an event, the prognosis is poor. Clients should never feel forced to work with a dog that terrifies or endangers them. They may feel sad about their decision to euthanize the dog (or in some cases place it in another home, if this is possible), but there is no reason to feel guilty if the clients behaved as previously mentioned. Clients who feel guilty are the ones who were unable to act in the safe, rational manner discussed here, and who, inadvertently and unintentionally, encouraged their dog's inappropriate behaviors.

B-26 PROTOCOL FOR TEACHING CHILDREN (AND ADULTS) TO PLAY WITH DOGS AND CATS

One of the reasons that we have pets is so that we can cuddle and play with them. Such interactions should be the source of much joy, but they often lead to injury to the pet or to the person. Rough play can worsen a behavioral problem that is developing. Some basic guidelines for appropriate play with cats and dogs can minimize these problems and may also lead people to more fully appreciate the intricacies of canine and feline communication.

Puppies and kittens, like young children, are energetic, can quickly progress to lack of control and exhaustion in their play, and make mistakes in both the objects and the intensity of their play behaviors. Unlike human children, puppies and kittens do not have hands with opposable thumbs (a purely primate trait). Instead, they have a jaw and tooth structure that allows them to carry and manipulate a variety of objects. Hence, much play between young cats and dogs involves the use of the mouth. Kittens and puppies will also box, rear, and pounce on each other as part of play. Young animals transfer these behaviors to people unchanged.

Boxing, Mounting, Rearing, and Pouncing

Boxing, mounting, rearing, and pouncing are normal kitten and puppy behaviors. These behaviors function to allow closeness and energetic play between animals and may help shape adult social behaviors and communication skills. By their second month of life, both puppies and kittens begin to pay more attention to people and use the same behaviors that they use to communicate with other animals to communicate with humans. All social mammals play, so we are able to recognize signals from puppies and kittens that they wish to play and to act on these impulses. Human children do not exhibit exactly the same form of play that puppies and kittens do, in part, because humans can manipulate objects and each other with their hands. The tendency is for puppies and kittens to play with humans exactly as they would play with other puppies and kittens and for humans to mimic these puppy and kitten behaviors using their hands.

When dogs and cats are small and do not weigh much, these wrestling and boxing behaviors tend to be noninjurious. However, as the animal grows the pouncing and boxing can injure a child, or, in the case of a large-breed dog, an adult human. Very exuberant, large-breed dogs can knock a human toddler to the ground and fracture the skull. Tragic deaths and injuries are no less tragic because the animal "didn't mean to do it." In fact, accidental injury to a child caused by an animal that is wonderful will cause more guilt for the humans involved than will injury by a dangerous animal. Puppies and kittens remain youngsters until they are socially mature, which occurs at around 2 years of age. Accordingly, they cannot be expected to show the judgment and restraint that an older dog or cat might. Furthermore, it is impossible to intellectually ascertain whether a dog or cat understands how fragile infants, young children, or aged, frail humans can be. It is absolutely unfair to make the puppy or kitten solely responsible for the decisions about the directions that play will take. Human guidance must be provided.

Tackling, pawing, and mounting by young animals can be acceptable *if and only if* the people involved can do the following: (1) always stop the behavior by saying no or by withdrawing, (2) redirect the behavior to another focus (a toy), and (3) gently correct the behavior so that it decreases in the future, should the behavior be too rough. If the animal's response to a gentle correction of standing up or withdrawing a leg is to attack it more forcefully, there is already a problem. Either the animal is already displacing some undesirable tendencies related to aggression and control, or the person has already taught the animal to play too roughly. Appropriate correction for forceful tackles or pouncing includes stopping, saying no, startling the animal (blowing in the animal's face may work), and asking the pet to exhibit a more appropriate behavior. More appropriate behavior may involve sitting and waiting for a toy or distracting the pounce to a better focal object (e.g., a feather on a string for the cat that lurks around corners and chases shoelaces).

People should not correct animals by swatting them in the face or by thumping them on the rump. This only stimulates the animals to respond to the body part that has just whacked them and teaches puppies and kittens that rough play stimulates rough play. This is not the message that people wish to send.

People should also refrain from exhibiting what they perceive to be human versions of feline or canine correctional behaviors. These including hanging a kitten by its scruff; rolling a dog over forcefully and lying on it while growling in its face; shaking a dog by the jowls, scruff, or neck; swatting a dog across the ears; slapping a dog under the chin; and so on. First, these behaviors are not mimics of behaviors that adult dogs and cats exhibit toward puppies and kittens. Second, even to the extent that these behaviors do overlap with corrections of dog and cat behaviors, there is a real danger in overdoing them and causing the pet injury. This is particularly true for cats. Cats are tiny, and, although adult cats frequently bite at or carry young cats by the nape of the neck, cats have pressure sensors under their teeth and can use just the right amount of control—people do not have this ability. Finally, these forceful kinds of correctional behaviors exhibited by people toward their pets may encourage physical solutions for problem that are better solved by intellectual solutions. People should not have to manhandle a cat or dog to convince the animal to alter its behavior—they should be smart enough to redirect that behavior in ways that can be mutually satisfying. Through evolutionary history, humans have lived with dogs and, to a lesser extent, cats in a manner that has encouraged them to take their cues from us. We can capitalize on that perception and learn to encourage limits to robust play. The best emotional relationships with pets are founded on a basis that is devoid of fear and injury. We need to protect both our children and our pets so that they can have those relationships.

One final comment on physical discipline and pets is warranted. Not only will physical discipline cause the animal to respond in an escalated and aggressive manner, but it will also send the message to any other individuals watching (i.e., your children, friends, or spouse) that the way you solve conflicts is through physical intervention and violence. Ask yourself if this is the message that you wish to send, especially given that the method does not appear to work as well as kinder, more benevolent methods. The American Humane Association and the Latham Foundation have demonstrated that child abuse and pet abuse are linked. People who are abused as children will hone their abuse skills on their pets before continuing the cycle by abusing their own children. In turn, pets that are abused may act as a flag for child abuse. The concepts of abuse and discipline are changing as we learn more about ourselves and our pets. Harsh punishment of our pets may act as a guide to other problems that we have not previously understood.

Claws and Scratching

Kittens are not able to reliably retract their claws before 4 weeks of age but can learn to do so after that time. If they are allowed to snag at people with their claws, they will continue this behavior as adults. Cat scratch disease is a serious problem for people who have been scratched by cats. Most of the cats that communicate this bacterial disease are young kittens that are infested with fleas, but any cat can potentially be responsible. Cat bites are a very serious problem in human health because cats' teeth are curved, small, and sharp. A cat bite provides the ideal environment for infection.

Kittens that are hand- or bottle-reared play more roughly with their claws and teeth than those who have been naturally weaned by and kept with their mothers. Their mothers and other siblings do not tolerate rough play and correct the cats. Early correction as the cat begins to get bigger is invaluable and involves not only the tendency to modulate or control rough behaviors, but also the ability to use signals that communicate when the play is getting too rough. For this and other reasons, kittens should be kept with their mothers until 9 to 14 weeks of age. The mother will control all the play, partly through her withdrawal from the kittens, and they will never learn to play roughly. Part of the problem with bottle-fed or orphaned kittens is that they never learn to inhibit their aggression using either their claws or their teeth because there is no adult present who can read the early signals that the play is rougher than needed. However, a second part of the problem involves social development and the evolution of cat behavior. Cats that are weaned early exhibit predatory behavior earlier than do cats that are allowed to spend extended amounts of time with their mothers and siblings. Clients who adopt these orphaned kittens must be realistic and learn to read their kitten's signals well: (1) no rough play should be tolerated, (2) toys should always be substituted for swatting at people, (3) corrections should include distractions (like blowing in the cat's face) followed by a substitution, and (4) if the cat pursues aggressive acts, the cat should be unceremoniously dumped from the client's lap (just stand up and let it fall off—do not dangle any body parts in front of an aggressive cat) and ignored until it has calmed down. Once the cat has become calm, play can be reintroduced with a toy. Clients must not encourage the direction of predatory behaviors toward themselves.

Claws are less of a consideration for clients with dogs but can still be problematic for dogs that bat and swat with their feet. These dogs do well with Kong toys or Boomer balls (Kong Co., Lakewood, CO) that redirect the dog's foreleg movements to something that will not be injured. Caution is urged: dogs in hot pursuit of a toy can knock over a child or small human and may not even realize that damage has been done. Appropriate supervision is always necessary.

Finally, keeping any dog's or cat's nails trimmed should be mandatory and part of routine maintenance. Clients can start this as soon as they get their pet. It will get easier with time, render their pet easier to handle, and make it safer and more comfortable for the pet to run and for the person to interact with the pet. If people are afraid to use nail clippers, emery boards can produce well-manicured dog and cat claws.

Mouthing and Biting

Mouthing and biting are common complaints of people who have inadvertently played too roughly with their dog or cats. No puppy or kitten should be encouraged to mouth. Puppies and kittens do this naturally because they use their mouths much as humans use hands. It is a simple matter to abort this behavior when it first starts, but it can be very difficult to abort it if it has been ongoing for a long time.

The first thing clients should do when their puppy or kitten mouths them is to say "no" and freeze. If clients pull their hand away from the puppy or kitten, even if doing so to avoid a prick, they encourage the animal to pursue the "game." Say "no," stop, and gently extricate or remove the body part while holding the body of the animal. Then *quickly* offer the animal something on which it can chew (a stuffed toy or a ball) and tell the dog or cat that it is good. Repeat this as often as necessary. If the animal persists, make a sharp noise, whistle, or blow in the animal's face to startle it. Remember, the only reason to startle the animal is to stop the behavior so that a more appropriate one can be taught. Most people understand that they wish the animal to stop the behavior and can get them to do that; however, it is equally important to reward the cessation of the undesirable behavior with one that is more appropriate (e.g., chewing on a toy). Remember, puppies and kittens are very focused and will exhaust the average person almost instantly. Clients must be vigilant and, if they are not willing to be so, should consider placing the animal in a safe area (its own room, a crate, or a pen) until they feel they have the energy again to face the onslaught of play. (If clients do not feel that they can honestly face this for days, they should reconsider why they have this pet.) Puppies and kittens need energetic, positive attention. If they are not able to get attention through positive means, they will get it through ones clients consider negative. Clients are responsible for shaping the pet's behavior. Young puppies and kittens are just like young children—if the only interaction they get is negative, they will learn to crave that negative interaction, and, like children, they will intensify the negative behaviors to get ever-increasing amounts of response.

Clients often think that they do not have to correct puppy nipping because it is not injurious and does not hurt. This is *absolutely incorrect*. These dogs will get bigger; the bigger the dog, the more powerful the jaws, and the more damage that the dog will do if it bites. The time to learn to inhibit activity using the mouth is when the dog is young. If dogs are allowed to mouth, they will form a behavioral habit in which mouthing is acceptable. It is much harder to unlearn a behavior than to teach an appropriate one at the beginning.

People (often adult human males) often believe that they can teach their dogs to be protective by wrestling with them. This is anthropomorphic, wrong, and dangerous. If a dog is going to protect a family when a threat is present, they will do so regardless of whether they play roughly. All such "training" does is to teach the dog to treat the family roughly. This is not what clients want. Clients should use a toy, not their arm! Using a toy for real play helps a dog understand the contextual differences between play and threat. Dogs need this help, which is easy to provide.

Some puppies that are raised with other energetic dogs can play very roughly. Dogs of all ages can learn to distinguish between rough play between dogs and more gentle play with people. One of the first clues that puppies can use is that the clients do not use their mouth to grab the ruff of their neck. Clients should not tolerate rough play from a puppy or kitten because they assume that this is the way to play with other pets. As long as none of the animals in the house is injured during energetic play, they can play as roughly as they want with each other but must be encouraged through the use of corrections, toy substitution, and withdrawal of attention that this same quality of play will *not* be tolerated from the clients. Clients can help the dog understand this. If clients' pets vary widely in size or in skills related to judgment about how hard to play with youngsters, the clients are responsible for supervising the pets. Bigger pets can and do kill smaller ones by accident. Some older animals have problems with smaller ones and may exhibit predatory behavior toward them (see "Protocol for the Introduction of a New Pet to Other Household Pets"). It is not necessary that the pet have this problem for the animal to injure a younger or smaller puppy or kitten in play. Only when clients are certain that the animals play well and safely together should they be left alone, and then only for short periods of time. If a new puppy or kitten plays too roughly with people after playing with another pet, consider limiting their time together to short, supervised periods and working with the puppy or kitten on a leash or harness immediately after play with the other pet.

Teaching Tug

Clients often want to play an energetic game of tug with their pets. Many training manuals state not to do so because it will make the pet aggressive. This is not true. If the goal is to play appropriately, energetically, and interactively, clients can play tug with a pet if the following rules are observed:

1. The dog must sit and wait until the client is ready to start the game and until the toy is offered.
2. Clients must say "take it," and the dog must wait to take the toy until the request.
3. The client and the dog both pull on the toy, and the tugging is gentle and does not swing the dog around the room (which could injure its neck), and the dog is gentle and does not grab any body parts.
4. If the dog simply grazes any body parts, the client should act as if mortally wounded, stop the game, ask the dog to sit or, preferably, lie down, and the dog complies.
5. Again offer the toy as in Step 1.
6. The client decides when the game is over by announcing that it is time to stop ("stop," "enough," "that is it"), the dog sits ("sit"), and drops the toy into the client's waiting hand ("drop it"), and the client always wins.
7. The client releases the dog and it goes off to do something else without charging.

If all of these steps cannot be executed flawlessly, do not play tug. The client and the pet will be safer.

Do not forget, similar games can be taught to cats!

Remember, dogs and cats, like people, make mistakes. Clients must not lose their temper with an animal, particularly one that is a baby. Not only could a young pet be seriously injured by such irresponsibility, but also it sets the tone for future interactions and could teach that dog or cat to be fearful, aggressive, or simply to play too roughly.

B-27 PROTOCOL FOR CHOOSING COLLARS, HEAD COLLARS, AND HARNESSES

Identification

One of the main objectives that collars accomplish is identification. All cats and dogs should be labeled. There are three main ways to do this, and they are not exclusive: (1) tags on a collar provide information about the client (name, address, and phone number), veterinarian (primarily the phone number), and vaccination status (current rabies vaccine); (2) tattoos in ears or on thighs; or (3) microchipping. Tattoos are usually comprised of the client's Social Security number (in the United States) or some code and require at least sedation to execute. The dog or cat then usually wears another tag on its collar indicating the telephone number to call should the animal be separated from its people and need to find its home. Microchipping is becoming more broadly available, but in Europe and the United Kingdom the systems are less standardized than they are in the United States. Microchips are easy to install but require the widespread availability of microchip readers. Long-term effects of an implanted, digitally coded device have not been fully evaluated, but the risks appear small in preliminary tests. The general principle behind microchips is that a number is displayed when the chip is scanned and ownership data can be obtained by calling a central depot. The animal generally but not always wears a tag that indicates that a chip has been implanted. The chips are radioopaque, meaning that they will be displayed on a radiograph or x-ray film. Whatever method is chosen, two factors should be certain: (1) the tags are current, and (2) they are on a collar that fits comfortably. The latter means that the collar is either a breakaway collar through which one or two fingers can slip comfortably or that the collar is sufficiently snug to stay on the animal if it tilts its head, but should the collar become entangled, the animal can pull its head out of the collar. If clients are not cautious about the fit of collars, animals can strangle or collars can become imbedded in their skin, resulting in morbidity or mortality. Breakaway collars are particularly important for cats, who have elevated squeezing their bodies into small places into an art form.

All animals should be labeled. If they are lost or stolen, it may be their only hope of getting home again. If the township or county in which the pet lives requires a license tag, this could be the only thing that saves the pet from impoundment, quarantine, or destruction.

Control

Collars and harnesses are used primarily for control of dogs, but a few words about harnesses and leashes for cats may be helpful.

Cats should be restrained when they go to the veterinarian and, if they are indoor cats, when they are outside. They should also be restrained in a car so that they do not become projectile. Placing them in a crate can accomplish this, but more freedom and exercise can be an excellent idea. All kittens should be fitted with a harness so that they can be encouraged to explore the world. A harness is preferable to a collar because, fitted correctly, it will not injure the cat and the cat cannot slip out of it. The younger the cat is when the client fits it with a harness, the easier it will be to accustom the cat to it. Once the harness is on the cat, it should be taken for trips in cars, on walks, and for visits to the veterinarian. These activities should occur frequently; they will pay off later when the cat needs care that requires

tractability. If the cat can safely be taken outside, the cat's life and the interaction between the cat and client will be enriched.

Buckle Collars

Buckle collars can be good to accustom young puppies or kittens to leashes but should not be relied on for control of any animal. Any animal that walks calmly and without resistance when on a leash that is attached to a buckle collar is not doing so because of the collar. These animals are exquisitely behaved despite the collar. Any animal that pulls or lunges while on a buckle collar needs another type of restraint or training device. Buckle collars—provided that they break away or can slip off, if caught—should be fitted to all animals so that tags or embroidered identification can always accompany the pet. This means that they are used in addition to, not instead of, other devices.

Choker Collars

Dogs are routinely fitted with devices such as choker collars as part of a training program. Choker collars are usually either made from chain or a rolled, braided nylon. When used correctly, choker collars are actually one of the best examples of true negative reinforcement: when the dog pulls, the collar tightens and either the sound or the pressure indicates that the dog has engaged in an undesirable behavior; when the dog stops, that pressure is released (and in the case of a chain, the sound of slippage occurs) and the dog is unimpeded. It is the release from the negative stimulus (the tightening of the collar) that is the reward. Unfortunately, most people do not use choke collars correctly; to do so requires a lot of work and patience. Instead, many dogs "choke" when chokers are used. When they are allowed to pull on the collar and permitted to sustain the pull, these dogs learn to override the choker. In doing so they are also at risk for laryngeal, esophageal, and ocular damage (damage in the blood vessels in the eye). Despite still being the preferred and, in some cases, the required form of restraint in a show ring, choke collars are an idea whose time may have passed. When clients can overcome their own misconceptions about how the collars look or what they mean, they will, with ever-increasing frequency, choose a head collar or a no-pull harness for their dog. When used correctly the devices are safer, easier to use, and help teach the dog better behaviors. They are a winning solution that could and perhaps should eclipse the choker.

Head Collars

Head collars are very much like horse halters. They act as a basket that holds the dog's cheeks and jaws and stay on the dog by fastening high on the back of the neck. Generally, at least one strap fits over the bridge of the dog's nose and one fits over the back of the neck. The leash is attached in the middle of the halter to the nose strap, but under the chin. This is how a lead is attached to a horse halter but is a major change for many people who are accustomed to attaching a leash directly to something around a dog's neck. The two major versions of the head collar are the Halti (Safari Whitco, Bohemia, NY) and the Gentle Leader/Promise System Canine Head Collar (Premier Pet Products, Richmond, VA). The Halti is intended to be fitted with a second collar because it fits loosely. It also cannot be tightened to prohibit biting by pulling forward, but it fits some very jowly breeds well and snugly. The Gentle Leader/Promise System Canine Head Collar gives most dogs a better fit, requires no second collar, and can be used with a leash to correct inappropriate behaviors and prohibit biting.

Head collars are wonderful for most dogs. They spare the dog's larynx and esophagus and thus are an ideal choice for dogs with laryngeal damage, tracheal collapse, or cervical (neck) damage involving disks, bones, nerves, or muscles. Head collars also ride high on the back of the dog's neck so that when the leash is pulled forward or the dog pulls in the direction opposite to that of the leash, this part of the collar tightens a bit and applies a small amount of steady pressure on the area of the upper neck near the head. Not only is this generally very safe, but also this pressure uses the same kind of signal that dogs communicate to other dogs when they wish to control them or stop. Thus when the dog is corrected with a leash, the head collar communicates a "doggy" signal to the dog to stop. No translation is necessary, and the response is quick. For clients who are already working with a behavior modification program, this type of helpful, kind device can be a godsend. If the dog has a mouthing or biting problem, the Gentle Leader/Promise System Canine Head Collar can be gently pulled forward to firmly, safely, securely, and humanely close the dog's mouth. When used correctly the collar cannot injure the dog and will allow the client to control most of the dog's behaviors and stop the dog from biting.

The leverage provided by a head collar allows children and people with arthritis to walk even unruly dogs—*and to enjoy it*. If dogs get more exercise they are calmer; if people enjoy being with their pets more, they will be more motivated to work with them. Head collars provide a win-win situation and are increasingly becoming the collar of first choice for a puppy. They are certainly appropriate for all life stages and have another advantage over chokers: they encourage humane behavior from people. We can use all the kindness and humanity we can learn.

As is true for any device, injury can occur if these collars are used incorrectly. The most common complaint about head collars involves loose-lipped dogs that chew on their lips because the nose piece of the collar fits too tightly. Hair on the nose can also be damaged if this occurs. A good fit is important, and some practice might be needed to determine the best adjustment of the neck strap and the nose strap. Dogs fitted with head collars should be able to comfortably eat, drink, pant, and even bark and bite, if not corrected. These are not muzzles, they are not rubber bands around the dog's nose, and they are not cruel or inhumane. They are great. Now that these head collars are available in designer colors, people should accept them more readily.

No-pull Harnesses

No-pull harnesses fit under the dog's front legs and loop over the dog's shoulders so that when the dog pulls, its front legs are pulled back and it slows its pace. The two main versions of these harnesses are the Lupi (Safari Whitco, Bohemia, NY) and the Sporn or No-Pull Harness (Four Paws Products Ltd., Hauppauge, NY). The No-Pull harness has a special collar that is sewn with two different-sized metal tabs. The loose, leashlike part of the harness fits through one of the loops, under and around the legs, and is attached to the other loops, under the neck, with a clasp. The leash is then attached to the loose part of the harness over the dog's back. The back part of the harness can be tightened for a better, more responsive, fit. The Lupi does not use any clasps or tabs but relies on a system of concentric loops that are fitted around the dog's front legs and over its back. The leash is then af-

fixed to the back portion, which slips to tighten if the dog pulls. The Lupi is easier to fit to very hairy dogs or for people whose hands are very arthritic. Both of these fitting patterns sound complex and like topological puzzles. They are not. Once clients have the devices in their hands, the fit becomes self-explanatory.

Such harnesses are wonderful for dogs that pull or lunge. These are not appropriate devices to fit to dogs whose biggest problem is biting because they do not control the dog's mouth or head. Furthermore, reaching around the dog's head and neck to fit these harnesses could be dangerous if the dog is aggressive to people.

When fitted correctly these harnesses easily allow children or people with arthritis to pleasurably and calmly walk their dogs. These harnesses, like head collars, spare the dog's neck so that dogs, even if they have laryngeal, tracheal, esophageal, or spinal problems, can be safely exercised. Caution is urged against fitting no-pull harnesses too tightly; too tight a fit could impede circulation in the dog's front legs. Fortunately, this is difficult to accomplish.

Harnesses

Regular harnesses fit around the dog's chest and avoid any pressure on the neck when the leash is pulled. They are devices used solely to attach the dog to the leash and offer no chance for correction of undesirable behaviors. Many dogs do not pull or lunge when walked and just need to be protected from the world and to comply with leash laws. Regular harnesses are fine for such dogs. They also work well for small dogs that perform undesirable leash behaviors but are too small to cause what the client would consider to be a problem. In fact, some of the harnesses for smaller dogs have built-in "handles" so that the dog can be picked up by the client if the dog must be removed from a situation or placed in a car. These harnesses are not good choices for large dogs that are not absolutely perfectly behaved because they provide the client with little control. In fact, big, highly motivated dogs are able to use the harness to push into the situation from which their people are trying to drag them because their shoulders are unrestrained. Clients often choose harnesses because they want to protect the dog's neck. This is a good idea, but head collars and no-pull harnesses are a better solution.

Prong or Pinch Collars

Prong collars are subject to all of the same criticisms as are chokers. Furthermore, they can seriously damage the dog's neck because they can become imbedded in the skin if the dog learns to override them. Most dogs learn to override these collars, and people who use them often voluntarily comment that they need to use some degree of pain to control their animals under some circumstances. These collars are intended to use pain to encourage the dog to attend to the person. For aggressive dogs this response can worsen their aggression, and for dominantly aggressive dogs this response may not only worsen their aggression, but may also endanger the client. If people understood more about how dogs communicate and how these collars work, they would appreciate that responses other than pain are more desirable for changing an animal's behavior. These collars are no substitute for early intervention and the treatment of problem behaviors. Every situation that clients claim is controlled by the use of such a collar can be better, more safely, and more humanely treated with a head collar and some time investment.

Some dogs are fitted with prong collars because they make the dog look "tough." The problem here does not lie with the dog.

Shock Collars

No dog should wear a shock collar to correct an inappropriate behavior except on the qualified recommendation of a specialist in behavioral medicine. This is almost akin to saying no dog should wear a shock collar. Certainly, no client should self-prescribe a shock collar for a dog to control an unruly or aggressive behavior. Given the correct motivational and timing circumstances and the appropriate level of shock, dogs (and humans) can learn from the application of a painful shock. However, the application of shock (and shock collars are intended to be painful) is an absolutely inappropriate treatment for aggression and fear. The use of shock collars invariably makes such behaviors worse, renders the dog less predictable, and potentially endangers the client. Most people who use shock collars either want a "quick fix" or need to absolutely control the dog. The former approach does not work for dogs with problem behaviors, and the latter may be problematic in itself. There are some rare exceptions when shock collars can be used rationally to change or shape a dog's behavior. Under these conditions very few (one to three) shocks are usually sufficient to cause the change. If clients who use a shock collar find that they have to, or do, shock the dog more frequently, there is a problem that the collar cannot address. Such clients should seek professional help from a specialist in behavioral medicine immediately.

B-28 PROTOCOL FOR CATS WITH PICA OR INAPPROPRIATE INGESTION CONDITIONS, INCLUDING WOOL SUCKING

1. Ensure that the cat is receiving an adequate, complete feline diet (most cats are). Rule out any medical disorders, including intestinal parasitemia, dental disease, small intestine or large bowel disease, and so on.

2. If the cat favors plants or soil, consider changing the texture of the cat's diet by adding some roughage (bran, vegetables, or crunchy food) or growing a garden of chives, catnip, or plain grass for the cat. Often, feeding the cat more frequently (the same amount but divided) and in a more interesting setting (dry food around large rocks so that the cat must work to find the food) may help. These benign approaches may enrich the cat's environment, and if they do not help, no harm is done.

3. Prohibit the cat from access to the objects it is inappropriately ingesting. This may mean keeping a spotless house or putting the cat in a large crate with food, litter, and toys during times when direct supervision is not an option. When the cat is not in the crate, it should be continuously monitored. Put a bell on its collar or attach a harness and leash to the cat and monitor its behavior. If the cat begins to show any intention or appetitive behavior toward an object it would suck or ingest, correct the cat by startling it in a manner sufficient to abort the behavior. After the cat has calmed itself, engage it in another activity that the cat enjoys and that is directly competitive with the ingestion behavior. (See steps 4 to 6 below.)

4. Set expectations for the cat. Set feeding times, play times, and attention times. Make sure the cat gets 10 to 15 minutes of concerted attention (grooming, stroking, and talking to) at least twice a day on a regular schedule. Identify any sources of stress (washing machines, noisy children, another cat that is not a favorite of the patient) and minimize contact with them. This may mean giving this cat its own room (or sole access to a favored room) or providing it with company. These are very individual circumstances.

5. Enrich the environment with kitty condos and toys if the cat will use them.

6. Teach the cat to sit and request, by pawing, a food scrap that is within the dietary regimen chosen. The cat will do this first by accident and needs to be rewarded *instantly*. Keep practicing on a regular schedule. This helps the cat learn to relax in exchange for a reward.

7. Pharmacological intervention can be an important part of therapy and may facilitate the above. Before *any* drugs are used, a complete chemistry screening profile and blood cell count should be performed by the veterinarian. There are two reasons for this: (1) the cat may have an underlying condition that would preclude the use of drugs that are metabolized through renal and hepatic pathways and (2) if medication is prescribed, the animal's response must be monitored if therapy is long term. To assess the significance of any changes, it is important to know the baseline values.

Drugs that have been successful in such cases

1. Diazepam (Valium) 1 to 2 mg (or 0.2 to 0.4 mg/kg) orally every 12 to 24 hours
2. Amitriptyline (Elavil) 5 mg (or 0.5 to 1.0 mg/kg) orally every 12 to 24 hours
3. Clomipramine (Anafranil) 2.5 mg (or 0.5 mg/kg) orally every 24 hours
4. Buspirone (BuSpar) 5 to 10 mg (or 0.5 to 1.0 mg/kg) orally every 24 hours or half that every 12 hours

Drug side effects

1. **Diazepam.** Diazepam is a humanly abusable drug and is *not* the appropriate drug for every household. This drug should be carefully monitored and may necessitate frequent reexaminations attendant with refills of the prescription because of the abuse potential. Benzodiazepines are metabolized through renal and hepatic pathways. Any animal with a preexisting renal or hepatic condition must be monitored carefully. The primary side effects are ataxia and stupor. Decreasing the dose often alleviates these effects. Any vomiting, inappetence, or profound change in normal behavior should act as a warning to the practitioner that the dose should be changed or the drug discontinued. There have been isolated reports of sudden death in cats that received relatively small amounts of both brand-name and generic diazepam. Sufficient epidemiological data do not exist to postulate an underlying cause for this, but many individuals have shied away from use of diazepam in cats. There have been relatively few recent cases of sudden death despite two decades of diazepam treatment of cats. More information should be forthcoming in the next few years. If the cat just started to exhibit the condition *and* the client and practitioner can identify an event associated with the start of this activity, diazepam may be a perfectly acceptable first-choice drug. The intermediate metabolite is the active compound (the half-life of diazepam is on the order of seconds); a gross assay of when the cat achieves effective levels of the intermediate metabolite can be gleaned from its behavior. As the cat metabolizes the drug and the metabolite reaches steady-state levels, the cat usually staggers or acts a little ataxic for a few days. This behavior should spontaneously resolve; if it does not, the cat may be receiving too large a dose of drug. If the cat never exhibits the transient perception changes, the dose may not be high enough.

2. **Amitriptyline.** Amitriptyline is a TCA that acts by inhibiting serotonin reuptake. As a result, more serotonin—one of the neurotransmitters associated with upbeat moods and decreased anxiety—is available. TCAs are metabolized through renal and hepatic pathways. One of the major pathways used is the glucuronic acid route. Cats have less efficient glucuronidation than dogs; hence the half-lives of many drugs are longer in cats. Amitriptyline is no exception. Cats that are able to take this drug and experience none of the common side effects (vomiting, sedation, anorexia, and tachycardia) benefit from its use. About 50% of cats (this is a clinical estimate) experience GI upset when treated with amitriptyline. This upset is usually profound enough to preclude the use of the drug. All side effects appear reversible. Amitriptyline may be the first drug of choice for barbering cats, particularly because the behavioral effects are usually evident within 7 to 10 days.

3. **Clomipramine.** Clomipramine is a more potent TCA than amitriptyline. It has almost no effects on norepinephrine pathways compared with amitriptyline and thus may have fewer global side effects than amitriptyline. Cats may be more sensitive to its arrythmogenic cardiac effects than are dogs or people. Clomipramine acts by inhibiting serotonin reuptake. More serotonin—one of the neurotransmitters associated with upbeat moods and decreased anxiety—is available. TCAs are metabolized

through renal and hepatic pathways. One of the major pathways used is the glucuronic acid route. Cats have less efficient glucuronidation than dogs; hence there are longer half-lives for many drugs in cats. Clomipramine is no exception. Cats that are able to take this drug with none of the common side effects (vomiting, sedation, anorexia, or tachycardia) benefit from its use.

4. **Buspirone.** Buspirone is a newer, nonspecific anxiolytic drug that increases brain levels of both dopamine and serotonin. The side effects include the same renal and hepatic ones as for the other drugs, but overall, most animals do not appear to experience side effects in dosage ranges that are considered therapeutic. This is an advantage for cats. Buspirone may be the drug of first or second choice for barbering cats. It *is* expensive, whereas amitriptyline is not. If amitriptyline is ineffective or the patient experiences side effects when treated with amitriptyline, buspirone is an excellent replacement drug. Buspirone may not reach therapeutic levels for 3 to 4 weeks in some animals with a minimum of 1 week in most. This is the only reason it is not the drug of first choice.

5. There may be some newer, experimental agents that are not readily available. These either alter cholecystokinin (CCK) metabolism or CCK binding. CCK is the hormone that is largely responsible for the feeling of GI fullness. Experimental data published in the Proceedings of the National Academy of Science in 1991 may suggest that feline appetitive movements are associated with abnormal CCK metabolism. This is one active area of research interest, but practical administration of the drugs is not yet an option.

Sample Pharmacological Decision Algorithm for PICA, Inappropriate Ingestion, Wool Sucking

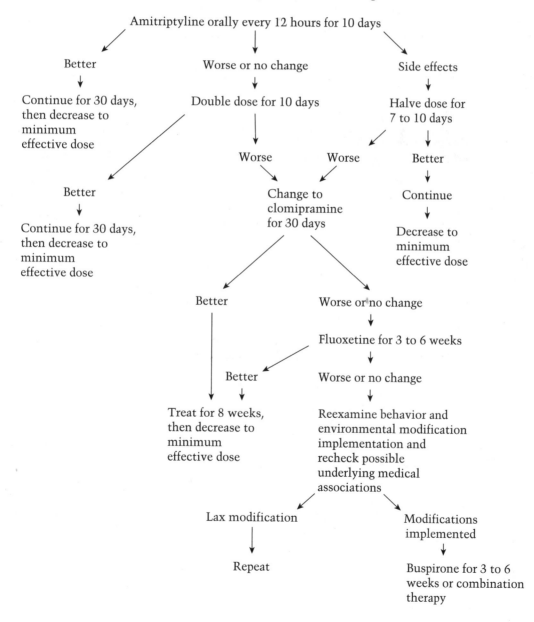

B-29 PROTOCOL FOR CATS WITH BARBERING, LICKING, OR OVERGROOMING CONDITIONS

1. Treat any underlying infectious condition. Assess the potential for atopic or endocrine disease (rare), but consider a biopsy if the condition is long standing. Biopsy may reveal fungi or dermatophytes that cultures fail to reveal.
2. Start a hypoallergenic diet for 8 to 12 weeks. This is very difficult in cats because part of their preference for certain foods or classes of foods is determined by the texture. It may not be possible to get the cats and the clients to cooperate. A second-best option is to remove all treats from the cat's diet and to feed only chicken- or turkey-based foods. These foods are available in kibble or wet forms, and commercial brands are readily available. They tend to contain two proteins (one is optimal), thus if clients can obtain other single-protein specialty diets, the latter are preferred.
3. Set expectations for the cat. Set feeding times, play times, and attention times. Make sure the cat gets 10 to 15 minutes of concerted attention (grooming, stroking, talking to) at least twice a day on a regular schedule. Identify any sources of stress (washing machines, noisy children, another cat that is not a favorite of the patient's) and minimize contact with them. This may mean giving this cat its own room (or sole access to a favored room) or providing it with company. These are very individual circumstances.
4. Enrich the environment with kitty condos and toys if the cat will use them.
5. Teach the cat to sit and request, by pawing, a food scrap that is within the dietary regimen chosen. The cat will do this first by accident and needs to be rewarded *instantly*. Keep practicing on a regular schedule. This helps the cat learn to relax in exchange for a reward.
6. Pharmacological intervention is almost always an important part of therapy and may facilitate the above. Before *any* drugs are used, a complete chemistry screening profile and blood cell count should be performed by the veterinarian. There are two reasons for this: (1) the cat may have an underlying condition that would preclude the use of drugs that are metabolized through renal and hepatic pathways and (2) if medication is prescribed, the animal's response must be monitored if therapy is long term. To assess the importance of any changes, it is important to know the baseline values.

Drugs that have been successful in such cases
1. Diazepam (Valium) 1 to 2 mg (or 0.2 to 0.4 mg/kg) orally every 12 to 24 hours
2. Amitriptyline (Elavil) 5 mg (or 0.5 to 1.0 mg/kg) orally every 12 to 24 hours
3. Clomipramine (Anafranil) 2.5 mg (or 0.5 mg/kg) orally every 24 hours
4. Buspirone (BuSpar) 5 to 10 mg (or 0.5 to 1.0 mg/kg) orally every 24 hours, or half that every 12 hours
5. Hydrocodone (Hycodan) 2.5 to 5.0 mg (or 0.25 to 0.5 mg/kg) orally every 12 to 24 hours

Drug side effects
1. **Diazepam.** Diazepam is a humanly abusable drug and is *not* the appropriate drug for every household. This drug should be carefully monitored and may necessitate frequent reexaminations attendant with refills of the prescription because of the abuse potential. Benzodiazepines are metabolized through renal and hepatic pathways. Any animal with a preexisting renal or hepatic condition must be monitored carefully. The primary side effects are ataxia and stupor. Decreasing the dose often alleviates this effect. Any vomiting, inappetence, or profound change in normal behavior should act as a warning to the practitioner that the dose should be changed or the drug discontinued. There have been isolated reports of sudden death in cats that received relatively small amounts of both brand-name and generic diazepam. Sufficient epidemiological data do not exist to postulate an underlying cause for this occurrence, but many individuals have shied away from use of diazepam in cats. There have been relatively few recent cases of sudden death despite two decades of diazepam treatment of cats. More information should be forthcoming in the next few years. If the cat just started to exhibit the condition *and* the client and practitioner can identify an event associated with the start of this activity, diazepam may be a perfectly acceptable first-choice drug. The intermediate metabolite is the active compound (the half-life of diazepam is on the order of seconds); a gross assay of when the cat achieves effective levels of the intermediate metabolite can be gleaned from its behavior. As the cat metabolizes the drug and the metabolite reaches steady-state levels, the cat usually staggers or acts a little ataxic for a few days. This behavior should spontaneously resolve; if it does not, the cat may be receiving too large a dose of the drug. If the cat never exhibits the transient perception changes, the dose may not be high enough.
2. **Amitriptyline.** Amitriptyline is a tricyclic antidepressant (TCA) that acts by inhibiting serotonin reuptake. As a result, more serotonin—one of the neurotransmitters associated with upbeat moods and decreased anxiety—is available. TCAs are metabolized through renal and hepatic pathways. One of the major pathways is the glucuronic acid route. Cats have less efficient glucuronidation than dogs; hence there are longer half-lives for many drugs in cats. Amitriptyline is no exception. Cats that are able to take this drug with none of the common side effects (vomiting, sedation, anorexia, or tachycardia) benefit from its use. About 50% of cats (this is a clinical estimate) experience gastrointestinal (GI) upset when treated with amitriptyline. This upset is usually profound enough to preclude the use of the drug. All side effects appear reversible. Amitriptyline may be the first drug of choice for barbering cats, particularly because the behavioral effects are usually evident within 7 to 10 days.
3. **Clomipramine.** Clomipramine is a more potent TCA than amitriptyline. It has almost no effects on norepinephrine pathways compared with amitriptyline and thus may produce fewer global side effects than amitriptyline. Cats may be more sensitive to its arrythmogenic cardiac effects than are dogs or people. Clomipramine acts by inhibiting serotonin reuptake. More serotonin—one of the neutrotransmitters associated with upbeat moods and decreased anxiety—is available. TCAs are metabolized through renal and hepatic pathways. One of the major pathways used is the glucuronic acid route. Cats have less efficient glucuronidation than dogs; hence the half-lives of many drugs are longer in cats. Clomipramine is no exception. Cats that are able to take this drug with none of the common side effects (vomiting, sedation, anorexia, or tachycardia) benefit from its use. Fluoxetine (Prozac) is another drug that may be useful if the cat cannot tolerate clomipramine; the mode of action is very similar.

4. **Buspirone.** Buspirone is a newer, nonspecific anxiolytic that increases brain levels of both dopamine and serotonin. The side effects include the same renal and hepatic ones as for the other drugs, but overall, most animals do not appear to experience side effects in dosage ranges that are considered therapeutic. This is an advantage for cats. Buspirone may be the drug of first or second choice for barbering cats. It *is* expensive, whereas amitriptyline is not. If amitriptyline is ineffective or the patient experiences side effects when treated with amitriptyline, buspirone is an excellent replacement drug. Buspirone may not reach therapeutic levels for 3 to 4 weeks in some animals and a minimum of 1 week in most. This is the only reason it is not the drug of first choice.

5. **Hydrocone.** Hydrocone acts by favorably affecting endorphin metabolism. It *is* a humanly abusable drug and may be both physiologically and psychologically addictive in people. Hence it does not belong in every household, even in the minuscule dosages appropriate for a cat. For some cats that mutilate in the course of barbering, this drug can be useful in blocking the cycle. Behavioral effects are noticed within 5 to 10 days. The most common side effects are lethargy (or wakefulness), changes in activity, and anorexia. Decreasing the dosage level may help alleviate these side effects, but it should be noted that cats do not tolerate morphine derivatives as well as dogs do. Frequent monitoring is necessary. These conditions, and the relatively high cost of the drug, make this the last drug of choice for general barbering; however, if mutilation is involved, this drug may be the best choice.

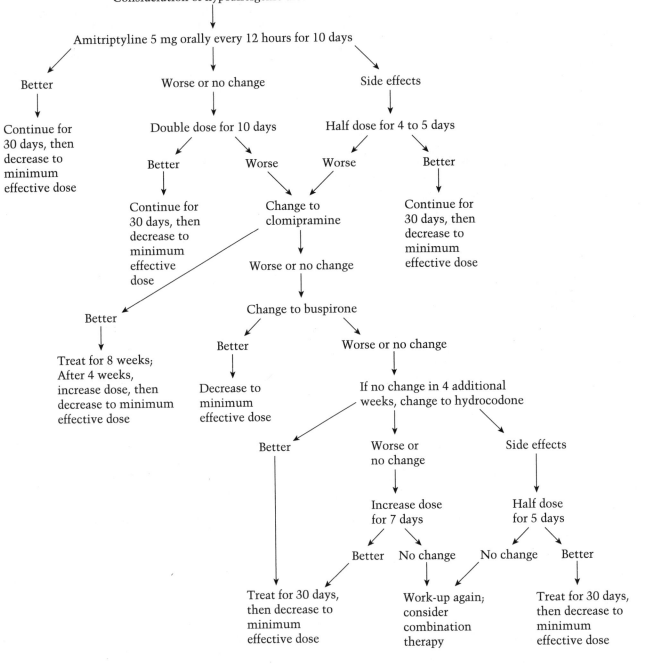

**Sample Decision Algorithm For
Feline Licking and Barbering, *Without* Mutilation**

Sample Decision Algorithm For
Feline Licking and Barbering, *With* Mutilation

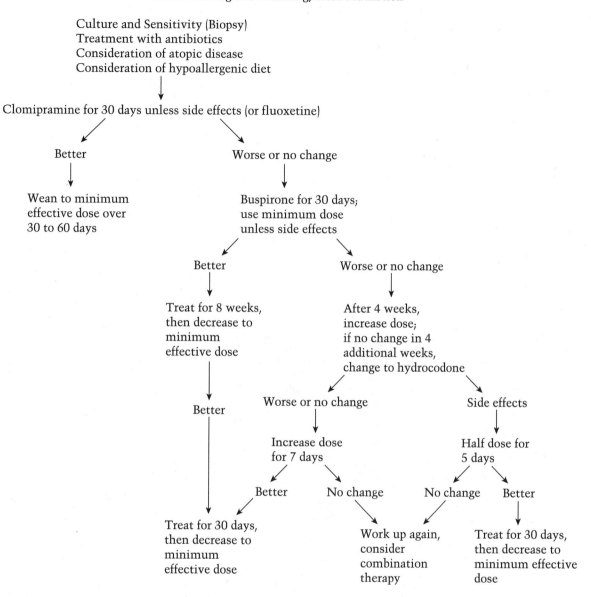

Culture and Sensitivity (Biopsy)
Treatment with antibiotics
Consideration of atopic disease
Consideration of hypoallergenic diet

↓

Clomipramine for 30 days unless side effects (or fluoxetine)

Better → Wean to minimum effective dose over 30 to 60 days

Worse or no change → Buspirone for 30 days; use minimum dose unless side effects

Better → Treat for 8 weeks, then decrease to minimum effective dose → **Better** → Treat for 30 days, then decrease to minimum effective dose

Worse or no change → After 4 weeks, increase dose; if no change in 4 additional weeks, change to hydrocodone

Worse or no change → Increase dose for 7 days → **Better** → Treat for 30 days, then decrease to minimum effective dose

No change → Work up again, consider combination therapy

Side effects → Half dose for 5 days → **No change** → Work up again, consider combination therapy

Better → Treat for 30 days, then decrease to minimum effective dose

**Sample Decision Algorithm For Treatment
of Behavioral Aspects of Acral Lick Dermatitis
All Forms**
Impression smear; CS; antibiotics (8 weeks minimum)

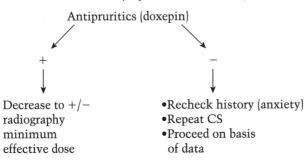

Injury

Antipruritics (doxepin)

+   −

Decrease to +/−
radiography
minimum
effective dose

•Recheck history (anxiety)
•Repeat CS
•Proceed on basis
 of data

**Sample Decision Algorithm For Treatment
of Behavioral Aspects of Acral Lick Dermatitis
All Forms**
Impression smear; CS; antibiotics (8 weeks minimum)

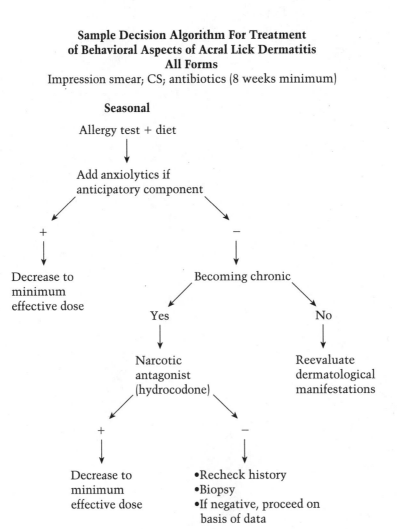

Seasonal

Allergy test + diet

Add anxiolytics if
anticipatory component

+   −

Decrease to
minimum
effective dose

Becoming chronic

Yes   No

Narcotic
antagonist
(hydrocodone)

Reevaluate
dermatological
manifestations

+   −

Decrease to
minimum
effective dose

•Recheck history
•Biopsy
•If negative, proceed on
 basis of data

**Sample Decision Algorithm For Treatment
of Behavioral Aspects of Acral Lick Dermatitis
All Forms**
Impression smear; CS; antibiotics (8 weeks minimum)

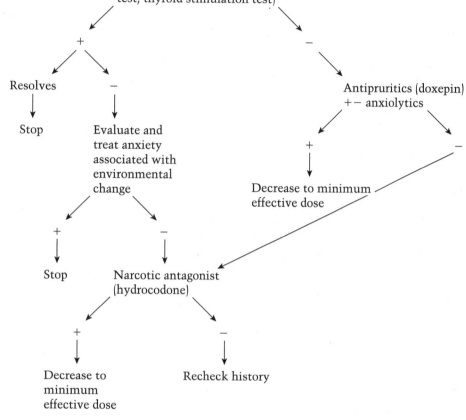

Gradual

•Biopsy/radiography
•Allergy test
•Endocrine evaluation
 (dexamethasone suppression
 test, thyroid stimulation test)

+ → Resolves → Stop

+ → − → Evaluate and treat anxiety associated with environmental change

Evaluate and treat anxiety → + → Stop

Evaluate and treat anxiety → − → Narcotic antagonist (hydrocodone)

− → Antipruritics (doxepin) +− anxiolytics

Antipruritics → + → Decrease to minimum effective dose

Antipruritics → − → Narcotic antagonist (hydrocodone)

Narcotic antagonist → + → Decrease to minimum effective dose

Narcotic antagonist → − → Recheck history

**Sample Decision Algorithm For Treatment
of Behavioral Aspects of Acral Lick Dermatitis
All Forms**
Impression smear; CS; antibiotics (8 weeks minimum)

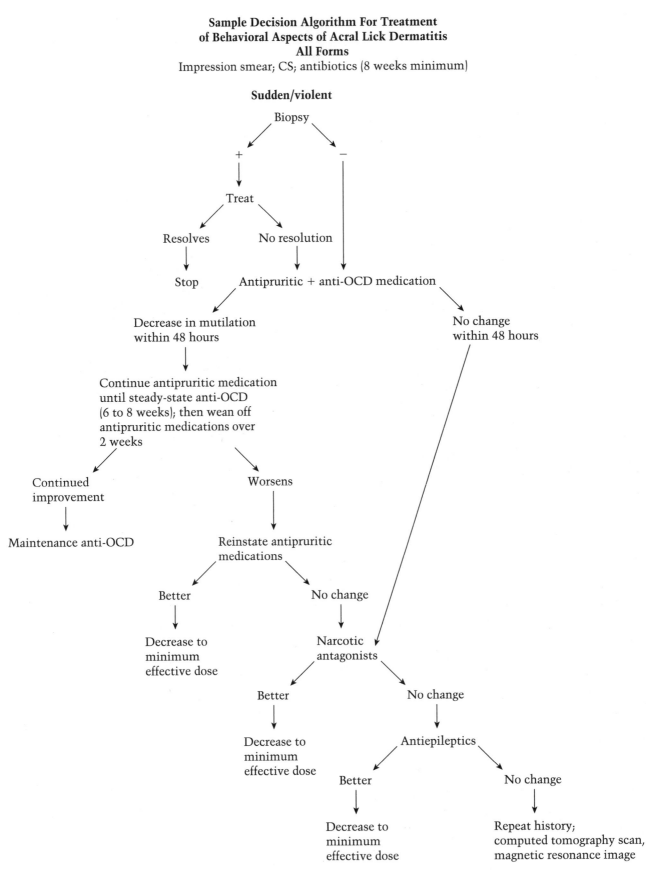

Sudden/violent
Biopsy
+   −
Treat
Resolves   No resolution
Stop   Antipruritic + anti-OCD medication

Decrease in mutilation
within 48 hours   No change
within 48 hours

Continue antipruritic medication
until steady-state anti-OCD
(6 to 8 weeks); then wean off
antipruritic medications over
2 weeks

Continued
improvement   Worsens

Maintenance anti-OCD   Reinstate antipruritic
medications

Better   No change

Decrease to
minimum
effective dose   Narcotic
antagonists

Better   No change

Decrease to
minimum
effective dose   Antiepileptics

Better   No change

Decrease to
minimum
effective dose   Repeat history;
computed tomography scan,
magnetic resonance image

**Sample Decision Algorithm For Treatment
of Behavioral Aspects of Acral Lick Dermatitis
All Forms**
Impression smear; CS; antibiotics (8 weeks minimum)

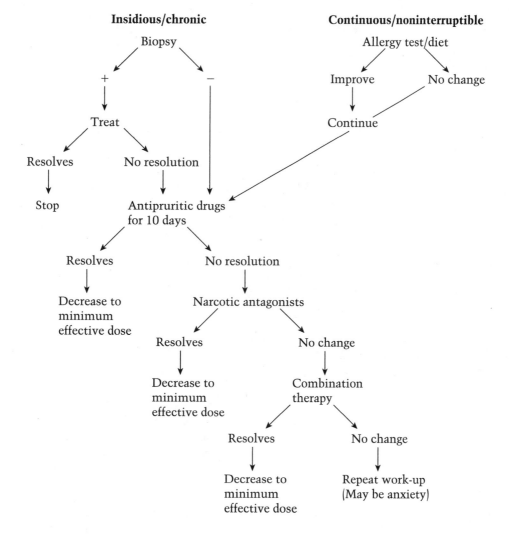

Appendix C

SOURCES OF INFORMATION AND PRODUCTS

Organizations: Dog Training and Competitive Events

International Network for Ethical Training, Sue Myles, Co-ordinator, 7338 Milton Ave., Whittier, CA 90602

The Association of Pet Dog Trainers, P.O. Box 954, Benicia, CA 94510; (707) 745-4237; fax (707) 745-8310. They publish a newsletter and have meetings (educational).

The Canadian Association of Pet Dog Trainers, c/o Debbie Amar, 1726 Bayview Ave., Toronto, Ontario, M4G 3C9, Canada. They publish a newsletter and have meetings (educational).

American Temperament Test Society, Inc. Fred McNabb, 13680 Van Nuys Blvd., Paima, CA 91331; (818) 896-1027

American Temperament Test Society (ATTS), P.O. Box 397, Fenton, MO 63026. Temperament Testing dogs, not puppy testing.

North American Flyball Association, 1 Gooch Park Dr., Barrie, Ontario, Canada L4M 4S6

American Dog Packing Association, 2154 Woodlyn Rd., Pasadena, CA 91104

United Schutzhund Clubs of America, 3704 Lemay Ferry Rd., St. Louis, MO 63125

National Association for Search and Rescue, P.O. Box 3709, Fairfax, VA 22308

SAR Dog Alert, P.O. Box 39, Somerset, CA 95684

Friskies Canine Frisbee Disc Championships, 4060 D Peachtree Rd., Suite 326G, Atlanta, GA 30319; (800) 786-9240

U.S. Agility Dog Association, P.O. Box 850955, Richardson, TX 75085-0955

Trans-National Club for Dog Agility, 401 Bluemont Circle, Manhattan, KS 66502-4531

The North American Agility Dog Council (NAADC), HCR 2, Box 277, St. Maries, ID 83861

National Council on Pet Population Study and Policy, c/o American Kennel Club, 51 Madison Ave., New York, NY 10010

Organizations: Dog Clubs/Humane and Kennel Organizations

American Kennel Club (AKC), 51 Madison Ave., New York, NY 10010; (212) 696-8234 (secretary); (21) 696-8276 (obedience department). Information on shows, field trials, obedience competitions, Breeder Referral Hotline, and Canine Good Citizen Program.

American Boarding Kennels Association, 4575 Galley Rd., Suite 400 A, Colorado Springs, CO 80915; (719) 591-1113. Information on how to choose a boarding kennel, etc.

American Humane Association, 63 Inverness Dr. East, Englewood, CO 80112; (303) 792-9900; fax (303) 793-5333. Source of Report on the Summit on Violence Towards Children and Animals, November 1–3, 1991, and other educational information about children and pets, pet problems, and neutering pets.

Humane Society of the United States, 2100 L St., Washington DC, 20037 (Department D; 20037-1525 for pamphlet about avoiding bites).

United Kennel Club, 100 East Kilgore Rd., Kalamazoo, MI 49001-5598; (616) 343-9020

Organizations: Animal Behavior

American Veterinary Society of Animal Behavior (AVSAB) c/o Dr. Debra Horwitz, Secretary/Treasurer, Veterinary Behavior Consultations, 253 S. Graeser Rd., St. Louis, MO 63141; (314) 567-3864

American College of Veterinary Behavior (Board Certification: President: Dr. Bonnie Beaver, Department of Animal Medicine and Surgery, CVM, Texas A & M University, College Station, TX 77843; (409) 845-2351; fax (409) 845-6978. Secretary: Dr. Kathy Haupt, Department of Physiology, CVM, Cornell University, Ithaca, NY 14853-6401; (607) 253-3450; fax (607) 253-3846.

Animal Behavior Consultant Newsletter, Mercer University, Department of Psychology, 1400 Coleman Ave., Macon, GA 31207-0001 (Attn. Dr. John Wright).

Companion Animal Behaviour Therapy Study Group, CABTSG Newsletter, c/o Mrs. Sarah Heath, BVSc, MRCVS, 33 Hayman Rd., Brackley, Northants, NN13 6JA, England

Animal Behavior Society (ABS), c/o Ira Perelle, c/o Animal Behavior Society, Mercy College, Dobbs Ferry, NY 10522. The ABS publishes a newsletter and scholarly journal, hosts annual research meetings, and certifies individuals as Applied Animal Behaviorists or Associate Applied Animal Behaviorists.

Association of Pet Behavior Counsellors, 257 Royal College St., London, NW1 9LU, England

International Society for Applied Ethology (ISAE), Dr. S.M. Rutter, ISAE Membership Secretary, Institute for Grassland and Environmental Research, North Wyke, Okehamptom, Devon, EX20 2SB, England, or Dr. J.C. Swanson, U.S. Regional Secretary, ISAE, Kansas State University, 134 Eber Hall, Manhattan, KS 66506. The ISAE publishes a scholarly journal and hosts annual research meetings.

Organizations: Miscellaneous

American Dog Owners Association, Inc., 1654 Columbia Turnpike, Castleton, NY 12033; (518) 477-8469; fax (518) 477-4034. Source of copies of brochure "1994 Update: Airline Transportation" (contains information on shipping dogs by air [accompanied or not] prepared by Ms. Priscilla Benkin. Ms. Benkin will answer questions from people who are (1) are not soliciting or raising money, (2) willing to cooperate with USDA investigations; (303) 381-6714 (call 8 to 9 AM or PM Mountain time).

USADA, APHIS Federal Building, Hyattsville, MD 20782. Agency is responsible for interstate transport of live animals in the United States.

American Veterinary Holistic Medical Association, 2214 Old Emmorton Rd., Bel Air, MD 21014 (301) 838-7777. Source of book list on pet massage therapies.

Canine Eye Registration Foundation (CERF), Veterinary Medical Data Program, South Campus Courts, Building C, Purdue University, West Lafayette, IN 47907; (314) 494-8179

National Dog Registry, P.O. Box 11, Woodstock, NY 12498. Tattoo registry and lost and found.

Orthopedic Foundation of America, University of Missouri, Columbia, MO 65211; (573) 442-0418

Organizations: Humane Conditions, Human-Animal Bond, Pet Therapy, Abuse, AIDS and Pets

The Delta Society, P.O. Box 1080, Renton, WA 98057-9906; (206) 226-7357. In addition to providing information and training for the Pet Partners Program, this organization has helped present a series of client information booklets published by ALPO (P.O. Box 14698, Baltimore, MD 21298-9276), including "My Pet Matters: A Guide to Responsible Pet Ownership."

Morris Animal Foundation, 45 Inverness Dr. East, Englewood, CO 80112-5480; (303) 790-2345; (800) 243-2345. This organization has funded and supported the development of residencies in behavioral medicine. It also provides client information, a variety of newsletters, humane education, and grants for veterinary research.

Therapy Dogs International, 260 Fox Chase Rd., Chester, NJ 07930

Tree House Animal Foundation, Inc., 1212 W. Carmen Ave., Chicago, IL 60640; (312) 784-5605. This organization pioneered rescue and placement of abused and abandoned animals and rehabilitates them in a relatively cageless environment in an effort to enhance the pets' social skills. They publish a quarterly newsletter, Tree House News, that frequently addresses problems related to behavior management.

HIV, AIDS, & Pet Ownership (booklet). Available from any PAWS Office (San Francisco, Philadelphia) or Tuskegee University, School of Veterinary Medicine, Tuskegee, AL 36088

Alpha Affiliates, 103 Washington St., Suite 362, Morristown, NJ 07960; (201) 539-2770; fax (201) 644-0610. Source of Alpha Bits newsletter, news and reviews of events and literature related to the human-animal interaction, including pet visitation and therapy.

Products: Odor Elimination Products

Odorzout, No Stink, Inc., 6020 W. Bell Rd., #E101, Glendale, AZ 85308; (800) 887-8465; Zeolite mineral absorbant system to be used with a vacuum cleaner.

Petzorb, ImmunoVet, 5910-G Breckenridge Parkway, Tampa, FL 33610-4253; (800) 762-7648. Polymer crystal absorbent system to be used with a vacuum cleaner.

X-O, X-O Plus, X-O Corporation, 8330 Moberly Ln., Dallas, TX 75227 (800) 442-9696; fax (214) 388-7140. Chemical binding and bacterial growth inhibitors.

Eliminodor, SmithKline Beecham Animal Health; West Chester, PA 19380. Chemical binding, decrease aerosolization, and bacterial growth inhibitors.

Oxyfresh, Oxyfresh USA, Inc., P.O. Box 3723, Spokane, WA 99220; (800) 999-9551, ext. 777. Chemical binding and bacterial growth inhibitors.

Nature's Miracle. Joe Weiss Co., 5312 Ironwood St., Rancho Palos Verdes, CA 90274. Enzymatic degradation of organic material.

The Equalizer. EVSCO, Buena, NJ 08310. Enzymatic degradation of organic material.

Outright, Branton Co. Bacterial/enzyme combinations.

AIP—Anti-Icky-Poo, Bug A Boo Chemicals (800) 326-3016. Distributed by MisterMax Products, 13256 Idyl Dr., Lakeside, CA 92040; (619) 443-7377; (800) 745-1671. Bacterial/enzyme combinations.

Yesterday's News Cat Litter, 28 Elizabeth St., Moncton, NB E1C 9T1, Canada; (506) 859-9118; (800) 267-5287; fax: (506) 859-8013. Soft, absorbant litter made from recycled newspaper.

KOE/AOE, Thornell Corporation, 160 Wheelock Rd., Penfield, NY 14526; (716) 586-5147. Odor neutralizing products: chemical binding and bacterial growth inhibitor.

Litters and Associated Gizmos

MONIpHOR litter, Animal Resources, Westport, CT 06881; (800) 624-6343. Color changes to show pH in range from 5.0-8.0.

Moisture Sensor. Available through MisterMax (800) 745-1671. Detects urine in carpets and pads.

Mountain Cat, (800) 535-9862. Flushable, wood-based litter with 10% cedar fiber (for which there are pluses and minuses).

Wheat Litter, (800) 437-4780. Flushable, all-natural, clumpable litter with enzymes that degrade scent.

Dog Training Devices and Other Gizmos

K-9 Pull Control, Dog Crazy, 8490 Production Ave., San Diego, CA 92121; (800) 459-7855. Slightly more complex, no-pull harness than the Lupi or Sporn, but unlike them, this restrains upper legs.

Halti, Lupi, Safari Whitco, 85 Orville Dr., Bohemia, NY 11716; (516) 563-6111; (800) 367-7387; Company of Animals, P.O. Box 23, Chertsey, Surrey, KT16 OPU, United Kingdom; (011) 441-93-246-6696.

Sporn/No-Pull Halter, Four Paws Products Ltd., 50 Wireless Blvd., Hauppauge, NY 11788; (516) 434-1100. Harness that fits over shoulders and around chest to discourage pulling.

Dog Stop, Company of Animals, P.O. Box 23, Chertsey, Surrey, KT16 OPU, United Kingdom; (011) 441-93-246-6696. Loud air horn that is hand held.

Barker Breaker, Super Barker Breaker, Scraminal, Critter Gitter, Amtek Pet Behavior Products, 11025 Sorrento Valley Court, San Diego, CA 92121; (619) 597-6681; (800) 762-7618. Handheld unit that uses audible and high-frequency sounds to deter behavior; super unit is remote.

Silencer Bark Collar, Austin Innovations, 2600 McHale Court, Suite 140, Austin, TX 78758; (512) 339-6765; (800) 966-2275. Audible tone produced each time dog barks.

Pet-Agree, Dazer, KII Enterprises, P.O. Box 306, Camillus, NY 13031; (315) 468-3596; (800) 262-3963. Unltrasonic, handheld deterrent.

Easy Trainer, Austin Innovations, 2600 McHale Court, Suite 140, Austin, TX 78758; (512) 339-6765; (800) 966-2275. Ultrasonic tone to deter undesired behavior, coupled with an audible tone to reinforce good behavior.

Tattle Tale, KII Enterprises, P.O. Box 306, Camillus, NY

13031; (315) 468-3596; (800) 262-3963. Vibration sensor that alerts client to pet's movement across a surface, while encouraging the pet to keep going.

Bark Eliminator, Bark Diminisher, 100/LR Training Collar, Tritronics, Inc., 1550 S. Research Loop, Tucson, AZ 85710; (800) 456-4343. A variety of bark-activated shock collars with a variety of delays and levels of shock.

Basic Trainer, Free Spirit, Innotek Incorporated, 9025 Coldwater Rd., Bldg. 100 A, Fort Wayne, IN 46825; (219) 489-0369; (800) 826-5527. Remote electronic shock collars.

Soft Paws, Soft Paws c/o Smart Practice, 3400 E. McDowell, Phoenix, AZ 85008; (602) 225-0599; (800) 522-0800. Nail caps in a variety of colors for dogs or cats. Nails still grow, but damage is eliminated; caps must be replaced every 4 to 6 weeks.

Kong toys, The Kong Company, 11111 W. 8th Ave., #D, Lakewood, CO; 80215-5516 (303) 233-9262. Balls, kongs, and other virtually indestructible toys that also bounce in a way that makes them "behave" more than standard toys.

Pavlov's Cat, Cat Scratch Feeder, Del West Enterprises, 9733 Caminito Doha, San Diego, CA 92131; (619) 689-9999. Toy and reward system that also encourages scratching in an appropriate spot.

Nylabone toys, TFH Publications, 1 TFH Plaza, 3rd and Union Ave., Neptune, NJ 07753; (908) 988-8400. Gummis or nearly indestructible nylon hard chew toys and frisbees for puppies and chewing dogs.

Quick Relief Remote Training Collar, Elexis Corporation, 700 NW 46th Street, Miami, FL 33166-5604; (305) 592-6069. Remote-controlled, handheld collar that relies on ultrasound; can be effective up to 60 feet.

Scat Mat, Contech Electronics, Inc., P.O. Box 115, Saanichton, BC, V0S 1M0, Canada; (604) 652-0755; (800) 767-8658; fax (604) (652-5352). Mats come in a variety of shapes and sizes and emit shocks when touched so that pets avoid areas where mats are placed.

Invisible Fencing, Invisible Fence Co., 355 Phoenixville Pike, Malvern, PA 19355; (610) 652-0999; (800) 538-3647. Electronic collar/fence combination that acts on a system of flags, audible cues, and shocks, combined with training to the fence, designed to allow animals to run free without being run over.

Scraminal, Critter Gitter, Amtek Pet Behavior Products, 11025 Sorrento Valley Court, San Diego, CA 92121; (619) 597-6681; (800) 762-7618. Motion detector that sounds alarm within 15 feet so that pet is discouraged from entering area.

Smart Bowl, AQCON, Inc., 340 Kingswood Road, Toronto, Ontario M4E 3N9, Canada; (416) 691-0558. Sets off alarm if an animal other than the one for whom the bowl is intended (and who is wearing a special collar) approaches it. Useful for medicated food or weight control.

Snappy Trainer, Innovative Pet Products, 8601 F5 West Cross Dr., Suite 209, Littleton, CO 80123-2200; (303) 797-0900; (800) 854-8800. Large "mousetrap"-like device that makes loud snapping noise to discourage lying on or digging in areas.

Sofasaver, Aris Enterprises, 10 W. 46th Street, 4th Floor, New York, NY 10036 (212) 840-2570. Large size mat for furniture that emits alarm when touched. LED displays let clients know if alarm was activated in their absence.

BeeperKid, Available from Frontgate, 2800 Henkle Dr., Lebanon, OH 45036-8894 (800) 626-6488. Sounds alarm if child or dog goes more than 15 feet from you; works by a two-piece electronic monitor.

Gentle Leader/Promise System Canine Head Collar (U.S.A.), Premier Pet Products, 2406 Krossridge Rd., Richmond, VA 23236; (804) 271-0200; (800) 933-5595. Head collar and training system designed for a humane approach to problems with walking on a leash, mouthing, and aggression.

Gentle Leader/Promise System Canine Head Collar (Canada), P.A.B.A. (Professional Animal Behavior Associates), Inc., P.O. Box 25111, London, Ontario, Canada, N6C-6A8; (519) 685-4756; fax (519)-685-6618.

Gentle Leader (U.K., Europe, and Asia), Canac Pet Products, Brecks Mill, Westbury Leigh, Wilts BA13 3SD, England; (01373) 864775; fax: (01373) 858166.

Aboistop, Vetoquinol Canada, 675 St. Pierre South, Jolliette, Quebec, J6E 3Z1, Canada; (514) 759-0497. Citronella collar to inhibit barking without client presence.

ABS (American version of Aboistop). Available from ImmunoVet, Vetoquinol U.S.A., Inc., 5910-G Breckenridge Parkway, Tampa, FL 336110-4253; (813) 621-9947; (800) 627-9447; fax (813) 621-0751. Citronella collar for inhibition of barking.

K9 Counterconditioning, Canine Communications, 1321 Longmeadow Dr., Glenview, IL 60025; (800) 952-6517. Tapes for reduction of noise fears/phobias.

Noiseshyness Cure Systems, Starfire, P.O. Box 3119, Warrenton, VA 22186; (703) 349-1039. Tapes and products for reduction of noise fears/phobias.

"The Ultimate Thunderstorm" and "Country Thunderstorm" (Nos. 4 and 11) Synotic Research, Inc., Environments Division, 3405 Barranca Circle, Austin, TX 78731-5711

"Sounds of Nature," Ovation Sound Effects (Vol. 5 [OVQD/1505]), Ovation Records, Glenview, IL 60025.

Easy Rider Car Seat Belt by Safari. Available from RC Steele, 1989 Transit Way, Box 910, Brockport, NY 14420-0910; (800) 872-3773. Safer alternatives to barriers, which still allow the dogs/cats to be thrown around, although not into clients' laps. Harness is designed to work with standard car seat belts; small size fits cats. Alternatively, a regular harness and a seat belt converter can be used (available from the same sources as seat belt harnesses).

Miscellaneous behavior modification and training devices, thunderstorm tapes, N.R.V.C., P.O. Box 1087, Niwot, CO 80544-1087

Yapper Zapper, Norwego, P.O. Box 216, 2640 Vuillet Rd., Highland, IL 62249; (618) 654-7130. Bark-activated water sprayer designed to be mounted on a cage or run.

Products: Books/Videos/Booklets

Frisbees: PRB & Associates, 4060-D Peachtree Rd., Suite 326M, Atlanta, GA 30319; (800) 786-9240.

Barish, Eileen. *Vacationing With Your Pet!* (1994), Pet-Friendly Publications, P.O. Box 8459, Scottsdale, AZ 85252; (800) 496-2665

Habgood D, Habgood R. *Frommer's on the Road Again With Man's Best Friend*, Macmillan/Howell Book House, $14.95, Regional guide books for the U.S.

"DogGone (The Newsletter about Fun Places To Go and Cool Stuff To Do With Your Dog)", $24 per year; to subscribe, call (407) 569-8434

Frommer's On the Road Again With Man's Best Friend: A Selective Guide to Bed and Breakfasts, Inns, Hotels and

Resorts That Welcome You and Your Dog, 1995, Howell Book House four books for four regions: West, Southeast, Mid-Atlantic, and New England.

SIRIUS Puppy Training Videos, related books, pamphlets, and audiocassettes, James and Kenneth Publishers, 2140 Shattuck Ave., #2406, Berkeley, CA 94704; (415) 658-8588

Nicki Meyer Educational Effort, Inc., 31 Davis Hill Rd., Weston, CT 06883; (203) 226-9877. Pamphlets designed for client use on how to crate train a dog ($0.20 each).

Gaines/Cycle Pet Care Center, P.O. Box 9001, Chicago, IL 60604-9001. Source of numerous free client education booklets on all aspects of caring for dogs and cats, with a particular emphasis on behavior. This is the source of the series on behavioral problems and their prevention, written by Voith and Borchelt, that appeared in The Compendium on Continuing Education, sponsored by Veterinary Learning Systems.

"Good Dog! The Consumer Magazine for Dog Owners," P.O. Box 10069, Austin, TX 78766; Subscriber information: (800) 968-1738; other: (803) 795-9555; fax (803) 795-2930. Magazine that eventually reviews every product, gizmo, and food usually related to dogs (and sometimes cats). Reviews are generally just listings of product information and not critical comparisons, but they always provide addresses, telephone numbers, and sources and have articles that focus on training, problem prevention, and other "hot" topics that clients really enjoy. (The stack of free ones that we get for the waiting room at VHUP is always gone within a day or two.)

"Living Safely With Dogs," 1995. The Coalition for Safe Children and Dogs, Inc. To order, call (412) 793-5797 or (412) 325-2518. Coloring book for children that illustrates dog signals. Teaches how to avoid bites and how to interact with dogs safely and appropriately.

Appendix D

BOOKS FOR THE PRACTITIONER'S SHELF AND
TO RECOMMEND TO CLIENTS

These books represent a small subset of those written by fanciers and specialists about animal behavior. Inclusion in this list is not an endorsement, nor is exclusion considered condemnation. I have attempted to provide a partial answer to two of the questions that I am so frequently asked by veterinarians: "Where can I read more?" and "Are there any books I can encourage my clients to read?" The descriptions are intended to provide some guidance about the books' contents and to encourage further perusal. The letter before the title indicates whether the book is best suited to veterinarian (V) or client (C) interest, or whether the book would be of interest to both (B).

C *Dogs and the Law*, by Anmarie Barrie. Neptune City, New Jersey, 1990, T.F.H. Books.

This book is intended to help clients understand liability and responsibility of pet ownership. There is information on the assumption of risk, differences that may pertain to assistance dogs, and recommendations of where to get that information. There are some general guidelines regarding vaccination, spaying, neutering, leash laws, vehicles, number of animals allowed on a property, and licensing of pets. Ms. Barrie outlines the basic codes that involve dog liability (e.g., which statute contains "dog-running-at-large"). This can be helpful to clients and veterinarians who want to check the most recent laws in their state. Dog law is evolving quite rapidly, and some of the specifics in this book will be superseded.

There is one very problematic chapter in this book: the one on buying and selling dogs. Ms. Barrie's assertion that if clients buy pets from a local breeder, they may not have the protection they would have from a standard pet store sales return is not true in many states. She unfortunately encourages people to buy pets from pet stores because of the return policy. This is unenlightened and ignores the potential problems of pet store dogs and cats.

V *Feline Behavior: A Guide for Veterinarians*, by Bonnie B. Beaver. Philadelphia, 1992, WB Saunders.

This is the second edition of Bonnie Beaver's original book on feline behavior that was published in 1980. She was one of the first to write a book about feline behavior and should be commended for developing the focus in the field. This book is appropriate only for veterinarians. It is very well referenced and has excellent sections on sensory and neurological function. It is illustrated with a series of good pictures of kittens at different developmental stages exhibiting behaviors that are discussed. For people who are interested in cat behavior, this book, in combination with those of Bradshaw, Bateson, and Turner, will form the core of the reference shelf.

B *Second-Hand Dog: How to Turn Yours Into a First-Rate Pet*, by Carol Lea Benjamin. New York, 1988, Howell Book House.

This book focuses on the recycled and previously rejected dog. It is a terrific book because Ms. Benjamin makes it clear that these dogs will not behave like dogs that were raised by good families in good homes with siblings. Ms. Benjamin explains that these dogs need to feel safe and to learn basic commands; this can be accomplished with the use of a stepwise program. She also explains that children should not interact in the same manner with these dogs that they might with another puppy because it is unknown how these dogs will react. Her advice on this issue will save heartbreak.

Ms. Benjamin has an excellent section on trainer's tips that can prevent biting. She points out that clients should not beat a dog with a newspaper or play very roughly with dogs. Much to her credit, Ms. Benjamin always tries to explain why dogs might *perceive* that what they did, albeit aggressive, could have been an appropriate response.

As in her other books, this one is accompanied by superb cartoon drawings that explain "come," "sit," "lie down," "stay," and quick verbal corrections for inappropriate behavior. Her litany is simple: if you love your dog, leash it, help it, do not ask it to make a mistake.

B *The Chosen Puppy: How to Select and Raise a Great Puppy from an Animal Shelter*, by Carol Lea Benjamin. New York, 1990, Howell Book House.

This is another charming book by Carol Lea Benjamin. It is designed for clients, not professionals. If any client is thinking of getting a puppy and there are children in the household, it would behoove the veterinarian to provide the client with a copy of this book. The text is brief and to the point. It focuses on puppies adopted from humane shelters. Ms. Benjamin explains why animals are often brought to humane shelters, and that animals that come from humane shelters may not have had many of the advantages of puppies that were home reared.

The section on body language of dogs is excellent. The issues are simplified, but the exceptional line drawings and labels help avoid misinterpretation problems. This book provides a wonderful foundation without flaws so that clients are not misinformed. Ms. Benjamin lists questions to ask when clients go to the humane shelter. She makes a point of providing instructions. One of her rules is that you are not allowed to "fall in love" with this puppy until the veterinarian tells you it is okay.

The book has illustrations on classic training techniques. Ms. Benjamin recommends the buckle-collar and only very mild corrections. Most management-related problems are discussed, and there are some very clever tricks that help to avoid behaviors such as unwanted barking.

This is a superb book; it is superior to many of the others listed here if the dog in question is a pup. One of the advantages is that this book is funny: the drawings are both humorous and illustrative, and they encourage clients to start right away. That makes this book worth its weight in gold.

C *Surviving Your Dog's Adolescence: A Positive Training Program*, by Carol Lea Benjamin. New York, 1993, Howell Book House.

Ms. Benjamin's other books include *Dog Training for Kids, Dog Tricks, Dog Problems, Second-Hand Dog: How to Turn Yours Into a First-Rate Pet, The Chosen Puppy, How to Select and Raise a Great Puppy from an Animal Shelter,* and her best-known book, *Mother Knows Best: The Natural Way to Train Your Dog.* Although this book covers many of the topics discussed in the other books, it focuses on the changes that occur in a dog's life when the dog reaches social maturity. The text is accompanied by wonderful line drawing cartoons that emphasize Ms. Benjamin's most important points.

The problems attendant with social maturity are divided into fairly broad categories. For each of these categories, Ms. Benjamin uses exemplary dogs and their stories to elaborate the problems. This allows clients to empathize with Ms. Benjamin and her dogs and to draw parallels to their own pets. This book is subject to the same problems as other books, with uncritical use of terminology and dogma related to pack orders and "alpha" status, but Ms. Benjamin's basic premise—that we should respect the dog and the dog's age-specific needs— should be lauded. Anything clinicians can do to encourage clients to view their dogs with respect, instead of as owned possessions, benefits everyone.

B *A Dog is Listening*, by Roger Caras. Simon & Schuster, 1992.

Roger Caras is president of the ASPCA and has been a commentator and a reporter on wildlife and pet issues for many years. This book is a testament to his ability to be empathic with other species.

Anyone who wants an empathic view of the variety of the behaviors to be expected from canine companions would really enjoy this book. After reading this book, clients will find many books that focus on training to be more meaningful.

V *The Natural History of Domesticated Animals*, by Juliet Clutton-Brock. Cambridge, 1987, Cambridge University Press, British Museum of Natural History.

Juliet Clutton-Brock was classically trained in the behavioral and evolutionary sciences, and it shows. This book covers standard companion animals, livestock and farm animals, and a category she calls *exploited captives:* large cats, elephants, camels and lamas, reindeer, Asiatic cattle, and so on. The latter comprise a category of animals that are seen in zoos or now are domesticated in a for-profit situation. Game ranching, lagomorphs, and ferrets are also discussed in the context of the evolution of the behavioral and physical attributes that have permitted exploitation for food and fur.

This book should be required reading for veterinarians and veterinary students sometime during their career. It provides anthropological, evolutionary, market and economic, and cultural perspectives on the forces driving the domestication of animals and the underlying basis for the behaviors for which animals were selected for domestication.

B *Dog Behavior—Why Dogs Do What They Do*, by Ian Dunbar. New Jersey, 1979, T. F. H. Publications.

This book is an excellent general introduction for anyone contemplating getting a dog or wanting to know about the basic biology of his or her dog. It includes chapters on puppy development, canine nonverbal communication, canine sensory systems, social systems of dogs, sexual behavior, and a section on the origin of dogs. The middle part of the book focuses on training puppies. Dr. Dunbar recommends working with puppies as soon as clients get them, or when the puppies are 6 weeks of age, whichever comes first (this means breeders should start the work). Some lovely black-and-white photographs demonstrate the points illustrated in the text. Dr. Dunbar focuses on working with the dog and understanding dog communication. He makes his points in a gentle way. Dr. Dunbar's techniques are rooted in appropriate rewards and timing. With the exception of recommending grabbing the scruff and muzzle in a correction, there are no major gaffes. It should be noted that even grabbing a scruff or a muzzle is not a major gaffe in a young puppy that does not resist it; however, if the dog begins to have problems, or the person is too rough, this is problematic. This book does not deal with problem dogs.

V *The Behaviour of Dogs and Cats*, by John Fisher, editor. London, 1993, Stanley Paul.

This is a compendium book written by members of the Association of Pet Behavior Counselors in England; the book is largely for veterinarians. It consists of chapters on the development of social behavior and its role in preventing or contributing to behavior problems, and chapters on the classic problems seen most frequently in practice. Unfortunately, cat problems are relegated to only one chapter, written by Dr. Peter Neville.

The best chapters in the book are the chapters by Roger Abrantes on the development of social behavior and by David Appleby on socialization and habituation. The chapters on phobias and canine aggression by Robin Walker are less than practical, although he should be lauded for stating that physical punishment and physical aggression should not be used to deal with aggressive situations. The chapter on separation anxiety by Margaret Goddard provides excellent information on why dogs become anxious. She discusses standard maintenance behaviors to prevent new dogs from becoming anxious; however, for truly anxious dogs with extreme separation anxiety, the techniques presented in the book will not correct the problem. The drug therapy discussed in this text has been superseded. John Fisher's chapter on training is quite good and explains many of the principles of gentle training in an intellectual manner. He expertly explains shaping—a progressive, gradual approach to getting the dog to comply. The book concludes with an excellent chapter by Ann McBride on pet loss, a topic about which all clinicians could be more knowledgeable.

B *The Dog's Mind: Understanding Your Dog's Behavior*, by Bruce Fogle. New York, 1990, Howell Book House.

This book would probably be better for the lay person

than the veterinarian, in part because it is lacking specific data. It is written at a level that clients will appreciate and that might make veterinarians seek more in-depth data. The book opens with chapters on the anatomy and physiology of the dog's mind and then moves on to behavior. It is a terrific overall review for clients who are interested in behavior. The primary problems are the uncritical acceptance of the terminology involved with packs and dominance and submissive relationships that have been previously discussed. Fogle also discusses some of the most common canine behavioral problems, including some treatment protocols and instructions for implementing behavior modification techniques. I have some concern that the average client might think this means that behavioral problems can be treated without the help of a specialist.

The average client will find the chapters on communication and behavioral patterns fascinating. The book is accompanied with line drawings that will help make it useful and enjoyable for an ambitious client.

B *Know Your Cat*, by Bruce Fogle. New York, 1991, Dorling Kindersley.

This book should be in every veterinary waiting room. As with his dog book, this book on cats does an excellent job of discussing and illustrating normal cat behavior and age-specific behavior. The photos of the cats being cats are amazing. Use this book to work with your clients.

B *Know Your Dog: An Owner's Guide to Dog Behavior*, by Bruce Fogle. New York, 1992, Dorling-Kindersley.

This little book is designed to teach both veterinarians and clients to interpret dog behavior. Although many of the descriptions of the behaviors rely on uncritical use of terminologies associated with packs and hierarchies, these are very minor faults. For each category of behaviors, there are multiple pictures accompanied by often numbered sets of descriptions that explain what each part of the dog's signaling behavior conveys. There is an excellent section on pregnancy and maternal behavior complete with full-color pictures of puppies being born and those same puppies later in life being disciplined and played with by their mother. There are excellent sections on what a dog's tail and ears can convey. One of the terrific things about this book is that these are actual pets, and the photos are not staged.

Another advantage of this book is the appendix that allows a client to evaluate a dog's character or personality. Although this could be overinterpreted, it is presented as a tool to give clients an indication about whether their dog will meet their expectations, and whether their dog could potentially have problems for which they could benefit from a consultation with either their veterinarian or a specialist in behavioral medicine.

This book should be in every waiting room. It will allow veterinarians to explain certain types of behavior through pictorial help.

B *ASPCA Complete Dog Training Manual*, by Bruce Fogle. New York, 1994, Dorling-Kindersley.

All people getting—or considering getting—puppies or a new dog should read this. The book starts by describing basic dog behavior and communication. There is a discussion of breed differences and personality types illustrated with excellent photos. There are pages of photos of every type of leash, collar, humane training gizmo, and reward toy known to humankind. A beautifully detailed section on crate training (with a seemingly ever-growing black Lab) should allay even the most anxious client's fears about crates. The book's focus is on basic manners training and obedience, but there is a short section on "bad habits" and problem behaviors. My only misgivings involve this section and the one on temperament. In both cases, I fear that clients will generalize extensively and not seek the help of a specialist early, when it will be most beneficial.

C *The Healing Touch*, by Michael W. Fox. New York, 1990, Newmarket Press.

Some clients and veterinarians will not like the "touchy-feely" tone of the book. If so, they should not read the text, but just look at the pictures. We are always telling clients to reward calm, relaxing behaviors. This book demonstrates a fine method of doing that.

C *Superdog—Raising the Perfect Canine Companion*, by Michael W. Fox. New York, 1990, Howell Book House.

This book is designed for clients, but the average veterinarian will also find it useful. One of the best chapters discusses the ability of dogs to reason. The human–companion animal bond has received much attention, as have the roles that dogs are intended to play (e.g., utilitarian, economic, companion). Dr. Fox outlines the evidence (pro and con) for the ability to comprehend and reason within these contexts.

The chapters on understanding canine communicatory behavior are not as in-depth as his other books, but they provide a good overview for the average client and a refresher for veterinarians. The chapters on the biochemistry of the ability to smell and a chapter on developmental periods are excellent. This book is designed to help clients create a better pet, thus it largely deals with working with dogs in specific situations (e.g., grooming, playing with children, basic companion animal commands). Dr. Fox seriously questions the validity of using choke collars and makes some very potent arguments against their use. He correctly states that collars are no substitute for working adequately with a dog.

B *The Complete Guide to Dog Law*, by Deidre E. Gannon. New York, 1994, Howell Book House.

This is a more rigorous treatment of aspects of law that deal with dogs than any of the other legal-oriented books mentioned here. Ms. Gannon, the author of Chapter 15, discussed the issues of dogs as property, contracts involving dogs, property damage done by dogs, and protection for dogs. Ms. Gannon, who has champion Argentine dogos, also cogently takes on the issue of dangerous dog laws and dog bans. Citations from the legal literature are included and explained.

V *Animal Minds*, by Donald R. Griffen. Chicago, 1992, University of Chicago Press.

When I was an undergraduate I had the pleasure of hearing two guest lectures from Dr. Griffen, who was then at Rockefeller University. Now professor emeritus and at Harvard, he persists in his unusual ability to ask insightful questions about the possibilities of cognition in animals. His discussions of the implications of string inference and the empirical method as they pertain to animal consciousness raise the concept beyond the standard, antiquated anthropomorphic approach. For anyone interested in a rigorous approach to cognitive ethology, this book is a must.

C *How to Raise a Sane and Healthy Cat*, by Sean Hammond and Carolyn Usrey. New York, 1994, Howell Book House.

Finally a "dog" book for cat lovers! This book is full of wonderfully sane and kind advice for cats and their people (including the address of a source for cat diapers). The sections on behavior problems and potential problems are great. The communication chapter is fun, useful, and accurate. The book also contains basic medical and first aid information, and the authors always recommend that clients seek competent help even for behavior problems. It's about time.

C *Child-Proofing Your Dog*, by Brian Kilcommons with Sarah Wilson. New York, 1994, Time Warner.

This short book provides some cogent advice and quick tricks relevant to our changing lifestyles, namely, how your "first" child, your dog (or cat) will react to the arrival of your "second" child, the human. The advent of a human addition can be problematic, and not all children should have pets. The book pays only scant attention to the fact that as babies become children they must learn to respect their pets and treat them kindly. There is no mention of the dog abuse–child abuse link, and this would be the perfect place to discuss it. Finally, most dogs that still do not accept children do not need to be killed—they can go to child-free homes, an option not discussed here.

B *Absent Friend: Coping with the Loss of a Treasured Pet*, by Laura and Martyn Lee. High Wycombe, Bucks, England, 1992, Henston Press.

This is the single best book I have ever read on the death of a pet. It is very much from the British standpoint—in Great Britain the pet-person relationship is a serious one. Accordingly, this book talks about Blue Cross, ambulances, protection leagues, defense leagues, pet crematoriums, pet rest cemeteries, and so on.

The time for clients to read this book for the first time is *not* when their pet is critically ill. Instead, this is a book that we mention during the last in our series of puppy classes at VHUP. The loss of a dog can happen at any age. Most people are very attached to their pets. They should be encouraged to experience whatever is necessary to help them resolve their potential loss. Thinking about it beforehand can help when the loss occurs. The last thing that people who have lost a treasured companion need is to feel that they are abnormal; this book will give them solace.

C *Dog Logic, Companion Obedience: Rapport-based Training*, by Joel M. McMannis. New York, 1992, Howell Book House.

This is an excellent *training* book, that is, a book that will teach clients how to actually put their dogs through the paces.

This is one of the kindest books on dog training that I have ever read. Although this book has the problems that many other training books do, namely, a reliance on critical assertions of roles and pack hierarchies, this does not overshadow the emphasis that the author places on kindly working with a dog. The author makes an effort early in the book to help prospective clients decide whether they want a dog, and what type of dog might be best for them. Rather than emphasizing breeds, Mr. McMannis emphasizes the reasons that dogs are brought to shelters. He discusses size, coat color, sex, age, and the reasons that people might want dogs as factors that should influence pet selection.

My one serious criticism of this book is the chapter on collars. Mr. McMannis' view of collars is restricted to pinch collars, choke collars, and electronic collars. I do not think that either pinch or choke collars are truly humane, rather, they can do serious long-term, possibly irreversible harm. Electronic collars are frequently abused, cause pain, and usually result in worsened behavior in aggressive or fearful dogs.

B *The Dog IQ Test*, by Melissa Miller. New York, 1993, Penguin Books.

This is not a book about how smart your dog is; this is a book about how much *you* know about dogs. It is not perfect and subscribes to some myths about behavior. However, it could be a powerful tool to open dialog between veterinarians and clients and should be read by and discussed with people who are thinking of getting a dog but may be hesitant. Whether the tests actually help clients find the type of dog best for them (and vice versa) is unclear; however, the quizzes are fun and will ensure that people enter into the dog-person/person-dog relationship informed.

C *How to Be Your Dog's Best Friend: A Training Manual for Owners*, by The Monks of New Skete. Boston, 1978, Little, Brown.

In his foreword, Michael Fox sums up the thrust of the approach of this book, "A reverence for all life entails responsible stewardship as well: love is not enough." That is the basis for this book.

This book falls prey to the same types of problems as do other books with an overgeneralization of alpha dog terminology, but it is accompanied by some excellent descriptions of actual behaviors, so that misconceptions are not as common as they might be with some other books.

My complaints about this book include some of the descriptions of discipline. The book advocates chin slaps, shakedowns, and alpha rollovers. Although the authors expertly describe the appropriate ways to use these types of commands, they do not discuss the risks attendant with them, particularly with dogs that already have behavioral problems. Furthermore, given their general philosophy, I have always been surprised that the authors do not discuss the potential for sending undesirable signals about the use of physical force attendant with such corrections. The authors do emphasize the use of these correctional postures in the context of canine communication, but the descriptions are not detailed enough. There are good photographs of ways dogs can be massaged. Applying the same logic as for massage, the authors correctly recommend the avoidance of all rough play, including slapping and sudden movements.

The short section on children and dogs is *excellent*. I honestly think that if more people read this, their *children* would also be better behaved. The main thrust of the section is that children often act unpredictably and excitably in front of dogs, and dogs who have not been specifically trained to discount these tendencies will react in a normal manner that might cause someone to be injured. A child always has the potential to inadvertently make an innocent dog responsible for a tragedy because of normal *child* behavior.

The final section of the book deals with specific behavior problems. Unfortunately, some of these "treatments" are potentially injurious to the dog and to everyone concerned. One problematic behavior that is well illustrated is kneeing the dog in the chest. Although the authors point out that this could be deadly for a puppy and should not be used on pups, they neglect to realize that by treating an attention-seeking behavior with attention, clients may be reinforcing the dog to seek more devious ways to get attention.

C *The Art of Raising a Puppy*, by The Monks of New Skete. Boston, 1991, Little, Brown.

One of the charming devices of this book is a preface that includes a long argument on why not to breed puppies. It is an incredibly clever device for a book that otherwise would make people enchanted to think that puppies would be something that everyone would want to raise.

The first few chapters concentrate on the developmental process during gestation and the behavioral developmental process during the early period of life. The descriptions about the "socialization" periods rely on uncritical acceptance of the intensity of socialization necessary to create a perfect dog. This is a minor failing when the descriptors of what happens during these periods are so good.

The book is illustrated with wonderful black-and-white photos that show the clients exactly how to do the exercises and how to do them in an age-specific manner. Appropriate collars and leashes are covered, although the emphasis is on training collars rather than the more creative and advanced view of head collars; however, pinch collars and harsher varieties of chokers are not recommended.

C *Dog Training the Mugford Way—Never Say No*, by Roger Mugford. London, 1992, Hutchinson, Stanley, Paul.

In 1979 Dr. Roger Mugford created the Animal Behaviour Centre in the United Kingdom for the purpose of helping animals with behavioral problems. Since then he has written popular books about correcting dogs' problems and about canine behavioral disorders and has created many useful devices, such as the Halti and the Lupi no-pull harness. It is interesting that his company name is The Company of Animals.

Dr. Mugford contends that we should value canine companions. We should treat them with respect, and we should treat them humanely. His book focuses on ways to do this.

Dr. Mugford carefully explains the differences between using a reward strategy versus a punishment strategy and when each would be appropriate. He accompanies these explanations with line drawings that explain conditional and unconditional stimuli and the role of behavior modification. This book has the requisite chapters on developmental periods and expectations of puppies versus adult dogs. Many specific questions about management-related problems, such as barking, pulling, and chasing after livestock, are addressed. Much to his credit, Dr. Mugford discourages physical punishment and the use of shock collars.

Dr. Mugford restricts most of his discussion of behavioral problems to milder problems or management-related problems. His advice on aggression is basic and cautious, so that clients are encouraged to seek competent help.

C *Do Cats Need Shrinks? Cat Behavior Explained*, by Peter Neville. Chicago, 1990, Contemporary Books.

This book describes normal cat behavior and how problems develop as a consequence of innate feline behaviors. Problems discussed include aggression, bonding problems, and nervousness; management-related problems include scratching, spraying, and marking. The discussion of these problems will appeal to average clients because it is done in a question-and-answer format: clients write letters and he answers them. The only problem is that sometimes the advice is so specific that it will be difficult for clients not to become their own veterinarians. Clients should be encouraged to understand that the real advantage of going to a behavioral specialist or to a veterinarian who is interested in behavior is that the behaviors that the cat is displaying can be used to understand the problem—the professional's role is, in part, interpretation. Dr. Neville apparently acknowledges this potential problem because the book has an excellent appendix that lists veterinarians who work seriously with animal behavior problems. Dr. Neville suggests throughout the book that clients seek help from their veterinarian if the pet is displaying any of the problems discussed.

C *Dog Law*, 2nd edition, by Mary Randolph. Berkeley, 1994, Nolo Press.

This recent update of Mary Randolph's *Dog Law* book addresses all questions clients commonly ask about the law and their dogs. These topics include buying a dog (Ms. Randolph does *not* sanction buying a pet in a pet store), landlord issues, traveling with dogs (great references that will help with safe pet travel), assistance dogs, providing for pets in your will, and aggressive and dangerous dogs. Her very reasoned approach to the pit bull issue should be lauded. This book is published by Nolo Press, which specializes in self-help legal books. The Press emphasizes that reading a book should help readers get competent legal advice, not substitute for it. To aid in this, Ms. Randolph has a chapter on how to learn about legal issues and interpret legal writings, and the Press offers a 25% refund if earlier editions of this book are returned.

C *How to Raise a Puppy You Can Live With*, 2nd edition, by Clarice Rutherford and David H. Neal. Loveland, Colorado, 1992, Alpine Publications.

This small book covers all of the periods of a puppy's development and explains what the puppy undergoes at the breeder and what it undergoes when it is placed in a new home. The authors make the point that the *breeders* should start exposing dogs to new environments and to mild stresses. The authors should be commended for this.

Good pictures and line drawings demonstrate basic training commands including "sit," "stay," "come," and "stand." The only problems with this book are that it uncritically accepts the terminology regarding packs. The authors recommend scruff shakes as discipline in this context, which is problematic.

The authors describe how to appropriately crate-train a dog and how to housebreak a dog. There is a short chapter on behavioral problems that really should be entitled, "Management Problems." The book emphasizes the extent to which clients are responsible for shaping and developing behaviors that they find acceptable. This point is illustrated in the short contract for clients contemplating getting a puppy that precedes the text of the book.

C *The Tellington Touch,* by Linda Tellington-Jones with Sybil Taylor. New York, 1992, Viking Penguin.

Some readers will have problems with the concepts espoused by this book; in truth, there are few studies that investigate any of them. Regardless, the text includes fine instructions on massage. For clients who need to learn to reward calm behaviors in their pet, this book could help. It is actually better, more refined, and less commercial than the video.

B *Dog Problems: The Gentle Modern Cure,* by David Weston and Ruth Ross. New York, 1992, Howell Book House.
Dog Training: The Gentle Modern Method, by David Weston. New York, 1990, Howell Book House.

These are great books. The authors have done a superb job of explaining why the kindest approaches work best, and they use food rewards! One of my favorite pictures is found in the first (1990) book: a child is holding a cookie to reward his impeccably behaved pet—that is twice his size. Any client who has problems with the concept of food rewards should read the authors' explanations of operant conditioning and dog learning found in Chapter 7 of the 1992 book.

Most of the problems in the 1992 book are management related or involve a preventive focus. Weston and Ross have adapted behavioral groupings to classify problem behaviors into the following behavioral systems: (1) investigatory, (2) ingestive, (3) eliminative, (4) care seeking, (5) shelter seeking, (6) agonistic, (7) group, (8) sexual, and (9) caregiving.

Weston and Ross cleverly color-code these systems and flag problem behaviors by a system using that color code. Superimposed on this is a system of symbols that tells whether the behavior is a *normal* behavior (e.g., a dog barking in response to other dogs barking) or a modified behavior (e.g., domestic dogs bark more readily than do their canid progenitors). The symbol and color code key is reprinted on all pages addressing problems. This is invaluable in helping clients structure their approach to the problem and for helping them to understand the factors that contribute to problems.

These books are not faultless. They use some unfortunate terminologies and do not emphasize that some behaviors (stereotypic behaviors, profound aggressions) are best dealt with by a specialist. However, they are so good in other respects that they would be the first books I would recommend to clients who want to improve their pet's behavior. They are beautifully illustrated with photos of the canine and human members of the Kintala Club in Australia. They are wonderfully suitable for clients who want manageable pets and those whose dogs compete in obedience.

For Veterinarians Interested in Animal Behavior

The following list of books is best suited for veterinarians with more than a passing interest in animal behavior. It is the list of recommended reading compiled in 1994 by the American College of Veterinary Behavior.

Alcock J: *Animal Behavior: An Evolutionary Approach,* 5th ed, 1993, Sinauer Associates.
Anderson RK, Hart BL, Hart LA: *The Pet Connection,* Center to Study Human-Animal Relationships and Environments, Minneapolis, 1984, University of Minnesota.
Archer J: *The Behavioral Biology of Aggression,* 1988, Cambridge University Press.
Arkow P: *Dynamic Relationships in Practice: Animals in the Helping Professions,* Alameda, Calif, 1984, Latham Foundations.
Arnold GW, Dudzinski M: *Ethology of Free-Ranging Domestic Animals,* 1979, Elsevier Scientific Publishing.
Beaver BV: *Feline Behavior,* 1992, WB Saunders.
Berger J: *Wild Horses of Great Britain,* 1986, University of Chicago Press.
Bradshaw WS: *The Behavior of the Domestic Cat,* 1992, CAB International.
Craig JV: *Domestic Animal Behavior: Causes and Implications for Animal Care and Management,* 1981, Prentice-Hall.
Drickamer LC, Vessey SH: *Animal Behavior: Mechanisms, Ecology, and Evolution,* 1992, William C. Brown.
Eibl-Eibesfeldt I: *Ethology: The Biology of Behavior,* 1970, Holt, Rinehart, & Winston.
Eisenberg JF, Kleiman D: *Advances in the Study of Mammalian Behavior,* 1983, American Society of Mammalogists (Gordon L. Kirkland, Jr., Vertebrate Museum, Shippensburg State College, Shippensburg, PA 17257).
Fox MF: *The Dog: Its Domestication and Behavior,* 1978, Garland STPM Press.
Frasier AF, Bloom DM: *Farm Animal Behaviour and Welfare,* 1990, Baillière Tindal.
Fuller JL, Simmel EC: *Behavior Genetics: Principles and Applications,* 1983, Lawrence Erlbaum Associates.
Geist V, Walther F: *The Behavior of Ungulates and Its Relation to Management,* 1974, International Union for Conservation of Nature and Natural Resources.
Goy RW, McEwen B: *Sexual Differentiation of the Brain,* 1980, MIT Press.
Hafez ESE: *The Behavior of Domestic Animals,* 1975, Williams & Wilkins.
Hart BL: *The Behavior of Domestic Animals,* 1985, WH Freeman.
Hart BL, Hart LA: *Canine and Feline Behavioral Therapy,* 1985, Lea & Febiger.
Hinde RA: *Non-Verbal Communication,* 1972, Cambridge University Press.
Houpt KK: *Animal Behavior for Veterinarians and Animal Scientists,* 1991, Iowa State University Press.
Katcher A, Beck A, eds: *New Perspectives on Our Lives with Companion Animals,* 1983, University of Pennsylvania Press.
Kilgour R, Dalton C: *Livestock Behaviour,* 1984, Westview Press.
Lehner PN: *Handbook of Ethological Methods,* 1979, Garland STPM Press.
Leyhausen P: *Cat Behavior: The Predatory and Social Behavior of Domestic and Wild Cats,* 1979, Garland STPM Press.
Lynch JJ, Hinch GN, Adams DB: *The Behaviour of Sheep: Biological Principles and Implications for Production,* 1992, CAB International.
Markowitz H: *Behavioral Enrichment in the Zoo,* 1982, Von Nostrand Reinhold.

Martin P, Bateson P: *Measuring Behaviour: An Introductory Guide*, 2nd ed, 1993, Cambridge University Press.

Monaghan P, Wood-Gush D: *Managing the Behaviour of Animals*, 1990, Chapman & Hall.

O'Farrell: *Manual of Canine Behaviour*, 1986, 1991, British Small Animal Veterinary Association.

Scott JP, Fuller JL: *Canine Behavior*, 1965, University of Chicago Press.

Sebeok T: *How Animals Communicate*, 1977, Indiana University Press.

Shair HN, Barr GA, Hofer M: *Developmental Psychobiology*, 1991, Oxford University Press.

Syme GJ, Syme LA: *The Social Structure in Farm Animals*, 1979, Elsevier Scientific Publishing.

Thorne CJ, ed: *The Waltham Book of Dog and Cat Behaviour*, 1992, Pergamon Press.

Turner DC, Bateson P, eds: *The Domestic Cat: The Biology of Its Behaviour*, 1988, Cambridge University Press.

Walther F: *Communication and Expression in Hoofed Mammals*, 1984, Indiana University Press.

Waring GH: *Horse Behavior*, 1983, Noyes Publications.

Wilson O: *Sociobiology: The New Synthesis*, 1975, Belknap Press.

Appendix E

MEDICAL CONDITIONS TO EXCLUDE BEFORE MAKING
A BEHAVIORAL DIAGNOSIS

••

Considerations About the Medical/Organic Underpinnings of Behavioral Problems

Behavior is the integrator between the internal and external environments. Clients often bring their pets to veterinarians because they believe that their pets are ill. That belief is often based on nothing more specific than the pet has changed the way it is acting. Not all alterations in behaviors are manifest as true behavioral disorders, and not all undesirable or annoying behaviors are truly "abnormal." There are truly abnormal behaviors, and a large part of this text focuses on them. Implicit in the intellectual construct of "abnormal" is that the behavioral presentation—or the phenotype—is driven by some underlying anomaly at the anatomical/neuroanatomical, neurochemical/physiological, receptor, and/or genetic levels. When this distinction is finally widely accepted, truly abnormal behaviors will be viewed as are metabolic disorders—as another form of an "organic" condition. When that is done, we will learn a lot more about, for example, the underlying neurochemistry of anxiety. We will also then be able to more clearly understand the relative impact of the environment on abnormal vs. undesirable behaviors. The field of behavioral medicine has not yet advanced to that stage, but it will come.

Congenital, inherited and genetic, infectious, inflammatory or immune-mediated, metabolic and hormonal, nutritional degenerative, neoplastic, toxic, and traumatic causes of changes in behavior or undesirable behaviors have all been noted. Known medical conditions with a neurologic or behavioral effect include epilepsy, narcolepsy, hydrocephalus, polyphagia, and some forms of stereotypic behaviors. This appendix outlines the *common* medical or organic conditions that may be confused with a behavioral diagnosis. These are the conditions that represent the diagnostic rule outs that should precede treatment. Unfortunately, there are few hard data that support the extent to which any underlying pathophysiological mechanism or cause is involved in any behavioral condition; however, it is just as foolish to assume that every behavioral complaint is purely "behavioral" as it is to assume that none are. There is no substitute for paying attention to the pattern of the pet's behavior. This will help suggest where diagnostic emphasis should be placed. Purely "behavioral" conditions seldom appear quickly, and the early, more subtle signs are often missed by the client and veterinarian alike.

Conditions Involving the Urogenital Systems

The pathophysiology of inappropriate elimination can involve inflammatory, neurogenic, and metabolic changes (Burrows et al., 1995; Leib and Matz, 1995; Lulich and Osborne, 1995; Lulich et al., 1995; Osborne et al., 1995). Common inflammatory conditions associated with complaints involving elimination include cystitis, urethritis, prostatitis, vaginitis, enteritis, and colitis.

Coordination of elimination involves the brainstem micturition center in the pons, spinal tracts, and local innervation of the urethra and detrusor. *Voluntary control* occurs at higher centers: the cerebrum, the basal ganglia, the thalamus, and the cerebellum. These centers exert control over the brainstem and affect voluntary relaxation of the external urethral sphincter and perineal muscles via the pudendal nerve. The role of higher centers is often overlooked, but dogs with lissencephaly (congenital lack of formation/differentiation of the cerebral cortex that has been reported in Fox Terriers, Irish Setters, and Lhasa Apsos) can be impossible to housebreak. These dogs have normal electroencephalograms (EEGs) and may show signs of aggression, growling, confusion, and hyperactivity. They have problems with housebreaking because they have no elimination inhibition—a voluntary condition. "Loss of housebreaking" in the absence of any other peripheral neurological or physiological sign in an animal that the behavioral history reveals was otherwise perfectly housebroken has been reported to herald a central brain lesion, usually in the cerebrum.

Urination. Neurogenic causes are less commonly reported but are broadly divided into two categories: upper motor neuron (UMN) disruption and lower motor neuron (LMN) disruption. UMN disruption disease is that resulting from lesions between the pons and the sacral cord. UMN disruption disease associated with the pons and the cerebellum should also be associated with brain signs. UMN disruption signs include those of reflex dyssynergia—a reflex bladder that automatically empties when it is full or at some pressure. The bladder has tone, but the animal is unable to act on that tone. UMN disruption signs are associated with large amounts of infrequently produced urine. Animals with UMN disruption have difficulty expressing urine from their bladders because of the increased urethral tone (Chrisman, 1982; Oliver and Lorenz, 1983). Bladders in which it is difficult to express urine can also be found in animals with conditions involving mechanical obstruction, urethral stricture, calculi or plugs, urethral spasm associated with urethritis, and bladder, prostatic, or urethral inflammation or neoplasia.

LMN disruption disease affects the sacral cord (S_1 to S_3 or L_4 to S_3), nerve roots, and pudendal and pelvic nerves. Signs of LMN disruption are associated with the storage phase of dysuria and include those associated with bladder atony (flaccid, neuropathic bladders), large urinary volumes, and overflow. Signs of LMN disruption are more frequently associated with dribbling of urine. These are nonreflex, or autonomous, bladders. Lesions disrupting the LMN of the reflex arc result in varying degrees of incontinence, depending on the extent to which the sphincter is competent. If the sphincter is competent, incontinence is partial. If the sphincter is minimal, any pressure causes leakage or dribbling. It is easy to express the bladder of an LMN-disrupted animal. Animals with LMN disruption disease may also have fecal obstructions, hind limb or tail deficits, loss of anal or bulbocavernosus reflexes, and loss of dermatosome sensation. Congenital lesions resulting in signs of LMN disruption have been reported in Manx cats and Bulldogs. Caution is urged in interpreting *any* elimination disorder associated with these breeds as purely behavioral. Any animal that has experienced trauma, neoplasia, degenerative processes, or repeated inflammation may be more at risk for LMN disruption disease.

Hypotonic bladders and those associated with reflex dyssynergia are often treated with the adrenergic antagonist phenoxybenzamine to maintain relaxation. Other agents that have noradrenergic or norepinephrinergic effects like tricyclic antidepressants and phenylpropanolamine have also been used to treat hypotonicity. Diazepam has been used to concomitantly decrease skeletal muscle reflexes.

Nonneurogenic causes of incontinence have been attributed to an ectopic ureter (more common in young females) or other functional abnormalities. Urinary incontinence (*sensu* Barsanti and Downey, 1984) is associated with the signs of polyuria, dysuria, pollakiuria (increased frequency of urination with normal or abnormal volume), and hematuria (feline urological syndrome [FUS]/feline lower urinary tract disease [FLUTD]). FLUTD has been associated with the presence of infectious conditions like viruses (e.g., cell-associated herpes virus [CAHV], syntia-forming virus [SFV], and feline calicivirus [FCV]). It is difficult to know if such associations are primary or secondary and opportunistic. FLUTD has also been associated with anatomical anomalies like vesicourachal diverticula (Osborne et al., 1995). Again, it is difficult to know if these are primary or secondary. Congenital or primary diverticula appear to be remnants of the urachus that are found in the vertex of the bladder. They appear to be a risk factor for macroscopic diverticula that may then tear or expand when exposed to pressure (i.e., urinary retention associated with painful urination). However, 25% of cats with hematuria, dysuria, and urethral obstruction also have such diverticula. They are more common in males than in females, and the mean age of the patient in which they are reported is 3.7 years. These findings are interesting because the age range overlaps with that of social maturity in cats, and male cats are more frequently represented in the urine-spraying population. Quantitative associations between these groups are largely unexplored.

Urinary incontinence with dysuria associated with the voiding phase and an abnormal urinalysis is more often caused by urethral spasm (neoplasia or infection). That associated with a normal urinalysis is more likely to be caused by a functional disorder of the bladder, should catheterization be accomplished without difficulty. Difficult catheterization may act as a flag for intraluminal (urolithiasis, polyps, blood clots, sloughed tissue) or extraluminal (tumor, prostatic disease, stricture, hernia) mechanical obstructions.

Urinary incontinence without dysuria that is associated with a normal neurological examination *and* with voluntary contraction is often a result of metabolic disease. This has been reported to be behavioral; however, the term *incontinence* is a misnomer in such situations. It is important to rule out metabolic disease when considering complaints involving inappropriate urination. The key here is to learn if the animal is truly polyuric/polydipsic (PU/PD). Animals that are truly PU/PD have decreased plasma osmolality and decreased urine-specific gravities (USGs) that deviate from the accepted range of up to 1.080 for dogs and cats. Isosthenuria occurs at a USG of 1.007 to 1.015 (U_{Osm} = 300 mOsm/kg) and true hyposthenuria occurs at a USG of <1.007 (U_{Osm} < 300 mOsm/kg) (DiBartola, 1995). Differential diagnoses for true PU/PD include diabetes mellitus, renal glucosuria, central diabetic insufficiency, nephrogenic diabetic insufficiency, renal insufficiency or failure, pyelonephritis, pyometra, hypercalcemia, hypokalemia, hyperadrenocorticism, hyperthyroidism, hypoadrenocorticism, hepatic insufficiency or portosystemic shunting, renal medullary washout, and primary polydipsia. Again, these conditions are unlikely to cause a purely behavioral disorder, but they can certainly be associated with one. It is extremely easy to understand that an animal with any of the previously mentioned conditions could develop a secondary preference for urination in what the owner would consider an undesirable area.

It is also important to note that polyuria, polydipsia, polyphagia, pica, and aphagia have also been associated with hypothalamic lesions.

Defecation. The pelvic nerve stimulates contraction of the smooth muscle of the descending colon and the rectum. The pudendal nerve stimulates *dis*inhibition of the sphincter tone, resulting in relaxation of the sphincter. The combined relaxation of the sphincter and the contraction of the rectum and colon result in fecal expression. Lesions that affect the cords S_1 to S_3, nerve roots, or pudendal or pelvic nerves result in no reflex—the sphincter remains dilated (dysautonomia).

In situations in which the neurological examination is nonremarkable and there are no central brain signs, failure to housebreak should be considered as a potential diagnosis. The age of the pet is also important because changes can occur with age that are neither primarily behavioral nor primarily neurological, but rather, associated with geriatric physiology. Finally, animals with irritable bowel syndrome may have other anxieties, and may be, otherwise, physically and neurologically nonremarkable. Documenting other behaviors that are associated with anxiety can lend credibility to a diagnosis of irritable bowel syndrome.

Hepatic Disease

Hepatic disease (liver dysfunction) has been associated with behavioral complaints that include pacing, spontaneous aggression, "hysteria," cortical blindness (hepatoencephalopathy [HE]), polyphagia/pica, intermittent deafness, and depression. The mechanism for depression has been postulated to be increased γ-aminobutyric acid (GABA) resorption from the gastrointestinal tract that can occur with liver failure (Maddison, 1992).

Cortical blindness and aggression (which may actually be caused by changes in perception, fear, and incoordination) have been associated with HE (Fenner, 1995). HE is caused by increased central brain ammonia (NH_3) concentrations that result from decreased hepatic catabolic properties associated with urea cycle deficits: animals are unable to appropriately metabolize the proteins in their foods, resulting in increased production and resorption of ammonia. Ammonia is detoxified in the brain—a process that decreases glutamate (the central excitatory amino acid [EAA] that acts as a neurotransmitter). This depletion results in depression and stupor. HE occurs in parenchymal liver disease (cirrhosis, acquired portosystemic shunts, toxicity, and neoplasia), congenital portosystemic shunts, and congenital urea cycle enzyme defects. Congenital portosystemic shunts and congenital urea cycle enzyme defects occur *only* in young animals, thus any animal with apparent *atypical* aggression (that which is both out-of-context and does not fit any of the patterns elucidated for known behavioral conditions) should be considered a candidate for HE.

Minimal work-ups should include complete behavioral histories, complete blood cell count, and serum biochemistry profiles. Serum bile acids, metabolic screens, blood ammonia concentrations, and ammonia tolerance tests are also useful. Ammonia has a high specificity and low sensitivity for liver disease; therefore if it is not elevated, the patient may still have liver disease. Particular caution is urged in the handling of samples in a manner that reduces artifactual results: red blood cells contain 2 to 3 times the ammonia found in plasma, thus all samples should be carefully separated in a timely manner. Ammonia tolerance tests are useful for diagnosing hepatic insufficiency and portosystemic shunts (concentrations remain elevated), but bile acid tolerance tests may be superior. Should these all be nonremarkable, the behavioral history should be reconsidered.

Liver enzyme anomalies, alone, are not sufficient either to diagnosis hepatic disease or to rule out behavioral conditions. Anticonvulsants increase alkaline phosphatase (ALP), aspartate aminotransferase (AST/SGOT), and γ-glutamyl transferase (GGT) and may affect alanine aminotransferase (glutamic pyruvic transaminase [SGPT]). Cats with hyperthyroidism have increased serum transaminases and increased ALP (Center, 1995).

ALP has a high sensitivity and low specificity for liver disease in dogs and relatively higher specificities and lower sensitivities for liver disease in cats. It is, however, affected by drug exposure and, in particular, by exposure to corticosteroids, anticonvulsants, and tricyclic antidepressants. The latter increases are not generally large in the absence of clinical signs, but they do occur.

AST is a microsomally induced enzyme in dogs that is found in the cytosol and associated mitochondrial membrane. It is a relatively sensitive, low-level indicator of hepatobiliary disease in cats. The use of glucocorticoids to treat dogs causes a mild increase is AST that resolves over a few weeks.

Alanine aminotransferase is relatively liver specific in dogs and cats and usually increases because of hepatocellular injury or increased membrane permeability. The magnitude of the increase correlates with the number of cells involved. Anticonvulsant medications can produce profound increases in ALT.

GGT is important for amino acid membrane transport, foreign compound detoxification, and glutathione metabolism. It has been implicated as a flag for hepatotoxicity and necrosis associated with atypical diazepam toxicity in cats (Center et al., 1996).

Inducers of mixed function oxidases (those found in the cytochrome p-450 system) include glucocorticoids and anticonvulsants, including carbamazepine. Accordingly, more drug may be needed with time to achieve a stable effect. Inhibitors of these endoplasmic reticular systems include phenothiazines, some antibiotics, and tricyclic antidepressants. Accordingly, less drug may be needed with time to achieve a stable effect.

Central Nervous System Disease

The pathophysiology of organic aggression in dogs includes intracranial neoplasia, cerebral hypoxia, seizure activity, neuroendocrine disturbances, and infectious causes, like rabies.

Rabies should be ruled out, particularly for patients in rabies-endemic areas, for any sudden-onset personality change not associated with social maturity (in which case it would be more gradual), changes in the social environment, and changes in the physical environment. Any animal that has a bite wound from another animal whose rabies or vaccination status is unknown or unable to be determined should be considered a potential rabies suspect. The rabies' incubation period, or the time between being bitten and showing signs of the condition, ranges from less than 25 days to greater than 12 months. Up to 13 days can pass before an animal that is shedding virus may show signs. This last number is the one that drives the 10- to 14-day quarantine periods recommended for most animals involved in bites as the biter.

Aggression in cats is often confused with normal feline behavior with increased motor activity. Hence, some hyperthyroid cats are considered *aggressive*. The most common organic causes of aggression in cats include infectious disease like rabies and toxoplasmosis, intracranial lesions, including neoplasia (meningiomas), and feline ischemic syndrome (Young, 1988). If any of these agents is found diffusely in the limbic system, it is problematic and can manifest as aggression.

Cerebral function is associated with learning, integration of the senses, and motor activity. Deficits in cerebral function can alter behavior through changes in perception and ability to act. The area of the brain that received more attention regarding specific behavioral changes is the limbic system, broadly composed of the amygdala, the cingulate gyri, the hippocampus, the hypothalamus, the septal nuclei, and the thalamus and reticulating activating system (RAS). The amygdala has been associated with some aggressive behavior, primarily that which is induced by fear. The cingulate gyrus has been associated with a lack of aggression and with the functional organization of some behaviors. Broad, contextual behaviors (e.g., personality, memory, attention) are thought to be controlled in the hippocampus. The hypothalamus, in addition to being responsible for most metabolic function and associated behaviors (eating, satiety), has been associated with rage, anger, fear, and some outburst forms of aggression. The septal nuclei are thought to be key for the integration and modulation of sensory stimuli and appear to act to suppress aggression that is affected by the amygdala and the hypothalamus. Most of the drugs used in behavioral therapy affect neurochemicals that originate in loci in the septal nuclei.

These are broad associations between neuroanatomical location and the suites of behaviors. Lesions in the frontal lobe and internal capsule are associated with loss of recognition, dementia, and the inability to learn. Compulsive pacing and circling are associated with lesions in the frontal lobe, internal capsule, and basal nuclei (particularly the caudate nucleus). Polyphagia, polydipsia, pica, and aphagia are associated with thalamic lesions. Thalamic lesions and those in subthalamic areas, the midbrain, and the frontal lobe have all been associated with sleepiness and coma.

Aggression, passivity, irritability, and hypersexuality have all been associated with lesions in the temporal lobe, limbic system, and hypothalamus. The neurochemical control of aggression has been most thoroughly investigated using rat and cat models.

The cat model utilizes the concept of (a) predatory attack involving stalking and silence and (b) affective defensive reactions that involve extensive autonomic response such as dilated pupils, piloerection, hissing, salivation, arching of the back, and circling. The model for these aggressions explored the relative roles of the ventromedial hypothalamus (VMH) and the lateral hypothalamus in aggressive behavior in the manner portrayed in the accompanying schematic.

	Ventromedial hypothalamus	Lateral hypothalamus
Stimulation	Affective defense	Predatory attack
Lesion	Increase aggression 2 weeks postlesion	Decrease or abolish aggression

Accordingly, the VMH inhibits aggression that is normally expressed by activation of the lateral hypothalamus. This work has been the basis for much of the development of neuroanatomical theories of aggression, but it should be remembered that these studies examined "normal" aggression and its role for consumption. Examination of the same experimental manipulations on eating produces the following schematic.

	Ventromedial hypothalamus	Lateral hypothalamus
Stimulation	Stop eating/decrease intake	Induce eating
Lesion	Hyperphagia	Hypophagia

These results dovetail nicely with those found for predatory and affective defensive reactions, but the overall portrait of *abnormal* aggression is likely to not be restricted to these two regions of the hypothalamus. Regardless, lesions of the hypothalamus may become apparent because of their resulting behavioral changes.

Modulation of aggression has been thought to occur in the temporal lobe region and the amygdala (Sarter and Markowitsch, 1985). Stimulation of this region results in a decrement in the amount of stimulation needed in the hypothalamus to induce an aggressive response. Experimental lesions of the amygdala abolish aggression. The medial amygdaloid nucleus (Ame) is primarily involved in social behavior, including in-context intraspecific aggression. The Ame is also rich in testosterone binding sites (Roselli et al., 1989). There is a functional interaction between testosterone and vasopressin in the regulation of social behavior, particularly offensive behavior (De Vries et al., 1983), and sexual differentiation in vasopressinergic innervation of the lateral septum is dependent on perinatal testosterone. This suggests a mechanism for the androgenization effect that has been postulated to be associated with aggression in some young females (O'Farrell and Peachey, 1991; vom Saal, 1981, 1989). Accordingly, it is fair to make the broad generalization that cortical limbic structures modulate aggression through tha-

lamic pathways. Any lesions in any of these global regions may result in a behavioral change. It is well established that pressure exerted on the hypothalamus by a pituitary tumor can cause a gradual increase in irritability or aggression. It is also thought that temporal lobe or psychomotor epilepsy may be associated either with preictal or postictal aggression (Holiday et al., 1970).

Unlike circling, (a relatively nonspecific sign that may indicate a lesion in the brainstem, cerebellum, or cerebrum), seizures tend to be signs of cerebral anomaly (Fenner, 1995). Causes of seizure disorders are numerous and can include (1) genetic mechanisms, (2) degenerative changes (i.e., storage diseases), (3) developmental anomalies (i.e., hydrocephaly, lissencephaly, porencephaly), (4) infectious conditions (i.e., bacterial, fungal, and viral conditions like distemper, rabies, and feline infectious peritonitis [FIP]), (5) metabolic conditions including hypoglycemia, hypocalcemia, vascular disorders, and hepatic shunts, (6) neoplastic conditions that are either primary or secondary (metastatic), (7) nutritional disorders like thiamine deficiencies, (8) toxic conditions (i.e., parasitemia, heavy metal toxicosis, organophosphate toxicity, strychnine poisoning), and (9) acute or chronic traumatic conditions (Chrisman, 1982; Fenner, 1995; Oliver and Lorenz, 1983). Given this vast array, it is likely that some personality changes that may be aggressive are attributable to some seizure disorders, but these are ones for which the patterns elucidated in the history will *not* fit the behavioral profiles.

Age can be a clue about the underlying cause of the seizure and has been used as *one* criteria that can *help* separate dominance aggression in dogs and status-related aggression in cats from rage or temporal lobe events. It is not an accident that many behavioral conditions in dogs and cats develop at social maturity. The same is true for human psychiatric conditions. Not all underlying causes of seizures occur uniformly through time, and the age at which the behavior changes may be important in diagnosis.

Seizures that begin in dogs and cats that are older than 5 years of age are more commonly attributable to (1) distemper/FIP, (2) steroid-responsive menigoencephalopathy, (3) granulomatous encephalopathy, (4) trauma, (5) toxicity, (6) hypoglycemia (insulinoma), (7) HE-acquired hepatopathy, (8) other metabolic disease, (9) acquired epilepsy, and (10) cerebral neoplasia.

Seizures that occur in dogs and cats that are aged 9 months (sexual maturity) to 5 years are often associated with (1) distemper/FIP encephalopathy, (2) viral, protozoal, or fungal encephalopathies, (3) steroid-responsive meningoencephalitis, (4) granulomatous meningoencephalitis, (5) trauma, (6) toxicity, (7) hypoglycemia, (8) HE-acquired hepatopathy/portocaval shunt, (9) other acquired metabolic disease, (10) acquired epilepsy, and (11) cerebral neoplasia.

Youngsters have a different profile for common underlying causes of seizure disorders: (1) congenital hydrocephalus, (2) lissencephaly, (3) lysosomal storage diseases, (4) distemper/FIP encephalitis, (5) viral, fungal, protozoal, and bacterial encephalitis, (6) trauma, (7) toxicity—primarily lead, (8) hypoglycemia, (9) HE-postsystemic shunt, (10) congenital defects and metabolic disease, and (11) thiamine deficiencies.

The age of the animal and the behavioral profile are important. Aggression associated with congenital hydrocephalus is likely to appear at a young age, to worsen with time (untreated), and to be associated with other signs of the condition including circling, head pressing, and anything from mild to severe cognitive changes. The advent of imaging techniques will help us begin to make finer distinctions about such changes.

Intracranial lesions have occasionally been noted to be causal in behavioral problems (Braund, 1984). Conditions that may be associated with lesions include aggression, apathy, disorientation, and excitability. The location of the lesion will determine the behavioral constellation seen. Primary tumors tend to be chronic and insidious, thus the changes may occur more slowly than is noted with metastatic tumors for which signs appear acutely. The general problems associated with intracranial neoplasia include stupor, coma, and seizure. In one of the few studies to examine the prevalence of behavioral signs with rostral, central neoplasia, Foster et al. (1988) found that of 43 patients, 9 (21%) had behavioral signs and 22 (51%) had seizures, but only 4 (9%) had both. This suggests that some separation on the basis of phenotype is possible and that the underlying mechanism driving the seizure is not the same as the underlying mechanism resulting in the behavioral signs (which were not specified in this study).

Voith (1984) proposed that seizure activity (i.e., psychomotor epilepsy, temporal lobe epilepsy, limbic epilepsy) be the putative diagnosis for aggressive outburst *only* if all of the following conditions are met: (1) the behavior is not species typical (i.e., either learned, a normal component of routine behavior (hunting in cats), or satisfying the criteria for a behavioral diagnosis), (2) EEG changes or other signs are consistently present, (3) the signs are inhibited with antiepileptic drugs, and (4) the signs are induced by epileptogenic drugs. These are rigorous criteria.

Unfortunately, EEGs performed on dogs and cats are difficult to interpret and are largely being abandoned as sole (and even in some cases as adjuvant) diagnostic tools in human neurology. It is safe to say that neuronal hyperexcitability has been noted in primary brain disease (hydrocephalus, congenital disease, meningoencephalopathy, cerebral injury, cerebral vascular disease, neoplasia), metabolic disease (hepatoencephalopathy, uremic encephalopathy, hypoglycemia, hypocalcemia and other nutritional diseases), and toxicity (e.g., organophosphate toxicity, strychnine poisoning). General changes in electroencephalographic parameters are noted for broad classes of conditions: inflammation produces low voltage, fast activity (LVFA) spiking; neuronal death produces high voltage, slow activity (HVSA) spiking, as do hypocalcemia and hepatoencephalopathy; space-occupying lesions produce intermittent, high amplitude slow waves, +/− high amplitude spikes; hypothyroidism has been associated with low voltage, moderate frequencies; and lead poisoning is associated with slow wave, intermittent high amplitudes. Changes in EEG activity are one more sign, but they do not advance our thinking about underlying cause or mechanism.

The most common types of seizure activity that have been associated with aggression are those that have been categorized as psychomotor and paroxysmal. They appear to be associated with aberrant activity in the limbic system and may be associated with running, hallucinations, furious rage, and atypical aggression. These can be relatively nonspecific signs and are associated with, for example, the changes that occur as a result of blood-brain barrier disruption that occurs in lead toxicosis. For conditions like lead toxicosis, seizuring is seldom the only presenting sign; for example, gastrointestinal upset and diarrhea are common in lead toxicosis.

Space-occupying lesions and vascular defects have also been associated with seizures and aggression, particularly in cats. Cerebral infarct in cats produces sudden neurological and behavioral changes that are often associated with aggression and attack behaviors. Cerebral infarcts, however, should be far less common than social situations that provoke normal but undesirable aggressions and abnormal, anxiety-related behavior. Notice that, in this example, the concurrent presence of other neurological signs is common.

Cranial cerebral trauma (CCT), which can result from fights between animals, may result in mentation and behavioral changes with or without seizure activity. Behavioral changes caused by CCT should be relatively sudden, represent a dramatic change, and follow a known or suspected event.

Sudden behavioral changes are rare with purely behavioral conditions but can be apparent even if the neurological condition is chronic. Van Winkle et al. (1994) report a sudden onset aggression in a 3-year-old male cat that was associated with underlying chronic polioencephalomalacia in the piriform lobes and hippocampus. This cat also exhibited hyperesthesia and seizure activity. It is an intriguing case because the neuroanatomical defect was chronic, but the aggression was sudden. Sudden-onset aggression, unless occurring in response to known, provocative stimuli, is not a common profile for aggression associated with a behavioral diagnosis.

A similar example involving a chronic pathologic condition accompanied by sudden behavioral changes was noted by Genovese et al. (1994). They report a 5-month history of aggression in a 7-year-old female, spayed Border Collie/mixed breed that was accompanied by failure to recognize the owner and circling to the right. Postmortem examination revealed chronic primary demyelination of the cerebral white matter that was believed to be viral in origin. Note that although the aggression was more gradual and intensified with time (a common behavioral profile), the age of onset was not associated with social maturity (common in aggressions associated with a behavioral diagnosis) and there were concomitant neurological signs. What is interesting in both of these cases is that the pathologic condition was thought to be *chronic*. Neurological disease does not have to be instantaneous to have behavioral ramifications.

Narcolepsy

Few animal patients are brought to veterinarians for complaints involving sleep disorders, although this may be one of the associations of cognitive dysfunction (Ruehl et al., 1995). The most obvious behavioral problem associated with sleeping is narcolepsy. Narcolepsy is characterized by cataplexy and is consistent with an EEG that is typical of rapid eye movement (REM) sleep and an electromyelogram (EMG) that indicates lack of muscle tone.

There is a REM sleep behavioral disorder (RBD) that may have an animal model in cats that have pontine/tegmental lesions (Schenck et al., 1993). This clinical disorder is characterized by attempts at dream enactment *(oneirism)* and is hallucinatory in nature. Affected cats also appear to hallucinate, although it could be argued that, at some level, hallucinations are a normal part of the feline behavioral repertoire. Cats that lack medullary inhibition of movement during REM sleep are active and can be perceived as *aggressive*. Both humans and cats with this disorder appear to respond to clonazepam.

Miscellaneous Conditions Associated with Stereotypic Behavior

Obsessive-compulsive, or stereotypic, behaviors are poorly understood, although, based on their heterogeneous response to medications that affect dopamine, norepinephrine, serotonin, and glutamate, it is difficult not to consider them to be *organic*. Some anecdotal observations have been made for these behaviors that attribute them to other infectious or anatomical causes. Fly snapping or biting has been reported to be associated with the presence of a remnant of the hyaloid artery, and cats that are FIV positive have been reported to lick objects and floors (Beaver, 1995). In the absence of hard data, including those that reflect the proportion of those so afflicted that *lack* the behaviors, it is best to consider these as incidental findings.

Fly biting has also been anecdotally reported to be associated with a diet excessively low in protein. The Cavalier King Charles Spaniel reported as affected became worse when exposed to red meats, poultry, and rabbit, suggesting that some degree of food hypersensitivity was involved (Brown, 1987). Regardless, stereotypic behavior of a hallucinatory nature is not commonly reported as a sequela to food hypersensitivity and restricted protein rations, although pica and coprophagia can be associated with severely restricted rations. Other signs of poor physical condition are usually present.

Many obsessive-compulsive behaviors are associated with self-injurious behavior or mutilation. The extent to which central deficits are involved in conditions like acral lick granuloma is unclear. The parietal lobe of the cortex (somaesthetic area) receives impulses from the surface of the body. The extent to which neurophysiological deficits in any step of this long pathway are involved in acral lick granuloma is underexplored. It is conceivable that some animals respond to specific serotonin reuptake inhibitors (SSRIs) because they ultimately affect cortical glutamate.

The more common and more frequently recognized pathologic condition associated with self-mutilation is a mutilating neuropathy. This neuropathy primarily affects sensory neurons. It is characterized by a decrease in the number of cells, degenerative fibers (myelinated and nonmyelinated) in the dorsal roots and the peripheral nerves, and decreased fiber density in the dorsolateral fasciculus of the cord. The deficit appears to be associated with problems with the growth or the differentiation of the sensory neurons. Substance P concentrations are adversely affected (Cunningham et al., 1981, 1983, 1984). Because this mediates nociception or pain, it has been postulated that these animals mutilate because of lack of feedback associated with the sensory stimuli.

Tetany is usually recognizable as such but could conceivably be confused with some stereotypic behaviors in some cases. Common causes of tetany could also cause twitching that resembles stereotypic behavior, thus exposure to toxins, hypocalcemia, hypomagnesemia, and abnormalities of acid base balance should be ruled out.

Withdrawal and depression in dogs and cats are sometimes difficult to recognize and always difficult to define. In any case, medical causes of generalized weakness and the associated depression should always be thoroughly explored. The most common of these include diabetes mellitus, hyperkalemia (especially that associated with neuropathies and lower motor neuron disease), hypothyroidism, and hyperadrenalcorticism.

Hormonal Conditions

Any hormonal condition can affect behavior, and hypothalamus-pituitary-adrenal (HPA) axis effects are bound to be complex. Alterations in this axis have been associated with clinical manifestations of fear and panic in humans. High levels of adrenocorticotropic hormone (ACTH) have been associated with increased aggression and low levels have been associated with decreased aggression (Kiley-Worthington, 1977). Again, it is unclear if this effect is not just a result of changes in overall activity.

Prolactin is the hormone associated with pseudocyesis, and it produces the same changes in this condition that is seen in normal pregnancy and lactation. Treatment involves inhibiting prolactin. Drugs that increase dopamine (i.e., bromocriptine) have this effect. So does ovariohysterectomy, although it should be performed in anestrus (Allen, 1986).

The hormone that has received the most attention for its potential complicity in behavioral conditions is thyroid hormone. Hyperthyroid cats are often frenzied. The postulated increase in their aggression is unlikely to be a specific proaggressive effect; it is more likely to be a correlate of the overall increased activity and metabolic rate. Hypothyroidism is far more controversial.

Hypothyroidism has been postulated to be associated with fear or aggression in dogs and with sudden shifts in these behaviors (Orwen, 1995). The canine prevalence of hypothyroidism is thought to be approximately 0.2%; the incidence of behavioral problems is considerably greater.

In humans, an association between thyroid dysfunction and depression has been suggested but is difficult to prove (Hatterer et al., 1993). There is decreased thyroid activity in depression that includes an exaggerated thyroid stimulation response to exogenous thyrotropin-releasing hormone (TRH) in approximately 10% of depressed human patients (Gold et al., 1988; Nemeroff et al., 1985). Thyrotropin response to TRH may be reduced in up to one third of depressed human subjects (Loosen and Prange, 1982). These patients appear to be nonresponders to traditional antidepressant medication but can be *converted* to responders with the addition of thyroxine. This effect has not been noted for the 90% of the human population demonstrating a normal TRH response. The extent to which transthyretin abnormalities are involved in this response is unknown, but cerebrospinal fluid levels of transthyretin were significantly lower than for neurologic controls in a small sample of patients with major depression that were refractory to treatment with antidepressants. Transthyretin is the protein associated with thyroid hormone transport, and it could be low in nonresponder-depressed patients with normal peripheral T_3-T_4 concentrations (Hatterer et al., 1993). The fact that this is an apparent transport protein defect suggests that the association with neurotransmitters associated with depression may be both direct and indirect.

That said, there is currently no good rationale for supplementation with exogenous thyroxin in the absence of specific behavioral clinical signs *and* aberrant levels or response of transthyretin in pets with behavioral problems. Such cavalier dispensation of potent medication is particularly problematic given the wide range of breed-specific reference ranges for T_3, T_4, free T_3, and free T_4 (Chastain and Panciera, 1995; Ferguson, 1992). Although still widely regarded as the most sensitive assay of canine thyroid function, the thyroid stimulating hormone (TSH) test is becoming increasingly hard to perform clinically because of the restricted availability of the hormone. Resting free T_4 levels, if grossly low, may provide a rough gauge to thyroid function because free T_4 is less likely than total T_4 to be affected by nonthyroidal illness or by drug therapy (Peterson and Ferguson, 1989). It is most accurately measured using dialysis methods; low free T_4 concentration by this method is consistent with a diagnosis of hypothyroidism (Nelson et al., 1991). Treatment with thyroid hormone is *not* benign and can cause clinical signs of toxicity (Overall, unpublished, 1996). In the absence of clinical signs of hypothyroidism (obesity, seborrhea, alopecia, weakness, lethargy, bradycardia, pyoderma) *and* low (*not* low-normal) free T_4 (or the equivalent TSH test result), there is no rational or competent reason to treat dogs with behavioral or any other diagnoses with thyroxin (Panciera, 1994). There may be a small population of dogs for which they might prove to not be true in the future, but they will be rare. These dogs, if they exist, may have anxiety conditions that are affected by cholecystokinin (CCK). In male rats, CCK-A (alimentary) receptor stimulation inhibits TSH secretion at the level of the anterior pituitary (Männistö et al., 1992).

This is not to say that dogs with thyroid disorders do not alter their behavior—they do, but the behavioral changes are nonspecific and should not be confused with a behavioral diagnosis. There may be nonresponders to antidepressant and antianxiety medication in the canine population that are analogous to those in the human population. If so, supplementation with thyroxin in addition to the antidepressant and/or antianxiety medications may help. However, most single-cause hypotheses (i.e., thyroid) for the underlying cause and treatment of complex behavioral phenomena like aggression and fear are simplistic and invariably wrong. In this case, supplementation is not benign and should not be executed in the absence of a diagnosis. Although the issue of hormonal interaction in behavioral conditions is a complex one, supplementation with thyroxin is largely a popular movement for which there are no rigorous data. Collection of these data would doubtless be enlightening.

Appendix F

TERMINOLOGY: NECESSARY AND SUFFICIENT CONDITIONS FOR BEHAVIORAL DIAGNOSES

The list in this Appendix follows the terminology cited in the Preface. The specific conditions have been discussed in the text; the original citations can be found there. The parenthetical codes are the codes used at VHUP in Medical Information and were developed by Ken Mullin, director of medical information. These codes represent an attempt to conform to the same classification system used in human medicine and were first used in the 1980s. As more has been learned, classification procedures have improved, and only the codes consistently used for diagnosis are included. Implicit in all diagnostic categories, unless explicitly stated, is that there is no known underlying physical or physiological reason for the behavioral problem and that physical and physiological causes have been ruled out. It is also important to remember that, as listed, these classifications represent diagnoses of problem behaviors and are not simply descriptions of a behavioral event (i.e., dominance aggression can *only* be a diagnosis for an abnormal behavior, but interdog aggression can be both a diagnosis and a description). The diagnoses below are listed alphabetically and are then followed by the necessary and sufficient criteria for making a particular diagnosis. These criteria are open to revision and discussion.

The implementation of "necessary and sufficient" criteria, as the terms are used in logical and mathematical applications, is a refinement over descriptive definitions of terms. The imposition of necessary and sufficient diagnostic criteria acts as a qualitative, and potentially quantitative, method of exclusion. The criteria allow for uniform and unambiguous assessment of aberrant, abnormal, and undesirable behaviors. I have tried to follow the terminology cited earlier in a manner that conforms with terminology from the human psychiatric literature while attempting to avoid psychological jargon.

A *necessary* criterion or condition is one that must be present for the listed diagnosis to be made. A *sufficient* criterion or condition is one that can be used to singularly identify the condition. Sufficiency is an outcome of knowledge—the more that is learned about the genetics, molecular response, neurochemistry, and neuroanatomy of any condition and its behavioral correlates (see Table 1 in the Preface), the more succinctly and accurately a sufficient condition can be defined. Definition of "necessary" and "sufficient" conditions is not synonymous with a compendium of signs associated with the condition. The number of signs present and their intensity may be a gauge for the severity of the condition, or serve as a "flag" when variable, nonoverlapping presentations of the same condition can occur. The diagnostic conditions for dominance aggression listed later in the chapter illustrate this difference.

This approach is similar to that taken by the American Psychiatric Association for the *Diagnostic and Statistical Manual of Mental Disorders* (4th edition) (DSM-IV, 1994). The conditions of interest in veterinary behavioral medicine need not be exact analogs of human conditions for this attempt at classification to be meritorious. The approach provides for a mechanism to collect behavioral data from a variety of populations across time and to compare those data. Comparisons of data predicated on the classification that follows should engender revisions and refinements of the classification. The classification itself is not important; the extent to which it provides a structured, logical, heuristic tool for the development of thought in the field *is* important.

On closer inspection, some of the categories that follow may be found not to exist, some categories currently overlap in our listing (and one of the purposes of such an approach is to create categories that are as discrete as possible), and some categories are not sufficiently fine or discrete and might be better if split. For most diagnoses the extent to which the condition is exhibited is not factored into the necessary and sufficient criteria in any quantitative manner. This is important because the intensity of a behavior, or the extent to which it occurs, could be the key issue in deciding when the behavior is a variant of "normal" or is a disorder. Notes have been added in troublesome areas.

A numerical listing of only the diagnostic codes and diagnoses follows the alphabetical listing.

Abnormal Ingestive Behavior Due to Psychological Disturbance (0000YX06.0)

Necessary: Consistently exhibited ingestion of abnormal amounts or types of food or nonfood material in a manner or frequency not consistent with previous behavior.

Sufficient: Incessant consumption of food or nonfood material, or incessant avoidance of food, in a manner that interferes with normal social functioning.

Concerns: This category is not sufficiently explicit and could include pica (see later discussion), polyphagia (00805510.X), aerophagia (see 0000X300.0), psychogenic water drinking (0000YX06.1), anorexia, and gorging. With the exceptions of pica and aerophagia, which truly differ from ingestion or lack of ingestion involving food, it is difficult, although not impossible, to rule out all physiological causal associations. It is logical that abnormal ingestion of food and abnormal ingestion of water should be separately classified because they are controlled by different, although overlapping, physiological systems.

Abnormal Maternal Behavior Due to Psychological Disturbance (0000YX08.0);

Necessary and sufficient: Excessive, deficient, or out-of-context, inappropriate behavior resembling any aspect of maternal care.

Concerns: This category is broad and includes maternal neglect, infanticide, cannibalism, excessive care leading to isolation or death of puppies, and pseudocyesis. It is unlikely that these conditions all share a common mechanistic pathway. Division and explicit identification of the more common categories may be more appropriate.

Aerophagia (0000X300.0)

Necessary: Ingestion through swallowing of air in amounts in excess of that required for normal drinking, eating, and breathing/panting.

Sufficient: Mechanically forced, volitional swallowing of air that is uncoupled with eating or drinking; behavior may be sufficiently frequent to interfere with normal activities; if questioned, clients are able to document trade-offs in the pet's time budget that have occurred as a result of the condition.

Concerns: Normal is a weak and often undefined term, but it may suffice here; this may be a subset of obsessive-compulsive disorder (OCD) in its full-blown form.

Aggression Caused by Psychological Disturbance (0000YX01.0)

Necessary and sufficient: Consistently displayed, abnormal, inappropriate, out-of-context threat, contest, or attack that does not meet the criteria for specific aggressions.

Concerns: This category could be the result of a poor history or uncritical diagnoses, or it could include undiagnosed neurological problems (e.g., epilepsy); idiopathic aggression is one subset of this classification.

Attention-seeking Behavior (0000YX05.2)

Necessary: Animal uses vocal or physical behaviors to obtain passive or active attention from people when the people are engaged in passive or active activities not directly involving the animal.

Sufficient: Whenever a person is not directly engaged in passive or active interaction or activity with the animal, the animal uses active or passive behaviors to direct some of the person's attention to itself and will interrupt human activity to do so.

Concerns: This may be an undesirable behavior, but it is common and may be a variant of normal; it is certainly a behavior that people unconsciously reinforce in their pets. In the extreme form the animal *must* solicit the behavior and, if prohibited from doing so, exhibits physical and physiological signs of anxiety. In this latter case the attention-seeking behavior is not only abnormal, but it is also probably a correlate, symptom, or subclass of one of the anxieties.

Aversion for Elimination [No Code Currently Available]

Necessary: Consistent avoidance of locations or substrates formerly used for elimination.

Sufficient: Consistent avoidance of locations or substrates formerly used for elimination accompanied by behaviors that are concurrent with active or passive avoidance or distaste that is amplified if the animal is forced to eliminate in the area or on the substrate that the animal finds aversive.

Concerns: The problems with this diagnosis involve evaluating the extent to which the behavior is a change. *Aversion* is a very specific term. This diagnosis does not involve casual disuse—it involves other behavioral changes associated with stimuli animals do not like. Other elimination disorders can be secondary to this one and may not resolve until this diagnosis is made and addressed.

Barking Due to Psychological Disturbance [0000YX04.0]

Necessary and sufficient: Repetitive vocalization unassociated with or in excess of provocative social stimuli.

Concerns: This diagnosis does not represent basic canine barking; this type of barking is often atonal and may be a manifestation of an anxiety disorder or OCD. Sonographic analysis provides information permitting a discrete and nonoverlapping distinction of this from "normal" barking.

Cognitive Dysfunction (01007890.0)

Necessary: Change in interactive, elimination, or navigational behaviors attendant with aging that are explicitly not related to primary failure of any organ system.

Sufficient: Unclear.

Concerns: This is a potential animal model for the age-dependent cognitive changes that occur in humans. The affiliated behaviors may be associated with Alzheimer's-like senile dementia of the Alzheimer type (SDAT) lesions. It is unclear whether this is associated with age-dependent changes in dopaminergic function, microembolic events, or if it is a form of old-age–onset separation anxiety. The latter could also be a subset of this dysfunction. The main method for evaluating cognitive dysfunction in people is not applicable to domestic pet animals. Refinements of cognitive tests based on learning and navigational skills should provide future enhancements.

Compulsive Licking/Obsessive-Compulsive Disorder—Grooming/Licking (0000YX05.6)

Necessary: Licking in excess of that required for grooming or exploration.

Sufficient: Licking in excess of that required for grooming or exploration that represents a change in the patient's behavior and interferes with other activities or functions (eating, drinking, playing, interacting with people) and cannot be aborted by interruption.

Concerns: The sufficient condition describes the hallmarks of all manifestations of obsessive-compulsive disorder: repetitive, out-of-context behaviors that are not interruptible by conventional stimuli (social or gustatory) for more than a short period, and that consistently interfere with the animal's ability to engage in what were formerly "normal" behaviors, or behaviors that are considered "normal" for that age or species. The condition of compulsive licking has more extreme intense behaviors associated with it than does excessive licking (0000YX000.2), and may be simply a subset of OCD. It is not clear whether the manifestation of OCD (grooming vs. locomotion) is indicative of varying underlying neuroanatomical or neurophysiological modalities. It is also possible that compulsive licking and excessive licking are merely two recognizable points on a blurry continuum.

Coprophagia (0000X610.0)

Necessary and sufficient: Ingestion of feces that is neither accidental nor incidental.

Concerns: Fecal ingestion can be a normal part of maternal behavior and may be a scavenging technique useful in nutrient-poor environments; the latter does *not* describe the average environment for any pet with coprophagia; in extreme cases the animals *must* have feces to ingest and actively engage in seeking out feces and may ingest their own as they are produced. In the latter case the coprophagia could be a component of or indicative of OCD or an anxiety disorder. These two scenarios are very different; that difference is not merely one of degree and is not adequately addressed under one heading.

Depression (No Code Available)

Necessary: Prolonged (>1 or 2 weeks) endogenous or reactive withdrawal from social stimuli, changes in appetite, and changes in sleep/wake cycles that are not incidental and not attributable solely to lethargy.

Sufficient: As above, accompanied by decreased motor activity and actual physical removal from normal social and environmental stimuli in the absence of any underlying neurological or physiological condition.

Concerns: The same criteria that allow human psychiatrists to define depression in people are not available to veterinarians. Many of the signs that would occur in depressed animals are nonspecific and may occur in other abnormal conditions, especially if the animal perceives that it is behaving abnormally.

Destruction Due to Psychological Disturbance (0000YX02.0)

Necessary: Destruction of any object when the destructive behavior is not associated with teething, playing, any medical condition, pica, or separation anxiety.

Sufficient: Destruction that occurs in client's presence and that is unassociated with any social, interactive, gustatory, olfactory, unattainable stimulus.

Concerns: The necessary and sufficient conditions hint that this form of destruction should be rare and may be a subset of OCD. This diagnosis could also be the result of a poor or incomplete history.

Dominance Aggression (0000YX01.1)

Necessary: Abnormal, inappropriate, out-of-context aggression (threat, challenge, or attack) consistently exhibited by dogs toward people under any circumstance involving passive or active control of the dog's behavior or the dog's access to the behavior.

Sufficient: Intensification of any aggressive response from the dog with any passive or active correction or interruption of the dog's behavior or the dog's access to the behavior.

Concerns: This is a very discrete definition of dominance aggression and has the advantage of not coupling the challenge to food (food-related aggression), toys (possessive aggression), or space (territorial aggression). These types of aggression can be correlates of dominance aggression and, when associated with it, may indicate a more severe situation (see Chapter 6 for a discussion of a canine control complex). The key elements are control and access—most of the problems with diagnosing the condition arise from the human's misunderstanding of canine social systems, canine signaling, and canine anxieties associated with endogenous uncertainty about contextually appropriate responses. This diagnosis cannot be made on the basis of a one-time event. Once it begins, the behavior becomes more visible and con-

sistent; however, data on early signs, patterns of change with experience, and changes in intensity are lacking. Note that the necessary and sufficient conditions are very different from the common descriptions of dominance aggression that specify that the dog will often react to being pushed on, to being corrected with a leash, or to being pushed away from a sofa or a person. The number of situations in which the dog reacts inappropriately or the intensity with which the animal reacts does not affect the necessary and sufficient conditions, although these factors may affect the prognosis, the ability to treat the condition, and the risk to people.

Excessive Grooming (0000X000.2)

Necessary: Grooming by means of licking, scratching, or rubbing that is unrelated to hygienic or maintenance needs and that is more frequent or more intensive than has been exhibited in the past under the same conditions.

Sufficient: Grooming unrelated to hygienic or maintenance needs that represents a change in previous behavior but that is interruptible and is not associated with profound changes in either the animal's time budget because of the amount of time that the grooming requires or in social interactions.

Comments: See compulsive licking (0000YX05.6). The same concerns apply.

Excitement Urination (01004X00.5)

Necessary: Urination that occurs only when the dog is engaged in active behavior and is concomitantly demonstrating physical and physiological signs of excitement (rapid motor activity that may occur vertically and horizontally, high-pitched greeting, panting and salivation associated with open-mouthed, relaxed greeting face) rather than fear.

Sufficient: Urination as above that occurs when the animal is not sitting or lying down, or approaching sitting or lying down, and about which the patient may exhibit no signs of awareness.

Concerns: This diagnosis can be difficult to distinguish from submissive urination, incomplete housebreaking, or intense need for micturition. Better inclusive descriptions of the behaviors, rather than the circumstances in which they occur, should obviate this problem.

Failure to Groom (0000X000.4)

Necessary: Change in normal rate of grooming with claws, mouth, or rubbing to an absence of any of these behaviors.

Sufficient: As above without any concomitant behavioral changes indicative of depression (anorexia, social withdrawal, changes in sleep/wake cycles).

Concerns: It is unclear whether this condition is always related to either physiological illness or is a symptom of depression (see previous discussion). Qualification of specific behaviors should help.

Fear Aggression (0000YX01.3)

Necessary: Aggression that consistently occurs concomitant with behavioral and physiological signs of fear as identified by withdrawal, passive, and avoidance behaviors associated with the sympathetic branch of the autonomic nervous system.

Sufficient: As above when the aggression is accompanied by urination or defecation or when the aggression is only active and interactive (rather than comprised of posturing) when the recipient of the aggression has disengaged from the behavior.

Concerns: The actual behaviors associated with fear, fear aggression, and any other aggression that is primarily driven by anxiety are poorly qualified and quantified (see Chapter 6 for discussion on dominance and interdog aggression, for example). In extreme cases the sufficient conditions above are clear; in less clear situations, which could be related to uncertainty on the patient's part, caution is urged in ruling out all other aggressions. The diagnosis that is most consistent and concordant with signs and criteria should be the one assigned to the patient. Note that consistent aggression is not required, although identification of the fearful stimuli permits assessment of the extent to which the behaviors are consistent and pose a predictable risk.

Fearful Behavior/Fear (01004X00.3)

Necessary and sufficient: Behavior that occurs concomitant with behavioral and physiological signs of fear as identified by withdrawal, passive, and avoidance behaviors associated with the sympathetic branch of the autonomic nervous system and in the absence of any aggressive behavior.

Concerns: Fear and anxiety have signs that overlap. Some nonspecific signs such as avoidance, shaking, and trembling can be characteristic of both. The physiological signs probably differ at some very refined level, and the neurochemistry of each is probably very different. Refinements in qualification and quantification of the observable behaviors will hopefully parallel these differences.

Fecal Incontinence Due to Psychological Disturbance (67205500X)

Necessary: Defecation in the absence of underlying physiological or physical conditions, fear, separation anxiety, and any other behavioral conditions that primarily involve elimination.

Sufficient: Unclear.

Concerns: This is another category that is too broad to be useful and uses a word—incontinence—that has a very specific definition. Caution is urged. Concerns should exist for diagnostic categories that rely on absence of other signs or conditions, rather than identification of the presence of specific characteristics or conditions.

Food-related Aggression (0000YX01.7)

Necessary: Consistent aggression that is exhibited in the presence, and only in the presence, of pet food, bones, rawhides, biscuits, blood, or human food, in the absence of torture or starvation.

Sufficient: As above with the aggression occurring *only* in the presence of a range or subset of the items listed.

Concerns: This is a very restrictive and specific diagnosis. The number or range of items involved, while possibly reflecting danger and risk, do not affect the diagnosis. It is possible that aggressions that are stimulated by different classes of food indicate varying neurochemical modalities and that these differences may represent subclasses of this diagnosis. This diagnosis highlights that food is not a possession, but rather something very different than a possession. This difference has been noted in neuroanatomical and neurochemical studies of aggression and is probably real. Certainly, a very good evolutionary case could be made for aggression related to food being potentially important. Although this type of aggression may be associated with dominance aggression (0000YX01.1) (i.e., an animal can have both diagnoses, but if so, the development of food-related aggression usually precedes the development of dominance aggression) it is absolutely, categorically different, on the basis of the necessary and sufficient criteria listed for each diagnosis. Food-related aggression can be a singular diagnosis, unrelated to any dominance aggression. Furthermore, if an event related to dominance aggression *only incidentally* involved food or food was only the vehicle for the aggression *once* and there is no pattern of other food-related responses, *and* the client has been able to take or interfere with the food item at other times, the issue is one of control (i.e., dominance aggression), not food.

Generalized Anxiety (Formerly Generalized Reactivity to Environmental Stress) (01004X00.0)

Necessary: Consistent exhibition of increased autonomic hyperreactivity, increased motor activity, and increased vigilance and scanning that interfere with a normal range of social interaction.

Sufficient: As above in the absolute absence of any provocational stimuli.

Concerns: The danger with this diagnosis is that it is very specific, but could easily and carelessly be made in the absence of critical thought or incomplete history. This should be a diagnosis of last resort, not first, and all of the signs should be concomitantly present under conditions where any of these signs would have subsided in a "normal" or non-symptomatic animal.

House Soiling Due to Psychological Disturbance (0000YX03.0)

Necessary: Elimination that is not related to an underlying physical or physiological condition and that represents a change from the animal's previous behavior.

Sufficient: As above and when there is no question that the animal is housebroken or has consistently exhibited appropriate elimination behaviors in the past.

Concerns: This category is not sufficiently explicit to permit any behavioral patterns to be ascertained or any mechanistic treatments to be implemented. Most behavioral conditions involving elimination are otherwise specified.

Hyperactivity Due to Psychological Disturbance (0000YX05.0)

Necessary: Motor activity in excess of that warranted by the animal's age and stimulation level that occurs in a consistent manner and does not respond to correction, redirection, or restraint.

Sufficient: As above concomitant with sympathetic signs (increased heart rate, increased respiratory rate, vasodilation), even when at rest, in the absence of other signs or significant laboratory data associated with thyroid disease, and the dog responds to treatment with amphetamine or methylphenidate with a paradoxical decrease in motor activity.

Concerns: Most dogs that clients call hyperactive—a diagnosis that does *not* depend on the dog's exercise level compared with his or her needs—are actually overactive, a diagnosis that *does* depend on the dog's exercise level compared with his or her needs. Hyperactivity is a very specific diagnosis for which specific behavioral signs have been poorly elucidated.

Hyperesthesia (22025720.0)

Necessary: Tactile response in excess of that warranted by external stimuli.

Sufficient: Repetitive, uninterruptible tactile response in excess of that warranted by external stimuli or that may occur in the absence of external stimuli and may be accompanied by locomotor activity and vocalization.

Concerns: Most of the diagnoses pertaining to this condition originate in the dermatological literature and are purely descriptive of the behaviors (e.g., twitchy cat syndrome). It is likely that in the extreme case that this is a subset of OCD, but also that there is a considerable range in both normal and abnormal tactile responses. Only by description and quantification of the behaviors can any progress be made in determining the range of normal and when the animal deviates from that.

Idiopathic Aggression (No Code Currently Available; Probably Should Be the Exclusive Listing Under 0000YX01.0)

Necessary and sufficient: Aggression that occurs in an unpredictable, toggle-switch manner in contexts not associated with stimuli noted for any other behavioral aggressive diagnosis and in the absence of any underlying causal physical or physiological condition.

Concerns: This is probably the only legitimate classification for 0000YX01.0. It must be distinguished from any neurological condition. Intensive characterization of attendant behaviors is necessary to rule out the most common condition with which this is confused: undiagnosed or subtle dominance aggression. This is the condition that has been labeled as *rage,* a term that should not be used because of our inability to adequately define the analogous emotional conditions in pets that are experienced and described by humans.

Inappropriate Elimination (0000YX03.4)

Necessary and sufficient: Elimination that is not related to an underlying physical or physiological condition and that represents a change from the animal's previous behavior.

Concerns: This category does not differ from house soiling (0000YX030) and is not sufficiently explicit to permit any behavioral patterns to be ascertained or any mechanistic treatments to be implemented. Most behavioral conditions involving elimination are otherwise specified. This diagnosis could include both abnormal behaviors and those that are normal but undesirable to clients. This category should also probably be abandoned in favor of or replaced by more specific categories that are not currently otherwise coded.

Inappropriate Greeting (0000YX05.4)

Necessary and sufficient: Consistent exhibition of behaviors (e.g., growling) not usually associated with greeting only in greeting circumstances.

Concerns: This may be a specific case of attention-seeking behavior (0000YX05.2). Any of the behaviors that could be involved in inappropriate greeting could also be associated with other conditions; qualitative and quantitative behavioral data are necessary to distinguish this condition—if in fact, it is a valid diagnostic category—from other conditions. Examples of conditions to be distinguished include growling related to territorial and protective aggression or spinning caused by OCD. This diagnostic category does not tend to be indicative of greeting behaviors that occur in situations where they should not, and it is unclear whether this circumstance occurs.

Inappropriate Play Behavior (0000YX05.3)

Necessary: Play behaviors (play-bows, yips, shoulder blocks) that occur in circumstances that are out of context; out-of-context conditions include circumstances in which the behaviors are directed toward inanimate objects, social circumstances in which play is not relevant (challenge), or behaviors that occur in contexts consistent with the solicitation of play but that involve actions that would discourage play (biting, pain).

Sufficient: Unclear.

Concerns: The normal, accepted, or in-context range of social play behaviors are relatively well defined when compared with abnormal, unacceptable, or out-of-context behaviors. Refinements are needed if this is to be a valid category. Those refinements must distinguish this from attention-seeking behavior (0000YX05.2)

Incomplete Housebreaking (No Classification Currently Available; Should Probably Be the Exclusive Diagnosis Under 0000YX03.4; Undiagnosed, Nonspecific House Soiling [0000YX03.3])

Necessary: Consistent and age-inappropriate elimination in undesirable locations or at undesirable times that is not associated with any lack of access or opportunity, other behavioral conditions, or any physical or physiological condition.

Sufficient: As above in an animal for whom this has always been true and for whom the complaint does not involve a change in behavior.

Concerns: The only way to reach this diagnosis is through exhaustive history and explication of actual behaviors. Diagnosis is confirmed by a response and adherence to a rigorous housebreaking paradigm.

Interanimal Aggression (0000YX01.2)
Intercat Aggression
Interdog Aggression

Necessary: Consistent, volitional, proactive aggression that is not contextual given the social signals, threat circumstances, or response received.

Sufficient: As above in the absence of any signal or interaction from the animal that is attacked.

Concerns: It is important to emphasize that, at some level, the behaviors involved with aggression are normal behaviors. This diagnostic category, although usually associated with changes in social hierarchy that are often related to the development of social maturity in one of the involved parties, does not depend on either hierarchy or social maturity: it depends on the contextual response. This is a subtle but important distinction that supports the contention that social shifts and occasional threats can be normal. A change in behavior is not necessary, although it may be usual, because if this is truly a diagnosis of an abnormal behavior some animals respond with aggression regardless of circumstances.

Location Preference for Elimination (No Code Currently Available; Suggested 0000YX03.5)

Necessary and sufficient: Consistent elimination in an area or a few areas that are restricted to one location and are not linked by some common sensory aspect.

Concerns: It is important to note that this is the normal condition for well-housebroken dogs or cats that use their litter boxes consistently; however, in those situations the location they prefer is also one that is acceptable to the clients. This becomes a diagnosis only when there is a client-pet preference mismatch. For examples of extremely restrictive preferences there may be other anxiety-related problems.

Marking Behavior (0000YX03.1)

Necessary: Urination or defecation that occurs in frequencies and locations, or both that are inconsistent solely with evacuation of bladder and bowel but consistent with social and olfactory stimuli.

Sufficient: Repeated urination or defecation associated with species-typical postures distinct from those used in simple elimination that occurs in frequencies, locations, or both that are inconsistent solely with evacuation of bladder and bowel but consistent with limited and identifiable social and olfactory stimuli.

Concerns: Social and olfactory stimuli can be difficult to evaluate; determining how they are perceived by the pet is a difficult task. Postures and associated behaviors should be sufficiently well described in a circumscribed manner that is not consistent with anxiety, excitement, incomplete housebreaking, or litter box aversions and preferences. Spraying could be a subclassification of this diagnosis, but may also be sufficiently distinct to stand alone. Marking functions can also be part of normal elimination that does not involve behavior that is distasteful to the client. As such, they would never be questioned under this category, illustrating the problem with the diagnostic label.

Maternal Aggression (No Classification Currently Available; May Be a Subset of 0000YX08.0)

Necessary: Consistent aggression (threat, challenge, or contest) directed toward puppies in the absence of pain, challenges, or threats to the mother by them.

Sufficient: Unprovoked, age-inappropriate attacks to puppies by the mother.

Concerns: When this is profound it is very easy to recognize. Puppies do not have to be injured or killed for this to occur. The extent to which discrete behaviors associated with aggression can be a component of "normal" maternal behavior has not been well quantified; such studies would be useful.

Neophobia (No Code Currently Available)

Necessary: Consistent, sustained, and extreme nongraded response to unfamiliar objects and circumstances manifest as intense, active avoidance, escape, or anxiety behaviors associated with the activities of the sympathetic branch of the autonomic nervous system.

Sufficient: Consistent, sustained, sudden, and profound, nongraded response to unfamiliar objects and circumstances manifest as intense, active avoidance, escape, or anxiety behaviors associated with the activities of the sympathetic branch of the autonomic nervous system; behaviors can include catatonia or mania concomitant with decreased sensitivity to pain or social stimuli; repeated exposure results in an invariant pattern of response.

Concerns: The stage at which a fear becomes a phobia is unknown but epistemologically important. Patterns related to the development of fears and phobias involve evaluation of frequency, intensity, and qualification of actual behaviors. Risks associated for the development of related behaviors are unknown for animals that already exhibit fear or anxiety. A phobic response is difficult to miss, but because of that, it is more complex than is commonly appreciated. This condition may be augmented by extreme deprivation during the relevant sensitive period. Regardless, there is likely to be a strong genetic component.

Nightmares (01004X00.7)

Necessary: Nocturnal activity or vocalization that occurs when the animal is asleep but not directly stimulated by external social or environmental factors.

Sufficient: Nocturnal activity or vocalization that occurs when the animal is asleep but not directly stimulated by external social or environmental factors in the absence of elimination, defecation, or tonic/clonic activity from which the animal can be aroused and will be fully sentient and normally responsive.

Concerns: In an extreme case, "nightmares" could be a manifestation of OCD. Some nightmares may be related to hallucinations but are difficult to evaluate directly in animals. It is important to rule out seizure or epileptic activity; behaviors associated with the range of normal sleep/wake cycles and activities may not have been sufficiently described to distinguish between some seizure activity, sleep disorders, and nightmares.

Noise Phobia (01004X00.6)

Necessary: Sudden and profound, nongraded, extreme response to noise manifest as intense, active avoidance, escape, or anxiety behaviors associated with the activities of the sympathetic branch of the autonomic nervous system.

Sufficient: Sudden and profound, nongraded, extreme response to noise manifest as intense, active avoidance, escape, or anxiety behaviors associated with the activities of the sympathetic branch of the autonomic nervous system; behaviors can include catatonia or mania concomitant with decreased sensitivity to pain or social stimuli; repeated exposure results in an invariant pattern of response.

Concerns: The stage at which a fear becomes a phobia is unknown but is epistemologically important. Patterns related to the development of fears and phobias involve evaluation of frequency, intensity, and qualification of actual behaviors. Risks associated for the development of related behaviors are unknown for animals that already exhibit fear or anxiety. A phobic response is difficult to miss, but because of that, is more complex than is commonly appreciated.

Obsessive-Compulsive Disorder (OCD) (0000X000.1)

Necessary: Repetitive, stereotypic motor, locomotor, grooming, ingestive, or hallucinogenic behaviors that occur out of context to their normal occurrence or in a frequency or duration that is in excess of that required to accomplish the ostensible goal.

Sufficient: As above in a manner that interferes with the animal's ability to otherwise normally function in its social environment.

Concerns: Whether animals can obsess is debatable. Given their responses to these abnormal behaviors, it appears that they perceive and experience concern and thus it may be likely that they can obsess. Such discussions should account for divergent evolutionary histories for animals that rely heavily on structured language and those that do not. Separate from the obsession issue is the issue of relative intensity—whether a behavior is excessive or a manifestation of OCD may be a determination of degree. Careful description and recording of behaviors and their durations could provide data that would permit evaluation of the extent to which such behaviors may lie on a continuum. Good histories and observation are important because in some peculiar forms, some OCDs could resemble seizurelike activity. By definition, some epileptic or seizure-like activity is stereotypic; this is one reason that this very explicit and specific diagnosis category is preferable to that of stereotypy.

Overactivity (0000YX05.1)

Necessary: Motor activity that is in excess of that exhibited when the animal experiences a regular exercise and interaction schedule.

Sufficient: As above in the absence of any signs of organic disease or true hyperactivity and that resolves with increased aerobic activity.

Concerns: Overactivity is a diagnosis that is contingent on context that includes the age of the animal, the age of the client, the breed of the animal, and the social and physical environment of the animal. It is more often a management-related concern than it is an abnormality. It must be distinguished from attention-seeking behavior and hyperactivity.

Pain Aggression (No Code Currently Available; Potentially, but Questionably, a Subcode of 0000X900.0 ["Psychosomatic" Pain or Disease])

Necessary and sufficient: Consistent aggressive behavior, in excess of that required to indicate concern and to effect restraint, demonstrated only in a context known or potentially associated with pain, but that may not be painful, itself.

Sufficient: As above in the absence of any behavioral and physiological signs of fear as identified by withdrawal, passive, and avoidance behaviors associated with the sympathetic branch of the autonomic nervous system.

Concerns: Pain is a difficult concept to assess in animals that can speak. Evaluation of pain in animals that do not speak is very difficult and subjective. This is a diagnosis of degree and correlation; conditions that are known to cause pain (i.e., fractured legs) could render the animal resistant to manipulation. Domestic animals do not have opposable thumbs and so may use their mouths to grasp and restrain. For this diagnosis to be made, fear must not be primary (although anticipation of pain and the attendant anxiety may be involved), and the behaviors must be in excess of those required to indicate the animal's concern.

Pica (No Code Currently Available; Probably Could Be a Subclass of 0000YX06.0; Abnormal Ingestive Behavior Caused by Psychological Disturbances)

Necessary: Consistently exhibits ingestion of nonfood material in a manner not consistent with past behavior.

Sufficient: Incessant consumption of nonfood material in a manner that interferes with normal social functioning.

Concerns: This category may be a subset of 0000YX06.0, abnormal ingestive behavior; however, it would be preferable to restrict the latter to abnormal ingestion of food items and separately specify pica and excessive water drinking (see 0000YX06.1, psychogenic water drinking).

Play Aggression (No Code Currently Available; Probably a Subclass of 0000YX05.3, Hyperactivity; Could Be a Specific Unnumbered Aggression [0000YX0._1])

Necessary: Consistent aggression that occurs in contexts in which play behaviors (play-bows, yips, shoulder blocks, and so on) would normally occur.

Sufficient: Out-of-context, consistent aggression in circumstances when play is relevant; or that occurs in contexts consistent with the solicitation of play, but that involves actions that would discourage play (biting, pain).

Concerns: The normal, accepted, or in-context range of social play behaviors is relatively well defined when compared with abnormal, unacceptable, or out-of-context behaviors. The difficulty lies in distinguishing rough play that the animals have learned in their interactions from other animals or people from truly abnormal behavior. Analysis of discrete behaviors should also distinguish this from attention-seeking behavior (0000YX05.2).

Possessive Aggression (0000YX01.8)

Necessary: Aggression that is consistently directed toward another individual who approaches or attempts to obtain a nonfood object or toy that the aggressor possesses or to which the aggressor controls access.

Sufficient: As above and in the absence of the object associated with the contentious behavior the aggressor is nonaggressive.

Concerns: As with food-related aggression, this is a very specific diagnosis. This diagnostic category includes only nonfood, nongustatory items. The stimuli and neurochemical changes associated with aggression toward objects and toward food are likely very different. Although this aggression may be correlated with the occurrence of canine dominance aggression (or feline status-related aggression), the latter is about control of activity or access—it is *not* about control of objects, and no diagnosis of dominance or status-related aggression should be made on the basis of a response to an object. For a diagnosis of possessive aggression to be made, the response to the object must be consistent, restrictive, and repeatable. If the animal also fulfills the criteria for status-related or dominance aggression, those diagnoses should be made in addition to, not instead of, the diagnosis of possessive aggression.

Predatory Aggression (0000YX01.6)

Necessary: Quiet aggression or behaviors congruent with subsequent predatory behavior (staring, salivating, stalking, body lowering and tail twitching), consistently exhibited in either circumstances associated with predation or toward victims that usually include infants or young or ill animals; death is not a necessary sequela, nor is ingestion, should death ensue.

Sufficient: Quiet, unheralded attacks, generally involving at least one fierce bite and shake, that include staring, salivating, stalking, body lowering and tail twitching, consistently exhibited toward species-contextual prey items (e.g., cats and birds), or toward individuals that exhibit uncoordinated movements and sudden sleep and wake cycles (human infants, young or ill animals, geriatric humans); death is not a necessary sequela, nor is ingestion, should death ensue.

Concerns: When the sufficient conditions are met, this diagnosis is unassailable; however, the necessary conditions provide for leeway in interpretation, and one seldom knows if an actual attack would occur. Although such an approach minimizes the cost of tragedy, it does not contribute greatly to our knowledge about the condition. Discrete analyses of the behaviors involved should elucidate different forms of this behavior and the role of the victims in determining the form that the aggression will take. The latter is important because predatory aggression can also be used to describe aggression to joggers and bicyclists. In the latter case territorial concerns are the obvious ones to rule out, but when predatory aggression involves sentient adult humans it is likely to be categorically different from that described above.

Protective Aggression (0000YX01.4)

Necessary: Aggression that is consistently demonstrated when an individual or class of individuals is approached by a third party in the absence of an actual, contextual threat from that third party.

Sufficient: As above when the aggression intensifies with decreasing distance or with vocal or physical cues that could indicate excitement or threat despite attempts at intervention, correction, or the desire to interact on the part of the individual being "protected."

Concerns: Protective and territorial aggression are often included in the same category. Until they are used separately, it is unlikely that the impetus will exist to learn if they are behaviorally discrete. It is important to acknowledge that some degree of in-context, innate "protectiveness" is desired in most pet dogs. Diagnosis of protective aggression must be made only after the relevance of the context in which it occurs has been evaluated.

Pseudocyesis (No Code Available; Probably a Subset of 0000YX08.0; Cyst Corpus Luteum [78827950.0])

Necessary: Maternal behavior exhibited in the absence of pregnancy.

Sufficient: Maternal or nesting behaviors exhibited in the absence of pregnancy that develop within 60 days of estrus and may be exhibited toward animate or inanimate objects.

Concerns: Note that aggression is not required and that the range of behaviors that could occur during this condition is sufficiently wide as to be missed in many households.

Psychogenic Pain or Distress (0000X900.0)

Necessary: Behavioral signs of pain (withdrawal, vocalization, selective use, decreased motor activity) that occur in the absence of known causal stimuli and in the absence of any other behavioral condition associated with such signs.

Sufficient: Unclear.

Concerns: The term *psychogenic* is problematic and may reflect more about the inability to understand the condition than about any underlying mechanism. Such terms should probably be lost from the diagnostic lexicon. Pain is difficult to evaluate under any circumstances. Evaluation of pain in animals that do not speak is very subjective. Accordingly, evaluation of pain that animals perceive but that might not truly exist could be folly. One of the only situations in which this diagnosis has been successfully and consistently used is change in the use of the paws, or increased attention to the paws after onychectomy. In such cases no physical signs associated with painful stimuli (infection, inflammation) are apparent; however, there are now numerous valid, recognized conditions in humans for which this is true.

They are no longer included under the heading of *psychogenic;* unless this diagnosis is used only as restrictively defined above and not to mean the animal is "crazy," its use should be abandoned.

Psychogenic Water Drinking (0000YX06.1)

Necessary: Consumption of water in excess to that necessary to meet daily fluid balance needs or in excess of that needed to thermoregulate or lubricate ingestion of food.

Sufficient: As above and the behaviors are exhibited to an extent that the animal alters its daily time budget; the behaviors interfere with the animal's ability to interact in its social and physical environment and represent a change in the animal's behavior.

Concerns: Most water drinking termed excessive by clients is normal and fluid balance is maintained. It is essential to rule out any underlying physical or physiological conditions before considering this diagnosis because water restriction can be injurious or fatal. Good histories and qualification of actual behaviors should reveal real differences from "normal" when this diagnosis is appropriate. In an extreme case, this diagnosis could be a subset of 0000X000.1 OCD. This diagnosis is a more specific subset of 0000YX06.0, Abnormal ingestive behavior. The term *psychogenic* is problematic and may reflect more about our inability to understand the condition than it does any underlying mechanism. Such terms should probably be eliminated.

Redirected Aggression (0000YX01.9)

Necessary: Aggression that is consistently directed toward a third party when the patient is thwarted or interrupted from exhibiting aggressive behaviors to the primary target.

Sufficient: Aggression that is instantly and consistently directed toward a third party when the patient is thwarted or interrupted from exhibiting aggressive behaviors to the primary target; the aggression is not accidental, and the patient actively pursues the third party, particularly if associated directly with the interruption of the patient's previous behaviors.

Concerns: This diagnosis describes an exchange in kind, the substitution of an identical activity, albeit with a different target, for the interrupted one; only the focus of the aggression has changed. It is not to be confused with displacement activity in which both target and behavior have been altered as a result of a frustrated, thwarted, interrupted, or corrected behavior. This diagnosis is very specific and is unassailably identified by discrete behavioral descriptions. The most common diagnostic error would be calling a behavior "redirected" aggression when the aggression was actually accidental and was the result of direct intervention in the absence of sufficient time for the aggressors to stop their activity (e.g., reaching between two fighting animals and being bitten because one animal was already in the process of biting the other and could not stop).

Roaming (0000YX05.7)

Necessary: Locomotor activity involving extended absences and variable distance that is in excess of that needed for the animal to relieve itself.

Sufficient: Locomotor activity involving extended absences and variable distance that is in excess of that needed for the animal to relieve itself; trajectory of movement may be determined by the presence of other animals, the estrous cycles of other animals, or behaviors related to patrolling.

Concerns: Roaming is almost always a variant of normal behavior. It can be a concern of clients because it can pose a risk to their pet's health and safety. Clients with pets that roam may be in violation of a leash or animal control law. Roaming is a description of a normal behavior, not a diagnosis of an abnormal one, and it should probably not be included in a diagnostic classification.

Satyriasis (0000X700.0)

Necessary: Excessive solicitation, mounting, and sexual thrusting by a male animal.

Sufficient: The exhibition of solicitation, mounting, and sexual thrusting (with or without intromission and ejaculation) by a male animal regardless of degree of provocation; may be directed interspecifically or intraspecifically, to animate or inanimate objects.

Concerns: The problem is distinguishing sexual from nonsexual or social mounting. Discrete descriptions of the mounting and associated behaviors should clearly distinguish the two. Satyriasis should be more affected by sexual dimorphism than is social mounting. Regardless, satyriasis is rare. The extent to which it is related to factors controlled solely by sex hormones, compared with central neurochemicals, is unclear and probably warrants investigation.

Self-Mutilation [0400YX00.0; May Be a Subset of 0000X000.1; See Also 0000X000.2 Excessive Grooming]; Self-trauma [Which Could Be Injury], (0Y004001.0)

Necessary: Barbering or removal of coat or abrasion, petechiation, or ulceration of any body part by use of teeth, claws, or an external substrate (e.g., rubbing against a wall).

Sufficient: Repeated and consistent (often stereotypic) barbering or removal of coat or abrasion, petechiation, or ulceration of any body part with teeth, claws, or an external substrate in excess of that necessary for normal grooming and maintenance behaviors and in the absence of any dermatological or physiological condition.

Concerns: In extreme situations this condition is minimally associated with anxiety related to environmental stimuli (or lack thereof), and is probably a subset of 0000X000.1. Physiological associations between sensation, pain, pruritus, anxiety, and perception probably become more complex the longer any self-mutilation behaviors are ongoing, rendering the physiological or neurochemical separation of these conditions very difficult.

Separation Anxiety (01004X00.1)

Necessary: Physical or behavioral signs of distress exhibited by the animal only in the absence of or lack of access to the client.

Sufficient: Consistent, intensive destruction, elimination, vocalization, or salivation exhibited only in the virtual or actual absence of the client (e.g., when denied access through a door or when left alone); behaviors are most severe within the first 15 to 20 minutes of separation, and many anxiety-related behaviors (autonomic hyperreactivity, increased motor activity, and increased vigilance and scanning) may become apparent as the client displays behaviors associated with the intention to leave.

Concerns: The extent to which animals exhibiting separation anxiety have other anxious behaviors or experience self-mutilation, phobias, or fears is unknown. No study has demonstrated that this condition is more common in animals whose clients are very attentive compared with those clients who do not fuss over their animals. This is an issue only because of the large degree of myth associated with the former. It is important to rule out other situations that could be associated with the signs that are common in separation anxiety: incomplete housebreaking, teething, play, and a response to a truly scary, unique event (e.g., a robbery).

Spraying (0000YX03.3)

Necessary: Elimination of feline urine through species-specific postures that include vertical stance, elevation and quivering of tail, and treading of feet that renders urine propelled against a vertical surface if one is available.

Sufficient: The detection of feline urine at a height that is equal to that of the cat; dripping could contribute to a secondary puddle on a lower, horizontal surface.

Concerns: Spraying is a wholly recognizable, unambiguous behavior (when observed), but it can be a variant of normal feline elimination behaviors. Cats also spray when they are distressed or anxious. The extent to which the behavior is related to normal baseline feline behaviors or to abnormal anxiety-related ones merits further exploration. Discrete qualification and quantification of ancillary or accompanying behaviors should distinguish at least two possible forms of this behavior.

Status-related Aggression (No Code currently Available; This Is the Feline Analog of 0000YX01.1)

Necessary: Abnormal, inappropriate, out-of-context aggression (threat, challenge, or attack) consistently exhibited by cats toward people under any circumstance involving passive or active control of the cat's behavior or the cat's access to the behavior.

Sufficient: Intensification of any aggressive response from the cat with any passive or active correction or interruption of the cat's behavior or the cat's access to the behavior.

Concerns: This is a very discrete definition of what has been called "the leave me alone bite." It is truly the analog (not homolog; canine and feline social systems are not truly homologous) of the canine condition and is defined in terms that are relevant to feline social systems. It is easier to recognize for cats than for the analogous situation in dogs that this diagnosis is not coupling the challenge to food (food-related aggression), toys (possessive aggression), or space (territorial aggression). However, these aggressions can be correlates of status-related aggression. The keys are control and access—most problems in diagnosing the condition arise from the human's misunderstanding of feline social systems, feline signaling, and feline anxieties.

Submissive Urination (01004X00.4)

Necessary: Urination that occurs in an otherwise housebroken animal only when the animal is exhibiting species-specific postures associated with deferential behavior.

Sufficient: Urination that occurs in an otherwise housebroken animal only when the animal is exhibiting species-specific postures associated with deferential behavior and that is worsened by approaches that solicit such deferential behaviors (e.g., reaching over, rolling over) in an animal that shows no signs of fear or aggression.

Concerns: Any confusion about whether this diagnosis is appropriate can be eliminated by evaluation of this history and concomitant behaviors. Discrete description of the posture in which this behavior occurs improves on the sufficient condition.

Substrate Preference for Elimination (0000YX03.2)

Necessary and sufficient: Consistent elimination in an area or areas that are linked by some common sensory aspect.

Concerns: It is important to note that this is the normal condition for well-housebroken dogs or for cats that use their litter boxes consistently; however, in those situations the substrate they prefer is also one that is acceptable to the clients. This becomes a diagnosis only when there is a client-pet preference mismatch. For examples of extremely restrictive preferences there may be other anxiety-related problems.

Tail Chasing (0000YX05.5)

Necessary: Repetitive locomotor activity directed toward following the trajectory established by the animal's tail.

Sufficient: Repetitive locomotor activity directed toward following the trajectory established by the animal's tail that is in excess of activity required for grooming and that cannot be externally or volitionally stopped.

Concerns: Tail chasing can be a normal behavior, and most puppies and kittens engage in it at some time. In that context it does not belong in a diagnostic scheme. Very extreme cases are recognizable as profoundly different from normal behavior and meet the sufficient conditions above. These are likely to be associated with an OCD and should probably be a subclass of that disorder along with self-mutilation, excessive grooming, and so on. The region of the body that becomes the animal's focus, and the pattern of the problematic behavior, if discretely qualified and quantified, would probably hint at related but differing underlying neurochemical modalities.

Territorial Aggression (0000YX01.5)

Necessary: Aggression that is consistently demonstrated in the vicinity of a mobile (e.g., car) or stationary (e.g., yard) circumscribed area when that area is approached by another individual in the absence of an actual, contextual threat from that individual.

Sufficient: As above when the aggression intensifies with decreasing distance, despite attempts at intervention, correction, or the desire to interact on the part of the approaching individual.

Concerns: Protective and territorial aggression are often included in the same category. Until the terms are used separately, it is unlikely that the impetus will exist to learn if they are behaviorally discrete. It is important to acknowledge that some degree of in-context, innate "territoriality" is desired in most pet dogs because people want their dogs to protect property. Diagnosis of territorial aggression must be made only after the relevance of the context in which it occurs has been evaluated.

Thunderstorm Phobia (01004X00.2)

Necessary: Sudden and profound, nongraded, extreme response to thunderstorms manifest as intense, active avoidance, escape, or anxiety behaviors associated with the activities of the sympathetic branch of the autonomic nervous system.

Sufficient: Sudden and profound, nongraded, extreme response to any aspect of thunderstorms (noise, dark, changes in barometric pressure, changes in ozone levels) manifest as intense, active avoidance, escape, or anxiety behaviors associated with the activities of the sympathetic branch of the autonomic nervous system; behaviors can include catatonia or mania concomitant with decreased sensitivity to pain or social stimuli; repeated exposure results in an invariant pattern of response.

Concerns: The stage at which a fear becomes a phobia is unknown but epistemologically important. Patterns related to the development of fears and phobias involve evaluation of frequency, intensity, and qualification of actual behaviors. Risks associated for the development of related behaviors are unknown for animals that already exhibit fear or anxiety. A phobic response is difficult to miss, but because of that is more complex than is commonly appreciated. Many animals with thunderstorm phobias may have generalized phobias, but this diagnosis entails other related cues that are associated with sensory systems (olfaction, vision) other than the auditory one. It is likely that all animals with noise phobias have a thunderstorm phobia, but the converse might not be true. Insufficient behavioral data exist to evaluate this idea. If it is true, thunderstorm phobias would be a subset of noise phobias.

Trichotillomania (0000X00.3)

Necessary: Pulling out of hair.

Sufficient: Consistent, repetitive, stereotypic removal of hair from follicles in the absence of conditions concomitant with self-mutilation (0400YX00.0); in this condition there is no injury to the skin.

Concerns: This diagnosis could be a subset of 0000X000.2 (excessive grooming) or of 0000X000.1 (OCD). It is likely that characterization of the behavior could reveal not only a discrete pattern unrelated to normal grooming behavior, but neurochemical or neuroanatomical correlates distinct from those found in either normal or abnormal grooming. The behaviors associated with this diagnosis should have a very unique underlying sensory modality.

Urinary Incontinence Due to Psychological Disorder (73005500.X)

Necessary: Nonvolitional lack of control of urination that is not associated with an underlying physical or physiological condition.

Sufficient: Unclear.

Concerns: Incontinence is a very specific term. Most of the behavioral conditions involving elimination do not imply incontinence. As written, this classification implies central lack of control that is not associated with neurological disease. It is possible that this is one sign of cognitive dysfunction, but most elimination behaviors associated with that condition appear to be associated with lack of inhibition, not with lack of control.

Numerical Listing—Cross-Reference

0000X000.1 Obsessive-compulsive disorder/OCD
0000X000.1 Self-mutilation (see discussion in text)
0000X000.2 Grooming, excessive
0000X000.3 Trichotillomania
0000X000.4 Failure to groom
0000X300.0 Aerophagia
0000X610.0 Coprophagia
0000X700.0 Satyriasis
0000X900.0 Pain or distress, psychogenic
0000X900.0 Aggression, pain (see discussion in text)
00004X03.6 Aversion for elimination; elimination, aversion for
0000YX01._ Aggression, play (see discussion in text)
0000YX01.0 Aggression due to psychological disturbance
0000YX01.0 Aggression, idiopathic (see discussion in text)

0000YX01.1 Aggression, dominance
0000YX01.1 Aggression, status-related (see discussion in text)
0000YX01.2 Aggression, interanimal
0000YX01.3 Aggression, fear
0000YX01.4 Aggression, protective
0000YX01.5 Aggression, territorial
0000YX01.6 Aggression, predatory
0000YX01.7 Aggression, food-related
0000YX01.8 Aggression, possessive
0000YX01.9 Aggression, redirected
0000YX02.0 Destruction due to psychological disturbance
0000YX03.0 House soiling due to psychological disturbance
0000YX03.1 Elimination, marking behavior
0000YX03.2 Elimination, substrate preference for
0000YX03._ Undiagnosed, nonspecific house-soiling (see discussion in text)
0000YX03.3 Spraying
0000YX03.4 Elimination, inappropriate
0000YX03.4 Housebreaking, incomplete (see discussion in text)
0000YX03.5 Elimination, location preference for
0000YX04.0 Barking due to psychological disturbance
0000YX05.0 Hyperactivity due to psychological disturbance
0000YX05.1 Overactivity
0000YX05.2 Attention-seeking behavior
0000YX05.3 Play behavior, inappropriate
0000YX05.4 Greeting, inappropriate
0000YX05.5 Tail chasing
0000YX05.6 Compulsive licking/obsessive-compulsive disorder—grooming/licking

0000YX05.7 Roaming
0000YX06.0 Abnormal ingestive behavior due to psychological disturbance (pica)
0000YX06._ Pica (possible subclass; see discussion in text)
0000YX06.1 Water drinking, psychogenic
0000YX08.0 Maternal behavior, abnormal, due to psychological disturbance (pseudocyesis)
0000YX08.0 Aggression, maternal (see discussion in text)
0000YX08.0 Pseudocyesis (see discussion in text and 78827950.0, cyst corpus luteum)
01004X00.0 Anxiety, generalized
01004X00.1 Anxiety, separation
01004X00.2 Phobia, thunderstorm
01004X00.3 Fearful behavior/fear
01004X00.4 Urination, submissive
01004X00.5 Urination, excitement
01004X00.6 Phobia, noise
01004X00.7 Nightmares
01007890.0 Cognitive dysfunction; senility
0400YX00.0 Self-mutilation
0Y004001.0 Self-injury
22025720.0 Hyperesthesia
67205500.X Incontinence, due to fecal, psychological disturbance
73005500.X Incontinence, urinary, due to psychological disturbance
78827950.0 Cyst corpus luteum
           Depression (no code)
           Neophobia (no code)
00805510.X Polyphagia

Appendix G

QUICK REFERENCE FOR TREATMENT PARADIGMS

This appendix is not meant as a substitute for reading the text, as a substitute for obtaining complete and rigorous behavioral history (i.e., collecting the data), or as a "quick fix" that removes from the practitioner the burden of careful thought. It is intended to be only an outline of the techniques or devices, behavioral modification programs, protocols, and behavioral drugs that might be best suited to the treatment of the problem. It is meant to be a heuristic device to help organize your thinking. I have listed only three or four medications for the relevant conditions; order of current preference is noted in parentheses. Obviously, no medication should be dispensed in the absence of a presumptive diagnosis, in the absence of a good behavioral history, without first performing a thorough physical examination, without first obtaining premedication baseline laboratory data, and without giving the client (and having him or her sign) an informed consent statement. Dosages and cautions about specific medications are listed in Chapter 13. The diagnoses listed follow the form in Appendix F. Listing is alphabetical for ease of use.

Abnormal ingestive behavior

Behavior modification approaches
  Banishment
  Crates
  Extinction
  Head collars
  Secondary reinforcers for good behavior
  Desensitization and counterconditioning
    Protocol for deference: Basic program
    Protocol for relaxation: Behavior modification tier 1
    Protocol for desensitizing and counterconditioning dogs to relinquish objects: Behavior modification tier 2
    Protocol for treating and preventing attention-seeking behavior
Possible medications
  Amitriptyline (1)
  Clomipramine (2)
  Fluoxetine (3)

Aerophagia

Behavior modification approaches
  Extinction
  Secondary reinforcers for good behavior
  Desensitization and counterconditioning
    Protocol for deference: Basic program
    Protocol for relaxation: Behavior modification tier 1
    Protocol for treating and preventing attention-seeking behavior
Possible medications
  Amitriptyline (1)
  Clomipramine (2)
  Fluoxetine (3)

Aggression, dominance

Behavior modification approaches
  Banishment
  Crates
  Extinction
  Head collars
  Secondary reinforcers for good behavior
  Desensitization and counterconditioning
    Protocol for deference: Basic program
    Protocol for relaxation: Behavior modification tier 1
    Protocol for treating and preventing attention-seeking behavior
    Protocol for dogs with dominance aggression
    Protocol for handling and surviving aggressive events
    Protocol for choosing collars, head collars, and harnesses
    Protocol for desensitizing dominantly aggressive dogs: Behavior modification tier 2
Possible medications
  Amitriptyline (1)
  Fluoxetine (2)
  Verapamil (?)

Aggression caused by lack of early experience (primarily felines)

Behavior modification approaches
  Extinction
  Flooding
  Habituation
  Limit play and attention
  Secondary reinforcers for good behavior
  Support in protected environment
  Desensitization and counterconditioning with passive reward structure
    Protocol for handling and surviving aggressive events
    Protocol for treating fearful behavior in dogs and cats
Possible medications
  None might be the preferred route, but consider
    Amitriptyline (1)
    Diazepam (use caution) (3)
    Fluoxetine (2)

Aggression, fear

Behavior modification approaches
  Citronella collar
  Crates
  Extinction
  Head collars
  Protect from provocative circumstances
  Secondary reinforcers for good behavior
  Desensitization and counterconditioning
    Protocol for deference: Basic program
    Protocol for relaxation: Behavior modification tier 1

Protocol for treating and preventing attention-seeking behavior

Protocol for dogs with fearful aggression

Protocol for handling and surviving aggressive events

Protocol for choosing collars, head collars, and harnesses

Protocol for desensitizing and counterconditioning a dog (or cat) from approaches from strangers: Behavior modification tier 2

Protocol for desensitization and counterconditioning to noises and activities that occur by the door

Possible medications

Amitriptyline (1)

Buspirone (2)

Fluoxetine (3)

Aggression, food-related

Behavior modification approaches

Banishment

Crates

Extinction

Head collars

Secondary reinforcers for good behavior

Desensitization and counterconditioning

Protocol for deference: Basic program

Protocol for relaxation: Behavior modification tier 1

Protocol for treating and preventing attention-seeking behavior

Protocol for handling and surviving aggressive events

Protocol for choosing collars, head collars, and harnesses

Protocol for dogs and interactions with food, rawhide, biscuits, and bones

Possible medications

Amitriptyline (1)

Buspirone (3)

Clomipramine (2)

Aggression, idiopathic

Behavior modification approaches

Crates

Head collars

Secondary reinforcers for good behavior

Desensitization and counterconditioning

Protocol for deference: Basic program

Protocol for relaxation: Behavior modification tier 1

Protocol for treating and preventing attention-seeking behavior

Protocol for handling and surviving aggressive events

Protocol for choosing collars, head collars, and harnesses

Possible medications

Amitriptyline (1)

Carbamazepine (3)

Fluoxetine (2)

Aggression, interanimal (intercat aggression, interdog aggression)

Behavior modification approaches

Banishment

Crates

Extinction

Flooding

Head collars

Secondary reinforcers for good behavior

Desensitization and counterconditioning

Protocol for deference: Basic program

Protocol for relaxation: Behavior modification tier 1

Protocol for handling and surviving aggressive events

Protocol for choosing collars, head collars, and harnesses

Protocol for desensitizing and counterconditioning a dog (or cat) from approaches from strangers: Behavior modification tier 2

Protocol for the introduction of a new pet to other household pets

Protocol for cats with intercat aggression

Protocol for dogs with interdog aggression

Possible medications

Amitriptyline (2)

Buspirone (cats who are victims)

Diazepam (1)

Fluoxetine (cats who are aggressors)

Aggression, maternal

Behavior modification approaches

Crates

Extinction

Head collars

Protect/avoid

Secondary reinforcers for good behavior

Desensitization and counterconditioning

Protocol for deference: Basic program

Protocol for relaxation: Behavior modification tier 1

Protocol for handling and surviving aggressive events

Protocol for choosing collars, head collars, and harnesses

Possible medications

None might be the best choice if nursing

Aggression, pain

Behavior modification approaches

Crates

Extinction

Head collars

Secondary reinforcers for good behavior

Treat any organic causes of pain

Desensitization and counterconditioning

Protocol for deference: Basic program

Protocol for relaxation: Behavior modification tier 1

Protocol for handling and surviving aggressive events

Protocol for choosing collars, head collars, and harnesses

Protocol for teaching children (and adults) to play with dogs and cats

Possible medications

First consider pain medications (e.g., butorphanol) (1)

Alprazolam (4)

Amitriptyline (2)

Clomipramine (3)

Aggression, play

Behavior modification approaches

Banishment

Crates

Secondary reinforcers for good behavior

Desensitization and counterconditioning

Protocol for deference: Basic program

Protocol for relaxation: Behavior modification tier 1

Protocol for treating and preventing attention-seeking behavior

Protocol for handling and surviving aggressive events

Protocol for choosing collars, head collars, and harnesses

Protocol for basic manners training and housebreaking for new dogs and puppies

Protocol for cats with play aggression

Protocol for teaching children (and adults) to play with dogs and cats
Possible medications
    Probably none

Aggression, possesive

Behavior modification approaches
    Banishment
    Crates
    Head collars
    Secondary reinforcers for good behavior
    Desensitization and counterconditioning
        Protocol for deference: Basic program
        Protocol for relaxation: Behavior modification tier 1
        Protocol for treating and preventing attention-seeking behavior
        Protocol for handling and surviving aggressive events
        Protocol for choosing collars, head collars, and harnesses
        Protocol for desensitizing and counterconditioning dogs to relinquish objects: Behavior modification tier 2
Possible medications
    Probably none unless accompanied by other aggressions

Aggression, predatory

Behavior modification approaches
    Banishment
    Caution
    Crates
    Head collars
        Protocol for introducing a new baby and a pet
        Protocol for the introduction of a new pet to other household pets
    Desensitization and counterconditioning
        Protocol for deference: Basic program
        Protocol for relaxation: Behavior modification tier 1
Possible medications
    None

Aggression, protective

Behavior modification approaches
    Banishment
    Crates
    Extinction
    Head collars
    Secondary reinforcers for good behavior
    Desensitization and counterconditioning
        Protocol for deference: Basic program
        Protocol for relaxation: Behavior modification tier 1
        Protocol for dogs with protective and/or territorial aggression
        Protocol for handling and surviving aggressive events
        Protocol for choosing collars, head collars, and harnesses
        Protocol for desensitizing and counterconditioning a dog (or cat) from approaches from strangers: Behavior modification tier 2
        Protocol for desensitization and counterconditioning to noises and activities that occur by the door: Behavior modification tier 2
Possible medications
    Amitriptyline (1)
    Buspirone (3)
    Clomipramine (2)

Aggression, redirected

Behavior modification approaches

    Banishment
    Crates
    Head collars
    Secondary reinforcers for good behavior
    Desensitization and counterconditioning
        Protocol for deference: Basic program
        Protocol for relaxation: Behavior modification tier 1
        Protocol for handling and surviving aggressive events
        Protocol for choosing collars, head collars, and harnesses
        Protocol for redirected aggression in cats (and dogs)
Possible medications
    Probably none unless accompanied by other aggressions
    Potentially tricyclic antidepressants (e.g., amitriptyline)

Aggression, status-related

Behavior modification approaches
    Banishment
    Crates
    Secondary reinforcers for good behavior
    Desensitization and counterconditioning
        Protocol for treating and preventing attention-seeking behavior
        Protocol for handling and surviving aggressive events
        Protocol for choosing collars, head collars, and harnesses
        Protocol for status-related aggression in cats
Possible medications
    Use caution, but potentially
        Amitriptyline (2)
        Diazepam (use caution; this can release aggression) (3)
        Fluoxetine (1)

Aggression, territorial

Behavior modification approaches
    Banishment
    Crates
    Extinction
    Head collars
    Secondary reinforcers for good behavior
    Desensitization and counterconditioning
        Protocol for deference: Basic program
        Protocol for relaxation: Behavior modification tier 1
        Protocol for dogs with protective and/or territorial aggression
        Protocol for handling and surviving aggressive events
        Protocol for choosing collars, head collars, and harnesses
        Protocol for desensitizing and counterconditioning a dog (or cat) from approaches from strangers: Behavior modification tier 2
        Protocol for desensitization and counterconditioning to noises and activities that occur by the door: Behavior modification tier 2
Possible medications
    Amitriptyline (1)
    Buspirone (3)
    Clomipramine (2)

Anxiety, generalized

Behavior modification approaches
    Crates
    Extinction
    Head collars
    Secondary reinforcers for good behavior
    Desensitization and counterconditioning
        Protocol for deference: Basic program
        Protocol for relaxation: Behavior modification tier 1

Protocol for choosing collars, head collars, and harnesses
Protocol for introducing a new baby and a pet
Protocol for treating and preventing attention-seeking behavior
Protocol for treating fearful behavior in cats and dogs
Protocol for desensitizing and counterconditioning a dog (or cat) from approaches from strangers: Behavior modification tier 2
Protocol for desensitization and counterconditioning to noises and activities that occur by the door: Behavior modification tier 2
Possible medications
Amitriptyline (1)
Buspirone (2)
Clomipramine (3)
Fluoxetine (4)
Some benzodiazepine (5)

Anxiety, separation
Behavior modification approaches
Crates (or no confinement)
Extinction
Head collars
Secondary reinforcers for good behavior
Desensitization and counterconditioning
Protocol for deference: Basic program
Protocol for relaxation: Behavior modification tier 1
Protocol for treating and preventing attention-seeking behavior
Protocol for dogs with separation anxiety
Protocol for desensitization and counterconditioning using gradual departures: Behavior modification tier 2
Protocol for teaching your dog to uncouple departures and departure cues
Protocol for desensitization and counterconditioning to noises and activities that occur by the door: Behavior modification tier 2
Possible medications
Amitriptyline (1)
Buspirone (3)
Clomipramine (2)
(All possibly preceded by diazepam or alprazolam 1 hour before departure if panic is involved)

Attention-seeking behavior
Behavior modification approaches
Banishment
Crates
Extinction
Head collars
Secondary reinforcers for good behavior
Desensitization and counterconditioning
Protocol for deference: Basic program
Protocol for relaxation: Behavior modification tier 1
Protocol for choosing collars, head collars, and harnesses
Protocol for treating and preventing attention-seeking behavior
Possible medications
None

Barking caused by psychological disturbance
Behavior modification approaches
Banishment
Citronella collars
Crates
Extinction

Head collars
Secondary reinforcers for good behavior
Desensitization and counterconditioning
Protocol for deference: Basic program
Protocol for relaxation: Behavior modification tier 1
Protocol for choosing collars, head collars, and harnesses
Protocol for desensitization and counterconditioning to noises and activities that occur by the door: Behavior modification tier 2
Possible medications
Amitriptyline (1)
Buspirone (3)
Clomipramine (2)

Cognitive dysfunction
Behavior modification approaches
Crates
Secondary reinforcers for good behavior
Desensitization and counterconditioning
Protocol for deference: Basic program
Protocol for relaxation: Behavior modification tier 1
Protocol for basic manners training and housebreaking for new dogs and puppies
Protocol for dogs with separation anxiety
Possible medications
Amitriptyline (1)
Clomipramine (3)
Selegiline (2)

Compulsive licking/OCD
Behavior modification approaches
Crates
Extinction
Head collars
Secondary reinforcers for good behavior
Desensitization and counterconditioning
Protocol for deference: Basic program
Protocol for relaxation: Behavior modification tier 1
Protocol for choosing collars, head collars, and harnesses
Protocol for treating and preventing attention-seeking behavior
Possible medications
Amitriptyline (1)
Clomipramine (2)
Fluoxetine (3)

Coprophagia
Behavior modification approaches
Banishment/prohibition
Crates
Head collars
Secondary reinforcers for good behavior
Desensitization and counterconditioning
Protocol for deference: Basic program
Protocol for relaxation: Behavior modification tier 1
Protocol for choosing collars, head collars, and harnesses
Protocol for treating and preventing attention-seeking behavior
Possible medications
Amitriptyline (1)
Clomipramine (2)
Fluoxetine (3)

Depression
Behavior modification approaches
Extinction

Secondary reinforcers for good behavior
Desensitization and counterconditioning
    Protocol for deference: Basic program
    Protocol for relaxation: Behavior modification tier 1
    Protocol for the introduction of a new pet to other household pets
    Protocol for introducing a new baby and a pet
Possible medications
    Amitriptyline (1)
    Buspirone (4)
    Clomipramine (3)
    Diazepam (2)

Elimination, aversion for substrate or location

Behavior modification approaches
    Banishment/sequestration
    Crates/baby gate
    Odor eliminators
    Secondary reinforcers for good behavior
    Desensitization and counterconditioning
        Cats
            Protocol for cats with elimination disorders
            Protocol for cats with intercat aggression
            Protocol for treating fearful behavior in dogs and cats
            Protocol for teaching children (and adults) to play with dogs and cats
        Dogs
            Protocol for treating fearful behavior in dogs and cats
            Protocol for basic manners training and housebreaking for new dogs and puppies
            Protocol for teaching children (and adults) to play with dogs and cats
Possible medications
    None, unless an underlying anxiety component (drugs are not used to housebreak a dog), but then consider
        Amitriptyline (1)
        Buspirone (2)
        Clomipramine (3)

Elimination, inappropriate

Behavior modification approaches
    Banishment/sequestration
    Crates/baby gate
    Odor eliminators
    Secondary reinforcers for good behavior
    Desensitization and counterconditioning
        Cats
            Protocol for cats with elimination disorders
            Protocol for cats with intercat aggression
            Protocol for treating fearful behavior in dogs and cats
            Protocol for teaching children (and adults) to play with dogs and cats
        Dogs
            Protocol for basic manners training and housebreaking for new dogs and puppies
            Protocol for treating fearful behavior in dogs and cats
            Protocol for teaching children (and adults) to play with dogs and cats
Possible medications
    None, *unless* an underlying anxiety component (drugs are not used to housebreak a dog), but then consider
        Amitriptyline (1)
        Buspirone (2)
        Clomipramine (3)

Elimination, location preference for

Behavior modification approaches
    Banishment/sequestration
    Crates/baby gate
    Odor eliminators
    Secondary reinforcers for good behavior
    Desensitization and counterconditioning
        Cats
            Protocol for cats with elimination disorders
            Protocol for cats with intercat aggression
            Protocol for teaching children (and adults to play with dogs and cats)
            Protocol for treating fearful behavior in dogs and cats
        Dogs
            Protocol for basic manners training and housebreaking for new dogs and puppies
            Protocol for dogs with interdog aggression
            Protocol for teaching children (and adults) to play with dogs and cats
            Protocol for treating fearful behavior in dogs and cats
Possible medications
    None, unless there is an underlying anxiety component, then consider
        Amitriptyline (1)
        Buspirone (2)
        Clomipramine (3)

Elimination, marking behavior

Behavior modification approaches
    Banishment/sequestration
    Crates/baby gate
    Odor eliminators
    Secondary reinforcers for good behavior
    Desensitization and counterconditioning
        Cats
            Protocol for cats with elimination disorders
            Protocol for cats with intercat aggression
            Protocol for treating fearful behavior in dogs and cats
        Dogs
            Protocol for deference: Basic program
            Protocol for relaxation: Behavior modification tier 1
            Protocol for basic manners training and housebreaking for new dogs and puppies
            Protocol for treating fearful behavior in dogs and cats
            Protocol for dogs with interdog aggression
Possible medications
    None, unless an underlying anxiety component (drugs are not used to housebreak a dog), but then consider
        Amitriptyline (1)
        Buspirone (4)
        Clomipramine (2)
        Diazepam (use caution; but it may work for cats that are very assertive or very fearful) (3)

Elimination, substrate preference for

Behavior modification approaches
    Banishment/sequestration
    Crates/baby gate
    Odor eliminators
    Secondary reinforcers for good behavior
    Desensitization and counterconditioning
        Cats
            Protocol for cats with elimination disorders
            Protocol for cats with intercat aggression
            Protocol for teaching children (and adults) to play with dogs and cat

Protocol for treating fearful behavior in dogs and cats

Dogs

Protocol for basic manners training and housebreaking for new dogs and puppies

Protocol for dogs with interdog aggression

Protocol for teaching children (and adults) to play with dogs and cats

Protocol for treating fearful behavior in dogs and cats

Possible medications

None, unless a strong aversion component involved, then consider

Amitriptyline (1)

Buspirone (2)

Clomipramine (3)

Failure to groom

Behavior modification approaches

Secondary reinforcers for good behavior

Desensitization and counterconditioning

Protocol for deference: Basic program

Protocol for relaxation: Behavior modification tier 1

Protocol for introducing a new baby and a pet

Protocol for treating fearful behavior in cats and dogs

Possible medications

Amitriptyline (2)

Buspirone (4)

Clomipramine (3)

Diazepam (1)

Fearful behavior

Behavior modification approaches

Crates

Extinction

Head collars

Secondary reinforcers for good behavior

Desensitization and counterconditioning

Protocol for deference: Basic program

Protocol for relaxation: Behavior modification tier 1

Protocol for choosing collars, head collars, and harnesses

Protocol for introducing a new baby and a pet

Protocol for treating fearful behavior in cats and dogs

Protocol for desensitizing and counterconditioning a dog (or cat) from approaches from strangers: Behavior modification tier 2

Protocol for desensitization and counterconditioning to noises and activities that occur by the door: Behavior modification tier 2

Possible medications

Amitriptyline (2)

Buspirone (3)

Clomipramine (4)

Diazepam (1)

Greeting, inappropriate

Behavior modification approaches

Citronella collars

Crates

Head collars

Secondary reinforcers for good behavior

Desensitization and counterconditioning

Protocol for deference: Basic program

Protocol for relaxation: Behavior modification tier 1

Protocol for choosing collars, head collars, and harnesses

Protocol for treating and preventing attention-seeking behavior

Protocol for desensitizing and counterconditioning a dog (or cat) from approaches from strangers: Behavior modification tier 2

Protocol for desensitization and counterconditioning to noises and activities that occur by the door: Behavior modification tier 2

Possible medications

None

Grooming, excessive

Behavior modification approaches

Crates

Extinction

Head collars

Secondary reinforcers for good behavior

Desensitization and counterconditioning

Protocol for deference: Basic program

Protocol for relaxation: Behavior modification tier 1

Protocol for choosing collars, head collars, and harnesses

Protocol for treating and preventing attention-seeking behavior

Possible medications

Amitriptyline (1)

Clomipramine (2)

Fluoxetine (4)

Hydrocodone (3)

Housebreaking, incomplete

Behavior modification approaches

Banishment/sequestration

Crates/baby gate

Odor eliminators

Secondary reinforcers for good behavior

Desensitization and counterconditioning

Protocol for deference: Basic program

Protocol for relaxation: Behavior modification tier 1

Protocol for basic manners training and housebreaking for new dogs and puppies

Protocol for treating fearful behavior in dogs and cats

Protocol for teaching children (and adults) to play with dogs and cats

Possible medications

None, unless anxiety component or decreased sphincter tone, then consider

Amitriptyline (2)

Phenylpropanolamine (1)

Hyperactivity caused by psychological disturbance

Make sure your diagnosis is accurate—hyperactivity is rare—attention-seeking behavior and overactivity are not.

Behavior modification approaches

Crates

Head collars

Increase aerobic exercise

Secondary reinforcers for good behavior

Desensitization and counterconditioning

Protocol for deference: Basic program

Protocol for relaxation: Behavior modification tier 1

Protocol for choosing collars, head collars, and harnesses

Protocol for treating and preventing attention-seeking behavior

Protocol for teaching children (and adults) to play with dogs and cats

Possible medications

Methylphenidate

Hyperesthesia

Behavior modification approaches
  Crates
  Secondary reinforcers for good behavior
  Desensitization and counterconditioning
    Protocol for treating fearful behavior in cats and dogs
    Protocol for handling and surviving aggressive events
    Protocol for treating and preventing attention-seeking behavior
Possible medications
  Amitriptyline (1)
  Clomipramine (2)
  Fluoxetine (3)

Incontinence, fecal caused by psychological disturbance

Behavior modification approaches
  Crates
  Diapers
  Secondary reinforcers for good behavior
  Desensitization and counterconditioning
    Protocol for deference: Basic program
    Protocol for relaxation: Behavior modification tier 1
    Protocol for basic manners training and housebreaking for new dogs and puppies
    Protocol for dogs with separation anxiety
Possible medications
  Amitriptyline (1)
  Clomipramine (2)
  Selegiline (3)

Incontinence, urinary caused by psychological disturbance

Behavior modification approaches
  Crates
  Diapers
  Secondary reinforcers for good behavior
  Desensitization and counterconditioning
    Protocol for deference: Basic program
    Protocol for relaxation: Behavior modification tier 1
    Protocol for basic manners training and housebreaking for new dogs and puppies
    Protocol for dogs with separation anxiety
Possible medications
  Amitriptyline (1)
  Clomipramine (2)
  Selegiline (3?)

Maternal behavior, abnormal caused by psychological disturbance

Behavior modification approaches
  Crates
  Do not rebreed
  Extinction
  Head collars
  Protect/avoid
  Secondary reinforcers for good behavior
  Desensitization and counterconditioning
    Protocol for deference: Basic program
    Protocol for relaxation: Behavior modification tier 1
    Protocol for handling and surviving aggressive events
    Protocol for choosing collars, head collars, and harnesses
    Protocol for treating fearful behavior in cats and dogs
Possible medications
  None might be the best choice if nursing

Neophobia

Behavior modification approaches
  Crates
  Extinction
  Head collars
  Protected environment
  Secondary reinforcers for good behavior
  Desensitization and counterconditioning
    Protocol for deference: Basic program
    Protocol for relaxation: Behavior modification tier 1
    Protocol for choosing collars, head collars, and harnesses
    Protocol for introducing a new baby and a pet
    Protocol for treating fearful behavior in cats and dogs
    Protocol for desensitizing and counterconditioning a dog (or cat) from approaches from strangers: Behavior modification tier 2
    Protocol for desensitization and counterconditioning to noises and activities that occur by the door: Behavior modification tier 2
Possible medications
  Amitriptyline (2)
  Buspirone (4)
  Clomipramine (3)
  Diazepam (1)

Nightmares

Behavior modification approaches
  Crates/bed
  Extinction
  Head collars
  Increased aerobic exercise
  Secondary reinforcers for good behavior
  Desensitization and counterconditioning
    Protocol for deference: Basic program
    Protocol for relaxation: Behavior modification tier 1
    Protocol for choosing collars, head collars, and harnesses
    Protocol for treating and preventing attention-seeking behavior
    Protocol for treating fearful behavior in cats and dogs
Possible medications
  Amitriptyline (2)
  Diazepam (before bedtime) (1)
  Imipramine (3)

Obsessive-compulsive disorder/OCD

Behavior modification approaches
  Companion
  Crates
  Distract
  Extinction
  Head collars
  Increase aerobic exercise
  Secondary reinforcers for good behavior
  Desensitization and counterconditioning
    Protocol for deference: Basic program
    Protocol for relaxation: Behavior modification tier 1
    Protocol for choosing collars, head collars, and harnesses
    Protocol for treating and preventing attention-seeking behavior
    Protocol for teaching children (and adults) to play with dogs and cats
Possible medications
  Amitriptyline (1)
  Clomipramine (2)
  Fluoxetine (3)

Overactivity

Behavior modification approaches
  Banishment when unwilling to monitor
  Companion
  Crates
  Extinction
  Head collars
  Increase aerobic exercise
  Secondary reinforcers for good behavior
  Desensitization and counterconditioning
    Protocol for deference: Basic program
    Protocol for relaxation: Behavior modification tier 1
    Protocol for choosing collars, head collars, and harnesses
    Protocol for treating and preventing attention-seeking behavior
Possible medications
  None

Phobia, noise

Behavior modification approaches
  Crates (or no confinement)
  Extinction
  Head collars
  Secondary reinforcers for good behavior
  Desensitization and counterconditioning
    Protocol for treating and preventing attention-seeking behavior
    Protocol for dogs with separation anxiety
    Protocol for deference: Basic program
    Protocol for relaxation: Behavior modification tier 1
    Protocol for desensitization and counterconditioning to noises and activities that occur by the door (consider use of taped sounds): Behavior modification tier 2
Possible medications
  Alprazolam (3)
  Buspirone (possibly preceded by diazepam or alprazolam 1 hour before departure if panic involved) (5)
  Clomipramine (possibly preceded by diazepam or alprazolam 1 hour before departure if panic involved) (4)
  Clorazepate (2)
  Diazepam (1)

Phobia, thunderstorm

Behavior modification approaches
  Crates (or no confinement)
  Extinction
  Head collars
  Secondary reinforcers for good behavior
  Desensitization and counterconditioning
    Protocol for treating and preventing attention-seeking behavior
    Protocol for dogs with separation anxiety
    Protocol for deference: Basic program
    Protocol for relaxation: Behavior modification tier 1
    Protocol for desensitization and counterconditioning to noises and activities that occur by the door (consider use of taped sounds): Behavior modification tier 2
Possible medications
  Alprazolam (3)
  Buspirone (possibly preceded by diazepam or alprazolam 1 hour before serious storm if possible) (5)
  Clomipramine (possibly preceded by diazepam or alprazolam 1 hour before serious storm if possible) (4)
  Clorazepate (2)
  Diazepam (1)

Pica

Behavior modification approaches
  Banishment/prohibition
  Crates
  Head collars
  Increase aerobic exercise
  Secondary reinforcers for good behavior
  Desensitization and counterconditioning
    Protocol for deference: Basic program
    Protocol for relaxation: Behavior modification tier 1
    Protocol for choosing collars, head collars, and harnesses
    Protocol for treating and preventing attention-seeking behavior
Possible medications
  Amitriptyline (1)
  Clomipramine (2)
  Fluoxetine (3)

Play behavior, inappropriate

Behavior modification approaches
  Banishment
  Companion (energetic)
  Crates
  Increase appropriate aerobic play
  Secondary reinforcers for good behavior
  Desensitization and counterconditioning
    Protocol for deference: Basic program
    Protocol for relaxation: Behavior modification tier 1
    Protocol for treating and preventing attention-seeking behavior
    Protocol for handling and surviving aggressive events
    Protocol for choosing collars, head collars, and harnesses
    Protocol for basic manners training and housebreaking for new dogs and puppies
    Protocol for cats with play aggression
    Protocol for teaching children (and adults) to play with dogs and cats
Possible medications
  Probably none

Roaming

Behavior modification approaches
  Banishment/sequestration
  Castration
  Crates/baby gate/leashes/fences
  Secondary reinforcers for good behavior
  Desensitization and counterconditioning
  Cats
    Protocol for cats with elimination disorders
    Protocol for cats with intercat aggression
  Dogs
    Protocol for deference: Basic program
    Protocol for relaxation: Behavior modification tier 1
    Protocol for treating fearful behavior in dogs and cats
    Protocol for dogs with interdog aggression
Possible medications
  None, unless an underlying anxiety component (drugs are not used to housebreak a dog), but then consider
    Amitriptyline (1)
    Buspirone (3)
    Clomipramine (2)

Satyriasis

Behavior modification approaches
  Banishment/sequestration

Castration
Crates/baby gate/leashes/fences
Secondary reinforcers for good behavior
Desensitization and counterconditioning
   Cats
      Protocol for cats with elimination disorders
      Protocol for cats with intercat aggression
   Dogs
      Protocol for deference: Basic program
      Protocol for relaxation: Behavior modification tier 1
      Protocol for treating fearful behavior in dogs and cats
      Protocol for dogs with interdog aggression
Possible medications
   Amitriptyline (1)
   Clomipramine (2)
   Fluoxetine (3)
   Progestins (4)

Self-mutilation

Behavior modification approaches
   Companion
   Distract
   Head collars
   Increase aerobic exercise
   Secondary reinforcers for good behavior
   Desensitization and counterconditioning
      Protocol for deference: Basic program
      Protocol for relaxation: Behavior modification tier 1
      Protocol for choosing collars, head collars, and harnesses
      Protocol for treating and preventing attention-seeking behavior
Possible medications
   Amitriptyline (1)
   Clomipramine (2)
   Fluoxetine (3)
   Hydrocodone (4)

Spraying

Behavior modification approaches
   Banishment/sequestration
   Crates/baby gate
   Odor eliminators
   Secondary reinforcers for good behavior
   Desensitization and counterconditioning
      Protocol for cats with elimination disorders
      Protocol for cats with intercat aggression
      Protocol for treating fearful behavior in dogs and cats
      Protocol for the introduction of a new pet to other household pets
Possible medications
   Amitriptyline (3)
   Buspirone (use in less confident cat) (1)
   Clomipramine (2)
   Diazepam (use caution, but it may work for cats that are very assertive or very fearful) (1)

Tail chasing

Behavior modification approaches
   Companion
   Crates
   Distract
   Extinction
   Head collars
   Increase aerobic exercise
   Secondary reinforcers for good behavior

Desensitization and counterconditioning
   Protocol for deference: Basic program
   Protocol for relaxation: Behavior modification tier 1
   Protocol for choosing collars, head collars, and harnesses
   Protocol for treating and preventing attention-seeking behavior
   Protocol for teaching children (and adults) to play with dogs and cats
Possible medications
   Amitriptyline (1)
   Clomipramine (2)
   Fluoxetine (3)

Trichotillomania

Behavior modification approaches
   Crates
   Head collars
   Increase aerobic exercise
   Secondary reinforcers for good behavior
   Desensitization and counterconditioning
      Protocol for deference: Basic program
      Protocol for relaxation: Behavior modification tier 1
      Protocol for choosing collars, head collars, and harnesses
      Protocol for treating and preventing attention-seeking behavior
Possible medications
   Amitriptyline (1)
   Clomipramine (2)
   Fluoxetine (3)
   Hydrocodone (4)

Urination, excitement

Behavior modification approaches
   Banishment/sequestration
   Crates/baby gate
   Odor eliminators
   Secondary reinforcers for good behavior
   Desensitization and counterconditioning
      Protocol for deference: Basic program
      Protocol for relaxation: Behavior modification tier 1
      Protocol for basic manners training and housebreaking for new dogs and puppies
      Protocol for treating fearful behavior in dogs and cats
      Protocol for teaching children (and adults) to play with dogs and cats
Possible medications
   None, unless anxiety component or decreased sphincter tone, then consider
      Amitriptyline (1)
      Phenylpropanolamine (2)

Urination, submissive

Behavior modification approaches
   Banishment/sequestration
   Crates/baby gate
   Odor eliminators
   Secondary reinforcers for good behavior
   Desensitization and counterconditioning
      Protocol for deference: Basic program
      Protocol for relaxation: Behavior modification tier 1
      Protocol for basic manners training and housebreaking for new dogs and puppies
      Protocol for treating fearful behavior in dogs and cats
      Protocol for teaching children (and adults) to play with dogs and cats

Possible medications
  None, unless anxiety component or decreased sphincter tone, then consider
    Amitriptyline (1)
    Phenylpropanolamine (2)

Water drinking, psychogenic

Behavior modification approaches
  Banishment/prohibition
  Crates
  Head collars
  Increased aerobic exercise
  Secondary reinforcers for good behavior
  Desensitization and counterconditioning

Protocol for deference: Basic program
Protocol for relaxation: Behavior modification tier 1
Protocol for choosing collars, head collars, and harnesses
Protocol for treating and preventing attention-seeking behavior
Protocol for teaching children (and adults) to play with dogs and cats
Possible medications
  Probably none unless profound anxiety component present, then consider
    Amitriptyline (1)
    Clomipramine (2)
    Fluoxetine (3)

Index